Radiologic Diagnosis of
DISEASES *of the* CHEST

Radiologic Diagnosis of
DISEASES *of the* CHEST

Nestor L. Müller, M.D., Ph.D.
Professor of Radiology
University of British Columbia
Vancouver Hospital and Health Sciences Centre
Vancouver, British Columbia

Richard S. Fraser, M.D.
Professor of Pathology
McGill University Health Centre
Royal Victoria Hospital
Montreal, Quebec

Neil C. Colman, M.D.
Associate Professor of Medicine
McGill University Health Centre
Montreal General Hospital
Montreal, Quebec

P.D. Paré, M.D.
Professor of Medicine
University of British Columbia
St. Paul's Hospital
Vancouver, British Columbia

SAUNDERS
An Imprint of Elsevier

SAUNDERS
An Imprint of Elsevier
The Curtis Center
Independence Square West
Philadelphia, PA 19106

Library of Congress Cataloging-in-Publication Data

Radiologic diagnosis of diseases of the chest / Nestor L. Müller . . . [et al.].—1st ed.

p.   cm.

Companion to: Fraser and Paré's diagnosis of diseases of the chest / Richard S. Fraser . . . [et al.]. 4th ed. 1999.

ISBN 0–7216–8808–X

1. Chest—Radiography.   I. Müller, Nestor Luiz   II. Fraser and Paré's
  diagnosis of diseases of the chest.
[DNLM: 1. Thoracic Diseases—radiography.   2. Lung Diseases—radiography.
WF 975 R1295 2001]

RC941.R264 2001   617.5′407572—dc21

DNLM/DLC   00–066129

Acquisitions Editor: Lisette Bralow
Project Manager: Gina Scala
Production Manager: Natalie Ware
Illustration Specialist: Walt Verbitski
Book Designer: Karen O'Keefe Owens

RADIOLOGIC DIAGNOSIS OF DISEASES OF THE CHEST   ISBN 0–7216–8808–X

Printed in the United States of America.

Last digit is the print number: 9   8   7   6   5   4   3   2

To our wives and our children:
Ruth, Alison, and Phillip Müller
Marie-Claire, Nicky, Russel, and Emily Fraser
Margo Zysman, Eli and Zofia Zysman-Colman
Lisa, Peter, and Jesse Paré

Preface

Following the seminal work of Fraser and Paré in the 1960s, it became widely accepted that the combination of a good clinical history and high-quality posteroanterior and lateral chest radiographs enabled the radiologist and the respiratory physician to diagnose or to significantly narrow the differential diagnosis of many chest diseases. Despite the value of radiographs in this regard, it was clear that this modality had important limitations. Partly because of the recognition of these limitations and partly because of the development of new technology, radiologic imaging of chest disease underwent a marked transformation in the 1980s and 1990s, particularly as the result of the availability and increased diagnostic accuracy of high-resolution computed tomography (CT) and spiral CT. The former has enabled the clinician to make a much better assessment of the pattern and distribution of pulmonary parenchymal and peripheral airway disease, while spiral CT has greatly improved the ability to image the central airways, mediastinum, and blood vessels. Magnetic resonance imaging (MRI) has also proved to have an important role in the assessment of mediastinal, chest wall, and vascular abnormalities. In this work, we document the use of these imaging modalities in the diagnosis of chest disease and provide descriptions and numerous illustrations of the characteristic findings of many specific abnormalities.

The book provides an imaging perspective to the fourth edition of *Fraser and Paré's Diagnosis of Diseases of the Chest*. It includes all the relevant radiologic information contained in the larger work; however, only the most essential etiologic, pathogenetic, clinical, and pathologic information is included. There are many new illustrations and tables, and much information is completely updated. This new work is intended mainly for radiologists, respiratory physicians, and internal medicine and radiology residents who are seeking a relatively concise review of the radiologic manifestations of chest disease. Although we believe that this book will provide a clear understanding of these manifestations, we invite our readers to inform us about differences of opinion they may have with its contents and areas that need improvement.

NESTOR L. MÜLLER, M.D., PH.D.
RICHARD S. FRASER, M.D.
NEIL C. COLMAN, M.D.
P.D. PARÉ, M.D.

Acknowledgments

First and foremost we would like to express our debt to Robert G. Fraser and J.A. Peter Paré for their seminal work in documenting the importance of radiologic findings in the diagnosis of chest disease. We would also like to express our gratitude to Ms. Jenny Silver for her outstanding secretarial assistance and to the many colleagues from around the world who loaned us illustrations. They are listed alphabetically below:

John D. Armstrong, Jr.
James Barrie
Colleen Bergin
Lynn Boderick
Maura Brown
W. G. Brown
A. Regina Buckley
Carole Dennie
Romeo Ethier
Jaime Fdez-Cuadrado
Christopher Flower
Tomás Franquet
Christopher Griffin
Thomas Hartman
R. Hedvigi
Immaculada Herraez

Laura Heyneman
Jung-Gi Im
Harumi Itoh
Juan Jimenez
Takeshi Johkoh
Eun-Young Kang
Ella Kazerooni
Kun-Il Kim
Glen Krinsky
J. Stephen Kwong
Kyung Soo Lee
Michael Lefcoe
Ann Leung
Andrew Mason
Fred Matzinger

John Mayo
Page McAdams
Georgeann McGuinness
Jacqueline Morgan-Parkes
David Naidich
Hiroshi Niimi
M.J. Palayew
Ned Patz
Steven Primack
Robert Pugatch
Martine Remy-Jardin
Cathy Staples
Robert Tarver
Pamela Woodard
Daniel Worsley

NOTICE

Medicine is an ever-changing field. Standard safety precautions must be followed, but as new research and clinical experience broaden our knowledge, changes in treatment and drug therapy may become necessary or appropriate. Readers are advised to check the most current product information provided by the manufacturer of each drug to be administered to verify the recommended dose, the method and duration of administration, and contraindications. It is the responsibility of the treating physician, relying on experience and knowledge of the patient, to determine dosages and the best treatment for each individual patient. Neither the publisher nor the editor assumes any liability for any injury and/or damage to persons or property arising from this publication.

THE PUBLISHER

Contents

The Normal Chest

The primary function of the airways is to conduct air to the alveolar surface, where gas transfer takes place between respired air and the blood of the alveolar capillaries. The greater part of the length and the smaller part of the volume of the respiratory system are concerned with this function. The trachea and bronchi (the walls of which contain cartilage) and membranous bronchioles carry out this function. The remainder of the respiratory system, comprising the large bulk of the lungs, is concerned with conduction and gas exchange, the terminal unit (the alveolus) being the only structure whose unique function is gas exchange. The lungs can be considered to comprise three zones, each with different but overlapping structural and functional characteristics.

The *conducting zone* is composed of airways whose walls do not contain alveoli and are thick enough that gas cannot diffuse into the adjacent lung parenchyma. This zone includes the trachea, bronchi, and membranous (non-alveolated) bronchioles. These airways, along with the pulmonary arteries and veins, lymphatic vessels, nerves, connective tissue of the peribronchial and perivascular spaces, interlobular septa, and pleura, constitute the nonparenchymatous portion of the lung.

The *transitional zone*, as its name implies, carries out conductive and respiratory functions. It consists of the respiratory bronchioles and alveolar ducts, each of which conducts air to the most peripheral portion of the lung. Alveoli that arise from the walls of these airways also serve in gas exchange.

The *respiratory zone* consists of the alveoli, whose primary function is the exchange of gases between air and blood. Together with the transitional zone, this tissue constitutes the lung *parenchyma*, the spongy respiratory portion of the lung. It has been estimated that approximately 87% of total lung volume is alveolar, of which 6% is composed of tissue and the remainder gas.[1]

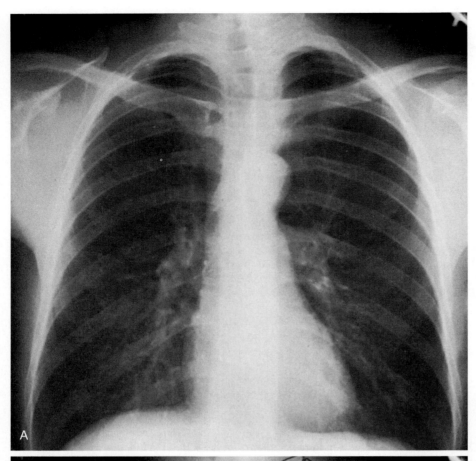

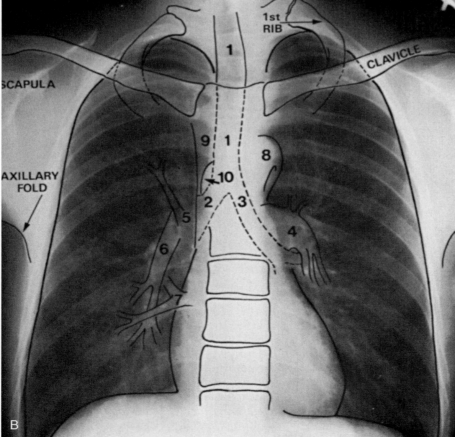

Figure 1–1. Normal Chest Radiograph, Posteroanterior Projection. Radiograph *(A)* of the chest of an asymptomatic 26-year-old man in the erect position. Diagrammatic overlay *(B)* shows the normal anatomic structures numbered or labeled: (1) trachea, (2) right main bronchus, (3) left main bronchus, (4) left pulmonary artery, (5) right upper lobe pulmonary vein, (6) right interlobar artery, (7) right lower and middle lobe vein, (8) aortic arch, (9) superior vena cava, and (10) azygos vein.

AIRWAYS

Trachea and Main Bronchi

The trachea is a midline structure; a slight deviation to the right at the level of the aortic arch is typical and should not be misinterpreted as evidence of displacement (Figs. 1–1 and 1–2). On a normal posteroanterior (PA) radiograph, the tracheal walls are parallel except on the left side just above the bifurcation, where the aorta commonly causes a smooth indentation. The upper limits of normal for coronal and sagittal diameters in men are 25 and 27 mm; in women, they are 21 and 23 mm.[2] The lower limit of normal for both dimensions is 13 mm in men and 10 mm in women.

The trachea divides into the left and right main bronchi at the carina. The right main bronchus divides into the right upper lobe bronchus and bronchus intermedius, and the left main bronchus divides into the left upper and lower lobe bronchi. The pattern of bronchial branching shows considerable variation in subsegmental airways and, to a lesser extent, in the lobar and segmental branches.[3] In most cases, however, these variations are of no clinical significance and are discovered only during bronchoscopy or at autopsy.

Lobar Bronchi and Bronchopulmonary Segments

Right Upper Lobe. The bronchus to the right upper lobe arises from the lateral aspect of the main bronchus, approximately 2 cm distal to the tracheal carina. It divides slightly more than 1 cm from its origin, most commonly into three branches designated anterior, posterior, and apical (Figs. 1–3 and 1–4).

Right Middle Lobe. The intermediate bronchus (bronchus intermedius) continues distally for 3 to 4 cm from the takeoff of the right upper lobe bronchus, then bifurcates to become the bronchi to the middle and lower lobes. The middle lobe bronchus arises from the anterolateral wall of the intermediate bronchus, almost opposite the origin of the superior segmental bronchus of the lower lobe; 1 to 2 cm beyond its origin, it bifurcates into lateral and medial branches (*see* Figs. 1–3 and 1–4).

Right Lower Lobe. The superior segmental bronchus arises from the posterior aspect of the lower lobe bronchus immediately beyond its origin. On a frontal radiograph, the location of the four basal segments of the lower lobe from the lateral to the medial aspect is *anterior-lateral-posterior-medial* (*see* Fig. 1–3). In the lateral projection, the relationship anterior-lateral-posterior is maintained—hence the mnemonic *ALP*. The relationship of one basal segment to

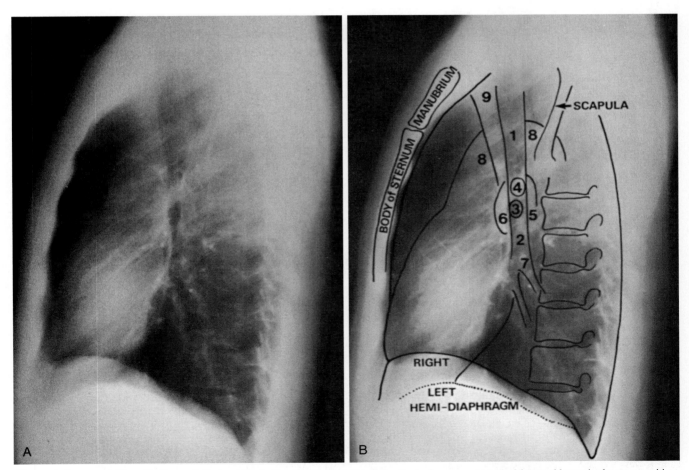

Figure 1–2. Normal Chest Radiograph, Lateral Projection. Radiograph *(A)* of the chest of an asymptomatic 26-year-old man in the erect position. Diagrammatic overlay *(B)* shows the normal anatomic structures numbered or labeled: (1) tracheal air column, (2) right intermediate bronchus, (3) left upper lobe bronchus, (4) right upper lobe bronchus, (5) left interlobar artery, (6) right interlobar artery, (7) confluence of pulmonary veins, (8) aortic arch, and (9) brachiocephalic vessels.

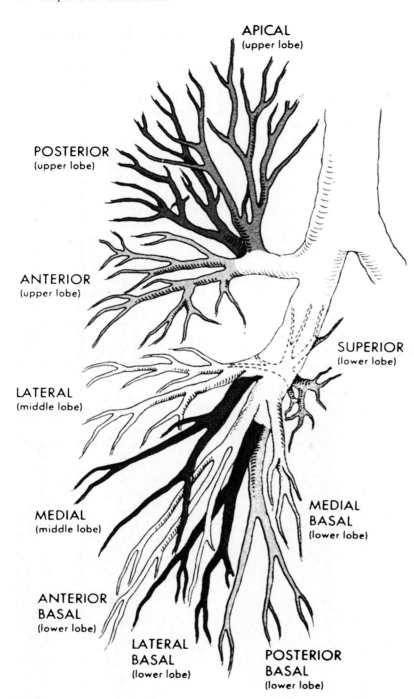

APICAL
(upper lobe)

POSTERIOR
(upper lobe)

ANTERIOR
(upper lobe)

LATERAL
(middle lobe)

SUPERIOR
(lower lobe)

MEDIAL
(middle lobe)

MEDIAL
BASAL
(lower lobe)

ANTERIOR
BASAL
(lower lobe)

LATERAL
BASAL
(lower lobe)

POSTERIOR
BASAL
(lower lobe)

Figure 1–3. Right Bronchial Tree (Frontal Projection). Schematic representation of the normal segments of the right bronchial tree in frontal projection. (From Lehman JS, Crellin JA: Med Radiogr Photogr 31:81, 1955. Courtesy of Eastman Kodak Company.)

another is recognized easily by use of the ALP designation, the medial basal segment being projected between the anterior and lateral segments in the lateral projection.

Left Upper Lobe. About 1 cm beyond its origin from the anterolateral aspect of the main bronchus, the bronchus to the left upper lobe either bifurcates or trifurcates, usually the former (Figs. 1–5 and 1–6). In the bifurcation pattern, the upper division almost immediately divides again into two segmental branches, the apicoposterior and anterior. The lower division is the lingular bronchus, which is analogous to the middle lobe bronchus of the right lung. The lingular bronchus extends anteroinferiorly for 2 to 3 cm before bifurcating into superior and inferior divisions.

Left Lower Lobe. The divisions of the left lower lobe bronchus are almost identical in name and anatomic distribution to those of the right lower lobe (*see* Figs. 1–5 and 1–6). The exception lies in the absence of a separate medial basal bronchus, the anterior and medial portions of the lobe being supplied by a single anteromedial bronchus. The mnemonic ALP applies as well to the left lower lobe as to the right for identification of the relationship of basilar bronchi to one another in frontal and lateral projections.

Bronchial Anatomy on Computed Tomography

Bronchi coursing horizontally within the plane of computed tomography (CT) section are seen along their long

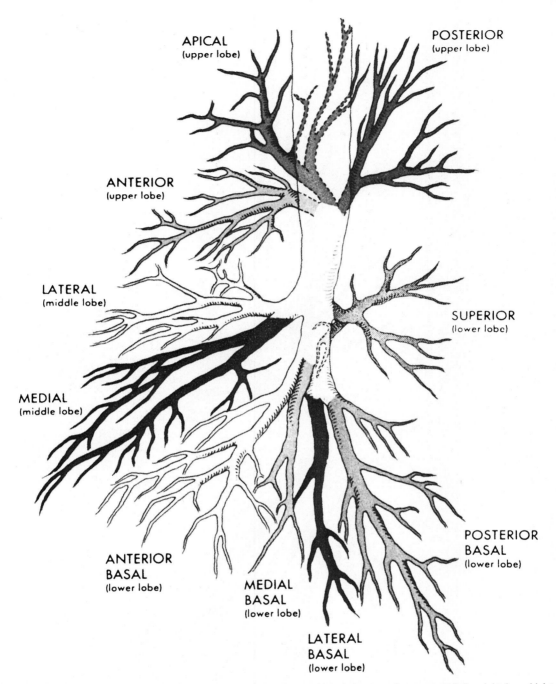

Figure 1–4. Right Bronchial Tree (Lateral Projection). Schematic representation of the normal segments of the right bronchial tree in lateral projection. (From Lehman JS, Crellin JA: Med Radiogr Photogr 31:81, 1955. Courtesy of Eastman Kodak Company.)

axes (Fig. 1–7). These bronchi include the right and left upper lobe bronchi, the anterior segmental bronchi of the upper lobes, the middle lobe bronchus, and the superior segmental bronchi of the lower lobes. Bronchi coursing vertically are cut in cross-section and are seen as circular lucencies. These bronchi include the apical segmental bronchus of the right upper lobe, the apicoposterior segmental bronchus of the left upper lobe, the bronchus intermedius, the lower lobe bronchi, and the basal segmental bronchi. Bronchi coursing obliquely are seen as oval lucencies and are less well visualized on CT scan. These include the

lingular bronchus, the superior and inferior segmental lingular bronchi, and the medial and lateral segmental bronchi of the right middle lobe.

Bronchioles

Bronchioles are airways whose walls lack cartilage but, at least focally, are composed of a connective tissue lamina propria that contains a branch of the pulmonary arterial system. Respiratory bronchioles are lined partly by alveoli; membranous bronchioles are nonalveolated. The membra-

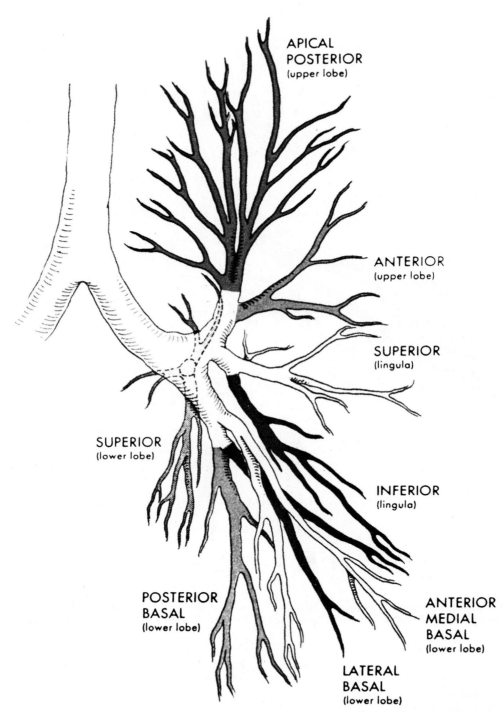

Figure 1–5. Left Bronchial Tree (Frontal Projection). Schematic representation of the normal segments of the left bronchial tree in frontal projection. (From Lehman JS, Crellin JA: Med Radiogr Photogr 31:81, 1955. Courtesy of Eastman Kodak Company.)

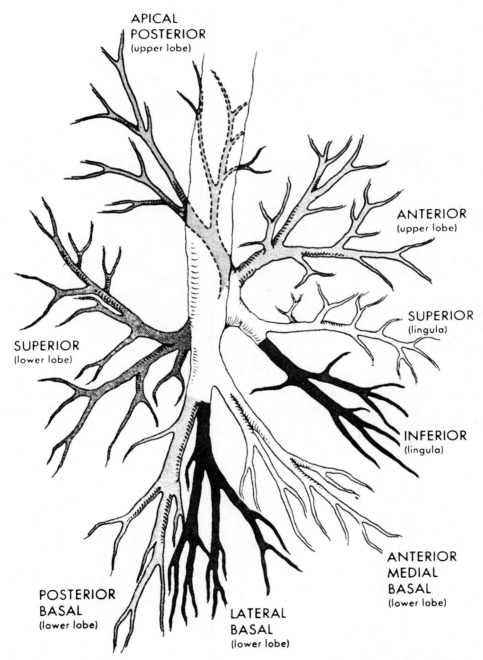

Figure 1–6. Left Bronchial Tree (Lateral Projection). Schematic representation of the normal segments of the left bronchial tree in lateral projection. (From Lehman JS, Crellin JA: Med Radiogr Photogr 31:81, 1955. Courtesy of Eastman Kodak Company.)

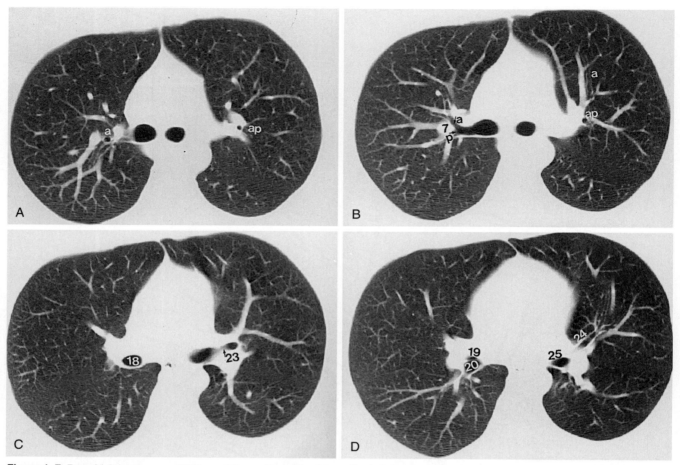

Figure 1–7. Bronchial Anatomy on CT Scan. CT scan *(A)* at a level immediately below the tracheal carina shows the apical segmental bronchus of the right upper lobe (a) and the apical posterior segmental bronchus (ap) of the left upper lobe. CT scan *(B)* at the level of the anterior (a) and posterior (p) segmental bronchi of the right upper lobe. Between the bronchi lies a branch of the right superior pulmonary vein (7). Also seen are right and left main bronchi and apicoposterior (ap) and anterior (a) segmental bronchi of the left upper lobe. Slightly more caudad *(C)*, the apicoposterior segmental bronchus joins the left upper lobe bronchus (23). Note the local anterior and posterior indentations of the left upper lobe bronchus by the pulmonary artery. On the right, the intermediate bronchus (18) is seen in cross-section. CT scan *(D)* at the level of the lingular (24) and left lower lobe (25) bronchi and the carina between the right lower lobe (20) and middle lobe (19) bronchi.

nous bronchiole immediately proximal to a respiratory bronchiole sometimes is called the *terminal bronchiole*. Approximately two to three additional generations of respiratory bronchiole are present after the most proximal branch. Terminal bronchioles measure about 0.6 mm in diameter, and distal respiratory bronchioles measure about 0.4 mm.[4] Because their walls are less than 0.1 mm thick, normal bronchioles cannot be visualized on the radiograph or CT scan.[5] Abnormalities of the bronchioles can be recognized frequently on high-resolution computed tomography (HRCT) scan, however, by their characteristic distribution near the center of the secondary pulmonary lobule (see farther on).

PULMONARY ARTERIAL AND VENOUS CIRCULATION

Pulmonary Arteries

The main pulmonary artery originates in the mediastinum at the pulmonary valve and extends cranially and slightly to the left for 4 to 5 cm before bifurcating within

the pericardium into the shorter left and longer right arteries (Figs. 1–8 and 1–9). The left pulmonary artery continues in more or less the same line as the pulmonary trunk until it reaches the hilum, where it arches over the left main bronchus. Subsequently the artery sometimes gives off a short ascending branch that divides into segmental branches to the upper lobe; more commonly, it continues directly into the vertically oriented left interlobar artery, from which the segmental arteries to the upper and lower lobes arise directly.[6] The left interlobar artery lies posterolateral to the upper lobe bronchus (Fig. 1–10).

The right pulmonary artery courses behind the ascending aorta before dividing behind the superior vena cava and in front of the right main bronchus into ascending (truncus anterior) and descending (interlobar) branches (*see* Fig. 1–10). Although variable, the common pattern is for the ascending artery to subdivide into the segmental branches that supply the right upper lobe and for the descending branch to contribute the segmental arteries to the middle and right lower lobes.[6]

The first portion of the right interlobar artery is horizontal and is interposed between the superior vena cava in

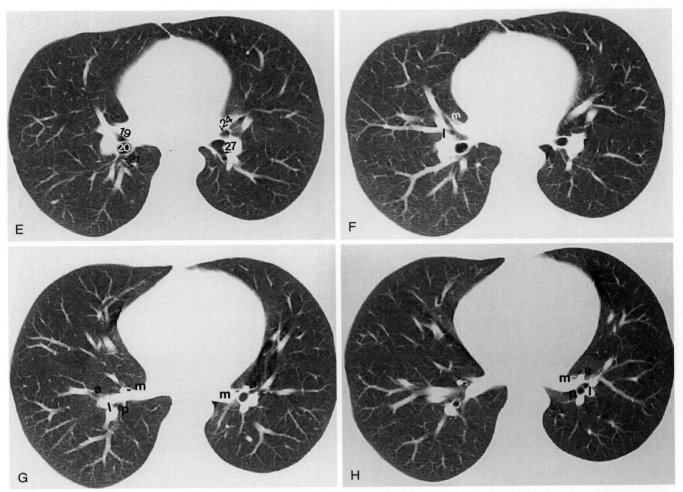

Figure 1–7. ***Continued*** CT scan *(E)* slightly more caudad shows the superior segmental bronchus (27) of left lower lobe; inferior lingular bronchus (24); and right superior segmental (21), lower lobe (20), and middle lobe bronchi (19). CT scan *(F)* at the level in which the right middle lobe bronchus divides into medial (m) and lateral (l) segmental bronchi. Also seen are the lobar bronchi in cross-section with the interlobar pulmonary arteries lateral to them. CT scan *(G)* at the level in which the inferior pulmonary veins join the left atrium shows right medial (m) and anterior (a) segmental bronchi anterior to the right inferior pulmonary vein and posterior segmental (p) and lateral segmental (l) bronchi posterior to the vein. On the left side, the medial segmental bronchus (m) and anterior segmental (a) bronchus can be seen as well as a common trunk between the posterior and lateral segmental bronchi. More commonly the anterior and medial bronchi originate as a common trunk to ventilate the anteromedial segmental bronchus of the left lower lobe. At a slightly lower level *(H)*, the medial (m) and anterior (a) segmental bronchi of the left lower lobe can be seen anterior to the inferior pulmonary vein, whereas the lateral (l) and posterior (p) bronchi are posterior to the vein.

front and the intermediate bronchus behind (*see* Fig. 1–10). It then turns sharply downward and backward, assuming a vertical orientation within the major fissure (thus its name) anterolateral to the intermediate and right lower lobe bronchi before giving the segmental branches—one or two to the middle lobe and usually single branches to each of the five bronchopulmonary segments of the lower lobe.

Although the course of the most proximal pulmonary arteries is fairly constant, the origin and branching pattern of lobar and segmental arteries show considerable variation.[7] Despite this variation, the pulmonary arterial system invariably is related intimately to the airways and divides with them, a branch always accompanying the adjacent airway down to the level of the distal respiratory bronchioles. In addition to these *conventional* vessels, many *supernumerary* (accessory) branches of the pulmonary artery arise at points other than corresponding airway divisions and penetrate the lung parenchyma directly.[8] These super-

numerary branches outnumber the conventional ones and originate throughout the length of the arterial tree, most frequently in a peripheral location.

The upper limit of normal of the transverse diameter of the interlobar artery (measured from its lateral aspect to the air column of the intermediate bronchus) is 16 mm in men and 15 mm in women.[9] Normal ranges in size of the pulmonary arteries also have been determined by CT scan. The upper limit of normal for the diameter of the main pulmonary artery at the level of the pulmonary artery bifurcation is 29 mm, and the upper limit of normal for the diameter of the right interlobar artery measured at the level of the origin of the middle lobe bronchus is 17 mm.[10] There is no significant difference between measurements in men and women.[10] Some of the most useful measurements are summarized in Table 1–1.

Another measurement that can be useful in the assessment of vascular disease is the pulmonary artery-to-bron-

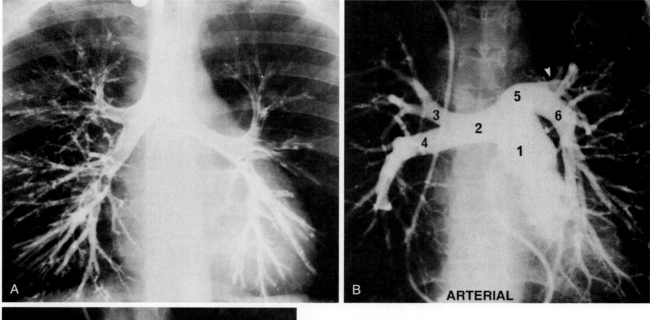

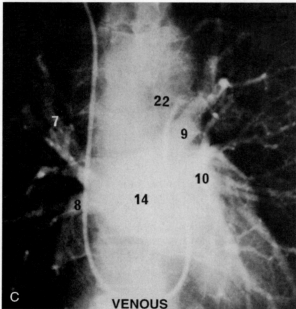

Figure 1–8. Normal Hilar Anatomy in Anteroposterior Projection. Anteroposterior tracheobronchogram *(A)* and anteroposterior angiogram during the arterial *(B)* and venous *(C)* phases for comparison of anatomic relationships. The main pulmonary artery (1) divides into shorter, higher left (5) and longer right (2) branches. The right branch divides into ascending (3) and descending (4) arteries within the pericardium, behind the superior vena cava (note course of the catheter), before appearing as hilar vessels *(B)*. The left pulmonary artery in this patient shows similar divisional features with relatively small ascending *(arrowhead)* and more prominent descending (6) branches. The venous phase of the angiogram *(C)* shows a close relationship between the right (7) and left (9) superior veins as they cross anterior to the hilar arterial vasculature. Note the typical course of the left superior vein in relation to the left main bronchus (22). On the right, three veins drain to the left atrium (14), whereas on the left, superior and inferior veins (10) join to form a common chamber before entering the atrium.

chus diameter ratio. In one study of 30 healthy individuals, the ratio on frontal radiographs was 0.85 ± 0.15 (mean ± standard deviation [SD]) above and 1.34 ± 0.25 below the right hilar angle in the erect position and 1.01 ± 0.13 above and 1.05 ± 0.13 below the right hilar angle in the supine position.[11] Calculation of these ratios is particularly helpful in the assessment of volume overload and congestive heart failure.[12] For example, in one study of 30 patients who had volume overload complicating chronic renal failure, the mean artery-to-bronchus ratio in the erect position was 1.62 ± 0.31 above the right hilar angle and 1.56 ± 0.28 below it;[11] in patients who had congestive heart failure, the ratio was 1.50 ± 0.25 above and 0.87 ± 0.20 below in the erect position and 1.49 ± 0.31 above and 0.96 ± 0.31 below in the supine position. The pulmonary artery-to-bronchus ratio was measured on HRCT in 30

patients who did not have cardiopulmonary disease.[13] In this study, the mean value ± SD was 0.98 ± 0.14, figures similar to those of 1.04 ± 0.13 reported on chest radiographs of healthy supine individuals.[11]

Pulmonary Veins

The pulmonary veins arise from venules that drain the alveolar capillaries and the capillary network of the pleura. In contrast to the pulmonary arteries, they are not associated with the airways. Although their final course is variable, there usually are two main superior and two main inferior vessels, the former draining the middle and upper lobes on the right side and the upper lobe on the left and the latter draining the lower lobes (Fig. 1–11). The right-sided veins course beneath the main pulmonary artery

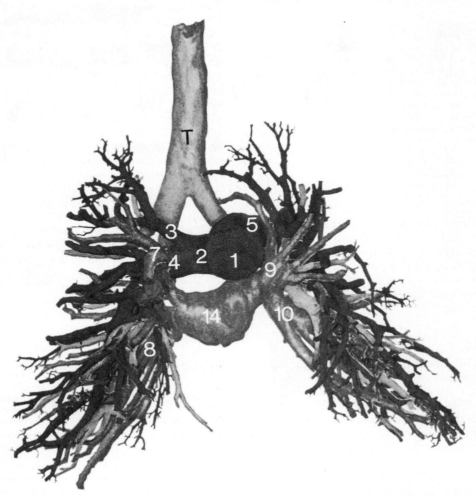

Figure 1–9. Anatomic Features of the Central Pulmonary Vasculature. Anterior cast of the trachea (T), bronchi, pulmonary arteries, and pulmonary veins. The intricate relationship of these structures to one another is apparent. Note that the right (7) and the left (9) superior veins relate most closely to the anterior aspect of the upper hila, whereas the right (8) and the left (10) inferior veins are situated posteromedial to the lower lobe bronchi. Numerical anatomic designations are used consistently throughout this section. 1, Main pulmonary artery; 2, right pulmonary artery; 3, truncus anterior; 4, right interlobar artery; 5, left pulmonary artery; 7, right superior pulmonary vein; 8, right inferior pulmonary vein; 9, left superior pulmonary vein; 10, left inferior pulmonary vein; 14, left atrium. (From Genereux GP: Am J Roentgenol 141:1241, 1983).

Figure 1–10. Anatomic Features of the Pulmonary Artery and Its Main Branches as Seen on CT Scan. CT scan *(A)* at the level of the main bronchi shows the ascending branch (3) of the right pulmonary artery and the main left pulmonary artery (5). CT scan *(B)* at the level of the bronchus intermedius shows the main pulmonary artery (1), right pulmonary artery (2), and right interlobar pulmonary artery (4). Also seen are the anterior segmental arteries of the right upper lobe *(straight arrow)* and the right upper lobe pulmonary veins *(curved arrows)*. On the left side, the left interlobar pulmonary artery (6) can be seen behind the left upper lobe bronchus, whereas the left superior pulmonary vein (9) lies in front of the bronchus.

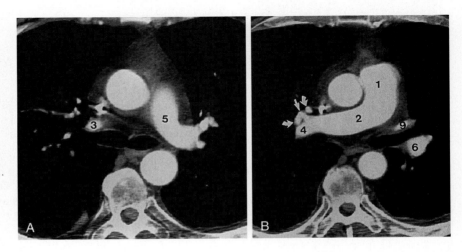

Table 1–1. NORMAL MEASUREMENTS

Trachea
    Range of diameters in men: 13–27 mm
    Range of diameters in women: 10–23 mm[2]
Right interlobar pulmonary artery on chest radiograph
    Upper limit of transverse diameter in men: 16 mm
    Upper limit of transverse diameter in women: 15 mm[9]
Pulmonary artery diameters on CT scan
    Upper limit of transverse diameter in men and women
        Right interlobar pulmonary artery: 17 mm
        Main pulmonary artery: 29 mm[10]
Pulmonary artery-to-bronchus diameter ratio
    Upright chest radiograph
        Above right hilum: 0.85 ± 0.15
        Below right hilum: 1.34 ± 0.25
        Supine radiograph: 1.04 ± 0.13[11]

posterior to the superior vena cava and enter the left atrium separately. The left-sided veins pass anterior to the descending aorta and enter the atrium separately as on the right or join within the pericardial cavity to enter the atrium as a common channel. As in the pulmonary arterial system, numerous supernumerary vessels join the veins as they course through the lung.[14]

Pulmonary Hila

The pulmonary hila are areas in the center of the thorax that connect the mediastinum to the lungs. The anatomic structures rendering the hila visible on radiographs are primarily the pulmonary arteries and veins, with lesser contributions from the bronchial walls, surrounding connective tissue, and lymph nodes.[15] As viewed on a conventional PA radiograph, the hila can be divided into upper and lower components by an imaginary horizontal line transecting the junction of the upper lobe and intermediate bronchi on the right and the upper and lower lobe bronchial dichotomy on the left.

On the *right* side, the upper hilar opacity relates to the ascending pulmonary artery and superior pulmonary vein (Fig. 1–12). The end-on opacity and radiolucency of the contiguous anterior (and occasionally posterior) segmental artery and bronchus can be identified in approximately 80% of normal individuals.[16] A short segment of the upper lobe bronchus beneath the ascending right pulmonary artery sometimes can be identified before it trifurcates into the segmental branches serving the upper lobe. The lower portion of the right hilum (Fig. 1–13) is formed by the vertically oriented interlobar artery, the right superior pulmonary vein superolaterally as it crosses the junction of the horizontal and vertical limbs of the interlobar artery, and the respective branches of these vessels. The horizontally oriented inferior pulmonary vein lies more inferiorly. The radiolucent lumen of the intermediate bronchus invariably can be identified medial to the interlobar artery. Occasionally, segmental bronchi and arteries in the middle and lower lobes can be seen in profile or end-on.

On the *left*, the upper hilar opacity is formed by the distal left pulmonary artery, the proximal portion of the left interlobar artery and its segmental arterial branches, and the left superior pulmonary vein and its major tributaries (Fig. 1–14). The proximal left pulmonary artery is almost always higher than the highest point of the right interlobar artery.

BRONCHIAL CIRCULATION

There is considerable variation in the number and origin of human bronchial arteries. In most individuals, there are two to four, a relatively common pattern being one on the right (originating from the third intercostal artery [the first right intercostal artery that arises directly from the aorta]) and two on the left (arising directly from the aorta on its anterolateral aspect, usually opposite the fifth and sixth thoracic vertebrae).[17–19] Their diameter at the hilum is about 1 to 1.5 mm. The intrapulmonary bronchial arteries are situated within the peribronchial connective tissue and

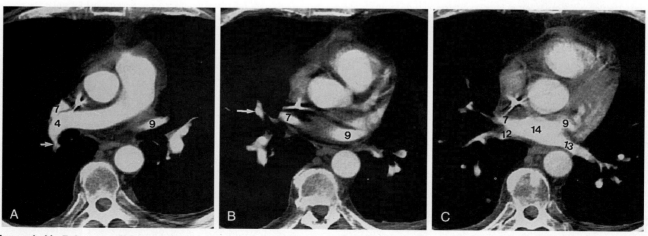

Figure 1–11. Pulmonary Veins on CT Scan. CT scan *(A)* at the level of bronchus intermedius shows the right superior pulmonary vein (7) immediately anterior to the descending branch of the right pulmonary artery (4). Also seen is the superior segmental artery of the right lower lobe *(straight arrow)*. On the left side, the superior pulmonary vein (9) can be seen anterior to the left main and upper lobe bronchi. At this level, the left interlobar artery can be seen to be bifurcating into lingular and left lower lobe branches. CT scan *(B)* at the level of the middle lobe bronchus shows right (7) and left (9) superior pulmonary veins converging toward the upper aspect of the left atrium. Also seen are the right middle lobe pulmonary artery *(arrow)* and branches of the right and left lower lobe arteries. A CT scan 5 mm more caudad *(C)* shows the right (7) and left (9) superior pulmonary veins and right (12) and left (13) inferior venous confluences entering the left atrium (14).

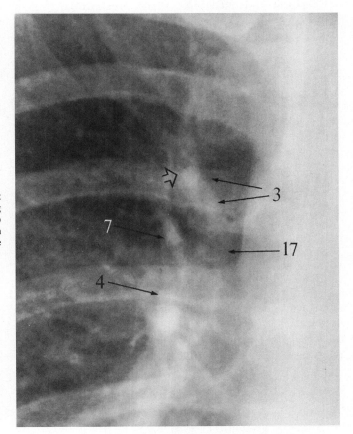

Figure 1–12. Right Upper Hilar Anatomy. Detail view of the right hilum from a conventional posteroanterior radiograph shows the ascending (3) and descending (4) arteries. The right superior pulmonary vein (7) crosses the hilum obliquely to form the typical V configuration. The lumen of the right upper lobe bronchus (17) and of the end-on bronchus and the opaque artery *(open arrow)* of the anterior segment are shown.

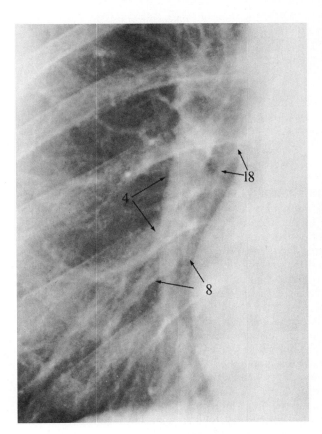

Figure 1–13. Right Lower Hilar Anatomy. On this detail view from a conventional posteroanterior radiograph, the interlobar (4) artery lies lateral to the intermediate bronchus (18). This vessel dominates the radiographic anatomy of the lower hilum. The horizontally oriented inferior pulmonary vein (8) lies posteroinferior to the hilum.

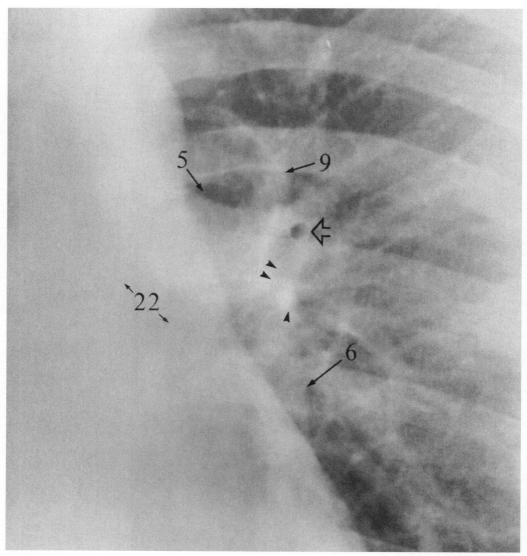

Figure 1–14. Left Hilar Anatomy. Detail view of the left hilum from a posteroanterior chest radiograph shows the left pulmonary artery (5), the interlobar artery (6), and the left superior pulmonary vein (9). The left main bronchus (22) and its superior *(two arrowheads)* and inferior *(single arrowhead)* divisions are overlapped by the hilar vessels. The end-on bronchus and opaque artery *(single open arrowhead)* of the anterior segment are seen.

branch with the airways. They continue as far as the terminal bronchioles.

The bronchial circulation is unique in that it has a dual venous drainage. One portion—related predominantly to the trachea and large bronchi—drains through the bronchial veins to the right side of the heart via the azygos and hemiazygos systems. A second portion, related to the major portion of the intrapulmonary bronchial flow,[19] is derived from extensive anastomoses with the pulmonary circulation at precapillary, capillary, and postcapillary sites and drains into the left atrium via the pulmonary veins (the bronchopulmonary anastomotic flow).[20]

LUNG PARENCHYMA

Secondary Lobule

The secondary lobule is the smallest discrete portion of the lung that is surrounded by connective tissue septa (Fig.

1–15).[21] Each lobule is supplied by a lobular bronchiole and pulmonary artery, which are located in the center of the lobule; the draining pulmonary veins are located in the interlobular septa. The lobule is irregularly polyhedral in shape and generally measures 1 to 2.5 cm in diameter. Interlobular septa are most numerous in the apical, anterior, and lateral aspects of the upper lobe and the lateral and anterior regions of the right middle lobe, lingula, and lower lobe.[22] In these areas, they measure approximately 100 μm in thickness and can be identified on visual inspection of the pleural or cut surfaces of the lung (Fig. 1–16).

The normal secondary lobule cannot be identified on the chest radiograph. Only when the interlobular septa are rendered visible as septal lines as a result of thickening by fluid or tissue (such as edema or carcinoma) can the lung between two lines be recognized as a secondary lobule. By contrast, normal interlobular septa are identified easily on HRCT scan as straight lines 1 to 2.5 cm in length and

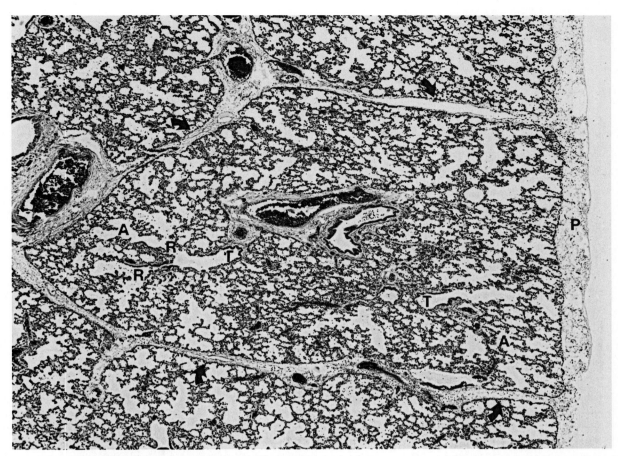

Figure 1–15. Secondary Lobule—Histologic Appearance. The bronchiole and pulmonary artery supplying the secondary lobule are located in the center of the lobule. The terminal (T) and respiratory (R) bronchioles are located near the center of the lobule. The more peripheral portions of the lobule contain alveolar ducts (A) and alveoli. The lobule is marginated by the interlobular septa *(arrows)* and pleura (P). (×6.)

slightly more than 0.1 mm in thickness that often extend to the pleural surface (Fig. 1–17).[23, 24] They are identified most commonly in the anterior and lateral aspects of the lungs, where they are best developed.[23, 24] Although less

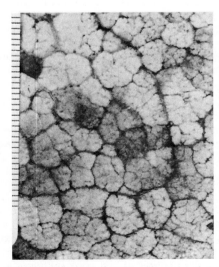

Figure 1–16. Secondary Lobule. Close-up view of the lower lobe visceral pleura shows the bases of numerous, irregularly shaped secondary lobules measuring 0.5 to 1.5 cm in greatest dimension.

well visualized in the more central regions of the lungs, they can be identified when they are thickened by edema or inflammatory or neoplastic tissue (Fig. 1–18).[25] The pulmonary parenchyma between the interlobular septa and the centrilobular pulmonary arteries (lobular core) contains small vessels and airways and their accompanying interstitium that are below the resolution of CT. This area is seen as a region of homogeneous attenuation slightly greater than air. Consolidation of a secondary lobule can be identified on HRCT scan as a focal area of opacification measuring 0.5 to 2 cm in diameter, which is marginated by the interlobular septa (Fig. 1–19).

There are two major reasons for considering the secondary lobule the fundamental unit of lung structure from a radiologic point of view: (1) It is the smallest anatomic unit that can be identified clearly on HRCT scan, and (2) assessment of the distribution of abnormalities within it can be helpful in the differential diagnosis of disease.[26–28] For example, pathologic processes related to the terminal or respiratory bronchioles are characterized on HRCT scan by predominant distribution near the center of the lobule.[5] Examples of specific abnormalities include localized areas of low attenuation in centrilobular emphysema and areas of increased attenuation in tuberculosis, hypersensitivity pneumonitis, sarcoidosis, asbestosis, and silicosis.[27, 29, 30] Various forms of bronchiolitis are characterized on HRCT

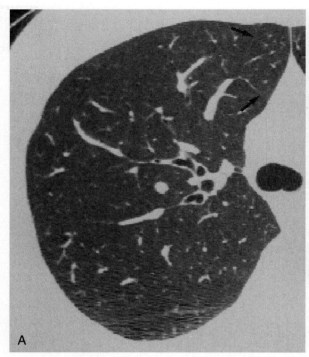

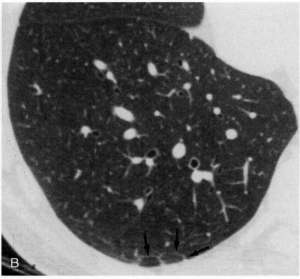

Figure 1–17. Normal Interlobular Septa. Views of the right upper *(A)* and right lower lobes *(B)* from HRCT scan in a 35-year-old woman show normal interlobular septa *(straight arrows).*

scan by the presence of nodular areas of attenuation or branching lines near the center of the lobule or by decreased attenuation of the lobule because of air trapping or vasoconstriction (Fig. 1–20).[5, 30, 31]

Acinus

The pulmonary acinus is the portion of lung distal to the terminal bronchiole and is composed of respiratory bronchioles, alveolar ducts, alveolar sacs, alveoli and their accompanying vessels, and connective tissue.[32, 33] Reported measurements of acinar diameter vary between 6 and 10 mm, depending to some extent on the technique by and pressure at which the lung is inflated.[34, 35]

NORMAL LUNG: RADIOGRAPHY

Radiographic Density

The radiopacity of the lungs is the result of the absorptive powers of each of its component parts—gas, blood, and tissue. The density of bloodless collapsed lung tissue is 1.065 gm/ml;[36] the density of blood is 1.052 gm/ml.[37] Because nonaerated lung *in vivo* consists of approximately half blood and half tissue,[38] the mean density of collapsed lung containing blood is approximately 1.06 gm/ml.[39] By comparison, water has a density of 1.0 gm/ml, and air has a density of 0. Using the average figures for total maximal tissue volume, derived from anatomic and physiologic estimates, and the predicted total lung capacity of a 20-year-old man 170 cm tall (6,500 ml),[40] the *average* density of lung is 740 gm ÷ 7,198 ml, or 0.103 gm/ml. A considerable portion of lung tissue—logically the air-containing parenchyma—must possess a density *less* than this to compensate for the relatively high density of the visible blood vessels.

Symmetry of radiographic density of the two lungs in a normal individual depends on proper positioning for radiography. If the patient is rotated, the lung closer to the film is uniformly more radiopaque (whiter) than the other lung (Fig. 1–21); conversely, the lung that is farthest away from the film is uniformly less radiopaque (more black), and a unilateral hyperlucent hemithorax is present that sometimes can hamper interpretation. In one investigation using phantoms, approximately 80% of this unilateral increase in radiographic density was found to be the result of asymmetric absorption of the primary x-ray beam, with the remaining 20% being due to scatter radiation.[41] Measurement of chest wall thickness showed that the x-ray beam traversed less tissue on the side of increased film blackening (or conversely more tissue on the side of increased opacity), chiefly as a result of the pectoral muscles. Because rotation to the right or to the left means different things to different people (is it rotation into the right anterior oblique or left posterior oblique?), it is preferable to relate the increased opacity or increased lucency to the side that is closest to or farthest removed from the film. The hemithorax closer to the film is more radiopaque than the contralateral hemithorax.

Provided that the patient is not rotated and the x-ray beam is centered properly, any discrepancy in the density of the two lungs must be interpreted as being abnormal. The cause varies from such benign conditions as scoliosis or congenital absence of the pectoral muscles to more significant disorders such as Swyer-James syndrome.

Pulmonary Markings

Correct interpretation of the chest radiograph requires a thorough knowledge of the pattern of linear markings throughout the normal lung. These markings are created by

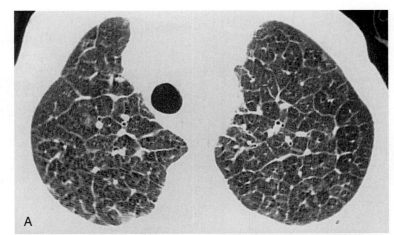

Figure 1–18. Interlobular Septal Thickening. HRCT (1-mm collimation) scan in a patient with interstitial pulmonary edema *(A)* shows thickening of the interlobular septa. Secondary pulmonary lobules are variable in size and have an irregular polyhedral shape. The patient was a 77-year-old woman with left heart failure. Incidental note is made of unrelated anterior mediastinal lymphadenopathy. Magnified view of a slice of upper lobe from another patient *(B)* shows mild-to-moderate interlobular septal thickening as a result of lymphangitic carcinomatosis. The architecture is similar to that of the HRCT image.

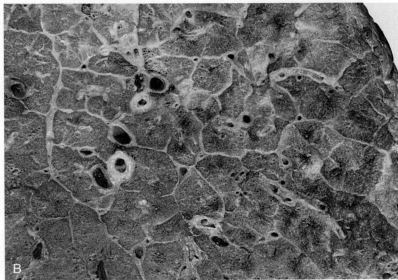

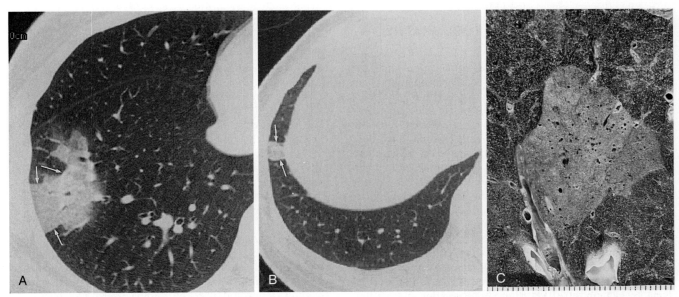

Figure 1–19. Consolidation of Secondary Pulmonary Lobules. HRCT scans *(A and B)* show consolidation of secondary pulmonary lobules, multiple *(A)* and solitary *(B)*. Note the sharp demarcation between the consolidated lobules outlined in the interlobular septa *(arrows)* and the normal adjacent lung parenchyma. Magnified view of lung from another patient *(C)* shows homogeneous consolidation of a portion of parenchyma demarcated by interlobular septa and the wall of a small bronchus. Histologic sections showed organizing pneumonia of uncertain origin. The appearance in each of these three cases suggests that the initial pathologic process was limited in its spread within the lung by the presence of the septa.

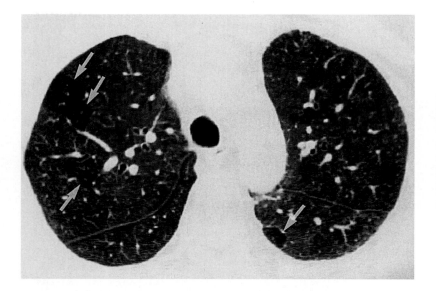

Figure 1–20. Decreased Attenuation of Pulmonary Lobule. HRCT scan shows sharply defined localized areas of decreased attenuation and vascularity *(arrows).* The areas of decreased attenuation have a size and configuration consistent with involvement of one or more adjacent secondary pulmonary lobules and reflect the presence of airway obstruction at the level of the lobular bronchioles. The decreased ventilation of the lobules leads to reflex vasoconstriction and decreased vascularity and attenuation on HRCT.

the pulmonary arteries, bronchi, veins, and accompanying interstitial tissue (*see* Figs. 1–1 and 1–2). The first two of these fan outward from both hila and gradually taper as they proceed distally. In the normal state, they are visible up to about 1 to 2 cm from the visceral pleural surface over the convexity of the lung, at which point it is composed predominantly of acini.

The posteroanterior chest radiograph of a normal erect individual invariably shows some discrepancy in size of pulmonary vessels in the upper lung zones compared with the lower, as a result of pressure-related differences in blood flow from the apex to base (a unit volume of lung at the base of the thorax having four to eight times the blood flow of a similar volume at the apex[42]). In a recumbent individual, a decrease in the influence of gravity renders this discrepancy in vascular size minimal.

NORMAL LUNG: COMPUTED TOMOGRAPHY

A cross-sectional CT image of the thorax is a two-dimensional representation of a three-dimensional slice; the third dimension—slice thickness, or CT collimation—can vary from 1 to 10 mm. All structures within the three-dimensional unit (volume = voxel) of the slice are represented as a two-dimensional unit (area = pixel) on the image. Thicker sections (5 to 10 mm collimation) allow assessment of the entire lung volume. This assessment usually can be performed during a single breath-hold when spiral CT technique is used. On such thick sections, vessels can be identified clearly within the lung parenchyma as they course through the slice (Fig. 1–22). Volume averaging within the plane of section results in decreased spatial resolution, however, and assessment of fine parenchymal detail requires the use of 1- to 2-mm collimation scans. The resulting thinner sections allow assessment of airways 1.5 to 2 mm in diameter and vessels down to the level of the interlobular septal veins and centrilobular arteries.[23, 24] Because of the thin section, however, vessels cut in cross-section may be difficult to distinguish from small nodules.[43]

The appearance of bronchi and vessels depends on their orientation: When imaged along their long axes, they ap-

pear as cylindrical structures that taper as they branch; when imaged at an angle to their longitudinal axes, they appear as rounded structures if perpendicular to the plane of the CT or as elliptical structures when oriented obliquely. The outer walls of pulmonary vessels form smooth, sharply defined interfaces with the surrounding lung. Central pulmonary vessels can be recognized readily as arteries by their location adjacent to bronchi. Central pulmonary veins can be identified as they course toward the left atrium. Although it is often impossible to distinguish peripheral pulmonary arteries from veins by conventional CT scan, differentiation frequently can be accomplished by HRCT; with this technique, veins can be identified as structures that separate secondary pulmonary lobules, extend into interlobular septa, and (sometimes) reach the pleura (Fig. 1–23);[44] by contrast, pulmonary arteries lie near the center of the secondary pulmonary lobule and do not abut the pleura.

The smallest normal airways that can be identified on CT scan are 1.5 to 2 mm in diameter;[23] smaller branches cannot be visualized because their walls are less than 0.1 mm thick and below the spatial resolution of current CT scanners. In normal individuals, no airways can be visualized within 1 cm of the costal or paravertebral pleura;[45] however, they can be identified within 1 cm of the mediastinal pleura (but not abutting it) in approximately 40%.[45] The smallest pulmonary artery that can be resolved by HRCT is approximately 0.2 mm in diameter and corresponds to the artery accompanying a terminal bronchiole.[23] The distance from this artery to the border of the secondary lobule or the pleural surface ranges from 3 to 5 mm (Fig. 1–24).

The outer diameter of a bronchus is approximately equal to that of the adjacent pulmonary artery.[13] The *apparent* bronchial wall thickness and the diameter of bronchi and vessels are markedly influenced by the display parameters (window level and window width) used. The results of studies with phantoms show that accurate assessment of the size of small parenchymal structures requires the use of a display level of −450 Hounsfield units (HU) (Fig. 1–25).[46, 47] For clinical practice, we recommend the use of

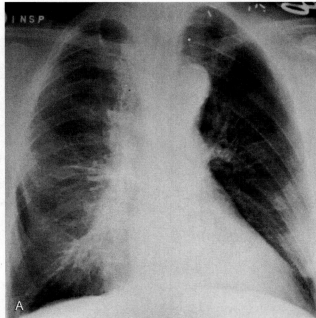

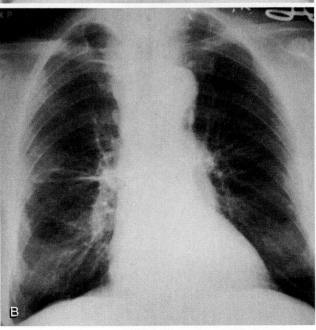

Figure 1–21. Alteration in Lung Density Owing to Improper Positioning. Radiograph *(A)* of the chest in posteroanterior projection was exposed with the patient rotated slightly into the right anterior oblique position to produce an overall increase in density of the right lung as compared with the left. When the positioning was corrected, the asymmetry disappeared *(B)*.

a window level of −600 to −700 HU and a window width of 1,000 to 1,500 HU because these settings provide the best depiction of airways and lung parenchyma. These display parameter settings result in an overestimation of the diameter of small structures and bronchial wall thickness and an underestimation of the diameter of the bronchial lumen.[46] Although a window level of −450 HU allows more accurate quantitative measurements, this setting seldom is used in clinical practice because the images are too dark and do not allow adequate visualization of small parenchymal structures and focal abnormalities.[5]

The pulmonary artery-to-outer bronchial diameter ratio (ABR) has been assessed by many workers. In one investigation of 30 patients who did not have cardiopulmonary

disease,[13] diameters were assessed at the level of subsegmental bronchi using a window level of −450 HU and a window width of 1,200 to 1,500 HU.[48] The mean ABR was 0.98 ± 0.14 (range, 0.53 to 1.39)—a value comparable to that reported on chest radiographs in supine healthy individuals (1.04 ± 0.13).[49] Because an increased ratio of inner bronchial diameter to pulmonary artery diameter is one of the CT criteria for the diagnosis of bronchiectasis,[45] this ratio is another parameter that has been investigated in normal individuals. The measurement has been found to be influenced by altitude, presumably as a result of a combination of hypoxic vasoconstriction and bronchodilation.[50, 51] In one investigation of 17 normal, nonsmoking individuals living at 1,600 m and 16 living at sea level, the

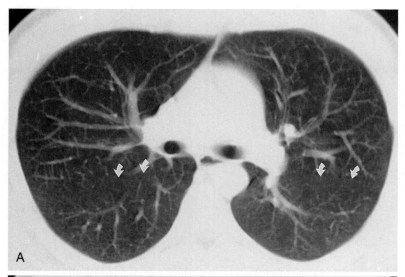

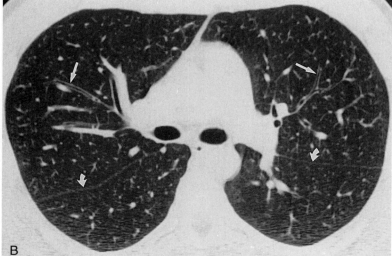

Figure 1–22. Comparison of Thick-Section CT and HRCT Scans. A 10-mm collimation CT scan *(A)* at the level of the bronchus intermedius shows normal lung parenchyma and airways as visualized on conventional CT scan. Pulmonary vessels can be identified easily as they course within the 10-mm thickness of the CT section. A 1-mm collimation HRCT scan *(B)* performed at the same level reveals sharper definition between vessels and bronchi and the adjacent lung parenchyma on the high-resolution image as compared with the conventional CT scan. Bronchi measuring approximately 2 mm in diameter *(straight arrows)* are identified clearly on the HRCT image but not on the conventional CT scan. Interlobar fissures *(curved arrows)* appear as sharply defined lines on the HRCT image compared with the broad areas of slightly increased attenuation on the corresponding conventional CT image. Both images were reconstructed using a high-resolution algorithm and photographed at window level of −700 and window width of 1,500 HU.

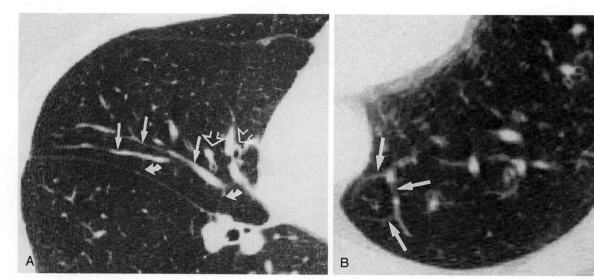

Figure 1–23. Pulmonary Veins and Interlobular Septa. View of the right lung from HRCT scan *(A)* reveals right middle lobe pulmonary veins *(straight arrows)* running almost horizontal to the plane of the CT section. Smaller feeding veins can be seen coming from interlobular septa near the right major fissure *(curved arrows)*. The larger veins also outline the margins of secondary pulmonary lobules. Right middle lobe pulmonary arteries and adjacent bronchi *(open arrows)* can be seen in cross-section. View of the left lower lobe from HRCT scan *(B)* shows pulmonary veins marginating a secondary pulmonary lobule *(arrows)*. An ectatic bronchiole can be seen near the center of the lobule.

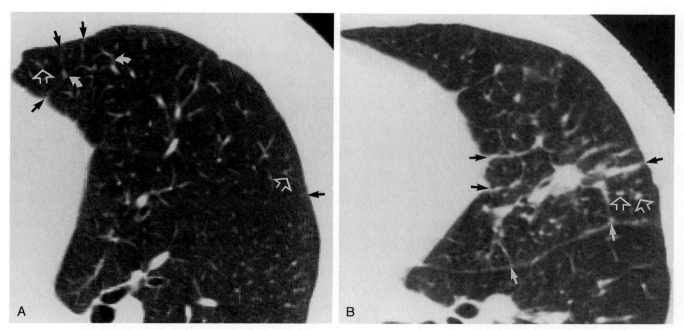

Figure 1–24. Normal and Abnormal Parenchyma. Magnified view of the left lung at the level of the lingula *(A)* from HRCT scan in a 60-year-old man shows normal interlobular septa *(straight arrows)* and peripheral veins *(curved arrows)* separating adjacent secondary pulmonary lobules. Small nodular and branching opacities *(open arrows)* located near the center of the secondary lobules and 3 to 5 mm from the pleura represent pulmonary arteries. HRCT scan *(B)* in a 61-year-old man with relatively mild parenchymal abnormalities caused by sarcoidosis shows thickening of the interlobular septa *(straight arrows)* and increased number and size of centrilobular opacities *(open arrows)*, findings consistent with a perilymphatic distribution of granulomas in the interlobular septal and bronchoarterial interstitium.

mean bronchoarterial ratio at a window level of −450 HU was 0.76 in the former and 0.62 in the latter.[50]

The attenuation of the lung parenchyma is determined by its relative proportions of blood, gas, extravascular fluid, and pulmonary tissue.[52, 53] Normal lung parenchyma has a fairly homogeneous attenuation that is slightly greater than that of air. A gradient is normally present, however, the attenuation being greater in the dependent than in the nondependent regions (Fig. 1–26).[53–55] This gradient is attributable primarily to the influence of gravity on blood flow and lung inflation.

CT scans of the chest usually are performed during suspended full inspiration. In selected cases, scans may be performed during or after forced expiration. As lung gas volume is reduced, lung attenuation increases, the increase being greater in the dependent than in the nondependent regions (Fig. 1–27).[56, 57] This increase is variable in different lung regions; for example, in one study, it ranged from 84 to 372 HU.[56] Focal areas of low attenuation frequently are seen on expiratory scans, particularly in the superior segments of the lower lobes and anterior aspects of the right middle lobe and lingula (Fig. 1–28).[56] Such areas presumably are the result of focal air-trapping.[56] The extent of air-trapping in normal individuals usually is limited to small, localized areas involving a few secondary lobules; this can be seen on expiratory HRCT in 90% of such individuals.[58] Air-trapping involving a total volume equal to or greater than that of a pulmonary segment also is seen in approximately 10% to 15% of normal individuals.[58, 59] It is the extent and not simply the presence of air-trapping that is important in determining the presence of airway obstruction.

Lung Density on Computed Tomography

The measurement of lung density with CT is based on the existence of an approximately linear relationship between the attenuation of an x-ray beam of 65 keV (120 kVp) and the density of materials of low atomic number (ranging from nitrogen to water).[52, 60] Attenuation on a CT scan is expressed in terms of the Hounsfield unit scale, in which water is 0 HU and air is −1,000 HU. The relationship between the physical density—weight of tissue per unit volume—and the Hounsfield scale can be expressed using a *scaled CT quotient*, which is obtained by adding 1,000 to the Hounsfield value, then dividing by 1,000. With this formulation, CT quotient values that range from air to water are approximately equal to physical density in grams per milliliter.[52, 53] For example, a CT attenuation value of −880 HU (approximately the mean value for normal lung at total lung capacity) represents a scaled CT quotient of 120 or a density equivalent of 0.12 gm/ml.

Differences in attenuation between dependent and nondependent lung regions were assessed in an HRCT study of six healthy men.[57] Mean differences in lung attenuation between dependent and nondependent lung regions at 10%, 50%, and 90% vital capacity with the subject supine were approximately 70, 51, and 40 HU for the apical portions of the lung and 130, 57, and 26 HU for the basal regions. With the subject prone, the values were approximately 126, 63, and 19 HU for the upper lung zones and 112, 64, and 48 HU for the lower lung zones. This attenuation gradient was significantly greater at a lung volume of 10% vital capacity than at a volume of 90% vital capacity in supine and prone positions.

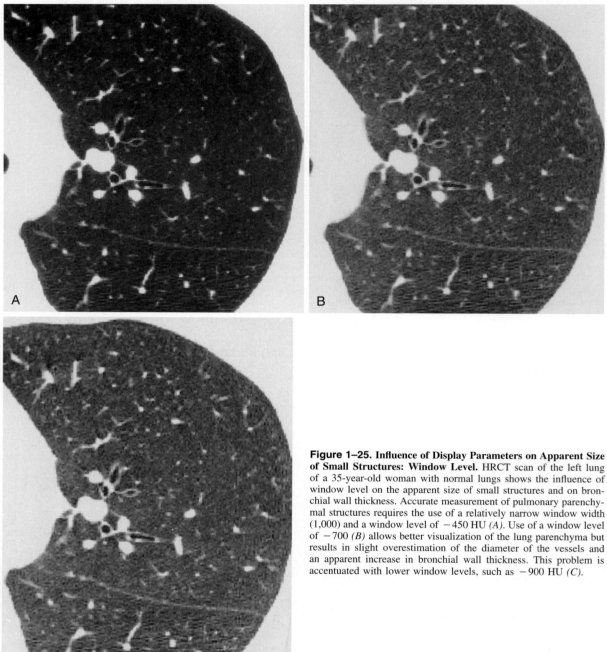

Figure 1–25. Influence of Display Parameters on Apparent Size of Small Structures: Window Level. HRCT scan of the left lung of a 35-year-old woman with normal lungs shows the influence of window level on the apparent size of small structures and on bronchial wall thickness. Accurate measurement of pulmonary parenchymal structures requires the use of a relatively narrow window width (1,000) and a window level of −450 HU *(A)*. Use of a window level of −700 *(B)* allows better visualization of the lung parenchyma but results in slight overestimation of the diameter of the vessels and an apparent increase in bronchial wall thickness. This problem is accentuated with lower window levels, such as −900 HU *(C)*.

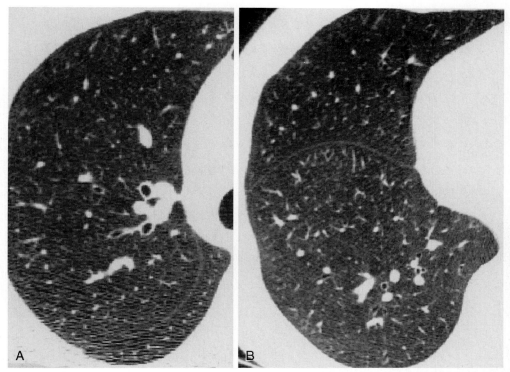

Figure 1–26. Normal Attenuation Gradient. HRCT scans through the right upper *(A)* and lower *(B)* lung zones show a normal increase in attenuation from the anterior to the posterior (dependent) lung regions. The attenuation gradient in the lower lung zones is slightly greater than in the upper zones.

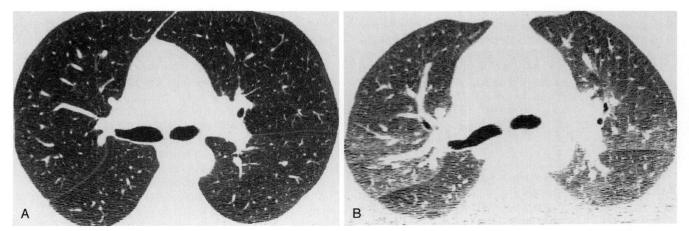

Figure 1–27. Increased Attenuation on Expiratory HRCT. Inspiratory *(A)* and expiratory *(B)* HRCT scans at the level of the main bronchi in a 35-year-old woman show the normal increase in attenuation seen at low lung volumes. The attenuation gradient from least dependent to most dependent lung regions is seen more readily on the expiratory CT scan. The increase in attenuation is not homogeneous inasmuch as a discontinuity is present at the level of the major fissures, the posterior aspect of the upper lobes having greater attenuation than the superior segments of the lower lobes.

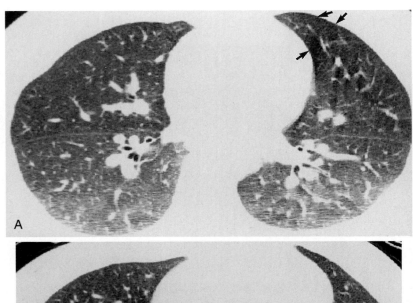

Figure 1–28. Expiratory HRCT Scans. HRCT scans (*A* and *B*) performed at the end of a maximal expiration in a 35-year-old woman with normal lungs show an attenuation gradient. Focal areas of decreased attenuation are present in the lingula *(straight arrows)* and in the lower lobes *(curved arrows)*, presumably a result of focal air trapping.

Attenuation values vary considerably in different regions of the lung and are influenced markedly by pulmonary volume. Values are affected by the type of CT scanner, kilovoltage, patient size, and particular region of lung being assessed.[61, 62] As a result, measurements of lung attenuation have a limited role in the radiologic assessment of the lung parenchyma. The principal exception is the use of attenuation values in the determination of the presence, distribution, and extent of emphysema.

PLEURA

Anatomy

The pleural space is enclosed by the visceral pleura, which covers the lungs, and by the parietal pleura, which lines the chest wall, diaphragm, and mediastinum. The two join at the hila. The visceral pleura consists of mesothelial cells overlying two layers of elastic tissue that separate a small amount of connective tissue and lymphatic vessels. Because the combined thickness of the normal parietal and visceral pleural layers is approximately 0.2 mm, the pleura over the convexity of the lungs and over the diaphragmatic and mediastinal surfaces is not visible on the chest radiograph or on conventional CT scan; however, it can be identified on HRCT scan.[63] Using HRCT, a 1- to 2-mm-thick line of soft tissue attenuation normally is seen between the lung and chest wall between the inner edges of the ribs in the intercostal spaces. This line represents the combined thickness of the visceral pleura, normal pleural fluid, parietal pleura, endothoracic fascia, and innermost intercostal muscle (Fig. 1–29).[63]

The pleura and endothoracic fascia along the inner aspects of the ribs normally are too thin to be visible on HRCT;[63] however, they may be identified as a thin, smooth line when there is increased extrapleural fat. The latter is most abundant over the posterolateral aspects of the fourth to eighth ribs, where it can be several millimeters thick in normal individuals.[64, 65] The pleura and endothoracic fascia also can be seen when a portion of rib is nearly horizontal, in which case the CT section may include only a portion of the upper and lower rib margins. The rib appears thinner than normal with a line representing the pleura and endothoracic fascia internal to it.

Interlobar Fissures

Fissures are invaginations of the pleura that extend from the outer surface of the lung into its substance. They are considered traditionally in two groups: those that separate the lungs into the three right-sided and two left-sided lobes (*normal* fissures) and those that occur within one of the lobes themselves (*accessory* fissures). The normal fissures

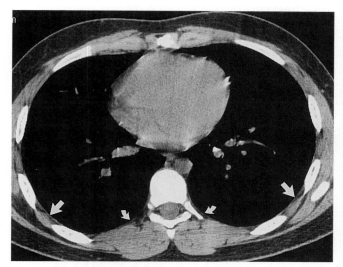

Figure 1–29. Normal Appearance of the Costal Pleura on HRCT Scan. In the intercostal spaces, a 1- to 2-mm-thick line is seen *(straight arrows)*. This line represents the combined thickness of the visceral pleura, normal pleural fluid, parietal pleura, endothoracic fascia, and innermost intercostal muscle. The combined thickness of normal visceral and parietal pleura and endothoracic fascia is too thin to be identified on CT scan over the inner aspect of the ribs, but it can be seen normally in the paravertebral regions as a line measuring 1 mm or less in thickness *(curved arrows)*.

are the *minor (horizontal) fissure* (located between the right middle and upper lobes), the *right major (oblique) fissure* (between the combined right upper and middle lobes and the right lower lobe), and the *left major (oblique) fissure* (between the left upper and lower lobes).

The completeness of fissures is variable. In one study of 100 fixed and inflated lung specimens (50 right and 50 left), an incomplete fissure (lobar fusion) was found between the right lower and upper lobes in 70% of cases and between the right lower and middle lobes in 47%.[66] In the left lung, fusion between the lower and upper lobes was less frequent than on the right: 40% of cases showed an incomplete fissure between the left lower lobe and the superior part of the upper lobe, and 46% showed an incomplete fissure between the lower lobe and lingula. Incompleteness of the minor fissure was far more common than that in any portion of either major fissure: Of the 50 right lungs examined, extensive fusion was present in 88%, especially medially; fusion is more common and usually more extensive between the middle and upper lobe (across the minor fissure) than between the middle and lower lobe (across the major fissure).

Radiography. As indicated, the major (oblique) fissures separate the upper (and on the right, the middle lobe) from the lower lobes. They begin at, or about, the level of the fifth thoracic vertebra and extend obliquely downward and forward, roughly paralleling the sixth rib, ending at the diaphragm a few centimeters behind the anterior pleural gutter (Fig. 1–30). The top of the left lower lobe usually is higher than that of the right, the right major fissure being at the same level as the left in only 25% of cases.[67]

The minor (horizontal) fissure separates the anterior segment of the right upper lobe from the middle lobe and lies in a roughly horizontal plane at about the level of the fourth rib anteriorly. Its orientation shows considerable variation, the anterior aspect generally being lower than the posterior and the lateral part lower than the medial.[66]

Computed Tomography. Interlobar fissures are manifested in three ways on CT scan: lucent bands, lines, and dense bands.[68] This variable appearance is related to the section thickness and the plane of the fissure on the cross-sectional CT image. On CT scans performed using 5- to 10-mm-thick sections, a perpendicular fissure (such as in the upper thorax) is likely to produce a linear configuration, whereas a more oblique orientation causes a well-defined, dense (ground-glass) band *(see* Fig. 1–30). Because the minor fissure and the plane of the CT scan are more or less tangential to one another, the fissure typically is manifested as a lucent area relatively devoid of vessels when compared with the same region in the left lung.

On HRCT scan, the major fissure can be seen as a single line, two parallel lines, or, less commonly, a band of increased attenuation. The minor fissure usually is visualized as a curvilinear line or band of increased attenuation that forms a quarter circle or semicircle in its highest aspect (located slightly cephalad to the level of the origin of the middle lobe bronchus) (Fig. 1–31).[69]

Accessory Fissures

Any portion of lung may be separated partly or completely from adjacent pulmonary tissue by an accessory fissure. The anatomic incidence of such fissures is much higher than generally is appreciated, amounting to about 50% of lungs.[70] Radiologically, they can be identified in approximately 10% of chest radiographs and 20% of conventional CT scans.[71] These fissures vary in their degree of development from superficial slits not more than 1 cm deep to complete fissures that extend all the way to the hilum. The most common are the azygos, inferior, and superior.

Azygos Fissure

Azygos fissure is created by downward invagination of the azygos vein through the apical portion of the right upper lobe (Fig. 1–32). It is manifested radiographically by a curvilinear shadow that extends obliquely across the upper portion of the right lung and terminates at a variable distance above the right hilum in a *teardrop* shadow caused by the azygos vein itself. Because the vein runs outside the parietal pleura, four pleural layers (two parietal and two visceral) form the fissure. The fissure is visible in about 0.5% of chest radiographs.[72]

Inferior Accessory Fissure

Inferior accessory fissure separates the medial basal segment from the remainder of the lower lobe (Fig. 1–33). Its incidence radiologically depends on the mode of examination. In one study of 500 radiographs, inferior accessory fissure was identified in 41 (8%), most commonly on the right.[72] In another investigation of 50 patients examined by conventional chest radiography and CT, the latter technique revealed the fissure in eight cases (16%); of these, only two were visible on the radiograph.[71]

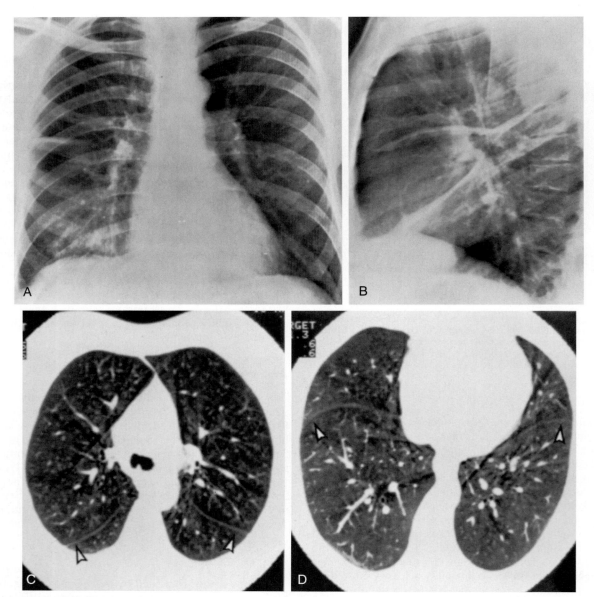

Figure 1–30. Interlobar Fissures, Right Lung. The presence of minimal interlobar effusion renders the fissures clearly visible on posteroanterior *(A)* and lateral *(B)* radiographs. CT scan *(C)* through the upper thorax reveals the lateral portion of the right and left major fissures *(arrowheads)* to be situated posterior to the anteromedial portion of the fissure, so-called lateral facing. CT scan *(D)* through the lower thorax shows that the lateral portion of the major fissures *(arrowheads)* is located anterior to the anteromedial aspect of the major fissures, so-called medial facing.

Superior Accessory Fissure

Superior accessory fissure separates the superior segment from the basal segments of the lower lobes, more commonly on the right. Although present in approximately 5% of lungs examined grossly, the fissure is seldom identified on radiograph or CT scan.[71]

Pulmonary Ligament

The pulmonary ligament consists of a double layer of pleura that tethers the medial aspect of the lower lobe to the adjacent mediastinum and diaphragm.[73] It is formed by the mediastinal parietal pleura as it reflects over the main bronchi and pulmonary arteries and veins onto the surface of the lung as the visceral pleura. Although the pulmonary ligament is anatomically extraparenchymal, it is contiguous laterally with a cleavage plane in the parenchyma of the lower lobe known as the *intersegmental (intersublobar) septum*, which separates the medial from the posterior basal segments.[74] The left pulmonary ligament is related closely to the esophagus and is bordered posteriorly by the descending aorta; the shorter right ligament can be situated anywhere along an arc that extends from the inferior vena cava anteriorly to the azygos vein posteriorly.

Although the pulmonary ligaments are never seen on conventional PA or lateral chest radiographs, the ligament on the left can be visualized on CT scan in 60% to 70% of individuals and the ligament on the right in 40% to 60%.[75, 76] The appearance is variable but usually consists of a small peak or pyramid on the mediastinal surface that represents the ligament and a thin linear opacity that extends from the apex of the peak to the lung, marking

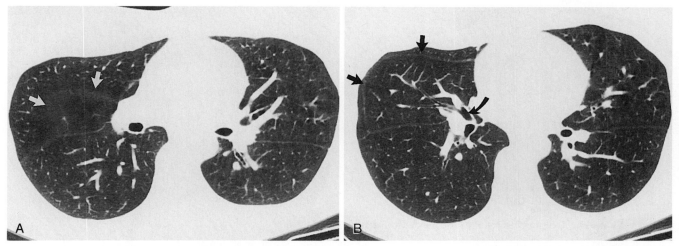

Figure 1–31. Normal Appearance of the Minor Fissure on HRCT Scan. The upper aspect *(A)* of the minor fissure is seen as a curvilinear band of increased attenuation *(arrows)*. The lower and steeper portion *(B)* of the minor fissure is seen as a thin line *(straight arrows)*. The right middle lobe bronchus can be seen at this level *(curved arrow)*.

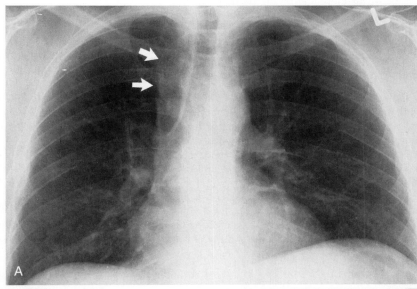

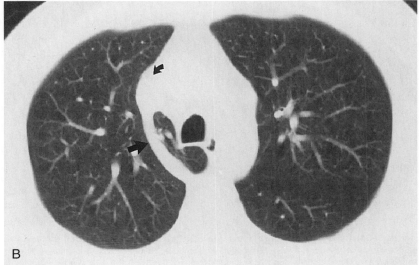

Figure 1–32. Azygos Fissure. On standard postero-anterior radiograph *(A)*, the fissure is identified as a curvilinear line *(arrows)* extending obliquely across the upper portion of the right lung. On CT scan *(B)*, the azygos arch *(straight arrows)* can be seen to end at the superior vena cava *(curved arrow)*. Lung tissue is visualized between the azygos vein and the trachea.

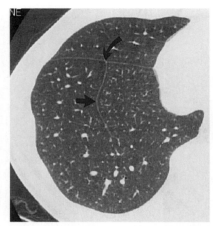

Figure 1–33. Inferior Accessory Fissure. HRCT scan shows the inferior accessory fissure as a linear arc convex laterally *(straight arrow)* and ending anteriorly at the level of the major fissure *(curved arrow).*

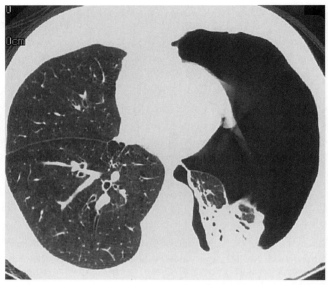

Figure 1–35. Pulmonary Ligament. HRCT scan in a patient with a large spontaneous pneumothorax reveals passive atelectasis of the left lung. The inferior aspect of the lung remains attached to the mediastinum medially by the pulmonary ligament.

the intersegmental septum (Fig. 1–34).[74] The presence and degree of development of the fissure may affect the radiographic appearance of pneumothorax (Fig. 1–35), lower lobe atelectasis, and medial pleural effusion.[73]

LYMPHATIC SYSTEM OF THE LUNGS, PLEURA, AND MEDIASTINUM

Parietal pleural lymphatics are distributed extensively over the costal and diaphragmatic surfaces. Visceral pleural lymphatics course within the connective tissue layer, where they form a plexus of channels whose major tributaries roughly follow the pleural lobular boundaries. Lymph flows toward the medial aspect of the lung and ultimately drains into hilar lymph nodes.

Within the lung, lymph flows along two major pathways, one in the peribronchovascular connective tissue and the other in the interlobular septal connective tissue (Fig. 1–36). In the latter, it flows centripetally toward the hilum,

eventually reaching the peribronchial and hilar lymph nodes; in the interlobular septa, it often drains into the pleural lymphatics. Anastomotic channels connect the interlobular lymphatics with those in the bronchoarterial sheath; they are up to 4 cm long and are particularly evident midway between the hilum and the periphery of the lung. (Distention of these communicating lymphatics and edema in their surrounding connective tissue result in Kerley A lines; the same processes in the interlobular lymphatics and connective tissue result in Kerley B lines).

Thoracic Duct and Right Lymphatic Duct

The thoracic duct is a continuation of the cisterna chyli, which is formed, in turn, by the junction of the two lumbar

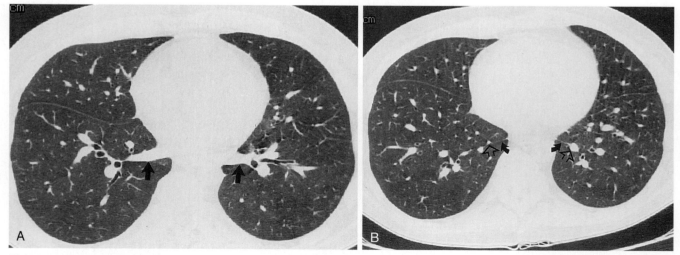

Figure 1–34. Pulmonary Ligaments and Their Relationship to the Inferior Pulmonary Veins. HRCT scan *(A)* shows the right and left inferior pulmonary veins *(straight arrows).* Immediately caudad to the veins *(B),* thin lines of attenuation can be seen extending to the mediastinum *(curved arrows).* These lines represent the intersegmental septa of the lower lobes, which are bounded at the mediastinum by the base of the pulmonary ligament and laterally by a vertically oriented vein *(open arrows).*

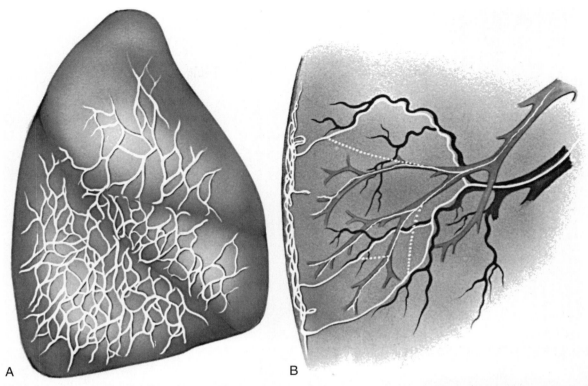

Figure 1–36. Lymphatic Drainage of the Pleura and Lungs. Drawing of the lateral aspect of the right lung *(A)* shows the pleural lymphatics to be much more numerous over the lower half of the lung than over the upper half. In coronal section through the midportion of the lung *(B)*, lymphatic channels from the pleura enter the lung at the interlobular septa and extend medially to the hilum along venous radicles (dark-shaded vessels), and lymphatic channels originating in the peripheral parenchyma extend medially in the bronchovascular bundles (light-shaded vessels). Communicating lymphatics *(dotted lines)* extend between the peribronchial and perivenous lymphatics.

lymphatic trunks on the anterior aspect of the vertebral column at the level of T12 to L2.[77] The duct enters the thorax through the aortic hiatus of the diaphragm. In most individuals, it lies to the right of the aorta and follows its course cephalad; in the lower portion of the thorax, it lies roughly in the midline or slightly to one side of the vertebral column. At about the level of the carina, the duct crosses the left main bronchus and runs cephalad in a plane parallel to the left lateral wall of the trachea and slightly posterior to it. The duct leaves the thorax between the esophagus and left subclavian artery and runs posterior to the left innominate vein. It joins the venous system most commonly at the internal jugular vein but sometimes drains into the subclavian, innominate, or external jugular veins. The radiologic anatomy of the right lymphatic duct has been documented poorly because it cannot be opacified easily and it is an inconstant channel.[78]

Lymph Nodes

Although pleuropulmonary lymphatics are not normally visible radiologically, their intrathoracic repository, the hilar and mediastinal lymph nodes, frequently are discernible. Enlargement of these structures is a common and often diagnostically important feature of disease arising within the thorax. Grossly enlarged mediastinal lymph nodes often can be suspected on plain radiographs by increased opacity and alteration of the normal mediastinal contour. Lymph nodes are identified on CT scan as round or oval structures

of soft tissue attenuation, with or without central or eccentric radiolucent fat, in a location that does not correspond to normal vascular or neural structures. When present, foci of calcification or lymphangiographic contrast medium serve as definitive markers. On magnetic resonance (MR) imaging, lymph nodes have soft tissue intensity and can be distinguished readily from vessels and fat; however, scattered calcifications cannot be identified.

Parietal and Visceral Groups of Thoracic Lymph Nodes

Intrathoracic lymph nodes can be classified into *parietal* and *visceral* groups;[79] the former reside outside the parietal pleura in extramediastinal tissue, where they drain the thoracic wall and other extrathoracic structures, whereas the latter are located within the mediastinum between the pleural membranes and drain primarily the intrathoracic tissues.

Parietal Lymph Nodes

Parietal lymph nodes can be subdivided into three groups.

Anterior Parietal (Internal Mammary) Lymph Nodes

Anterior parietal (internal mammary) lymph nodes are located in the upper portion of the thorax behind the anterior intercostal spaces bilaterally, either medial or lat-

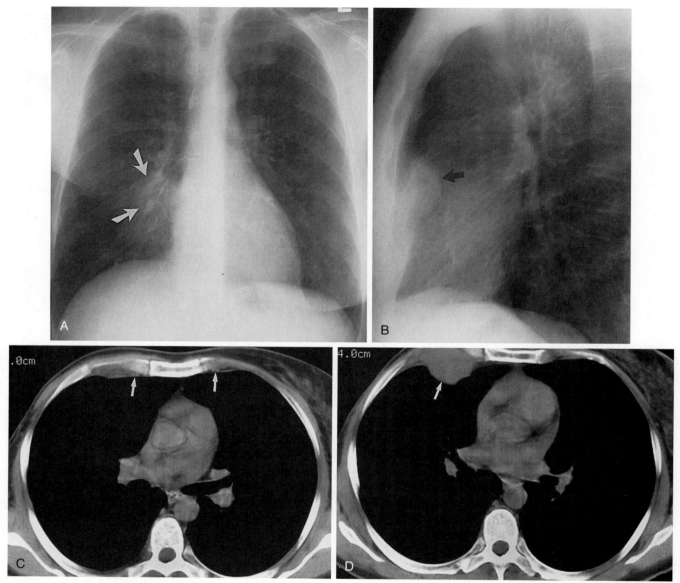

Figure 1–37. Enlargement of Internal Mammary Lymph Nodes. Posteroanterior radiograph *(A)* shows surgical absence of the right breast and poorly defined increased opacity over the right hilum *(arrows)*. Lateral chest radiograph *(B)* shows a smooth, homogeneous soft tissue opacity in the retrosternal area *(arrow)* caused by enlargement of the internal mammary lymph nodes. CT scan at the level of the bronchus intermedius *(C)* shows the right and left internal mammary artery and vein *(arrows)*; the enlarged internal mammary node is seen at a slightly lower level *(D; arrow)*. The patient was a 46-year-old woman with metastatic carcinoma of the breast.

eral to the internal mammary vessels (Fig. 1–37). They drain the anterior chest wall, breasts, and anterior diaphragm.

Posterior Parietal Lymph Nodes

Posterior parietal lymph nodes are found adjacent to the rib heads in the posterior intercostal spaces (*intercostal nodes*) or adjacent to the vertebrae (*juxtavertebral nodes*). Both groups drain the intercostal spaces, parietal pleura, and vertebral column. They communicate with other posterior mediastinal lymph nodes that relate to the descending aorta and the esophagus.

Diaphragmatic Lymph Nodes

Diaphragmatic lymph nodes are composed of the *anterior (prepericardiac)* group, located immediately behind

the xiphoid and to the right and left of the pericardium anteriorly; the *middle (juxtaphrenic)* group, which is in proximity to the phrenic nerves as they meet the diaphragm; and the *posterior (retrocrural)* nodes, which reside behind the right and left crura of the diaphragm.

Visceral Lymph Nodes

The visceral lymph nodes can be divided into three groups.

Anterior Mediastinal Lymph Nodes

Anterior mediastinal lymph nodes are congregated along the anterior aspect of the superior vena cava, right and left innominate veins, and ascending aorta (Fig. 1–38). Some

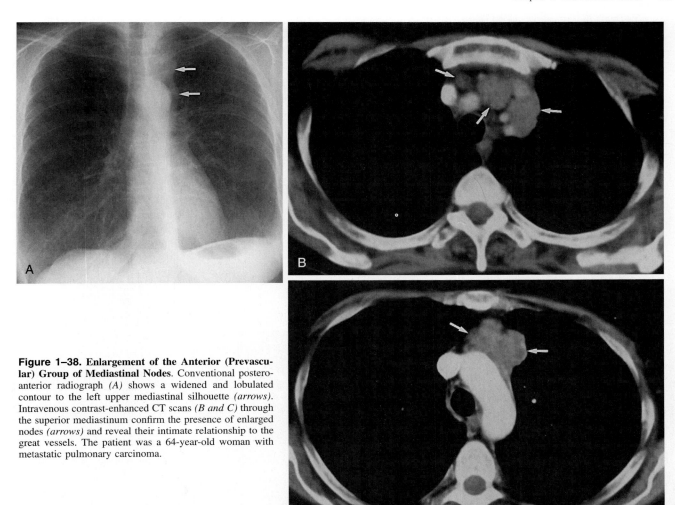

Figure 1–38. Enlargement of the Anterior (Prevascular) Group of Mediastinal Nodes. Conventional postero-anterior radiograph *(A)* shows a widened and lobulated contour to the left upper mediastinal silhouette *(arrows)*. Intravenous contrast-enhanced CT scans *(B and C)* through the superior mediastinum confirm the presence of enlarged nodes *(arrows)* and reveal their intimate relationship to the great vessels. The patient was a 64-year-old woman with metastatic pulmonary carcinoma.

are situated posterior to the sternum in the lower thorax, and others reside behind the manubrium anterior to the thymus.

Posterior Mediastinal Lymph Nodes

Posterior mediastinal lymph nodes are located adjacent to the esophagus *(paraesophageal nodes)* and along the anterior and lateral aspects of the descending aorta *(para-aortic nodes)*.

Tracheobronchial Lymph Nodes

Tracheobronchial lymph nodes constitute the most important group of visceral lymph nodes and consist in turn of several subgroups. The *paratracheal* nodes are located in front and to the right and left of the trachea (Fig. 1–39); occasionally a retrotracheal component is present.

The *tracheal bifurcation* lymph nodes are situated in the precarinal *(see* Fig. 1–39) and subcarinal (Fig. 1–40) fat as well as around the circumference of the right and left main bronchi. The nodes in mediastinal fat between the left pulmonary artery and aortic arch and lateral to the ligamentum arteriosum are designated *aortopulmonary window* (subaortic) nodes.

Radiologically, the *hilar* nodes include the proximal lobar nodes (i.e., the nodes immediately distal to the mediastinal pleural reflection), the nodes adjacent to the bronchus intermedius, and the nodes lying adjacent to the lobar bronchi (interlobar nodes).[80] These nodes (Fig. 1–41) are normally too small to be detected on conventional radiographs or unenhanced CT studies; however, they are well visualized on contrast-enhanced CT scan and with MR imaging. They are located around the main bronchi and vessels, particularly at their points of division, and receive afferent channels from all lobes of the lungs; their efferent drainage is to the precarinal, subcarinal, carinal, and paratracheal nodes. Intraparenchymal lymphoid nodules resembling lymph nodes but not related to airways are sometimes large enough to be visualized macroscopically and radiologically.[81, 82]

Classification of Regional Nodal Stations

The mediastinal and pulmonary lymph nodes are classified according to their relationship to major anatomic structures. The preferred classification scheme is the lymph node map proposed by the American Joint Committee on Cancer and the Union Internationale Contre le Cancer (Table 1–2, Fig. 1–42).[80] In this classification, the lymph

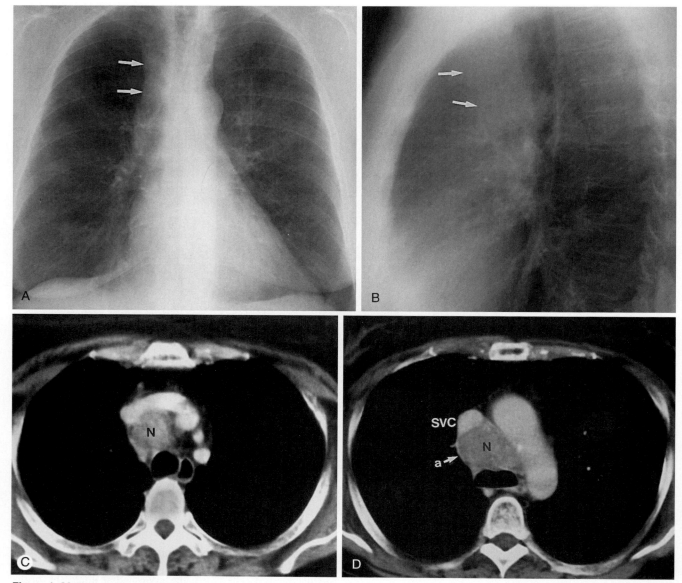

Figure 1–39. Enlargement of the Paratracheal Nodes. Posteroanterior *(A)* and lateral *(B)* chest radiographs show increased opacity to the right and anterior to the trachea *(arrows)*. Intravenous contrast-enhanced CT scan *(C)* at the level of the great vessels shows enlarged paratracheal lymph nodes (N). CT scan *(D)* at the level of the tracheal carina shows anterior displacement of the superior vena cava (SVC) and lateral displacement of the azygos vein (a) by enlarged precarinal nodes (N). The patient was a 59-year-old woman with metastatic pulmonary carcinoma.

node groups are classified based on their relationship to anatomic structures that can be identified readily by the radiologist on CT scan or MR imaging and by the surgeon at mediastinoscopy or thoracotomy. These structures include the left brachiocephalic vein, aortic arch, trachea, azygos vein, ligamentum arteriosum, left pulmonary artery, and bronchi. Guides to this classification on CT scan have been published based on the demonstration of enlarged lymph nodes.[83, 84]

Lymph Node Size

On CT scan or MR imaging, lymph nodes are usually ovoid in shape. Assessment of their size usually is based on the measurement of the smallest nodal diameter (short axis) as seen on the transverse CT image because it shows much less variability than the long axis (Fig. 1–43).[85–87]

The short-axis diameter above which a node should be considered enlarged depends on its location. Strictly speaking, upper paratracheal and left paraesophageal nodes should be considered enlarged when the short-axis diameter is greater than 7 mm. The threshold value for anterior mediastinal nodes is 8 mm; for lower paratracheal and right paraesophageal, 10 mm; and for subcarinal nodes, 11 mm.[85] A more pragmatic and commonly used approach, although less accurate, is to consider all mediastinal lymph nodes as being normal in size unless they exceed 10 mm in short-axis diameter.[84]

Magnetic Resonance Imaging Versus Computed Tomography in the Assessment of Mediastinal Lymph Nodes

PA and lateral chest radiographs often suffice for the identification of gross hilar and mediastinal lymph node

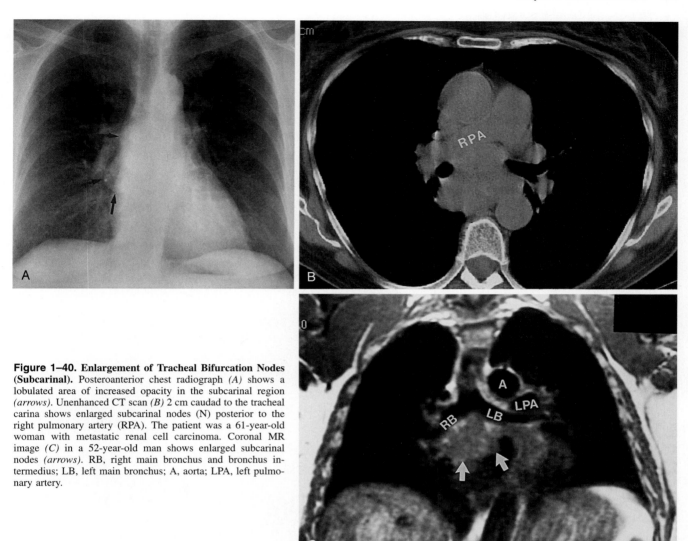

Figure 1–40. Enlargement of Tracheal Bifurcation Nodes (Subcarinal). Posteroanterior chest radiograph *(A)* shows a lobulated area of increased opacity in the subcarinal region *(arrows)*. Unenhanced CT scan *(B)* 2 cm caudad to the tracheal carina shows enlarged subcarinal nodes (N) posterior to the right pulmonary artery (RPA). The patient was a 61-year-old woman with metastatic renal cell carcinoma. Coronal MR image *(C)* in a 52-year-old man shows enlarged subcarinal nodes *(arrows)*. RB, right main bronchus and bronchus intermedius; LB, left main bronchus; A, aorta; LPA, left pulmonary artery.

enlargement, the main findings being increased opacity and alteration of the normal mediastinal or hilar contour. When enlargement is less pronounced or when more precise demonstration of abnormal anatomy is necessary, CT scan or MR imaging is required.[88, 89] Each technique has advantages and disadvantages. Proper evaluation of mediastinal and hilar lymph nodes on CT scans requires attention to the CT imaging technique and detailed knowledge of mediastinal vascular anatomy. Mediastinal nodes usually can be well visualized on CT scans without the need for intravenous contrast material; however, contrast material is necessary for optimal assessment of hilar lymph nodes.[90] MR imaging is capable of showing greater soft tissue contrast than CT and has an intrinsic flow sensitivity that allows easy distinction between vascular structures and soft tissue, including lymph nodes.[91, 92] Calcification within nodes is not visible on MR imaging but is detected readily on CT scan.[93]

Perhaps the greatest limitation of CT and MR imaging is the similarity of the soft tissue signal characteristics of benign and malignant lymph nodes. Several groups of workers have shown that these two conditions can be distinguished in most cases using positron emission tomography (PET) with labeled substances such as 2-(^{18}F)-fluoro-2-deoxy-D-glucose (FDG), which is accumulated preferentially in primary lung cancers and metastatic deposits in lymph nodes.[94–96] FDG-PET imaging may detect tumor in normal-sized lymph nodes and exclude tumor in enlarged nodes; in one prospective study of 99 patients who had newly diagnosed or suspected pulmonary carcinoma, FDG-PET imaging had a sensitivity of 83% and a specificity of 94% for the detection of mediastinal lymph node metastases, whereas CT had a sensitivity of 63% and a specificity of 73%.[95] Similar results have been reported in other studies.[96–98]

THORACIC INLET

The thoracic inlet represents the junction between structures at the base of the neck and those of the thorax. It parallels the first rib and is higher posteriorly than anteriorly (Fig. 1–44). On the basis of this anatomic observation, it is evident that an opacity on a PA chest radiograph that

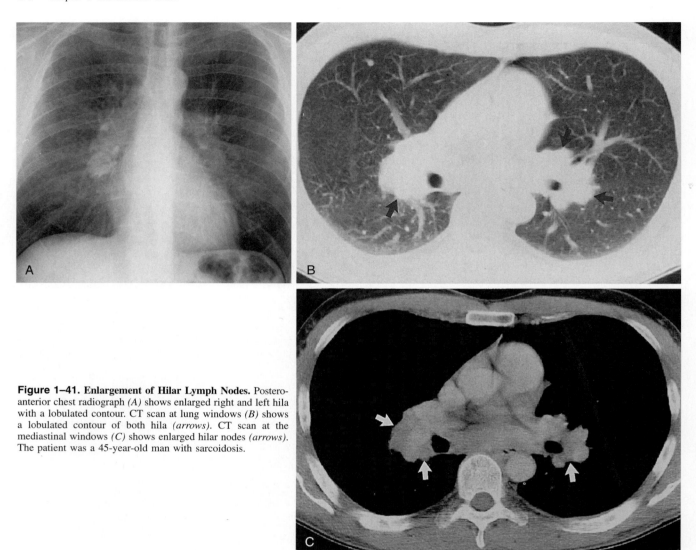

Figure 1–41. Enlargement of Hilar Lymph Nodes. Postero-anterior chest radiograph *(A)* shows enlarged right and left hila with a lobulated contour. CT scan at lung windows *(B)* shows a lobulated contour of both hila *(arrows)*. CT scan at the mediastinal windows *(C)* shows enlarged hilar nodes *(arrows)*. The patient was a 45-year-old man with sarcoidosis.

is effaced on its superior aspect and that projects at or below the level of the clavicles must be situated anteriorly, whereas one that projects above the clavicles is retrotracheal and posteriorly situated (Fig. 1–45). These characteristic findings together have been termed the *cervicothoracic sign*.[99]

From front to back, structures occupying the thoracic inlet include the right and left brachiocephalic veins (which join behind the right side of the manubrium to form the superior vena cava), the common carotid arteries (lying immediately anterior to the subclavian arteries and medial to the subclavian veins), the trachea (situated immediately behind the great vessels), the esophagus (located behind the trachea and in front of the spine), and the recurrent laryngeal nerves on either side of the esophagus (Fig. 1–46).

MEDIASTINUM

The mediastinum separates the thorax vertically in two compartments and can be defined anatomically as the parti-

tion between the lungs (Fig. 1–47).[100] Anatomically, it can be divided into three compartments: anterior (prevascular), middle (cardiovascular), and posterior (postvascular).[100]

The *anterior mediastinal compartment* is bounded anteriorly by the sternum and posteriorly by the pericardium, aorta, and brachiocephalic vessels. It merges superiorly with the anterior aspect of the thoracic inlet and extends down to the level of the diaphragm. The compartment contains the thymus gland, branches of the internal mammary artery and vein, lymph nodes, the inferior sternopericardial ligament, and variable amounts of fat.

The *middle mediastinal compartment* contains the pericardium and its contents, the ascending and transverse portions of the aorta, the superior and inferior vena cava, the brachiocephalic (innominate) arteries and veins, the phrenic nerves and cephalad portion of the vagus nerves, the trachea and main bronchi and their contiguous lymph nodes, and the main pulmonary arteries and veins. The *posterior mediastinal compartment* is bounded anteriorly by the pericardium and the vertical part of the diaphragm, laterally by the mediastinal pleura, and posteriorly by the

Table 1–2. LYMPH NODE MAP DEFINITIONS

Nodal Station	Anatomic Landmarks
N2 nodes — all N2 nodes lie within the mediastinal pleural envelope	
1. Highest mediastinal nodes	Nodes lying above a horizontal line at the upper rim of the brachiocephalic (left innominate) vein, where it ascends to the left, crossing in front of the trachea at its midline
2. Upper paratracheal nodes	Nodes lying above a horizontal line drawn tangential to the upper margin of the aortic arch and below the inferior boundary of No. 1 nodes
3. Prevascular and retrotracheal nodes	Prevascular and retrotracheal nodes may be designated *3A* and *3P*; midline nodes are considered to be ipsilateral
4. Lower paratracheal nodes	Lower paratracheal nodes on the right lie to the right of the midline of the trachea between a horizontal line drawn tangential to the upper margin of the aortic arch and a line extending across the right main bronchus at the upper margin of the upper lobe bronchus and contained within the mediastinal pleural envelope; the lower paratracheal nodes on the left lie to the left of the midline of the trachea between a horizontal line drawn tangential to the upper margin of the aortic arch and a line extending across the left main bronchus at the level of the upper margin of the left upper lobe bronchus, medial to the ligamentum arteriosum and contained within the mediastinal pleural envelope. Researchers may wish to designate the lower paratracheal nodes as No. *4S* (superior) and No. *4I* (inferior) subsets for study purposes; the No. *4S* nodes may be defined by a horizontal line extending across the trachea and drawn tangential to the cephalic border of the azygos vein; the No. *4I* nodes may be defined by the lower boundary of No. 4S and the lower boundary of No. 4, as described above
5. Subaortic (aortopulmonary window)	Subaortic nodes are lateral to the ligamentum arteriosum or the aorta or left pulmonary artery and proximal to the first branch of the left pulmonary artery and lie within the mediastinal pleural envelope
6. Para-aortic nodes (ascending aorta or phrenic)	Nodes lying anterior and lateral to the ascending aorta and the aortic arch or the innominate artery, beneath a line tangential to the upper margin of the aortic arch
7. Subcarinal nodes	Nodes lying caudad to the carina of the trachea but not associated with the lower lobe bronchi or arteries within the lung
8. Paraesophageal nodes (below carina)	Nodes lying adjacent to the wall of the esophagus and to the right or left of the midline, excluding subcarinal nodes
9. Pulmonary ligament nodes	Nodes lying within the pulmonary ligament, including those in the posterior wall and lower part of the inferior pulmonary vein
N1 nodes — all N1 nodes lie distal to the mediastinal pleural reflection and within the visceral pleura	
10. Hilar nodes	Proximal lobar nodes, distal to the mediastinal pleural reflection and the nodes adjacent to the bronchus intermedius on the right; radiographically, the hilar shadow may be created by enlargement of hilar and interlobar nodes
11. Interlobar nodes	Nodes lying between the lobar bronchi
12. Lobar nodes	Nodes adjacent to the distal lobar bronchi
13. Segmental nodes	Nodes adjacent to the segmental bronchi
14. Subsegmental nodes	Nodes around the subsegmental bronchi

From Mountain CF, Dresler CM: Regional lymph node classification for lung cancer staging. Chest 111:1720, 1997.

bodies of the thoracic vertebrae. It contains the descending thoracic aorta, esophagus, thoracic duct, azygos and hemiazygos veins, autonomic nerves, fat, and lymph nodes. Some of the more useful measurements of mediastinal structures are summarized in Table 1–3.

Thymus

The thymus is located in the anterosuperior portion of the mediastinum and in adults generally extends from a point above the manubrium to the fourth costal cartilage. Posteriorly, it relates to the trachea, aortic arch and its branches, and pericardium covering the ascending aorta and main pulmonary artery (Fig. 1–48; *see* Fig. 1–47).

On conventional radiographs, the thymus is visible only in infants and young children, in whom it fills much of the anterior mediastinal space. In one CT study of 154 normal individuals, the thymus was recognized in all individuals younger than age 30 years, in 73% of individuals between the ages of 30 and 49 years, and in 17% of individuals older than age 49 years.[101] The maximal size was observed in individuals between 12 and 19 years of age, with regression occurring between 20 and 60 years and usually associated with fatty replacement of the parenchyma; by the age of 60 years, the thymus was estimated to weigh 50% less than at age 19 years. Of glands, 62% had an arrowhead configuration, whereas 32% had separate right and left lobes.

The most reliable measurement of thymic size on CT scan is the thickness (short-axis or transverse dimension of a lobe) (Fig. 1–49). In the study of 154 subjects mentioned previously, the thickness displayed a statistically significant decrease between the 6- to 19-year-old and 40- to 49-year-old groups; the thickness of the right and left lobes in these two age categories was 10 mm ($\pm$ 3.9 mm SD) and 11 mm ($\pm$ 4.0 mm SD) and 6 mm ($\pm$ 2.3 mm SD) and 6 mm ($\pm$ 2.0 mm SD).[101] It generally is accepted that the maximum thickness of the normal thymus in individuals younger than age 20 is 1.8 cm, whereas in individuals age 20 or older, it is 1.3 cm.[102, 103]

Text continued on page 40

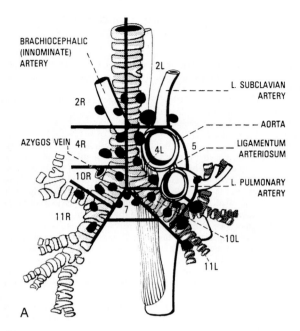

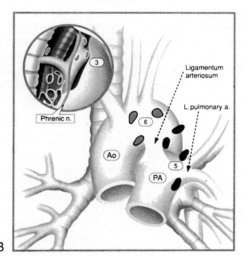

Superior Mediastinal Nodes

● **1** Highest Mediastinal

● **2** Upper Paratracheal

● **3** Pre-vascular and Retrotracheal

● **4** Lower Paratracheal
(including Azygos Nodes)

N₂ = single digit, ipsilateral
N₃ = single digit, contralateral or supraclavicular

Aortic Nodes

● **5** Subaortic (A-P window)

● **6** Para-aortic (ascending
aorta or phrenic)

Inferior Mediastinal Nodes

● **7** Subcarinal

● **8** Paraesophageal
(below carina)

● **9** Pulmonary Ligament

N₁ Nodes

○ **10** Hilar

● **11** Interlobar

● **12** Lobar

● **13** Segmental

● **14** Subsegmental

Figure 1–42. Regional Lymph Node Stations for Lung Cancer Staging. (From Mountain CF, Dresler CM: Chest 111:1719, 1997.)

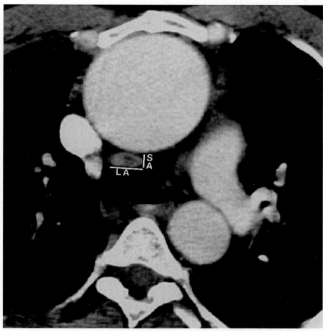

Figure 1–43. Mediastinal Nodes: Long-Axis and Short-Axis Measurements. Intravenous contrast-enhanced CT scan shows normal precarinal node in a patient with aneurysm of the ascending aorta. The node is ovoid rather than round. Initial studies measured the maximal diameter of the node in the cross-sectional image (long-axis [LA]). Because there is less variability in the normal range of short-axis (SA) diameters, most authors recommend using the SA diameter when measuring mediastinal lymph nodes. The LA measurement of the node illustrated is 15 mm, and the SA is 7 mm.

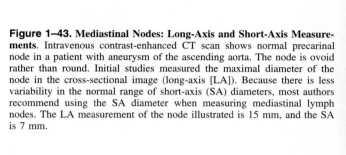

Figure 1–44. Normal Thoracic Inlet. Detail view from posteroanterior chest radiograph in a 40-year-old man shows the normal appearance of the thoracic inlet. Because the thoracic inlet parallels the first rib *(arrows)*, it is higher posteriorly than anteriorly.

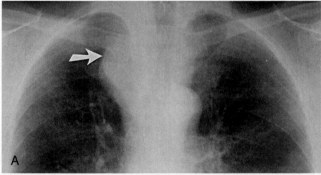

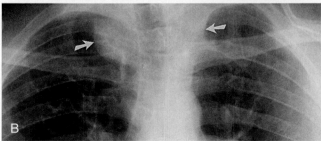

Figure 1–45. Cervicothoracic Sign. Posteroanterior chest radiograph *(A)* from a 69-year-old man with a large thyroid goiter shows a mass *(arrow)* in the thoracic inlet displacing the trachea to the left. The mass is effaced above the level of the clavicle because it is anterior and lateral to the trachea and continuous with the soft tissues of the neck. Posteroanterior chest radiograph *(B)* in a 34-year-old patient shows bilateral paraspinal soft tissue opacities *(arrows)* well seen above the level of the clavicles. These are well seen at this level because they are situated posterior to the trachea. The patient had bilateral paraspinal extension and involvement of the T3 vertebral body by hydatid disease.

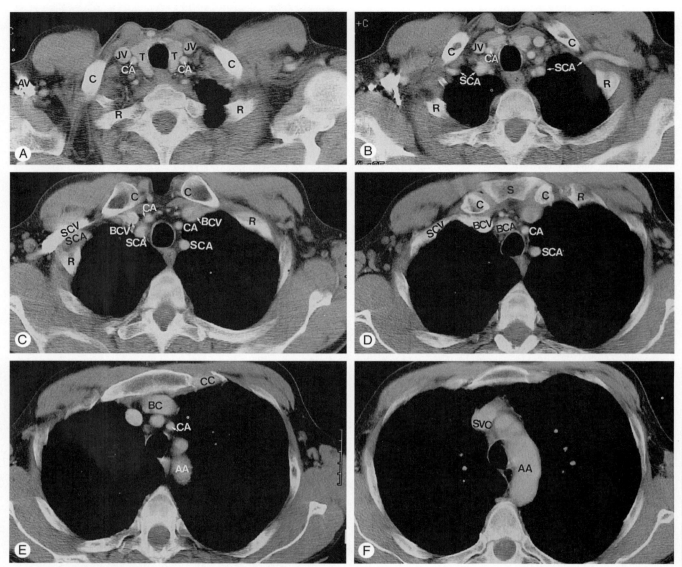

Figure 1–46. Normal CT Scan of the Thoracic Inlet. Contrast-enhanced CT scan in a 51-year-old man shows the normal anatomy of the thoracic inlet. CT scan *(A)* at the level of the posterior aspect of the first rib (R) shows left lung apex, clavicles (C), thyroid gland (T), jugular veins (JV), and carotid arteries (CA). Contrast material was injected in a right antecubital vein resulting in marked enhancement of the right axillary vein (AV). The thyroid gland surrounds the anterior and lateral aspects of the trachea in the lower neck, whereas the esophagus lies immediately posterior to the trachea. CT scan *(B)* at the level of the lateral aspect of the first ribs shows subclavian arteries (SCA), carotid arteries, jugular veins, and inferior aspect of the thyroid gland. CT scan *(C)* at the level of the anteromedial aspect of the first ribs shows the right subclavian vein (SCV) lying anterior to the subclavian artery, the proximal portions of the subclavian arteries, and the carotid arteries. The right and left brachiocephalic veins (BCV) can be seen anterior to the carotid arteries. The medial portion of the clavicle can be seen anterior to the first ribs outlining the region of the suprasternal notch. The esophagus is situated immediately posterior to the trachea. CT scan *(D)* at the level of the anterior aspect of the first ribs shows the left costochondral junction, the upper aspect of the sternum (S), and the clavicles at the level of the sternoclavicular joint. At this level, the right subclavian vein (SCV) can be seen joining the brachiocephalic vein (anterolateral to the brachiocephalic artery [BCA]). The left brachiocephalic vein is seen anterolateral to the left carotid artery. At this level, as with the higher levels, the left subclavian artery and surrounding fat can be seen to form the left lateral margin of the thoracic inlet. CT scan *(E)* at the level of the first costal cartilages (CC) shows the left brachiocephalic vein crossing the midline anterior to the brachiocephalic and carotid arteries. Also seen is the left subclavian artery as it originates from the uppermost aspect of the aortic arch (AA). CT scan *(F)* at the level of the aortic arch (AA) shows the origin of the brachiocephalic and left carotid arteries from the aorta. At this level the left brachiocephalic vein can be seen joining the superior vena cava (SVC).

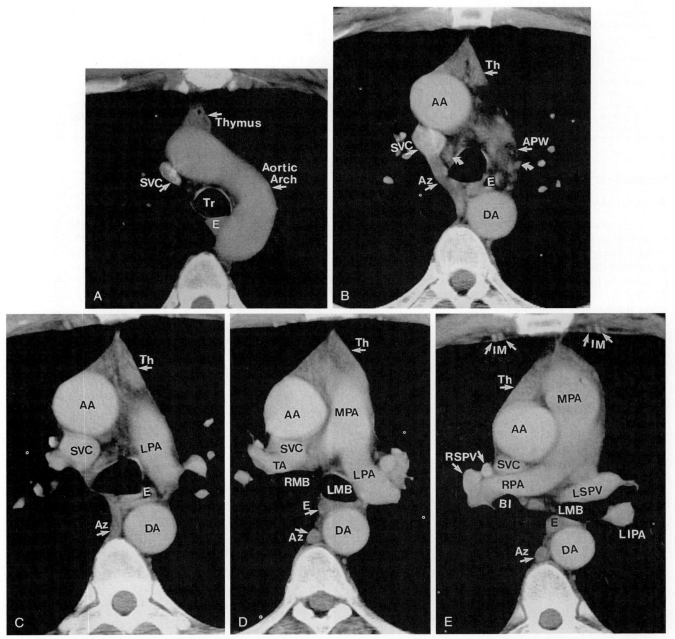

Figure 1–47. Normal CT Anatomy of the Mediastinum. Image at the level of the aortic arch *(A)* shows the thymus, superior vena cava (SVC), trachea (Tr), and esophagus (E). The paravertebral region and posterior gutters are not part of the mediastinum. Image immediately caudad to the aortic arch *(B)* shows the region of the aortopulmonary window (APW), ascending (AA) and descending aorta (DA), azygos vein (Az) draining into the superior vena cava (SVC), esophagus (E), and normal-sized mediastinal lymph nodes *(curved arrows)*. Note triangular shape of the thymus (Th). Image at the level of the tracheal carina *(C)* shows the left pulmonary artery (LPA), superior vena cava (SVC), ascending (AA) and descending aorta (DA), thymus (Th), esophagus (E), and azygos vein (Az). Image at the level of the right (RMB) and left (LMB) main bronchi *(D)* shows the thymus (Th), ascending (AA) and descending aorta (DA), superior vena cava (SVC), truncus anterior (TA), esophagus (E), and azygos vein (Az). Image at the level of the bronchus intermedius (BI) *(E)* shows the right and left internal mammary arteries and veins (IM); thymus (Th); main (MPA), right (RPA), and left interlobular (LIPA) pulmonary arteries; superior vena cava (SVC); left superior pulmonary vein (LSPV); confluence of right upper lobe veins to form the right superior pulmonary vein (RSPV); esophagus (E); and azygos vein (Az).

Table 1–3. NORMAL MEASUREMENTS OF MEDIASTINAL STRUCTURES

Thymus
 Thickness (transverse dimension of a lobe)
  Patients <20 yr old: 1.8 cm
  Patients ≥20 yr old: 1.3 cm[102]
Aorta
 Ascending aorta: 3.6 cm (range, 2.4–4.7 cm)
 Descending aorta: 2.6 cm (range, 1.6–3.7 cm)[121]
Heart
 Transverse diameter: 11.5–15.5 cm
 Cardiothoracic ratio (posteroanterior radiograph): ≤0.5[109]
Lymph nodes
 Short axis (smallest diameter of node seen in cross-section)
  Upper limit of normal: 10 mm[84]

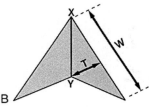

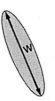

Figure 1–49. Measurement of Thymic Size. The two thymic lobes are measured separately. The width (W) corresponds to the long axis of the lobe as seen on the transverse CT scan, and the thickness (T) corresponds to the short-axis diameter *(A).* When the two lobes are confluent, the thymus has a triangular or arrowhead shape *(B).* The thymus is divided in half by a line through the anterior apex of the gland and perpendicular to it (X-Y). The width (W) and thickness (T) of each lobe are then measured. (Measurements as described by Baron RL, et al: Radiology 142:121, 1982.)

Mediastinal Lines and Interfaces

Anterior Junction Line

As the two lungs approximate anteromedially, they are separated by four layers of pleura and a variable quantity of intervening mediastinal adipose tissue, forming a *septum* of variable thickness (the anterior junction line—anterior mediastinal line) (Fig. 1–50). On a PA chest radiograph, this line typically is oriented obliquely from upper right to lower left behind the sternum.

Aortopulmonary Window

The aortopulmonary window consists of a space situated between the arch of the aorta and left pulmonary artery. It is occupied largely by mediastinal fat; its medial boundary is the ductus ligament, and its lateral boundary is the mediastinal and visceral pleura over the left lung, creating

the aortopulmonary window interface (Fig. 1–51). Within this space are situated fat, the left recurrent laryngeal nerve, and lymph nodes. The lateral border (aortopulmonary window interface) is normally concave or straight.

Tracheal Interfaces

The trachea normally is bordered on its right lateral aspect by pleura covering the right upper lobe; its anterior and posterior aspects are bordered to a variable extent. Contact of the right lung in the supra-azygos area with the right lateral wall of the trachea creates a thin stripe of soft tissue density usually visible on frontal chest radiographs, which has been designated the *right paratracheal stripe.* This stripe is formed by the right wall of the trachea, contiguous parietal and visceral pleura, and a variable quantity of mediastinal fat.[104] The thickness of the stripe

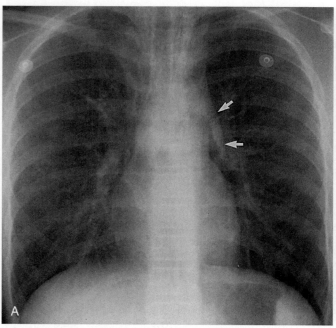
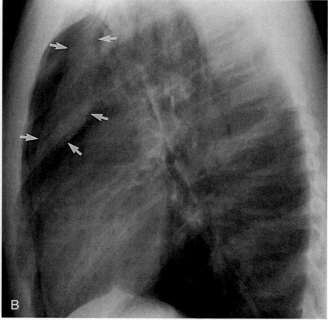

Figure 1–48. Normal Thymus Delineated by Pneumomediastinum. Posteroanterior *(A)* and lateral *(B)* chest radiographs in a 10-year-old boy with pneumomediastinum show the normal location of the thymus, which is outlined by surrounding air *(arrows).* The left lobe of the thymus is larger than the right lobe.

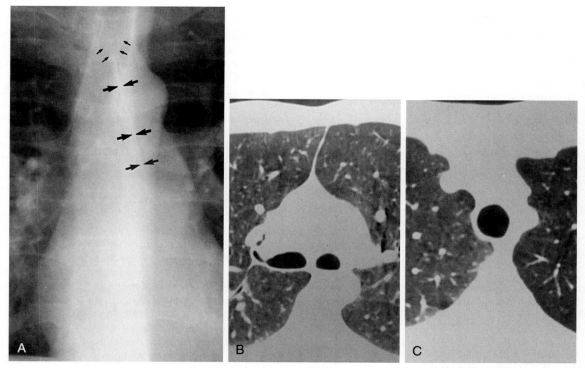

Figure 1–50. Anterior Junction Line and Superior Recess. Posteroanterior chest radiograph *(A)* in a 38-year-old man shows the anterior junction line *(large arrows)* extending from the right to the left caudally from the level of the aortic arch. Immediately above the arch is a V-shaped area of increased opacity *(small arrows)* representing the anterior mediastinal triangle. CT scan at the level of the main bronchi *(B)* shows the right and left lungs to abut each other anterior to the mediastinum. The anterior junction line is formed by apposition of the visceral and mediastinal pleurae of the right and left lungs. CT scan above the level of the aortic arch *(C)* shows that at this level the lungs are separated by the great vessels and mediastinal fat, which accounts for the anterior mediastinal triangle seen on the radiograph.

must be measured above the level of the azygos vein; an increase in width on serial films is a more important sign of abnormality than is a single measurement. In one series of 1,259 normal individuals, the maximal width of the stripe was 4 mm.[104]

Widening of the paratracheal stripe (≥5 mm) may be due to paratracheal lymph node enlargement, mediastinal hemorrhage, or disease of the pleura or tracheal wall. It is not a particularly sensitive sign, being present in only approximately 30% of patients who have paratracheal lymph node enlargement shown on CT scan.[88] The *posterior tracheal stripe* is a vertically oriented opacity formed by the posterior wall of the trachea where it comes in contact with right upper lobe parenchyma.

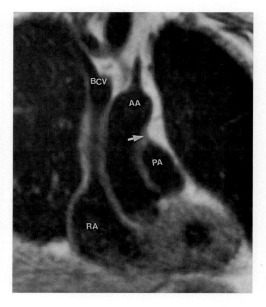

Figure 1–51. Aortopulmonary Window. MR image in an 83-year-old man shows the structures responsible for the left mediastinal border. Fat can be seen lateral to the aortic arch (AA) and main pulmonary artery (PA) and outlines the region of the aortopulmonary window. The ligament of the ductus arteriosus *(arrow)* can be seen to delineate the medial margin of the aortopulmonary window. Also noted are the left carotid artery, right brachiocephalic vein (BCV), superior vena cava, and right atrium (RA).

Posterior Junction Line

The apices of the right and left upper lobes contact the mediastinum behind the esophagus anterior to the first and second vertebral bodies. In so doing, they create a V-shaped triangular opacity that constitutes the *posterior mediastinal triangle*; marginating the triangle are the *right* and *left superior recesses*. Caudally, the lungs intrude deeper into a prespinal location posterior to the esophagus and anterior to the third through fifth vertebral bodies, where they form a pleural apposition that, along with any intervening mediastinal tissue, forms the *posterior junction line*. On a PA radiograph, the posterior junction line usually projects through the air column of the trachea; it may be straight or slightly convex to the left. When intervening mediastinal tissue is abundant or a narrowed retroesophageal space precludes lung apposition, the posterior junction line can appear as a distinct stripe.[105]

Azygoesophageal Recess

The azygos vein ascends in the posterior mediastinum in relation to the right side or front of the vertebral column. The esophagus usually is located slightly anterior and to the left of the vein in the prevertebral region, although they are sometimes in contact. The *azygoesophageal recess* is formed by contact of the right lower lobe with the esophagus and the ascending portion of the azygos vein (Fig. 1–52).[106, 107]

The recess frequently is identified on a well-penetrated PA radiograph as an interface that extends from the diaphragm below to the level of the azygos arch above. Typically, it is seen as a continuous, shallow or deep arc concave to the right; however, in young adults, a straight or slightly dextroconvex interface may be seen.[108] Focal right-sided convexity of the azygoesophageal recess interface should raise the suspicion of an underlying pathologic process, such as hiatal hernia, esophageal tumor or duplication cyst, azygos vein dilation, or subcarinal lymph node enlargement.[107]

HEART

On a frontal radiograph of the normal chest, the position of the heart in relation to the midline of the thorax depends largely on the patient's build. Assuming radiographic exposure with lungs fully inflated, the heart shadow is almost exactly midline in position in asthenic individuals, projecting only slightly more to the left; in individuals of stockier build, it lies a little more to the left of midline.[109]

In normal individuals, the transverse diameter of the heart measured on standard PA radiographs is usually in the range of 11.5 to 15.5 cm;[109] it is less than 11.5 cm in approximately 5% and only rarely exceeds 15.5 cm (in heavy subjects of stocky build). The custom of trying to assess cardiac size by relating it to the transverse diameter of the chest (cardiothoracic ratio), although helpful, has potential pitfalls. On a PA radiograph, a cardiothoracic ratio of 50% is accepted widely as the upper limit of normal; however, the ratio exceeds 50% in at least 10% of normal individuals.[109] Measurement of the ratio is especially fallacious in individuals who have a small heart: In an individual who has an 8-cm transverse cardiac diameter in a 24-cm thorax, the heart would have to enlarge 4 cm before the cardiothoracic ratio reaches 50%.[109] In our view, it is preferable to evaluate cardiac size subjectively; alternatively, it is reasonable to assume that a heart whose transverse diameter exceeds 16 cm is enlarged.

When the influence of systole and diastole is controlled (by exposure of ≥1 second), the major influences on cardiac size and contour are fourfold: (1) the *height of the diaphragm*, which, in turn, is influenced by the degree of pulmonary inflation—the lower the position of the diaphragm, the longer and narrower is the cardiovascular silhouette; (2) *intrathoracic pressure*, which influences not only cardiac size, but also the appearance of the pulmonary vascular pattern; (3) *body position*—assuming equality of all other factors, the heart is broader when a subject is recumbent than when he or she is erect; and (4) *PA versus anteroposterior radiograph*—the heart is magnified more, and this appears larger on radiographs performed using anteroposterior projection of the x-ray beam.

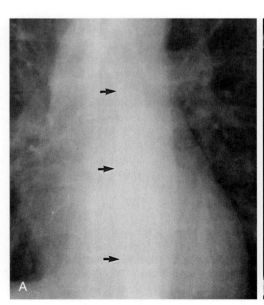 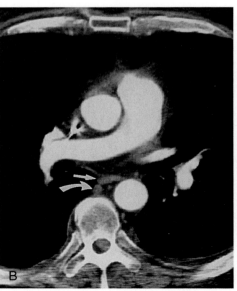

Figure 1–52. Azygoesophageal Recess. Posteroanterior chest radiograph *(A)* in a 36-year-old man shows normal azygoesophageal recess interface *(arrows)* extending from the level of the tracheal carina to the diaphragm to form a shallow arc convex to the right. CT scan *(B)* shows that the interface is due to contact between the right lung and the posterior mediastinum (more specifically, between the right lung and the esophagus *[straight arrow]* and azygos vein *[curved arrow]*).

FORAMINA OF MORGAGNI

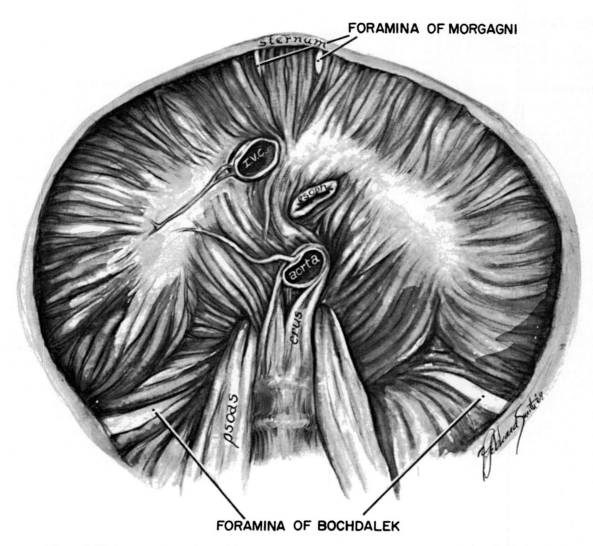

Figure 1–53. Anatomy of the Normal Diaphragm Viewed from Below. See the text. I.V.C., inferior vena cava.

FORAMINA OF BOCHDALEK

Accumulations of fat are common in the cardiophrenic recesses bilaterally and produce an obtuse angular configuration of the inferior mediastinum at its junction with the diaphragm. Their density may be slightly less than that of the heart, allowing identification through them of the approximate position of the cardiac borders. These pleuropericardial fat shadows should not be misinterpreted as cardiac enlargement or as mediastinal or diaphragmatic masses.

DIAPHRAGM

The diaphragm is a musculotendinous structure that separates the thoracic and abdominal cavities (Fig. 1–53). Its costal muscle fibers arise anteriorly from the xiphoid process and around the convexity of the thorax from ribs 7 to 12; posteriorly the crural fibers arise from the lateral margins of the first, second, and third lumbar vertebrae on the right side and from the first and second lumbar vertebrae on the left. These fibers converge toward the central tendon and are inserted into it nearly perpendicular to its margin.

On the chest radiograph, the upper surface of the dome-shaped diaphragm normally is visualized as it forms an interface with the lung; the soft tissues of the abdomen obscure its inferior surface. In approximately 95% of normal adults, the level of the cupola of the right hemidiaphragm is projected in a plane ranging from the anterior end of the fifth rib to the sixth anterior interspace; in approximately 5%, it is projected at or below the level of the seventh rib.[110] In approximately 90% of adults, the plane of the right diaphragmatic dome is about half an interspace higher than the left; both are at the same height, or the left is higher than the right in approximately 10% of normal subjects.[111]

On CT scan, the diaphragm can be visualized only where its upper surface interfaces with the lung and the inferior surface interfaces with intra-abdominal fat.[112] Although it is not visualized where it abuts structures of similar soft tissue attenuation, such as the liver and spleen, its position can be inferred because at all levels the lungs and pleura lie adjacent and peripheral to it, whereas the abdominal viscera lie central to it (Fig. 1–54).[112] The posterior or lumbar portion of the diaphragm is well visualized

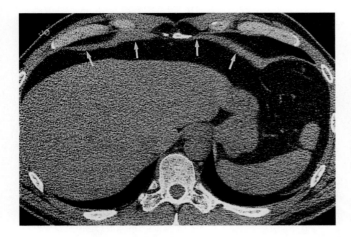

Figure 1–54. Anterior Portion of the Diaphragm. CT scan at the level of the xiphoid shows continuity between the anterior (xiphoid) and lateral (costal) diaphragmatic fibers *(arrows).* The diaphragm is well visualized in areas where it is outlined by lung and peritoneal or retroperitoneal fat. Where it abuts structures of similar soft tissue attenuation, such as the liver and spleen, it is not visualized; however, its position can be inferred because of its relation to the lungs and pleura (adjacent and peripheral to it) and the abdominal viscera (central to it).

where the fibers arising from the crura and arcuate ligament arch forward to insert into the central tendon (Fig. 1–55).

CHEST WALL

On a frontal radiograph of the thorax, the soft tissues, including the skin, subcutaneous fat, and muscles, are usually distinguishable over the shoulders and along the thoracic wall. In the absence of pulmonary or pleural disease, deformity of the spine, or congenital anomalies of the ribs themselves, the rib cage should be symmetric. The upper and lower borders of the ribs normally are defined sharply except in the middle and lower thoracic regions; here the thin flanges created by the vascular sulci on the inferior aspects of the ribs posteriorly are viewed *en face,* resulting in a less distinct inferior margin. On the lateral view, the ribs farther from the film are magnified more than those adjacent to the film (the *big rib* sign);[113, 114] on a left lateral radiograph, the right ribs appear bigger than the left ribs.

Calcification of the rib cartilage is common and probably never of pathologic significance. The first rib cartilage is usually the first to calcify, often shortly after the age of 20. Fairly consistent differences in the pattern of costal calcification are observed in the two sexes (Fig. 1–56), particularly in older individuals.[115] In men, the upper and lower borders of cartilage calcify first, with calcification

extending in continuity with the end of the rib; calcification of the central area follows.[116] By contrast, calcification in women tends to occur first in a central location, in the form of a solid tongue or as two parallel lines extending into the cartilage from the end of the rib.

Because of their oblique orientation, only a small portion of any given rib is seen on a single CT section.[117, 118] Identification of a specific rib can be made by identifying the thoracic spine level adjacent to the posterior end of the rib.[117] The first rib can be identified readily because it lies adjacent to the medial end of the clavicle at the level of the sternoclavicular joint. The second, third, and fourth ribs usually can be identified at the same level by counting posteriorly along the rib cage (Fig. 1–57).[118] By proceeding sequentially caudally, each next vertebra and corresponding rib can be identified.

Occasionally, the inferior aspect of the clavicle has an irregular notch or indentation 2 to 3 cm from the sternal articulation; its size and shape vary from a superficial saucer-shaped defect to a deep notch 2 cm wide by 1.0 to 1.5 cm deep. These rhomboid fossae (Fig. 1–58) give rise to the costoclavicular or rhomboid ligaments that radiate downward to bind the clavicles to the first rib.[119] The fossae are seen in about 10% of clavicles studied anatomically but rarely are detected radiologically.[120]

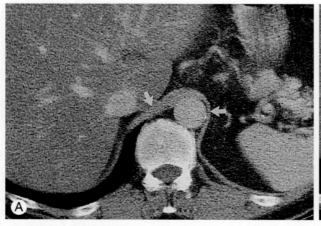
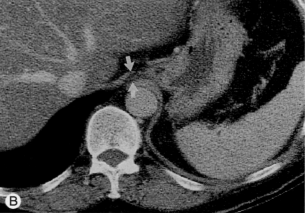

Figure 1–55. Lumbar Portion of the Diaphragm. CT scan (A) shows right and left crura *(arrows)* extending anterior to the aorta. Posterolaterally, the crural fibers merge smoothly and indistinguishably from fibers arising from the medial arcuate ligaments. CT scan at a slightly more cephalad level (B) shows discontinuity of the right and left crura at the level of the esophageal hiatus *(arrows).*

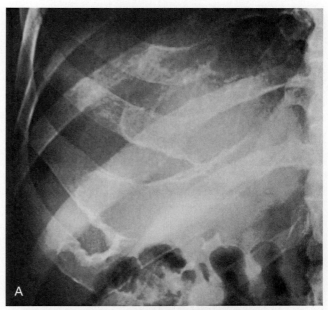

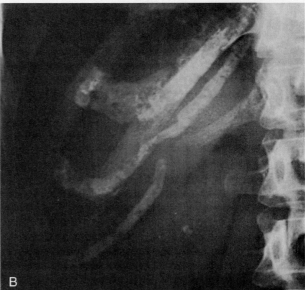

Figure 1–56. Patterns of Rib Cartilage Calcification in Men and Women. Marginal calcification in a man *(A)*. Central calcification in a woman *(B)*. See the text.

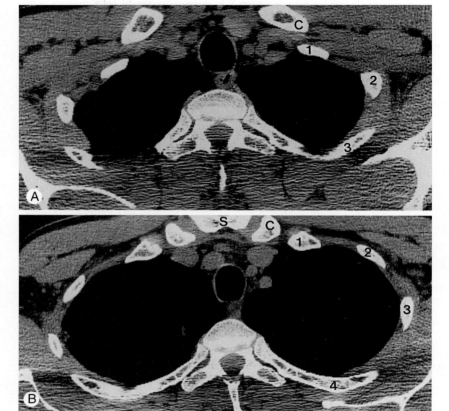

Figure 1–57. Ribs in Cross-Section. HRCT scan at the level of the thoracic inlet *(A)* shows right and left clavicles (C) and first (1), second (2), and third (3) ribs. HRCT scan at the level of the sternoclavicular joint *(B)* shows the upper part of the sternum (S) and the medial end of the clavicles (C). The first costal cartilage (1) and the second (2), third (3), and fourth (4) ribs can be identified by counting posteriorly along the rib cage. The fourth rib can be seen to articulate with the fourth thoracic vertebra.

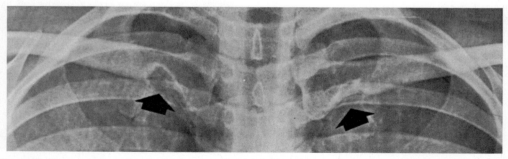

Figure 1–58. Rhomboid Fossae. An irregular notch is present in the inferior aspect of both clavicles approximately 2 cm from the sternal end *(arrows)*. These fossae give origin to the costoclavicular or rhomboid ligaments.

Congenital anomalies of the ribs are relatively uncommon. Supernumerary ribs arising from the seventh cervical vertebra were identified in 1.5% of 350 normal individuals in one study;[111] nearly all were bilateral, but many had developed asymmetrically.

References

1. Stone KC, Mercer RR, Freeman BA, et al: Distribution of lung cell numbers and volumes between alveolar and nonalveolar tissue. Am Rev Respir Dis 146:454, 1992.
2. Breatnach E, Abbott GC, Fraser RG: Dimensions of the normal human trachea. Am J Roentgenol 141:903, 1984.
3. Atwell SW: Major anomalies of the tracheobronchial tree with a list of the minor anomalies. Dis Chest 52:611, 1967.
4. Horsfield K, Cumming G: Morphology of the bronchial tree in man. J Appl Physiol 24:373, 1968.
5. Müller NL, Miller RR: Diseases of the bronchioles: CT and histopathologic findings. Radiology 196:3, 1995.
6. Jefferson KE: The normal pulmonary angiogram and some changes seen in chronic nonspecific lung disease: I. The pulmonary vessels in the normal pulmonary angiogram. Proc Roy Soc Med 58:677, 1965.
7. Cory RAS, Valentine EJ: Varying patterns of the lobar branches of the pulmonary artery. Thorax 14:267, 1959.
8. Elliot FM, Reid L: Some new facts about the pulmonary artery and its branching pattern. Clin Radiol 16:193, 1965.
9. Chang CH (Joseph): The normal roentgenographic measurement of the right descending pulmonary artery in 1,085 cases. Am J Roentgenol 87:929, 1962.
10. Kuriyama K, Gamsu G, Stern RG, et al: CT-determined pulmonary artery diameters in predicting pulmonary hypertension. Invest Radiol 19:16, 1984.
11. Woodring JH: Pulmonary artery-bronchus ratios in patients with normal lungs, pulmonary vascular plethora, and congestive heart failure. Radiology 179:115, 1991.
12. Ravin CE: Gleaning physiologic information from the conventional chest radiograph (editorial). Radiology 179:17, 1991.
13. Kim SJ, Im J-G, Kim IO, et al: Normal bronchial and pulmonary arterial diameters measured by thin-section CT. J Comput Assist Tomogr 19:365, 1995.
14. Hislop A, Reid L: Fetal and childhood development of the intrapulmonary veins in man: Branching patterns and structure. Thorax 28:313, 1973.
15. Müller NL, Webb WR: Radiographic imaging of the pulmonary hila. Invest Radiol 20:661, 1985.
16. Fraser RG, Fraser RS, Renner JW, et al: The roentgenologic diagnosis of chronic bronchitis: A reassessment with emphasis on parahilar bronchi seen end-on. Radiology 120:1, 1976.
17. Newton TH, Preger L: Selective bronchial arteriography. Radiology 84:1043, 1965.
18. Liebow AA: Patterns of origin and distribution of the major bronchial arteries in man. Am J Anat 117:19, 1965.
19. Deffebach ME, Charan NB, Lakshminarayan S, et al: The bronchial circulation: Small, but a vital attribute of the lung. Am Rev Respir Dis 135:463, 1987.
20. Murata K, Itoh H, Todo G, et al: Bronchial venous plexus and its communication with pulmonary circulation. Invest Radiol 21:24, 1986.
21. Miller WS: The Lung. Springfield, IL, Charles C Thomas, 1937.
22. Reid L, Rubino M: The connective tissue septa in the foetal human lung. Thorax 14:3, 1959.
23. Murata K, Itoh H, Todo G, et al: Centrilobular lesions of the lung: Demonstration by HRCT and pathologic correlation. Radiology 161:641, 1986.
24. Webb WR, Stein MG, Finkbeiner WE, et al: Normal and diseased isolated lungs: HRCT. Radiology 166:81, 1988.
25. Kang E-Y, Grenier P, Laurent F, et al: Interlobular septal thickening: Patterns at high-resolution computed tomography. J Thorac Imaging 11:260, 1996.
26. Bergin C, Roggli V, Coblentz C, et al: The secondary pulmonary lobule: Normal and abnormal CT appearances. Am J Roentgenol 151:21, 1988.
27. Bessis L, Callard P, Gotheil C, et al: HRCT of parenchymal lung disease: Precise correlation with histologic findings. Radiographics 12:45, 1992.
28. Colby TV, Swensen SJ: Anatomic distribution and histopathologic patterns in diffuse lung disease: Correlation with HRCT. J Thorac Imaging 11:1, 1996.
29. Murata K, Khan A, Herman PG: Pulmonary parenchymal disease: Evaluation with HRCT. Radiology 170:629, 1989.
30. Gruden JF, Webb WR, Warnock M: Centrilobular opacities in the lung on HRCT: Diagnostic considerations and pathologic correlation. Am J Roentgenol 162:569, 1994.
31. Worthy SA, Müller NL: Small airway diseases. Radiol Clin North Am 36:163, 1998.
32. Pump KK: The morphology of the finer branches of the bronchial tree of the human lung. Dis Chest 46:379, 1964.
33. Raskin SP: The pulmonary acinus: Historical notes. Radiology 144:31, 1982.
34. Gamsu G, Thurlbeck WM, Macklem PT, et al: Roentgenographic appearance of the human pulmonary acinus. Invest Radiol 6:171, 1971.
35. Lui YM, Taylor JR, Zylak CJ: Roentgen-anatomical correlation of the individual human pulmonary acinus. Radiology 109:1, 1973.
36. Hogg JC, Nepszy S: Regional lung volume and the pleural pressure gradient estimated from lung density in dogs. J Appl Physiol 27:198, 1969.
37. Altman PL, Dittmer DS: Respiration and Circulation. Bethesda, MD, Federation of American Societies of Experimental Biology, 1971, p 27.
38. Staub NC: Pulmonary edema. Physiol Rev 54:678, 1974.
39. Wandtke JC, Hyde RW, Fahey PJ, et al: Measurement of lung gas volume and regional density by computed tomography in dogs. Invest Radiol 21:108, 1986.
40. Goldman HI, Becklake MR: Respiratory function tests: Normal values at median altitudes and the prediction of normal results. Am Rev Tuberc 79:457, 1959.
41. Joseph AEA, Lacey GJ, Bryant THE, et al: The hypertransradiant hemithorax: The importance of lateral decentering, and the explanation for its appearance due to rotation. Clin Radiol 29:125, 1978.
42. Glazier JB, DeNardo GL: Pulmonary function studied with the xenon 133 scanning technique: Normal values and a postural study. Am Rev Respir Dis 94:188, 1966.
43. Primack SL, Remy-Jardin M, Remy J, et al: HRCT of the lungs: Pitfalls in the diagnosis of infiltrative lung disease. Am J Roentgenol 167:413, 1996.
44. Itoh H, Murata K, Konishi J, et al: Diffuse lung disease: Pathologic basis for the high-resolution computed tomography findings. J Thorac Imaging 8:176, 1993.
45. Kim JS, Müller NL, Park CS, et al: Cylindrical bronchiectasis: Diagnostic findings at thin-section CT. Am J Roentgenol 168:751, 1997.
46. Webb WR, Gamsu G, Wall SD, et al: CT of a bronchial phantom: Factors affecting appearance and size measurements. Invest Radiol 19:394, 1984.
47. McNamara AE, Müller NL, Okazawa M, et al: Airway narrowing in excised canine lungs measured by high-resolution computed tomography. J Appl Physiol 73:307, 1992.
48. Kim SJ, Im JG, Kim IO, et al: Normal bronchial and pulmonary arterial diameters measured by thin section CT. J Comput Assist Tomogr 19:365, 1995.
49. Woodring JH: Pulmonary artery-bronchus ratios in patients with normal lungs, pulmonary vascular plethora, and congestive heart failure. Radiology 179:115, 1991.
50. Kim JS, Müller NL, Park CS, et al: Broncho-arterial ratio on thin-section CT: Comparison between high-altitude and sea level. J Comput Assist Tomogr 21:306, 1997.
51. Herold CJ, Wetzel RC, Robotham JL, et al: Acute effects of increased intravascular volume and hypoxia on the pulmonary circulation: Assessment with HRCT. Radiology 183:665, 1992.
52. Hedlund LW, Vock P, Effmann EL: Evaluating lung density by computed tomography. Semin Respir Med 5:76, 1983.
53. Hedlund LW, Vock P, Effmann EL: Computed tomography of the lung: Densitometric studies. Radiol Clin North Am 21:775, 1983.
54. Rosenblum LJ, Mauceri RA, Wellenstein DE, et al: Density patterns in the normal lung as determined by computed tomography. Radiology 137:409, 1980.
55. Genereux GP: Computed tomography and the lungs: Review of

anatomic and densitometric features with their clinical application. Assoc Radiol 36:88, 1985.

56. Webb WR, Stern EJ, Kanth N, et al: Dynamic pulmonary CT: Findings in healthy adult men. Radiology 186:117, 1993.

57. Verschakelen JA, Van Fraeyenhoven L, Laureys G, et al: Differences in CT density between dependent and nondependent portions of the lung: Influence of lung volume. Am J Roentgenol 161:713, 1993.

58. Park CS, Müller NL, Worthy SA, et al: Airway obstruction in asthmatic and healthy individuals: Inspiratory and expiratory thin-section CT findings. Radiology 203:361, 1997.

59. Worthy SA, Park CS, Kim JS, et al: Bronchiolitis obliterans after lung transplantation: High resolution CT findings in 15 patients. Am J Roentgenol 169:673, 1997.

60. Rhodes CG, Wollmer P, Fazio F, et al: Quantitative measurement of regional extravascular lung density using positron emission and transmission tomography. J Comput Assist Tomogr 5:783, 1981.

61. Müller NL, Staples CA, Miller RR, et al: "Density mask": An objective method to quantitate emphysema using computed tomography. Chest 94:782, 1988.

62. Zerhouni EA, Boukadoum M, Siddiky MA, et al: A standard phantom for quantitative CT analysis of pulmonary nodules. Radiology 149:767, 1983.

63. Im J-G, Webb WR, Rosen A, et al: Costal pleura: Appearance at HRCT. Radiology 171:125, 1989.

64. Vix VA: Extrapleural costal fat. Radiology 112:563, 1974.

65. Sargent EN, Boswell WD Jr, Ralls PW, et al: Subpleural fat pads in patients exposed to asbestos: Distinction from non-calcified pleural plaques. Radiology 152:273, 1984.

66. Raasch BN, Carsky EW, Lane EJ, et al: Radiographic anatomy of the interlobar fissures: A study of 100 specimens. Am J Roentgenol 138:1043, 1982.

67. Yamashita H: Roentgenologic Anatomy of the Lung. New York, Igaku-Shoin, 1978, pp 46–58.

68. Glazer HS, Anderson DJ, DiCroce JJ, et al: Anatomy of the major fissure: Evaluation with standard and thin-section CT. Radiology 180:839, 1991.

69. Berkmen YM, Auh YH, Davis SD, et al: Anatomy of the minor fissure: Evaluation with thin-section CT. Radiology 170:647, 1989.

70. von Hayek H: The Human Lung. New York, Hafner, 1960.

71. Godwin JD, Tarver RD: Accessory fissures of the lung. Am J Roentgenol 144:39, 1985.

72. Felson B: The lobes and interlobar pleura: Fundamental roentgen considerations. Am J Med Sci 230:572, 1955.

73. Rabinowitz JG, Cohen BA, Mendleson DS: The pulmonary ligament. Radiol Clin North Am 22:659, 1984.

74. Berkmen YM, Drossman SR, Marboe CC: Intersegmental (intersublobar) septum of the lower lobe in relation to the pulmonary ligament: Anatomic, histologic, and CT correlations. Radiology 185:389, 1992.

75. Rost RC, Proto AV: Inferior pulmonary ligament: Computed tomographic appearance. Radiology 148:479, 1983.

76. Godwin JD, Bock P, Osborne DR: CT of the pulmonary ligament. Am J Roentgenol 141:237, 1983.

77. Rosenberger A, Abrams HL: Radiology of the thoracic duct. Am J Roentgenol 11:807, 1971.

78. Abramson DI: Blood Vessels and Lymphatics. New York, Academic Press, 1962, p 703.

79. Leigh TF, Weens HS: The Mediastinum. Springfield, IL, Charles C Thomas, 1959, pp 16–27.

80. Mountain CF, Dresler CM: Regional lymph node classification for lung cancer staging. Chest 111:1718, 1997.

81. Kradin RL, Spirn PW, Mark EJ: Intrapulmonary lymph nodes—clinical, radiologic, and pathologic findings. Chest 87:662, 1985.

82. Miyake H, Yamada Y, Kawagoe T, et al: Intrapulmonary lymph nodes CT and pathologic features. Clin Radiol 54:640, 1999.

83. Cymbalista M, Waysberg A, Zacharias C, et al: CT demonstration of the 1996 AJCC-UICC regional lymph node classification for lung cancer staging. Radiographics 19:899, 1999.

84. Ko JP, Drucker EA, Shepard J-AO, et al: CT depiction of regional nodal stations for lung cancer staging. Am J Roentgenol 174:775, 2000.

85. Glazer GM, Orringer MB, Gross BH, et al: The mediastinum in non-small cell lung cancer: CT-surgical correlation. Am J Roentgenol 152:1101, 1984.

86. Quint LE, Glazer GM, Orringer MB, et al: Mediastinal lymph node detection and sizing at CT and autopsy. Am J Roentgenol 147:469, 1986.

87. Kiyono K, Sone S, Sakai F, et al: The number and size of normal mediastinal lymph nodes: A postmortem study. Am J Roentgenol 150:771, 1988.

88. Müller NL, Webb WR, Gamsu G: Paratracheal lymphadenopathy: Radiographic findings and correlation with CT. Radiology 156:761, 1985.

89. Platt JF, Glazer GM, Orringer MB, et al: Radiologic evaluation of the subcarinal lymph nodes: A comparative study. Am J Roentgenol 151:279, 1988.

90. Remy-Jardin M, Duyck P, Remy J, et al: Hilar lymph nodes: Identification with spiral CT and histologic correlation. Radiology 196:387, 1995.

91. Musset D, Grenier P, Carette MF, et al: Primary lung cancer staging: Prospective comparative study of MR imaging with CT. Radiology 160:607, 1986.

92. Webb WR, Gamsu G, Stark DD, et al: Magnetic resonance imaging of the normal and abnormal pulmonary hila. Radiology 152:89, 1984.

93. Levitt RG, Glazer HS, Roper CL, et al: Magnetic resonance imaging of mediastinal and hilar masses: Comparison with CT. Am J Roentgenol 145:9, 1985.

94. Erasmus JJ, Page McAdams H, Patz EF Jr: Non-small cell lung cancer: FDG-PET imaging. J Thorac Imaging 14:247, 1999.

95. Valk PE, Pounds TR, Hopkins DM, et al: Staging non–small cell lung cancer by whole-body positron emission tomographic imaging. Ann Thorac Surg 60:1573, 1995.

96. Patz EF Jr, Lowe VJ, Goodman PC, et al: Thoracic nodal staging with PET imaging with [18]FDG in patients with bronchogenic carcinoma. Chest 108:1617, 1995.

97. Sazon DAD, Santiago SM, Hoo GWS, et al: Fluorodeoxyglucose-positron emission tomography in the detection and staging of lung cancer. Am J Respir Crit Care Med 153:417, 1996.

98. Dwamena BA, Sonnad SS, Angobaldo JO, et al: Metastases from non-small cell lung cancer: Mediastinal staging in the 1990s—meta-analytic comparison of PET and CT. Radiology 213:530, 1999.

99. Felson B: The mediastinum. Semin Roentgenol 4:31, 1969.

100. Bannister LH: The respiratory system. In Williams PL (ed): Gray's Anatomy. New York, Churchill Livingstone, 1995, pp 1627–1682.

101. Baron RL, Lee JKT, Sagel SS, et al: Computed tomography of the normal thymus. Radiology 142:121, 1982.

102. Francis IR, Glazer GM, Bookstein FL, et al: The thymus: Reexamination of age-related changes in size and shape. Am J Roentgenol 145:249, 1985.

103. Nicolaou S, Müller NL, Li DKB, et al: Thymus in myasthenia gravis: Comparison of CT and pathologic findings and clinical outcome after thymectomy. Radiology 201:471, 1996.

104. Savoca CJ, Austin JHM, Goldberg HI: The right paratracheal stripe. Radiology 122:295, 1977.

105. Proto AV, Simmons JD, Zylak CJ: The posterior junction anatomy. CRC Crit Rev Diagn Imaging 20:121, 1983.

106. Heitzman ER, Scrivani JV, Martino J, et al: The azygos vein and its pleural reflections: I. Normal roentgen anatomy. Radiology 101:249, 1971.

107. Heitzman ER, Scrivani JV, Martino J, et al: The azygos vein and its pleural reflections: II. Applications in the radiological diagnosis of mediastinal abnormality. Radiology 101:259, 1971.

108. Onitsuka H, Kuhns LR: Dextroconvexity of the mediastinum in the azygoesophageal recess. Radiology 135:126, 1980.

109. Simon G: Principles of Chest X-Ray Diagnosis. 3rd ed. London, Butterworth, 1971.

110. Lennon EA, Simon G: The height of the diaphragm in the chest radiograph of normal adults. Br J Radiol 38:937, 1965.

111. Felson B: Chest Roentgenology. Philadelphia, WB Saunders, 1973.

112. Naidich DP, Megibow AJ, Ross CR, et al: Computed tomography of the diaphragm: Normal anatomy and variants. J Comput Assist Tomogr 7:4, 1983.

113. Naidich JB, Naidich TP, Roger AH, et al: The big rib sign: Localization of basal pulmonary pathology in lateral projection utilizing differential magnification of the two hemithoraces. Radiology 131:1, 1979.

114. Kurihara Y, Yakushiji YK, Matsumoto J, et al: The ribs: Anatomic and radiologic considerations. Radiographics 19:105, 1999.

115. Stewart JH, McCormick WF: A sex- and age-limited ossification pattern in human costal cartilages. Am J Clin Pathol 81:765, 1984.
116. Sanders CF: Sexing by costal cartilage calcification. Br J Radiol 39:233, 1966.
117. Wechsler RJ, Steiner RM: Cross-sectional imaging of the chest wall. J Thorac Imaging 4:29, 1989.
118. Bhalla M, McCauley DI, Golimbu C, et al: Counting ribs on chest CT. J Comput Assist Tomogr 14:590, 1990.
119. Goldenberg DB, Brogdon BG: Congenital anomalies of the pectoral girdle demonstrated by chest radiography. J Can Assoc Radiol 18:472, 1967.
120. Parsons FG: On the proportions and characteristics of the modern English clavicle. J Anat 51:71, 1917.
121. Aronberg DJ, Glazer HS, Madsen K, et al: Normal thoracic aortic diameters by computed tomograph. J Comput Assist Tomogr 8:247, 1984.

CHAPTER 2

Methods of Radiologic Investigation

The cornerstone of radiologic diagnosis is the chest radiograph. As a general rule, establishing the *presence* of a disease process on the chest radiograph should constitute the first step in radiologic diagnosis; if this first examination does not show clearly the nature and extent of the abnormality, additional studies such as computed tomography (CT) or magnetic resonance (MR) imaging can be carried out to *complement* the radiograph.

CONVENTIONAL RADIOGRAPHY

Projections

The most satisfactory basic or routine radiographic views for evaluation of the chest are posteroanterior (PA) and lateral projections with the patient standing; such projections provide the essential requirement for proper three-dimensional assessment. In patients who are too ill to

stand, anteroposterior upright or supine projections offer alternative but considerably less satisfactory views. The anteroposterior projection is of inferior quality because of the shorter focal-film distance, the greater magnification of the heart, and the restricted ability of many of such patients to suspend respiration or to achieve full inspiration.

Situations in which the performance of routine radiography is likely to be cost-effective have been the subject of considerable study.[1] Table 2–1 summarizes our recommendations on the use of chest radiographs based on a review of the literature and the recommendations of the American College of Chest Radiology[2] and the American Thoracic Society.[3]

Basic Radiographic Techniques

Diagnostic accuracy in chest disease is related partly to the quality of the radiographic images themselves. Careful

---

Table 2–1. RECOMMENDATIONS FOR THE USE OF CHEST RADIOGRAPHY

Indications for chest radiography
 Signs and symptoms related to the respiratory and cardiovascular systems
 Follow-up of previously diagnosed thoracic disease for the evaluation of improvement, resolution, or progression
 Staging of intrathoracic and extrathoracic tumors
 Preoperative assessment of patients scheduled for intrathoracic surgery
 Preoperative evaluation of patients who have cardiac or respiratory symptoms, or patients who have a significant potential for thoracic pathology that may lead to increased perioperative morbidity or mortality
 Monitoring of patients who have life support devices and patients who have undergone cardiac or thoracic surgery or other interventional procedures
Routine chest radiographs are not indicated in the following situations
 Routine screening of unselected populations
 Routine prenatal chest radiographs for the detection of unsuspected disease
 Routine radiographs solely because of hospital admission
 Mandated radiographs for employment
 Repeated radiograph examinations after long-term facility admission

Based on recommendations from American College of Radiology: ACR Standard for the Performance of Pediatric and Adult Chest Radiography. Reston, VA, Standards: American College of Radiology, 1997, p 27; and American Thoracic Society: Chest x-ray screening statements. Am Thorac News 10:14, 1984.

attention to several variables is necessary to ensure such quality.

Patient Positioning. Positioning must be such that the x-ray beam is centered properly, the patient's body is not rotated, and the scapulas are rotated sufficiently anteriorly so as to be projected away from the lungs. On properly centered radiographs, the medial ends of the clavicles are projected equidistant from the spinous processes of the thoracic vertebrae.

Patient Respiration. Respiration must be suspended, preferably at full inspiration.

Film Exposure. Exposure factors should be such that the resultant radiograph permits faint visualization of the thoracic spine *and* the intervertebral disks on the PA radiograph so that lung markings behind the heart are clearly visible; exposure should be as short as possible, consistent with the production of adequate contrast.

For a PA chest radiograph, the mean radiation dose at skin entrance should not exceed 0.3 mGy per exposure, and the exposure time should not exceed 40 msec.[2] An optimally exposed radiograph presents the lung at midgray level (average optical density, 1.6 to 1.9). (Optical density is the measurement of the ability of the film to stop light [film blackness] and is equal to the logarithm of light incident on the film over light transmitted by the film [D = log Io/It].) The focus-film distance should be at least 180 cm (72 inches) to minimize magnification.[2] (Focus-film distance is the distance between the focal spot of the x-ray tube and the radiograph.)

Kilovoltage. A high-kilovoltage technique appropriate to the film speed should be used;[2] for PA and lateral chest radiographs, we recommend using 115 to 150 kVp. (The abbreviation kVp is the peak voltage applied across the x-ray tube.)

Grids and Filters. When using a grid, one that has at least a 10:1 aluminum interspace with a minimum of 103 lines per inch is recommended by the American College of Radiology.[2] It is also possible to use an air gap technique, in which a space of 15 cm (6 inches) is interposed between the patient and the x-ray film;[4, 5] because the gap reduces radiation scatter by distance dispersion, no grid is required. When this technique is used, a constant focus-film distance of 10 feet is recommended.

Other techniques that have been developed to compensate for the large range of densities within the thorax include rapidly customized patient-specific filters[6] and scanning equalization radiography.[7, 8] The latter technique incorporates a feedback system that modulates the x-ray beam intensity according to the patient's body habitus. The best known of these systems is marketed as AMBER (Advanced Multiple-Beam Equalization Radiography, Optische Industries Oldelft, Delft, The Netherlands).[9] This system markedly improves visualization of mediastinal detail on PA radiographs[10] and detection of nodules overlying the mediastinum or diaphragm.[11] The AMBER system decreases the contrast in the periphery of the lung,[12] requires a higher radiation dose than conventional radiography, and cannot be used for bedside examinations.

Digital Radiography

Digital radiography has many advantages over conventional-screen film systems.[10, 13] One of the most important

advantages is its wide exposure latitude, which is 10 to 100 times greater than the widest dynamic range of screen-film systems. During digital image processing, the systems automatically determine the range of clinically appropriate gray levels and produce an image within that range. As a result, the final image is virtually independent of absolute x-ray exposure levels. (A potential disadvantage is that patients may receive unnecessarily high radiation doses, which may not be detected because they do not result in perceivable alterations in image quality.) The wider latitude of digital systems allows them to be used under a much broader range of exposure conditions than conventional systems and makes them an ideal choice in applications in which exposures are highly variable or difficult to control, such as bedside radiography. Another major advantage of digital radiography is that it produces what are essentially electronic images; as a result, an image may be transmitted to any location, displayed at multiple sites simultaneously, and efficiently archived for later reference. The images may be displayed on video monitors (soft copy) or printed onto film or paper (hard copy). Two main types of digital radiography systems are available commercially: systems based on photostimulable storage phosphor image receptors and systems based on selenium-coated receptors.

Storage Phosphor Radiography

Storage phosphor imaging (computed radiography) has been used mainly for bedside chest radiography because its wide dynamic range allows it to achieve consistent images over a wide range of x-ray exposures (Fig. 2–1).[14] Storage phosphor systems have a dynamic range of approximately 1:10,000 as compared with 1:100 for standard films;[15] that is, they are capable of producing diagnostic images over a much broader range of exposures, which results in a considerable decrease in the repeat rate for bedside chest radiographs.[16]

In the storage phosphor technology, a reusable photostimulable phosphor, rather than film, is used to record the image. Plates coated with the phosphor are loaded into special cassettes that are outwardly similar to screen-film cassettes. During exposure, the receptor stores the x-ray energy, then is scanned by a laser beam, which results in the creation of visible or infrared radiation, the intensity of which corresponds to the absorbed x-ray energy. The resultant luminescence is measured and recorded digitally.[17]

Selenium Detector Digital Radiography

Similar to the photostimulable storage phosphor systems, selenium-based chest imaging systems use a receptor, which allows production of a digital image that can be adjusted after processing and displayed on a monitor or on film. The main advantage of selenium-based detectors is a considerably greater quantum efficiency than that of conventional screen-film systems and photostimulable phosphor detectors.[18, 19]

COMPUTED TOMOGRAPHY

The CT image is a two-dimensional representation of a three-dimensional cross-sectional slice, the third dimension

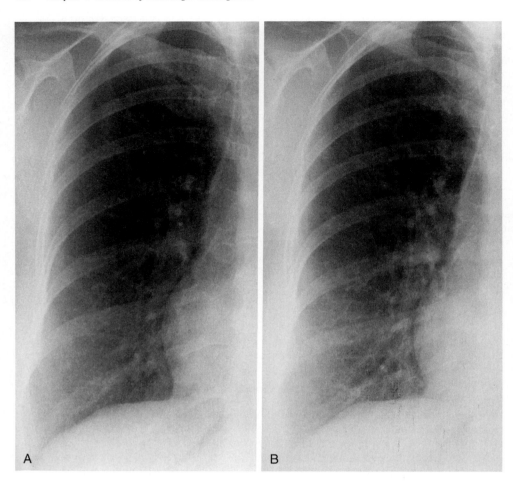

Figure 2–1. Storage Phosphor and Conventional Radiography. Views of the normal right lung in a 54-year-old woman obtained using storage phosphor technology *(A)* and conventional radiography *(B)* demonstrate comparable visualization of parenchymal detail.

being the section or slice thickness. The slice thickness also is known as the collimation width and is defined by collimators between the x-ray tube and the patient. The CT image is composed of multiple picture elements (typically 512 × 512) known as *pixels*. A pixel is a unit area (i.e., each square on the image matrix); it reflects the attenuation of a unit volume of tissue, or voxel, which corresponds to the area of the pixel multiplied by the section thickness. The x-ray attenuations of the structures within a given voxel are averaged to produce the image.

Technical Considerations

Several operator-dependent parameters greatly influence the information provided by chest CT. The main parameters are slice thickness, slice spacing, field of view, reconstruction algorithm, and image display settings (window width and level). In selected cases, intravenous contrast medium may be used to distinguish vessels from soft tissue lesions or to detect intravascular abnormalities, such as thromboemboli (Fig. 2–2).

The optimal slice thickness is determined by the size of the structure being assessed and by the number of scans required to evaluate the patient. It has been well established that thin sections (1- to 2-mm collimation) are required for adequate assessment of the pulmonary parenchyma and peripheral bronchi (Fig. 2–3).[20, 21] Adequate assessment of the chest can be obtained by performing these scans at 10-mm intervals. Although only 10% to 20% of the lung

parenchyma is sampled, the improved spatial resolution allows better assessment of normal and abnormal findings than is possible with thicker sections.[22] This approach is not acceptable in all situations, however; for example, when assessing pulmonary metastases, it is essential to evaluate the entire chest, preferably by using continuous spiral CT through the chest with 3- to 5-mm-thick sections. Volumetric scanning during a single breath-hold using 3- to 5-mm collimation is recommended for the assessment of abnormalities involving the trachea and central bronchi.[23] The optimal slice thickness is dictated by the indication for performing the CT scan.

CT scanning should be performed using a field-of-view just large enough to encompass the patient (35 to 40 cm). In general, the largest matrix available (usually 512 × 512) should be used in image reconstruction to reduce pixel size. Using a field-of-view of 40 cm and a 512 × 512 matrix results in a pixel size of 0.78 mm. Targeting the image prospectively or retrospectively to a smaller field-of-view decreases pixel size and increases spatial resolution. For example, targeting the image to a single lung using a field-of-view of 25 cm results in a pixel size of 0.49 mm. The maximal spatial resolution usually is obtained using a field-of-view of 13 cm, which results in a pixel size of 0.25 mm.[24] Although small fields-of-view increase spatial resolution, they should be used only in selected cases as an ancillary technique because they allow assessment of only a small portion of the chest.

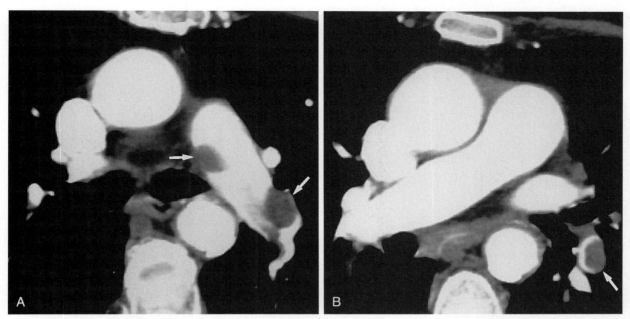

Figure 2–2. Spiral CT in Pulmonary Thromboembolism. A 3-mm collimation spiral CT scan after intravenous administration of contrast medium *(A and B)* shows several emboli in the left main and interlobar pulmonary arteries *(arrows)*. The patient was an 84-year-old woman with acute shortness of breath.

CT numbers in the thorax range from $-1,000$ Hounsfield units (HU) for air in the trachea to approximately 700 HU for dense bones. The display of the CT image on the monitor (soft copy) or film (hard copy) is determined by the window level and width and is limited to 256 shades of gray. No single window setting can display adequately all of the information available on a chest CT scan. To display the large number of attenuation values (HU) within a limited number of shades of gray, a CT number is selected that corresponds to approximately the mean attenuation value of the tissue being examined. This center CT attenuation value is called the *window level*. The computer

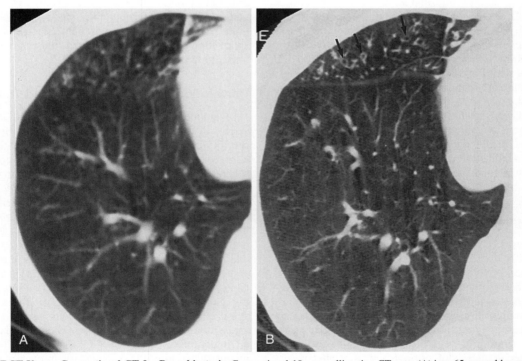

Figure 2–3. HRCT Versus Conventional CT for Bronchiectasis. Conventional 10-mm collimation CT scan *(A)* in a 65-year-old woman shows small focal areas of ground-glass attenuation and consolidation in the right middle lobe. HRCT scan (1.5-mm collimation) *(B)* performed immediately after conventional CT scan shows right middle lobe bronchiectasis *(arrows)*. Even in retrospect the bronchiectasis cannot be seen on the conventional CT scan.

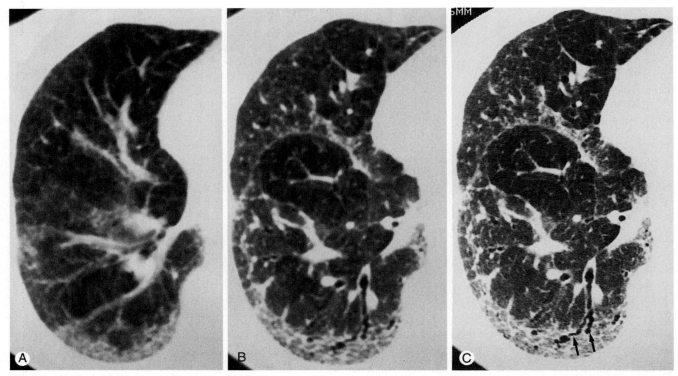

Figure 2–4. Influence of Section Thickness and Reconstruction Algorithm on Image Quality. A 10-mm collimation CT scan *(A)* in a 71-year-old patient shows poorly defined areas of increased attenuation in the right lung. The pattern and distribution of abnormalities are visualized better on the 1.5-mm collimation CT scan *(B)*. Both images *(A* and *B)* were reconstructed by using a standard reconstruction algorithm. HRCT scan (1.5-mm collimation CT scan reconstructed by using a high-spatial frequency algorithm) *(C)* allows optimal assessment of fine parenchymal detail. The edges of vessels and bronchi are defined more sharply than on the standard algorithm. The abnormalities consist of a fine reticular pattern and areas of ground-glass attenuation involving mainly the subpleural regions. Note the irregular dilation of the posterior basal bronchi of the right lower lobe as they enter into an area of fibrosis (traction bronchiectasis *[arrows]*). The diagnosis of idiopathic pulmonary fibrosis was confirmed by open-lung biopsy.

is instructed to assign one shade of gray to a certain number of CT attenuation values above and below the window level. The range of CT numbers above and below the window level is called the *window width*. To depict the lungs adequately, a window level of −600 to −700 HU and a window width of 1,000 to 1,500 HU most commonly are recommended.[25] Window levels of 30 to 50 HU and window widths of 350 to 500 HU usually provide the best assessment of the mediastinum, hila, and pleura. These figures represent guidelines only, and there are no universally accepted ideal window settings for the lung parenchyma or the mediastinum; different windows may provide optimal assessment of particular abnormalities in individual cases.

High-Resolution Computed Tomography

In most cases, CT scan data are reconstructed using a standard or soft tissue algorithm, which smoothes the image and reduces visible image noise; such an algorithm is preferred in the assessment of abnormalities of the mediastinum and chest wall. Use of a high spatial frequency reconstruction algorithm is required for optimal assessment of the lung parenchyma, however.[24, 26] This algorithm reduces image smoothing and increases spatial resolution, allowing better depiction of normal and abnormal parenchymal interfaces and better visualization of small vessels, airways, and subtle interstitial abnormalities.[26, 27] The com-

bination of thin-section CT scan (1- to 2-mm collimation) and a high spatial frequency reconstruction algorithm provides for the optimal assessment of interstitial and air-space lung disease and is referred to as *high-resolution CT* (HRCT) (Fig. 2–4).[20, 25]

Conventional and Spiral Computed Tomography

A conventional CT scan of the chest consists of a series of cross-sectional slices obtained during suspended respiration. After each slice is obtained, the patient is allowed to breathe while the table is moved to the next scanning position. This method of obtaining a series of cross-sectional images is known as *incremental CT scanning*. Although each image can be obtained in approximately 1 second, there is a delay of 5 to 10 seconds between images recorded. Spiral (helical) CT is an important technical advance that allows continuous scanning while the patient is moved continuously through the CT gantry.[28] With this technique, patient progress through the gantry and x-ray source rotation occur simultaneously during data acquisition. The x-ray beam traces a helical or spiral curve in relation to the patient. Each rotation of the x-ray tube can be considered as generating data specific to an angled plane of section.[29] Cross-sectional images can be reconstructed after the data specific to each plane of section have been estimated. This mathematical calculation is performed by interpolation of the spiral data above and below each plane of section. Most current spiral CT scanners reorder the projection data and perform interpolation from views separated by 180 degrees to optimize resolution in the longitudinal axis.[30] The position and spacing of these images can be chosen retrospectively for arbitrary table positions and at small increments.

A spiral CT scan of the entire chest may be completed during a single breath-hold or several successive short breath-holds. The continuous nature of the data acquisition allows true volumetric scanning and the production of multiple overlapping images resulting in increased spatial resolution in the longitudinal axis. These overlapping reconstructions allow the production of high-quality multiplanar reformations without additional radiation exposure (Fig. 2–5). Because spiral CT allows major portions or the entire chest to be scanned during a single breath-hold, it virtually eliminates motion artifacts due to respiratory motion that otherwise degrade image quality.

Major recent developments in spiral CT include the introduction of faster rotational times (subsecond CT scans) and multiple detector arrays (multisection CT).[31, 31a] Faster rotational times make it possible to increase the anatomic coverage for any given section thickness, and result in a marked reduction in cardiac motion artifacts and improvement in the evaluation of the pulmonary and systemic vessels. Multiple detector arrays allow simultaneous acquisition of data from each of several detectors, rather than from a single detector row, as was the case with previous CT scanners. The advantages of multisection CT scanners include improved temporal resolution, improved spatial resolution in the z axis, increased efficiency in x-ray tube use, and decreased image noise.[31a] The improved temporal resolution permits imaging of the entire chest with thin sections during a single breath-hold, to optimize the intravascular contrast enhancement, and to reduce the amount of intravenous contrast. The increased spatial resolution in the z axis (cephalocaudad plane) results in considerable improvement in the multiplanar and three-dimensional reconstructions.

Computed Tomography Tracheobronchography and Bronchoscopy

Multiplanar image displays allow better appreciation of the spatial relationships of various structures than a series

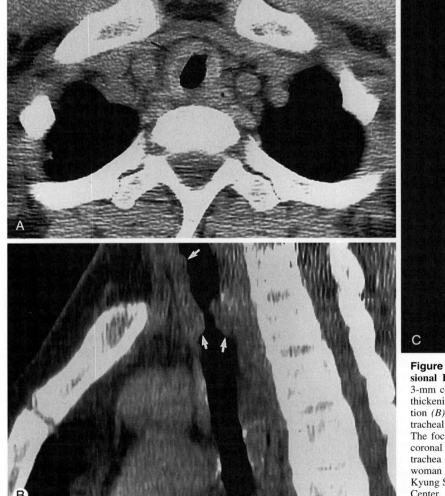
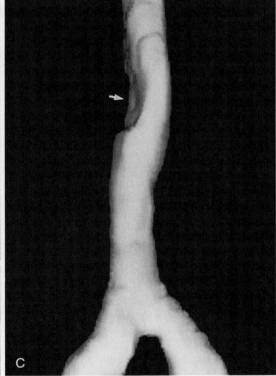

Figure 2–5. Spiral CT with Sagittal and Three-Dimensional Reconstructions in Endotracheal Tuberculosis. A 3-mm collimation spiral CT scan *(A)* shows circumferential thickening of the trachea *(arrows)*. The sagittal reconstruction *(B)* allows better assessment of the focal nature of the tracheal thickening with narrowing of the lumen *(arrows)*. The focal narrowing of the trachea also is well seen on the coronal three-dimensional reconstruction *(arrow in C)* of the trachea and main bronchi. The patient was a 27-year-old woman with endotracheal tuberculosis. (Case courtesy of Dr. Kyung Soo Lee, Department of Radiology, Samsung Medical Center, Seoul, Korea.)

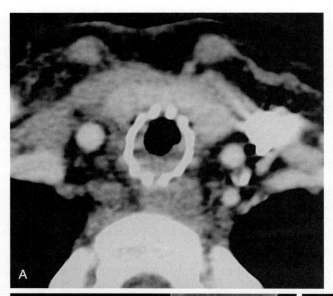

Figure 2–6. CT Tracheobronchography. A patient previously treated with tracheal endoprosthesis for post-tracheotomy tracheal stenosis developed progressive shortness of breath. Spiral CT scan *(A)* shows tracheal endoprosthesis and recurrent tracheal narrowing resulting from soft tissue internal to the prosthesis. CT tracheo-bronchography performed using volume-rendering technique *(B)* shows the extent of tracheal narrowing and the relationship to the endoprosthesis. The endoprosthesis obscures the anatomic detail of the trachea. Electronic subtraction of the prosthesis *(C)* allows better assessment of the extent of tracheal stenosis *(arrows)*. (Case courtesy of Dr. Martine Remy-Jardin, Department of Radiology, Hopital Calmette, Lille, France.)

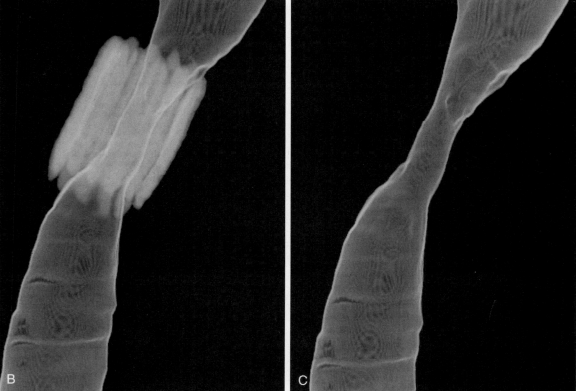

of individual cross-sectional images.[32] Use of graphics-based software systems and volume-rendering techniques allows depiction of the luminal surface of the airways that resemble the images seen by bronchography or during bronchoscopy (Fig. 2–6).[32, 33] It has been recommended that the CT technique that depicts the interior of the trachea and bronchi in a manner that resembles conventional bron-chography be called *CT tracheobronchography*.[34, 35] The technique by which luminal surface views provided from the virtual environment of the CT database resemble those of bronchoscopy is known as *virtual bronchoscopy*[33] or, preferably, *CT bronchoscopy* (Fig. 2–7).[35, 36]

Indications

Table 2–2 summarizes the most common indications for the use of CT as based on published data.[37, 38] The main indications for the use of HRCT (1- to 2-mm collimation, high spatial frequency reconstruction algorithm) include the following.[20, 25]

Diagnosis of Bronchiectasis. *See* Figure 2-3 for comparison of CT and HRCT in diagnosis of bronchiectasis.

Detection of Parenchymal Lung Disease. HRCT is useful in assessment of patients who have symptoms or pulmonary function abnormalities suggestive of parenchy-

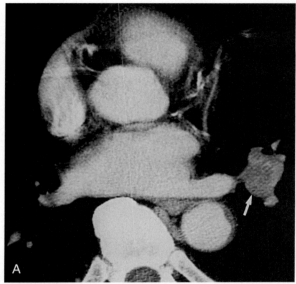

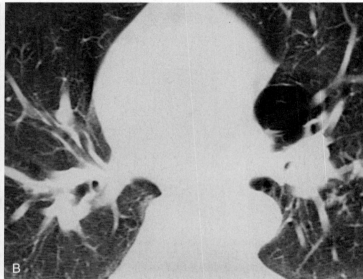

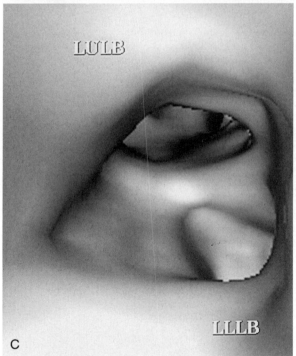

Figure 2–7. CT Bronchoscopy. Spiral CT scan *(A)* after intravenous administration of contrast medium shows left lower lobe tumor *(arrow)*. Lung windows *(B)* show extrinsic compression of the left lower lobe bronchus. CT bronchoscopy (internal rendering technique) *(C)* shows left upper lobe bronchus (LULB) and obstruction of the left lower lobe bronchus (LLLB) by soft tissue mass. (Case courtesy of Dr. David Naidich, Department of Radiology, New York University Medical Center, New York, New York.)

Table 2–2. MOST COMMON INDICATIONS FOR CHEST COMPUTED TOMOGRAPHY

Evaluation of suspected mediastinal abnormalities identified on standard chest radiographs
Determination of the presence and extent of neoplastic disease
Search for diffuse or central calcification in pulmonary nodule
Diagnosis of pulmonary thromboembolism
Guidance to percutaneous biopsy of mediastinal, pleural, or pulmonary nodules or masses
Localization of loculated collections of fluid within the pleural space when standard radiographic or ultrasonic techniques prove inadequate
Assessment of abnormalities of the thoracic aorta
Diagnosis of bronchiectasis and assessment of the nature and extent of interstitial lung disease, small airway disease, and emphysema using HRCT

HRCT, high-resolution computed tomography.

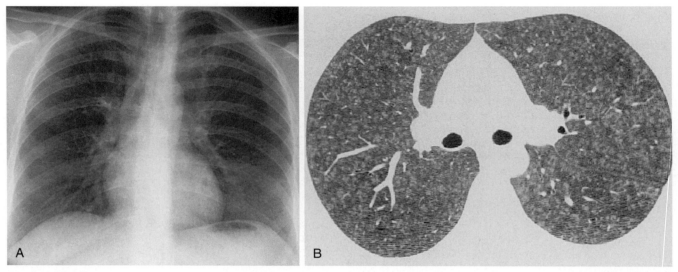

Figure 2–8. HRCT in Chronic Diffuse Lung Disease. Posteroanterior chest radiograph *(A)* in a 35-year-old woman with progressive shortness of breath shows subtle bilateral areas of increased opacity. HRCT scan *(B)* shows small rounded opacities in a centrilobular distribution. Although the radiographic findings were nonspecific, the HRCT appearance is most suggestive of hypersensitivity pneumonitis. The diagnosis was proved by open-lung biopsy.

mal lung disease but normal or questionable radiographic findings (Fig. 2–8).

Differential Diagnosis of Diffuse Lung Disease. HRCT is recommended in assessment of patients in whom the combination of clinical and radiographic findings does not provide a confident diagnosis and further radiologic assessment is considered warranted. This indication in particular includes patients who have chronic interstitial and air-space disease and immunocompromised patients who have acute parenchymal abnormalities; in such patients, the differential diagnosis can be narrowed or a specific diagnosis often made on HRCT when the radiographic findings are nonspecific.

MAGNETIC RESONANCE IMAGING

With the exception of the hydrogen nucleus, which consists of a single proton, atomic nuclei contain both protons and neutrons. The constituent *nucleons* (the generic term for a proton or neutron) each possess an intrinsic angular moment or *spin*; however, because pairs of protons or neutrons align in such a way that their spins cancel out, a *net* spin exists for a nucleus only when it contains an odd (unpaired) proton or an odd neutron. This intrinsic spin has an associated magnetic moment so that each nucleus may be considered to act as a small bar magnet. When these nuclei are exposed to a magnetic field, they experience a torque, their axis of spin rotating about the field direction as the nuclei attempt to line up parallel to the magnetic field. Any nucleus with a net spin possesses a characteristic resonant or *precessional* frequency that is determined by the magnetic field strength and a constant (the gyromagnetic ratio, which takes into account the magnetic properties of the nuclear species in question). For a nuclear magnetic interaction to occur, the pulse of radio-frequency (RF) radiation must be at precisely the same frequency as the precessional frequency of the nucleus (also known as the *Larmor frequency*).

To induce the MR phenomenon, a short RF pulse is applied through a coil surrounding the patient, the RF radiation being equivalent to the application of a second, smaller magnetic field. The RF signal changes the state of the protons in the magnetic field from one of equilibrium to one of excitation. This excited state is inherently unstable and naturally decays toward the equilibrium state over a period of time. As the nuclei relax to their original alignment in the magnetic field, they radiate to their surroundings the absorbed energy at their characteristic or Larmor frequency. The re-emitted energy provides a signal that can be detected by a receiver coil surrounding the patient; if there are a sufficient number of these signals and if they can be spatially resolved, an image of the distribution of the emitting nuclei can be formed.

Currently, most medical MR imaging uses hydrogen protons as the nuclei of interest because they are abundant in the body. The greater the number of hydrogen protons present, the more intense the MR signal. Several factors influence the nature of the energy emitted during MR imaging.

Relaxation Times

The signal strength during emission diminishes exponentially with a characteristic *relaxation time* that is determined, in part, by the general environment of the nuclei. The greater the facility to pass energy to neighboring nuclei, the more rapidly the irradiated nuclei can return to their original energy state; hence, a shorter relaxation time. There are two such relaxation times, designated *T1* and *T2*.

T1. Once nuclei have been energized by an RF pulse, T1 is the time constant corresponding to the exponential restoration of the magnetization *parallel* to the external field; T1 represents the time required for the component of the net magnetization vector parallel to the external field to return to its initial value after it has been perturbed by the RF pulse. T1 also is known as the spin-lattice or *longitudinal relaxation time*. In a pure liquid, the return to equilibrium is exponential, and after three T1 periods have elapsed, 95% of the original magnetization will have been restored. The T1 relaxation time tends to be long for fluids (e.g., cerebrospinal fluid, hydatid cyst contents) and shorter for fat. Any process that increases tissue water content (e.g., edema) lengthens the T1.

T2. T2 corresponds to the exponential decay of the magnetization *perpendicular* to the external field and also is known as the *spin-spin relaxation time.* After an RF pulse has tipped the nuclear magnetization vector toward the transverse plane, the components of this vector all precess together or *in phase* and appear to be stationary in the rotating reference frame. The precession does not remain in phase, however; subtle local alterations of the magnetic field strength cause some nuclei to precess at different rates from others, the RF waves from individual nuclei dephase and cancel each other out, and the sum of nuclear magnetization vectors in the transverse plane decays to zero. The time constant for this dephasing or decay is called *T2* or *spin-spin relaxation time* and provides additional data about the local environment in which the hydrogen nuclei reside. During the measuring pulse, the precessing protons are brought into phase with the frequency of the radio signal.

The T2 relaxation time is the result of random molecular motion, which leads to signal dephasing. The latter in turn is related to the local molecular environment, T2 times being characteristically long for homogeneous environments (e.g., fluid) and short for complex tissues (e.g., muscle). An increase in tissue water as a result of congestive heart failure or a pulmonary neoplasm results in lengthening of the T2 relaxation time.[39]

The MR signal is influenced by motion of water or blood during the imaging sequence. To generate an MR signal, protons need to be excited by the RF pulse, then need to be refocused. Four interactions occur between flowing protons and the pulse sequence: (1) signal loss related to flow through the imaging plane during the pulse sequence, (2) signal loss as a result of phase encoding misregistration, (3) signal loss as a result of destructive phase interference in the voxel, and (4) signal gain related to inflow of blood that has not yet received any RF pulses (unsaturated spins).[39] As a result of these four effects and depending on the velocity of blood flow and the image sequence used, the MR signal of flowing blood may be increased (*white blood* signal), decreased (*black blood* signal), or intermediate. Many specialized MR pulse sequences have been devised that have special sensitivity to flow and that may allow its quantification.[40, 41]

Magnetic Resonance Pulse Sequences

The RF pulse duration determines the extent to which the net magnetization rotates with respect to its original alignment. For example, a 90-degree pulse rotates the net magnetization 90 degrees; similarly, a 180-degree pulse rotates the net magnetization 180 degrees. An appropriate sequence of RF pulses may be used to emphasize the T1 or T2 portion of the MR signal or to improve the efficiency of data accumulation.[42]

The spin-echo sequence is the most commonly used MR technique in assessment of the chest. The separation of the successive 90-degree pulses on spin-echo MR is known as the *repetition time (TR).* Short repetition times are required to allow distinction between tissues that have different T1 relaxation times. The short repetition times are known as *T1-weighted sequences.* In 1.5-tesla MR scanners, T1-weighted sequences have TRs ranging from 600 to 1,000 msec.[39] Because chest MR images are cardiac (electrocardiogram) gated to decrease motion artifacts, this corresponds to one R-R interval.

The MR signal decays as an exponential function of the T2 relaxation time. To distinguish tissues with different T2 characteristics, a long echo time is required ($\geq$80 msec). To maximize T2 differences and to minimize the effect of T1 relaxation, T2-weighted images require long TR intervals. T2-weighted images on cardiac-gated MR imaging are obtained using two to three R-R intervals and a TE of 80 msec or more. In practice, a double echo sequence commonly is used (i.e., a TR corresponding to two or three R-R intervals using a short echo delay [TE of $\leqq$20 msec] and a long echo delay [TE of $\geq$80 msec]). The sequence that minimizes the T1 effect (long TR) and the T2 effect (short TE) is referred to as the *proton density sequence.* The signal on the proton density–weighted image is influenced primarily by the proton density or relative water content. Although this sequence provides the best signal-to-noise ratio, it has limited contrast (i.e., limited ability to distinguish various tissues) because it minimizes the effects of T1 and T2 relaxation times. The intensity of the MR image depends on four parameters: nuclear density, two relaxation times called T1 and T2, and motion of the nuclei within the imaged volume.

The depiction of blood vessels on MR imaging can be improved by using gadolinium enhancement (MR angiography) and fast gradient-recalled echo (GRE) sequences.[43, 44] The use of gadolinium enhancement and high-speed imaging gradients makes it possible to obtain three-dimensional images of the mediastinal and pulmonary vessels during a single breath-hold.[43, 44] On these angiographic MR images, flowing blood results in high signal intensity (white blood MR angiography) (Fig. 2–9). Visualization of the vessel walls is optimized by using sequences in which flowing blood results in signal void (black blood angiography).[37]

The advantages of MR imaging over CT include (1) lack of ionizing radiation; (2) direct coronal, sagittal, or oblique as well as transverse imaging; (3) intrinsic contrast in blood vessels as a result of flow; and (4) increased soft tissue contrast owing to multiple MR parameters as compared with only electron density on CT (Fig. 2–10). The main limitation of MR imaging in the assessment of chest disease is the presence of physiologic motion, which severely degrades image quality. Although this quality has improved greatly with the use of cardiac gating and respiratory compensation, the use of MR imaging in the assessment of the lung parenchyma still is hampered by the low signal-to-noise ratio related to the low proton density of the lungs and the loss in signal caused by magnetic field inhomogeneity created by the difference in the diamagnetic susceptibilities between air and water.

Indications

Evaluation of the Heart and Great Vessels. MR imaging has a well-established role in the assessment of

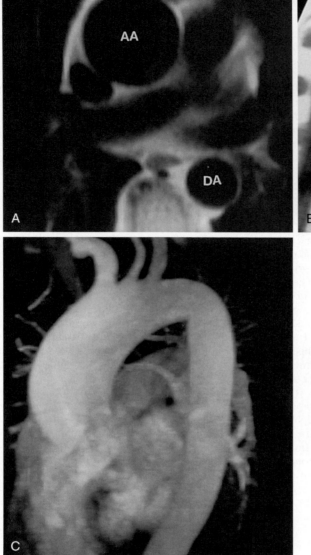

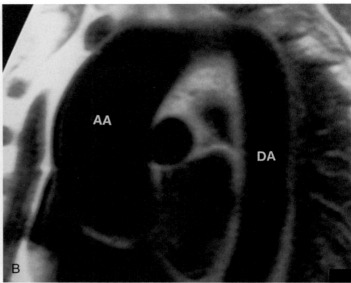

Figure 2–9. MR Angiography. Cross-sectional T1-weighted spin-echo image *(A)* shows aneurysm of the ascending aorta (AA) measuring 6 cm in diameter. The descending thoracic aorta (DA) is normal. Sagittal T1-weighted spin-echo image *(B)* shows the extent of the aneurysm. MR angiogram *(C)* allows better assessment of the extent of the aneurysm and its relationship to the great vessels. The MR angiogram was obtained using cine-gradient-echo (GRE) technique during a single breath-hold and with intravenous gadolinium enhancement. (Case courtesy of Dr. Glen Krinsky, New York University Medical Center, New York, New York.)

congenital abnormalities of the heart and great vessels. It is superior to echocardiography in the assessment of adult congenital heart disease because it permits unobstructed views of all atrial, ventricular, and great vessel abnormalities.[45, 46] It is usually reserved for patients who have nondiagnostic or equivocal findings on echocardiography, however.[46] MR imaging allows excellent evaluation of central pulmonary artery abnormalities. Cine gradient-echo sequences permit assessment of cardiac wall motion and can detect high-velocity jets related to ventricular septal defects, valvular regurgitation, or focal stenoses.[45, 47] Velocity-encoded cine sequences can be used to calculate blood flow.[48]

Although comparable to conventional CT in the assessment of aortic aneurysms[49] and aortic dissection,[50] MR imaging has been shown to be inferior to spiral CT.[51] In one study in which spiral CT, multiplanar transesophageal echocardiography, and MR imaging were compared, the three techniques were found to have 100% sensitivity in the detection of thoracic aortic dissection;[51] however, spiral CT had a higher specificity. The sensitivity in detecting aortic arch vessel involvement was 93% for spiral CT, 60% for transesophageal echocardiography, and 67% for MR imaging, with specificities of 97%, 85%, and 88%.

Evaluation of the Mediastinum and Hila. Currently, MR imaging is a secondary imaging modality in the mediastinum and hila used mainly as a problem-solving technique in cases in which CT findings are equivocal. In patients who have pulmonary carcinoma, MR imaging has been shown to be superior to CT in the assessment of mediastinal and vascular invasion.[52] It can be helpful in the diagnosis of bronchogenic cysts in cases in which the CT findings are not diagnostic (*see* Fig. 2–10);[53] these lesions characteristically show a homogeneous high signal inten-

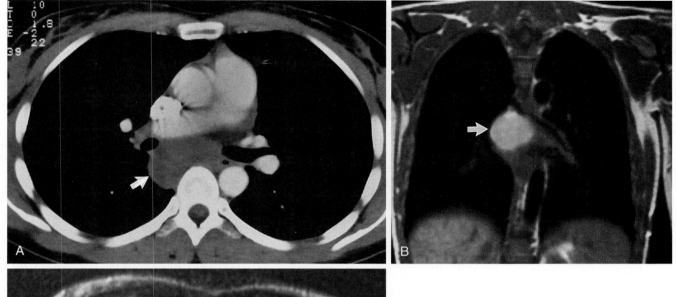

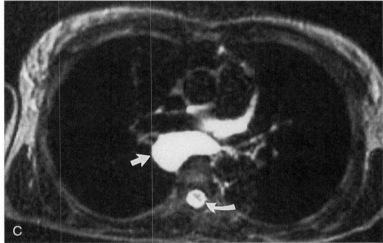

Figure 2–10. Soft Tissue and Fluid Characterization on CT and MR Imaging. Contrast-enhanced CT scan *(A)* shows a large, smoothly marginated subcarinal lesion *(arrow)*. The attenuation value is consistent with either a soft tissue lesion or a cyst filled with proteinaceous material. Coronal T1-weighted (TR/TE, 923/20) spin-echo MR image *(B)* shows a subcarinal mass with high signal intensity *(arrow)*. Transverse T2-weighted (TR/TE, 2,769/100) *(C)* spin-echo MR image obtained at the same level as the CT scan *(A)* shows an area of homogeneous high signal intensity *(straight arrow)*. The high signal intensity on the T2-weighted image is diagnostic of fluid. The signal in the subcarinal mass *(straight arrow)* in the T2-weighted image *(C)* is identical to that of cerebrospinal fluid *(curved arrow)*.

sity on T2-weighted MR images as a result of their fluid content.

Evaluation of the Chest Wall. MR imaging allows excellent assessment of primary chest wall tumors[54] and chest wall extension by lymphoma[55] and pulmonary carcinoma, particularly lesions located in the superior sulcus region.[56, 57] Assessment of tumor invasion of fat and vessels is made most readily with the use of T1-weighted sequences. T2-weighted sequences are optimal for differentiation of tumor and edema from surrounding muscle.[39] MR imaging is ideally suited for the evaluation of neurogenic tumors because it provides excellent assessment of the tissue characteristics of the mass as well as the presence or absence of intraspinal extension.[58, 59] The technique is the imaging modality of choice in the assessment of paraspinal lesions.

RADIONUCLIDE IMAGING

The most commonly used scintigraphic techniques in pulmonary nuclear medicine are ventilation-perfusion ($\dot{V}/\dot{Q}$) lung scans and gallium 67 citrate scans. Recent studies have shown that positron emission tomography (PET) with 2-[F-18]-fluoro-2-deoxy-D-glucose (FDG) can be helpful in distinguishing benign from malignant lung neoplasms and in staging pulmonary carcinoma.

Ventilation-Perfusion Scanning

Technique

The radiopharmaceuticals of choice for perfusion lung scanning are either technetium-99m labeled human albumin microspheres (Tc-99m HAM) or macroaggregated albumin (Tc-99m MAA). The latter vary in size from 10 to 150 μm, with greater than 90% of particles measuring between 10 and 90 μm. Tc-99m HAM particles are more uniform in size and range from 35 to 60 μm.

Perfusion scintigraphy is sensitive but nonspecific for diagnosing pulmonary diseases. Virtually all parenchymal lung diseases, including neoplasms, infections, chronic obstructive pulmonary disease, and asthma, can cause decreased pulmonary arterial blood flow within the affected lung zone. Thromboemboli characteristically cause abnormal perfusion with preserved ventilation (mismatched defects) (Fig. 2–11), whereas parenchymal lung disease most often causes ventilation and perfusion abnormalities in the

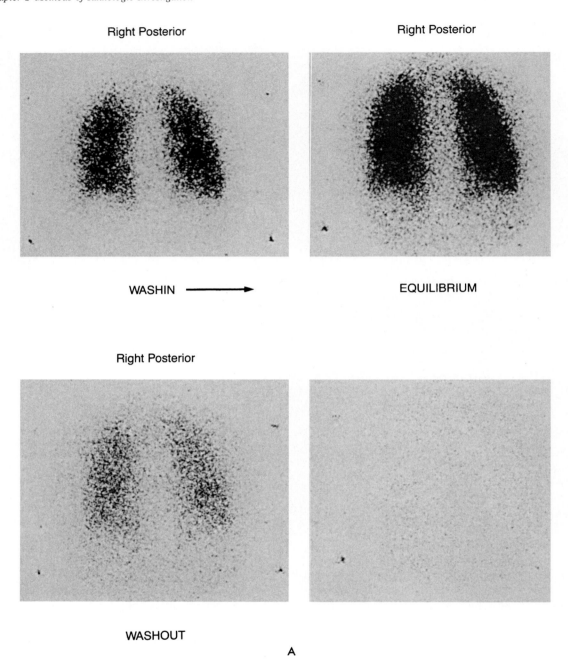

Right Posterior

Right Posterior

WASHIN ⟶

EQUILIBRIUM

Right Posterior

WASHOUT

A

Figure 2–11. *See legend on opposite page*

same lung region (matched defects); combined ventilation and perfusion scintigraphy is performed routinely to improve diagnostic specificity.

Most experience with ventilation imaging has been with xenon 133. Alternative ventilation imaging techniques, such as xenon 127, krypton 81m, technetium-99m aerosols, technegas, or pertechnegas, have not been evaluated as extensively.[60] The available data suggest, however, that there is no major diagnostic difference between the agents.

Indications

Diagnosis and Follow-up of Acute Thromboembolism. The $\dot{V}/\dot{Q}$ lung scan has been shown to be a safe, noninvasive technique to evaluate regional pulmonary perfusion and ventilation and has been used widely in the evaluation of patients with suspected thromboembolism (Tables 2–3 and 2–4).[61, 62]

Prediction of Pulmonary Function After Surgery. Quantitative $\dot{V}/\dot{Q}$ lung scanning has been shown to be a useful method for determining regional lung function in patients who are to undergo pulmonary resection or lung transplantation. Its major use is in the prediction of postoperative function after lobectomy or pneumonectomy. The predicted postoperative forced expiratory volume in 1 second (FEV_1) after these two procedures is calculated by multiplying the preoperative value by the percentage of radionuclide activity in the lobes or lung that will remain

Anterior

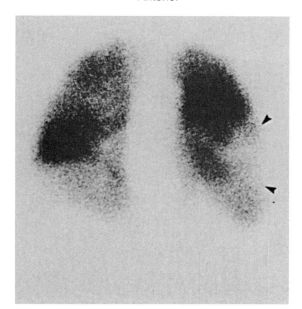

Posterior

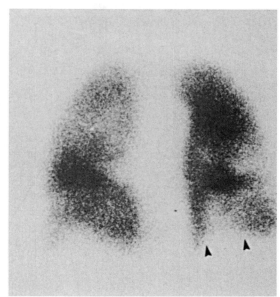

Right Posterior Oblique

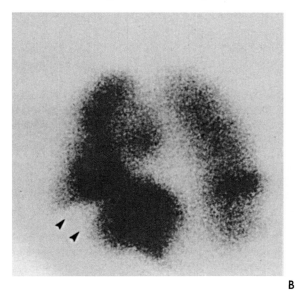

Left Posterior Oblique

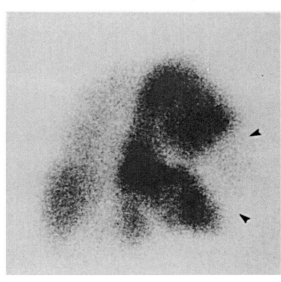

B

Figure 2–11. The Value of Ventilation-Perfusion Lung Scans in the Diagnosis of Thromboembolism. Xenon inhalation lung scan *(A)* discloses normal ventilation parameters during the washin, equilibrium, and washout phases. Corresponding technetium-99m labeled macroaggregated albumin perfusion lung scans *(B)* in anterior, posterior, and right and left posterior oblique projections identify multiple segmental filling defects throughout both lungs *(arrowheads)*. These findings, in concert with the ventilation study, are virtually diagnostic (high probability) of pulmonary thromboembolism. The patient was a 65-year-old man with acute dyspnea.

after surgery.[63] An expected postoperative FEV_1 less than 0.8 liter or 35% of predicted usually precludes lung resection.

Gallium 67 Lung Scanning

The radiopharmaceutical of choice for imaging pulmonary infection and noninfectous inflammatory conditions is gallium 67 citrate, a ferric analogue that has a physical half-life of 78 hours. The optimal time to perform thoracic

imaging is 48 to 72 hours after injection. The precise mechanism by which gallium localizes at sites of inflammation is not understood completely but has been postulated to be related to increased vascular permeability, direct bacterial uptake of gallium (binding to siderophores), binding to lactoferrin secreted by activated leukocytes, and direct binding to circulating leukocytes.[64]

Increased gallium activity within the chest is a sensitive

Table 2–3. SENSITIVITY, SPECIFICITY, AND POSITIVE PREDICTIVE VALUE OF VENTILATION-PERFUSION LUNG SCANNING FOR DETECTING ACUTE PULMONARY THROMBOEMBOLISM USING THE ORIGINAL PIOPED INTERPRETATION CRITERIA

Ventilation-Perfusion Interpretation	Sensitivity (%)	Specificity (%)	PPV (%)
High	40	98	87
High, intermediate	82	64	49
High, intermediate, low	98	12	32

PIOPED, Prospective Investigation of Pulmonary Embolism Diagnosis; PPV, positive predictive value.
Data from The PIOPED Investigators: JAMA 263:2753, 1990.

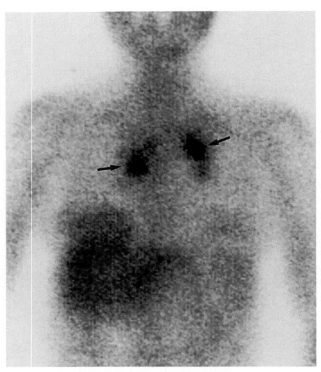

Figure 2–12. Gallium 67 Scintigraphy in Sarcoidosis. An anterior gallium 67 citrate image of the chest shows bilateral symmetric perihilar increased activity *(arrows)* in a patient with active sarcoidosis. (Courtesy of Dr. Daniel Worsley, Department of Radiology, Vancouver Hospital and Health Sciences Centre, Vancouver, BC, Canada.)

but relatively nonspecific indicator of pulmonary infection or inflammation. A variety of conditions, including adult respiratory distress syndrome, pneumonia, drug reactions, pneumoconiosis, idiopathic pulmonary fibrosis, and sarcoidosis, may cause increased radiogallium accumulation within the lungs. Neoplastic disease, such as lymphoma, leukemia, mesothelioma, or metastatic carcinoma, may be associated with increased activity, although its distribution is usually focal.

Gallium 67 scintigraphy has been used most commonly in patients who have sarcoidosis, in which the typical scintigraphic appearance consists of bilateral, perihilar, or peritracheal activity (Fig. 2–12).[64] Parenchymal activity also can be seen, with or without hilar activity; although it may be diffuse, it is usually most marked within the mid lung zones with relative sparing of the upper and lower lung zones.

Positron Emission Tomography

PET is a functional imaging technique in which tomographic images are obtained after administration of positron-emitting radiopharmaceuticals. Once emitted, positrons travel only several millimeters before losing enough energy to be susceptible to annihilation with an electron. During annihilation, the rest mass energy of the positron and electron is converted to energy, and two 511 keV gamma rays are emitted in opposite directions 180 degrees apart. The annihilation photons are detected simultaneously (coincidence detection) at opposite sides of a ring-type gantry.[65] Similar to CT and MR imaging, PET is based on the principle that a three-dimensional representation of an object can be obtained from multiple annular projections. The optimal tomographic resolution of modern PET im-

aging systems is approximately 3 mm. The disadvantages of FDG-PET imaging relate predominantly to its inherent complexities and cost.

Malignant cells have increased glucose transport and metabolism related to their rapid proliferation and increased content of messenger RNA.[66, 67] These biochemical alterations can be imaged by PET after administration of the glucose analogue FDG. The mechanism of uptake and initial phosphorylation of FDG is similar to glucose. Once FDG is phosphorylated (FDG-6-phosphate), it is not metabolized further and remains within the cell. The amount of FDG-6-phosphate within the cell can be imaged with PET systems and is proportional to glucose uptake and metabolism.

Current indications for FDG-PET imaging in patients who have suspected pulmonary carcinoma include distinction of benign from malignant pulmonary nodules, assessment of the presence or absence of metastases from non–small cell carcinoma in mediastinal lymph nodes, and

Table 2–4. EFFECT OF SELECTED RISK FACTORS ON THE PREVALENCE OF PULMONARY THROMBOEMBOLISM

Ventilation-Perfusion	0 Risk Factors*	1 Risk Factor*	≥2 Risk Factors*
High	63/77 (82%)	41/49 (84%)	56/58 (97%)
Intermediate	52/207 (25%)	40/107 (37%)	77/173 (45%)
Low, very low	14/315 (4%)	19/155 (12%)	37/179 (21%)

*Risk factors include immobilization, trauma to the lower extremities, surgery, and central venous instrumentation within 3 months of enrollment.
Results are based on data published in Worsley DF, Alavi A, Palevsky HI: Radiology 199:481, 1996.

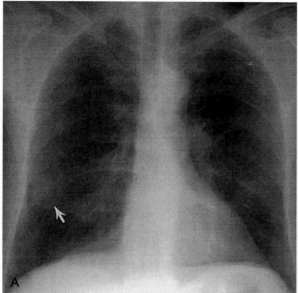

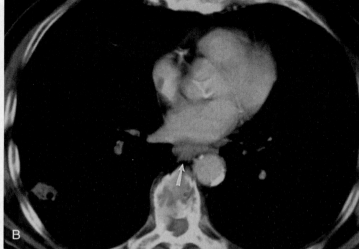

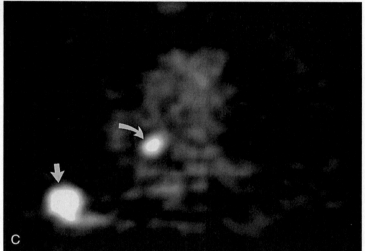

Figure 2–13. Positron Emission Tomography (PET). Posteroanterior chest radiograph *(A)* shows a poorly defined right lower lobe nodule *(arrow)*. CT scan *(B)* confirms the presence of the right lower lobe nodule and shows enlarged paraesophageal lymph node *(arrow)*. PET image *(C)* shows marked 2-(^{18}F)-fluoro-2-deoxy-D-glucose (FDG) uptake in the right lower lobe nodule *(straight arrow)* and in the paraesophageal node *(curved arrow)*. This case was surgically proven large cell pulmonary carcinoma. (Case courtesy of Dr. Ned Patz, Duke University Medical Center, Durham, NC.)

differentiation between parenchymal scarring and recurrent tumor in patients who have had previous therapy for a pulmonary carcinoma (Fig. 2–13).

The reported sensitivity and specificity of FDG-PET imaging for distinguishing malignant from benign lesions range from approximately 80% to 100% and 50% to 97%.[68–70] False-positive results have been reported in conditions of active inflammation, such as aspergillosis, tuberculosis, and sarcoidosis. An additional advantage of FDG-PET in the evaluation of solitary pulmonary nodules is the ability to stage non–small cell pulmonary carcinoma.[71–73] Several studies have shown that PET imaging is superior to CT in the detection of mediastinal nodal metastases from non–small cell lung cancer.[71, 72] One group of investigators performed a meta-analytic comparison of the diagnostic performance of PET imaging and CT, based on a review of English-language reports published in the 1990s.[72] The analysis included the results of 14 studies that used PET and 29 studies that used CT. The mean sensitivity and specificity of PET in detecting mediastinal nodal metastases were 79% and 91%, respectively, compared to 60% and 77%, respectively, for CT. Recent studies suggest that whole-body PET imaging may also be superior to CT

and bone scintigraphy in the detection of extrathoracic metastases.[73, 73a]

ULTRASONOGRAPHY

With respect to thoracic disease, ultrasonography has its greatest value in the assessment of congenital and acquired heart disease, particularly in establishing the nature of valvular deformity, the volume of cardiac chambers, the thickness of their walls, and the effectiveness of cardiac contraction (ejection fraction). The role of ultrasound in the assessment of abnormalities of the aorta has increased considerably with the advent of transesophageal echocardiography. The procedure is also valuable for detecting pericardial effusion, assessing its size, and differentiating it from cardiomegaly and has been used to detect intravascular air bubbles in cases of pulmonary air embolism. Because it is portable, does not use ionizing radiation, and frequently provides useful diagnostic information, ultrasound is used commonly in the diagnosis of pleural, diaphragmatic, and infradiaphragmatic abnormalities. Except for these important applications, the role of ultrasound in the diagnosis of noncardiovascular chest disease is limited by the physical composition of the intrathoracic structures. Neither air nor bone transmits sound; instead, air and bone reflect or absorb incoming sonic energy and prevent the collection of information about acoustic interfaces behind ribs or lung tissue. Sonography is limited to assessment of pulmonary masses or consolidation abutting the mediastinum, chest wall, or diaphragm and to documenting the presence and nature of pleural fluid.

Indications

Assessment of Pleural Effusion and Distinction of an Effusion from a Solid Pleural Lesion. Differentiation of liquid from solid pleural collections, a process that may be exceedingly difficult on chest radiographs, usually is achieved easily with ultrasonography.[74, 75] Although lateral decubitus chest radiographs readily show a free-flowing pleural effusion, they are not helpful in distinguishing loculated effusions from empyema or solid pleural masses. Because of its portability, bedside sonography has become a major imaging modality, not only in determining the presence of pleural fluid, but also as a guide to aspiration and drainage.[76, 77]

Most pleural fluid collections are identified readily at ultrasound as anechoic or hypoechoic collections, often delineated by echogenic aerated lung (Fig. 2–14). Although transudates and exudates have similar radiologic appearances, they may have different ultrasound characteristics.[78, 79] In one study of 50 patients, 15 of 19 (79%) effusions containing septations at ultrasound represented exudates.[78] In another investigation of 320 patients, effusions that had complex septated, complex nonseptated, or homogeneously

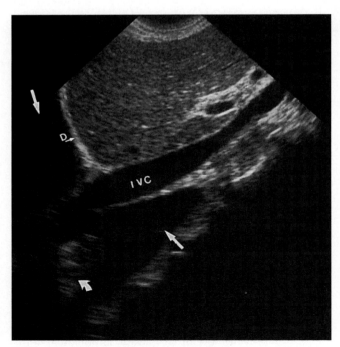

Figure 2–14. Pleural Effusion on Ultrasound. Ultrasound shows a large echo-free right pleural effusion *(straight arrows)*. Also noted are an atelectatic right lung *(curved arrow)*, the diaphragm (D), the inferior vena cava (IVC), and the liver. The effusion was shown on needle aspiration to be a transudate.

echogenic patterns were always exudates.[79] Other findings indicative of exudative effusion include the presence of a thickened pleura or an associated pulmonary parenchymal lesion. Although these findings are helpful, hypoechoic effusions may be transudates or exudates.[78, 79] Although sonography is more accurate than plain radiography in differentiating pleural fluid from solid pleural lesions, optimal assessment requires that sonography be guided by the radiographic findings: In one analysis, the combined use of the two modalities was more accurate (98%) than either radiography (68%) or sonography (92%) alone.[76]

Assessment of the Diaphragm. Ultrasonography provides excellent assessment of diaphragmatic and peridiaphragmatic masses and fluid collections and allows easy distinction of small pleural effusion from infradiaphragmatic fluid collections. The procedure has been shown to be helpful in the diagnosis of traumatic tears of the right hemidiaphragm because the liver provides an optimal acoustic window to assess the right hemidiaphragm.[80] The presence of bowel gas usually precludes optimal sonographic assessment of the left hemidiaphragm.

Guide to Needle Biopsy and Catheter Placement. Ultrasonography allows excellent visualization of pulmonary, pleural, or mediastinal lesions in contact with the chest wall or in a juxtadiaphragmatic location, permitting real-time monitoring while performing fine-needle biopsy.[81] The procedure is used frequently as a guide to placement of a catheter for pleural sclerotherapy or drainage of empyema.[82, 83] Ultrasonography allows pleural drainage to be performed at the bedside in critically ill patients.

TRANSTHORACIC NEEDLE ASPIRATION AND BIOPSY

Transthoracic needle aspiration (TTNA) consists of sucking fluid and cells into a syringe through a narrow-gauge needle inserted percutaneously into a parenchymal lesion. Most radiologists use 20- to 22-gauge needles because of the relatively low incidence of complications and a good yield.[84] Transthoracic needle biopsy (TTNB) is a procedure whereby a core of lung, lymph node, or tumor tissue can be obtained by the use of a cutting or core biopsy needle. The optimal technique for performing TTNA or TTNB as well as a range of instruments available with their purported advantages and disadvantages has been reviewed.[85–87]

The two main indications for fine-needle aspiration are the diagnosis of pulmonary malignancy and determination of the cause of serious pneumonia when noninvasive diagnostic methods have failed. TTNB offers no advantage over TTNA in the diagnosis of pulmonary carcinoma[88, 89] and has higher complication rates. The larger samples provided by cutting needle biopsies are more likely to be diagnostic in benign lesions,[90, 91] however, including those characterized by more diffuse disease, such as vasculitis and infection.[92, 93] There is substantial evidence that TTNB under CT guidance is useful in the examination of hilar and mediastinal masses for the staging of pulmonary carcinoma;[94, 95] however, it is not appropriate for the examination of normal-sized nodes and may not enable precise histologic classification of lymphoma.[96] It is safer, less costly, and better tolerated than thoracotomy or mediastinoscopy.[85]

Most TTNAs and TTNBs can be done under fluoroscopic guidance, an approach that is suitable when the lesion is visible in two 90-degree planes.[97] When this approach is not possible, CT is useful for determining the optimal approach; it offers superb resolution of anatomic structures (lessening the risk of vascular complications), permits documentation of needle position within the lesion, helps avoid biopsy of necrotic areas in larger lesions, and is helpful in planning the simplest and safest route for needle placement.[85] Ultrasound guidance also is useful in avoiding the necrotic centers of some lung masses[98] and may be used when a lesion abuts the pleura.

The most common complication of TTNA or TTNB is pneumothorax. Most operators using 20- to 23-gauge needles have reported pneumothorax rates of 20% to 40% for TTNA and TTNB.[84, 99] The risk of pneumothorax increases with larger needle diameter, increased number of passes, smaller size lesion, and the presence of underlying obstructive lung disease.[87, 99, 100] Factors that increase the likelihood of pneumothorax requiring chest tube drainage include obstructive lung function, emphysema along the needle path, and location of the lesion along an interlobar fissure.[100a]

The most important risk factor for pneumothorax is the presence of obstructive lung disease; in one study, patients who had normal spirometric test results and radiographs that did not show any findings suggestive of air-flow obstruction had a 7% pneumothorax rate;[101] by contrast, pneumothorax developed in approximately 45% of patients who had radiographic and spirometric findings of obstructive lung disease, many requiring chest tube placement.

Although severe hemorrhage is more likely to occur with the use of larger biopsy needles,[85, 100] small needles have been associated with fatal hemorrhage in patients who have a coagulopathy.[102] Overall, hemoptysis occurs in 10% to 15% of patients.[103, 104] Other rarer complications of TTNB include cerebral air embolism,[105, 106] lobar or lung torsion,[107] and seeding of the needle tract by malignant cells.[108]

References

1. Robin ED, Burke CM: Routine chest x-ray examinations. Chest 90:258, 1986.
2. American College of Radiology: ACR Standard for the Performance of Pediatric and Adult Chest Radiography. Reston, VA, Standards: American College of Radiology, 1997, p 27.
3. American Thoracic Society: Chest x-ray screening statements. Am Thorac News 10:14, 1984.
4. Watson W: Gridless radiography at high voltage with air gap technique. X-ray Focus 2:12, 1958.
5. Jackson FI: The air-gap technique, and an improvement by anteroposterior positioning for chest roentgenography. Am J Roentgenol 92:688, 1964.
6. Hasegawa BH, Naimuddin S, Dobbins JT, et al: Digital beam attenuator technique for compensated chest radiography. Radiology 159:537, 1986.
7. Plewes DB: A scanning system for chest radiography with regional exposure control: Theoretical considerations. Med Phys 10:646, 1984.
8. Plewes DB, Vogelstein EE: A scanning system for chest radiography with regional exposure control: Practical implementation. Med Phys 10:654, 1984.
9. Vlasbloem H, Schultze Kool LJ: AMBER: A scanning multiple-beam equalization system for chest radiography. Radiology 169:29, 1988.
10. MacMahon H, Vyborny C: Technical advances in chest radiography. Am J Roentgenol 163:1049, 1994.
11. Schultze Kool LJ, Busscher DLT, Vlasbloem H, et al: Advanced multiple-beam equalization radiography in chest radiology: A simulated nodule detection study. Radiology 169:35, 1988.
12. Chotas HG, van Metter RL, Johnson GA, et al: Small object contrast in AMBER and conventional chest radiography. Radiology 180:853, 1991.
13. Ravin CE, Chotas HG: Chest radiography. Radiology 204:593, 1997.
14. Wandtke JC: Bedside chest radiography. Radiology 190:1, 1994.
15. Schaefer CM, Greene R, Llewellyn HJ, et al: Interstitial lung disease: Impact of postprocessing in digital storage phosphor imaging. Radiology 178:733, 1991.
16. Sagel SS, Jost RG, Glazer HS, et al: Digital mobile radiography. J Thorac Imaging 5:36, 1990.
17. Sonoda M, Takano M, Miyahara J, et al: Computed radiography utilizing scanning laser stimulated luminescence. Radiology 148:833, 1983.
18. Chotas HG, Floyd CE Jr, Ravin CE: Technical evaluation of a digital chest radiography system that uses a selenium detector. Radiology 195:264, 1995.
19. Garmer M, Hennigs SP, Jager HJ, et al: Digital radiography versus conventional radiography in chest imaging: Diagnostic performance of a large-area silicon flat-panel detector in a clinical CT-controlled study. Am J Roentgenol 174:75, 2000.
20. Müller NL: Clinical value of high resolution CT in chronic diffuse lung disease. Am J Roentgenol 157:1163, 1991.
21. McGuinness G, Naidich DP: Bronchiectasis: CT/clinical correlations. Semin Ultrasound CT MR 16:395, 1995.
22. Leung AN, Staples CA, Müller NL: Chronic diffuse infiltrative lung disease: Comparison of diagnostic accuracy of high-resolution and conventional CT. Am J Roentgenol 157:693, 1991.
23. Naidich DP, Harkin TJ: Airways and lung: Correlation of CT with fiberoptic bronchoscopy. Radiology 197:1, 1995.
24. Mayo JR, Webb WR, Gold R, et al: High resolution CT of the lungs: An optimal approach. Radiology 163:507, 1987.
25. Webb WR, Müller NL, Naidich DP (eds): High Resolution CT of the Lung. Philadelphia, Lippincott-Raven, 2001.
26. Zwirewich CV, Terrif B, Müller NL: High-spatial-frequency (bone) algorithm improves quality of standard CT of the thorax. Am J Roentgenol 153:1169, 1989.
27. Mayo JR: The high resolution CT technique. Semin Roentgenol 26:104, 1991.
28. Kalender WA, Seissler W, Klotz E, et al: Spiral volumetric CT with single-breath-hold technique, continuous transport, and continuous scanner rotation. Radiology 176:181, 1990.
29. Bressler Y, Skraba CZ: Optimal interpolation in helical scan computed tomography. Proc ICASSP 3:1472, 1989.
30. Crawford CR, King K: Computed tomography scanning with simultaneous patient translation. Med Phys 17:967, 1990.
31. Fishman EK: High-resolution three-dimensional imaging from subsecond helical CT data sets: Applications in vascular imaging. Am J Roentgenol 169:441, 1997.
31a. Rydberg J, Buckwalter KA, Caldemeyer KS, et al: Multisection CT: Scanning techniques and clinical applications. Radiographics 20:1787, 2000.
32. Remy-Jardin M, Remy J, Artaud D, et al: Volume rendering of the tracheobronchial tree: Clinical evaluation of bronchographic images. Radiology 208:761, 1998.
33. Higgins WE, Ramaswamy K, Swift RD, et al: Virtual bronchoscopy for three-dimensional pulmonary image assessment: State of the art and future needs. Radiographics 18:761, 1998.
34. Rogers LF: A day in the Court of Lexicon: Virtual endoscopy. Am J Roentgenol 171:1185, 1998.
35. Johnson CD, Hara AK, Reed JE: Virtual endoscopy: What's in a name? Am J Roentgenol 171:1201, 1998.
36. Hopper KD, Iyriboz TC, Mahraj RPM, et al: CT bronchoscopy: Optimization of imaging parameters. Radiology 209:872, 1998.
37. Naidich DP, Webb WR, Müller NL, et al (eds): Computed Tomography and Magnetic Resonance of the Thorax. Philadelphia, Lippincott-Raven, 1999.
38. Remy-Jardin M, Remy J: Spiral CT angiography of the pulmonary circulation. Radiology 212:615, 1999.

39. Mayo JR: Magnetic resonance imaging of the chest: Where we stand. Radiol Clin North Am 32:795, 1994.

40. Firmin DN, Nayler GL, Kilner PJ, et al: Application of phase shifts in NMR for flow measurement. Magn Reson Med 14:230, 1990.

41. Boxerman JL, Mosher TJ, McVeigh ER, et al: Advanced MR imaging techniques for evaluation of the heart and great vessels. Radiographics 18:543, 1998.

42. Harms SE, Morgan TJ, Yamanashi WS, et al: Principles of nuclear magnetic resonance imaging. Radiographics 4(Suppl):26, 1984.

43. Ho VB, Prince MR: Thoracic MR aortography: Imaging techniques and strategies. Radiographics 18:287, 1998.

44. Alley MT, Shifrin RY, Pelc NJ, et al: Ultrafast contrast-enhanced three-dimensional MR angiography: State of the art. Radiographics 18:273, 1998.

45. Higgins CB, Sakuma H: Heart disease: Functional evaluation with MR imaging. Radiology 199:307, 1996.

46. Higgins CB, Caputo GR: Role of MR imaging in acquired and congenital cardiovascular disease. Am J Roentgenol 161:13, 1993.

47. Sechtem U, Pflugfelder PW, White RD, et al: Cine MR imaging: Potential for the evaluation of cardiovascular function. Am J Roentgenol 148:239, 1987.

48. Kondo C, Caputo GR, Semelka R, et al: Right and left ventricular stroke volume measurements with velocity-encoded cine MR imaging: In vitro and in vivo validation. Am J Roentgenol 157:9, 1991.

49. Glazer HS, Gutierrez FR, Levitt RG, et al: The thoracic aorta studies by MR imaging. Radiology 157:149, 1985.

50. Kersting-Sommerhoff BA, Higgins CB, White RD, et al: Aortic dissection: Sensitivity and specificity of MR imaging. Radiology 166:651, 1988.

51. Sommer T, Fehske W, Holzknecht N, et al: Aortic dissection: A comparative study of diagnosis with spiral CT, multiplanar transesophageal echocardiography, and MR imaging. Radiology 199:347, 1996.

52. Webb WR, Gatsonis C, Zerhouni EA, et al: CT and MR imaging in staging non-small cell bronchogenic carcinoma: Report of the radiologic diagnostic oncology group. Radiology 178:705, 1991.

53. Nakata H, Egashira K, Watanabe H, et al: MRI of bronchogenic cysts. J Comput Assist Tomogr 17:267, 1993.

54. Fortier MV, Mayo JR, Swensen SJ, et al: MR imaging of chest wall lesions. Radiographics 14:597, 1994.

55. Bergin CJ, Healy MV, Zincone GE, et al: MR evaluation of chest wall involvement in malignant lymphoma. J Comput Assist Tomogr 14:928, 1990.

56. Heelan RT, Demas BE, Caravelli JF, et al: Superior sulcus tumors: CT and MR imaging. Radiology 170:637, 1989.

57. McLoud TC, Filion RB, Edelman RR, et al: MR imaging of superior sulcus carcinoma. J Comput Assist Tomogr 13:233, 1989.

58. Flickinger FW, Yuh WT, Behrendt DM: Magnetic resonance imaging of mediastinal paraganglioma. Chest 94:652,1988.

59. Siegel MJ, Jamroz GA, Glazer HS, et al:. MR imaging of intraspinal extension of neuroblastoma. J Comput Assist Tomogr 10:593,1986.

60. James JM, Herman KJ, Lloyd JJ, et al: Evaluation of 99Tcm Technegas ventilation scintigraphy in the diagnosis of pulmonary embolism. Br J Radiol 64:711, 1991.

61. Hull RD, Raskob GE, Ginsberg JS, et al: A noninvasive strategy for the treatment of patients with suspected pulmonary embolism. Arch Intern Med 154:289, 1994.

62. PIOPED Investigators: Value of the ventilation/perfusion scan in acute pulmonary embolism. JAMA 263:2753, 1990.

63. Ali MK, Mountain CF, Ewer MS, et al: Predicting loss of pulmonary function after pulmonary resection for bronchogenic carcinoma. Chest 77:337, 1980.

64. Line BR: Scintigraphic studies of inflammation in diffuse lung disease. Radiol Clin North Am 29:1095, 1991.

65. Patz EF, Goodman PC: Positron emission tomography imaging of the thorax. Radiol Clin North Am 32:811, 1994.

66. Weber G: Enzymology of cancer cells: Part 1. N Engl J Med 296:486, 1977.

67. Weber G: Enzymology of cancer cells: Part 2. N Engl J Med 296:541, 1977.

68. Gupta NC, Frank AR, Dewan NA, et al: Solitary pulmonary nodules: Detection of malignancy with PET with 2-[F-18]-fluoro-2-deoxy-D-glucose. Radiology 184:441, 1992.

69. Patz EF, Lowe VJ, Hoffman J, et al: Focal pulmonary abnormalities: Evaluation with F-18 fluorodeoxyglucose PET scanning. Radiology 88:487, 1993.

70. Sazon DAD, Santiago SM, Hoo GWS, et al: Fluorodeoxyglucose-positron emission tomography in the detection and staging of lung cancer. Am J Respir Crit Care Med 153:417, 1996.

71. Wahl RL, Quint LE, Greenough RL, et al: Staging of mediastinal non-small cell lung cancer with FDG PET, CT and fusion images: Preliminary prospective evaluation. Radiology 191:371, 1994.

72. Dwamena BA, Sonnad SS, Angobaldo JO, et al: Metastases from non-small cell lung cancer: Mediastinal staging in the 1990s—meta-analytic comparison of PET and CT. Radiology 213:530, 1999.

73. Valk PE, Pounds TR, Hopkins DM, et al: Staging non-small cell lung cancer by whole-body positron emission tomographic imaging. Ann Thorac Surg 60:1573, 1995.

73a. Marom EM, Page McAdams H, Erasmus JJ, et al: Staging non-small cell lung cancer with whole-body PET. Radiology 21:803, 1999.

74. Müller NL: Imaging of the pleura. Radiology 186:297, 1993.

75. McLoud TC, Flower CDR: Imaging the pleura: Sonography, CT, and MR imaging. Am J Roentgenol 156:1145, 1991.

76. Lipscomb DJ, Flower CDR, Hadfield JW: Ultrasound of the pleura: An assessment of its clinical value. Clin Radiol 32:289, 1981.

77. O'Moore PV, Mueller PR, Simeone JF, et al: Sonographic guidance in diagnostic and therapeutic interventions in the pleural space. Am J Roentgenol 149:1, 1987.

78. Hirsch JH, Rogers JV, Mack LA: Real-time sonography of the pleural opacities. Am J Roentgenol 136:297, 1981.

79. Yang PC, Luh KT, Chang DB, et al: Value of sonography in determining the nature of pleural effusion: Analysis of 320 cases. Am J Roentgenol 159:29, 1992.

80. Somers JM, Gleeson FV, Flower CD: Rupture of the right hemidiaphragm following blunt trauma: The use of ultrasound in diagnosis. Clin Radiol 42:97, 1990.

81. Ikezoe J, Morimoto S, Arisawa J, et al: Percutaneous biopsy of thoracic lesions: Value of sonography for needle guidance. Am J Roentgenol 154:1181, 1990.

82. Morrison MC, Mueller PR, Lee MJ, et al: Sclerotherapy of malignant pleural effusion through sonographically placed small-bore catheters. Am J Roentgenol 158:41, 1992.

83. Klein JS, Schultz S, Heffner JE: Interventional radiology of the chest: Image-guided percutaneous drainage of pleural effusions, lung abscess, and pneumothorax. Am J Roentgenol 164:581, 1995

84. Li H, Boiselle PM, Shepard JO, et al: Diagnostic accuracy and safety of CT-guided percutaneous needle aspiration biopsy of the lung: Comparison of small and large pulmonary nodules. Am J Roentgenol 167:105, 1996.

85. Salazar AM, Westcott JL: The role of transthoracic needle biopsy for the diagnosis and staging of lung cancer. Clin Chest Med 14:99, 1993.

86. Klein JS, Zarka MA: Transthoracic needle biopsy: An overview. J Thorac Imaging 12:232, 1997.

87. Moore EH: Needle-aspiration lung biopsy: A comprehensive approach to complication reduction. J Thorac Imaging 12:259, 1997.

88. Tao LC, Pearson FG, Delarue NC, et al: Percutaneous fine-needle aspiration biopsy: 1. Its value to clinical practice. Cancer 45:1480, 1980.

89. Poe RH, Tobin RE: Sensitivity and specificity of needle biopsy in lung malignancy. Am Rev Respir Dis 122:725, 1980.

90. Arakawa H, Nakajima Y, Kurihara Y, et al: CT-guided transthoracic needle biopsy: A comparison between automated biopsy gun and fine needle aspiration. Clin Radiol 51:503, 1996.

91. Klein JS, Salomon G, Stewart EA: Transthoracic needle biopsy with a coaxially placed 20-gauge automated cutting needle: Results in 122 patients. Radiology 198:715, 1996.

92. Gruden JF, Klein JS, Webb WR: Percutaneous transthoracic needle biopsy in AIDS: Analysis in 32 patients. Radiology 189:567, 1993.

93. Staroslesky AN, Schwarz Y, Man A, et al: Additional information from percutaneous cutting needle biopsy following fine-needle aspiration in the diagnosis of chest lesions. Chest 113:1522, 1998.

94. Adler OB, Rosenberger A, Peleg H: Fine-needle aspiration biopsy of mediastinal masses: Evaluation of 136 experiences. Am J Roentgenol 140:893, 1983.

95. Gardner D, van Sonnenberg E, D'Agostino HB, et al: CT-guided transthoracic needle biopsy. Cardiovasc Intervent Radiol 14:17, 1991.

96. Welch TJ, Sheedy PF II, Johnson CD, et al: CT-guided biopsy: Prospective analysis of 1,000 procedures. Radiology 171:493, 1989.

97. van Sonnenberg E, Casola G, D'Agostino HB, et al: Interventional radiology in the chest. Chest 102:608, 1992.

98. Pan JF, Yang PC, Chang DB, et al: Needle aspiration biopsy of malignant lung masses with necrotic centers. Chest 103:452, 1993.

99. Cox JE, Chiles C, McManus CM, et al: Transthoracic needle aspiration biopsy: Variables that affect risk of pneumothorax. Radiology 212:165, 1999.

100. Perlmutt LM, Johnston WW, Dunnick NR: Percutaneous transthoracic needle aspiration: A review. Am J Roentgenol 152:451, 1989.

100a. Ko JP, Shepard JO, Drucker EA, et al: Factors influencing pneumothorax rate at lung biopsy: Are dwell time and angle of pleural puncture contributing factors? Radiology 218:491, 2001.

101. Fish GD, Stanley JH, Miller KS, et al: Postbiopsy pneumothorax: Estimating the risk by chest radiography and pulmonary function tests. Am J Roentgenol 150:71, 1988.

102. Milner LB, Ryan K, Gullo J: Fatal intrathoracic hemorrhage after percutaneous aspiration lung biopsy. Am J Roentgenol 132:280, 1979.

103. Mehnert JH, Brown MJ: Percutaneous needle core biopsy of peripheral pulmonary masses. Am J Surg 136:151, 1978.

104. McEvoy RD, Begley MD, Antic R: Percutaneous biopsy of intrapulmonary mass lesions: Experience with a disposable cutting needle. Cancer 51:2321, 1983.

105. Aberle DR, Gamsu G, Golden JA: Fatal systemic arterial air embolism following lung needle aspiration. Radiology 165:351, 1987.

106. Kodama F, Ogawa T, Hashimoto M, et al: Fatal air embolism as a complication of CT-guided needle biopsy of the lung. J Comput Assist Tomogr 23:949, 1999.

107. Graham RJ, Heyd RL, Raval VA, et al: Lung torsion after percutaneous needle biopsy of lung. Am J Roentgenol 159:35, 1992.

108. Müller NL, Bergin CJ, Miller RR, et al: Seeding of malignant cells into the needle track after lung and pleural biopsy. Can Assoc Radiol J 37:192, 1986.

Radiologic Signs of Chest Disease

The differential diagnosis of radiologic abnormalities is based on considerations such as density, size, number, homogeneity, sharpness of definition, anatomic location, and presence or absence of calcification or cavitation. This chapter describes the basic radiologic signs that are seen in chest disease and that are useful in differential diagnosis. These signs can be considered in four major categories: increased lung density, decreased lung density, atelectasis, and pleural abnormalities.

INCREASED LUNG DENSITY

Most diseases that increase lung density involve the air spaces and interstitial tissue to a variable extent; however, it is helpful to recognize three general radiographic patterns, depending on which component appears predominant: (1) *air-space disease*, the air being replaced by liquid, cells, or a combination of the two (consolidation); (2) *interstitial disease*; and (3) *combined air-space and interstitial disease*. This division is useful if one accepts the proviso that the term *air-space pattern* indicates *predominant* involvement of the parenchymal air spaces and that a linear, reticular, or nodular pattern indicates *predominant* involvement of the interstitium.

Predominantly Air-Space Disease

Parenchymal consolidation is defined as the replacement of gas within the air spaces by liquid, cells, or a combination of the two. Such air-space disease is characterized on radiographs and computed tomography (CT) scans by the presence of one or more fairly homogeneous opacities associated with obscuration of the pulmonary vessels and little or no volume loss (Fig. 3–1).[3, 4] The margins of the opacities are defined poorly except where the consolidation abuts the pleura. Air-containing bronchi (air bronchograms)

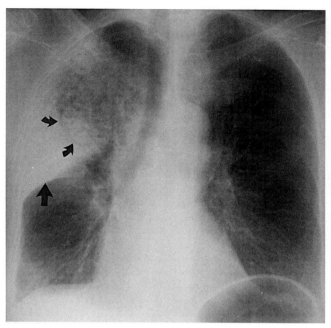

Figure 3–1. Air-Space Consolidation. Posteroanterior chest radiograph in a 64-year-old woman shows extensive air-space consolidation in the right upper lobe. The findings consist of confluent fluffy opacities with poorly defined margins except where the consolidation abuts the horizontal fissure *(straight arrow)*. Note presence of air bronchograms *(curved arrows)*. Incidental note is made of a small right pleural effusion. The patient had lobar pneumonia caused by *Streptococcus pneumoniae.*

are visualized frequently; localized small lucencies corresponding to patent membranous bronchioles (air bronchiolograms) or nonconsolidated lung parenchyma and localized round areas of consolidation measuring 10 mm in diameter or less (air-space nodules) also may be identified.

Distribution Characteristics

The air-space consolidation may be focal, patchy, or distributed widely throughout both lungs (Table 3–1). Focal consolidation may be segmental or nonsegmental in distribution; occasionally, it involves an entire lobe or lung. Segmental consolidation with or without associated volume loss typically results from endobronchial obstruction (e.g., pulmonary carcinoma) or from pulmonary infarction (e.g., thromboembolism or angioinvasive aspergillosis) (Fig. 3–2). A segmental distribution can be seen after aspiration and with pneumonia caused by *Staphylococcus aureus*, *Streptococcus pyogenes*, or a variety of gram-negative bacteria. These organisms more commonly cause multifocal or patchy bilateral consolidation (bronchopneumonia), however. A similar distribution may be seen in severe fungal pneumonia, particularly in immunocompromised patients (Fig. 3–3).

On high-resolution computed tomography (HRCT) scan, areas of air-space consolidation often can be seen to be marginated by interlobular septa (Fig. 3–4).[5] Single or multiple spared lobules may be present within areas of massive consolidation.[5] Involvement of a secondary lobule or a cluster of lobules with adjacent normal parenchyma is

particularly common in bronchopneumonia,[6] which is also known as *lobular pneumonia.*

Causes of nonsegmental consolidation include pneumonia, focal hemorrhage, neoplasm, irradiation, Loeffler's syndrome, and chronic eosinophilic pneumonia. Nonsegmental pneumonia most commonly is caused by *Streptococcus pneumoniae* and, less often, by *Klebsiella pneumoniae*, *Legionella* species, and *Mycobacterium tuberculosis* (*see* Fig. 3–1). The consolidation in Loeffler's syndrome is typically migratory, whereas that in chronic eosinophilic pneumonia characteristically involves the peripheral lung regions. Nonsegmental consolidation that progresses over several months should raise the possibility of bronchioloalveolar carcinoma or lymphoma. Consolidation of an entire lobe may be secondary to bronchial obstruction (e.g., pul-

Table 3–1. AIR-SPACE CONSOLIDATION

Common Causes	Helpful Diagnostic Features
Acute	
Pulmonary edema	Hydrostatic pulmonary edema tends to involve mainly the central lung regions (butterfly distribution) and commonly is associated with cardiomegaly and septal (Kerley B) lines. Increased permeability pulmonary edema (adult respiratory distress syndrome) tends to be patchy or to involve mainly the peripheral lung regions. Cardiomegaly and septal lines are uncommon
Pneumonia	Consolidation may be homogeneous and lobar (nonsegmental) in distribution (e.g., *Streptococcus pneumoniae*), inhomogeneous and patchy (segmental) in distribution (e.g., gram-negative organisms, *Staphylococcus aureus)*, or diffuse (e.g., *Pneumocystis carinii)*
Hemorrhage	May be focal (e.g., pulmonary contusion, bronchiectasis) or diffuse (e.g., Goodpasture's syndrome, bleeding diathesis). When secondary to pulmonary embolism, may resemble a truncated cone (Hampton's hump)
Aspiration	Aspiration of gastric contents (aspiration pneumonia) tends to involve mainly the dependent lung regions. Aspiration of lipids (lipid pneumonia) can usually be diagnosed on HRCT by the presence of localized areas of fat density.
Chronic	
Bronchiolitis obliterans organizing pneumonia	Findings consist of patchy, nonsegmental, unilateral or bilateral areas of consolidation that progress over several weeks or months. Frequently has a predominantly peribronchial or subpleural distribution on HRCT
Chronic eosinophilic pneumonia	Characteristic homogeneous nonsegmental peripheral consolidation pneumonia involving mainly the upper lobes
Neoplasm	Postobstructive pneumonitis involving a segment, lobe, or entire lung is a common manifestation of endobronchial pulmonary carcinoma. Nonsegmental consolidation is seen with bronchioloalveolar carcinoma and lymphoma
Alveolar proteinosis	An uncommon cause of chronic air-space consolidation that may be patchy or involve mainly the perihilar regions. HRCT shows ground-glass attenuation with associated smooth thickening of interlobular septa (crazy-paving pattern)

HRCT, high-resolution computed tomography.

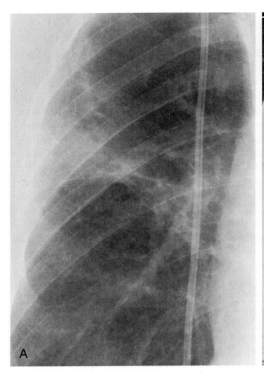

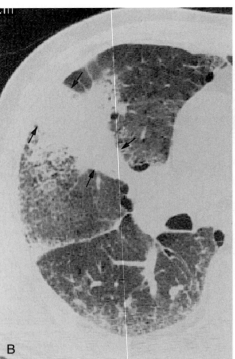

Figure 3–2. Subsegmental Consolidation. A view of the right lung from posteroanterior chest radiograph *(A)* shows a wedge-shaped, pleural-based area of consolidation in the right upper lobe. HRCT scan *(B)* also shows a subsegmental area of dense consolidation *(arrows)* that extends into the adjacent parenchyma. The appearance is consistent with a subsegmental hemorrhagic infarct. The patient was an immunocompromised 54-year-old woman with proven angioinvasive aspergillosis.

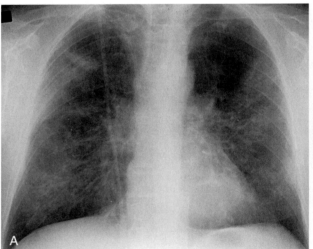

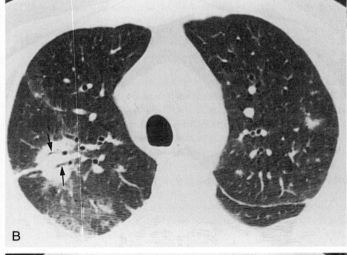

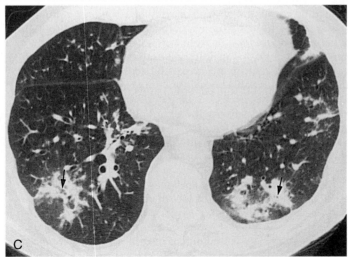

Figure 3–3. Bronchopneumonia. Posteroanterior chest radiograph *(A)* shows patchy bilateral areas of consolidation. HRCT scans *(B and C)* show the predominant peribronchial distribution of the areas of consolidation. Air bronchograms are identified clearly within the areas of consolidation *(arrows)*. The patient was a 55-year-old man with acute myelogenous leukemia and pathologically proven bronchopneumonia caused by *Aspergillus*.

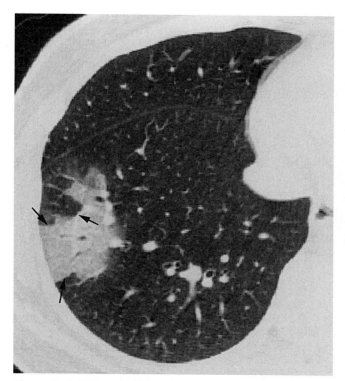

Figure 3–4. Pulmonary Hemorrhage. HRCT scan in a 29-year-old woman shows focal area of consolidation in the right lower lobe resulting from pulmonary hemorrhage. Several of the margins are outlined clearly by interlobular septa *(arrows)*, a feature leading to sharp demarcation between involved and uninvolved secondary pulmonary lobules.

monary carcinoma), in which case it is associated typically with atelectasis and a lack of air bronchograms, or to bacterial pneumonia (typically, *S. pneumoniae* or *K. pneumoniae*), in which case it is associated with normal or, occasionally, increased lung volume and air bronchograms.

Extensive or diffuse bilateral consolidation is seen most commonly in hydrostatic pulmonary edema, adult respiratory distress syndrome, diffuse pulmonary hemorrhage, and *Pneumocystis carinii* pneumonia. In hydrostatic pulmonary edema, the consolidation tends to involve mainly the perihilar regions (*butterfly* distribution) and commonly is associated with thickening of the interlobular septa (septal lines) and cardiomegaly. The consolidation in adult respiratory distress syndrome tends to have a patchy and predominantly peripheral distribution and is associated typically with a normal heart size. *Pneumocystis carinii* pneumonia, seen most commonly in patients who have acquired immunodeficiency syndrome, typically progresses from a subtle perihilar haze to diffuse bilateral consolidation.

Predominantly Interstitial Disease

Radiologic Patterns of Diffuse Interstitial Disease

Interstitial lung disease is associated with five radiologic patterns: septal, reticular, nodular, reticulonodular, and ground-glass. Although each of these patterns can be visualized on HRCT and correlated with specific histopathologic findings,[9, 10, 25] superimposition of structures makes interpretation considerably more difficult on the chest radiograph.

Septal Pattern

A septal pattern results from thickening of the interlobular septa (i.e., the tissue that separates the secondary pulmonary lobules). Normally, no septal lines can be identified on the radiograph, and only a few can be seen on HRCT, mostly in the anterior and lower aspects of the lower lobes.[15, 22] When thickened, interlobular septa (septal lines) are visualized on the radiograph as short (1 to 2 cm) lines perpendicular to and continuous with the pleura (Kerley B lines) or as longer (2 to 6 cm) lines oriented toward the hila (Kerley A lines) (Fig. 3–5). On HRCT scan, septal lines can be seen as short lines that extend to the pleura in the lung periphery and as polygonal arcades outlining one or more pulmonary lobules in more central lung regions (Fig. 3–6).[15, 22]

The presence of septal lines as the predominant radiologic abnormality effectively restricts the diagnostic considerations to hydrostatic pulmonary edema or malignancy (either lymphangitic spread of carcinoma or lymphoma), usually with simultaneous involvement of bronchoarterial interstitium. The distinction between edema and cancer often can be determined on the basis of clinical findings; however, in cases in which there is doubt, the HRCT appearance may be helpful in differentiation: Interlobular septal thickening as a result of pulmonary edema is usually smooth, whereas malignancy frequently is associated with a nodular component (Fig. 3–7).[9, 23] Although septal thickening may be seen in idiopathic pulmonary fibrosis, sarcoidosis, and alveolar proteinosis, it is usually not the main abnormality.[22] Apparent thickening of interlobular septa on HRCT scan occasionally results from disease affecting the perilobular alveoli on both sides of a normal septum, particularly in idiopathic pulmonary fibrosis,[23, 24] adult respiratory distress syndrome,[21, 23] and alveolar proteinosis.[21] The most common causes of interlobular septal thickening are listed in Table 3–2.

Table 3–2. SEPTAL PATTERN

Common Causes	Characteristic Radiographic and HRCT Findings
Hydrostatic pulmonary edema	Most common cause. Predominantly lower lung zone distribution. Smooth interlobular septal thickening on HRCT
Lymphangitic carcinomatosis	May be focal or diffuse. Smooth or nodular septal thickening. Lymph node enlargement seen at presentation in 30% of cases
Sarcoidosis	Septal thickening seldom evident on radiograph but commonly seen on HRCT. Septal involvement usually mild compared with peribronchovascular nodularity seen in sarcoidosis. Thickening may be smooth or nodular. Usually associated with bilateral hilar and mediastinal lymph node enlargement
Idiopathic pulmonary fibrosis	Irregular septal thickening usually mild and associated with other findings of fibrosis, including intralobular lines, traction bronchiectasis, and honeycombing
Asbestosis	Irregular septal thickening usually mild and associated with other findings of fibrosis and pleural plaques or diffuse pleural thickening

HRCT, high-resolution computed tomography.

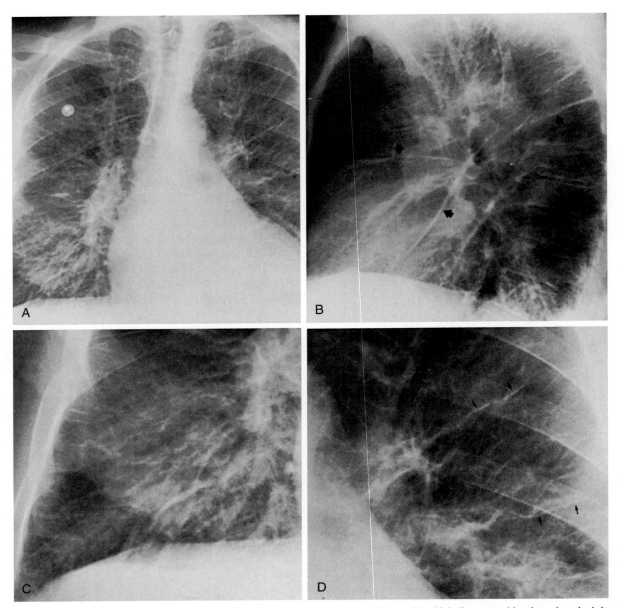

Figure 3–5. Interstitial Pulmonary Edema. Posteroanterior *(A)* and lateral *(B)* radiographs reveal multiple linear opacities throughout both lungs that are seen to better advantage in magnified views of the right lower *(C)* and left upper *(D)* lungs. These lines consist of a combination of long septal lines (Kerley A), predominantly in the midlung zones *(arrows* in *D)*, and shorter peripheral septal lines (Kerley B). In lateral projection *(B)*, the interlobar fissures are prominent *(arrows)*, representing subpleural edema. Twenty-four hours later, the edema had cleared completely.

Reticular Pattern

A reticular pattern is characterized by innumerable, interlacing line shadows that suggest a mesh (Fig. 3–8).[4] On the chest radiograph, the pattern may be the result of summation of smooth or irregular linear opacities, cystic spaces, or both. Although distinction between these abnormalities often is difficult on the radiograph, it can be made readily on HRCT scan. The most common causes of a reticular pattern are listed in Table 3–3.

Although pulmonary edema often leads to a predominant linear pattern characterized by the presence of septal (Kerley B) lines, a fine reticular pattern also is seen frequently. Other causes of a reticular pattern that develops acutely are viral and mycoplasma pneumonia.

Chronic diseases associated with a fine reticular pattern include interstitial pulmonary edema associated with mitral stenosis, asbestosis, idiopathic pulmonary fibrosis, and pulmonary fibrosis associated with connective tissue disease. The last two conditions are characterized initially on the chest radiograph by a fine reticular pattern involving mainly the lower lung zones. As disease progresses, the reticular pattern becomes coarser and the process more diffuse. HRCT scan shows intralobular linear opacities (reflecting thickening of the interstitium within the secondary lobule), irregular thickening of the interlobular septa, and honeycombing predominantly in the subpleural lung regions and in the lower lung zones (Fig. 3–9).[9, 25]

Cystic air spaces can be defined as enlarged foci of air-containing lung surrounded by a wall of variable thickness and composition.[4] Cystic air spaces may be present without associated fibrosis, as in lymphangioleiomyomatosis (Fig.

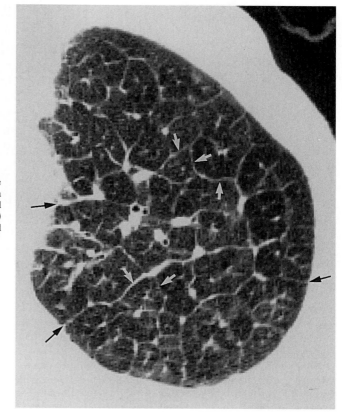

Figure 3–6. Interlobular Septal Thickening. HRCT scan targeted to the left upper lobe shows interlobular septal thickening. The thickened septa can be identified as lines *(black arrows)* perpendicular to the pleura and extending to it and, more centrally, as polygonal arcades *(white arrows)* outlining the secondary pulmonary lobules. The patient was a 77-year-old woman with interstitial pulmonary edema resulting from left heart failure.

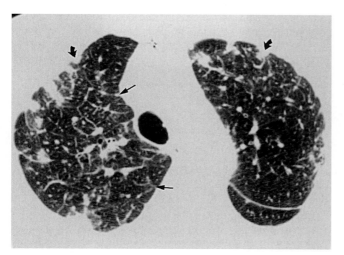

Figure 3–7. Lymphangitic Carcinomatosis. HRCT scan shows thickening of the interlobular septa *(straight arrows)* and several nodules *(curved arrows)* with irregular margins predominantly in the subpleural lung regions. Lymphangitic carcinomatosis secondary to adenocarcinoma was proved at transbronchial biopsy.

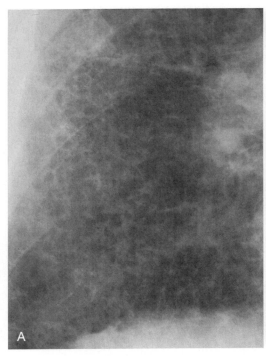
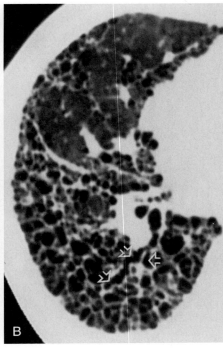

Figure 3–8. Reticular Pattern. Close-up view of the right lower lung zone from posteroanterior chest radiograph *(A)* shows a reticular pattern. HRCT scan *(B)* shows honeycombing throughout the right lower lobe. Note associated dilation and distortion of the bronchi (traction bronchiectasis) *(arrows)*. Although the honeycombing is diffuse in the right lower lobe, it shows a subpleural predominance in the right middle lobe. This pattern and distribution are consistent with end-stage fibrosis in idiopathic pulmonary fibrosis.

3–10),[26] or may represent end-stage fibrosis (honeycombing), as in idiopathic pulmonary fibrosis, Langerhans's cell histiocytosis, asbestosis, and sarcoidosis.[4, 27] Common causes of a cystic pattern are listed in Table 3–4.

Honeycombing refers to the presence of cystic spaces 0.3 to 1 cm in diameter whose walls consist of a variable amount of fibrous tissue *(see* Fig. 3–8). The most common diseases in which the abnormality is identified are idiopathic pulmonary fibrosis, connective tissue disease, and sarcoidosis;[29] however, the process can be seen in the advanced stage of pulmonary fibrosis of any cause.[27, 29] The spaces represent mainly respiratory bronchioles and alveolar ducts that have become dilated as a result of traction by the adjacent fibrous tissue.[5, 28] The presence, distribution, and extent of honeycombing are assessed much more readily on HRCT scan than on the chest radiograph.[30]

The presence and severity of honeycombing vary considerably in different regions of the lung in different diseases, an important observation in differential diagnosis.

Table 3–3. RETICULAR PATTERN

Common Causes	Characteristic Radiographic and HRCT Findings
Acute	
Hydrostatic pulmonary edema	Reticular pattern usually seen in association with septal (Kerley) lines. Prominence of upper lobe vessels, pleural effusions, and cardiomegaly common
Mycoplasma pneumonia	Often in association with segmental consolidation. HRCT shows centrilobular nodules and branching linear opacities (*tree-in-bud* pattern)
Chronic	
Idiopathic pulmonary fibrosis and pulmonary fibrosis associated with collagen vascular disease	Lower lung zone predominance. HRCT shows intralobular linear opacities, irregular thickening of interlobular septa, and honeycombing involving mainly the subpleural regions and lower lung zones
Asbestosis	Lower lung zone predominance. Almost always in association with pleural plaques or diffuse pleural thickening. HRCT shows subpleural lines, intralobular lines, and irregular interlobular septal thickening in a predominantly subpleural distribution
Chronic hypersensitivity pneumonitis	Usually has middle or lower lung zone predominance. HRCT commonly shows intralobular lines, poorly defined centrilobular nodules, and extensive areas of ground-glass attenuation
Sarcoidosis	Coarse reticulation is seen with chronic fibrosis. Involves mainly perihilar region of middle and upper lung zones

HRCT, high-resolution computed tomography.

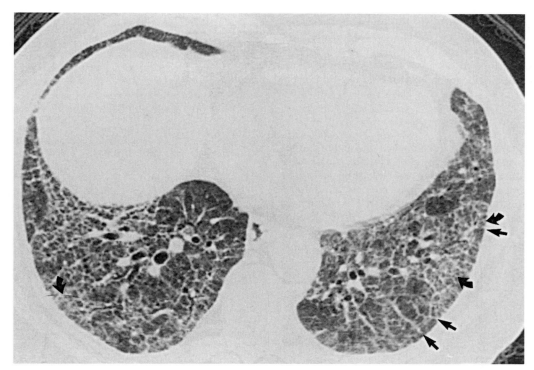

Figure 3–9. Reticular Pattern on HRCT. HRCT scan through the lower lung zones shows a diffuse fine reticular pattern resulting from a combination of irregular thickening of interlobular septa and intralobular lines. The interlobular septa are 1 to 2 cm in length and separated by 1 to 2 cm *(straight arrows)*, which corresponds to the diameter of the secondary lobule, whereas the intralobular linear opacities are smaller and separated by only a few millimeters *(curved arrows)*. The patient was a 58-year-old woman with idiopathic pulmonary fibrosis.

Langerhans's cell histiocytosis and sarcoidosis usually show a predilection for the middle and upper lung zones, whereas idiopathic pulmonary fibrosis and pulmonary fibrosis associated with connective tissue disease usually involve mainly the lower lung zones. On HRCT scan, the cystic spaces in Langerhans's cell histiocytosis have a random or diffuse distribution in the middle and upper lung zones with relative sparing of the lung bases, whereas the cysts in sarcoidosis have a predominantly peribronchovascular and perihilar distribution.[27] The honeycombing in idiopathic pulmonary fibrosis and connective tissue diseases involves mainly the subpleural lung regions and the

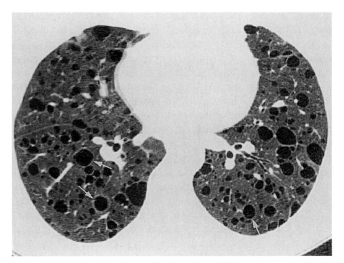

Figure 3–10. Cystic Spaces in Lymphangioleiomyomatosis. HRCT scan through the lung bases shows numerous cystic spaces with thin walls *(arrows)*. The lung parenchyma between the cysts is normal, and there is no evidence of fibrosis. The patient was a 50-year-old woman with lymphangioleiomyomatosis.

Table 3–4. CYSTIC PATTERN

Common Causes	Characteristic Radiographic and HRCT Findings
Idiopathic pulmonary fibrosis and pulmonary fibrosis associated with collagen vascular disease	Cystic pattern characteristic of end-stage fibrosis (honeycombing). Lower lung zone and subpleural predominance
Langerhans' pulmonary histiocytosis	Cysts often have bizarre shapes. Commonly associated with nodules. Diffuse but shows relative sparing of costophrenic angles on radiographs and basal regions on HRCT
Sarcoidosis	Cystic spaces are seen in association with extensive fibrosis and usually represent central conglomeration of ectatic bronchi (traction bronchiectasis). Middle and upper lung zone predominance. Subpleural honeycombing occasionally may be present
Lymphangioleiomyomatosis	Smooth thin-walled cysts. Diffuse distribution on radiograph and HRCT
Bronchiectasis	Bronchial dilation readily diagnosed on HRCT
Lymphocytic interstitial pneumonia	Cysts random in distribution usually few in number and associated with areas of ground-glass attenuation

HRCT, high-resolution computed tomography.

lower lung zones.[27] In lymphangioleiomyomatosis, the cysts are thin walled and are surrounded by normal lung parenchyma.[27, 31] They usually are distributed diffusely throughout the lungs, allowing ready distinction from Langerhans's cell histiocytosis and idiopathic pulmonary fibrosis.[27]

Nodular Pattern

A nodular pattern is produced when the parenchymal interstitium is expanded in a roughly spherical fashion by a cellular infiltrate, fibrous tissue, or both (Fig. 3–11). In the setting of interstitial lung disease, nodules are defined as round opacities less than 1 cm in diameter.[1, 25] The most common causes of a nodular pattern are listed in Table 3–5.

A purely nodular pattern in a febrile patient presenting with acute disease is most suggestive of hematogenous infection, particularly miliary tuberculosis (Fig. 3–12). The nodules usually measure less than 3 mm in diameter and typically are distributed diffusely throughout the lungs (although they may have a lower lung zone predominance).[32] A similar pattern may be seen in miliary fungal disease (e.g., histoplasmosis, coccidioidomycosis), silicosis, coal workers' pneumoconiosis, intravenous talcosis, metastatic carcinoma (particularly from the thyroid), and bronchioloalveolar carcinoma.[25, 34, 35]

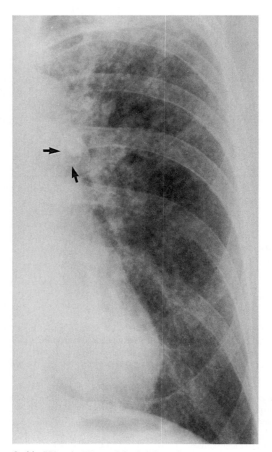

Figure 3–11. Silicosis. View of the left lung from a posteroanterior chest radiograph in a patient with silicosis shows well-defined nodules, most numerous in the upper lobes. Eggshell calcification of hilar and mediastinal nodes *(arrows)* is a finding virtually diagnostic of silicosis.

Table 3–5. SMALL NODULAR PATTERN

Common Causes	Characteristic Radiographic and HRCT Findings
Acute	
Miliary tuberculosis or histoplasmosis	Diffuse throughout both lungs. Random distribution on HRCT
Endobronchial tuberculosis	Patchy or asymmetric bilateral distribution. Centrilobular nodules and branching lines (*tree-in-bud* appearance) on HRCT
Viral infection	Diffuse or patchy. Centrilobular nodules on HRCT
Subacute or Chronic	
Sarcoidosis	Usually has perihilar and upper lobe predominance. Usually associated with bilateral hilar and mediastinal lymphadenopathy. HRCT shows nodular thickening along bronchial and perivascular interstitium
Hypersensitivity pneumonitis	Generalized or middle and lower lung zone predominance. HRCT shows poorly defined centrilobular nodules and areas of ground-glass attenuation
Silicosis and coal workers' pneumoconiosis	Upper lung zone predominance. HRCT often shows centrilobular predominance
Metastatic carcinoma	Diffuse or lower lung zone predominance. HRCT shows random distribution in relation to lobular structures

HRCT, high-resolution computed tomography.

The nodules in silicosis and coal workers' pneumoconiosis tend to involve mainly the middle and upper lung zones (*see* Fig. 3–11),[1] whereas those resulting from hematogenous processes, such as miliary tuberculosis and metastases, are diffuse or involve mainly the lower lung zones (where blood flow is greater).[15, 32] On HRCT scan, nodules resulting from hematogenous processes tend to have a random distribution in relation to lobular structures.[15, 34] By contrast, the nodules in silicosis and coal workers' pneumoconiosis frequently show a predominantly centrilobular distribution, a localization that corresponds to the accumulation of dust and fibrous tissue adjacent to respiratory bronchioles (Fig. 3–13).[35, 36]

In hypersensitivity pneumonitis, the centrilobular nodules typically have ill-defined margins and are distributed diffusely throughout the lungs. Centrilobular nodules reflect the presence of a bronchiolocentric process and are seen in various forms of bronchiolitis (*see* Chapter 15) (Fig. 3–14). Centrilobular nodules in a patchy distribution and often associated with branching linear opacities giving an appearance resembling a tree-in-bud are most suggestive of infectious bronchiolitis (Fig. 3–15).[39, 40] A tree-in-bud pattern has been described in viral, mycoplasma, and bacterial pneumonias and in endobronchial spread of tuberculosis.[37, 38, 40]

The nodules in sarcoidosis characteristically are located predominantly in the central peribronchovascular interstitium of the upper and middle lung zones.[10, 19] They also are seen along the interlobular septa and in the subpleural regions, including interlobar fissures but to a lesser extent than in the peribronchovascular interstitium. Such a perilymphatic distribution also is characteristic of lymphangitic carcinomatosis; however, as distinct from sarcoidosis, the

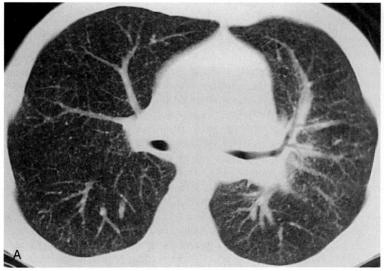

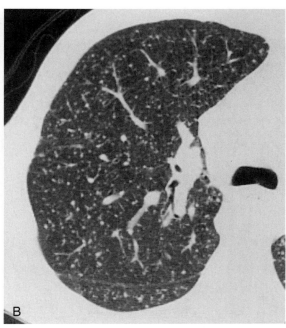

Figure 3–12. Miliary Nodules on CT. Conventional 10-mm collimation CT scan *(A)* in a patient with miliary tuberculosis shows 1- to 2-mm-diameter nodules throughout both lungs. HRCT scan *(B)* targeted to the right lung in the same patient shows the sharp margins of the miliary nodules better.

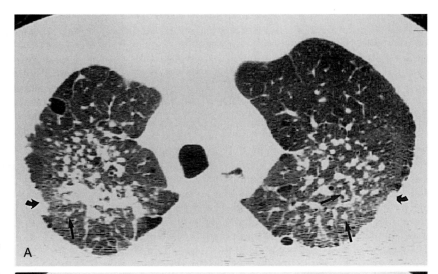

Figure 3–13. Silicosis. HRCT scans at the level of the upper *(A)* and middle *(B)* lung zones show numerous sharply defined nodules. Many have a centrilobular distribution *(straight arrows)*. Subpleural nodules *(curved arrows)* and evidence of emphysema also are present. The patient was a 58-year-old man with longstanding silicosis.

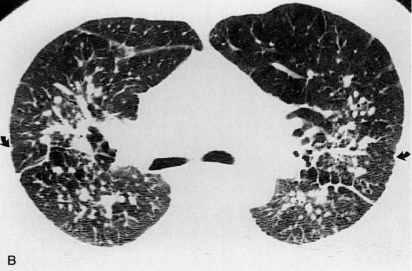

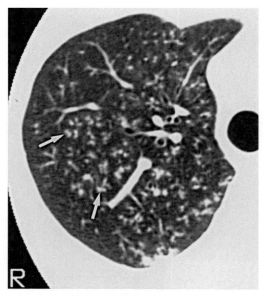

Figure 3–14. Centrilobular Nodules Caused by Bronchiolitis. HRCT (1.5-mm collimation) scan shows small nodules and branching structures *(arrows)*. These abnormalities are situated approximately 5 mm away from vessels that are too large to be within the secondary pulmonary lobule and represent borders of secondary pulmonary lobules. Structures and abnormalities located 5 mm away from these borders must be centrilobular in location. The patient was a 28-year-old man with bronchiolitis related to inhalation of foreign material.

predominant abnormality is thickening of the interlobular septa.[15, 17]

The usefulness of the anatomic localization of small nodules on HRCT scan in the differential diagnosis was assessed in a study of 58 patients.[40] Four radiologists categorized the nodules according to their location and distribution into four groups: perilymphatic, random, centrilobular, and diffuse throughout the lungs and centrilobular but patchy in distribution. All four observers agreed in 79% of cases (46 of 58) with regard to nodule localization and three of the four agreed in an additional 17% (10 of 58). The observers were correct in 218 (94%) of 232 localizations in the 58 cases. Nodules that had a perilymphatic distribution included those related to sarcoidosis and lymphangitic carcinomatosis, nodules that had a random distribution included miliary infection or metastases, nodules that had a diffuse centrilobular distribution included hypersensitivity pneumonitis and respiratory bronchiolitis, and nodules that had a centrilobular but patchy distribution were the result of infectious bronchiolitis.[40]

Reticulonodular Pattern

The presence of interconnecting linear opacities results in a reticular pattern.[4] Orientation of some linear opacities parallel to the x-ray beam causes an additional nodular component, resulting in a reticulonodular pattern. The latter also can be produced by the presence of nodules superimposed on a reticular pattern, as in sarcoidosis (Fig. 3–16), Langerhans' cell histiocytosis, and lymphangitic carcinomatosis.

Ground-Glass Pattern

A ground-glass pattern is considered to be present when there is a hazy increase in opacity unassociated with obscuration of underlying vascular markings.[4] (If vessels are obscured, the term *consolidation* should be used.) The abnormality is a frequent and important finding on HRCT scan but often is difficult to recognize on the chest radiograph. With HRCT, ground-glass attenuation reflects the presence of abnormalities below the resolution limit. Ground-glass attenuation may be seen in a number of situations, including interstitial disease, air-space disease, and increased capillary blood volume resulting from congestive heart failure or blood flow redistribution.[41–43]

Acute lung diseases characteristically associated with a ground-glass pattern include *P. carinii* pneumonia (Fig. 3–17),[43, 44] pulmonary hemorrhage,[45] and (occasionally) pulmonary edema.[18, 20] *Pneumocystis carinii* pneumonia is particularly associated with ground-glass attenuation; in an individual infected with human immunodeficiency virus, the abnormality is highly suggestive of this diagnosis.[46]

Ground-glass opacification is frequently the main abnormality seen in the subacute phase of hypersensitivity pneumonitis (Fig. 3–18).[47, 48] It is also the predominant finding in patients who have desquamative interstitial pneumonia, in which it reflects the presence of mild interstitial thickening and filling of the air spaces with macrophages.[49, 51] The areas of ground-glass attenuation in pulmonary alveolar proteinosis usually have a patchy or geographic distribution;[20, 50] although the abnormality consists mainly of filling of air spaces with proteinaceous material, on HRCT scan, interlobular septal thickening frequently is identified in the areas of ground-glass attenuation.[20, 50] The most common causes of a ground-glass pattern are listed in Table 3–6.

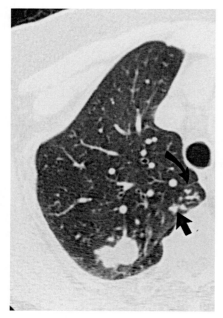

Figure 3–15. Centrilobular Nodules in Tuberculosis. HRCT scan shows a lobulated, 2-cm-diameter nodule in the posterior segment of the right upper lobe. Note the centrilobular distribution of smaller nodules *(straight arrow)* and normal interlobular septum *(curved arrow)*. The patient was an 80-year-old woman with reactivation tuberculosis (large nodule) and endobronchial spread (smaller nodules).

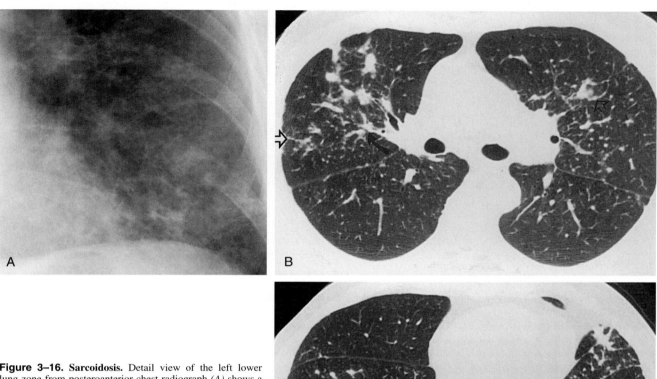

Figure 3–16. Sarcoidosis. Detail view of the left lower lung zone from posteroanterior chest radiograph *(A)* shows a reticulonodular pattern. HRCT scans *(B* and *C)* show nodular thickening along the bronchi *(straight arrows)*, pulmonary vessels *(curved arrows)*, and interlobular septa *(open arrows)*. Although several nodules with irregular margins can be seen in the subpleural lung regions, the abnormalities in sarcoidosis usually involve mainly the central perihilar regions. The patient was a 60-year-old-man.

Table 3–6. GROUND-GLASS OPACIFICATION

Common Causes	Helpful Diagnostic Features
Pneumocystis carinii pneumonia	Patchy or diffuse ground-glass attenuation in patient with AIDS is highly suggestive
Hypersensitivity pneumonitis	May be diffuse or have a lower lung zone predominance. Often associated with lobular areas of decreased attenuation and air-trapping owing to bronchiolar obstruction. Often associated with poorly defined centrilobular nodules
Idiopathic interstitial pneumonias	Ground-glass attenuation may be the predominant or only abnormality seen in patients with desquamative interstitial pneumonia, nonspecific interstitial pneumonia, or acute interstitial pneumonia. In patients with usual interstitial pneumonia, it usually is seen in association with predominantly subpleural and lower lung zone reticular pattern and honeycombing
Pulmonary hemorrhage	May be focal (e.g., caused by bronchiectasis), or diffuse (e.g., Goodpasture's syndrome)

AIDS, acquired immunodeficiency syndrome.

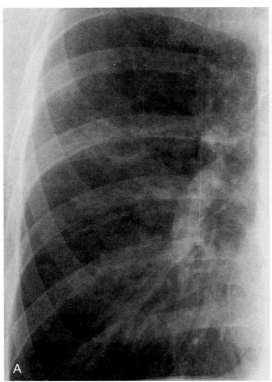

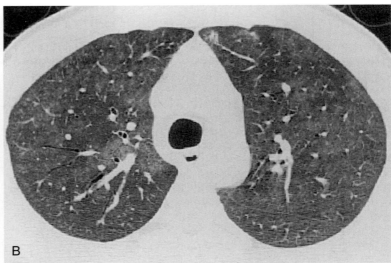

Figure 3–17. *Pneumocystis carinii* **Pneumonia.** View of the right lung from posteroanterior chest radiograph *(A)* in a 28-year-old patient with acquired immunodeficiency syndrome shows mild hazy increase in opacity (ground-glass opacity). HRCT scan *(B)* reveals extensive bilateral areas of ground-glass attenuation. The latter can be recognized readily by comparing the attenuation of the involved lung with the attenuation within the bronchi *(black bronchus* sign).

Limitations of the Pattern Approach

Modifying Factors

The pattern of parenchymal abnormality seen on the chest radiograph and HRCT scan may be modified by associated underlying parenchymal lung disease, particularly emphysema, and by the secondary effects sometimes

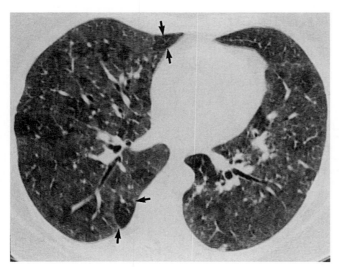

Figure 3–18. Hypersensitivity Pneumonitis. HRCT scan in a 59-year-old woman shows extensive bilateral areas of ground-glass attenuation. Focal areas of lung parenchyma without ground-glass attenuation have a size and configuration of secondary pulmonary lobules *(arrows).* This pattern of diffuse ground-glass attenuation with sparing of individual secondary pulmonary lobules is characteristic of the subacute stage of hypersensitivity pneumonitis.

produced by the diffuse interstitial disease itself. For example, on the radiograph, lobar pneumonia superimposed on emphysema may simulate interstitial lung disease (Fig. 3–19), whereas conglomerate interstitial fibrosis may simulate air-space disease.

Nonspecific Radiographic Findings

The usefulness of recognizing patterns of parenchymal abnormality on the chest radiograph cannot be overemphasized. Identification of the correct pattern, whether airspace, linear, reticular, nodular, or reticulonodular, in the appropriate clinical context often allows one to narrow the differential diagnosis to a relatively small number of entities and, occasionally, to make a specific diagnosis with a high degree of confidence. Nonetheless, in some cases, it is impossible to determine the main pattern of abnormality on the chest radiograph, an observation that has led to the recognition of the "I don't know pattern."[52] It is preferable to recognize the nonspecificity of the radiologic findings in some patients rather than to choose the wrong pattern for differential diagnosis. Experienced readers may disagree in the interpretation of a radiograph pattern; for example, in one review of 360 chest radiographs in patients who had biopsy-proven diffuse *infiltrative* disease,[1] two expert readers agreed that the predominant pattern was either nodular or linear in only 70% of cases. The presence of ground-glass opacity may be readily missed on the chest radiograph.[8, 12]

Comparison of Chest Radiography and High-Resolution Computed Tomography

Several groups of investigators have compared the diagnostic accuracy of HRCT with that of chest radiography in

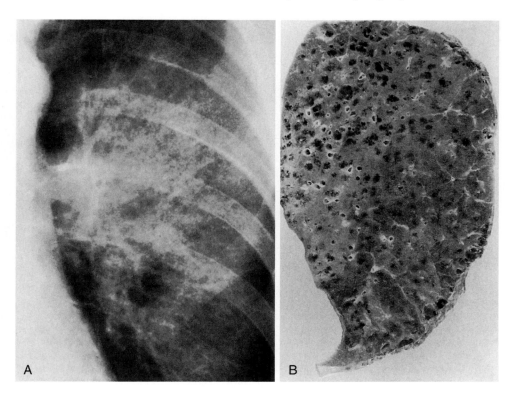

Figure 3–19. Acute Air-Space Pneumonia Superimposed on Emphysema. View of the left midlung zone from posteroanterior radiograph *(A)* reveals a poorly defined opacity in the superior segment of the left lower lobe. Instead of the homogeneous opacity characteristic of acute air-space pneumonia, this consolidation contains many small radiolucencies. A slice of an upper lobe *(B)* from another patient shows essentially homogeneous consolidation of the apical and posterior lung parenchyma. Within this region, there are numerous well-defined emphysematous spaces unaffected by the pneumonia. Such incomplete consolidation is responsible for the appearance in the radiograph of the first patient *(A)*.

the differential diagnosis of chronic diffuse interstitial and air-space lung disease.[2, 11, 53] In one investigation of 118 patients, radiographs and CT scans were assessed independently by three observers without knowledge of clinical or pathologic data.[2] The observers made a confident diagnosis in 23% of radiographic and 49% of CT interpretations, the diagnosis being correct in 77% and 93% of readings. A confident diagnosis was made more than twice as often on the basis of HRCT scans than on the basis of chest radiographs, and the CT-based diagnosis was correct more often. In a second study of 140 patients, three independent observers listed the three most likely diagnoses and recorded the degree of confidence they had in their choice.[11] The percentages of high-confidence diagnosis by each of the three observers that were correct with chest radiography were 29%, 34%, and 19%, as compared with 57%, 55%, and 47% with HRCT. Interobserver agreement for the proposed diagnosis also was significantly better with HRCT than with conventional radiography.[11]

The diagnostic accuracy of radiography and CT improves considerably when the findings are analyzed in the context of clinical findings, pulmonary function tests, and laboratory data. The value of such combined information in classifying chronic diffuse lung disease was assessed in one investigation of 208 patients.[53] When clinical, chest radiograph, and CT scan findings were evaluated independently, a correct diagnosis with a high degree of confidence was made in 29% of the cases on the basis of clinical data, 9% on the basis of radiographic images, and 36% on the basis of the HRCT findings. Combining the clinical and radiographic data allowed a correct diagnosis with a high degree of confidence in 54% of cases. Combining the information provided by the clinical, radiographic, and CT findings allowed a high-confidence diagnosis in 174 of the 208 patients (84%). This diagnosis was correct in 166 cases (95%). In the appropriate clinical context, a specific diagnosis often can be made with confidence and may preclude the need for lung biopsy.

General Signs in Diseases that Increase Lung Density

In addition to the basic patterns and signs already described, several additional radiologic features may aid in determining the nature of a pathologic process within the lungs.

Characteristics of the Border of a Pulmonary Lesion

The margin of a pulmonary nodule may be smooth, lobulated, or spiculated (Fig. 3–20). These margin characteristics are helpful in predicting whether the nodule is more likely to be benign or malignant. In general, smooth margins suggest benignity, and spiculation suggests malignancy; lobulation is seen with approximately equal frequency in benign and malignant nodules.[54–56] In a review of the CT findings of 634 solitary pulmonary nodules, 52 of 66 (79%) that had sharply defined, smooth, nonlobulated margins were benign, and 14 (21%) were malignant.[55] Of 218 nodules that had spiculated margins, 184 (84%) represented a primary pulmonary carcinoma, and 9 represented a metastasis; only 25 (11%) were benign. Of 359 nodules (58%) that had smooth but lobulated margins, 202 were benign, whereas 148 were malignant (either primary pulmonary carcinoma or metastasis). In another multicenter study of patients who had lung nodules not considered to be calcified, 130 nodules seen on radiographs were classi-

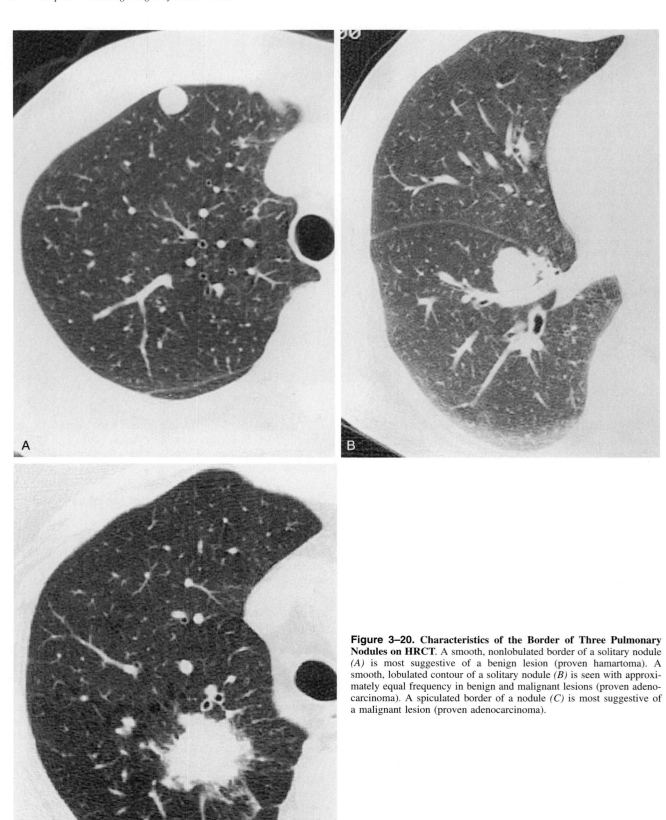

Figure 3–20. Characteristics of the Border of Three Pulmonary Nodules on HRCT. A smooth, nonlobulated border of a solitary nodule *(A)* is most suggestive of a benign lesion (proven hamartoma). A smooth, lobulated contour of a solitary nodule *(B)* is seen with approximately equal frequency in benign and malignant lesions (proven adenocarcinoma). A spiculated border of a nodule *(C)* is most suggestive of a malignant lesion (proven adenocarcinoma).

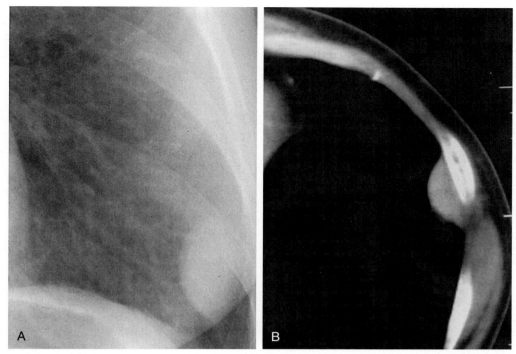

Figure 3–21. Extrapulmonary Sign. View of the left lower hemithorax from posteroanterior chest radiograph *(A)* shows the characteristic features of an extrapulmonary mass: a smooth convex border, where it abuts the lung and tapers superiorly and inferiorly; the lateral margin, where it abuts the soft tissues of the chest wall, is obscured. CT scan *(B)* shows tapering anterior and posterior margins. The patient was a 46-year-old woman with benign fibrous tumor of the pleura.

fied as having smooth margins; 48, as having lobulated margins; and 91, as having spiculated margins.[56] Of the nodules that had smooth margins, 80 (62%) were benign, 28 (22%) represented metastases, 9 were carcinoid tumors, and 13 (10%) were primary pulmonary carcinomas. Of the 48 nodules that had lobulated margins, 20 (42%) were benign, and 28 were malignant. Only 11 of the 91 nodules (12%) that had spiculated margins were benign. Correlation of HRCT with pathologic findings has shown that spiculation may result from irregular fibrosis or infiltration of carcinoma in the lymphatics (lymphangitic spread) or lung parenchyma adjacent to the tumor.[54]

A discussion of *satellite lesions* is included here because they are closely related to the margins of a pulmonary lesion. These abnormalities can be defined as small, nodular opacities in close proximity to a larger lesion, usually a solitary peripheral nodule. They usually indicate an infectious cause; in two studies, they were observed in about 10% of patients who had tuberculoma,[57, 58] as compared with only 1% of patients who had carcinoma.[58] The confidence that any single sign has identified accurately the nature of a lung nodule, whether benign or malignant, depends on the prevalence of malignancy in any given population. For example, a nodule in an adolescent patient is likely to be benign, regardless of its margin characteristics. A growing noncalcified nodule in an older smoking patient is likely to be malignant in the presence of a well-defined smooth border.

The contour of an opacity that relates to the pleura, either over the convexity of the thorax or contiguous to the mediastinum or diaphragm, can provide a useful clue as to whether the process is intrapulmonary or extrapulmonary in origin. A mass that originates within the pleural space or extrapleurally displaces the pleura and underlying lung inward, such that the angle formed by the margins of the mass and the chest wall is obtuse; by contrast, an intrapulmonary mass tends to form an acute angle with the contiguous pleura (Fig. 3–21). When viewed *en face*, the extrapulmonary mass is defined indistinctly because of the obtuse angle of its margins, whereas an intrapulmonary mass tends to be defined more sharply. Similar to all other radiologic signs, this sign is fallible: Occasionally an extrapulmonary mass relates to the lung with an acute angle and an intrapulmonary mass with an obtuse angle.

Silhouette Sign

The mediastinal and diaphragmatic contours are rendered radiographically visible by their contrast with contiguous air-containing lung. When a soft tissue opacity is situated in any portion of lung adjacent to a mediastinal or diaphragmatic border, that border no longer can be seen radiographically (Fig. 3–22). This situation constitutes a positive silhouette sign.[7] The corollary is that an opacity within the lungs that does *not* obliterate the mediastinal or diaphragmatic contour cannot be situated within lung contiguous to these structures (Fig. 3–23). These contours are apparent only when structures have been exposed adequately; for example, in an underexposed radiograph, massive consolidation of the right lower lobe may prevent identification of the right border of the heart, merely because the number of x-ray photons is of insufficient penetration to reproduce the heart shadow through the lower

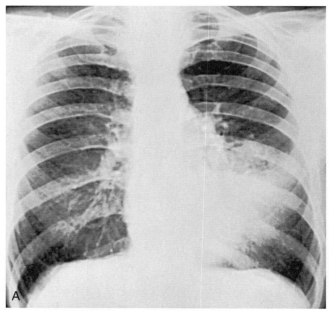

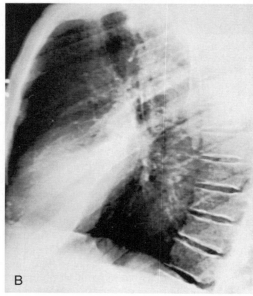

Figure 3–22. Silhouette Sign. Posteroanterior *(A)* and lateral *(B)* radiographs reveal obliteration of the left heart border by a shadow of homogeneous density situated within the lingula; such obliteration inevitably indicates lingular disease (provided that there is adequate radiographic exposure). Squamous cell carcinoma of the lingular bronchus with distal obstructive pneumonitis was diagnosed.

lobe density, despite the presence of air-containing lung contiguous to the heart.

Although the silhouette sign is most useful in the differentiation of middle lobe and lingular disease from lower lobe disease, it may provide precise anatomic information in many other sites. Obliteration of the aortic arch on the left side by airlessness of the apical-posterior segment of the left upper lobe, obliteration of the ascending arch of the aorta and of the superior vena cava by consolidation of the anterior segment of the right upper lobe, and obliteration of the posterior paraspinal line by contiguous airless lung in the left posterior gutter may be shown.

Cavitation

A cavity is defined radiologically as a gas-containing space within the lung surrounded by a wall whose thickness is greater than 1 mm.[3] In most cases, the cavity is formed by necrosis of the central portion of a lesion and drainage of the resultant partially liquefied material through the bronchi.[3] Neither the presence of a fluid level nor the size of the cavity is necessary to the definition of cavity. The terms *cavity* and *abscess* are not synonymous. An intrapulmonary abscess without communication with the bronchial tree is radiographically opaque; only when the abscess cavity communicates with the bronchial tree, allowing air to replace necrotic material, should the term *cavity* be applied.

In many cases, the radiologic appearance of the cavity gives some indication of its cause, particularly as to whether it is benign or malignant (Fig. 3–24). The specific radiologic features that should be noted with respect to this distinction include the thickness of the cavity wall, the character of its inner lining (whether irregular or smooth), the presence and nature of its contents, the number of lesions, and, when multiple, the number that have cavitated. The following discussion indicates the findings that are suggestive of a specific cause for each of these features; there are occasional exceptions to the rule in each category.

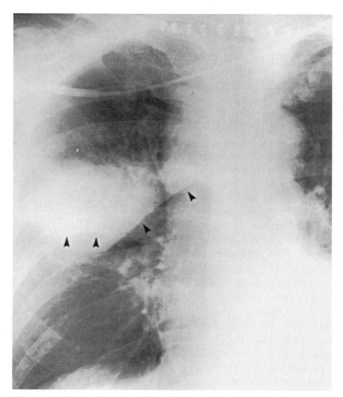

Figure 3–23. Application of the Silhouette Sign for Disease Localization. Detail view of the right hemithorax from anteroposterior chest radiograph shows an area of air-space consolidation in the right lung caused by acute bacterial pneumonia. The process does not obliterate any portion of the right mediastinal contour and is delineated sharply by the superomedial portion of the right major fissure *(oblique arrowheads)* and the lateral aspect of the minor fissure *(vertical arrowheads)*. These three features localize the pneumonia to the posterior and lateral portions of the right upper lobe.

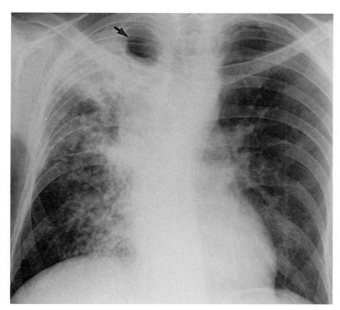

Figure 3–24. Tuberculous Cavity with Bronchogenic Spread. Postero-anterior chest radiograph shows a 3-cm-diameter cavity in the apical segment of the right upper lobe *(arrow)*, extensive consolidation in the right upper lobe, and 3- to 7-mm-diameter nodules throughout the right lung. The findings are characteristic of tuberculosis with associated endobronchial spread. The patient had positive smear and culture for *Mycobacterium tuberculosis.*

Cavity Wall. The cavity wall is usually thick in acute lung abscess (Fig. 3–25), primary and metastatic carcinoma, and Wegener's granulomatosis and often thin in chronic infection, such as coccidioidomycosis. Assessment of cavity wall thickness perhaps is most useful in distinguishing between a benign and a malignant lesion. In one study of 65 solitary cavities in the lung, all lesions in which the thickest part of the cavity wall was 1 mm or less were benign;[59] of the lesions whose thickest measurement was 4 mm or less, 92% were benign; of cavities that were 5 to 15 mm in their thickest part, benign and malignant lesions were equally divided; when the cavity wall was greater than 15 mm in thickness, 92% of lesions were malignant.

Character of Inner Lining. The inner lining is usually nodular in carcinoma, shaggy in acute lung abscess, and smooth in most other cavitary lesions.

Nature of Cavitary Contents. When material is identified within a cavity, it usually represents pus or partially liquefied necrotic neoplasm and appears as a flat, smooth air-fluid level without specific radiologic features. Occasionally, intracavitary material has characteristics that are strongly suggestive of a specific disease. Examples include the intracavitary fungus ball, which may form a mobile mass (Fig. 3–26), and the collapsed membranes of a ruptured *Echinococcus* cyst, which float on top of the fluid within the cyst and create the characteristic *water-lily* sign[60] or the *sign of the camalote* (a water plant found in South American rivers). The sign of the camalote is seen on the radiograph or CT scan in approximately 75% of patients who have ruptured pulmonary echinococcal cysts.[60] Another rare but characteristic intracavitary mass is that associated with pulmonary gangrene, in which irregular pieces

of sloughed necrotic lung parenchyma float like icebergs in the cavity fluid; although this complication can be seen with infection by virtually any organism, it is most common with *K. pneumoniae.*[61, 62]

Multiplicity of Lesions. Some cavitary disease is characteristically solitary (e.g., primary pulmonary carcinoma, acute lung abscess, and post-traumatic lung cyst). Other diseases are characteristically multiple (e.g., metastatic neoplasm, Wegener's granulomatosis, and septic thromboemboli).[63–65]

Bubble Lucencies (Pseudocavitation). On CT scan, particularly HRCT, round or oval areas of low attenuation usually measuring 5 mm or less in diameter (Fig. 3–27) may be visible within a pulmonary nodule.[54, 66] Such *bubble lucencies* (pseudocavitation) can be identified on HRCT scan in approximately 60% of bronchioloalveolar carcinomas; in 30% of acinar adenocarcinomas; and, less commonly, in other malignant lung tumors.[54, 66] Uncommonly, bubble lucencies also can be identified in benign lesions. In one study, bubble lucencies were found in only 1 of 11 (9%) of such nodules.[54] Correlation with pathologic findings has shown that the lucencies usually represent patent bronchi, localized bronchiectasis, irregular emphysema, or small air-containing cystic spaces associated with papillary tumor growth.[54, 67]

Calcification and Ossification

The presence or absence of calcification in pulmonary lesions, and, when present, its site, as detected by chest radiograph or CT scan is an important diagnostic sign. The most common form of pulmonary calcification is a single, often densely calcified nodule situated anywhere in the lungs, which represents a healed focus of granulomatous inflammation.

Calcification within a solitary pulmonary nodule is the most reliable piece of evidence that a lesion is benign.[68, 69] Although calcification can be seen in malignant tumors, its pattern allows distinction of benign from malignant nodules in most cases.[69, 70] Four patterns of calcification characteristically are associated with benign lesions: diffuse, central, laminated, and popcorn (Fig. 3–28).[70] The diffuse or laminated forms are virtually diagnostic of a granuloma. A small central nidus of calcification is seen most commonly with granulomatous lesions, although it also occurs in some hamartomas. Popcorn calcification is characteristic of hamartoma. Such benign patterns of calcification rarely are seen in malignant tumors. In one study of 634 nodules assessed with CT, 153 were diagnosed correctly as benign based on the presence of central or diffuse calcification;[55] although focal areas of calcification were identified in 13% of the primary lung tumors, only one carcinoid tumor had a benign pattern of calcification. The other malignant tumors had neither central nor diffuse calcification. Calcification in malignant tumors may be seen in several circumstances: (1) most important from a differential diagnosis point of view, the isolated instance of a peripheral primary carcinoma engulfing a calcified granuloma, in which case the calcification usually is eccentric; (2) a solitary metastasis of osteogenic sarcoma or chondrosarcoma, in which there is bone formation in the osteoid or calcification of the malignant cartilage;[71] and (3) occasional primary pul-

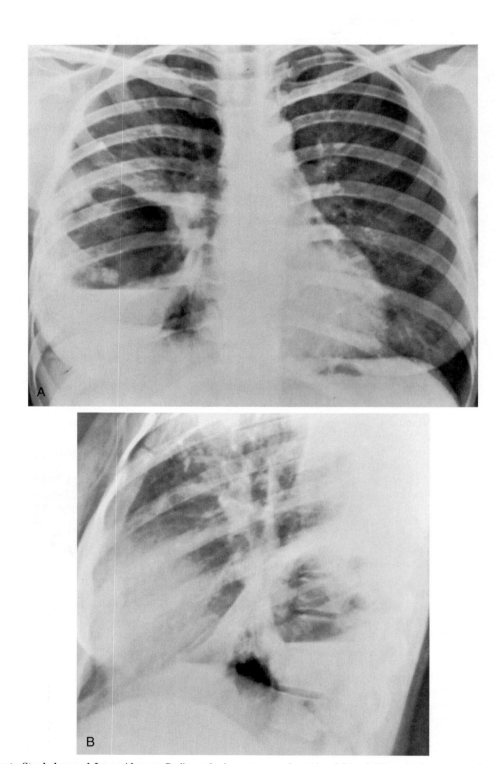

Figure 3–25. Acute Staphylococcal Lung Abscess. Radiographs in posteroanterior *(A)* and lateral *(B)* projection reveal a large cavity in the right lower lobe. The thickness of its wall and shaggy irregular nature of its inner lining suggest an acute lung abscess.

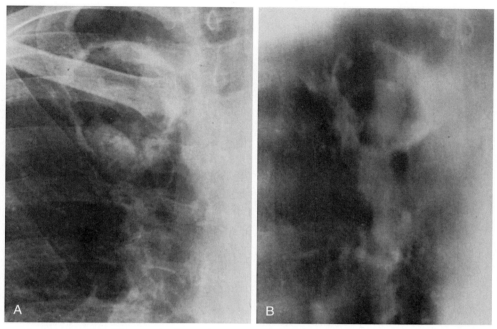

Figure 3–26. Intracavitary Fungus Ball (Mycetoma). Views of the upper half of the right lung with the patient upright *(A)* and supine *(B)* reveal a thin-walled but irregular cavity in the paramediastinal zone. Situated within it is a smooth oblong shadow of homogeneous density whose relationship to the wall of the cavity changes from the erect *(A)* to the supine *(B)* position. The cavity was of tuberculous origin, and the loose body was composed mainly of mycelial threads characteristic of *Aspergillus* hyphae.

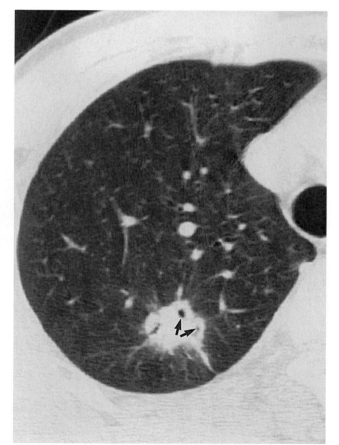

Figure 3–27. Bubble Lucencies. HRCT scan through a 2-cm-diameter nodule in the right upper lobe shows focal lucencies measuring less than 5 mm in diameter *(arrows)*. The patient underwent right upper lobectomy. Pathologic assessment showed bronchioloalveolar carcinoma. The bubble lucencies were shown to represent patent bronchi within the tumor.

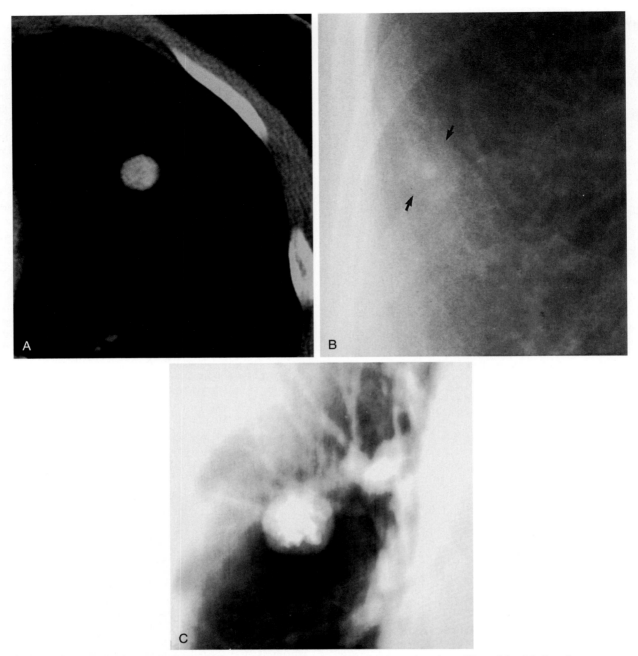

Figure 3–28. Benign Patterns of Calcification. CT scan *(A)* shows diffuse calcification in a tuberculoma. View of the right lung from posteroanterior chest radiograph *(B)* shows a tuberculoma *(arrows)* with a central nidus of calcification. View from the right upper lobe *(C)* shows a large central area of so-called popcorn ball calcification characteristic of hamartoma.

monary carcinoid tumors, in which there is ossification of the stroma.[55, 72]

Lymph node calcification usually is amorphous and irregular in distribution. It results most commonly from healed granulomatous infection, usually tuberculosis or histoplasmosis, in which case it constitutes part of Ranke's complex. A ring of calcification around the periphery of a lymph node *(eggshell* calcification) is an uncommon form of lymph node calcification. The abnormality is seen most often after silica *(see* Fig. 3–11) or coal dust exposure; other rare causes include sarcoidosis, Hodgkin's disease

(after mediastinal irradiation), blastomycosis, histoplasmosis, amyloidosis, and tuberculosis (Fig. 3–29).

DECREASED LUNG DENSITY

The diseases that cause a decrease in lung density result in increased radiolucency (hyperlucency) on the chest radiograph and decreased attenuation on CT scan. Here we are dealing only with the diseases of the lung that cause increased radiolucency. Any assessment of chest radiographs must take into consideration the contribution that

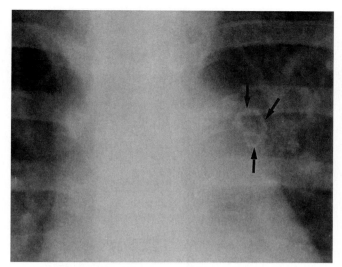

Figure 3–29. Eggshell Calcification in Tuberculosis. View from antero-posterior chest radiograph in a 4-year-old girl shows eggshell calcification in an aortopulmonary window node *(arrows)*. Smaller calcified nodes can be seen lateral to the aortic arch and in the left hilum. The patient had been treated for primary tuberculosis 2 years previously.

abnormalities of extrapulmonary tissue might make to reduced density, however. Certain pleural diseases (e.g., pneumothorax) and some congenital and acquired abnormalities of the chest wall (e.g., congenital absence of the pectoral muscles and mastectomy) produce unilateral radiolucency that easily might be mistaken for pulmonary disease unless this possibility is borne in mind. Because it eliminates the influence of superimposition of density from the chest wall, CT scan is superior to the chest radiograph in showing focal and diffuse reductions in lung density. Decreased lung density may result from (1) obstructive overinflation without lung destruction (e.g., asthma); (2) increased air with decreased blood and tissue (e.g., emphysema); (3) reduction in the quantity of blood and tissue in the absence of pulmonary overinflation (e.g., Swyer-James syndrome and pulmonary thromboembolism without infarction); or (4) a combination of these three components (proximal interruption [absence] of the right or left pulmonary artery).

Alteration in Pulmonary Volume

General Excess of Air

Lung diseases that cause decreased density are characterized by overinflation, with the exception of unilateral interruption (absence) of the pulmonary artery, unilateral hyperlucent lung (Swyer-James syndrome), partly obstructing endobronchial lesions, and pulmonary thromboembolism without infarction. Radiologic signs that may be observed in association with a general increase in intrapulmonary air relate to the diaphragm, the retrosternal space, and the cardiovascular silhouette (Fig. 3–30); the most important of these are signs related to the diaphragm. In patients who have severe emphysema, the diaphragm is depressed often to the level of the 7th rib anteriorly and the 11th interspace or 12th rib posteriorly; the normal dome configuration is concomitantly flattened. Although such

flattening often is evaluated subjectively, direct measurement is more accurate. Flattening of the diaphragm is best assessed on the lateral chest radiograph by drawing a straight line from the sternophrenic junction to the posterior costophrenic junction. The dome of the hemidiaphragm should be 2.6 cm or more above this line; measurements less than this indicate overinflation.[73] Flattening of the diaphragm also can be assessed on the posteroanterior (PA) radiograph by drawing a line from the costophrenic to the costovertebral angle and measuring the height of the dome of each hemidiaphragm;[73] this measurement is less sensitive than that performed on a lateral radiograph.[73, 74]

The severity of diaphragmatic flattening is valuable in differential diagnosis. It is invariably most marked in emphysema; the overinflation in this disease may render the diaphragmatic contour concave rather than convex upward (*see* Fig. 3–30). In asthma, the upper surface is nearly always convex (this applies in adults only; severe air trapping in infants and children may be associated with remarkable depression and flattening of diaphragmatic domes).

Another helpful sign in the detection of overinflation is an increase in the retrosternal air space on the lateral chest radiograph.[75] Direct measurement is preferred to subjective assessment; a distance greater than 2.5 cm between the posterior sternum and the most anterior margin of the ascending aorta is indicative of overinflation.[75, 76]

Local Excess of Air

Isolated overinflation of a segment or of one or more lobes occurs in two different sets of circumstances: with and without air trapping. Distinction between the two is of major diagnostic importance.

Overinflation *with air trapping* results from obstruction of the egress of air from affected lung parenchyma. It may be seen in neonatal lobar hyperinflation (congenital lobar emphysema),[77, 78] in congenital bronchial atresia,[79, 80] or distal to an endobronchial lesion as a result of check-valve obstruction. Such obstructive hyperinflation may develop in association with tumors of the main, lobar, or segmental bronchi, and its recognition may be useful in its diagnosis;[81] however, in our experience and that of others, it is a rare manifestation. For example, in one study of the radiographic patterns of 600 cases of bronchogenic carcinoma, overinflation distal to a partly obstructing endobronchial lesion was not seen in any case.[82–84] By contrast, in our experience, the volume of lung behind a partly obstructing endobronchial lesion almost invariably is reduced at total lung capacity. Despite this smaller volume, the density of affected parenchyma typically is *less* than that of the opposite lung as a result of decreased perfusion (oligemia) secondary to hypoxic vasoconstriction in response to alveolar hypoventilation. The overall effect is an increase in radiolucency despite the reduction in volume (Fig. 3–31).

Overinflation *without air trapping* is a compensatory process: Parts of the lung assume a larger volume than normal in response to loss of volume elsewhere in the thorax. This process may occur after surgical removal of lung tissue or as a result of atelectasis (Fig. 3–32) or parenchymal scarring. The remaining lung contains more than its normal complement of air.

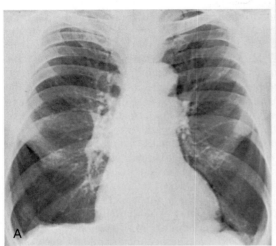

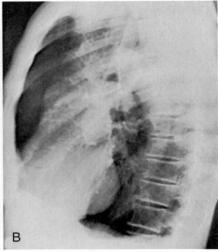

Figure 3–30. Diffuse Emphysema. Posteroanterior chest radiograph *(A)* shows a low position and somewhat flattened contour of both hemidiaphragms. The lungs are oligemic. In lateral projection *(B)*, the superior aspect of the diaphragm is concave rather than convex, and the retrosternal air space is deepened.

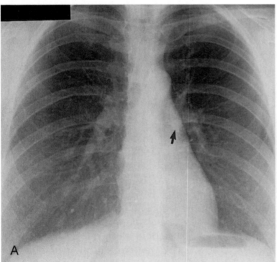

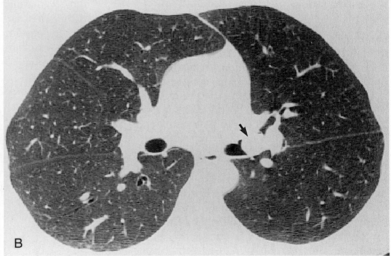

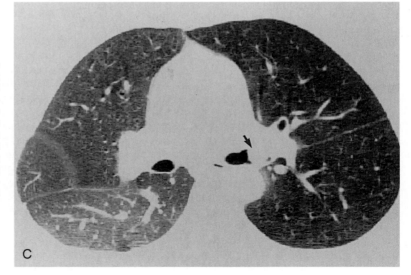

Figure 3–31. Decreased Vascularity and Lung Volume Caused by Endobronchial Tumor. Posteroanterior chest radiograph *(A)* in a 35-year-old woman reveals increased radiolucency of the left hemithorax and decreased vascularity. An endobronchial tumor *(arrow)* is present in the distal left main bronchus. Also note decrease in size of the left lung. HRCT scan *(B)* shows the endobronchial tumor *(arrow)*, decreased vascularity of the left lung, and slight decrease in attenuation. Note the decrease in size of the left lung with shift of the mediastinum and anterior junction line to the left. HRCT scan at end expiration *(C)* shows air-trapping in the left lung with shift of the mediastinum and anterior junction line to the right.

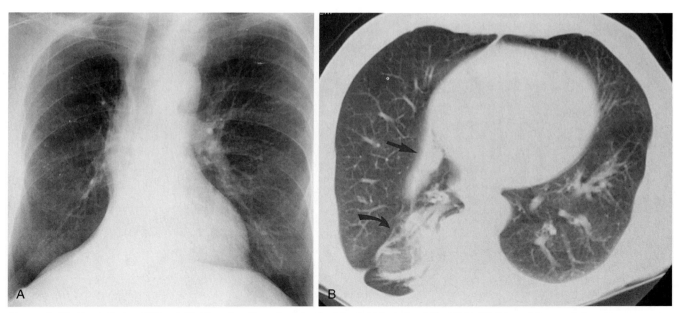

Figure 3–32. Overinflation Without Air-Trapping Secondary to Combined Atelectasis of the Right Middle and Lower Lobes. Posteroanterior chest radiograph *(A)* shows increased radiolucency of the right hemithorax as a result of compensatory overinflation of the right upper lobe secondary to combined atelectasis of the right middle and lower lobes. CT scan *(B)* shows right middle *(straight arrow)* and lower *(curved arrow)* lobe atelectasis and hyperinflation of the right upper lobe. There is decreased vascularity and attenuation of the right lung when compared with the left. The patient was a 69-year-old man with long-standing right middle and lower lobe atelectasis of unknown cause.

Bullae, Blebs, and Pneumatoceles

Bulla. A bulla is a sharply demarcated, air-containing space measuring 1 cm or more in diameter and possessing a smooth wall 1 mm or less in thickness. The space may be unilocular or separated into several compartments by thin septa (Fig. 3–33).

Bleb. A bleb is a localized collection of air in the immediate subpleural lung or within the pleura. It develops most frequently over the lung apices and seldom exceeds 1 cm in diameter. Pathogenesis has been hypothesized to be dissection of gas from ruptured alveoli into the adjacent interstitial tissue and into the interstitial layer of the visceral pleura, where it accumulates in the form of a cyst.[85, 86]

Pneumatocele. A pneumatocele is a thin-walled, gas-filled space within the lung that characteristically increases in size over a period of days to weeks and almost invariably

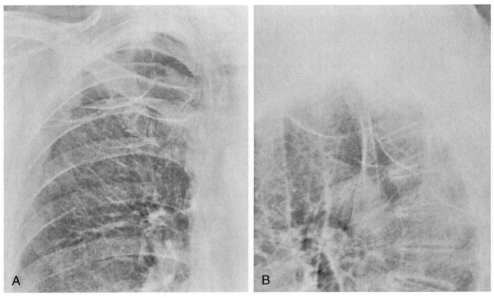

Figure 3–33. Bullae. Views of the upper half of the right lung in posteroanterior *(A)* and lateral *(B)* projections reveal several spaces in the lung apex sharply separated from contiguous lung by curvilinear, hairline shadows. The appearance suggests multiple bullae rather than a single space separated into compartments by thin septa.

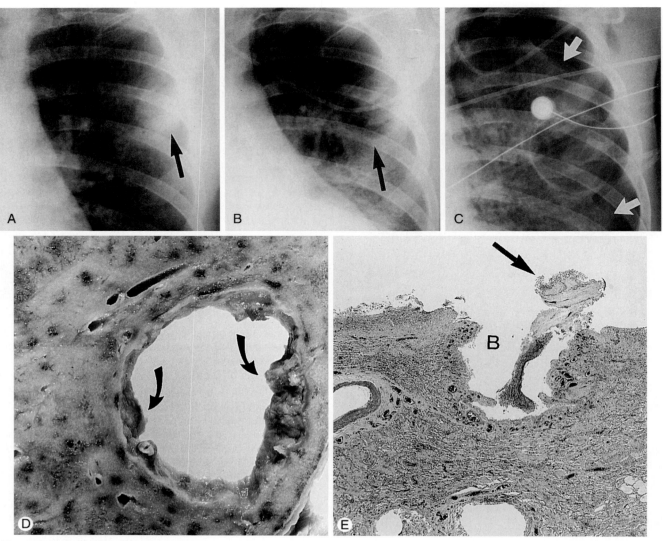

Figure 3–34. Pulmonary Pneumatocele. Chest radiograph *(A)* from a 28-year-old man with acute myelocytic leukemia and leukopenia shows an ill-defined opacity in the peripheral parenchyma of the left upper lobe. Twelve days later *(B)*, the opacity has been replaced by a smooth, thin-walled cavity approximately 4 cm in diameter. The following day *(C)*, the lesion measured 5.5 cm even in the presence of partial collapse of the left lung as a result of pneumothorax *(arrows)*. At autopsy *(D)*, the cavity was seen to have a shaggy inner lining related to the presence of necrotic tissue *(arrows)*. A section through an airway *(B)* entering the cavity *(E)* showed a partially obstructing flap of mucus and inflammatory exudate; this was mobile in the gross specimen and was hypothesized to permit entry of air into the cavity during inspiration and to prevent its egress on expiration. The cause of the cavity was believed to be most likely anaerobic organisms related to aspiration. *(A to E from Quigley MJ, Fraser RS: Am J Roentgenol 150:1275, 1988.)*

resolves; it typically occurs in association with infection. The pathogenesis is believed to relate to check-valve obstruction of an airway lumen or to local necrosis of a bronchial wall with dissection of air into the adjacent bronchovascular interstitial tissue (Fig. 3–34).[87] It usually is caused by *S. aureus* infection in infants and children or *P. carinii* in patients who have acquired immunodeficiency syndrome (Fig. 3–35). The abnormality also can occur after trauma.

Alteration in Pulmonary Vasculature

Just as overinflation may reflect an abnormality of the conducting airways of the lung, so may alteration in the vascular pattern indicate an abnormality of perfusion. Vascular loss may be central or peripheral. In the former

instance, it is produced by vascular obstruction (e.g., massive pulmonary thromboembolism) and in the latter by peripheral vascular obliteration (e.g., emphysema). Other causes include congenital cardiac malformations (e.g., tetralogy of Fallot) and diseases that affect the peripheral pulmonary vasculature (e.g., primary pulmonary hypertension).

ATELECTASIS

The term *atelectasis* is derived from the Greek words *ateles* (incomplete) and *ektasis* (stretching). In this text, we use it specifically to denote diminished gas within the lung associated with reduced lung volume. (Although the term *collapse* often is used synonymously with atelectasis, it should be reserved for complete atelectasis.[3])

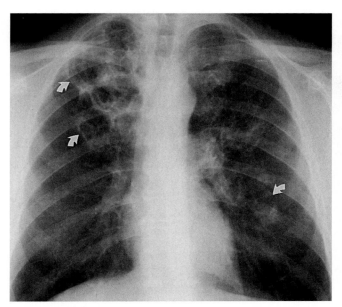

Figure 3–35. Pneumatoceles in *Pneumocystis carinii* pneumonia. Posteroanterior chest radiograph in a 53-year-old man with acquired immunodeficiency syndrome shows numerous cystic lesions *(arrows)* involving mainly the right upper lobe. The pneumatoceles had not been present on a chest radiograph performed 3 months previously when *P. carinii* was identified in bronchoalveolar lavage fluid.

Mechanisms of Atelectasis

Atelectasis can be classified into five types: resorption, passive, compressive, adhesive, and cicatrization (Table 3–7).

Resorption Atelectasis

Resorption atelectasis occurs when air flow to a region of lung is interrupted as a result of airway obstruction (Fig. 3–36). The end result of such airway obstruction is not necessarily a collapsed lobe or lung, particularly if the obstructing process is prolonged (e.g., as with pulmonary carcinoma). In this situation, *obstructive pneumonitis* frequently leads to consolidation severe enough to limit loss of volume. The characteristic radiographic picture of obstructive pneumonitis (i.e., homogeneous opacification of a segment, lobe, or lung without air bronchograms) is highly suggestive of an obstructing endobronchial lesion (Fig. 3–37).

Passive Atelectasis

Passive atelectasis denotes loss of volume as the lung retracts in the presence of pneumothorax (Fig. 3–38). Provided that the pleural space is free (i.e., without adhesions), atelectasis of any portion of lung is proportional to the amount of air in the adjacent pleural space.

Compressive Atelectasis

Compressive atelectasis results from compression of the lung by an adjacent space-occupying process. Any intrathoracic space-occupying process, such as a bronchogenic cyst, a bulla, or a peripheral neoplasm, induces airlessness of a thin layer of contiguous lung parenchyma (Fig. 3–39). This atelectasis is local rather than general, as in pneumothorax. Although some authors have considered the presence of atelectasis in patients with pleural effusion as a form of passive atelectasis,[88] it would seem more reasonable to consider this a form of compressive atelectasis.

On CT scan, atelectasis is seen commonly in the dependent lung regions as an ill-defined area of increased attenuation or subpleural curvilinear opacities (Fig. 3–40).[89–91] The former measures from a few millimeters to 1 cm or more in thickness and has been called *dependent opacity* or *dependent density*.[89, 90] Subpleural curvilinear opacities, also known as *subpleural lines*, are linear areas of increased attenuation measuring several centimeters in length and located within 1 cm of the pleura and parallel to it.[92] Both manifestations of dependent atelectasis characteristically disappear when the patient changes position (*see* Fig. 3–40); differentiation of dependent atelectasis from true interstitial or air-space disease can be established easily by scanning the patient in the supine and prone positions.[89, 93]

Round Atelectasis

Round atelectasis (rounded atelectasis, folded lung) is a distinct form of atelectasis characteristically associated with focal or diffuse pleural thickening.[95, 96] On conventional radiographs, the lesion appears as a fairly homogeneous, round, oval, wedge-shaped, or, less commonly, irregularly shaped subpleural mass.[95, 96] It usually measures 2.5 to 5 cm in greatest diameter, although it may reach 10 cm in diameter[97, 98] and involve an entire lobe.[99]

The characteristic CT features consist of bronchi and vessels curving and converging toward a round or oval mass that abuts an area of pleural thickening and that is associated with evidence of volume loss in the affected

Table 3–7. MECHANISMS OF ATELECTASIS

Atelectasis	Mechanisms
Resorption atelectasis	Occurs when communication between the trachea and alveoli is obstructed; the obstruction may be in a major bronchus or in multiple small bronchi or bronchioles
Passive atelectasis	Denotes the loss of volume owing to lung elastic recoil in the presence of a nonloculated pneumothorax
Compressive atelectasis	Denotes loss of volume accompanying an intrathoracic space-occupying process, such as pleural effusion, pulmonary mass, or bulla
Adhesive atelectasis	Adhesive atelectasis is related to a deficiency of surfactant. As with passive, compressive and cicatrization atelectasis, it is associated with patent large airway communications
Cicatrization atelectasis	Results from contraction of interstitial fibrous tissue as it matures. Can be focal (e.g., tuberculosis) or diffuse (e.g., idiopathic pulmonary fibrosis)

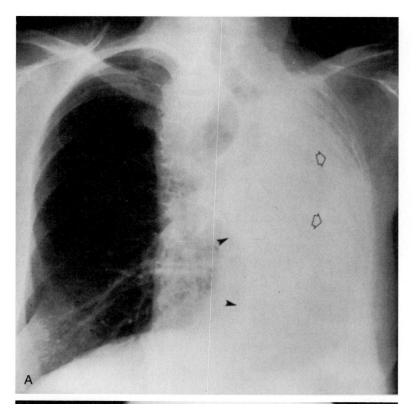

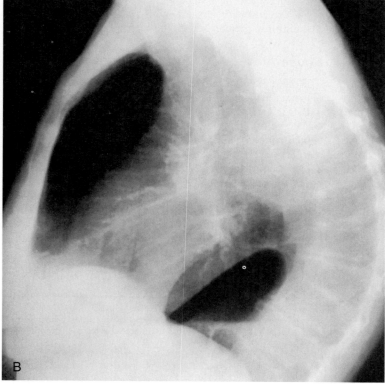

Figure 3–36. Total Atelectasis of the Left Lung. Postero-anterior *(A)* and lateral *(B)* chest radiographs disclose an opaque and shrunken left hemithorax. The right lung is markedly overinflated and has displaced the mediastinum to the left posteriorly *(arrowheads)* and anteriorly *(open arrows)*. The cardiac silhouette is obscured except for its anterior surface, which is visible in lateral projection; curvilinear calcification in the upper left hemithorax identifies the aortic arch. The patient was a 73-year-old woman with total atelectasis of the left lung caused by a centrally obstructing carcinoma.

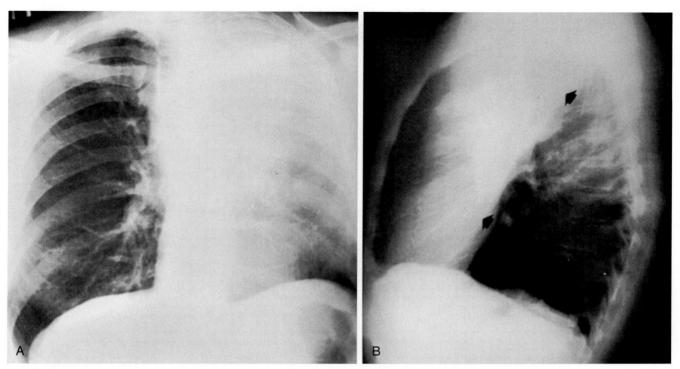

Figure 3–37. Obstructive Pneumonitis—Left Upper Lobe. Posteroanterior *(A)* and lateral *(B)* radiographs show homogeneous opacification of the left upper lobe; there is no air bronchogram. The major fissure *(arrow)* is not displaced forward, and the only signs indicating loss of volume are slight mediastinal shift and hemidiaphragmatic elevation. Collapse was prevented by the accumulation of fluid and alveolar macrophages within distal air spaces and chronic inflammatory cells and fibrous tissue within the interstitium—obstructive pneumonitis. The patient had squamous cell carcinoma originating in the left upper lobe bronchus.

Figure 3–38. Passive Atelectasis: Spontaneous Pneumothorax. Posteroanterior radiograph after spontaneous pneumothorax reveals the small volume occupied by a whole lung when totally collapsed. The well-defined air bronchogram indicates airway patency.

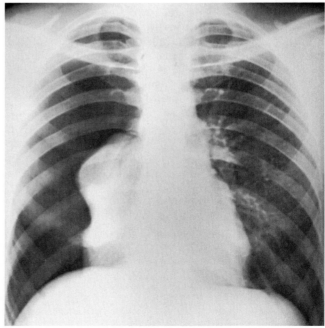

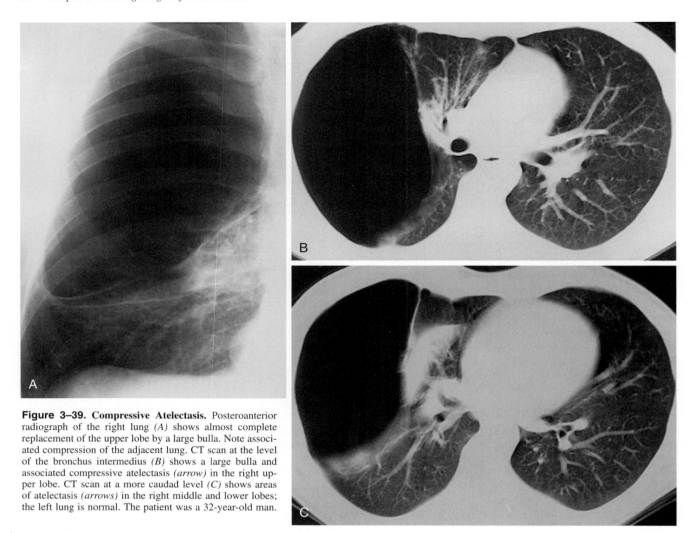

Figure 3–39. Compressive Atelectasis. Posteroanterior radiograph of the right lung *(A)* shows almost complete replacement of the upper lobe by a large bulla. Note associated compression of the adjacent lung. CT scan at the level of the bronchus intermedius *(B)* shows a large bulla and associated compressive atelectasis *(arrow)* in the right upper lobe. CT scan at a more caudad level *(C)* shows areas of atelectasis *(arrows)* in the right middle and lower lobes; the left lung is normal. The patient was a 32-year-old man.

lobe (Fig. 3–41).[101, 102] The hilar (central) aspect of the mass usually has indistinct margins as a result of blurring by the entering vessels.[101, 102] Air bronchograms are identified within the mass in approximately 60% of cases.[101, 102] Vessels and bronchi curve into the periphery of the mass, forming the basis for the *comet tail* sign. Although this sign is seen commonly, bronchi and blood vessels sometimes are oriented obliquely or in the cephalocaudad plane and are not readily apparent on conventional cross-sectional CT images. Multiplanar reconstructions using spiral

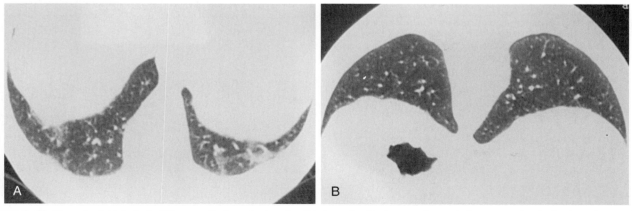

Figure 3–40. Dependent Atelectasis. CT scan with the patient supine *(A)* shows localized areas of ground-glass attenuation in the dependent portions of both lower lobes. Repeat scan with the patient prone *(B)* is normal. Reversibility from supine to prone positions allows distinction of passive dependent atelectasis from air-space or interstitial lung disease.

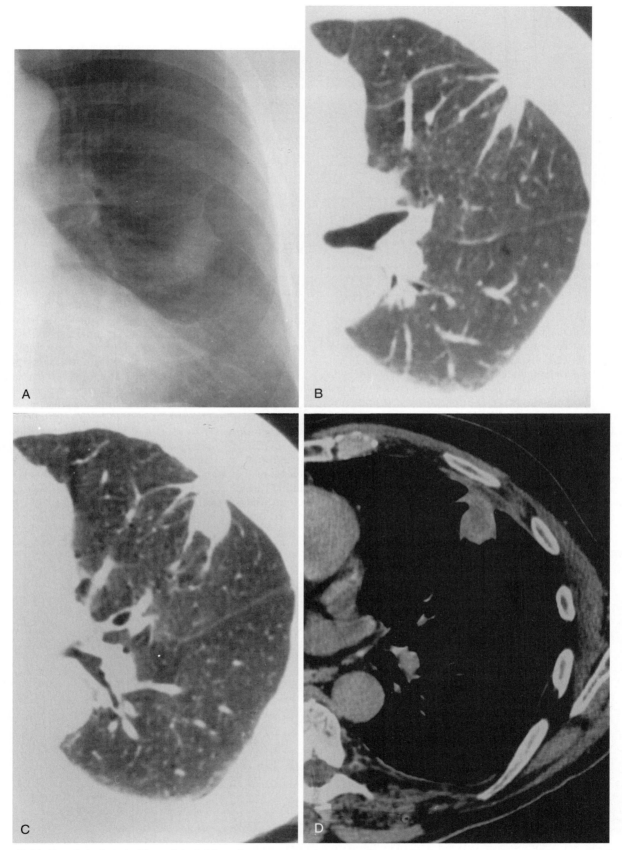

Figure 3–41. Round Atelectasis. View of the left lung from posteroanterior chest radiograph *(A)* shows oval soft tissue nodule measuring 3 cm in maximal diameter. CT scans *(B* and *C)* show vessels converging toward the nodule. There is evidence of volume loss with the vessels and the left major fissure curving toward the area of round atelectasis. CT photographed at soft tissue windows *(D)* shows that the nodule abuts a focal area of pleural thickening. The patient was a 70-year-old man who had a history of asbestos exposure.

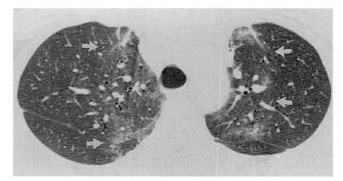

Figure 3–42. Adhesive Atelectasis in Radiation Pneumonitis. HRCT scan shows areas of ground-glass attenuation in a distribution conforming to the radiation portals for treatment of Hodgkin's disease *(arrows)*. Evidence of loss of volume is present with bronchi and vessels closer to the mediastinum than normal, particularly on the left side. The patient was a 28-year-old woman who had undergone radiation therapy 5 months previously.

CT or multiplanar imaging using magnetic resonance (MR) imaging may be helpful in determining better the course of the vessels and airways in these cases.[98, 103]

Most cases of round atelectasis are seen in patients who have been exposed to asbestos.[100] Other causes include pleural effusion secondary to tuberculosis, therapeutic pneumothorax, congestive heart failure, infections other than tuberculosis, pulmonary infarction, and malignancy.[100, 104]

Adhesive Atelectasis

The term *adhesive atelectasis* is used to describe atelectasis caused, at least in part, by surfactant deficiency.[94]

The best examples of this form of disease are respiratory distress syndrome of newborn infants and acute radiation pneumonitis (Fig. 3–42); other causes include adult respiratory distress syndrome, pneumonia, prolonged shallow breathing, and pulmonary thromboembolism.[94, 105]

Cicatrization Atelectasis

In a static system, the volume attained by the lung depends on the balance between the applied force and the opposing elastic forces. It follows that when the lung is stiffer than normal (i.e., when compliance is decreased), lung volume is decreased. This situation classically occurs with pulmonary fibrosis and is termed *cicatrization atelectasis*.

Localized cicatrization atelectasis is exemplified best by chronic infection, often granulomatous in nature, and epitomized by long-standing fibrocaseous tuberculosis (Fig. 3–43). The bronchi and bronchioles within the affected lung are dilated, presumably as a result of the increased elastic recoil from the surrounding pulmonary fibrosis, a phenomenon known as *traction bronchiectasis and bronchiolectasis*.[106] The radiologic signs are as might be expected—a segment or lobe occupying a volume smaller than normal, with a density rendered inhomogeneous by dilated, air-containing airways, with irregular thickened strands extending from the atelectatic segment to the hilum. Compensatory signs of chronic loss of volume usually are evident, including local mediastinal shift (frequently manifested by sharp deviation of the trachea when segments of the upper lobe are involved), displacement of the hilum (which may be severe in upper lobe disease), and compensatory overinflation of the remainder of the affected lung.

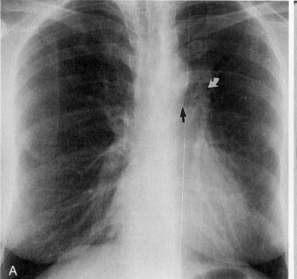
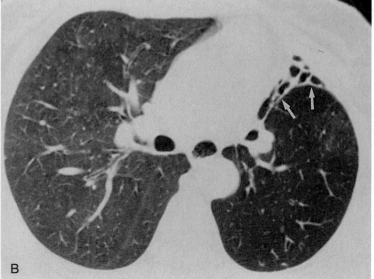

Figure 3–43. Severe Cicatrization Atelectasis Caused by Tuberculosis. Posteroanterior chest radiograph *(A)* in a 41-year-old woman shows volume loss of the left upper lobe with elevation of the left main bronchus *(straight black arrow)* and left hilum *(curved white arrow)* and shift of the mediastinum. There is decreased vascularity of the left lung compared with the right. Although the left upper lobe is collapsed, it has not resulted in any increase in opacity. HRCT scan *(B)* confirms the presence of complete atelectasis of left upper lobe. All that remains are markedly ectatic bronchi outlined by the major fissure *(arrows)*, which is displaced cephalad, anteriorly and medially. There is marked hyperinflation of the left lower lobe and decreased size of the left hemithorax. The findings are the result of previous tuberculosis.

Table 3–8. RADIOLOGIC SIGNS OF ATELECTASIS

Direct
    Displacement of interlobar fissures
    Crowding of vessels and bronchi
Indirect
    Local increase in opacity
    Elevation of hemidiaphragm
    Displacement of mediastinum
    Compensatory overinflation of remaining lung
    Displacement of hila
    Approximation of ribs
    Absence of an air bronchogram (in cases of resorption atelectasis
      only)
    Absence of visibility of the interlobar artery (in cases of lower lobe
      atelectasis only)

Generalized fibrotic disease of the lungs may be associated with loss of volume. For example, elevation of the diaphragm and overall reduction in lung size are seen commonly in idiopathic pulmonary fibrosis. A gradual reduction in thoracic volume in cases of diffuse interstitial disease is a useful indicator of the fibrotic nature of the underlying pathologic process.

Radiologic Signs of Atelectasis

The radiologic signs of atelectasis may be classified into direct and indirect types (Table 3–8). Direct types include displacement of the interlobar fissures and crowding of bronchi and vessels within the area of atelectasis; indirect types include pulmonary opacification and signs related to shift of other structures to compensate for the loss of volume.

Direct Signs

Displacement of Interlobar Fissures. Displacement of the fissures that form the boundary of an atelectatic lobe is one of the most dependable and easily recognized signs of atelectasis (Fig. 3–44). For each lobe, the position and configuration of the displaced fissures are predictable for a given loss of volume; these factors are considered further on in relation to patterns of specific lobar and segmental atelectasis.

Crowding of Vessels and Bronchi. As the lung loses volume, the vessels and bronchi in the atelectatic area become crowded together. This finding is one of the earliest signs of atelectasis and can be recognized most readily when comparison is made with previous radiographs.[107] Increased opacification of the atelectatic lobe may result in obscuration of the vessels; however, except in patients who have resorptive atelectasis, crowded air bronchograms are visible within the area of atelectasis on the radiograph or CT scan (*see* Fig. 3–44).

Indirect Signs

Apart from the presence of a local opacity, the main indirect radiologic signs of atelectasis are signs that are related to mechanisms that compensate for the reduction in intrapleural pressure—diaphragmatic elevation, mediastinal shift, approximation of ribs, and overinflation of the remainder of the lung (*see* Fig. 3–44).

Patterns of Atelectasis

Total Pulmonary Atelectasis

Atelectasis of an entire lung usually is secondary to complete obstruction of a main bronchus and is associated

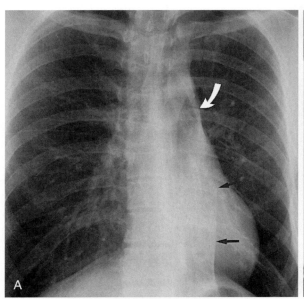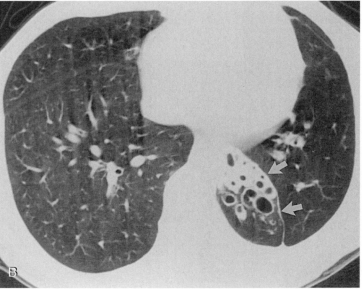

Figure 3–44. Left Lower Lobe Atelectasis. Posteroanterior chest radiograph *(A)* shows caudad and medial displacement of the left major fissure *(black arrows)* characteristic of left lower lobe atelectasis. Crowding of ectatic bronchi within the atelectatic lobe also can be seen. Indirect signs of left lower lobe atelectasis include overinflation of the left upper lobe, overinflation of the right lung with displacement of the anterior junction line *(curved white arrow)* to the left, and shift of the mediastinum. HRCT scan *(B)* shows caudad and medial displacement of the major fissure *(straight white arrows)* and left lower lobe bronchiectasis. Although the lobe is markedly atelectatic, there is little opacification of the lung parenchyma, presumably as a result of reflex vasoconstriction. The patient was a 23-year-old man who had a history of childhood viral pneumonia.

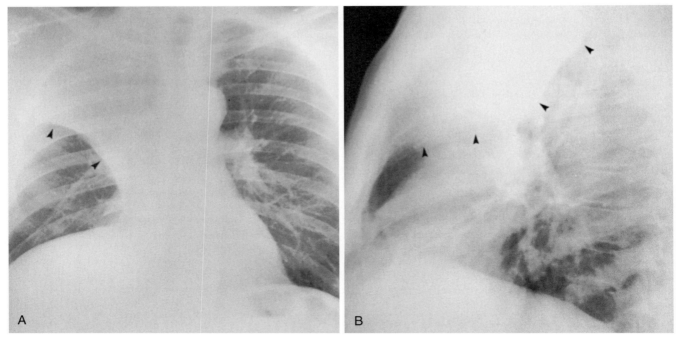

Figure 3–45. Right Upper Lobe Atelectasis (Moderate). Posteroanterior *(A)* and lateral *(B)* radiographs show a homogeneous opacity *(arrowheads)* occupying the anterosuperior portion of the right hemithorax. In lateral projection, the opacity is defined sharply on its posterior and anteroinferior margins. The right hemidiaphragm is elevated, and there is slight displacement of the trachea to the right. The patient was a 51-year-old man with a large squamous cell carcinoma in the right upper lobe. The atelectasis was caused by bronchial compression from involved lymph nodes.

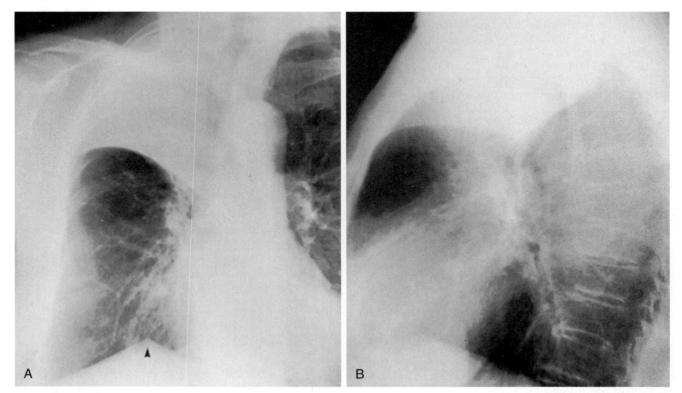

Figure 3–46. Juxtaphrenic Peak in Upper Lobe Atelectasis. Posteroanterior *(A)* and lateral *(B)* chest radiographs in a patient with right upper lobe atelectasis show the normally smooth contour of the right hemidiaphragm to be interrupted by a triangular opacity *(arrowhead)*, apex pointing cephalad. This juxtaphrenic peak is due to an inferior accessory fissure that can be seen extending obliquely cephalad and medial from the juxtaphrenic peak.

with increased opacity of the atelectatic lung (*see* Fig. 3–36). In patients who have partial obstruction or pneumothorax, however, loss of volume may occur with normal or increased radiolucency of the atelectatic lung.

Lobar Atelectasis

The patterns created by atelectasis of the right and left upper lobes differ and are described separately. The lower lobes have almost identical patterns and are considered together.

Right Upper Lobe

The minor fissure and the upper half of the major fissure approximate by shifting upward and forward (Fig. 3–45). On lateral projection, both fissures appear gently curved, the minor fissure assuming a concave configuration inferiorly, whereas the major fissure may be convex, concave, or flat;[109] the minor fissure shows roughly the same curvature in PA projection.

Another sign commonly associated with right or left upper lobe atelectasis (less commonly with middle lobe atelectasis) is the *juxtaphrenic peak*.[110] This sign consists of a small, sharply defined triangular opacity that projects upward from the medial half of the hemidiaphragm at or near the highest point of the dome (Fig. 3–46). The peak usually is related to cephalad displacement of an inferior accessory fissure.[111, 112]

Right upper lobe atelectasis caused by large hilar tumors may be associated with a characteristic downward bulge in the medial portion of the minor fissure. This feature, combined with the concave appearance of the lateral aspect of the minor fissure, results in a reverse S configuration of the minor fissure and is known as *Golden's S sign* (Fig. 3–47).[107, 113] On radiographs[94, 107] and CT scan,[108] this sign strongly suggests the presence of pulmonary carcinoma as the cause of atelectasis. Although initially described for right upper lobe atelectasis, Golden's S sign is applicable to atelectasis of any lobe.[94, 107]

On CT scan, the medial margin of the atelectatic right upper lobe abuts the mediastinum and is associated with superior and medial displacement of the minor fissure (*see* Fig. 3–47). With elevation of the minor fissure, the overinflated middle lobe shifts upward laterally alongside the atelectatic upper lobe. Compensatory overinflation of the

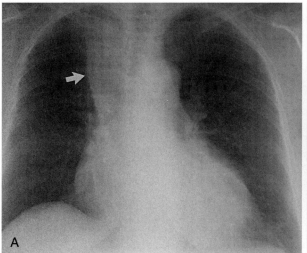

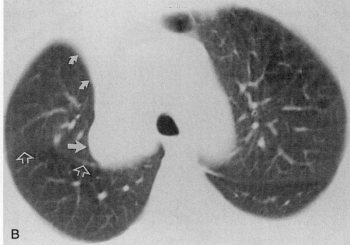

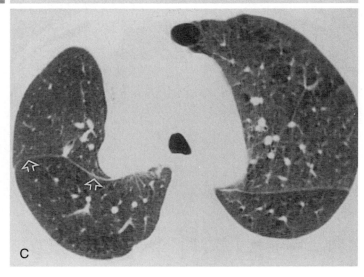

Figure 3–47. Right Upper Lobe Atelectasis with Golden's S Sign. Posteroanterior chest radiograph *(A)* shows right upper lobe atelectasis with elevation and medial displacement of the minor fissure. Note focal convexity resulting from a central tumor (Golden's S sign) *(arrow)*. CT scan at the level of the tracheal carina *(B)* shows upward and medial displacement of the minor fissure *(curved arrows)* with a localized convexity (Golden's S sign) *(straight arrow)* and upward and forward displacement of the right major fissure *(open arrows)*. The reorientation of the major fissure is easier to appreciate on HRCT scan *(C; open arrows)*. The patient was a 55-year-old woman with right upper lobe obstruction by squamous cell carcinoma.

right lower lobe results in superior, anterior, and medial displacement of the major fissure.[99]

Left Upper Lobe

The major difference between atelectasis of the left and right upper lobes is related to the absence of a minor fissure on the left; all lung tissue anterior to the major fissure is involved (Fig. 3–48). This fissure—which is slightly more vertical than the major fissure on the right—is displaced forward in a plane roughly parallel to the anterior chest wall, a relationship particularly evident on the lateral radiograph. As volume loss increases, the fissure moves further anteriorly and medially, until on lateral projection the shadow of the lobe is no more than a broad linear opacity contiguous with and parallel to the anterior chest wall. The contiguity of the atelectatic lobe with the anterior mediastinum obliterates the left cardiac border in frontal projection (the *silhouette sign*).

As the apical segment moves downward and forward, the space it vacates is occupied by the overinflated superior segment of the lower lobe; the apex of the hemithorax contains aerated lung (*see* Fig. 3–48).[114] Sometimes this lower lobe segment inserts itself medially between the apex of the atelectatic upper lobe and the mediastinum, creating a sharp interface with the medial edge of the atelectatic lobe and allowing visualization of the aortic arch. The overinflated superior segment is seen as a crescent of hyperlucency, hence the term *Luftsichel* (*air crescent*) in the German literature.[115] This finding is seen more often on the left (*see* Fig. 3–48) than on the right.

On CT scan, the atelectatic left upper lobe can be seen to abut the anterior chest wall and mediastinum (Fig. 3–49). The major fissure is shifted cephalad and anteriorly. The posterior margin of the atelectatic left upper lobe has a V-shaped contour or a small peak from the lung apex to the hilum as a result of tethering of the major fissure by the hilum. A focal convexity in the hilar region indicates the presence of a central obstructing tumor (Golden's S sign) (*see* Fig. 3–49).

Right Middle Lobe

The diagnosis of right middle lobe atelectasis is one of the easiest to make on a lateral radiograph and one of the most difficult to make on PA projection (Fig. 3–50). With progressive loss of volume, the minor fissure and the lower half of the major fissure approximate and are almost in contact when collapse is complete. In PA projection, there may be no discernible increase in opacity, the only evidence of disease being obliteration of part of the right cardiac border as a result of contiguity of the right atrium with the medial segment of the atelectatic lobe (the silhouette sign). The difficulty in detecting atelectasis in this projection is related to the obliquity of the atelectatic lobe in a superoinferior plane and the thickness of the collapsed

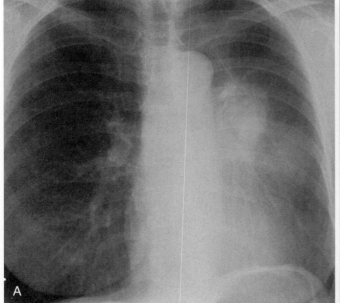

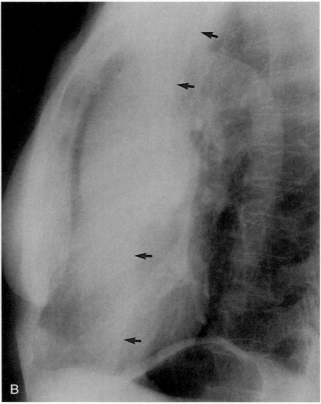

Figure 3–48. Left Upper Lobe Atelectasis with *Luftsichel* sign. Posteroanterior chest radiograph *(A)* shows elevation of the left hilum and left main bronchus and poorly defined increased opacity in the left perihilar region. A crescent of aerated lung outlines the aortic arch (*Luftsichel* sign). The lateral radiograph *(B)* reveals anterior displacement of the major fissure *(arrows)*. The overinflated superior segment of the left lower lobe outlines the aortic arch and accounts for the area of increased lucency lateral to the aortic arch on the posteroanterior radiograph.

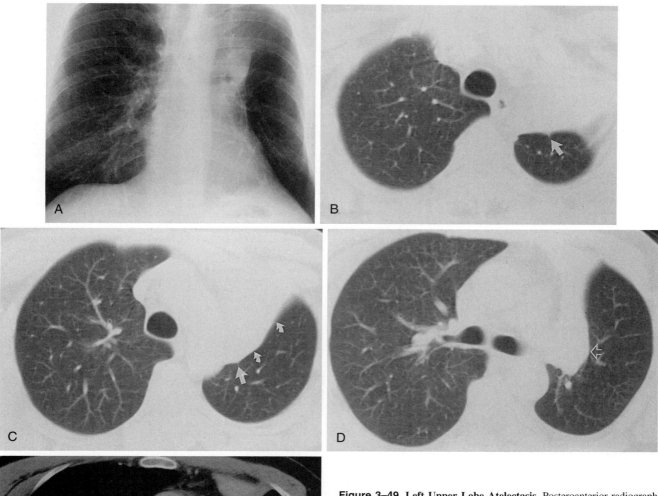

Figure 3–49. Left Upper Lobe Atelectasis. Posteroanterior radiograph *(A)* shows elevation of the left hilum and opacification of the left upper lobe. CT scan near the lung apex *(B)* reveals anterior and cephalad displacement of the major fissure. The slightly peaked appearance of the posterior surface of the major fissure *(straight arrow)* is caused by tethering from the hilar structures. CT scan at the level of the aortic arch *(C)* shows anterior and medial displacement of the interlobar fissure *(curved arrows)* and with a focal peak *(straight arrow)*. Peaked appearance of the posterior fissural surface *(arrow)* and lack of air bronchograms are indicative of resorptive atelectasis. CT scan at the level of the left main bronchus *(D)* shows focal convexity *(open arrow)* characteristic of a central obstructive tumor (Golden's S sign). CT scan photographed at soft tissue windows *(E)* shows central tumor *(arrows)* associated with complete obstruction of the left upper lobe bronchus. The patient was a 58-year-old man with squamous cell carcinoma.

lobe itself. The CT appearance of right middle lobe atelectasis is characteristic and consists of a broad triangular or trapezoidal opacity with the apex directed toward the hilum *(see* Fig. 3–50).

Lower Lobes

The configuration of atelectatic lower lobes is modified by the fulcrum-like effect exerted on the lung by the hilum and pulmonary ligament,[116] the fissures approximating in such a manner that the upper half of the major fissure swings downward and the lower half backward (Fig. 3–51; *see* Fig. 3–44). This displacement is appreciated best in lateral projection when the lobe is only partly atelectatic and the major fissure is tangential to the x-ray beam and visible as a well-defined interface. During its downward displacement, the upper half of the fissure usually becomes clearly evident in PA projection as a well-defined interface extending obliquely downward and laterally from the region of the hilum *(see* Figs. 3–44 and 3–51).[117, 118] On CT scan, an atelectatic lower lobe can be seen to lose volume in a posteromedial direction, pulling down the major fissure

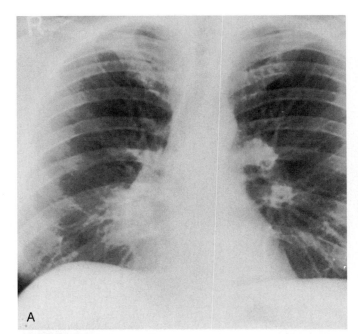

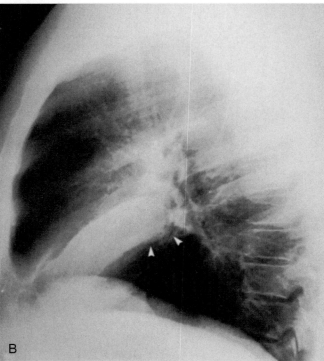

Figure 3–50. Right Middle Lobe Atelectasis. Posterior radiograph *(A)* shows a vague opacity in the right lower hemithorax obliterating the right cardiac border, whereas a lateral projection of the same patient *(B)* shows the characteristic triangular opacity of middle lobe atelectasis. The convex inferior configuration of the major fissure at the hilum *(arrowheads)* is indicative of an underlying mass. The opacity of the middle lobe possesses a sharp oblique orientation downward. CT scans *(C)* show the typical triangular opacity with its apex pointing peripherally. Contiguity between the visceral and parietal pleura over the anterolateral aspect of the lobe has been lost. The right middle lobe bronchus was obstructed by carcinoma.

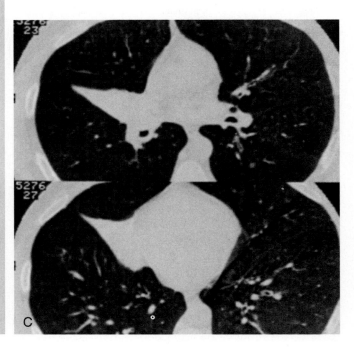

(see Fig. 3–44). The lateral portion of the major fissure shows a greater degree of mobility because the medial aspect is fixed to the mediastinum by the hilar structures and the pulmonary ligament.

Segmental Atelectasis

Segmental atelectasis usually results from bronchial obstruction and is associated with obstructive pneumonitis. A homogeneous opacity that conforms to the anatomic distribution of a bronchopulmonary segment and in which

no air bronchogram is identifiable should alert the physician immediately to the presence of an obstructing endobronchial lesion (Fig. 3–52).

Linear (Platelike) Atelectasis

Linear (platelike) atelectasis is characterized by linear opacities ranging from 1 to 3 mm in thickness and 4 to 10 cm in length; they are situated in the mid and lower lung zones, most commonly the latter (Fig. 3–53). Although usually oriented in a roughly horizontal plane, the linear

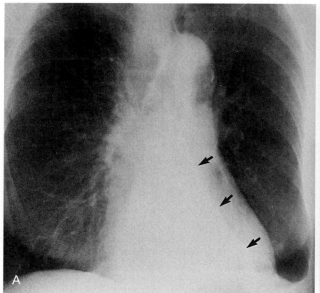

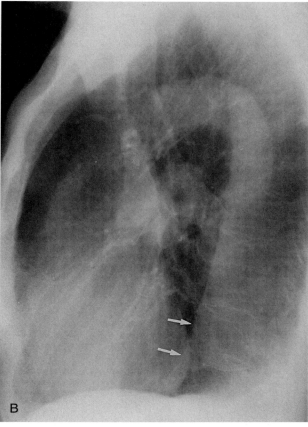

Figure 3–51. Left Lower Lobe Atelectasis. Posteroanterior chest radiograph *(A)* shows caudad and medial shift of the left major interlobar fissure *(arrow)*. Note the caudad displacement of the left hilum, compensatory overinflation of the left upper lobe and right lung, and shift of the mediastinum. Lateral radiograph *(B)* reveals posterior displacement of the interlobar fissure. The atelectatic left lower lobe is associated with increased opacity in the paravertebral region. A small left pleural effusion is also evident. The patient was a 74-year-old man with left lower lobe atelectasis due to a mucus plug.

opacities may be oriented obliquely depending on the zone of lung affected; in midlung zones particularly, they may be angled more than 45 degrees to the horizontal. The linear opacities may be single or multiple, unilateral or bilateral. The opacities almost invariably are associated with conditions that diminish diaphragmatic excursion, such as intra-abdominal surgery or inflammatory disease.

PLEURAL ABNORMALITIES

Pleural Effusion

Conventional PA and lateral chest radiographs are considerably less sensitive than the lateral decubitus view in the detection of pleural effusions. Although 10 ml of fluid can be detected on the lateral decubitus view, accumulation of at least 175 ml of fluid is necessary to cause blunting of the lateral costophrenic sulcus on a PA radiograph.[120] Although most effusions greater than 200 ml are evident on the PA radiograph, 500 ml of fluid may be present without any blunting of the costophrenic sulcus on this view (Fig. 3–54).[120] Because the posterior costophrenic sulcus is deeper than the lateral sulcus, small effusions are detected more readily on a lateral radiograph than on the frontal view.[123, 124]

Ultrasonography, CT, and MR imaging allow more effective detection of small or loculated effusions and distinction of effusions from pleural thickening.[121] Because of its ready availability and utility for bedside imaging, ultrasonography has become a particularly important imaging

modality, not only in determining the presence of pleural fluid, but also as a guide to therapeutic and diagnostic aspiration (*see* Fig. 3–54).[125, 126] Ultrasonography has been shown to be superior to lateral decubitus radiography in the quantification of pleural fluid.[127]

Typical Configuration of Free Pleural Fluid

Normally the opacity produced by an effusion on a PA radiograph is high laterally and curves gently downward and medially with a smooth, meniscus-shaped upper border, terminating along the midcardiac border. In lateral projection, because the fluid has ascended along the anterior and posterior thoracic wall to roughly an equal extent, the upper surface of the fluid density is semicircular, being high anteriorly and posteriorly and curving smoothly downward to its lowest point in the midaxillary line. Comparison of the maximal height of the fluid density in the PA and lateral projections shows that this height is identical posteriorly, laterally, and anteriorly (Fig. 3–55) (i.e., the top of the fluid accumulation is *horizontal*); the meniscus shape is caused by the fact that the layer of fluid is of insufficient depth to cast a discernible shadow when viewed *en face*.[128, 129]

The first place fluid accumulates in the erect patient is between the inferior surface of the lower lobe and the diaphragm; in effect, the lung floats on a layer of fluid. A subpulmonary location of fluid is *usual* in the normal pleural space[119, 123] (although it would be reasonable to consider subpulmonary accumulation of a large amount of

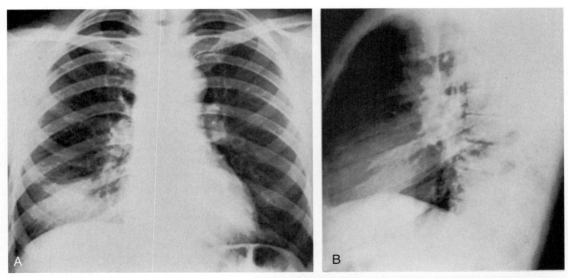

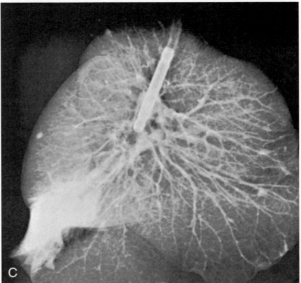

Figure 3–52. Segmental Atelectasis and Consolidation, Posterior Basal Segment, Right Lower Lobe. Posteroanterior *(A)* and lateral *(B)* radiographs show a homogeneous opacity localized to the posterior bronchopulmonary segment of the right lower lobe; no air bronchogram is present. The process is consolidative and atelectatic, the latter evidenced by posterior displacement of the major fissure. A lateral radiograph of the resected lung *(C)* shows the precise segmental nature of the disease; as a result of preoperative chemotherapy, the bronchial obstruction had been relieved partly so that the operative specimen shows a well-defined air bronchogram. Squamous cell carcinoma of the posterior basal bronchus was diagnosed.

fluid as atypical). Subpulmonary effusion causes a configuration in the erect patient that closely simulates diaphragmatic elevation (thus the designation *pseudodiaphragmatic contour*). It may be unilateral or bilateral, the former more commonly on the right.[130] Several signs are helpful in detection of subpulmonary effusion.

1. In PA projection (Fig. 3–56), the peak of the pseudodiaphragmatic configuration is lateral to that of the normal hemidiaphragm, being situated near the junction of the middle and lateral thirds rather than near the center, and slopes down sharply toward the lateral costophrenic sulcus.[123, 128]

2. On the left side, the pseudodiaphragmatic contour is separated farther than normal from the gastric air bubble, and effusion should be suspected when there is a greater than 2 cm distance between the two.[119] Care is needed to detect interposition of the spleen or the left lobe of the liver and to exclude the presence of gross ascites, which occasionally can simulate subpulmonic effusion.[131]

3. On lateral projection, a characteristic configuration frequently is seen anteriorly where the convex upper margin of the fluid meets the major fissure. In these cases, the contour anterior to the fissure is flattened, this portion of the pseudodiaphragmatic contour descending abruptly to the anterior costophrenic sulcus.[123, 128]

4. Pulmonary vessels, which normally are visible below the diaphragmatic contour, cannot be seen through the pseudodiaphragmatic contour of a subpulmonic effusion. Care should be taken to exclude underexposed radiographs, lower lobe consolidation, and ascites, all of which may cause similar findings.[132]

Distribution of Pleural Effusion in the Supine Patient

In the supine patient, free pleural fluid layers posteriorly and produces a hazy increase in opacity without obscuration of the bronchovascular markings.[119, 128] With small pleural effusions, the increase in opacity is limited to the lower lung zones; as the amount of fluid increases, there is

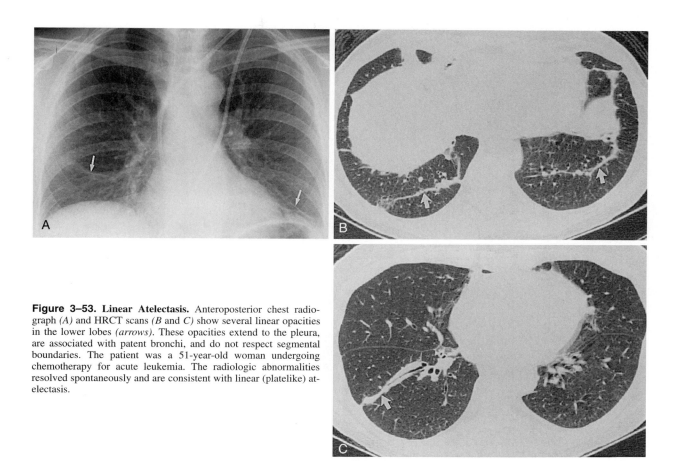

Figure 3–53. Linear Atelectasis. Anteroposterior chest radiograph *(A)* and HRCT scans *(B* and *C)* show several linear opacities in the lower lobes *(arrows)*. These opacities extend to the pleura, are associated with patent bronchi, and do not respect segmental boundaries. The patient was a 51-year-old woman undergoing chemotherapy for acute leukemia. The radiologic abnormalities resolved spontaneously and are consistent with linear (platelike) atelectasis.

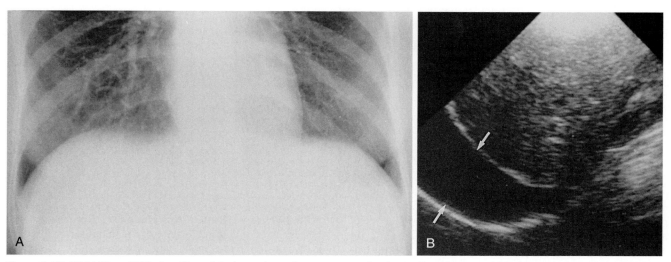

Figure 3–54. Right Pleural Effusion. View of the lower thorax from anteroposterior chest radiograph *(A)* is essentially normal except for questionable minimal blunting of the right costophrenic sulcus. Ultrasound *(B)* shows right pleural effusion *(arrows)*.

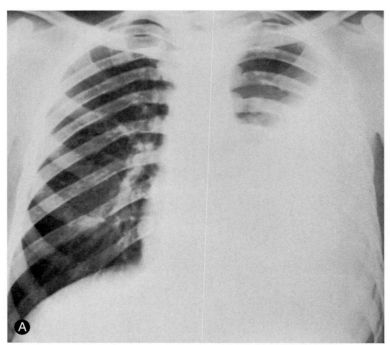

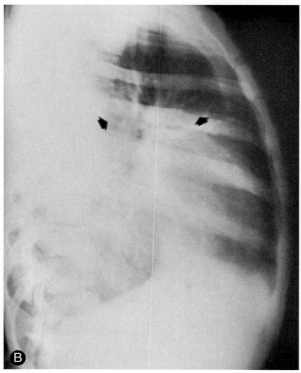

Figure 3–55. Large Pleural Effusion: Typical Arrangement. Posteroanterior *(A)* and lateral *(B)* radiographs exposed in the upright position show uniform opacification of the lower two thirds of the left hemithorax. The upper level of the fluid is meniscus shaped in posteroanterior and lateral projections *(arrows on B)*. Only the right hemidiaphragm is visualized in the lateral projection, the left being obscured by fluid (the silhouette sign).

progressive cephalad extension of the increased opacity until the entire hemithorax is involved (Fig. 3–57).[133] An apical fluid cap is seen on supine radiographs in approximately 50% of patients who have large effusions.[133]

Compared with lateral decubitus radiographs, supine radiographs have a relatively low sensitivity and specificity in the diagnosis of pleural effusions.[122] In one prospective analysis of anteroposterior supine radiographs, pleural effusions were identified correctly on supine radiographs in 24 of 36 cases (sensitivity 67%) and excluded correctly in 18 of 26 cases (specificity 70%). The most helpful diagnostic findings were increased opacity of the hemithorax, blunting of the costophrenic angle, and obscuration of the hemidiaphragm.[122]

Pleural effusions are characterized on CT scan by attenuation values between those of water (0 HU) and soft tissue (approximately 100 HU); except when small,[134] effusions usually can be distinguished readily from pleural thickening or pleural masses (Fig. 3–58).[135] On CT scan of a supine patient, free pleural fluid accumulates first in the

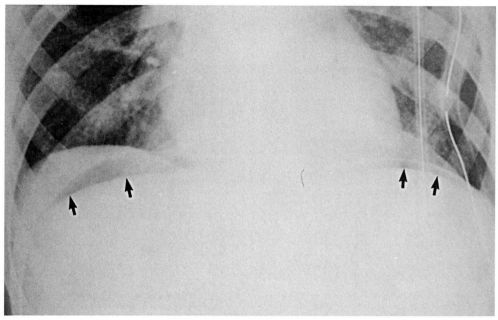

Figure 3–56. Subpulmonic Effusion. View of the lower chest from upright anteroposterior chest radiograph reveals the presence of pneumoperitoneum *(arrows)* and of a small right subpulmonic pleural effusion. Note the characteristic distribution of subpulmonic effusion with a flat upper surface medially and a steep lateral drop-off. On the left side, the normal thickness of the hemidiaphragm is approximately 1 mm.

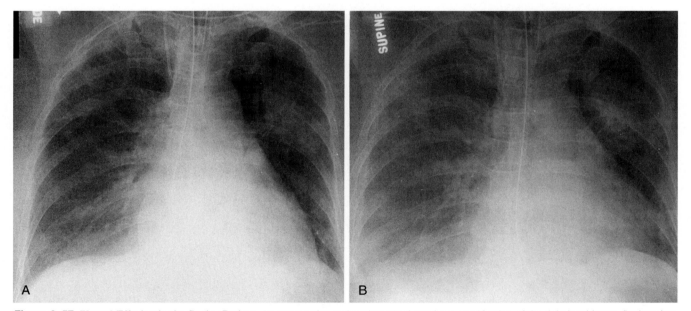

Figure 3–57. Pleural Effusion in the Supine Patient. Anteroposterior supine view *(A)* shows hazy opacification of the right hemithorax. Supine view of the chest 24 hours later *(B)* shows further increase in opacity of the right hemithorax, obscuration of the lateral border of the right hemidiaphragm, blunting of the right costophrenic sulcus, and fluid extending cephalad along the lateral chest wall. The patient was a 60-year-old woman who developed a large right pleural effusion after liver transplantation.

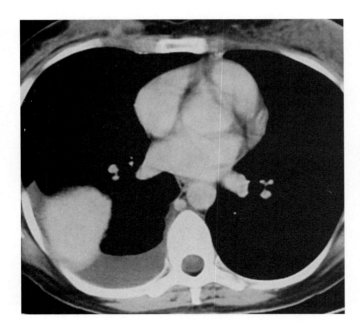

Figure 3–58. Pleural Effusion. Contrast-enhanced CT scan shows a small right pleural effusion. The near-water density of pleural fluid allows ready distinction from the pleural-based mass. The patient was a 35-year-old woman with right pleural effusion associated with a localized fibrous tumor of the pleura.

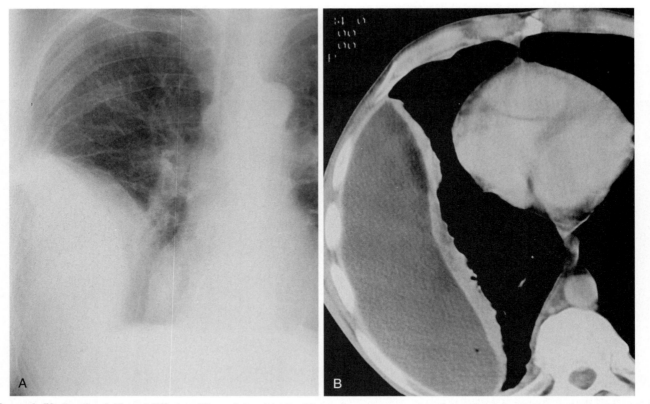

Figure 3–59. Loculated Pleural Effusion. View of the right hemithorax from posteroanterior chest radiograph *(A)* shows sharply demarcated, homogeneous opacity with convex borders with the lung and displacing the adjacent parenchyma. Contrast-enhanced CT scan *(B)* shows right pleural effusion associated with enhancement and thickening of the visceral and parietal pleura and compressive atelectasis of the adjacent lung. The findings are characteristic of a loculated empyema. Visualization of enhancing thickened visceral and parietal pleura surrounding pleural fluid is known as the *split-pleura* sign.

posterior pleural recesses. Because the lung tends to maintain its shape as it loses volume, the fluid has a concave or meniscoid anterior margin. As the effusion increases in size, fluid extends cephalad and anteriorly and may extend into the major and right minor fissures.

Loculation of Pleural Fluid

A loculated effusion may occur anywhere in the pleural space—between the parietal and visceral pleura over the periphery of the lung or between visceral layers in the interlobar fissures. Loculation is caused by adhesions between contiguous pleural surfaces and tends to occur during or after episodes of pleuritis; it often is associated with pyothorax or hemothorax. Over the convexity of the thorax, a loculated effusion appears as a smooth, sharply demarcated, homogeneous opacity protruding into the hemithorax and compressing contiguous lung (Fig. 3–59).

Interlobar loculated effusions typically are elliptical when viewed tangentially on the chest radiograph, their extremities blending imperceptibly with the interlobar fissure (Fig. 3–60). In some conditions, particularly cardiac decompensation, the effusion may simulate a mass and be misdiagnosed as a pulmonary neoplasm;[137, 138] however, its distinctive configuration on PA or lateral projection should establish the diagnosis in most cases. Occasionally, CT or sonography is required for definitive diagnosis (Fig. 3–61).

These fluid accumulations tend to be absorbed spontaneously when the heart failure resolves and have been called *vanishing tumor (phantom tumor, pseudotumor)*.

Radiologic Signs of Pleural Thickening

Several radiologic features are helpful in differentiating the various causes of pleural thickening on radiographs and CT scans.[141] Evidence of underlying parenchymal disease usually is seen in patients who have had tuberculosis or empyema. Extensive calcification of the fibrothorax also favors these conditions and seldom is seen with asbestos-related diffuse pleural thickening.[139] Pleural plaques are identified radiologically as circumscribed areas of pleural thickening, typically 3 to 10 mm in thickness and 1 to 5 cm in length (Fig. 3–62). They usually are associated with a history of asbestos exposure. Diffuse asbestos-related pleural thickening is considered to be present when there is a smooth uninterrupted pleural opacity extending over at least one fourth of the chest wall with or without associated obliteration of the costophrenic sulci (Fig. 3–63).[121, 140] Pleural thickening secondary to hemorrhagic effusion, tuberculosis, and empyema usually is unilateral, whereas that related to asbestos usually is bilateral, whether manifested as diffuse thickening or as plaques.[89, 141]

When pleural fibrosis is extensive, it seldom involves the mediastinal pleura (*see* Fig. 3–63).[141] This feature is

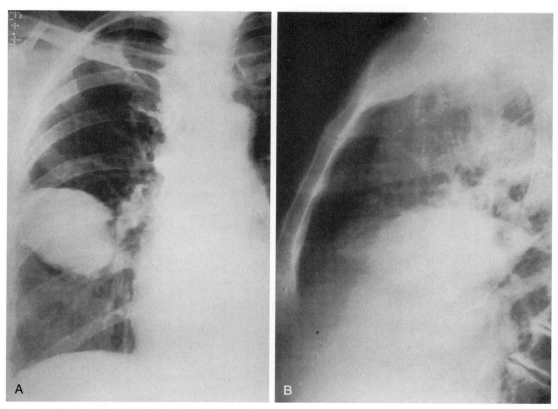

Figure 3–60. Pleural Effusion Localized to the Minor Fissure. View of the right hemithorax from a posteroanterior radiograph *(A)* shows a sharply circumscribed, homogeneous opacity in the right midlung zone. In lateral projection *(B)*, the true nature of the opacity can be appreciated: The mass is elliptical in shape, its pointed extremities being situated anteriorly and posteriorly in keeping with the position of the minor fissure. This unusual collection of pleural fluid developed during a recent episode of cardiac decompensation. With appropriate therapy, it disappeared completely in 3 weeks (*vanishing tumor*).

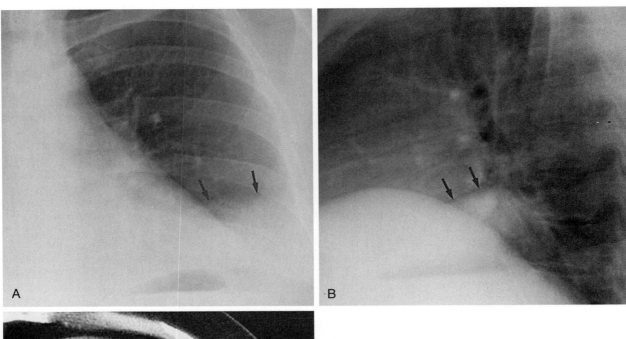

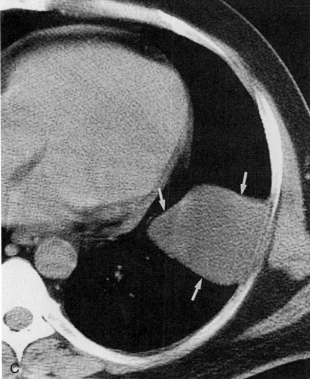

Figure 3–61. **Loculated Interlobar Effusion.** View of the left hemithorax from posteroanterior *(A)* chest radiograph shows poorly defined opacity *(arrows)* in the left lower chest. View from lateral radiograph *(B)* reveals that the opacity lies in the region of the interlobar fissure *(arrows)*. CT scan *(C)* shows characteristic appearance of fluid within the left major fissure *(arrows)*. The fluid collection tapers medially. Diagnosis of a transudate was made by fine-needle aspiration under ultrasound guidance. Follow-up chest radiographs 6 months later showed resolution of the fluid collection.

helpful in the differential diagnosis of benign from malignant causes of pleural thickening. For example, in one study, only 1 (12%) of 8 patients who had fibrothorax had mediastinal pleural thickening compared with 8 (72%) of 11 who had mesothelioma (Fig. 3–64).[141] (The *mediastinal pleura* is defined as the pleura that abuts the mediastinum, the posterior extent of which is demarcated by the anterior aspect of the vertebrae.[121, 142]) The parietal pleura abutting the paravertebral sulci is not part of the anatomic mediastinal pleura and most commonly is referred to as the *paravertebral pleura*.[136, 141]

Radiologic Signs of Pneumothorax

Pneumothorax in the Upright Patient

A radiologic diagnosis of pneumothorax can be made only by identifying the visceral pleural line. The visceral pleural line is visualized as a sharply defined line of increased opacity that can be distinguished readily from the black line owing to the Mach effect, which may be seen outlining a skin fold (Fig. 3–65).

In the erect patient, pneumothorax is first evident near the apex of the chest; a subpulmonic location has been

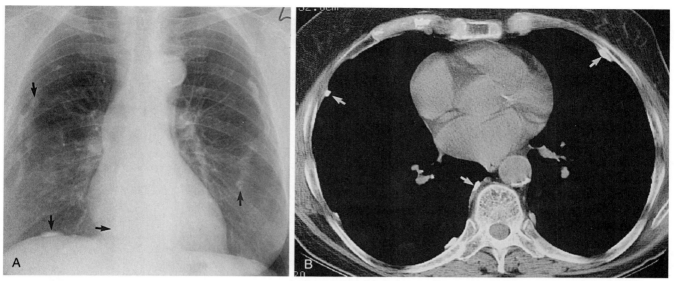

Figure 3–62. Calcified Asbestos-Related Pleural Plaques. Posteroanterior chest radiograph *(A)* and CT scan *(B)* show multiple bilateral, discrete, calcified pleural plaques *(arrows)* involving the costal, diaphragmatic, and paravertebral pleura. The patient was a 79-year-old man with previous occupational asbestos exposure.

reported occasionally in patients who have chronic obstructive pulmonary disease[143] or penetrating thoracic injury.[149] The visceral pleural line usually is readily identifiable, even on radiographs exposed at total lung capacity. In most cases, the inspiratory chest radiograph is the only imaging modality required for diagnosis. When pneumothorax is strongly suspected clinically but a pleural line is not identified (possibly because it is obscured by an overlying rib), gas in the pleural space can be detected by one of two procedures: (1) radiography in the erect position in full expiration (the rationale being that lung volume is reduced, while the volume of gas in the pleural space is constant, making it easier to detect the pneumothorax) and (2) radiography in the lateral decubitus position with a horizontal x-ray beam (the rationale being that air rises to the highest point in the hemithorax and is visible more clearly over the lateral chest wall than over the apex, where overlying bone shadows may obscure fine linear shadows). Although

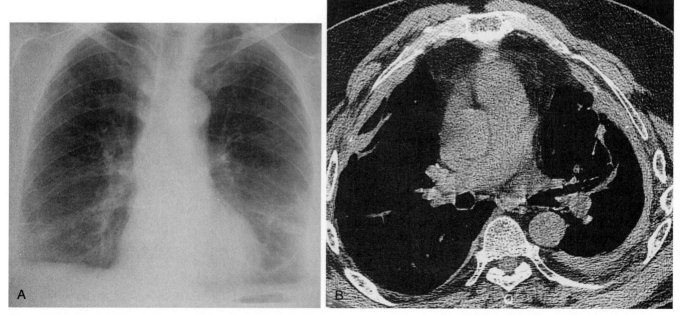

Figure 3–63. Pleural Fibrosis. Posteroanterior chest radiograph *(A)* shows extensive bilateral pleural thickening. The blunted costophrenic angles are angulated sharply rather than meniscus shaped, a finding helpful in distinguishing pleural thickening from pleural effusion. Curved bands of increased opacity extend from the left lung to the pleural thickening, a feature most commonly related to asbestos. CT scan *(B)* reveals marked bilateral pleural thickening with small areas of calcification. Although there is marked thickening of the costal and paravertebral pleura, the mediastinal pleura is free. The patient was a 53-year-old man with a history of exposure to asbestos.

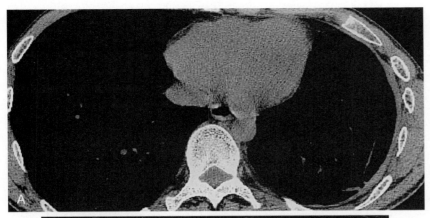

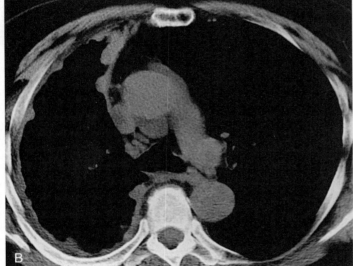

Figure 3–64. Benign Versus Malignant Pleural Thickening. Benign pleural thickening is shown *(A)*; CT scan shows smooth thickening of the left costal pleura with no associated pleural effusion or involvement of the mediastinal pleura. The patient was a 32-year-old man with surgically proven benign fibrothorax, presumably caused by previous pleurisy. Malignant pleural thickening is shown *(B)*; CT scan shows right pleural thickening that is diffuse and nodular in nature. At surgical biopsy, this thickening was shown to represent a mesothelioma. In both cases, the size of the affected hemithorax is decreased, a finding that is not helpful in distinguishing benign from malignant pleural thickening.

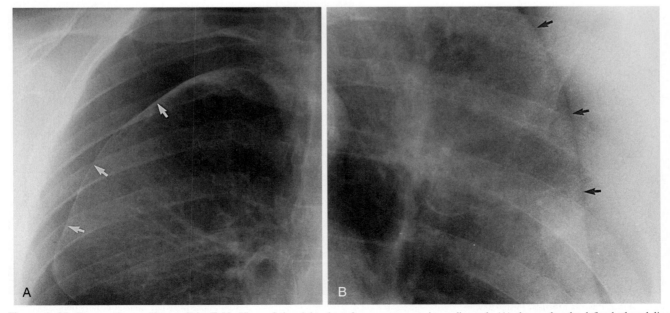

Figure 3–65. Pneumothorax Versus Skin Fold. View of the right chest from posteroanterior radiograph *(A)* shows sharply defined pleural line *(arrows)* characteristic of a pneumothorax. View of the left chest from anteroposterior radiograph *(B)* shows a skin fold. The black line *(arrows)* seen at the edge of the skin fold is due to Mach effect.

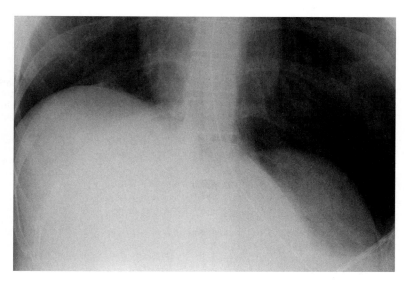

Figure 3–66. Pneumothorax with Deep Sulcus Sign. View of the lower chest from an anteroposterior chest radiograph with the patient supine shows a radiolucent left costophrenic sulcus and a sharply defined left hemidiaphragm. These findings are characteristic of a pneumothorax in a supine patient.

upright expiratory radiographs are obtained in most patients in whom pneumothorax is suspected clinically, the lateral decubitus view provides an excellent alternative when an upright expiratory radiograph cannot be obtained or when the upright view provides equivocal findings.[144–146]

Pneumothorax in the Supine Patient

When patients who have suspected pneumothorax must be examined in the supine position, as is often the case in the intensive care unit, gas within the pleural space rises to the vicinity of the diaphragm, the highest point in the hemithorax in this position. Depending on the size of the pneumothorax, the result can be an exceptionally deep radiolucent costophrenic sulcus (*deep sulcus sign*) (Fig. 3–66),[149] a lucency over the right or left upper quadrant,[147] or a much sharper than normal appearance of the hemidiaphragm with or without the presence of a visceral pleural line visible above it.[149] Other findings include visualization of the anterior costophrenic sulcus, increased sharpness of the cardiac border, collection of air within the minor fissure, and depression of the ipsilateral hemidiaphragm.[148–150] When a pneumothorax is suspected in a supine patient, confirmation can be obtained most readily by performing a lateral decubitus view with the involved hemithorax uppermost.[144–146] CT has also been shown to be useful and is superior to frontal chest radiography.[148]

References

1. McLoud TC, Carrington CB, Gaensler EA: Diffuse infiltrative lung disease: A new scheme for description. Radiology 149:353, 1983.
2. Mathieson JR, Mayo JR, Staples CA, et al: Chronic diffuse infiltrative lung disease: Comparison of diagnostic accuracy of CT and chest radiography. Radiology 171:111, 1989.
3. Glossary of terms for thoracic radiology: Recommendations of the nomenclature committee of the Fleischner Society. Am J Roentgenol 143:509, 1984.
4. Austin JHM, Müller NL, Friedman PJ, et al: Glossary of terms for CT of the lungs: Recommendations of the nomenclature committee of the Fleischer Society. Radiology 200:327, 1996.
5. Itoh H, Murata K, Konishi J, et al: Diffuse lung disease: Pathologic basis for the high-resolution computed tomography findings. J Thorac Imaging 8:176, 1993.
6. Heitzman ER, Markarian B, Berger I, et al: The secondary pulmonary lobule: A practical concept for interpretation of chest radiographs. Radiology 93:513, 1969.
7. Felson B: Chest Roentgenology. Philadelphia, WB Saunders, 1973.
8. Genereux GP: The Fleischner lecture: Computed tomography of diffuse pulmonary disease. J Thorac Imaging 4:50, 1989.
9. Müller NL, Miller RR: State of the art: Computed tomography of chronic diffuse infiltrative lung disease: I. Am Rev Respir Dis 142:1206, 1990.
10. Müller NL, Miller RR: State of the art: Computed tomography of chronic diffuse infiltrative lung disease: II. Am Rev Respir Dis 142:1440, 1990.
11. Grenier P, Valeyre D, Cluzel P, et al: Chronic diffuse interstitial lung disease: Diagnostic value of chest radiography and high-resolution CT. Radiology 179:123, 1991.
12. Müller NL: Clinical value of high-resolution CT in chronic diffuse lung disease. Am J Roentgenol 157:1163, 1991.
13. Colby TV, Swensen SJ: Anatomic distribution and histopathologic patterns in diffuse lung disease: Correlation with HRCT. J Thorac Imaging 11:1, 1996.
14. Stein MG, Mayo J, Müller N, et al: Pulmonary lymphangitic spread of carcinoma: Appearance on CT scans. Radiology 162:371, 1987.
15. Hirakata K, Nakata H, Nakagawa T: CT of pulmonary metastases with pathological correlation. Semin Ultrasound CT MR 16:379, 1995.
16. Bessis L, Callard P, Gotheil C, et al: High-resolution CT of parenchymal lung disease: Precise correlation with histologic findings. Radiographics 12:45, 1992.
17. Munk PL, Müller NL, Miller RR, et al: Pulmonary lymphangitic carcinomatosis: CT and pathologic findings. Radiology 166:705, 1988.
18. Webb WR, Stein MG, Finkbeiner WE, et al: Normal and diseased isolated lungs: High-resolution CT. Radiology 166:81, 1988.
19. Müller NL, Kullnig P, Miller RR: The CT findings of pulmonary sarcoidosis: Analysis of 25 patients. Am J Roentgenol 152:1179, 1989.
20. Murch CR, Carr DH: Computed tomography appearances of pulmonary alveolar proteinosis. Clin Radiol 40:240, 1989.
21. Kang EY, Grenier P, Laurent F, et al: Interlobular septal thickening: Patterns at high-resolution CT. J Thorac Imaging 11:260, 1996.
22. Johkoh T, Müller NL, Ichikado K, et al: Perilobular pulmonary opacities: High-resolution CT findings and pathologic correlation. J Thorac Imaging 14:172, 1999.
23. Johkoh T, Itoh H, Müller NL, et al: Crazy-paving appearance at thin-section CT: Spectrum of disease and pathologic findings. Radiology 211:155, 1999.
24. Nishimura K, Kitaichi M, Izumi T, et al: Usual interstitial pneumonia: Histologic correlation with high-resolution CT. Radiology 182:337, 1992.
25. Webb WR, Müller NL, Naidich DP: High-Resolution CT of the Lung. 2nd ed. Philadelphia, Lippincott-Raven, 2001, pp 71–192.
26. Müller NL, Chiles C, Kullnig P: Pulmonary lymphangiomyomatosis: Correlation of CT with radiographic and functional findings. Radiology 175:335, 1990.

27. Primack SL, Hartman TE, Hansell DM, et al: End-stage lung disease: CT findings in 61 patients. Radiology 189:681, 1993.
28. Hogg JC: Chronic interstitial lung disease of unknown cause: A new classification based on pathogenesis. Am J Roentgenol 156:225, 1991.
29. Genereux GP: The end-stage lung: Pathogenesis, pathology, and radiology. Radiology 116:279, 1975.
30. Staples CA, Müller NL, Vedal S, et al: Usual interstitial pneumonia: Correlation of CT with clinical, functional, and radiologic findings. Radiology 162:377, 1987.
31. Templeton PA, McLoud TC, Müller NL, et al: Pulmonary lymphangioleiomyomatosis: CT and pathologic findings. J Comput Assist Tomogr 13:54, 1989.
32. Kwong JS, Carignan S, Kang EY, et al: Miliary tuberculosis: Diagnostic accuracy of chest radiography. Chest 110:339, 1996.
33. Coppage L, Shaw C, Curtis AM: Metastatic disease to the chest in patients with extrathoracic malignancy. J Thorac Imaging 2:24, 1987.
34. Murata K, Takahashi M, Mori M, et al: Pulmonary metastatic nodules: CT-pathologic correlation. Radiology 182:331, 1992.
35. Remy-Jardin M, Degreef JM, Beuscart R, et al: Coal worker's pneumoconiosis: CT assessment in exposed workers and correlation with radiographic findings. Radiology 177:363, 1990.
36. Bégin R, Bergeron D, Samson L, et al: CT assessment of silicosis in exposed workers. Am J Roentgenol 148:509, 1987.
37. Im J-G, Itoh H, Shim Y-S, et al: Pulmonary tuberculosis: CT findings—early active disease and sequential change with antituberculous therapy. Radiology 186:653, 1993.
38. Aquino SL, Gamsu G, Webb WR, et al: Tree-in-bud pattern: Frequency and significance on thin-section CT. J Comput Assist Tomogr 20:594, 1996.
39. Müller NL, Miller RR: Diseases of the bronchioles: CT and histopathologic findings. Radiology 196:3, 1995.
40. Gruden JF, Webb WR, Naidich DP, et al: Multinodular disease: Anatomic localization at thin section CT—multireader evaluation of a simple algorithm. Radiology 210:711, 1999.
41. Remy-Jardin M, Remy J, Giraud F, et al: Computed tomography assessment of ground-glass opacity: Semiology and significance. J Thorac Imaging 8:249, 1993.
42. Leung AN, Miller RR, Müller NL: Parenchymal opacification in chronic infiltrative lung diseases: CT-pathologic correlation. Radiology 188:209, 1993.
43. Bergin CJ, Wirth RL, Berry GJ, et al: *Pneumocystis carinii* pneumonia: CT and HRCT observations. J Comput Assist Tomogr 14:756, 1990.
44. Moskovic E, Miller R, Pearson M: High resolution computed tomography of *Pneumocystis carinii* pneumonia in AIDS. Clin Radiol 42:239, 1990.
45. Primack SL, Miller RR, Müller NL: Diffuse pulmonary hemorrhage: Clinical, pathologic, and imaging features. Am J Roentgenol 164:295, 1995.
46. Hartman TE, Primack SL, Müller NL, et al: Diagnosis of thoracic complications in AIDS: Accuracy of CT. Am J Roentgenol 162:547, 1994.
47. Silver SF, Müller NL, Miller RR, et al: Hypersensitivity pneumonitis: Evaluation with CT. Radiology 173:441, 1989.
48. Hansell DM, Moskovic E: High-resolution computed tomography in extrinsic allergic alveolitis. Clin Radiol 43:8, 1991.
49. Hartman TE, Primack SL, Swensen SJ, et al: Desquamative interstitial pneumonia: Thin-section CT findings in 22 patients. Radiology 187:787, 1993.
50. Godwin JD, Müller NL, Takasugi JE: Pulmonary alveolar proteinosis: CT findings. Radiology 169:609, 1988.
51. Müller NL, Colby TV: Idiopathic interstitial pneumonias: High-resolution CT and histologic findings. Radiographics 17:1016, 1997.
52. Felson B: A new look at pattern recognition of diffuse pulmonary disease. Am J Roentgenol 133:183, 1979.
53. Grenier P, Chevret S, Beigelman C, et al: Chronic diffuse infiltrative lung disease: Determination of the diagnostic value of clinical data, chest radiography, and CT with Bayesian analysis. Radiology 191:383, 1994.
54. Zwirewich CV, Vedal S, Miller RR, et al: Solitary pulmonary nodule: High-resolution CT and radiologic-pathologic correlation. Radiology 179:469, 1991.
55. Siegelman SS, Khouri NF, Leo FP, et al: Solitary pulmonary nodules: CT assessment. Radiology 160:307, 1986.

56. Zerhouni EA, Stitik FP, Siegelman SS, et al: CT of the pulmonary nodule: A cooperative study. Radiology 160:319, 1986.
57. Bleyer JM, Marks JH: Tuberculosis and hamartomas of the lung: Comparative study of 66 proved cases. Am J Roentgenol 77:1013, 1957.
58. Steele JD: The Solitary Pulmonary Nodule. Springfield, IL, Charles C Thomas, 1964.
59. Woodring JH, Fried M, Chuang VP: Solitary cavities of the lung: Diagnostic implications of cavity wall thickness. Am J Roentgenol 135:1269, 1980.
60. Lewall DB, McCorkell SJ: Rupture of echinococcal cysts: Diagnosis, classification, and clinical implications. Am J Roentgenol 146:391, 1986.
61. Danner PK, McFarland DR, Felson B: Massive pulmonary gangrene. Am J Roentgenol 103:548, 1968.
62. Penner C, Maycher B, Long R: Pulmonary gangrene: A complication of bacterial pneumonia. Chest 105:567, 1994.
63. Cordier JF, Valeyre D, Guillevin L, et al: Pulmonary Wegener's granulomatosis: A clinical and imaging study of 77 cases. Chest 97:906, 1990.
64. Huang RM, Naidich DP, Lubat E, et al: Septic pulmonary emboli: CT-radiographic correlation. Am J Roentgenol 153:41, 1989.
65. Kuhlman JE, Fishman EK, Teigen C: Pulmonary septic emboli: Diagnosis with CT. Radiology 174:211, 1990.
66. Kuhlman JE, Fishman EK, Kuhajda FP, et al: Solitary bronchioloalveolar carcinoma: CT criteria. Radiology 167:379, 1988.
67. Weisbrod GL, Chamberlain D, Herman SJ: Cystic change (pseudocavitation) associated with bronchioloalveolar carcinoma: A report of four patients. J Thorac Imaging 10:106, 1995.
68. Good CA: The solitary pulmonary nodule: A problem of management. Radiol Clin North Am 1:429, 1963.
69. Gurney JW: Determining the likelihood of malignancy in solitary pulmonary nodules with Bayesian analysis: I. Theory. Radiology 186:405, 1993.
70. O'Keefe ME Jr, Good CA, McDonald JR: Calcification in solitary nodules of the lung. Am J Roentgenol 77:1023, 1957.
71. Maile CW, Rodan BA, Godwin JD, et al: Calcification in pulmonary metastases. Br J Radiol 55:108, 1982.
72. Zwiebel BR, Austin JHM, Grimes MM: Bronchial carcinoid tumors: Assessment with CT of location and intratumoral calcification in 31 patients. Radiology 179:483, 1991.
73. Reich SB, Weinshelbaum A, Yee J: Correlation of radiographic measurements and pulmonary function tests in chronic obstructive pulmonary disease. Am J Roentgenol 144:695, 1985.
74. Kilburn KH, Warshaw RH, Thornton JC: Do radiographic criteria for emphysema predict physiologic impairment? Chest 197:1225, 1995.
75. Sutinen S, Christoforidis AJ, Klugh GA, et al: Roentgenologic criteria for the recognition of nonsymptomatic pulmonary emphysema: Correlation between roentgenologic findings and pulmonary pathology. Am Rev Respir Dis 91:69, 1965.
76. Pratt PC: Role of conventional chest radiography in diagnosis and exclusion of emphysema. Am J Med 82:998, 1987.
77. Franken EA, Buehl I: Infantile lobar emphysema: Report of two cases with the usual roentgenographic manifestations. Am J Roentgenol 98:354, 1966.
78. Kennedy CD, Habibi P, Matthew DJ, et al: Lobar emphysema: long-term imaging follow-up. Radiology 180:189, 1991.
79. Simon G, Reid L: Atresia of an apical bronchus of the left upper lobe: Report of three cases. Br J Dis Chest 57:126, 1963.
80. Jederlinic PJ, Sicilian LS, Baigelman W, et al: Congenital bronchial atresia: A report of 4 cases and a review of the literature. Medicine (Baltimore) 65:73, 1986.
81. Woodring JH: Pitfalls in the radiologic diagnosis of lung cancer. Am J Roentgenol 154:1165, 1990.
82. Byrd RB, Miller WE, Carr DT, et al: The roentgenographic appearance of squamous cell carcinoma of the bronchus. Mayo Clin Proc 43:327, 1968.
83. Byrd RB, Miller WE, Carr DT, et al: The roentgenographic appearance of large cell carcinoma of the bronchus. Mayo Clin Proc 43:333, 1968.
84. Byrd RB, Miller WE, Carr DT, et al: The roentgenographic appearance of small cell carcinoma of the bronchus. Mayo Clin Proc 43:337, 1968.
85. Grimes OF, Farber SM: Air cysts of the lung. Surg Gynecol Obstet 113:720, 1961.
86. Feraru F, Morrow CS: Surgery of subpleural blebs: Indications and contraindications. Am Rev Respir Dis 79:577, 1959.

87. Quigley MJ, Fraser RS: Pulmonary pneumatocele: Pathology and pathogenesis. Am J Roentgenol 150:1275, 1988.
88. Reed JC: Chest Radiology: Plain Film Patterns and Differential Diagnoses. 3rd ed. St. Louis, Mosby-Year Book, 1997, pp 185–210.
89. Aberle DR, Gamsu G, Ray CS, et al: Asbestos-related pleural and parenchymal fibrosis: Detection with high-resolution CT. Radiology 166:729, 1988.
90. Gamsu G, Aberle DR, Lynch D: Computed tomography in the diagnosis of asbestos-related thoracic disease. J Thorac Imaging 4:61, 1989.
91. Bergin CJ, Castellino RA, Blank N, et al: Specificity of high-resolution CT findings in pulmonary asbestosis: Do patients scanned for other indications have similar findings? Am J Roentgenol 163:551, 1994.
92. Yoshimura H, Hatakeyama M, Otsuji H, et al: Pulmonary asbestosis: CT study of curvilinear shadow. Radiology 158:653, 1986.
93. Primack SL, Remy-Jardin M, Remy J, et al: High-resolution CT of the lung: Pitfalls in the diagnosis of infiltrative lung disease. Am J Roentgenol 167:413, 1996.
94. Woodring JH, Reed JC: Types and mechanisms of pulmonary atelectasis. J Thorac Imaging 11:92, 1996.
95. Schneider HJ, Felson B, Gonzalez LL: Rounded atelectasis. Am J Roentgenol 134:225, 1980.
96. Cho S-R, Henry DA, Beachley MC, et al: Round (helical) atelectasis. Br J Radiol 54:643, 1981.
97. Hayashi K, Kohzaki S, Uetani M, et al: Rounded atelectasis with emphasis on its wide spectrum. Nippon Acta Radiol 53:1020, 1993.
98. Batra P, Brown K, Hayashi K, et al: Rounded atelectasis. J Thorac Imaging 11:187, 1996.
99. Lee KS, Ahn JM, Im JG, et al: Lobar atelectasis: Typical and atypical radiographic and CT findings. Postgrad Radiol 15:203, 1995.
100. Hillerdal G: Rounded atelectasis: Clinical experience with 74 patients. Chest 95:836, 1989.
101. McHugh K, Blaquiere RM: CT features of rounded atelectasis. Am J Roentgenol 153:257, 1989.
102. Carvalho PM, Carr DH: Computed tomography of folded lung. Clin Radiol 41:86, 1990.
103. Verschakelen JA, Demaerel P, Coolen J, et al: Rounded atelectasis of the lung: MR appearance. Am J Roentgenol 152:965, 1989.
104. Stancato-Pasik A, Mendelson DS, Marom Z: Rounded atelectasis caused by histoplasmosis. Am J Roentgenol 155:275, 1990.
105. Iannuzzi M, Petty TL: The diagnosis, pathogenesis, and treatment of adult respiratory distress syndrome. J Thorac Imaging 1:1, 1986.
106. Westcott JL, Cole SR: Traction bronchiectasis in end-stage pulmonary fibrosis. Radiology 161:665, 1986.
107. Proto AV, Tocino I: Radiographic manifestations of lobar collapse. Semin Roentgenol 15:117, 1980.
108. Reinig JW, Ross P: Computed tomography appearance of Golden's "S" sign. CT. J Comput Tomogr 8:219, 1984.
109. Khoury MB, Godwin JD, Halvorsen RA Jr, et al: CT of obstructive lobar collapse. Invest Radiol 20:708, 1985.
110. Kattan KR, Eyler WR, Felson B: The juxtaphrenic peak in upper lobe collapse. Semin Roentgenol 15:187, 1980.
111. Cameron DC: The juxtaphrenic peak (Katten's [sic] sign) is produced by rotation of an inferior accessory fissure. Australas Radiol 37:332, 1993.
112. Davis SD, Yankelevitz DF, Ward A, et al: Juxtaphrenic peak in upper and middle lobe volume loss: Assessment with CT. Radiology 198:143, 1996.
113. Golden R: The effect of bronchostenosis upon the roentgen-ray shadows in carcinoma of the bronchus. Am J Roentgenol Radiat Ther 13:21, 1925.
114. Zdansky E: Bemerkung zur atelektatischen Retraktion des linken Oberlappens. [Atelectatic retraction of the left upper lobe.] Fortschr Roentgenstr 100:725, 1964.
115. Webber M, Davies P: The Luftsichel: An old sign in upper lobe collapse. Clin Radiol 32:271, 1981.
116. Cohen BA, Robinowitz JG, Mendleson DS: The pulmonary ligament. Radiol Clin North Am 22:659, 1984.
117. Fisher MS: Significance of a visible major fissure on the frontal chest radiograph. Am J Roentgenol 137:577, 1981.
118. Friedman PJ: Radiology of the superior segment of the lower lobe: A regional perspective, introducing the B(6) bronchus sign. Radiology 144:15, 1982.
119. Hessén I: Roentgen examination of pleural fluid: A study of the localization of free effusion: The potentialities of diagnosing minimal quantities of fluid and its existence under physiological conditions. Acta Radiol 86(Suppl), 1951.
120. Collins JD, Burwell D, Furmanski S, et al: Minimal detectable pleural effusions. Radiology 105:51, 1972.
121. Müller NL: Imaging of the pleura. Radiology 186:297, 1993.
122. Ruskin JA, Gurney JW, Thorsen MK, et al: Detection of pleural effusions on supine chest radiographs. Am J Roentgenol 148:681, 1987.
123. Raasch BN, Carsky EW, Lane EJ, et al: Pleural effusion: Explanation of some typical appearances. Am J Roentgenol 139:899, 1982.
124. Henschke CI, Davis SD, Romano PM, et al: The pathogenesis, radiologic evaluation, and therapy of pleural effusions. Radiol Clin North Am 27:1241, 1989.
125. Lipscomb DJ, Flower CDR, Hadfield JW: Ultrasound of the pleura: An assessment of its clinical value. Clin Radiol 32:289, 1981.
126. O'Moore PV, Mueller PR, Simeone JF, et al: Sonographic guidance in diagnostic and therapeutic interventions in the pleural space. Am J Roentgenol 149:1, 1987.
127. Eibenberger KL, Dock WI, Ammann ME, et al: Quantification of pleural effusions: Sonography versus radiography. Radiology 191:681, 1994.
128. Fleischner FG: Atypical arrangement of free pleural effusion. Radiol Clin North Am 1:347, 1963.
129. Davis S, Gardner F, Ovist G: The shape of a pleural effusion. BMJ 1:436, 1963.
130. Dunbar JS, Favreau M: Infrapulmonary pleural effusion with particular reference to its occurrence in nephrosis. J Can Assoc Radiol 10:24, 1959.
131. Kafura PJ, Barnhard JH: Ascites simulating subpulmonary pleural effusion. Radiology 101:525, 1971.
132. Schwartz MI, Marmorstein BL: A new radiologic sign of subpulmonic effusion. Chest 67:176, 1975.
133. Woodring JH: Recognition of pleural effusion on supine radiographs: How much fluid is required? Am J Roentgenol 142:59, 1984.
134. Pugatch RD, Faling LJ, Robbins AH, et al: Differentiation of pleural and pulmonary lesions using computed tomography. J Comput Assist Tomogr 2:601, 1978.
135. Maffessanti M, Tommasi M, Pellegrini P: Computed tomography of free pleural effusions. Eur J Radiol 7:87, 1987.
136. Im JG, Webb WR, Rosen A, et al: Costal pleura: Appearance at high-resolution CT. Radiology 171:125, 1989.
137. Feldman DJ: Localized interlobar pleural effusion in heart failure. JAMA 146:408, 1951.
138. Weiss W, Boucot KR, Gefter WI: Localized interlobular effusion in congestive heart failure. Ann Intern Med 38:1177, 1953.
139. Friedman AC, Fiel SB, Radecki PD, et al: Computed tomography of benign pleural and pulmonary parenchymal abnormalities related to asbestos exposure. Semin Ultrasound CT MR 11:393, 1990.
140. McLoud TC, Woods BO, Carrington CB, et al: Diffuse pleural thickening in an asbestos-exposed population: Prevalence and causes. Am J Roentgenol 144:9, 1985.
141. Leung AN, Müller NL, Miller RR: CT in differential diagnosis of diffuse pleural disease. Am J Roentgenol 154:487, 1990.
142. Platzer W: Pernkopf Anatomy: Atlas of Topographic and Applied Human Anatomy. Vol 2. Thorax, Abdomen, and Extremities. Baltimore, Urban & Schwarzenberg, 1989, p 63.
143. Christensen EE, Dietz GW: Subpulmonic pneumothorax in patients with chronic obstructive pulmonary disease. Radiology 121:33, 1976.
144. Carr JJ, Reed JC, Choplin RH, et al: Conventional film and computed radiography of experimentally induced pneumothoraces in cadavers: Implications for detection in patients. Radiology 183:193, 1992.
145. Beres RA, Goodman LR: Pneumothorax: Detection with upright versus decubitus radiography. Radiology 186:19, 1993.
146. Beres RA, Goodman LR: Pneumothorax detection: Clarifications and additional thoughts. Radiology 186:25, 1993.
147. Rhea JT, van Sonnenberg E, McLoud TC: Basilar pneumothorax in the supine adult. Radiology 133:595, 1979.
148. Tocino IM, Miller MH, Fairfax WR: Distribution of pneumothorax in the supine and semirecumbent critically ill adult. Am J Roentgenol 144:901, 1985.
149. Schulman A, Dalrymple RB: Subpulmonary pneumothorax. Br J Radiol 51:494, 1978.
150. Spizarny Dl, Goodman LR: Air in the minor fissure: A sign of right-sided pneumothorax. Radiology 160:329, 1986.

Developmental and Hereditary Lung Disease

For purposes of discussion, developmental anomalies of the lungs can be divided into two major groups, depending on the *predominant* structure affected: (1) anomalies originating in the primitive foregut or its lung bud (bronchopulmonary anomalies) and (2) anomalies arising from the sixth aortic arch or venous radicals and their derivatives (pulmonary vascular anomalies). Despite the convenience of this division and the use of specific terms for various anatomic patterns of disease, considerable overlap exists between conditions in both groups,[1, 2] and multiple lesions occasionally are identified in the same patient.[3] Although strictly speaking not developmental in nature, many abnormalities of pulmonary mesenchymal tissue that have a proven or possible hereditary basis also are discussed in this chapter.

DEVELOPMENTAL ANOMALIES AFFECTING THE AIRWAYS AND LUNG PARENCHYMA

Pulmonary Agenesis, Aplasia, and Hypoplasia

Arrested development of the lung can be classified into three types:[4] (1) *agenesis*, in which there is complete absence of one or both lungs, with no trace of bronchial or vascular supply or of parenchymal tissue; (2) *aplasia*, in which there is suppression of all but a rudimentary bronchus that ends in a blind pouch, with no evidence of pulmonary vasculature or parenchyma; and (3) *hypoplasia*, in which the gross morphology of the lung essentially is unremarkable but in which there is a decrease in the number or size of airways, vessels, and alveoli. Although most evidence suggests that patients who have unilateral pulmonary agenesis usually die in the neonatal period, survival into adulthood, sometimes without symptoms, is possible.[5, 6] The number of individuals who survive with hypoplasia, especially the less severe forms, is much greater.

The radiographic findings in cases of agenesis, aplasia, or severe hypoplasia are similar and are characterized principally by total or almost total absence of aerated lung in one hemithorax (Table 4–1). The markedly reduced volume is indicated by approximation of the ribs, elevation of the ipsilateral hemidiaphragm, and shift of the mediastinum. In most cases, the contralateral lung is greatly overinflated and displaced, along with the anterior mediastinum, into the involved hemithorax;[7] this displacement of air-containing lung to the side of the agenesis may lead to some confusion in diagnosis. Computed tomography (CT) may be required to establish the degree of underdevelopment[8] or to differentiate agenesis from other conditions that may mimic it closely radiographically, including total atelectasis from any cause, severe bronchiectasis with collapse, and

Table 4–1. PULMONARY AGENESIS, APLASIA, AND HYPOPLASIA: MAIN RADIOLOGIC FEATURES

Partial or complete absence of aerated lung
Markedly reduced lung volume
Complete absence of lung (agenesis)
Rudimentary bronchus, no artery, no lung (aplasia)
Small bronchus and pulmonary artery, small lung (hypoplasia)
No air-trapping on expiratory radiograph

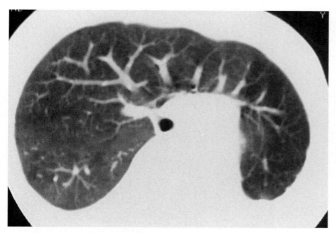

Figure 4–1. Pulmonary Agenesis. CT scan at the level of the bronchus intermedius in an 18-year-old man shows absence of the left lung with compensatory overinflation of the right lung. No left bronchus or pulmonary artery was identified on CT.

advanced fibrothorax (Fig. 4–1).[135] The diagnosis of pulmonary agenesis also can be made with magnetic resonance (MR) imaging.[136] In patients who have aplasia, CT can show the rudimentary bronchus as well as absence of the ipsilateral pulmonary artery;[8] in patients with hypoplasia, CT can show the patent bronchus, the pulmonary artery, and the hypoplastic lung.[8]

The main differential diagnosis of hypoplastic lung is Swyer-James syndrome (*see* Chapter 15). Although both conditions are associated with unilateral reduction in lung volume, patients who have Swyer-James syndrome show air-trapping on radiographs or high-resolution computed tomography (HRCT) scans performed at the end of maximal expiration.[9, 10]

Bronchopulmonary Sequestration

Bronchopulmonary sequestration is a pulmonary malformation in which a portion of pulmonary tissue is segregated from the remainder of the normal lung and receives its blood supply from a systemic artery. The anomaly may be intralobar or extralobar. An intralobar anomaly lies contiguous with normal lung parenchyma and within the same visceral pleural envelope; an extralobar anomaly is enclosed within its own pleural membrane, usually in close proximity to the normal lung but sometimes within or below the diaphragm.

Most authors believe that extralobar and intralobar sequestration represent an anomaly of embryonic tracheobronchial branching characterized by persistence and localized development of a separate branch fragment and retention of its initial systemic vascular supply.[12] Others consider that the intralobar form of disease is an acquired abnormality, however, the initial event being bronchial obstruction, possibly as a result of infection, followed by fibrosis and cyst formation in the distal lung.[13, 14] The inflammatory process is hypothesized to interrupt the pulmonary blood flow into the affected lung segment; hypertrophy of systemic arteries in the pulmonary ligament then results in the anomalous vascular supply.

Intralobar Sequestration

Intralobar sequestration accounts for approximately 75% of bronchopulmonary sequestrations.[14, 15] Although most commonly diagnosed in children and young adults, it may be recognized at any age. Most patients are asymptomatic until an acute respiratory infection develops; in many cases, this infection does not occur until adulthood.[17, 21] Signs and symptoms are usually those of acute lower lobe pneumonia, the basic defect becoming apparent only through radiologic observation of the sequence of changes during resolution of the infection.

The abnormal tissue invariably derives its arterial supply from the aorta or one of its branches, most commonly the descending thoracic aorta and less often the abdominal aorta or one of its branches.[14, 15] In 95% of cases, the venous drainage is through the pulmonary venous system, producing a left-to-left shunt; in 5% of cases, the drainage is into the inferior vena cava or azygos system.[14, 15]

The most common radiographic presentation is a homogeneous opacity in the posterior basal segment of a lower lobe (usually the left and almost invariably contiguous with the hemidiaphragm) (Fig. 4–2); less commonly, intralobar sequestration presents as a cystic mass or prominent vessels (Fig. 4–3; Table 4–2).[11, 14, 16] Definitive diagnosis is based on the demonstration of the anomalous systemic arterial supply to the sequestered lobe. This diagnosis traditionally has been made with aortography, a procedure that allows assessment of the origin of the arterial supply, the presence of one or more tributary vessels, and the assessment of the venous drainage.[14, 15] Identification of the systemic arterial supply also can be made in most cases by CT (*see* Figs. 4–2 and 4–3).[14, 16] The demonstration of the origin and course of the anomalous systemic vessel supplying the sequestered lung has improved considerably with the advent of spiral CT and the use of multiplanar re-formations.[14, 18]

Although MR imaging has been performed in only a few cases, it allows excellent visualization of vessels in multiple imaging planes and may obviate the need for angiography.[14, 134] MR imaging may show vessels not visualized at arteriography.[20]

Extralobar Sequestration

Extralobar pulmonary sequestration accounts for approximately 25% of cases of sequestration.[14, 15] The abnor-

Table 4–2. BRONCHOPULMONARY SEQUESTRATION: MAIN RADIOLOGIC FEATURES

	Intralobar	Extralobar
Arterial supply	Aorta	Aorta
Venous drainage	Pulmonary veins	Systemic veins
Findings	Homogeneous opacity or cystic mass	Homogeneous opacity
Location	Lower lobe adjacent to diaphragm	Lower lobe adjacent to diaphragm
Side	Left in ⅔ of cases	Left in 90% of cases
Congenital anomalies	Uncommon	Very common
Typical age of diagnosis	Children, young adults	First 6 months of life

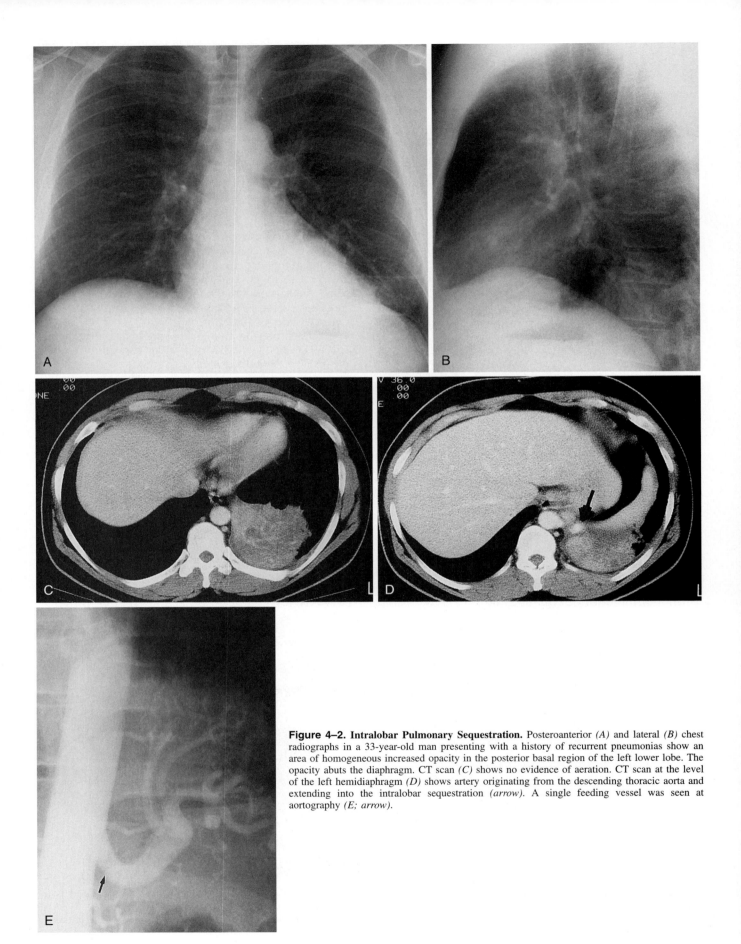

Figure 4–2. Intralobar Pulmonary Sequestration. Posteroanterior *(A)* and lateral *(B)* chest radiographs in a 33-year-old man presenting with a history of recurrent pneumonias show an area of homogeneous increased opacity in the posterior basal region of the left lower lobe. The opacity abuts the diaphragm. CT scan *(C)* shows no evidence of aeration. CT scan at the level of the left hemidiaphragm *(D)* shows artery originating from the descending thoracic aorta and extending into the intralobar sequestration *(arrow)*. A single feeding vessel was seen at aortography *(E; arrow)*.

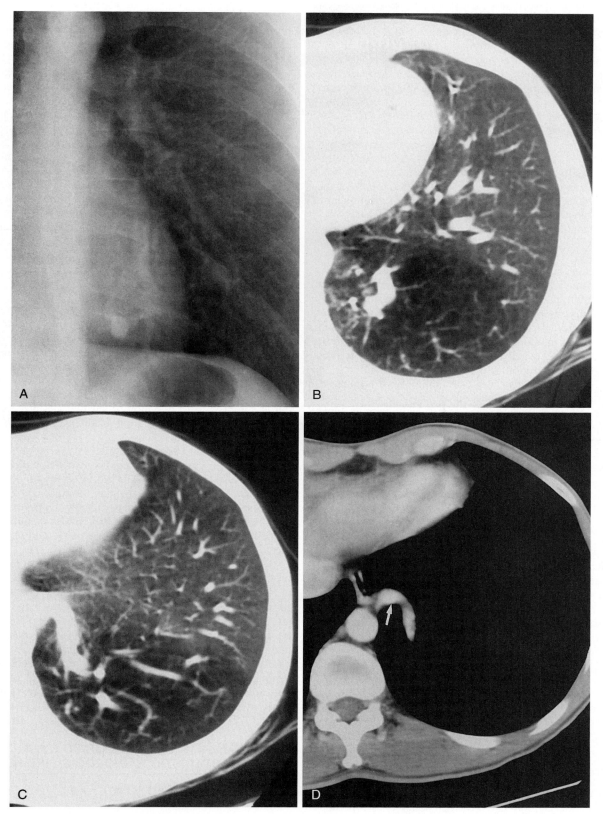

Figure 4–3. Intralobar Pulmonary Sequestration. Posteroanterior chest radiograph *(A)* in a 35-year-old man shows enlarged vessels in the left lower lobe. CT scans *(B* and *C)* show an area of decreased attenuation in the posterior left lung with associated anterior displacement of the left lower lobe vessels. Contrast-enhanced CT scan *(D)* shows that the feeding vessel *(arrow)* originates from the descending thoracic aorta.

mality often is associated with other congenital anomalies, particularly eventration or paralysis of the ipsilateral hemidiaphragm, which is present in approximately 60% of cases, and left-sided diaphragmatic hernia, present in approximately 30%.[15, 24] Because of symptoms related to associated congenital anomalies, most cases are discovered in early childhood (approximately 60% in the first 6 months of life).[24]

The systemic arterial supply is commonly from the abdominal aorta or one of its branches usually through a single feeding vessel; occasionally the vessels are multiple and small.[17, 24] In contrast to intralobar sequestration, drainage is usually through the systemic venous system—the inferior vena cava, the azygos or hemiazygos veins, or the portal venous system[23, 24]—resulting in a left-to-right shunt.

Radiographic findings typically consist of a sharply defined, triangular-shaped opacity in the posterior costophrenic angle usually adjacent to the left hemidiaphragm (*see* Table 4–2).[15, 24] Extralobar sequestration may appear as a small bump on the left hemidiaphragm.[24] Less commonly, the abnormality presents as a mass in the upper thorax, mediastinum, paravertebral region, or (rarely) subdiaphragmatic region.[22, 24] Aortography usually shows the anomalous systemic arterial supply;[15, 24] multiple feeding vessels can be shown in about 20% of cases.[24] Identification of the venous drainage, usually into a systemic vein, may require selective catheterization of the feeding vessels.[24]

The CT findings consist most commonly of a homogeneous opacity or well-circumscribed mass.[16, 24] Cystic areas are seen occasionally.[16] In one study of eight patients, areas of low attenuation in the surrounding nonsequestered lung were described in seven.[16] CT is of limited value in showing the vascular supply; in one review of 24 cases of sequestration, an anomalous systemic artery was identified on CT scan in 13 of 16 (81%) that were intralobar but in only 3 of 8 (37%) that were extralobar.[16]

Congenital Bronchogenic Cysts

Intrathoracic cysts derived from the foregut may be classified into three major categories according to their presumed embryologic derivation:[25] (1) *paravertebral (neuroenteric) cysts*, arising from a primordial foregut that has herniated through a split in the notochord—they often are associated with spinal anomalies; (2) *esophageal cysts (esophageal duplication)*, resulting from failure of the originally solid esophagus to produce completely a hollow tube; and (3) *bronchogenic cysts*, resulting from abnormal budding of the developing tracheobronchial tree. Approximately 65% to 90% of bronchogenic cysts occur in the mediastinum; almost all the remainder are present in the lungs.[26, 27] Rare examples are found in the pericardium, thymus, diaphragm, retroperitoneum, or cervical region.[27–29]

Pulmonary Bronchogenic Cysts

Most patients with pulmonary bronchogenic cysts are asymptomatic. Symptoms—of which hemoptysis is perhaps the most common—almost always are secondary to infection in and around the cyst.[36, 37] The typical appearance of an intrapulmonary bronchogenic cyst is a sharply circumscribed, round or oval nodule or mass, usually in the medial

third of the lungs. There is a predilection for the lower lobes—in one report of 32 cases, almost two thirds were in this location—with equal distribution in the two lungs.[31] Characteristically, the lesions usually do not communicate with the tracheobronchial tree until they become infected, a complication that occurs in about 75% of cases recognized clinically. When communication is established, the cyst contains air, with or without fluid.[31]

In approximately 50% of cases, a confident diagnosis can be made on CT scan based on the presence of nonenhancing homogeneous attenuation at or near water density (0 to 20 HU) and a smooth, thin wall.[8, 19] In approximately 50% of cases, the cysts have higher than water density as a result of the presence of proteinaceous material or calcium.[32, 33] When infected, the cysts may have inhomogeneous enhancement and resemble an abscess.[34] The cysts may be air filled and multilocular.[27] MR imaging is superior to CT in diagnosis.[34, 35] The characteristic findings consist of homogeneous high-signal intensity (approximating that of cerebrospinal fluid) on T2-weighted spin-echo images.

Mediastinal Bronchogenic Cysts

Mediastinal bronchogenic cysts occur most commonly in the paratracheal and subcarinal regions.[27, 31] Less common locations include hilar region, periesophageal region, thymus, pericardium, and anterolateral surface of a thoracic vertebral body.[27] Many patients are asymptomatic;[38, 41] however, in one surgical review of 69 patients, almost two thirds complained of a symptom attributable to the cyst.[42] Symptoms include dyspnea on effort, stridor, persistent cough, and chest pain.[30, 43]

Mediastinal bronchogenic cysts usually present as clearly defined masses of homogeneous density in the right paratracheal region (Fig. 4–4) or just inferior to and slightly to the right of the carina, overlapping the right hilar shadow (Table 4–3). Most are oval or round; the shape may vary with inspiration and expiration. In contrast to pulmonary bronchogenic cysts, the mediastinal variety rarely communicates with the tracheobronchial tree.[39]

A diagnosis of a benign cyst can be made confidently on CT scan when it shows a homogeneous attenuation at or near water density (0 to 20 HU) (*see* Fig. 4–4).[27, 32] In approximately 50% of patients, the cysts have higher attenuation (130 HU) and are indistinguishable from soft tissue lesions. Similar to pulmonary cysts, this increase in attenuation is the result of a high protein level or calcium oxalate in the mucoid cyst contents.[32, 40] The difficulty in distinguishing a soft tissue lesion from a cystic one may be resolved by MR imaging. With this procedure, bronchogenic cysts show variable signal intensity on T1-weighted

Table 4–3. BRONCHOGENIC CYST: CHARACTERISTIC RADIOLOGIC FINDINGS

65–90% occur in the mediastinum
Most commonly paratracheal or subcarinal in location
Sharply circumscribed, round, or oval
50% have water density on CT
No enhancement after intravenous contrast
Virtually all have homogeneous high-signal intensity on T2-weighted MR images

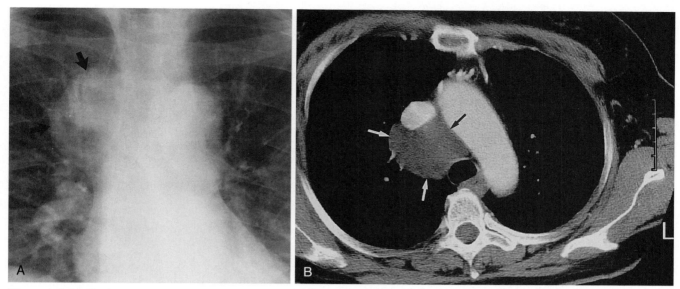

Figure 4–4. Mediastinal Bronchogenic Cyst. View from a posteroanterior chest radiograph *(A)* in a 60-year-old woman shows a right paratracheal mass *(arrows)*. Contrast-enhanced CT scan *(B)* shows that the lesion *(arrows)* has homogeneous water density characteristic of a bronchial cyst. The attenuation value was 9 HU.

images but characteristically have homogeneous high signal intensity on T2-weighted sequences (Fig. 4–5).[34, 35]

Congenital Cystic Adenomatoid Malformation

The term *congenital cystic adenomatoid malformation* refers to a group of several pathologically distinct abnormalities characterized by architecturally abnormal pulmonary tissue with or without gross cyst formation. When present, the cysts usually can be shown to communicate with normal airways. Most often, the vascular supply is by way of the pulmonary circulation; however, some lesions have a systemic blood supply.[44, 45]

As might be expected, most cases are discovered in the very young; in one review of 142 patients from the literature and 17 new cases, 62% of affected individuals presented between birth and 1 month of age;[46] an additional 24% of cases became manifest after 1 month, mostly in the first 5 years of life. Cases have been discovered in adults up to 61 years of age.[47, 49] Most patients present with increasing respiratory distress in the neonatal period, the severity being related chiefly to the volume of lung involved. A few patients present later in life with cough and fever, with or without recurrent respiratory infection;[49] most of these patients are older than 1 month of age. Spontaneous pneumothorax occurs occasionally.[49]

In older children and adults, the lesion usually appears radiologically as a lower lobe soft tissue mass containing numerous air-containing cysts. It is space-occupying, expanding the ipsilateral hemithorax and shifting the mediastinum to the contralateral side. Occasionally, one cyst expands preferentially, creating a single lucent area (Fig. 4–6).[48, 49] The cysts may contain fluid, air, or both. Fluid levels are seen occasionally; only rarely does fluid fill the cysts completely, resulting in complete radiographic opacification.[48] CT is superior to chest radiography in showing the cystic and solid components of the abnormality.[49, 50]

Congenital Bronchial Atresia

Congenital bronchial atresia consists of atresia or stenosis of a lobar, segmental, or subsegmental bronchus at or near its origin. The apicoposterior segmental bronchus of the left upper lobe is affected most commonly, followed by segmental bronchi of the right upper lobe, middle lobe, and lower lobe.[52] Most patients are asymptomatic. Some present with a history of recurrent pneumonia.[53, 54] Pectus excavatum has been noted in some individuals.[53]

Chest radiographs reveal an area of pulmonary hyperlucency in 90% of cases, a hilar mass in 80%, and a combination of both findings in 70% (Table 4–4).[54] The hyperlucency results from a combination of oligemia and an increase in the volume of air within the affected segment.[54] Adjacent normal lung is compressed and displaced; the mediastinum may or may not show displacement. Accumulation of secretions and mucoid impaction distal to the bronchial atresia result in ovoid, round, branching opacities near the hilum in most cases.[51]

CT is the most sensitive imaging technique for confirming the diagnosis.[51] It allows excellent visualization of the mucoid impaction, segmental hyperlucency, and decreased vascularity,[8, 56] a combination of findings that generally is considered diagnostic.[19] Mucoid impaction is recognized readily by the presence of branching soft tissue densities in a bronchial distribution, usually associated with bronchial dilation (Fig. 4–7).[55] Although a similar appearance has

Table 4–4. CONGENITAL BRONCHIAL ATRESIA: CHARACTERISTIC RADIOLOGIC FINDINGS

Usually apicoposterior segment left upper lobe
Hyperlucency, decreased vascularity, and air-trapping of affected segment
Hilar mass (bronchocele) or branching soft tissue opacities (mucoid impaction)
Findings best seen on CT

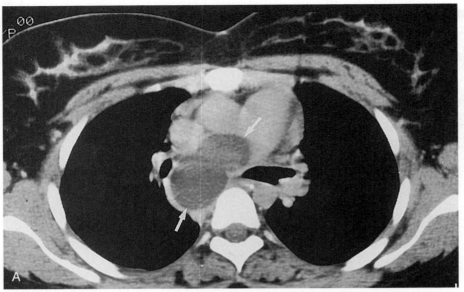

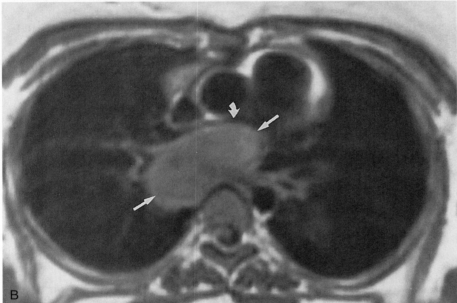

Figure 4–5. Mediastinal Bronchogenic Cyst. Contrast-enhanced CT scan *(A)* in a 26-year-old woman shows a dumbbell-shaped mass *(arrows)* with inhomogeneous attenuation in the subcarinal region. The attenuation values within the mass were greater than 20 HU. Transverse T1-weighted (TR/TE, 645/20) MR image *(B)* shows a slightly inhomogeneous mass *(straight arrows)* with a signal similar to that of chest wall muscle. There is marked narrowing of the right pulmonary artery *(curved arrow)*. Transverse T2-weighted (TR/TE, 2,581/90) spin-echo MR image *(C)* shows homogeneous high-signal intensity mass *(arrows)* characteristic of a fluid-filled cyst. At surgery, the lesion was shown to be a mediastinal bronchial cyst associated with a partial pericardial defect.

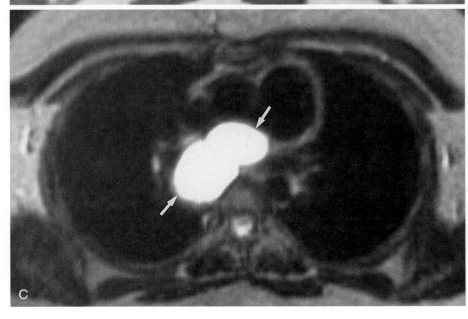

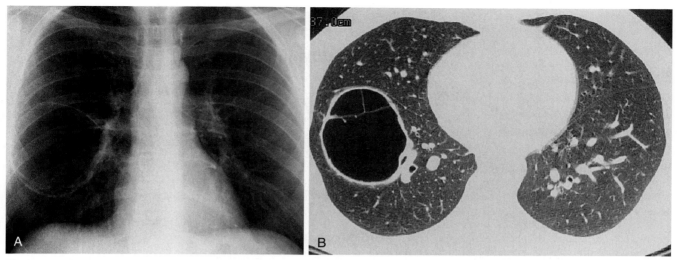

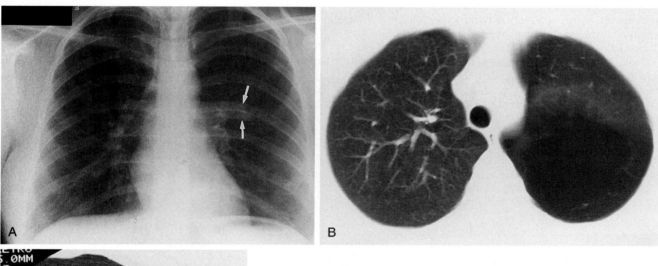

Figure 4–6. Congenital Cystic Adenomatoid Malformation. Posteroanterior chest radiograph *(A)* in a 31-year-old man shows large cystic lesion in the right lower lobe. HRCT scan *(B)* shows a few septations within the thin-walled cyst. At surgery, this was shown to be a type I cystic adenomatoid malformation.

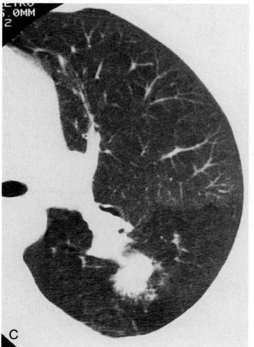

Figure 4–7. Bronchial Atresia. Posteroanterior chest radiograph *(A)* in a 14-year-old girl shows marked lucency and decreased vascularity in the left upper lobe. An ill-defined opacity is visible near the left hilum *(arrows)*. Conventional 10-mm collimation CT scan *(B)* shows marked decrease in attenuation and vascularity in the region of the apicoposterior segment of the left upper lobe. HRCT scan *(C)* shows focal opacity near the origin of the apicoposterior segmental bronchus and decreased attenuation of the adjacent lung.

been reported on MR imaging,[57, 58] CT is the imaging modality of choice.

DEVELOPMENTAL ABNORMALITIES AFFECTING THE PULMONARY VESSELS

Hypogenetic Lung (Scimitar) Syndrome

Hypogenetic lung (scimitar) syndrome is a rare congenital anomaly characterized principally by hypoplasia of the right lung and anomalous pulmonary venous drainage from it to the inferior vena cava.[59–61] The incidence is estimated to be 1 to 3 per 100,000 births.[62] The anomalous pulmonary vein most commonly drains into the inferior vena cava below the level of the right hemidiaphragm.[60, 61] Hypoplasia of the right pulmonary artery and partial or complete arterial supply to the right lung by systemic arteries originating from the descending thoracic or upper abdominal aorta also are usually present.[60] Greater than 50% of patients have cardiorespiratory symptoms, similar in many respects to symptoms experienced by patients who have large left-to-right shunts with pulmonary arterial hypertension.[60] Some patients have repeated bronchopulmonary infections or hemoptysis.

The anomalous vein usually is visible radiographically as a broad, gently curved shadow descending to the diaphragm just to the right of the heart; this shadow is shaped like a Turkish sword or scimitar, accounting for the designation, *scimitar* syndrome (Fig. 4–8).[64, 65]

The diagnosis can be made on the chest radiograph, the characteristic findings consisting of a small right lung with small hilum and diminished vascularity, a shift of the heart and mediastinum to the right, and the characteristic appearance of the anomalous draining vein coursing parallel to the right atrium.[63] If radiographic findings are not definitive, the diagnosis usually can be made with CT.[62, 66–68] The procedure also allows identification of associated abnormalities, such as bilobed right lung with absence of the minor fissure and horseshoe lung.[62, 68] The diagnosis also may be made using MR imaging.[69]

Pulmonary Arteriovenous Malformation

The term *pulmonary arteriovenous malformation* is used here to describe a spectrum of abnormal vascular communications between pulmonary arteries and pulmonary veins.[70] This spectrum ranges from microscopic communications that are too small to be visualized radiologically to complex aneurysms with multiple feeding arteries and draining veins, which may involve the entire blood supply of a segment or lobe and may have arterial communication with the neighboring chest wall or adjacent lung segments.[70] Eighty per cent to 90% consist of a single feeding artery and draining vein (simple arteriovenous malformation), and the remaining are complex with two or more feeding arteries or draining veins.[132, 133]

Approximately 70% of patients with pulmonary lesions have arteriovenous communications in the skin, mucous membranes, or other organs.[133] This disorder, known as *hereditary hemorrhagic telangiectasia* (Rendu-Osler-Weber disease), has an autosomal dominant non–sex-linked inheritance.[71] Although it is assumed that the vascular defect is present at birth, only 10% of cases are identified during childhood.[133]

The most common clinical manifestation is hemoptysis. Dyspnea is present in 60% of cases.[72] Other findings include cyanosis and finger clubbing. Symptoms of central nervous system disease may be the result of metastatic abscess, hypoxemia, cerebral thromboemboli, cerebral vas-

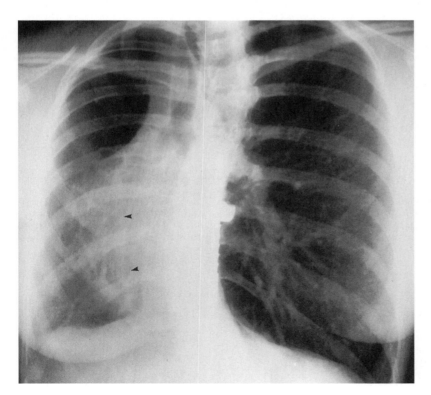

Figure 4–8. Hypogenetic Lung (Scimitar) Syndrome. Posteroanterior chest radiograph shows a small right hemithorax. The pulmonary vasculature of the right lung is diminutive and disorganized, whereas that of the left lung is normal. A large vascular shadow consistent with an anomalous vein *(arrowheads)*, coursing caudally from the midlung zone toward the cardiophrenic angle, can be identified through a dextroposed cardiac silhouette.

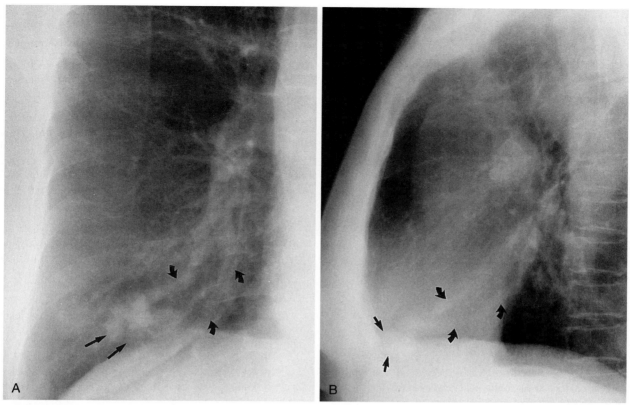

Figure 4–9. Pulmonary Arteriovenous Malformation. Views of the right lung from posteroanterior *(A)* and lateral chest radiographs *(B)* in a 71-year-old woman show a serpiginous soft tissue opacity in the right middle lobe *(straight arrows)*. The associated large feeding artery and draining vein *(curved arrows)* are diagnostic of arteriovenous malformation.

cular thrombosis from secondary polycythemia, and cerebral hemorrhage from a concomitant intracerebral arteriovenous aneurysm.[72, 76]

Pulmonary arteriovenous malformations are seen more commonly in the lower lobes than in the middle or upper lobes and are multiple in about one third of cases.[133] The characteristic radiographic appearance is a round or oval homogeneous mass of unit density, somewhat lobulated in contour but sharply defined, in the medial third of the lung, ranging from less than 1 cm to several centimeters in diameter (Fig. 4–9; Table 4–5). A feeding artery and draining vein often can be identified, the artery relating to the hilum and the vein deviating from the course of the artery toward the left atrium.

The characteristic CT finding consists of a homogeneous, circumscribed nodule or serpiginous mass connected with blood vessels.[73, 74] Optimal investigation of the malformations by CT requires the use of spiral volumetric CT.

This modality allows assessment of the entire lung in one or two breath-holds, minimizing the risk of missing small lesions. The procedure also enables image reconstruction of various levels within the lesion, facilitating depiction of the center of the malformation (Fig. 4–10).[73, 74] Despite the value of spiral CT, pulmonary angiography is performed routinely before treatment of arteriovenous malformations. Pulmonary angiography provides absolute confirmation of the presence of the malformation, analysis of the feeding arterial and draining venous structures, and detection of other malformations.[73, 75]

Anomalies of the Heart and Great Vessels
Anomalies Resulting in Increased Pulmonary Blood Flow

The most common anomaly resulting in increased pulmonary blood flow in the adult is atrial septal defect; less common causes include ventricular septal defect and patent ductus arteriosus. The left-to-right shunt results in some degree of increased pulmonary blood flow, which may be recognizable radiologically by an increase in size and amplitude of pulsation of the central and peripheral pulmonary arteries (Fig. 4–11).

Anomalies Resulting in Decreased Pulmonary Blood Flow

The most common cause of general pulmonary oligemia as a result of diminished flow is a congenital anomaly of

Table 4–5. PULMONARY ARTERIOVENOUS MALFORMATION: CHARACTERISTIC RADIOLOGIC FEATURES

Single (²⁄₃) or multiple (¹⁄₃ of cases)
Most commonly in lower lobes
Round, oval, or lobulated
Feeding artery and draining vein sometimes evident on radiograph
Spiral CT is diagnostic

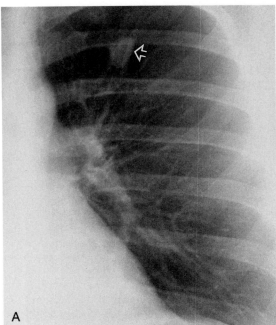

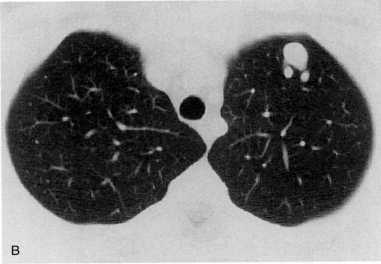

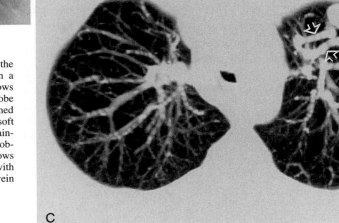

Figure 4–10. Arteriovenous Malformation. View of the left lung from posteroanterior chest radiograph *(A)* in a 33-year-old man with Rendu-Osler-Weber disease shows slightly lobulated soft tissue opacity in the left upper lobe *(arrow)*. A 5-mm collimation spiral CT scan performed without intravenous contrast material *(B)* shows the soft tissue opacity with the associated feeding artery and draining vein. Maximal intensity projection reconstruction obtained using the volumetric spiral CT data *(C)* allows better depiction of the vascular nature of the lesion with demonstration of the feeding artery and draining vein *(arrows)*.

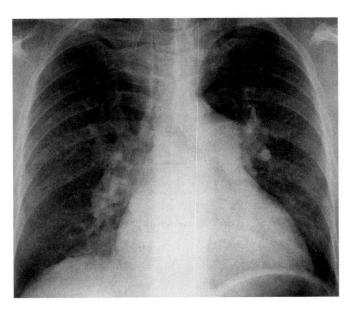

Figure 4–11. Increased Size of Pulmonary Vessels: Atrial Septal Defect. Posteroanterior chest radiograph in a 56-year-old man shows enlargement of the central pulmonary arteries and increased size of the peripheral vessels. Note mild cardiomegaly and decreased size of the aortic arch, findings frequently seen in patients with long-standing atrial septal defect. The patient had proven atrial septal defect with associated pulmonary arterial hypertension.

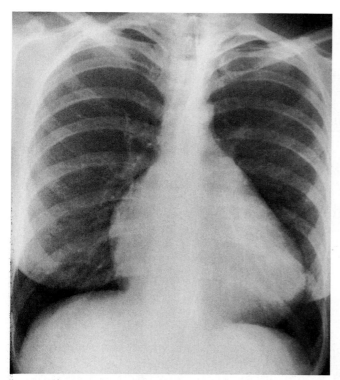

Figure 4–12. Diffuse Oligemia Without Overinflation: Ebstein's Anomaly. The peripheral pulmonary markings are diminished in caliber, and the hila are diminutive; the lungs are not overinflated. The contour of the markedly enlarged heart is consistent with Ebstein's anomaly.

the right ventricular outflow tract (isolated pulmonic stenosis, tetralogy of Fallot with pulmonary atresia, type IV persistent truncus arteriosus, and Ebstein's anomaly) (Fig. 4–12). The caliber of the pulmonary vessels generally reflects the severity of the reduction in flow, the hila usually being diminutive and the peripheral vessels correspondingly small (except with valvular pulmonic stenosis, in which poststenotic dilation may enlarge the main or left pulmonary artery) (Fig. 4–13).

Systemic Arterial Supply to the Lung

Systemic arterial supply to the lung may be congenital or acquired, and the supplied lung may be normal or abnormal.[77] The congenital form is seen in association with a variety of other anomalies, most often bronchopulmonary sequestration and occasionally hypogenetic lung syndrome, congenital cystic adenomatoid malformation, absence of the main pulmonary artery, and proximal interruption of a pulmonary artery.[61, 138] The anomaly may not be associated with symptoms or may result in cardiac decompensation secondary to a left-to-left shunt.[78] Rarely, it causes hemoptysis.[79]

The chest radiograph shows normal or increased vascular markings.[81, 83] The increased blood flow from the systemic artery causes dilation of the draining inferior pulmonary veins, which may result in a tubular shadow visible radiographically in the left lower lobe.[79, 80] The dilated vein and the increased vascularity in the lower lobe are recognized readily on CT scan (Fig. 4–14).[79, 80] Ipsilateral

rib notching may be present.[82] Pulmonary angiography, CT, or MR imaging can be used to determine whether there is an absence of pulmonary arterial supply to the involved lung.

HEREDITARY ABNORMALITIES OF PULMONARY CONNECTIVE TISSUE

Marfan's Syndrome

Marfan's syndrome is characterized by abnormally long extremities (particularly the fingers and toes), subluxation of the lens, and cardiovascular abnormalities (particularly aortic dilation and dissection).[84, 85] Its incidence has been estimated to be about 5 per 100,000.[85] Marfan's syndrome shows an autosomal dominant pattern of inheritance with variable penetrance.[86] Aortic dissection often is manifested by the sudden onset of chest pain; in a patient who has Marfan's syndrome, this complaint should lead to its rapid diagnosis or exclusion (pneumothorax being the most likely differential diagnosis).

The most common chest radiograph manifestations are a long thin thorax, scoliosis, and pectus excavatum;[87] in one series of 50 patients, 34 (68%) had pectus deformity and 22 (44%) had scoliosis (Table 4–6).[85] The most frequently reported pulmonary abnormality is spontaneous pneumothorax,[87–89] a complication that arises in about 5% to 10% of patients (values that are several hundred times greater than those of the general population).[87, 88] Other pulmonary manifestations include apical bullae (Fig. 4–15) and, less commonly, diffuse emphysema, bronchiectasis, or upper lobe fibrosis.[87–89]

Cardiovascular disease develops in most patients who have Marfan's syndrome and is the cause of death in more than 90%.[90, 91] The most common abnormalities are aortic aneurysm, aortic dissection, and aortic and mitral valve insufficiency.[91] The first two of these conditions usually involve the ascending aorta (Fig. 4–16). Serial chest radiographs may show progressive aortic enlargement and commonly show cardiomegaly as a result of aortic regurgitation.[92] The diagnosis usually is confirmed by CT. Diagnostic features of aortic dissection include the presence of an intimal flap and a false lumen.[91, 92] Aortic aneurysms and dissection as well as the associated cardiovascular abnormalities can be recognized readily on MR imaging and echocardiography.[93, 94]

Lymphangioleiomyomatosis

Lymphangioleiomyomatosis (lymphangiomyomatosis) is a rare condition characterized by a predominantly peribronchovascular proliferation of smooth muscle cells asso-

Table 4–6. MARFAN'S SYNDROME: CHARACTERISTIC RADIOLOGIC FEATURES

Long, thin thorax
Scoliosis, pectus excavatum
Aortic enlargement caused by aneurysm or dissection
Cardiomegaly caused by aortic regurgitation
Apical bullae
Spontaneous pneumothorax

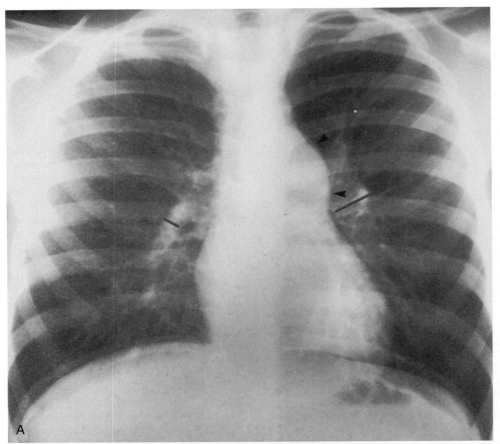

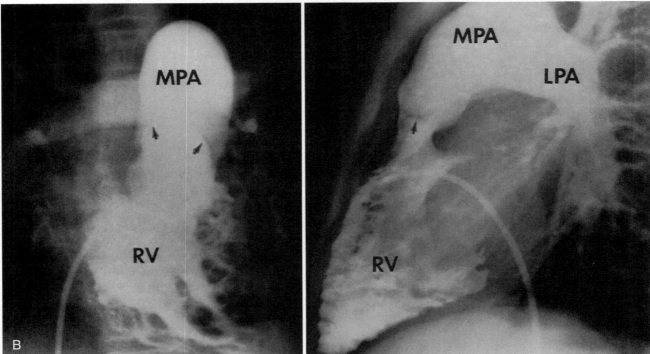

Figure 4–13. Valvular Pulmonary Stenosis with Poststenotic Arterial Dilation. Posteroanterior chest radiograph *(A)* shows a prominent main pulmonary artery *(arrowheads)* and a sharp discrepancy between the size of the right and left interlobar arteries at comparable levels *(oblique bars)*. The midlung vasculature is normal on both sides. These features should suggest pulmonary valvular stenosis with poststenotic dilation of the main and proximal left interlobular pulmonary arteries. Right ventricular (RV) angiogram *(B)* in anteroposterior *(left)* and lateral *(right)* projection reveals dilation of the right ventricle. The pulmonic valves *(arrows)* are thickened and domed, indicating stenosis. Note poststenotic dilation of the main pulmonary artery (MPA) and the proximal portion of the left interlobar artery (LPA).

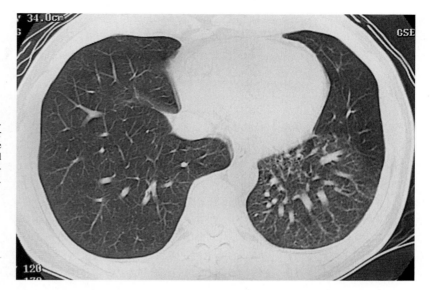

Figure 4–14. Systemic Arterial Supply to the Lung. CT scan shows increased vascularity of the left lower lobe caused by enlargement of the pulmonary veins. The systemic arterial supply to the left lower lobe originated from the descending thoracic aorta. The patient was a 54-year-old woman. The diagnosis was confirmed at surgery.

ciated with airway and vascular obstruction and cyst formation.[137] The disease is confined to women and is most common during the childbearing years, the average age at presentation being 30 to 35.[95] Lymphangioleiomyomatosis also can occur in postmenopausal women[96] and has been reported in a patient 72 years old.[97] In such individuals, it is possible that the onset of slowly progressive disease precedes clinical recognition.[97]

The presenting complaint usually is shortness of breath, sometimes gradual and sometimes acute, in which case there is usually an associated pneumothorax.[95] The latter manifestation can be troublesome because of either bilaterality or recurrence;[110, 111] for example, in one investigation of six patients, four had a total of 25 episodes.[100] Cough, hemoptysis, and chest pain are uncommon presenting symptoms but have been found to occur in 35% to 45% of patients at some time in the course of the disease.[95] Chylothorax is a common manifestation;[101] occasionally, chyle is coughed up (chyloptysis) or passed in the urine (chyluria).

The most common radiographic finding of lymphangioleiomyomatosis (seen in 80% to 90% of patients) is a bilateral reticular pattern (Fig. 4–17; Table 4–7).[102–104] In approximately 80% of cases, it involves all lung zones to a similar degree; in the remainder, it is more marked in the lower lung zones.[102] Cysts can be identified on the radiograph in 50% to 60% of cases.[103, 104] Evidence of hyperinflation with increase in the retrosternal air space or flattening of the diaphragm is seen at presentation in many patients.[102–104] Pneumothorax has been reported in 30% to 40% of cases[102, 104] and unilateral or bilateral pleural effusions in 10% to 20%.[102, 104] The pulmonary parenchymal abnormalities may precede, accompany, or follow the pleural manifestations.[102] In 2% to 20% of cases, the chest radiograph is normal.[102–104]

The characteristic HRCT finding consists of numerous air-filled cysts surrounded by normal lung parenchyma (Fig. 4–18).[102, 103] This pattern was observed in 107 of 108 patients reported in five studies.[102–106] Cysts can be seen in patients who have normal radiographs[102] or who have radiographs showing only reticular opacities.[102, 103] They usually measure between 0.2 and 2 cm in diameter, although they may be 6 cm.[102, 103] The size varies with the severity of disease; most patients with relatively mild involvement have cysts less than 1 cm in diameter.[102] Most

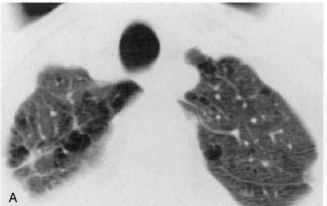

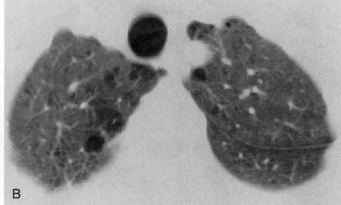

Figure 4–15. Marfan's Syndrome. CT scans *(A and B)* in a 29-year-old man with Marfan's syndrome show bilateral apical bullae. The bullae were found incidentally at CT being performed for assessment of aortic dissection.

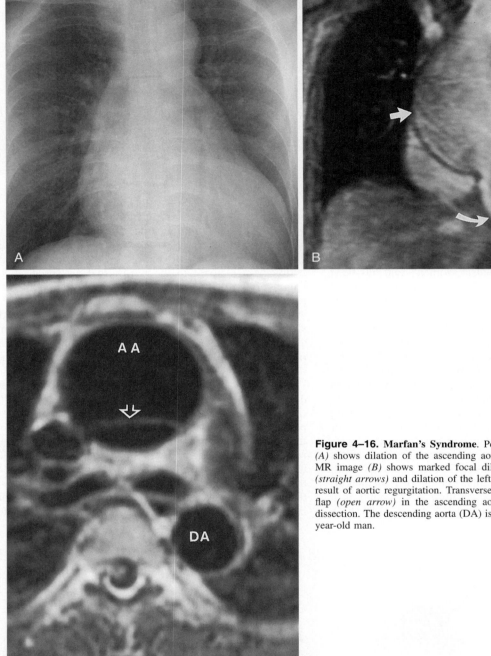

Figure 4–16. Marfan's Syndrome. Posteroanterior chest radiograph *(A)* shows dilation of the ascending aorta and cardiomegaly. Coronal MR image *(B)* shows marked focal dilation of the descending aorta *(straight arrows)* and dilation of the left ventricle *(curved arrows)* as a result of aortic regurgitation. Transverse MR image *(C)* shows intimal flap *(open arrow)* in the ascending aorta (AA) diagnostic of aortic dissection. The descending aorta (DA) is normal. The patient was a 32-year-old man.

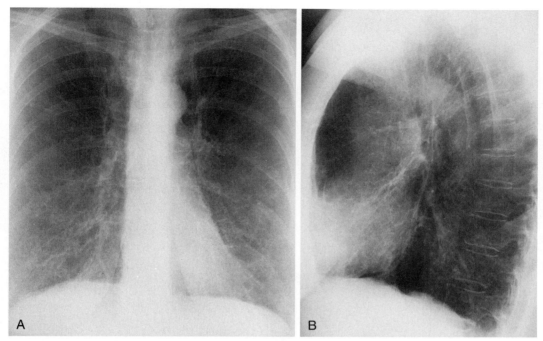

Figure 4–17. Lymphangioleiomyomatosis. Posteroanterior *(A)* and lateral *(B)* chest radiographs show a diffuse bilateral reticular pattern. A few individual cysts can be identified. The lung volumes are increased. The patient was a 40-year-old woman.

cysts are round and have smooth walls ranging from faintly perceptible to 4 mm in thickness.[102, 103] They are distributed diffusely throughout the lungs, without central, peripheral, or lower lung zone predominance.[102] In most cases, the parenchyma between the cysts appears normal; occasionally, there is a slight increase in interstitial markings,[105, 106] interlobular septal thickening,[103, 106] or patchy areas of ground-glass attenuation (presumably the result of pulmonary hemorrhage).[102] Rarely a few small nodular opacities can be seen.[104]

The cysts can be distinguished easily from honeycombing related to idiopathic pulmonary fibrosis by their diffuse distribution and the presence of relatively normal intervening parenchyma.[102, 103] The main differential diagnosis on HRCT is with Langerhans's cell histiocytosis.[102, 107] The latter is characterized by air-filled cysts involving the mid and upper lung zones with relative sparing of the lung bases;[107, 108] most patients who have Langerhans's cell histiocytosis have nodules, a finding that is seen rarely in lymphangioleiomyomatosis.[108, 109]

Tuberous Sclerosis

Tuberous sclerosis is an autosomal dominant disorder of mesodermal development that affects males and females

Table 4–7. LYMPHANGIOLEIOMYOMATOSIS: CHARACTERISTIC RADIOLOGIC FEATURES

Reticular pattern on the radiograph
Thin-walled, air-filled cysts on HRCT
Parenchyma between cysts normal on HRCT
Hyperinflation in late stage of disease
Pneumothorax in 30–40% of patients
Pleural effusion in 10–20% of patients

HRCT, high-resolution computed tomography.

equally. Approximately 25% of patients have positive family histories.[99] The disease is characterized classically by the triad of mental retardation, epilepsy, and adenoma sebaceum; however, a variety of other abnormalities can be seen, including retinal phakoma, angiomyolipomas of the kidneys, rhabdomyomas of the heart, sclerotic lesions of bones, and subungual fibromas. These various manifestations usually appear in infancy or early childhood, and 75% of patients so affected die before they reach age 20.[113]

Pulmonary involvement is uncommon, occurring in about 1% to 2.5% of patients[114, 115] and being seen almost exclusively in women.[98, 115] Clinical manifestations are similar to those of lymphangioleiomyomatosis. Respiratory symptoms usually are first noted between 20 and 45 years of age.[115] Dyspnea is the most common complaint; hemoptysis and cough are seen occasionally.[115] Extrathoracic manifestations of tuberous sclerosis are seen in virtually all patients and include most commonly seizures, renal angiomyolipomas, cerebral calcification, skin lesions, and retinal hamartomas.[115]

The radiographic and CT manifestations of thoracic involvement are similar to those of lymphangioleiomyomatosis (Fig. 4–19). The former consist of a diffuse reticular pattern with or without identifiable cystic or bullous changes.[103, 115] HRCT shows thin-walled cysts throughout both lungs,[103, 115, 116] sometimes in patients who have normal chest radiographs.[115] Similar to lymphangioleiomyomatosis, pneumothorax is common, having been reported in 50% of patients who have tuberous sclerosis and pulmonary involvement.[115, 117] Chylous pleural effusion is distinctly unusual.[112, 115] The diagnosis of tuberous sclerosis should be considered when bilateral renal angiomyolipomas are seen on CT images through the upper abdomen. These tumors have a characteristic appearance of mixed fat and soft tissue attenuation on CT scan (*see* Fig. 4–19). Al-

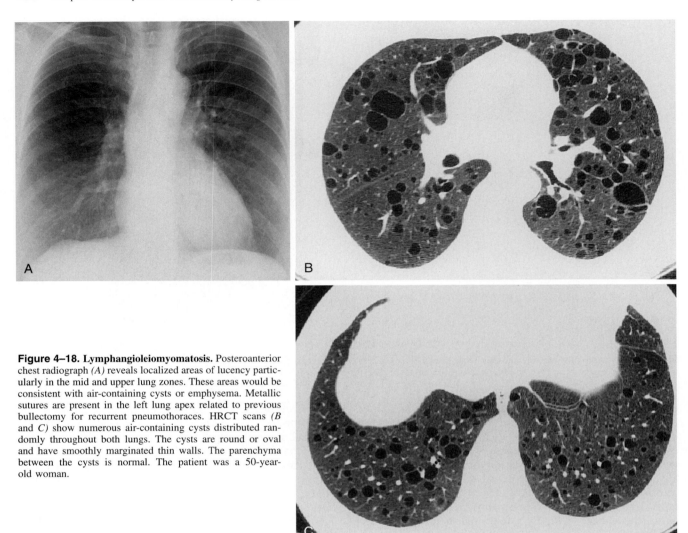

Figure 4–18. Lymphangioleiomyomatosis. Posteroanterior chest radiograph *(A)* reveals localized areas of lucency particularly in the mid and upper lung zones. These areas would be consistent with air-containing cysts or emphysema. Metallic sutures are present in the left lung apex related to previous bullectomy for recurrent pneumothoraces. HRCT scans *(B* and *C)* show numerous air-containing cysts distributed randomly throughout both lungs. The cysts are round or oval and have smoothly marginated thin walls. The parenchyma between the cysts is normal. The patient was a 50-year-old woman.

though such tumors are characteristic of tuberous sclerosis, unilateral or bilateral renal angiomyolipomas are seen in 15% of patients who have lymphangioleiomyomatosis.[115]

Neurofibromatosis

Neurofibromatosis (von Recklinghausen's disease) is a relatively common familial disorder with a frequency of about 1 in 3,000. Although it is inexorably progressive, only about 20% of affected patients develop disabling disease.[118] The most prominent manifestations are cutaneous café au lait spots and neurofibromas of the cutaneous and subcutaneous peripheral nerves, nerve roots, and viscera.[118] The most common pulmonary manifestations consist of diffuse interstitial fibrosis and bullae, either alone or in combination. The prevalence of interstitial fibrosis is about 5% to 10%;[120, 121] bullae have been seen in almost 20% of patients in some series.[120]

Clinically the diagnosis is made readily by the presence on the skin of multiple sessile or pedunculated neurofibromas. Pulmonary disease typically does not become evident until the patient reaches adulthood. Respiratory symptoms usually are mild, the most common complaint being dyspnea on exertion.[121] Pulmonary hypertension has been reported in some patients.[131]

Radiologically, the interstitial disease is characterized by a reticular pattern that involves both lungs symmetrically with some basal predominance.[121, 122] Bullae tend to develop in the upper lobes;[120] they seldom develop in the lower lobes.[119] The bullae may contain mycetomas.[122] Cutaneous neurofibromas (Fig. 4–20) are seen as nodular opacities on the chest radiograph and may mimic intrapulmonary nodules such as might be found with metastases from malignant peripheral nerve sheath tumors; in these cases, CT may be helpful.[123, 124] Plexiform neurofibromas can result in erosion of the inferior or superior margins of one or more ribs.[122] Other relatively common chest wall abnormalities include scoliosis and *twisted ribbon* deformity of the ribs.[125, 126] Although scoliosis itself is a nonspecific finding, the presence of acute angle lower thoracic scoliosis involving five or fewer vertebrae is characteristic of neurofibromatosis.[122, 126] Additional characteristic findings include scalloping of vertebral bodies owing to dural ectasia[127] and lateral thoracic meningoceles.[128]

Paraspinal masses may be caused by neural tumors. When the latter arise from the intercostal nerves, they may

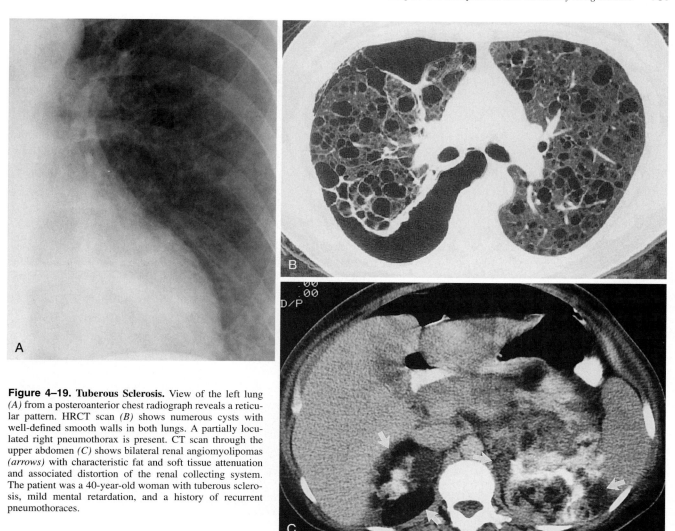

Figure 4–19. Tuberous Sclerosis. View of the left lung *(A)* from a posteroanterior chest radiograph reveals a reticular pattern. HRCT scan *(B)* shows numerous cysts with well-defined smooth walls in both lungs. A partially loculated right pneumothorax is present. CT scan through the upper abdomen *(C)* shows bilateral renal angiomyolipomas *(arrows)* with characteristic fat and soft tissue attenuation and associated distortion of the renal collecting system. The patient was a 40-year-old woman with tuberous sclerosis, mild mental retardation, and a history of recurrent pneumothoraces.

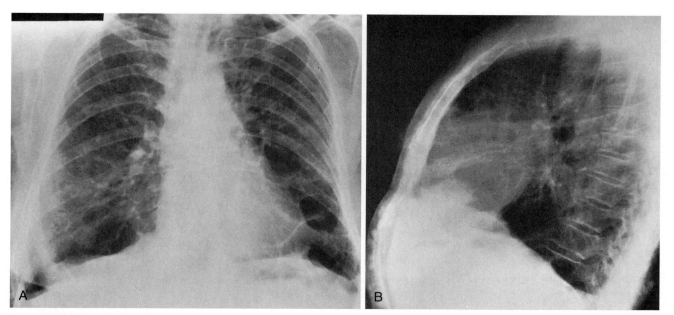

Figure 4–20. Neurofibromatosis—Pulmonary and Cutaneous Manifestations. Posteroanterior chest radiograph *(A)* shows numerous bullae in the lower portion of both lungs. Along the anterior and posterior chest walls in lateral projection *(B)* are numerous nodular opacities representing cutaneous neurofibromas.

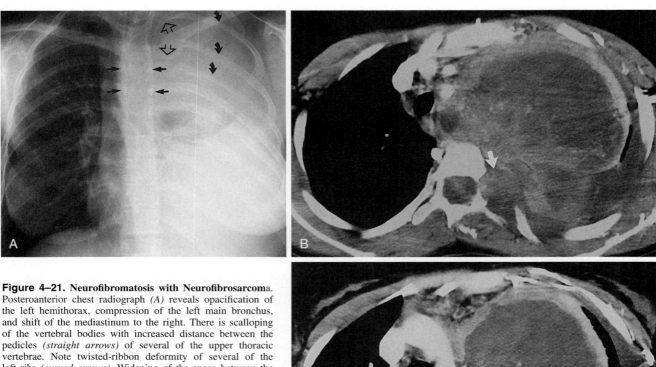

Figure 4–21. Neurofibromatosis with Neurofibrosarcoma. Posteroanterior chest radiograph *(A)* reveals opacification of the left hemithorax, compression of the left main bronchus, and shift of the mediastinum to the right. There is scalloping of the vertebral bodies with increased distance between the pedicles *(straight arrows)* of several of the upper thoracic vertebrae. Note twisted-ribbon deformity of several of the left ribs *(curved arrows)*. Widening of the space between the posterior left third and fourth ribs *(open arrows)* indicates the origin of the neurogenic tumor. Contrast-enhanced CT scans *(B and C)* show a large inhomogeneous mass occupying most of the left hemithorax associated with shift of the mediastinum to the right. Also present is a left pleural effusion. At surgery, the mass was shown to be a neurofibrosarcoma arising from an intercostal nerve in the left paraspinal region *(white arrow)*. Widening of the spinal canal and erosion of the adjacent pedicle and rib can be seen. The patient was an 18-year-old woman.

be seen as extrapleural soft tissue masses running parallel to and occasionally eroding a rib;[128] occasionally, such tumors become large. Tumors of the vagus or phrenic nerves may result in mediastinal masses. Rarely, plexiform neurofibromas originating from the sympathetic chain or phrenic or vagus nerves are seen as masses infiltrating contiguous mediastinal structures;[129, 130] these tumors have a lower attenuation than chest wall muscle, with CT attenuation values ranging from 15 to 30 HU.[129, 130] Malignant degeneration of neurogenic tumors has been reported in 1% to 29% of patients with neurofibromatosis (Fig. 4–21).[122] The development of a malignant peripheral nerve sheath tumor should be suspected when there is a rapid increase in size of a pre-existing mass or when it is associated with pain.[122]

References

1. Clements BS, Warner JO, Shinebourne EA: Congenital bronchopulmonary vascular malformations: Clinical application of a simple anatomical approach in 25 cases. Thorax 42:409, 1987.
2. Panicek DM, Heitzman ER, Randall PA, et al: The continuum of pulmonary developmental anomalies. Radiographics 7:747, 1987.
3. Williams S, Burton EM, Day S, et al: Combined sequestration, bronchogenic cyst, and dysgenetic lung simulating congenital lobar emphysema. South Med J 89:1220, 1996.
4. Boyden EA: Developmental anomalies of the lungs. Am J Surg 89:79, 1955.
5. Maltz DL, Nadas AS: Agenesis of the lung: Presentation of eight new cases and review of the literature. Pediatrics 42:175, 1968.
6. Mardini MK, Nyhan WL: Agenesis of the lung: Report of four patients with unusual anomalies. Chest 87:522, 1985.
7. Soulen RL, Cohen RV: Plain film recognition of pulmonary agenesis in the adult. Chest 60:185, 1971.
8. Mata JM, Cáceres J, Lucaya J, et al: CT of congenital malformations of the lung. Radiographics 10:651, 1990.
9. Greenspan RH, Sagel S, McMahon J, et al: Timed expiratory chest films in detection of air-trapping. Invest Radiol 8:264, 1973.
10. Moore ADA, Godwin JD, Dietrich PA, et al: Swyer-James syndrome: CT findings in eight patients. Am J Roentgenol 158:1211, 1992.
11. Felker RE, Tonkin ILD: Imaging of pulmonary sequestration. Am J Roentgenol 154:241, 1990.
12. Gerle RD, Jaretzi A III, Ashley CA, et al: Congenital bronchopulmonary-foregut malformation: Pulmonary sequestration communicating with the gastrointestinal tract. N Engl J Med 278:1413, 1968.
13. Stocker JT, Malczak HT: A study of pulmonary ligament arteries: Relationship to intralobar pulmonary sequestration. Chest 86:611, 1984.
14. Frazier AA, Rosado de Christenson ML, Stocker JT, et al: Intralobar sequestration: Radiologic-pathologic correlation. Radiographics 17:725, 1997.
15. Savic B, Birtel FJ, Tholen W, et al: Lung sequestration: Report of seven cases and review of 540 published cases. Thorax 34:96, 1979.
16. Ikezoe J, Murayama S, Godwin JD, et al: Bronchopulmonary sequestration: CT assessment. Radiology 176:375, 1990.
17. Ranniger K, Valvassori GE: Angiographic diagnosis of intralobar pulmonary sequestration. Am J Roentgenol 92:540, 1964.

18. Frush DP, Donnelly LF: Pulmonary sequestration spectrum: A new spin with helical CT. Am J Roentgenol 169:679, 1997.
19. Rappaport DC, Herman SJ, Weisbrod GL: Congenital bronchopulmonary diseases in adults: CT findings. Am J Roentgenol 162:1295, 1994.
20. Doyle AJ: Demonstration of blood supply to pulmonary sequestration by MR angiography. Am J Roentgenol 258:989, 1992.
21. Durnin RE, Lababidi Z, Butler C, et al: Bronchopulmonary sequestration. Chest 57:454, 1970.
22. Sippel JM, Ravichandran PS, Antonovic R, et al: Extralobar pulmonary sequestration presenting as a mediastinal malignancy. Ann Thorac Surg 63:1169, 1997.
23. Shuford WH, Sybers RG: Bronchopulmonary sequestration with venous drainage to the portal vein. Am J Roentgenol 106:118, 1969.
24. Rosado de Christenson ML, Frazier AA, Stocker JT, et al: Extralobar sequestrations: Radiologic-pathologic correlation. Radiographics 13:425, 1993.
25. Kirwan WO, Walbaum PR, McCormack RJM: Cystic intrathoracic derivatives of the foregut and their complications. Thorax 28:424, 1973.
26. St Georges R, Deslauriers J, Duranceau A: Clinical spectrum of bronchogenic cysts of the mediastinum and lung. Ann Thorac Surg 52:6, 1991.
27. Suen HC, Mathisen DJ, Grillo HC, et al: Surgical management and radiological characteristics of bronchogenic cysts. Ann Thorac Surg 55:476, 1993.
28. Menke H, Roher HD, Gabbert H, et al: Bronchogenic cyst: A rare cause of a retroperitoneal mass. Eur J Surg 163:311, 1997.
29. Rozenblit A, Iqbal A, Kaleya R, et al: Case report: Intradiaphragmatic bronchogenic cyst. Clin Radiol 53:918, 1998.
30. Okubo K, Sone S, Ogushi F, et al: A case of bronchogenic cyst with high production of antigen CA 19-9. Cancer 63:1994, 1989.
31. Rogers LF, Osmer JC: Bronchogenic cyst: A review of 46 cases. Am J Roentgenol 91:273, 1964.
32. Nakata H, Nakayama C, Kimoto T, et al: Computed tomography of mediastinal bronchogenic cysts. J Comput Assist Tomogr 6:733, 1982.
33. Mendelson DS, Rose JS, Efremidis SC, et al: Bronchogenic cysts with high CT numbers. Am J Radiol 140:463, 1983.
34. Naidich DP, Rumancik WM, Ettenger NA, et al: Congenital anomalies of the lungs in adults: MR diagnosis. Am J Roentgenol 151:13, 1988.
35. Nakata H, Egashira K, Watanabe H, et al: MRI of bronchogenic cysts. J Comput Assist Tomogr 17:267, 1993.
36. Kent DC: Bleeding into pulmonary cyst associated with anticoagulant therapy. Am Rev Respir Dis 92:108, 1965.
37. Brünner S, Poulsen PT, Vesterdal J: Cysts of the lung in infants and children. Acta Paediatr 49:39, 1960.
38. Aktogu S, Yuncu G, Halilcolar H, et al: Bronchogenic cysts: Clinicopathological presentation and treatment. Eur Respir J 9:2017, 1996.
39. Nunzio MC, Evans AJ: Case report: The computed tomographic features of mediastinal bronchogenic cyst rupture into the bronchial tree. Br J Radiol 67:589, 1994.
40. Yernault J-C, Kuhn G, Dumortier P, et al: "Solid" mediastinal bronchogenic cyst: Mineralogic analysis. Am J Roentgenol 146:73, 1986.
41. Patel SR, Meeker DP, Biscotti CV, et al: Presentation and management of bronchogenic cysts in the adult. Chest 106:79, 1994.
42. Ribet ME, Copin MC, Gosselin B: Bronchogenic cysts of the mediastinum. J Thorac Cardiovasc Surg 109:1003, 1995.
43. Davis JG, Simonton JH: Mediastinal carinal bronchogenic cysts. Radiology 7:391, 1956.
44. Hutchin P, Friedman PJ, Saltzstein SL: Congenital cystic adenomatoid malformation with anomalous blood supply. J Thorac Cardiovasc Surg 62:220, 1971.
45. Rashad F, Grisoni E, Gaglione S: Aberrant arterial supply in congenital cystic adenomatoid malformation of the lung. J Pediatr Surg 23:1007, 1988.
46. Miller RK, Sieber WK, Yunis EJ: Congenital adenomatoid malformation of the lung: A report of 17 cases, and review of the literature. *In* Sommers SC, Rosen PP (eds): Pathology Annual, Part I. New York, Appleton-Century-Crofts, 1980, p 387.
47. Hulnick DH, Naidich DP, McCauley DI, et al: Late presentation of congenital cystic adenomatoid malformation of the lung. Radiology 151:569, 1984.
48. Stocker JT, Madewell JE, Drake RM: Congenital cystic adenomatoid malformation of the lung: Classification and morphologic spectrum. Hum Pathol 8:155, 1977.
49. Patz EF, Müller NL, Swensen SJ, et al: Congenital cystic adenomatoid malformation in adults: CT findings. J Comput Assist Tomogr 19:361, 1995.
50. Kim WS, Lee KS, Kim IO, et al: Congenital cystic adenomatoid malformation of the lung: CT-pathologic correlation. Am J Roentgenol 168:47, 1997.
51. Kinsella D, Sissons G, Williams MP: The radiological imaging of bronchial atresia. Br J Radiol 65:681, 1992.
52. Meng RL, Jensik RJ, Faber LP, et al: Bronchial atresia. Ann Thorac Surg 25:184, 1978.
53. van Klaveren RJ, Morshuis WJ, Lacquet LK, et al: Congenital bronchial atresia with regional emphysema associated with pectus excavatum. Thorax 47:1082, 1992.
54. Jederlinic PJ, Sicilian LS, Baigelman W, et al: Congenital bronchial atresia: A report of 4 cases and review of the literature. Medicine 66:73, 1986.
55. Cohen AM, Solomon EH, Alfidi RJ: Computed tomography in bronchial atresia. Am J Roentgenol 135:1097, 1980.
56. Al-Nakshabandi N, Lingawi S, Müller NL: Congenital bronchial atresia. Can Assoc Radiol J 51:47, 2000.
57. Finck S, Milne ENC: A case report of segmental bronchial atresia: Radiologic evaluation including computed tomography and magnetic resonance imaging. J Thorac Imaging 3:53, 1988.
58. Rossoff LJ, Steinberg H: Bronchial atresia and mucocele: A report of two cases. Respir Med 88:789, 1994.
59. Ellis K: Developmental abnormalities in the systemic blood supply to the lungs. Am J Roentgenol 156:669, 1991.
60. Mathey J, Galey JJ, Logeais Y, et al: Anomalous pulmonary venous return into inferior vena cava and associated bronchovascular anomalies (the scimitar syndrome). Thorax 23:398, 1968.
61. Woodring JH, Howard TA, Kanga JF: Congenital pulmonary venolobar syndrome revisited. Radiographics 14:349, 1994.
62. Dupuis C, Charaf LAC, Breviè GM, et al: The "adult" form of the scimitar syndrome. Am J Cardiol 70:502, 1992.
63. Kiely B, Filler J, Stone S, et al: Syndrome of anomalous venous drainage of the right lung to the inferior vena cava: A review of 67 reported cases and three new cases in children. Am J Cardiol 20:102, 1967.
64. Roehm JOF Jr, Jue KL, Amplatz K: Radiographic features of the scimitary syndrome. Radiology 86:856, 1966.
65. Cirillo RL: The scimitar sign. Radiology 206:623, 1998.
66. Godwin JD, Tarver RD: Scimitar syndrome: Four new cases examined with CT. Radiology 159:15, 1986.
67. Olson MA, Becker GJ: The scimitar syndrome: CT findings in partial anomalous pulmonary venous return. Radiology 159:25, 1986.
68. Gilkeson RC, Basile V, Sands MJ, et al: Chest case of the day. Am J Roentgenol 169:266, 1997.
69. Baran R, Kir A, Tor MM, et al: Scimitar syndrome: Confirmation of diagnosis by a noninvasive technique (MRI). Eur Radiol 6:92, 1996.
70. Burke CM, Safai C, Nelson DP, et al: Pulmonary arteriovenous malformations: A critical update. Am Rev Respir Dis 134:334, 1986.
71. Guttmacher AE, Marchuk DA, White RI Jr: Hereditary hemorrhagic telangiectasia. N Engl J Med 333:918, 1995.
72. Moyer JH, Glantz G, Brest AN: Pulmonary arteriovenous fistulas: Physiologic and clinical considerations. Am J Med 32:417, 1962.
73. Remy J, Remy-Jardin M, Wattinne L, et al: Pulmonary arteriovenous malformations: Evaluation with CT of the chest before and after treatment. Radiology 182:809, 1992.
74. Remy J, Remy-Jardin M, Giraud F, et al: Angioarchitecture of pulmonary arteriovenous malformations: Clinical utility of three-dimensional helical CT. Radiology 191:657, 1994.
75. Coley SC, Jackson JE: Pulmonary arteriovenous malformations. Clin Radiol 53:396, 1998.
76. Hunter DD: Pulmonary arteriovenous malformation: An unusual cause of cerebral embolism. Can Med Assoc J 93:662, 1965.
77. Tadavarthy SM, Klugman J, Castaneda-Zuniga WR, et al: Systemic-to-pulmonary collaterals in pathologic states. Radiology 144:55, 1982.
78. Kirks DR, Kane PE, Free EA, et al: Systemic arterial supply to normal basilar segments of the left lower lobe. Am J Roentgenol 126:817, 1976.
79. Matzinger FR, Bhargava R, Peterson RA, et al: Systemic arterial supply to the lung without sequestration: an unusual cause of hemoptysis. Can Assoc Radiol J 45:44, 1994.

80. Hirai T, Ohtake Y, Mutoh S, et al: Anomalous systemic arterial supply to normal basal segments of the left lower lobe: A report of two cases. Chest 109:286, 1996.

81. Miyake H, Hori Y, Takeoka H, et al: Systemic arterial supply to normal basal segments of the left lung: Characteristic features on chest radiography and CT. Am J Roentgenol 171:387, 1998.

82. Piessens J, De Geest H, Kesteloot H, et al: Anomalous collateral systemic pulmonary circulation to a normal lung. Chest 59:222, 1971.

83. Painter RL, Billig DM, Epstein I: Brief recordings: Anomalous systemic arterialization of the lung without sequestration. N Engl J Med 279:866, 1968.

84. Mainardi CL, Kang AH: Collagen disease: A new perspective. Am J Med 71:913, 1981.

85. Pyeritz RE, McKusick VA: The Marfan syndrome: Diagnosis and management. N Engl J Med 300:772, 1979.

86. Ramirez F: Fibrillin mutations in Marfan syndrome and related phenotypes. Curr Opin Genet Dev 6:309, 1996.

87. Tanoue LT: Pulmonary involvement in collagen vascular disease: A review of the pulmonary manifestations of the Marfan syndrome, ankylosing spondylitis, Sjögren's syndrome, and relapsing polychondritis. J Thorac Imaging 7:62, 1992.

88. Hall JR, Pyeritz RE, Dudgeon DL, et al: Pneumothorax in the Marfan syndrome: Prevalence and therapy. Ann Thorac Surg 37:500, 1984.

89. Wood JR, Bellamy D, Child AH, et al: Pulmonary disease in patients with Marfan syndrome. Thorax 39:780, 1984.

90. Murdoch JL, Walker BA, Halpern BL, et al: Life expectancy and causes of death in the Marfan syndrome. N Engl J Med 286:804, 1972.

91. Posniak HV, Olson MC, Demos TC, et al: CT of thoracic aortic aneurysms. Radiographics 10:839, 1990.

92. Fisher ER, Stern EJ, Godwin JD, et al: Acute aortic dissection: Typical and atypical imaging features. Radiographics 14:1263, 1994.

93. Sommer T, Fehske W, Holzknecht N, et al: Aortic dissection: A comparative study of diagnosis with spiral CT, multiplanar transesophageal echocardiography, and MR imaging. Radiology 199:347, 1996.

94. Mayo JR: Magnetic resonance imaging of the chest: Where we stand. Radiol Clin North Am 32:795, 1994.

95. Taylor JR, Ryu J, Colby TV, et al: Lymphangioleiomyomatosis: Clinical course in 32 patients. N Engl J Med 323:1254, 1990.

96. Baldi S, Papotti M, Valente ML, et al: Pulmonary lymphangioleiomyomatosis in postmenopausal women: Report of two cases and review of the literature. Eur Respir J 7:1013, 1994.

97. Sinclair W, Wright JL, Churg A: Lymphangioleiomyomatosis presenting in a postmenopausal woman. Thorax 40:475, 1985.

98. Jao J, Gilbert S, Messer R: Lymphangiomyoma and tuberous sclerosis. Cancer 29:1188, 1972.

99. Valensi QJ: Pulmonary lymphangiomyoma, a probable *forme fruste* of tuberous sclerosis: A case report and survey of the literature. Am Rev Respir Dis 108:1411, 1973.

100. Carrington CB, Cugell DW, Gaensler EA, et al: Lymphangioleiomyomatosis: Physiologic-pathologic-radiologic correlations. Am Rev Respir Dis 116:977, 1977.

101. Corrin B, Liebow AA, Friedman PJ: Pulmonary lymphangiomyomatosis. Am J Pathol 79:347, 1975.

102. Müller NL, Chiles C, Kullnig P: Pulmonary lymphangiomyomatosis: Correlation of CT with radiographic and functional findings. Radiology 175:335, 1990.

103. Lenoir S, Grenier P, Brauner MW, et al: Pulmonary lymphangiomyomatosis and tuberous sclerosis: Comparison of radiographic and thin-section CT findings. Radiology 175:329, 1990.

104. Kitaichi M, Nishimura K, Itoh H, et al: Pulmonary lymphangioleiomyomatosis: A report of 46 patients including a clinicopathologic study of prognostic factors. Am J Respir Crit Care Med 151:527, 1995.

105. Rappaport DC, Weisbrod GL, Herman SJ, et al: Pulmonary lymphangioleiomyomatosis: High-resolution CT findings in four cases. Am J Roentgenol 152:961, 1989.

106. Templeton PA, McLoud TC, Müller NL, et al: Pulmonary lymphangioleiomyomatosis: CT and pathologic findings. J Comput Assist Tomogr 13:54, 1989.

107. Moore ADA, Godwin JD, Müller NL, et al: Pulmonary histiocytosis X: Comparison of radiographic and CT findings. Radiology 172:249, 1989.

108. Brauner MW, Grenier P, Mouelhi MM, et al: Pulmonary histiocytosis X: Evaluation with high-resolution CT. Radiology 172:255, 1989.

109. Bonelli FS, Hartman TE, Swensen SJ, et al: Accuracy of high-resolution CT in diagnosing lung diseases. Am J Roentgenol 170:1507, 1998.

110. Graf-Deuel E, Knoblauch A: Simultaneous bilateral spontaneous pneumothorax. Chest 105:1142, 1994.

111. Berkman N, Bloom A, Cohen P, et al: Bilateral spontaneous pneumothorax as the presenting feature in lymphangioleiomyomatosis. Respir Med 89:381, 1995.

112. Stovin PGI, Lum LC, Flower CDR, et al: The lungs in lymphangiomyomatosis and in tuberous sclerosis. Thorax 30:497, 1975.

113. Harris JO, Waltuck BL, Swenson EW: The pathophysiology of the lungs in tuberous sclerosis: A case report and literature review. Am Rev Respir Dis 100:379, 1969.

114. Lie JT, Miller RD, Williams DE: Cystic disease of the lungs in tuberous sclerosis: Clinicopathologic correlation, including body plethysmographic lung function tests. Mayo Clin Proc 55:547, 1980.

115. Castro M, Shepherd CW, Gomez MR, et al: Pulmonary tuberous sclerosis. Chest 107:189, 1995.

116. Kullnig P, Melzer G, Smolle-Jüttner FM: High-resolution-computer-tomographie des thorax bei lymphangioleiomyomatose und tuberöser sklerose. Rofo Fortschr Geb Rontgenstr Neuen Bildgeb Verfahr 151:32, 1989.

117. Dwyer JM, Hickie JB, Garvan J: Pulmonary tuberous sclerosis: Report of three patients and a review of the literature. QJM 40:115, 1971.

118. Riccardi VM: von Recklinghausen neurofibromatosis. N Engl J Med 305:1617, 1981.

119. Burkhalter JL, Morano JU, McCay MB: Diffuse interstitial lung disease in neurofibromatosis. South Med J 79:944, 1986.

120. Massaro D, Katz S: Fibrosing alveolitis: Its occurrence, roentgenographic and pathologic features in von Recklinghausen's neurofibromatosis. Am Rev Respir Dis 93:934, 1966.

121. Webb WR, Goodman PC: Fibrosing alveolitis in patients with neurofibromatosis. Radiology 122:289, 1977.

122. Rossi SE, Erasmus JJ, McAdams HP, et al: Thoracic manifestations of neurofibromatosis I. Am J Roentgenol 173:1631, 1999.

123. Patel YD, Moorhouse HT: Neurofibrosarcomas in neurofibromatosis: Role of CT scanning and angiography. Clin Radiol 33:555, 1982.

124. Schabel SI, Schmidt GE, Vujic I: Overlooked pulmonary malignancy in neurofibromatosis. Can Assoc Radiol J 31:135, 1980.

125. Casselman ES, Miller WT, Lin SR, et al: Von Recklinghausen's disease: Incidence of roentgenographic findings with a clinical review of the literature. Crit Rev Diagn Imaging 9:387, 1978.

126. Hunt JC, Pugh DG: Skeletal lesions in neurofibromatosis. Radiology 76:1, 1961.

127. Casselman ES, Mandell GA: Vertebral scalloping in neurofibromatosis. Radiology 131:89, 1979.

128. Klatte EC, Franken EA, Smith JA: The radiographic spectrum in neurofibromatosis. Semin Roentgenol 11:17, 1976.

129. Bourgouin PM, Shepard JAO, Moore EH, et al: Plexiform neurofibromatosis of the mediastinum: CT appearance. Am J Roentgenol 151:461, 1988.

130. Gossios KJ, Guy RL: Case report: Imaging of widespread plexiform neurofibromatosis. Clin Radiol 47:211, 1993.

131. Porterfield JK, Pyeritz RE, Traill TA: Pulmonary hypertension and interstitial fibrosis in von Recklinghausen neurofibromatosis. Am J Med Genet 25:531, 1986.

132. White RI, Mitchell SE, Barth KH, et al: Angioarchitecture of pulmonary arteriovenous malformations: An important consideration before embolotherapy. Am J Roentgenol 140:681, 1983.

133. Gossage JR, Kanj G: Pulmonary arteriovenous malformations: A state of the art review. Am J Respir Crit Care Med 158:643, 1998.

134. Naidich DP, Rumancik WM, Lefleur RS, et al: Intralobar pulmonary sequestration: MR evaluation. J Comput Assist Tomogr 11:531, 1987.

135. Wu CT, Chen MR, Shih SL, et al: Case report: Agenesis of the right lung diagnosed by three-dimensional reconstruction of helical chest CT. Br J Radiol 69:1052, 1996.

136. Newman B, Gondor M: MR evaluation of right pulmonary agenesis and vascular airway compression in pediatric patients. Am J Roentgenol 168:55, 1997.

137. Sullivan EJ: Lymphangioleiomyomatosis: A review. Chest 114:1689, 1998.

138. Ellis K: Developmental abnormalities in the systemic blood supply to the lungs. AJR 156:669, 1991.

CHAPTER 5

Pulmonary Infection

PATTERNS OF PULMONARY INFECTION

Organisms can enter the lung and cause infection by three routes: the tracheobronchial tree, the pulmonary vasculature, and directly from the mediastinum or neck or across the diaphragm or chest wall. Although there is overlap, infection acquired by each of these routes results in fairly characteristic pulmonary abnormalities.

Infection via the Tracheobronchial Tree

Infection of the lower respiratory tract acquired via the airways may be confined predominantly to the airways themselves (tracheitis, bronchitis, or bronchiolitis) or to the lung parenchyma (pneumonia). The latter can be subdivided, in turn, into three types, each with fairly typical

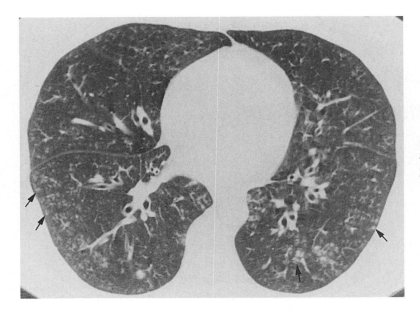

Figure 5–1. Acute Bronchiolitis—*Mycoplasma pneumoniae.* HRCT scan shows small nodular opacities *(arrows)* in a centrilobular distribution involving mainly the lower lobes. The patient was a 40-year-old woman.

pathologic and radiologic characteristics: lobar (nonsegmental*) pneumonia, bronchopneumonia (lobular pneumonia*), and interstitial pneumonia. These patterns can be recognized with sufficient frequency and are associated with different causative organisms in enough cases that their recognition is useful diagnostically. For example, lobar pneumonia is usually of bacterial origin, most commonly *Streptococcus pneumoniae* or *Klebsiella pneumoniae*, whereas diffuse interstitial pneumonia most commonly results from *Pneumocystis carinii*.[2, 3, 3a]

Tracheitis, Bronchitis, and Bronchiolitis

Infection involving predominantly the airways may be limited to the trachea, bronchi, or bronchioles or affect two or three of these sites simultaneously. Viral and mycoplasmal organisms are the most frequent pathogenic agents.

Acute tracheitis and bronchitis usually are associated with a normal radiograph or nonspecific radiographic findings; occasionally, acute bronchitis leads to bronchial wall thickening, bronchial dilation, and peribronchial inflammation apparent on the chest radiograph and high-resolution computed tomography (HRCT) scan.[7, 8] Bronchiolitis also may be associated with a normal radiograph[9] or may result in accentuation of lung markings or a reticulonodular pattern.[10, 11] On HRCT scan, inflammation of the bronchiolar wall and filling of the bronchiolar lumen with exudate results in a pattern of small centrilobular nodules and branching lines (Fig. 5–1).[8, 12] The pattern of centrilobular nodular and branching linear opacities has been referred to aptly as resembling a *tree-in-bud* and is seen most commonly in infectious bronchiolitis and endobronchial spread of tuberculosis or other mycobacterial infection.[13, 15] These abnormalities may be evident on HRCT scan in patients

who have normal radiographs.[8] The distribution may be focal[7, 8] or diffuse.[12]

Lobar Pneumonia

Lobar (nonsegmental air-space) pneumonia most commonly is caused by *S. pneumoniae*, but it can occur with other organisms, such as *K. pneumoniae*. Lobar consolidation involving single or, less commonly, multiple lobes is the most common pattern of presentation of community-acquired pneumococcal pneumonia in patients requiring hospitalization.[3a] The most important pathogenetic feature of this form of infection appears to be rapid production of edema fluid with relatively mild cellular reaction. Consolidation tends to occur initially in the periphery of the lung beneath the visceral pleura.[14] As it forms, the edema fluid flows directly between adjacent alveoli, acini, and bronchopulmonary segments. Such flow seems to be through the pores of Kohn and small peripheral collateral channels but not along the bronchovascular bundles. Because the airways largely are spared, there is little, if any, associated volume loss.

Radiographically, lobar pneumonia is manifested by nonsegmental, homogeneous consolidation involving predominantly or exclusively one lobe (Fig. 5–2, Table 5–1).[16] The larger bronchi often remain patent and air containing, creating an air bronchogram. The amount of inflammatory exudate may be such that it results in expansion of a lobe and a *bulging fissure* sign (Fig. 5–3).[17]

Table 5–1. LOBAR (NONSEGMENTAL) PNEUMONIA

Affects predominantly one lobe	Less common causes
Consolidation crosses segmental boundaries	*Mycobacterium tuberculosis*
	Actinomyces and *Nocardia*
Common organisms	species
Streptococcus pneumoniae	*Pseudomonas aeruginosa*
Klebsiella pneumoniae	*Escherichia coli*
Legionella pneumophila	

---

*Because it is often identified early in its course and is treated effectively with antibiotics, lobar pneumonia seldom involves a whole lobe nowadays; although the term *nonsegmental air-space pneumonia* has been advocated to reflect this,[1] *lobar pneumonia* is used much more commonly. Because bronchopneumonia affects the secondary pulmonary lobules (at times, in a patchy fashion), it also has been referred to as *lobular pneumonia*.

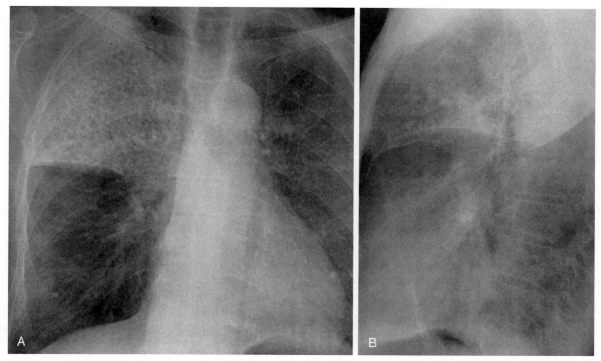

Figure 5–2. Lobar Pneumonia. Posteroanterior *(A)* and lateral *(B)* chest radiographs in a 79-year-old man show diffuse consolidation of the right upper lobe. Small foci of consolidation are present in the right lower lobe and in the left lung. Sputum cultures grew *Streptococcus pneumoniae.*

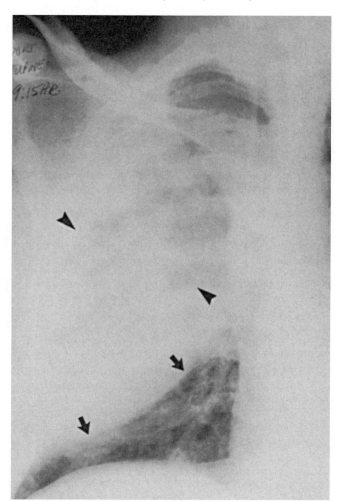

Figure 5–3. Acute *Klebsiella* Pneumonia with Bulging Fissure. View of the right lung from posteroanterior chest radiograph reveals massive air-space consolidation involving most of the upper lobe. The downward-displaced bulging minor fissure *(arrows)* indicates lobar expansion; numerous central radiolucencies (between *arrowheads*) suggest parenchymal necrosis.

Table 5–2. BRONCHOPNEUMONIA (LOBULAR PNEUMONIA)

Patchy, inhomogeneous consolidation	Less common causes
Usually involves several lobes	*Streptococcus pneumoniae*
Common organisms	*Mycobacterium tuberculosis*
Staphylococcus aureus	*Aspergillus fumigatus*
Escherichia coli	Viruses
Pseudomonas aeruginosa	*Mycoplasma pneumoniae*
Anaerobes	
Haemophilus influenzae	

Bronchopneumonia

Bronchopneumonia is exemplified by infection by *Staphylococcus aureus*, most gram-negative bacteria, and some fungi. It differs pathogenetically from lobar pneumonia by the relatively rapid exudation of polymorphonuclear leukocytes in addition to edema fluid. Because the exudate develops first in relation to small membranous and respiratory bronchioles, there is typically a bronchiolocentric distribution of consolidation. With the progression of disease, the inflammatory reaction spreads to involve entire lobules.

The radiologic manifestations of bronchopneumonia depend on the severity of the disease. Mild bronchopneumonia results in peribronchial thickening and poorly defined air-space opacities. More severe disease results in inhomogeneous, patchy areas of consolidation that usually involve several lobes (Table 5–2; Fig. 5–4).[18, 19] Consolidation involving the terminal and respiratory bronchioles and adjacent alveoli results in poorly defined centrilobular nodular opacities measuring 4 to 10 mm in diameter (air-space nodules);[11, 20] extension to involve the entire secondary lobule (lobular consolidation) may be seen.[4] Because it involves the airways, bronchopneumonia frequently results in loss of volume of the affected segments or lobes.[19] When confluent, bronchopneumonia may resemble lobar pneumonia; distinction from the latter can be made in many cases by the presence of associated volume loss and the lobular or segmental distribution of the abnormalities in other areas. Because it usually is associated with tissue destruction, bronchopneumonia can be complicated by several abnormalities, including pulmonary abscess, pulmonary gangrene, and pneumatocele formation.

Pulmonary Abscess

Pulmonary abscesses vary in size from those that can be seen only with the microscope to those that occupy a large area of a pulmonary lobe. The radiologic manifestations consist of single or multiple cavities (Fig. 5–5) that may be isolated or occur within areas of consolidation. In one review of the radiographic findings in 50 patients, the internal margins of the abscesses were smooth in 88% of cases and shaggy in 12%.[21] Air-fluid levels were present in 72%, and adjacent parenchymal consolidation was present in 48%. Anaerobic bacteria are often the cause.[22, 23] Other relatively common agents are *S. aureus* and *Pseudomonas aeruginosa*.

Pulmonary Gangrene

Pulmonary gangrene is a relatively uncommon complication of bronchopneumonia characterized by the development of fragments of necrotic lung within an abscess cavity. The radiologic manifestations initially consist of small lucencies within an area of consolidated lung, usually developing within lobar consolidation associated with enlargement of the lobe and outward bulging of the fissure.[24] The small lucencies rapidly coalesce into a large cavity containing fluid and sloughed lung.[24, 25] Lateral decubitus views show that the necrotic lung is freely mobile within the cavity. Most cases are secondary to *K. pneumoniae*; other causative organisms include *S. pneumoniae*, *Haemophilus influenzae*, *Bacteroides fragilis*, other *Bacteroides*, and *S. aureus*.[24]

Pneumatocele

Pneumatoceles are thin-walled, gas-filled spaces that usually develop in association with infection; characteristi-

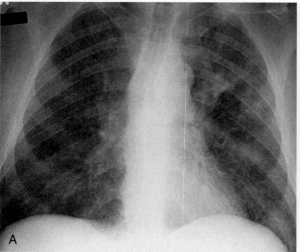
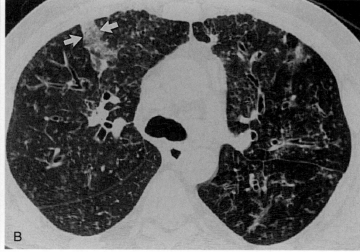

Figure 5–4. *Haemophilus influenzae* **Pneumonia.** Anteroposterior chest radiograph *(A)* in a 50-year-old man shows poorly defined nodular opacities and patchy areas of consolidation. HRCT scan *(B)* shows that the small nodules are in a centrilobular distribution consistent with bronchiolitis. An area of lobular consolidation *(arrows)* characteristic of early bronchopneumonia also is present. Sputum and blood cultures grew *H. influenzae*.

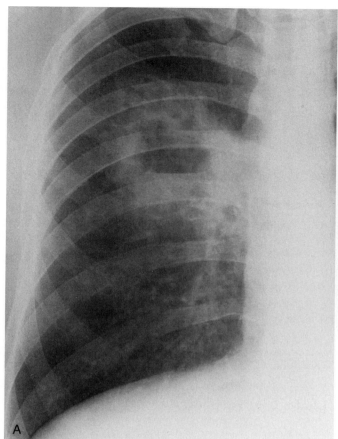

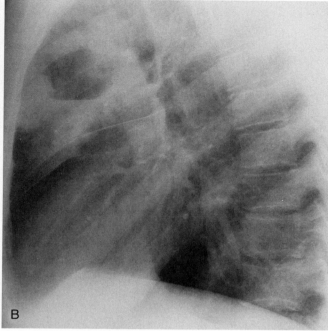

Figure 5–5. Lung Abscess. Views of the right lung from posteroanterior *(A)* and lateral *(B)* chest radiographs show a large abscess with an air-fluid level in the anterior segment of the right upper lobe. The internal margin of the abscess is irregular. There is minimal surrounding consolidation. The patient was a 38-year-old alcoholic man who customarily slept on his stomach. Gram stain of the sputum revealed gram-positive and gram-negative bacteria; no cultures were taken. The abscess resolved after treatment with antibiotics.

cally, they increase in size over days to weeks and almost invariably resolve. Of the several mechanisms proposed for their formation, the most likely is drainage of a focus of necrotic lung parenchyma followed by check-valve obstruction of the airway subtending it; the *valve*, which may be inflammatory exudate, necrotic airway wall, or both, enables air to enter the parenchymal space during inspiration but prevents its egress during expiration.[26] The complication usually is caused by *S. aureus* in infants and children or *P. carinii* in patients who have acquired immunodeficiency syndrome (AIDS).[27]

Interstitial Pneumonia

Interstitial pneumonia is caused typically by viruses and *P. carinii* and is characterized by edema and an inflammatory cellular infiltrate situated predominantly in the interstitial tissue of the alveolar septa and surrounding small airways and vessels. The radiographic manifestations of interstitial pneumonia resulting from viral or mycoplasmal infection consist of a reticular or reticulonodular pattern (Fig. 5–6).[28–30] Septal (Kerley B) lines may be seen.[31] Associated bronchiolitis may result in centrilobular linear and nodular opacities, best seen on HRCT scan;[12, 495] bronchitis may be manifested by peribronchial thickening and accentuation of lung markings (Table 5–3).[10]

Pneumonia caused by *P. carinii* typically presents radiographically as a bilateral, symmetric fine granular or poorly defined reticulonodular pattern (Fig. 5–7).[32–34] With more severe infection, the findings progress to more homoge-

neous parenchymal opacification ranging from *ground-glass* opacities to consolidation.[33] On HRCT scan, the predominant abnormality consists of extensive bilateral areas of ground-glass attenuation (Fig. 5–8); small nodules, reticular opacities, and interlobular septal thickening are seen in 20% to 40% of patients.[35, 36] Similar radiographic and HRCT findings may be seen in patients who have cytomegalovirus pneumonia.[37, 38]

Limitations of the Pattern Approach

There is variation in the radiologic manifestations of pneumonia caused by specific organisms, and sometimes it is not possible to fit an individual case into the categories of lobar pneumonia, bronchopneumonia, and interstitial pneumonia. Many factors can modify the radiologic manifestations of pulmonary infection,[5] including the age and immunologic status of the patient and the state of the underlying lung. Of greatest importance with regard to the last of these is emphysema, a condition that can result in a spongelike appearance to consolidated lung parenchyma.

Table 5–3. INTERSTITIAL PNEUMONIA

Reticulonodular pattern	Less common causes
Peribronchial thickening	*Streptococcus pneumoniae*
Common organisms	*Mycobacterium tuberculosis*
Viruses	Fungi
Mycoplasma pneumoniae	
Pneumocystis carinii	

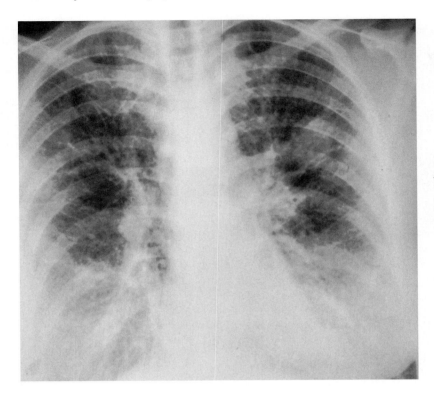

Figure 5–6. Acute Interstitial Pneumonia—*Myco-plasma pneumoniae*. Posteroanterior chest radiograph shows thickening of the bronchovascular bundles and a ground-glass opacity throughout both lungs. Also shown are a focal area of consolidation in the left upper lobe and bilateral hilar lymph node enlargement. The patient was a previously healthy 17-year-old girl.

The severity and cause of pneumonia are influenced by the immunologic status, with immunosuppressed patients being prone to develop widespread pneumonia, often by opportunistic organisms. There is evidence that typical patterns of parenchymal consolidation may not be seen in the presence of agranulocytosis.[6]

Infection via the Pulmonary Vasculature

Infection by way of the pulmonary vasculature usually occurs in association with an extrapulmonary focus of infection. When the infection is associated with sepsis, it typically takes the form of innumerable nodules 1 to 5 mm

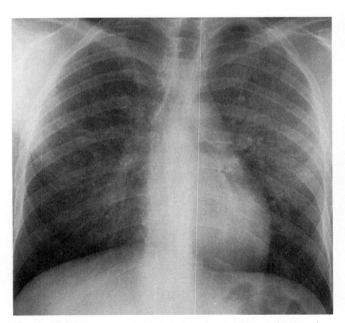

Figure 5–7. *Pneumocystis carinii* Pneumonia. Posteroanterior chest radiograph shows bilateral ground-glass opacities and poorly defined reticulonodular pattern. The patient was a 24-year-old man who had acquired immunodeficiency syndrome and *P. carinii* pneumonia.

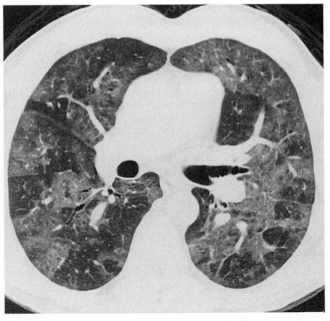

Figure 5–8. *Pneumocystis carinii* Pneumonia. HRCT shows a characteristic appearance consisting of bilateral areas of ground-glass attenuation and areas of normal-appearing lung causing a geographic pattern. The patient was a 46-year-old man who had acquired immunodeficiency syndrome and *P. carinii* pneumonia.

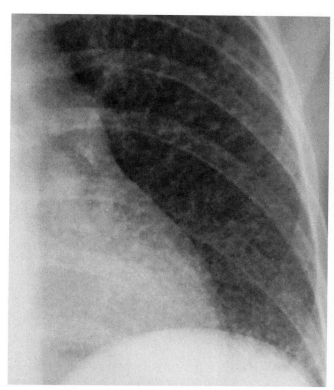

Figure 5–9. Miliary Tuberculosis. View of the left lung from antero-posterior chest radiograph in a 22-year-old woman shows numerous sharply defined nodules 1 to 3 mm in diameter. The nodules are most numerous in the lung base. The diagnosis of miliary tuberculosis was proved by bone marrow biopsy.

in diameter (miliary infection); such a pattern most often is seen in disseminated tuberculosis. When infection via the pulmonary vasculature is associated with infected (septic) thromboemboli, multiple but substantially less numerous abscesses are characteristic.

The radiologic appearance of miliary disease associated with tuberculosis is distinctive, consisting of discrete, pinpoint opacities, usually distributed evenly throughout both lungs;[39, 40] sometimes, there is a slight basal predominance reflecting the gravity-induced increased blood flow (Fig. 5–9). When first visible, the nodules measure 1 to 2 mm in diameter (hence the term *miliary*, which refers to the similarly sized millet seed); in the absence of adequate therapy, nodules may increase to 3 to 5 mm in diameter, a finding seen in approximately 10% of cases.[40]

Disease associated with septic thromboemboli is characterized radiologically by the presence of nodules usually 1 to 3 cm in diameter (Fig. 5–10); they frequently are cavitated. Computed tomography (CT) scan also frequently shows subpleural wedge-shaped areas of consolidation, often with central areas of necrosis or frank cavitation.[41, 42] In approximately two thirds of patients who have multiple septic thromboemboli, at least some of the nodules can be seen on CT scan to have vessels leading into the nodule, the so-called feeding vessel sign (Fig. 5–11).[41, 42]

Infection via Direct Spread from an Extrapulmonary Site

Spread of infection to the lung may occur across the chest wall or diaphragm or from the mediastinum after thoracic trauma or by extension of disease from an extrapulmonary source, such as an intra-abdominal abscess or a focus of mediastinitis secondary to esophageal rupture.[43] In these situations, the pulmonary disease usually is localized to an area contiguous with the extrapulmonary source of infection and often takes the form of an abscess. The source of such infection may not be immediately apparent (e.g., an adrenal abscess or pyelonephritis with retroperitoneal or nephrobronchial fistula).[44, 45]

BACTERIA

Aerobic Bacteria

Gram-Positive Cocci

Streptococcus pneumoniae

S. pneumoniae is the most commonly identified pathogenic organism in patients admitted to the hospital for pneumonia, accounting for about 40% of all isolated species.[47, 48] Risk factors for the development of pneumococcal pneumonia include the extremes of age,[49, 52]1 chronic heart or lung disease, immunosuppression, alcoholism,[50] institutionalization,[51] and prior splenectomy.[53] The characteristic clinical presentation is abrupt in onset, with fever, shaking chills, cough, and intense pleural pain. Many patients give a history of an upper respiratory tract infection before the onset of the more dramatic symptoms. Cough may be nonproductive at first but soon produces bloody, *rusty*, or greenish material. In the elderly, these classic features of disease may be absent, and pneumonia may be confused with or confounded by other common medical problems, such as congestive heart failure, pulmonary thromboembolism, or malignancy.[60]

The characteristic radiographic pattern of acute pneumococcal pneumonia consists of homogeneous, nonsegmental consolidation involving one lobe (Fig. 5–12). Because the consolidation begins in the peripheral air spaces of the lung, it almost invariably abuts against a visceral pleural surface, either interlobar or over the convexity of the lung (*see* Fig. 5–2). Occasionally, infection is manifested as a round (spherical) focus of consolidation that simulates a mass; although this pattern can be seen in adults (Fig. 5–13), it is more common in children.[55]

Although homogeneous lobar consolidation is the most common radiographic manifestation of acute pneumococcal pneumonia, other patterns may be seen. For example, although 20 (67%) of 30 patients in one prospective survey had the typical pattern, 6 (20%) had patchy areas of consolidation, and 4 (13%) had mixed air-space and interstitial opacities (Fig. 5–14).[56] In another review of 132 patients who had severe community-acquired pneumonia treated in the intensive care unit, 28 (65%) of 43 patients with *S. pneumoniae* pneumonia had typical lobar consolidation, and 35% had bronchopneumonia; none had reticular or reticulonodular opacities.[57]

Complications, such as cavitation, pulmonary gangrene, and pneumatocele formation, are rare (Fig. 5–15). It is probable that many of these are related to mixed infections; associated anaerobic microorganisms in particular are likely to be undetected because of lack of appropriate culture methods.[54] The reported incidence of pleural effu-

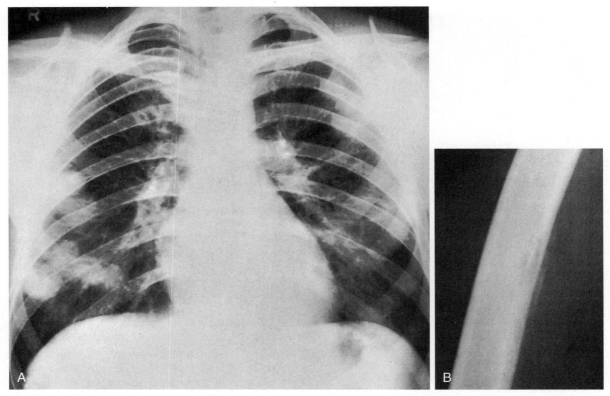

Figure 5–10. Septic Embolism. Posteroanterior chest radiograph *(A)* shows several sharply defined nodules 2 to 3 cm in diameter situated predominantly in the right lower lobe and the left upper lobe. The nodules are homogeneous in density and show no evidence of cavitation (although cavitation occurred eventually in most). Lateral view of the midshaft of the right femur *(B)* shows an irregular area of rarefaction in the cortex, associated with the subperiosteal new bone formation along the posterior aspect. *Staphylococcus aureus* was cultured from the sputum and from pus obtained from the thigh at incision and drainage.

sion varies with the radiographic technique used to detect it, the severity of infection, and the presence or not of bacteremia. Pleural effusion is evident on posteroanterior and lateral radiographs in about 10% of patients overall;[59] in patients who have severe pneumonia requiring treatment in the intensive care unit, it is approximately 30%,[57] and in patients who have bacteremia, incidence is 50%.[58]

Staphylococcus aureus

S. aureus is an uncommon cause of community-acquired pneumonia, accounting for only about 3% of all cases;[47, 522] it is, however, an important cause of nosocomial pneumonia, especially in the intensive care unit. In this setting, *S. aureus* is one of the more common pathogenic organisms, being found in 15% or more of all cases.[62, 63, 523] The clinical presentation usually is abrupt, with pleural pain, cough, and expectoration of purulent yellow or brown sputum, sometimes streaked with blood.

The parenchymal consolidation in acute staphylococcal bronchopneumonia typically is segmental in distribution. Depending on the severity of involvement, the process may be patchy or homogeneous; the latter represents confluent bronchopneumonia (Fig. 5–16). Because an inflammatory exudate fills the airways, segmental atelectasis may accompany the consolidation; for the same reason, an air bronchogram seldom is observed, and its presence should cast some doubt on the diagnosis. The airway involvement is

easier to appreciate on HRCT scan than on the radiograph (Fig. 5–17). With HRCT, bronchiolar involvement is manifested by centrilobular nodular and branching linear opacities (*tree-in-bud* pattern).

In a review of the radiographic abnormalities of 26 adults who had staphylococcal pneumonia, 14 (54%) had homogeneous consolidation, 12 (46%) had patchy consolidation, and 2 (8%) had a mixed picture.[19] The consolidation involved a single lobe in 36% of cases, involved more than one lobe in 54%, and was bilateral in 35%. In a second series of 31 adults, 15 (60%) had multilobar consolidation, and 12 (39%) had bilateral pneumonia;[18] the consolidation involved predominantly or exclusively the lower lobes in 16 patients (64%).

Abscesses develop in 15% to 30% of patients (Fig. 5–18).[18, 19] Characteristically, patients have an irregular shaggy inner wall. Although usually solitary, abscesses may be multiple. Pneumatocele formation also is common, occurring in about 50% of children[64] and 15% of adults.[19] They usually appear during the first week of the pneumonia and disappear spontaneously within weeks[65] or months.[66] Pleural effusions occur in 30% to 50% of patients; of these, approximately half represent empyemas.[18, 19] Spontaneous pneumothorax occurs occasionally; because the complication is associated with pneumatoceles, it is less common in adults than in children.[19]

In pneumonia related to hematogenous spread of organisms, the radiologic appearance is one of multiple nodules

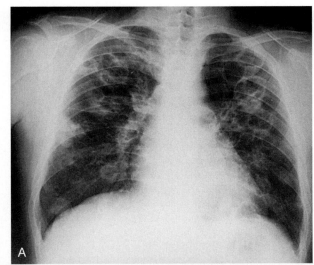

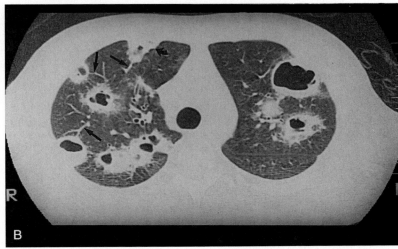

Figure 5–11. Septic Embolism. Chest radiograph *(A)* shows multiple bilateral cavitating nodules. CT scan *(B)* shows that several of the cavitating nodules are in a subpleural location. Some of the nodules have vessels leading into them *(feeding vessel* sign) *(straight arrows).* Note wedge-shaped subpleural consolidation *(curved arrow).* Blood cultures grew *Nocardia.* The patient was positive for human immunodeficiency virus. (Case courtesy of Dr. Tomás Franquet, Department of Radiology, Hospital de Sant Pau, Barcelona, Spain.)

or masses throughout the lungs *(see* Fig. 5–10). Sometimes the nodules have poorly defined borders or are confluent. Abscesses may erode into bronchi and produce air-containing cavities, frequently with fluid levels.[67] On CT scan, most abnormalities are in a subpleural location. In approximately two thirds of cases, some of the nodules have a vessel coursing into their substance *(feeding vessel* sign).[41, 42] Most nodules cavitate eventually. Septic infarcts result in subpleural wedge-shaped areas of consolidation; these were reported in 11 (73%) of 15 patients in one series.[41]

Gram-Negative Bacilli

Gram-negative bacilli are important causes of nosocomial and, under certain conditions, community-acquired lung infection. More than 50% of ventilator-associated pneumonias are caused by these organisms; when only lung superinfection is considered, they are responsible for about two thirds of cases.[68, 69]

Enterobacteriaceae

Klebsiella pneumoniae

Acute pneumonia caused by *K. pneumoniae* occurs predominantly in men in their 50s, many of whom are chronic alcoholics.[72] Chronic bronchopulmonary disease and, to a lesser extent, diabetes mellitus and debilitation appear to predispose to the infection.[52] The onset of acute pneumonia usually is abrupt, with prostration, pain on breathing, cyanosis, moderate fever, and severe dyspnea. Expectoration often is greenish, purulent, and blood streaked and occasionally brick red and gelatinous *(currant jelly sputum).*[52]

As an acute air-space pneumonia, *Klebsiella* pneumonia shows the same general radiographic features as pneumococcal pneumonia: homogeneous lobar parenchymal consolidation containing an air bronchogram. Compared with pneumococcal pneumonia, acute *Klebsiella* pneumonia has a greater tendency for the formation of voluminous inflammatory exudate leading to lobar expansion with resultant bulging of interlobar fissures *(see* Fig. 5–3),[17, 353] a greater tendency for abscess and cavity formation (Fig. 5–19),[61, 74] and a greater frequency of pleural effusion and empyema.[77, 78]

Bulging of interlobar fissures has been reported in approximately 30% of patients who have *Klebsiella* pneumonia,[17, 78] compared with 10% or less of patients with pneumococcal pneumonia.[17] Because of the greater prevalence of pneumococcal pneumonia, lobar expansion in any patient is more likely to be due to *S. pneumoniae* than to

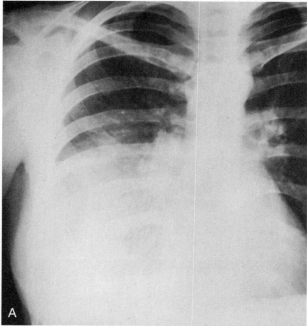

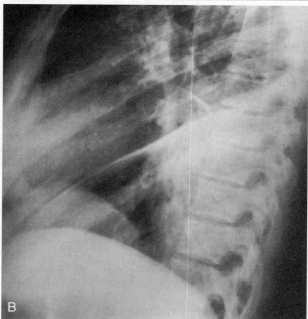

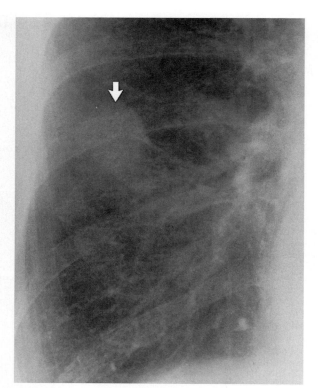

Figure 5–13. Round Pneumonia Resulting from *Streptococcus pneumoniae.* View of the right lung from posteroanterior chest radiograph shows a focal round area of consolidation *(arrow)* in the right lower lobe. Sputum cultures grew *S. pneumoniae*. The findings resolved after treatment with antibiotics.

Figure 5–12. Lobar Pneumonia: *Streptococcus pneumoniae.* Postero-anterior *(A)* and lateral *(B)* radiographs reveal extensive consolidation of the right lower lobe, a portion of the anterior segment being the only volume of lung unaffected. An air bronchogram is visible in the lateral projection. There is little loss of volume. Sputum culture produced a heavy growth of *Streptococcus pneumoniae*.

Klebsiella. Pleural effusion is seen in 60% to 70% of cases.[78, 79] Occasionally, acute *Klebsiella* pneumonia undergoes only partial resolution and passes into a chronic phase with cavitation and persistent positive cultures; in this circumstance, the radiographic picture simulates that seen in tuberculosis.

The pattern of nonsegmental air-space consolidation is seen more commonly in patients who have community-

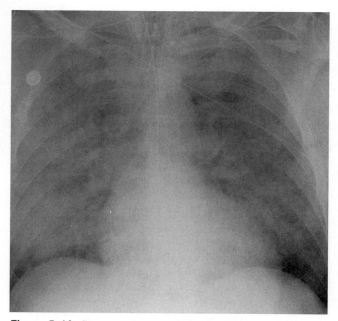

Figure 5–14. *Streptococcus pneumoniae* Pneumonia. A 50-year-old man presented with a 2-day history of high fever and progressive shortness of breath. Anteroposterior chest radiograph performed shortly after admission shows extensive bilateral areas of consolidation. Sputum and blood cultures grew *S. pneumoniae*. The disease resolved within 2 weeks after treatment with antibiotics.

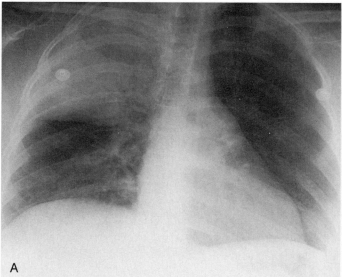

A

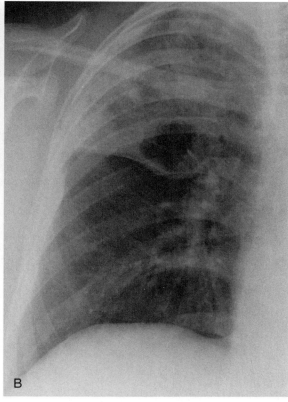

B

Figure 5–15. *Streptococcus pneumoniae* **Pneumonia.** Posteroanterior chest radiograph *(A)* in a 20-year-old woman shows extensive consolidation of the right upper lobe. Sputum cultures grew *S. pneumoniae*. Chest radiograph performed 1 week later, when the patient had markedly improved clinically *(B)*, shows focal lucency in the right upper lobe with bulging of the minor fissure. This subsequently resolved without complications. The appearance is consistent with a pneumatocele.

acquired than nosocomial *Klebsiella* pneumonia. Approximately 75% of patients with community-acquired infection have lobar pneumonia, most commonly involving the right upper lobe.[75, 76] By contrast, in one study of 15 patients who had *Klebsiella* infection, 13 of whom were considered to have hospital-acquired pneumonia, consolidation confined to one lobe occurred in 7 of 15 patients, patchy bilateral consolidation consistent with bronchopneumonia occurred in 7, and patchy unilateral consolidation occurred

in 1;[79] none of the 15 patients developed lobar expansion or cavitation.

Escherichia coli

Escherichia coli accounts for about 5% to 20% of cases of pneumonia acquired in a hospital or a nursing home.[73, 80] The typical history is one of abrupt onset of fever, chills,

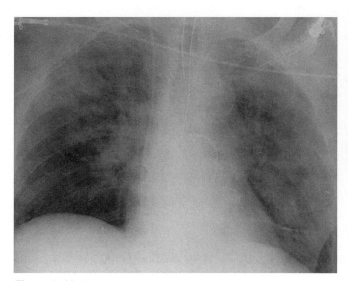

Figure 5–16. Staphylococcal Pneumonia. Anteroposterior chest radiograph in a 72-year-old man shows poorly defined bilateral areas of consolidation. Sputum and blood cultures grew *Staphylococcus aureus*.

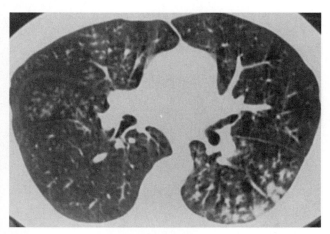

Figure 5–17. Staphylococcal Bronchiolitis and Bronchopneumonia. HRCT scan in a 32-year-old woman shows centrilobular nodular and branching linear opacities in the right middle and upper lobes and in the left lower lobe. This pattern (which often is referred to as *tree-in-bud*) and distribution are characteristic of bronchiolitis (early bronchopneumonia). In the left lower lobe, the process has progressed to parenchymal consolidation. Cultures from a bronchoscopic specimen grew *Staphylococcus aureus*.

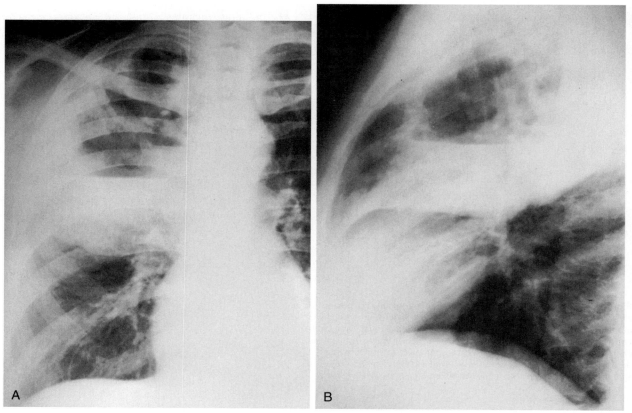

Figure 5–18. Acute Lung Abscess: *Staphylococcus aureus.* Posteroanterior *(A)* and lateral *(B)* radiographs reveal massive consolidation of the whole of the right upper lobe, a large ragged cavity being evident in its center. Volume of the lobe is increased, as indicated by the posterior bulging of the major fissure. Sputum culture produced a heavy growth of *S. aureus.*

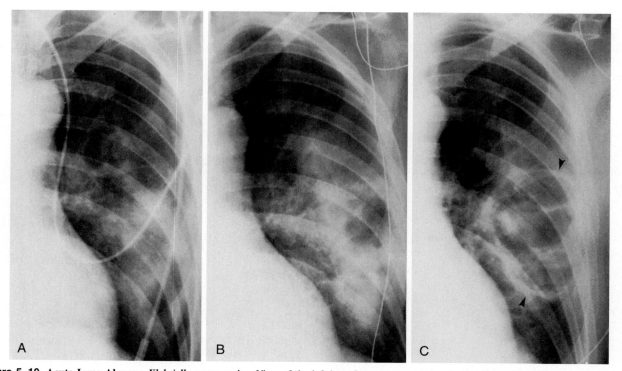

Figure 5–19. Acute Lung Abscess: *Klebsiella pneumoniae.* View of the left lung from posteroanterior chest radiograph *(A)* shows a poorly defined area of air-space consolidation in the lower lobe. Three days later *(B)*, the consolidation is more extensive, and several radiolucencies have appeared, indicating necrosis and bronchial communication. Five days later *(C)*, the cavities have coalesced to form a smoothly contoured, multiloculated abscess *(arrowheads).* The patient was a 45-year-old alcoholic man.

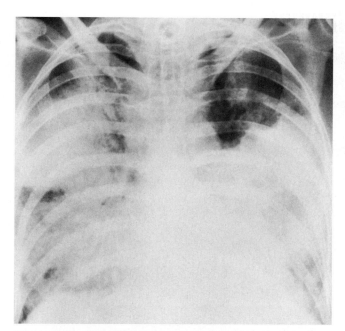

Figure 5–20. Acute Bronchopneumonia: *Pseudomonas aeruginosa.* This 38-year-old woman was admitted to the hospital in a deep coma as a result of an overdose of barbiturates. Several days after admission, anteroposterior radiograph showed massive air-space consolidation of all lobes of both lungs, the superior portion of the left upper lobe being least involved. An air bronchogram was present in all areas. The patient died 3 days after the radiograph was taken. *P. aeruginosa* was recovered in pure culture from the sputum and directly from the lung at autopsy.

dyspnea, pleuritic pain, cough, and expectoration of yellow sputum in a patient with pre-existing chronic disease.

The radiographic manifestations usually are those of bronchopneumonia; rarely a pattern of lobar pneumonia has been described.[82] Involvement usually is multilobar, with a strong lower lobe anatomic bias. Cavitation is uncommon, occurring in only one of seven patients in one series. Pleural effusion is frequent.[83]

Pseudomonas aeruginosa

Pneumonia caused by *P. aeruginosa* is the most common and most lethal form of nosocomial pulmonary infection.[85] The organism is the cause of approximately 20% of nosocomial pneumonia in adult patients in the intensive care unit.[71] Many risk factors for the infection have been identified in this setting, including chronic obstructive pulmonary disease (COPD) (relative risk, 29.9), mechanical ventilation longer than 8 days (relative risk, 8.1), and prior use of antibiotics (relative risk, 5.5).[86] Risk factors noted in other studies include the use of corticosteroids, malnutrition, and prolonged hospitalization.[70]

Although *P. aeruginosa* pneumonia is generally a nosocomial infection, it is sometimes community acquired,[87] particularly in patients who have advanced AIDS. The clinical presentation is typically abrupt, with chills, fever, severe dyspnea, and cough productive of copious yellow or green, occasionally blood-streaked sputum. Pleural pain is infrequent. Bradycardia is the rule. The organism is an important cause of chronic airway colonization and pneumonia in patients who have cystic fibrosis.

The radiologic manifestations of *P. aeruginosa* pneumonia are usually those of bronchopneumonia, consisting of multifocal bilateral areas of consolidation.[88] These areas may be lobular, subsegmental, or segmental in distribution and patchy or confluent (Fig. 5–20).[88] The consolidation frequently involves all lobes,[88] although it tends to involve predominantly the lower lobes. Less common radiographic manifestations include multiple nodular opacities[90] and (occasionally) a reticular pattern.[88] The nodules usually are secondary to bacteremia[89] but occasionally follow aspiration.[90]

The reported incidence of abscess formation in acute *P. aeruginosa* pneumonia is variable.[83, 91] In one review of 56 patients who had ventilator-associated *P. aeruginosa* documented at bronchoscopy,[88] 12 patients (23%) developed cavitation (in two, evident on CT scan but not on chest radiograph). The cavities may be small or large,[88] may be single or multiple, and may have thin or thick walls (Fig. 5–21).[88] Pneumatocele formation was reported in 4 of 56 patients in one series.[88]

Unilateral or bilateral pleural effusions, usually small, were identified on chest radiograph in 16 (84%) of 19 patients in one early study[84] but in only 13 (23%) of 56 patients in a more recent series.[88] Empyema is seen in a small percentage of cases;[88] rarely, enlargement of the cardiopericardial silhouette occurs secondary to purulent pericarditis.[92]

Gram-Negative Coccobacilli

Haemophilus influenzae

H. influenzae is responsible for about 5% to 20% of community-acquired pneumonias in patients in whom an

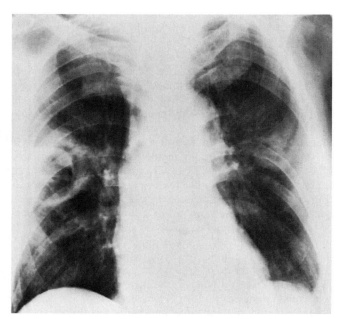

Figure 5–21. Lung Abscess: *Pseudomonas aeruginosa.* This 78-year-old man had had an esophageal resection with esophagogastric anastomosis for esophageal ulcer and stricture 10 days before this anteroposterior radiograph. Abscesses are present in both lungs, situated in the superior segment of the lower lobes. Repeated sputum cultures revealed heavy growth of *P. aeruginosa.*

organism can be identified successfully.[57, 81, 99] Risk factors include COPD,[95] alcoholism, diabetes mellitus, anatomic or functional asplenia, immunoglobulin defect,[94, 96] old age,[98] and AIDS.[97]

The radiologic manifestations of pulmonary *H. influenzae* infection are variable. In 50% to 60% of patients, the pattern is that of bronchopneumonia, consisting of areas of consolidation in a patchy or segmental distribution (*see* Fig. 5–4).[57, 100] The consolidation may be unilateral or bilateral and tends to involve mainly the lower lobes.[57, 100] In 30% to 50% of patients, the pattern is that of acute nonsegmental air-space consolidation similar to that of *S. pneumoniae*; this pattern may be seen alone or in combination with a pattern of bronchopneumonia.[57, 100] A reticular or reticulonodular interstitial pattern, by itself or in combination with air-space consolidation, occurs in 15% to 30% of cases.[57, 100] Cavitation has been reported in 15% or less of cases,[57, 100] and pleural effusion has been reported in approximately 50%;[93, 100] empyema is uncommon.

Legionella Species

The precise incidence of *Legionella pneumophila* pneumonia in the United States is uncertain. Prospective studies on consecutive patients hospitalized with pneumonia show an incidence of 2% to 25%,[101, 103] making the organism one of the more common in this setting. Among patients who have nosocomial pneumonia, the reported incidence of *Legionella* species has varied from 1% to 40%.[101]

Legionnaires' disease shows a propensity for older men, the male-to-female ratio being in the order of 2 or 3:1.[102] Most cases occur in patients who have pre-existing disease. Malignancy, renal failure, and transplantation are the most common underlying conditions associated with nosocomial infection;[105, 107] COPD and malignancy often are present in patients who become infected in the community.[104] The severity of disease varies from a mild respiratory illness to a fulminating one.[101] The usual presenting symptoms are fever (sometimes high and unremitting[105]), malaise, myalgia, rigors, confusion, headaches, and diarrhea. The most common respiratory complaints are a nonproductive cough without prior upper respiratory tract symptoms and, as the pneumonia progresses, dyspnea.[105] In time, cough may become productive and can be associated with hemoptysis. Pleural pain develops in about one third of patients.[105]

The characteristic radiographic pattern is one of air-space consolidation that is initially peripheral and sublobar, similar to that seen in acute *S. pneumoniae* pneumonia (Fig. 5–22). In many cases, the area of consolidation subsequently enlarges to occupy all or a large portion of a lobe or to involve contiguous lobes on the ipsilateral side.[109, 111, 112] Progression of the pneumonia usually is rapid,[109] most of a lobe becoming involved within 3 or 4 days, often despite the institution of appropriate antibiotic therapy (*see* Fig. 5–22);[110] such a behavior seldom is seen in acute air-space pneumonia caused by *S. pneumoniae*.[111, 113] There is a tendency for bilateral involvement as the disease progresses.[109, 111] No difference has been found in the radiographic findings between community-acquired and nosocomial infection.[103, 112]

In immunocompetent patients, abscess formation with subsequent cavitation is infrequent.[114] For example, cavita-

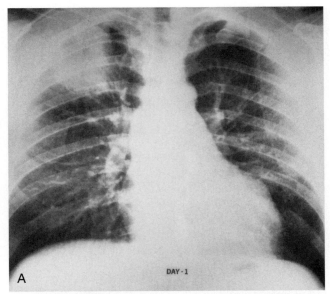
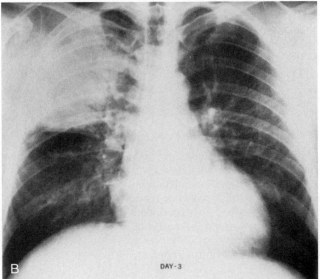

Figure 5–22. Acute Legionnaires' Pneumonia. On the day of admission of this 69-year-old man, posteroanterior radiograph *(A)* showed homogeneous consolidation of the axillary portion of the right upper lobe; an air bronchogram was apparent. Radiographs 2 days later *(B)* showed marked worsening. *Legionella pneumophila* was recovered from the sputum.

tion was identified in only 3 (4%) of 70 cases in one series[115] and 9 (6%) of 154 in a second.[112] In the latter study, there was no difference in the prevalence of abscess formation between nosocomial (7 of 122 cases) and community-acquired (2 of 32 cases) pneumonia.[112] By contrast, cavitation is seen fairly frequently in immunocompromised patients;[116, 117] for example, in one series of 10 patients who had received renal transplants, it was identified in 7, the interval between the first evidence of infection and cavitation ranging from 4 to 14 days (Fig. 5–23).[106] Pleural effusion may occur at the peak of the illness; it was described in 35% to 63% of cases in two series.[105, 526] Hilar lymph node enlargement,[2, 110] lobar expansion, and hydropneumothorax[118] are rare manifestations.

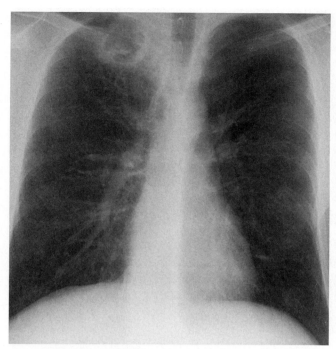

Figure 5–23. Abscess Formation: *Legionella pneumophila.* Posteroanterior chest radiograph in a 25-year-old renal transplant patient shows a 3-cm-diameter cavity in the right lung apex. Cultures of a fine-needle aspiration biopsy specimen revealed *L. pneumophila.* The abnormality resolved after treatment with antibiotics.

Occasionally, the focus of pneumonia is round, simulating a mass (Fig. 5–24).[119] Single or multiple nodules, which sometimes undergo rapid growth, may be seen in addition to consolidation involving part or all of one or more lobes.[120] Most investigators have found the radiographic pattern associated with infection by various *Legionella* species to be similar to that of *L. pneumophila* (Fig. 5–25).[108, 121, 122]

Anaerobic Bacteria

More than 30 genera and 200 species of anaerobes have been identified in human infection; such infection of the lung usually is polymicrobial.[46] Among the most important agents are the gram-negative bacilli *Bacteroides, Fusobacterium, Porphyromonas,* and *Prevotella*; the gram-positive bacilli *Actinomyces, Eubacterium,* and *Clostridium*; the gram-positive cocci *Peptostreptococcus* and *Peptococcus*; and the gram-negative cocci *Veillonella.*[124–127]

Among all patients admitted to hospital with pneumonia, anaerobic bacteria are isolated in approximately 20% to 35%,[128, 129] the organisms being second only to *S. pneumoniae* as a cause of community-acquired pneumonia. They also are important in nosocomial infection; for example, in one careful and extensive study of 159 patients with this complication, including patients in intensive care units, wards, and chronic care units, anaerobic organisms were found to be the cause of the infection in 59 (35%).[130] About 25% of patients have a history of impaired consciousness associated with such factors as general anesthesia, acute cerebrovascular accident, epileptic seizure, or drug inges-

tion.[123, 133, 134] Alcoholism has been reported in 40% to 75% of patients.[133, 134]

The clinical features of anaerobic pulmonary infection are variable. Acute pneumonitis may be indistinguishable from that caused by infection with *S. pneumoniae*;[137] infection complicated by lung abscess or empyema may have a protracted, insidious course. For example, in one series of 87 presumed anaerobic lung abscesses, illness before admission to a hospital ranged from a few days to 10 months.[132] Overall the mean duration appears to be about 2 to 3 weeks.[131, 135] Patients may be virtually asymptomatic; most do not appear seriously ill when first seen, although occasionally the disease runs a fulminant course leading to death. Fever is present in 70% to 80% of patients[133] but is usually low grade.

In the initial stages of infection, cough is frequently nonproductive, and the expectorated material, if any, is seldom putrid. When cavitation occurs—usually 7 to 10 days or more after the onset of pneumonia[123]—expectoration increases and becomes putrid in 40% to 75% of cases.[131, 133] Foul-smelling sputum always indicates the presence of anaerobic organisms; however, in the absence of abscess formation, such putrid expectoration is present in only 5% of patients.

The typical radiographic pattern is that of bronchopneumonia ranging from localized segmental areas of consolida-

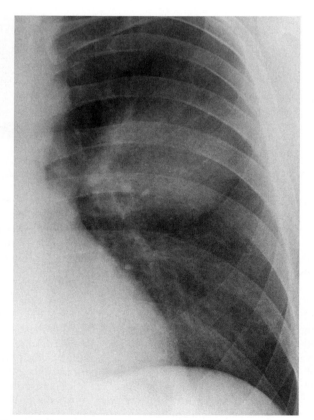

Figure 5–24. Round Pneumonia Resulting from *Legionella pneumophila.* View of the left lung from posteroanterior chest radiograph in a 34-year-old man shows a round area of consolidation. The patient presented with a 3-day history of fever and pleuritic chest pain. Sputum cultures grew *L. pneumophila.* The findings resolved within 2 weeks after treatment with erythromycin.

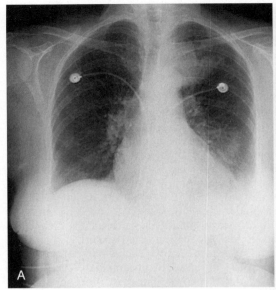

Figure 5–25. Pneumonia Resulting from *Legionella micdadei.* Anteroposterior chest radiograph *(A)* in a 66-year-old woman shows focal dense area of consolidation in the left upper lobe and poorly defined localized patchy areas of consolidation in the lower lobes. Contrast-enhanced CT scan *(B)* shows dense, masslike consolidation in the left upper lobe immediately adjacent to the aortic arch. CT scan at the level of the dome of the right hemidiaphragm *(C)* shows subsegmental areas of consolidation in the lower lobes. Cultures from bronchoscopy specimens grew *L. micdadei.*

tion to patchy bilateral consolidation to extensive confluent multilobar consolidation (Fig. 5–26). The distribution of pneumonia from aspiration of material contaminated by anaerobic organisms reflects gravitational flow; the posterior segments of the upper lobes or superior segments of the lower lobes tend to be involved with aspiration in the recumbent position and the basal segments of the lower lobes when aspiration occurs in an erect patient.[131, 135]

Cavitation has been reported in 20% to 60% of cases.[136, 137] In one study of 69 patients, approximately 50% had pulmonary parenchymal abnormalities, 30% had empyema without apparent parenchymal abnormalities, and 20% had combined parenchymal and pleural disease at presentation.[136] The parenchymal abnormalities consisted of consolidation without cavitation in approximately 50% of cases and lung abscess (defined as a circumscribed cavity with relatively little surrounding consolidation) or necrotizing pneumonia (defined as areas of consolidation containing single or multiple cavities) in the remaining 50% of cases. Occasionally, hilar or mediastinal lymph node enlargement is associated with an abscess, a combination of findings that may resemble that seen in patients who have pulmonary carcinoma (Fig. 5–27).[138]

MYCOBACTERIA

Mycobacterium tuberculosis

Tuberculosis is one of the most important infectious diseases. In 1996, 21,337 cases were reported in the United States (rate, 8 per 100,000).[141] Rates are much higher in many developing countries, particularly those in South East Asia and Africa.[142] It has been estimated that between 1997 and 2020, close to 1 billion people worldwide will be infected by *M. tuberculosis*, and 70 million will die from tuberculosis.[142]

Although any mycobacterial disease other than that caused by *M. leprae* theoretically can be designated *tuberculosis*, the term usually implies disease caused by *M. tuberculosis*. Such disease should be distinguished from simple infection by the organism in the absence of clinical or radiologic manifestations. Tuberculosis has been estimated to develop in only 5% to 15% of individuals who are infected.[143, 144]

In most cases, tuberculous infection is acquired from an individual who has active (often cavitary) disease after inhalation of droplet nuclei carrying the organisms.[139, 140] The risk of infection is related to the degree of conta-

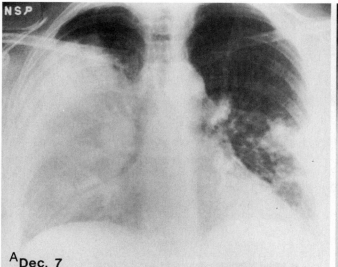

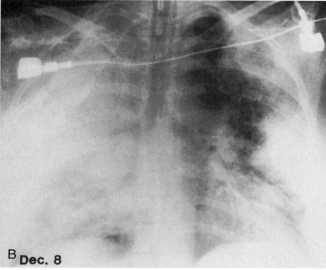

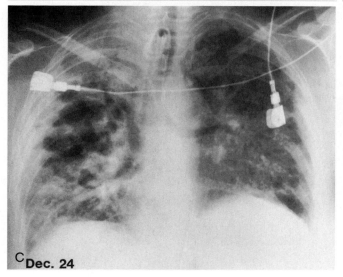

Figure 5–26. Anaerobic Pneumonia—Massive Air-Space Pneumonia with Abscess Formation. The first examination *(A)* on this extremely ill 45-year-old alcoholic woman revealed massive, homogeneous consolidation of the right lower lobe and patchy consolidation of the left lung. Twenty-four hours later *(B)*, acute pneumonia had extended throughout most of the right lung and much of the left. During the next 2 weeks on antibiotic therapy, most of the pneumonia in the left lung had resolved *(C)*. A large, ragged, thick-walled cavity had appeared in the right lung, however. A heavy growth of bacilli was present on anaerobic culture.

giousness of the primarily infected individual, the adequacy of antimicrobial defense of the exposed individual, the frequency of contact between the two, and the environment in which the contact takes place. Disease may be associated with progression of the primary focus of infection (*primary tuberculosis*) or with the development of new disease months or years after healing of the initial infection has occurred (*postprimary tuberculosis*). The latter is often the result of reactivation of an endogenous focus of infection acquired earlier in life;[145, 146] an exogenous source is responsible at times (i.e., reinfection)[147, 148] and may be predominant in areas in which tuberculosis is common.[524]

Primary Pulmonary Tuberculosis

Clinical Manifestations

Primary pulmonary tuberculosis traditionally has been thought to occur predominantly in children, in whom it is particularly prevalent in regions in which the annual risk of infection is high. With the reduction in the incidence of tuberculosis since the early part of the twentieth century in

many regions, however, and the resulting increase in the number of nonsensitized individuals, the primary form of disease appears to have become more common in adults than it was previously.[149] Based on data derived from molecular studies, it appears that 30% to 40% of cases of tuberculosis in some populations are recently acquired.[164, 165]

The initial focus of parenchymal disease in primary tuberculosis is termed the *Ghon focus*. It either enlarges as the disease progresses or, more commonly, undergoes healing. In the latter event, fibroblasts at the periphery of the necrotic foci proliferate and form collagen. Although this process sometimes results in conversion of the entire area into a dense fibrous scar, more often the central necrotic material persists and becomes separated from the surrounding lung parenchyma by a well-developed fibrous capsule. Dystrophic calcification is common in the necrotic material at this stage and often is of sufficient degree to be visible radiographically. Despite the fact that the disease is inactive, viable organisms may remain within the encapsulated necrotic areas and serve as a focus for reactivation in later life.

During the early phase of infection, spread of organisms

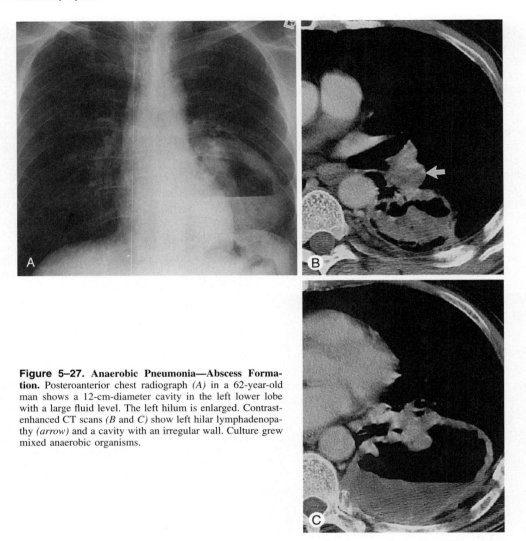

Figure 5–27. Anaerobic Pneumonia—Abscess Formation. Posteroanterior chest radiograph *(A)* in a 62-year-old man shows a 12-cm-diameter cavity in the left lower lobe with a large fluid level. The left hilum is enlarged. Contrast-enhanced CT scans *(B* and *C)* show left hilar lymphadenopathy *(arrow)* and a cavity with an irregular wall. Culture grew mixed anaerobic organisms.

to regional lymph nodes via lymphatic channels is common and results in granulomatous inflammation adjacent to the lymphatic vessels and in the nodes themselves. The combination of a Ghon focus and affected lymph nodes is known as the *Ranke complex.* The course of the disease in lymph nodes is similar to that in the parenchyma, consisting initially of granulomatous inflammation and necrosis followed by fibrosis and calcification; however, the degree of inflammatory reaction typically is greater in lymph nodes than in the parenchyma, making this site of infection more obvious radiographically.

Most children who have primary tuberculosis are asymptomatic. By comparison, 82% of 103 adults who had primary disease in another review were found to be symptomatic;[154] the symptoms consisted of fever in 40% of patients, cough in 37%, weight loss in 24%, and hemoptysis in 8%.[154] Other reported manifestations include sweating, chest pain, and lethargy.[151]

Radiologic Manifestations

As indicated, most individuals infected with *M. tuberculosis* do not have radiologic abnormalities. When infection

leads to primary thoracic disease, it usually involves one or more of four structures: (1) the pulmonary parenchyma, (2) the mediastinal and hilar lymph nodes, (3) the tracheobronchial tree, and (4) the pleura (Table 5–4).

Parenchymal Involvement

The largest study of the radiologic manifestations of primary tuberculosis in children is based on a review of 252 consecutive cases, for which chest radiographs were

Table 5–4. PRIMARY PULMONARY TUBERCULOSIS: APPROXIMATE PREVALENCE OF RADIOLOGIC MANIFESTATIONS

Radiologic Findings	Children (%)	Adults (%)
Hilar and mediastinal lymphadenopathy	95	30
Parenchymal consolidation	70	90
Cavitation	2	6
Miliary disease	3	5
Pleural effusion	5	30

available in 191.[153] Air-space consolidation was identified in approximately 70% of these cases; it affected the right lung more often than the left, was bilateral in 15% of cases, and showed no significant predilection for any particular lung region. A previous study based on a smaller number of cases had shown a slight upper lobe predominance.[151]

In a review of the chest radiographs of 103 adults who had primary disease, evidence of air-space consolidation was found in approximately 90%.[154] The consolidation involved the right upper lobe most commonly (30% of cases) and the right middle lobe least commonly (10% of cases); each of the remaining lobes and lingula were involved in approximately 20% of cases. The consolidation usually is homogeneous, dense, and anatomically confined to a segment (Fig. 5–28) or, more commonly, a lobe.[155] In approximately 25% of cases, it is multifocal, and in 10% it is bilateral.[153, 154] Cavitation has been reported in approximately 2% of children and 6% of adults.[153, 154] Radiologic evidence of miliary disease has been reported in about 3% of children and 6% of adults.[151, 154]

Lymph Node Involvement

Evidence of lymph node enlargement is identified on the chest radiograph in about 90% to 95% of children who have primary disease.[151, 153] Most have hilar involvement, most commonly on the right; approximately 50% have hilar and mediastinal (usually the right paratracheal region) disease.[153]

Lymph node enlargement is seen less commonly in adults than in children; for example, in two studies of 103 and 19 adults who had primary tuberculosis, it was evident radiographically in only 10 (10%) of the 103 adults[154] and 6 (32%) of the 19 adults.[154] As with children, the lymph node enlargement most commonly is unilateral and hilar (*see* Fig. 5–28) or paratracheal (Fig. 5–29); it may be the only abnormality, and in children and adults, unilateral lymph node enlargement should suggest the disease. The presence of bilateral lymph node enlargement or lymph node enlargement without parenchymal consolidation does not exclude tuberculosis; with the exception of patients who have AIDS, this picture is uncommon in adults.[154]

On CT scan, affected lymph nodes often have relatively low attenuation of the central region and show peripheral (rim) enhancement after intravenous administration of contrast material (Fig. 5–30).[155, 158] In one study of 23 patients, such rim enhancement usually was seen in nodes larger than 2 cm in diameter;[157] smaller nodes usually showed inhomogeneous enhancement throughout. In a subsequent study, the attenuation values of enlarged lymph nodes before and after intravenous administration of contrast material were assessed in 38 patients.[158] Approximately 50% of nodes had low attenuation (<30 HU), and 50% had soft

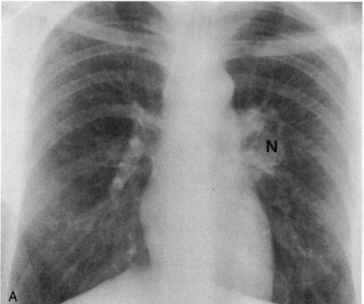

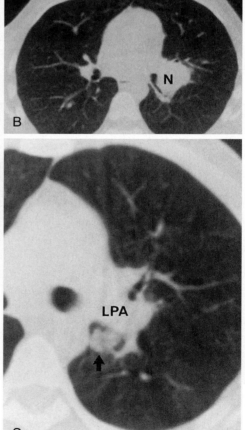

Figure 5–28. Primary Pulmonary Tuberculosis. Posteroanterior chest radiograph *(A)* shows left hilar lymph node enlargement (N). CT scan through the left hilum *(B)* confirms the presence of enlarged lymph nodes (N). CT scan at a slightly higher level *(C)* shows the primary focus in the superior segment of the lower lobe *(arrow)* behind the left pulmonary artery (LPA). The patient was a 25-year-old man.

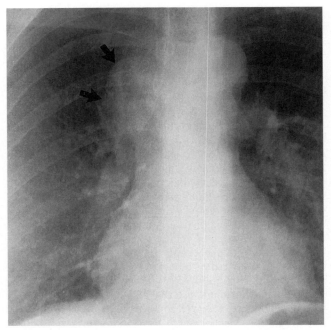

Figure 5–29. Primary Tuberculosis. View of the mediastinum from posteroanterior chest radiograph in a 46-year-old woman shows right paratracheal lymphadenopathy *(arrows).* Cultures from lymph node biopsy grew *Mycobacterium tuberculosis.*

tissue attenuation (>35 HU). Four patterns of contrast enhancement were identified: (1) peripheral rim enhancement (57%), (2) inhomogeneous enhancement (21%), (3) homogeneous enhancement (16%), and (4) homogeneous nonenhancement (5%). The authors concluded that although neither the nodal attenuation values nor the patterns of enhancement were diagnostic of tuberculosis, the pres-

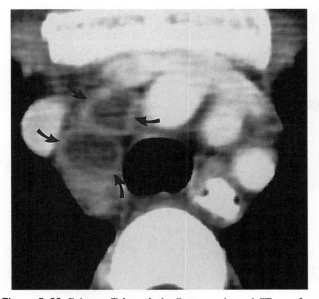

Figure 5–30. Primary Tuberculosis. Contrast-enhanced CT scan 2 cm above the level of the aortic arch shows enlarged right paratracheal lymph nodes *(curved arrows)* with low attenuation center and rim enhancement. Cultures from lymph node biopsy grew *Mycobacterium tuberculosis.* The patient was a 29-year-old woman.

ence of peripheral rim enhancement with relative low attenuation centers should suggest the diagnosis in the appropriate clinical setting. Low attenuation nodes with peripheral enhancement also have been described in other infections caused by organisms such as *M. avium* complex and *Histoplasma capsulatum* and, less commonly, in lymph node enlargement secondary to pulmonary carcinoma or lymphoma.[36, 160]

Airway Involvement

Atelectasis, usually lobar and right-sided, has been reported in 10% to 30% of children who have primary tuberculosis.[151, 153] It usually is the result of bronchial compression by enlarged lymph nodes; less commonly, endobronchial disease is responsible.[151, 161] Occasionally, enlarged lymph nodes result in obstructive overinflation of a lobe or lobes.[151, 153] Atelectasis is less common in adults than in children; when it occurs, it tends to involve the anterior segment of the upper lobes and may simulate pulmonary carcinoma radiographically.[162]

Pleural Involvement

Pleural effusions have been reported in 5% to 10% of children[151, 153] and 30% to 40% of adults[152, 154] who have primary tuberculosis. They usually are seen in association with parenchymal abnormalities; however, in about 5% of adults, the effusion is the only radiographic manifestation of the disease.[154]

Calcification

Follow-up chest radiographs in children who have had primary tuberculosis have shown evidence of calcification in the pulmonary lesion in about 10% to 15% of cases and in the lymph nodes in about 5% to 35%.[151, 153] Although a calcified Ranke complex constitutes reasonable evidence of primary tuberculosis (Fig. 5–31), the same radiographic finding can occur as a sequela to histoplasmosis or other fungal infection. The presence and character of splenic calcifications can be useful in determining the cause of associated pulmonary calcification: Such calcifications are more common in the spleen in histoplasmosis than in tuberculosis and tend to be multiple, small, and punctate in histoplasmosis and relatively few and larger in tuberculosis.[163]

Postprimary Tuberculosis

Clinical Manifestations

The term *postprimary (secondary, reactivation) tuberculosis* is used to describe a clinical and radiologic form of disease that is correlated pathogenetically with the presence of acquired hypersensitivity and immunity. Many cases occur in adults as a result of reactivation of a focus of infection acquired earlier in life. Although previously it was believed that this mechanism was responsible for most cases of pulmonary tuberculosis, epidemiologic evidence based on DNA fingerprinting has shown that 30% to 40% of such cases are recently acquired in selected populations.[164, 165]

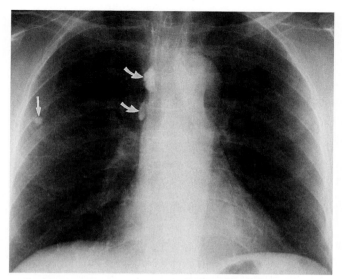

Figure 5–31. Calcified Ghon's Focus and Lymph Nodes (Ranke's Complex). Posteroanterior chest radiograph in a 35-year-old woman shows calcified right upper lobe nodule *(straight arrow)* and right paratracheal lymph nodes *(curved arrows)*.

Table 5–5. POSTPRIMARY TUBERCULOSIS: APPROXIMATE PREVALENCE OF RADIOLOGIC MANIFESTATIONS

Radiologic Finding	Prevalence (% of Patients)
Location in apical or posterior segment of upper lobe	85
Focal consolidation	50–70
Cavitation	20–45
Focal nodular opacities (2- to 10-mm-diameter) on chest radiograph	20–25
Centrilobular nodules on HRCT	80–95
Evidence of endobronchial spread on chest radiograph	10–20
Evidence of endobronchial spread on HRCT	35–95

HRCT, high-resolution computed tomography.

In contrast to primary tuberculosis, in which fibrosis and healing are the rule, postprimary tuberculosis tends to progress, foci of inflammation and necrosis enlarging to occupy ever greater portions of lung parenchyma. During this process, communication with airways is frequent, resulting in expulsion of necrotic material and cavity formation.

The most common symptoms of postprimary tuberculosis are nonspecific and may not direct the attention of the patient or the physician to the lungs; they include fatigue, weakness, anorexia, weight loss, and a low-grade fever (sometimes associated with rigors).[185, 186] Direct questioning often elicits a history of unproductive or mildly productive cough.

Radiologic Manifestations

A characteristic manifestation of postprimary tuberculosis is its tendency to localize in the apical and posterior segments of the upper lobes.[166, 171] For example, in one study of 423 adults who had local pulmonary tuberculosis, the lesions were predominantly in the apical and posterior segments of an upper lobe in 85% and in the superior segment of one or other lower lobe in 9.5%.[168] In about 70% to 90% of cases, the abnormalities involve more than one segment.[166, 167]

Air-Space Consolidation

Focal areas of consolidation are seen on chest radiograph and HRCT scan in approximately 50% to 70% of patients who have postprimary tuberculosis (Table 5–5).[166, 167] On the radiograph, the areas of consolidation have ill-defined margins and show a tendency to coalesce, often with small satellite foci in the adjacent lung (Fig. 5–32). HRCT-pathologic correlations have shown that these areas of consolidation tend to be lobular in distribution; that is,

they involve entire secondary lobules, while sparing adjacent lobules (Fig. 5–33).[13, 169] There is frequently an accentuation of the bronchovascular markings leading to the ipsilateral hilum. Associated hilar or mediastinal lymph node enlargement is relatively uncommon, being identified on chest radiographs in only 5% of 56 patients in one series[156] and in 9% of 158 patients in another.[166] On HRCT scan, mediastinal lymph node enlargement (defined as a lymph node >10 mm in short-axis diameter) was identified in 7 (8%) of 89 patients in one series[167] and in 9 (31%) of 29 patients in a second series.[13] As in primary disease, enlarged lymph nodes usually show inhomogeneous enhancement or low attenuation centers with rim enhance-

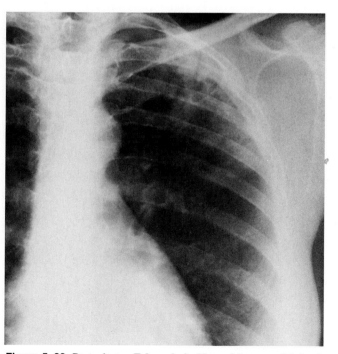

Figure 5–32. Postprimary Tuberculosis. View of the upper left hemithorax from posteroanterior radiograph in a 49-year-old woman shows poorly defined focal areas of consolidation and small satellite foci in the left upper lobe. *Mycobacterium tuberculosis* was recovered from the sputum.

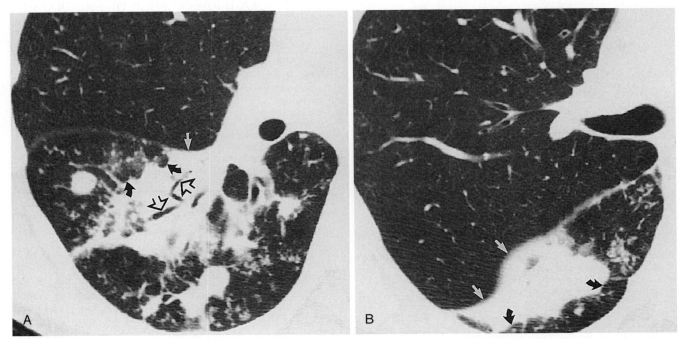

Figure 5–33. Air-Space Consolidation in Postprimary Tuberculosis. HRCT scans *(A and B)* in a 26-year-old woman show focal area of consolidation with air bronchograms *(open arrows)* in the superior segment of the right lower lobe. The consolidation is marginated by the right major interlobar fissure *(straight arrows)* and by interlobular septa *(curved arrows)* with sparing of the adjacent secondary lobules. Several satellite nodules also are evident. Sputum cultures grew *Mycobacterium tuberculosis*.

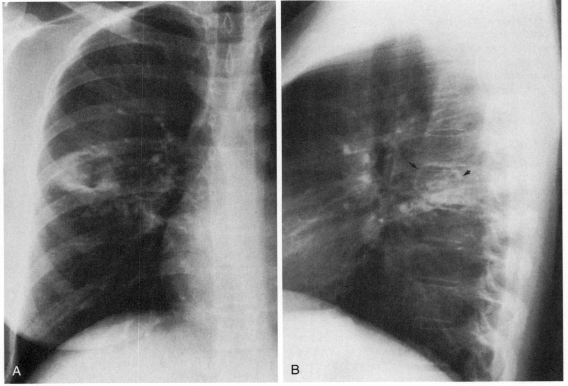

Figure 5–34. Cavitary Tuberculosis (Postprimary). Posteroanterior *(A)* and lateral *(B)* radiographs show a poorly defined, thin-walled cavity in the superior segment of the right lower lobe *(arrows in B)*. Both lungs were otherwise normal. *Mycobacterium tuberculosis* was recovered from the sputum.

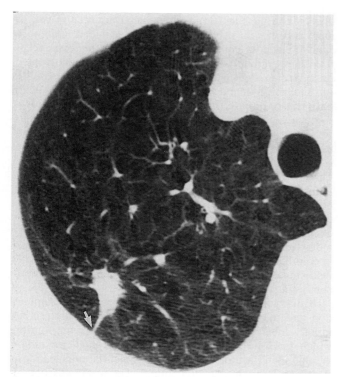

Figure 5–35. Tuberculoma. View of the right upper lobe from HRCT scan in a 59-year-old smoker shows 1.5-cm-diameter nodule with spiculated margins and a pleural tag *(arrow)*. Emphysema also is present. The resected nodule was found to be a granuloma from which cultures grew *Mycobacterium tuberculosis*.

ment after intravenous administration of contrast material.[157, 159]

In most cases, the consolidation is limited to one segment or portions of several segments of a lobe.[171] Occasionally, disease evolves to affect an entire lobe (tuberculous lobar pneumonia) or, after endobronchial spread of disease, several lobes[156, 171] (tuberculous bronchopneumonia). Rarely, disease affects all lobes and leads to respiratory failure.[172]

Cavitation

Cavitation is identified on chest radiograph in 20% to 45% of patients (Fig. 5–34).[156, 166, 169] It is appreciated more frequently on HRCT scan;[169, 170] for example, in one study of 41 patients, cavitation was identified in 58% on HRCT scan compared with 22% on radiographs.[169] Approximately 80% to 85% of cavities are located in the apical or posterior segments of the upper lobes and 10% to 15% in the superior segments of the lower lobes.[171] Cavities may be single or multiple and thin or thick walled. Approximately 20% have an air-fluid level.[166, 174, 175]

With adequate therapy, a cavity may disappear. Sometimes, the cavity wall becomes paper thin, and it appears as an air-filled cystic space. Such persistent cavitation after chemotherapy does not indicate active disease.[173, 174]

Nodular Opacities

Nodular opacities can be classified into four types: (1) a single nodule usually greater than 1 cm in diameter (tuberculoma), with or without adjacent smaller nodules; (2) multiple nodules usually less than 1 cm in diameter

limited to one or two regions of the lung (focal nodular opacities), with or without associated branching linear opacities; (3) multiple nodules 2 to 10 mm in diameter involving several lobes usually in an asymmetric or patchy distribution (representing endobronchial spread of tuberculosis); and (4) innumerable nodules 1 to 3 mm in diameter diffusely throughout both lungs (miliary tuberculosis).

Tuberculoma. A tuberculoma may be a manifestation of primary or postprimary tuberculosis; in the latter form, tuberculomas have been described as the main or only abnormality seen on chest radiographs in approximately 5% of patients.[156, 166] The lesions are manifested by round or oval opacities situated most commonly in an upper lobe, the right more often than the left.[176] They usually measure 1 to 4 cm in diameter and typically are smooth and sharply defined;[176, 177] occasionally, tuberculomas have indistinct, lobulated, or spiculated margins (Fig. 5–35).[171, 179] Small discrete nodules in the immediate vicinity of the main lesion—*satellite* lesions—can be identified in 80% of cases.[176] Similar to granulomas caused by other infectious organisms, tuberculomas often show little or no enhancement on CT scan after intravenous administration of contrast material.[171, 180]

Most tuberculomas remain stable for a long time,[527] and many calcify. Calcification is usually diffuse but may be central (Fig. 5–36) or punctate.[155, 178] CT is superior to radiography in the detection of any of these patterns.[181]

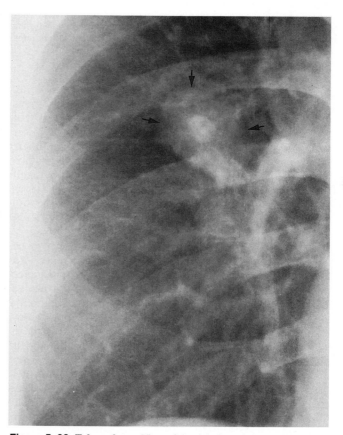

Figure 5–36. Tuberculoma. View of the right lung from posteroanterior chest radiograph in a 54-year-old man shows a tuberculoma *(arrows)* with central calcification. The patient had been treated previously for postprimary tuberculosis.

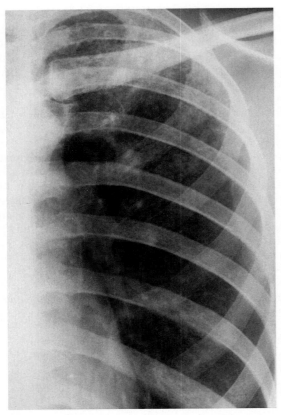

Figure 5–37. Small Nodular Opacities in Postprimary Tuberculosis. View of the left upper chest from posteroanterior radiograph in a 52-year-old woman shows poorly defined small nodular opacities involving the apicoposterior segment of the left upper lobe. Sputum cultures grew *Mycobacterium tuberculosis*.

Focal Nodular Opacities. Nodular opacities measuring 2 to 10 mm in diameter and localized to one or two regions of the lungs, usually the apical or posterior segments of the upper lobes or the superior segment of the lower lobes, have been described as the main or only radiologic manifestation in 20% to 25% of patients who have postprimary tuberculosis (Fig. 5–37).[156, 166] More commonly, small nodular opacities are seen in association with focal areas of consolidation, a combination of findings that is seen on radiograph and on HRCT scan in approximately 80% of patients.[156, 167]

On HRCT scan, the opacities have been shown to be centrilobular in distribution and often associated with branching linear opacities (Fig. 5–38),[13, 167] an appearance that has been likened to that of a *tree-in-bud*.[13] As indicated earlier, these abnormalities are common: Centrilobular nodules measuring 2 to 5 mm in diameter or branching centrilobular linear opacities were identified on HRCT scan in 97% of 29 patients in one series[13] and in 92% of 89 patients in a second.[167] Pathologically, the nodules have been shown to reflect the presence of intrabronchiolar and peribronchiolar inflammatory exudate, whereas the branching linear opacities correlate with the presence of caseous material filling or surrounding terminal or respiratory bronchioles or alveolar ducts.[13, 169]

Endobronchial Spread of Tuberculosis. Endobronchial spread of tuberculosis can be inferred when multiple nod-

ules measuring 2 to 10 mm in diameter are seen in two or more lobes or in a lobe other than the one containing a cavity or area of consolidation (Fig. 5–39) (the one exception being miliary disease; see farther on). Radiographic findings consistent with endobronchial spread of tuberculosis have been reported in 10% to 20% of patients with postprimary disease.[156, 166] Studies using HRCT have shown a much higher prevalence; for example, HRCT findings consistent with endobronchial spread were seen in 34% of 89 patients in one study,[167] in 98% of 41 patients in a second study,[13] and in 97% of 31 patients in a third study.[173] The most common findings on HRCT scan consist of 2- to 4-mm-diameter centrilobular nodules and branching linear opacities with sharply defined margins. Other abnormalities, in decreasing order of frequency, are 4- to 8-mm-diameter nodules with poorly defined margins (also commonly located in a centrilobular distribution), lobular areas of consolidation, and thickening of the interlobular septa.[13, 171] Occasionally, CT scan may show narrowing of the bronchial lumen (Fig. 5–40).

Miliary Tuberculosis. The interval between dissemination and the development of radiographically discernible miliary tuberculosis is probably 6 weeks or more, during which time the foci of infection are too small for radiographic identification. When first visible, the nodules measure 1 to 2 mm in diameter (Fig. 5–41); in the absence of adequate therapy, they may grow to 3 to 5 mm in diameter, a finding seen in approximately 10% of cases.[40] By this time, they may have become almost confluent, presenting a *snowstorm* appearance.

The diagnostic accuracy for the identification of miliary tuberculosis on chest radiograph was assessed in a retrospective study, which included radiographs of 71 patients who had culture-proven, biopsy-proven, or autopsy-proven miliary tuberculosis. Included as controls were 44 normal chest radiographs and 22 radiographs of patients who had localized pulmonary tuberculosis.[40] Three independent radiologists had a 60% to 70% sensitivity in identifying miliary tuberculosis and a 97% to 100% specificity in excluding it. In 30% of patients, nodules could not be seen on the radiograph at the time of diagnosis, even in retrospect.

HRCT can be helpful in the diagnosis of miliary tuberculosis in patients who have normal or nonspecific radiographic findings.[182, 183] Findings consist of nodules, usually sharply defined, measuring 1 to 4 mm in diameter and having a diffuse random distribution throughout both lungs (Fig. 5–42).[183, 189] Other abnormalities that may be seen on CT scan include nodular thickening of the interlobular septa and interlobar fissures, nodular irregularity of vessels, and areas of ground-glass attenuation.[183, 184, 189] Although some nodules may be seen in relation to vessels, interlobular septa, or pleural surfaces, most have a random distribution in relation to the structures of the secondary pulmonary lobule.[183]

Bronchiectasis

Bronchiectasis is seen on HRCT scan in 30% to 60% of patients who have postprimary tuberculosis.[167, 170, 173] The prevalence is greater in patients who have healed disease; for example, in two studies, it was seen on HRCT scan in 56% of 32 patients and 63% of 89 patients who had active

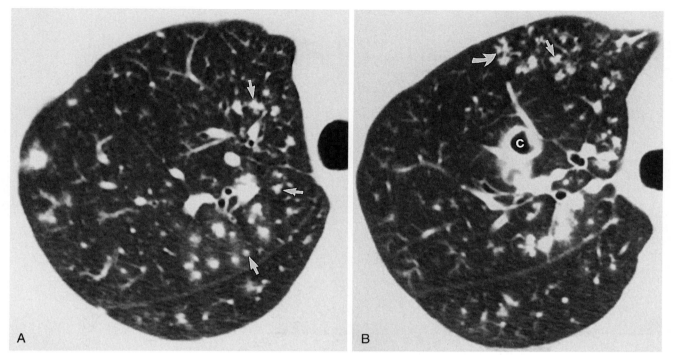

Figure 5–38. Small Nodular Opacities in Postprimary Tuberculosis. Views of the right upper lobe *(A and B)* from HRCT scan in a 29-year-old woman show a cavity *(C)* and several nodular opacities measuring 2 to 7 mm in diameter. Most nodules are located near the center of the secondary lobule *(straight arrows).* Also shown are centrilobular branching linear opacities. The combination of small nodules and branching centrilobular linear opacities gives an appearance that has been likened to a *tree-in-bud (curved arrow).*

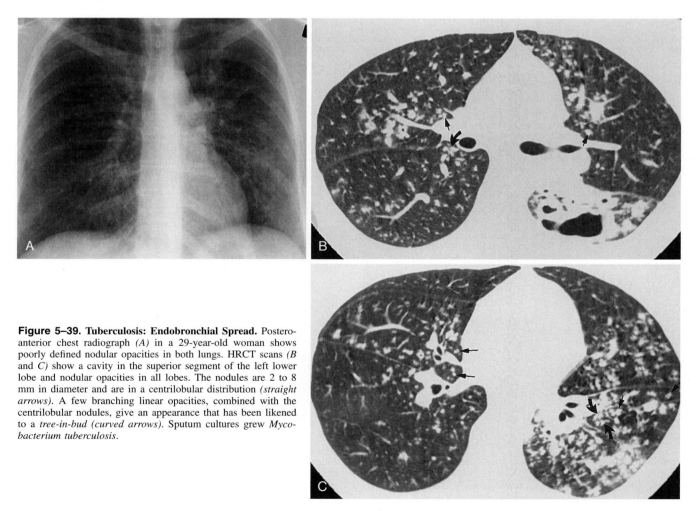

Figure 5–39. Tuberculosis: Endobronchial Spread. Postero-anterior chest radiograph *(A)* in a 29-year-old woman shows poorly defined nodular opacities in both lungs. HRCT scans *(B and C)* show a cavity in the superior segment of the left lower lobe and nodular opacities in all lobes. The nodules are 2 to 8 mm in diameter and are in a centrilobular distribution *(straight arrows).* A few branching linear opacities, combined with the centrilobular nodules, give an appearance that has been likened to a *tree-in-bud (curved arrows).* Sputum cultures grew *Mycobacterium tuberculosis.*

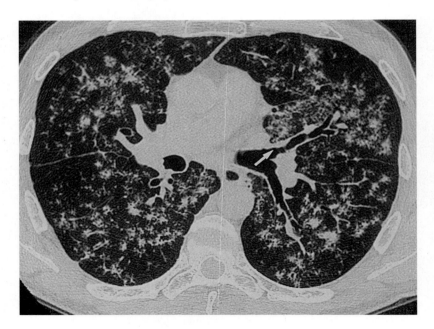

Figure 5–40. Tuberculosis—Endobronchial Spread. HRCT scan shows numerous bilateral centrilobular nodules. Focal narrowing of the left upper lobe bronchus *(arrow)* is due to involvement of the bronchial wall by tuberculosis. (Case courtesy of Dr. Inmaculada Herraez, Department of Radiology, Hospital de Leon, Leon, Spain.)

disease compared with 71% of 34 patients and 86% of 57 patients who had inactive disease.[167, 173] The bronchiectasis is bilateral in approximately 60% of cases and unilateral in the remainder.[170] Bronchiectasis usually affects one or two lobes and involves mainly the upper lobes.[170] In most patients, the abnormality is not readily apparent on radiography.

Extrapulmonary Tuberculosis

Extrapulmonary tuberculosis can develop in several ways, perhaps the most common of which is hematogenous dissemination during primary infection. Although the foci of infection established by such dissemination usually are not apparent at the time of the primary disease, they may reactivate and cause clinically evident disease months or years later, as in postprimary pulmonary tuberculosis. Such

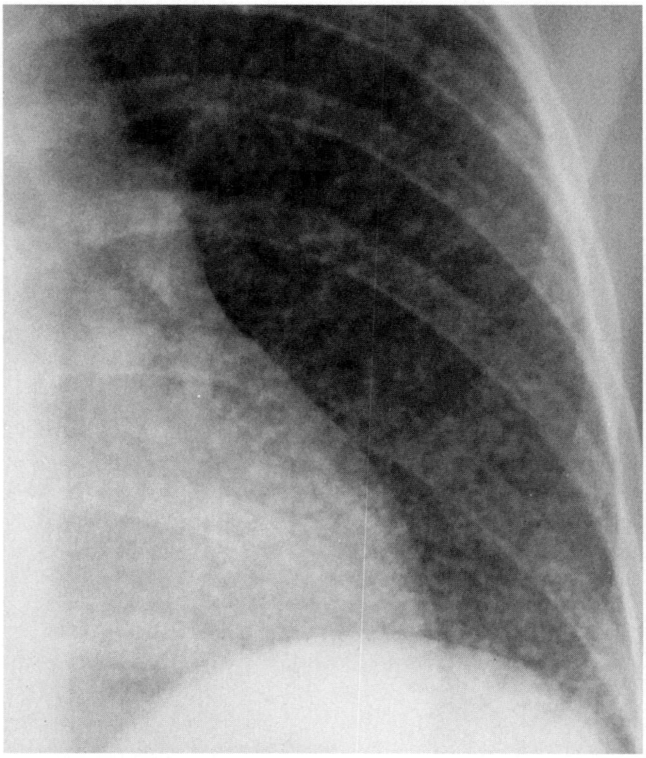

Figure 5–41. Miliary Tuberculosis. View of the left lung from antero-posterior chest radiograph in a 22-year-old woman shows numerous sharply defined nodules 1 to 3 mm in diameter. The diagnosis of miliary tuberculosis was proved by bone marrow biopsy.

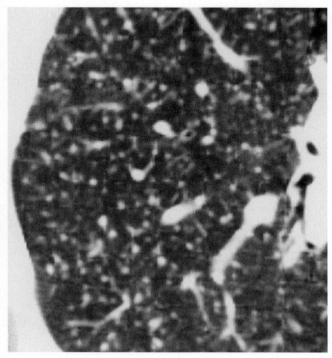

Figure 5–42. Miliary Tuberculosis. View of the right lung from HRCT scan in a 32-year-old man shows multiple nodules measuring approximately 2 mm in diameter in random distribution throughout the lung. The diagnosis of miliary tuberculosis was proved by open-lung biopsy.

reactivation can occur in any tissue or organ in the body but most often involves the kidneys, adrenal glands, fallopian tubes, epididymis, and bones (particularly the thoracic spine). Extrapulmonary disease also can develop during progressive primary or postprimary pulmonary tuberculosis (in both situations, particularly as miliary disease).

Before the onset of the AIDS epidemic, approximately 15% of cases of tuberculosis involved extrapulmonary sites in the absence of pulmonary disease.[187] Because the risk of developing extrapulmonary disease is much greater in patients who have AIDS,[188] the incidence of this form of infection is increasing.

Tuberculosis of the spine (Pott's disease) is the most common form of skeletal disease and usually affects the lower thoracic or upper lumbar vertebrae. The early radio-

graphic manifestations consist of irregularity of the vertebral end plates, decreased height of the intervertebral disk space, and sclerosis of the adjacent bone. With progression of disease, there is a tendency to anterior wedging of the vertebral body, leading to kyphosis and development of paravertebral abscesses (the latter associated with displacement of the paraspinal interface[190]) (Fig. 5–43). CT is superior to the radiograph in showing the extent of the abnormalities, development of paraspinal abscesses, and involvement of the spinal canal.[191–193] With this technique, paravertebral abscesses show peripheral rim enhancement and low attenuation centers after intravenous administration of contrast material (*see* Fig. 5–43);[192, 193] in most cases, amorphous calcification also is seen.[193] The extent of the abnormalities is well demonstrated on magnetic resonance (MR) imaging.[194]

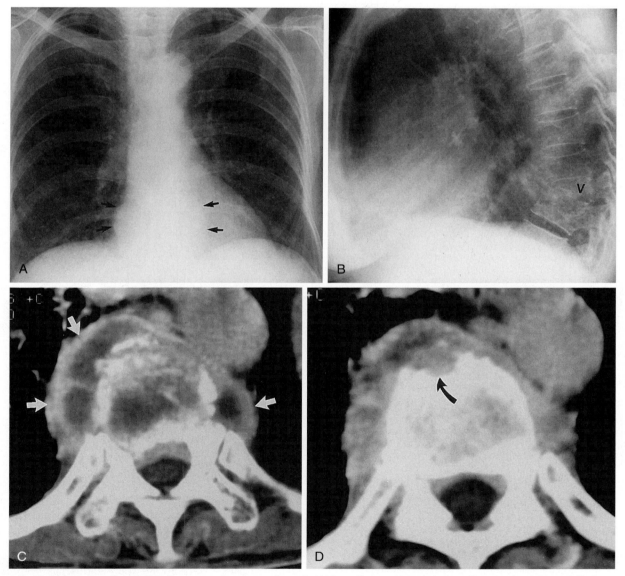

Figure 5–43. Tuberculous Spondylitis. Posteroanterior chest radiograph *(A)* in a 62-year-old man shows miliary lung nodules and displacement of the paraspinal interfaces *(arrows)*. Lateral chest radiograph *(B)* shows destruction of the T10 vertebral body (V), leading to localized kyphosis. Contrast-enhanced CT scans *(C* and *D)* show destruction of the T10 vertebral body, paraspinal abscess formation with low attenuation centers and rim enhancement *(straight arrows)*, and cortical erosion of the adjacent T9 vertebral body *(curved arrow)*. Cultures of needle biopsy specimens taken from the paraspinal abscess grew *Mycobacterium tuberculosis.*

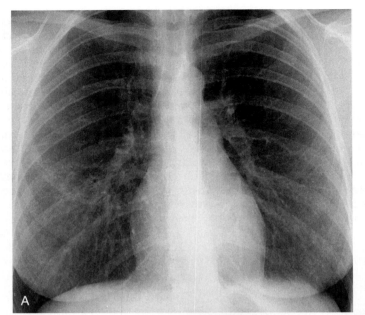

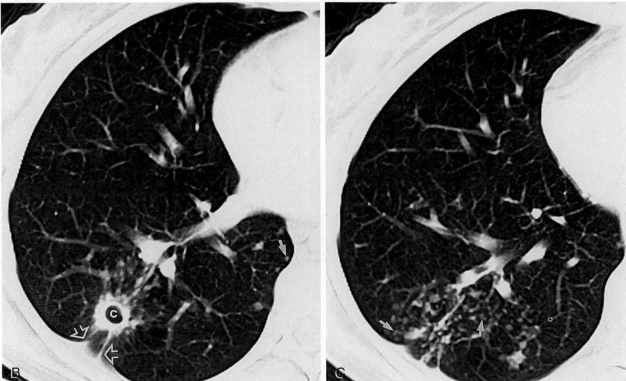

Figure 5–44. Pulmonary *Mycobacterium avium* Complex Infection. Posteroanterior chest radiograph *(A)* in a 28-year-old woman shows poorly defined small nodular opacities in the right lower lobe. Views of the right lung from HRCT scan *(B* and *C)* show a cavity (c) in the right lower lobe and associated pleural tags *(open arrows)* and several centrilobular nodular opacities *(closed arrows)*. Three sputum cultures grew *M. avium* complex. The radiologic findings are indistinguishable from findings of tuberculosis.

Nontuberculous (Atypical) Mycobacteria

The majority of nontuberculous mycobacterial pulmonary infections are caused by a few species, most commonly *M. avium-intracellulare* and *M. kansasii;* however, new or previously nonpathogenic species are being seen more frequently, particularly in immunocompromised patients.[196, 197] The clinical presentation of nontuberculous mycobacterial infection of the lung is similar to that of tuberculosis. The most common findings are cough, low-grade fever, and weight loss.

M. avium-intracellulare is the most common nontuber-

culous mycobacterium to cause human disease. As with many other nontuberculous mycobacteria, such infection often is associated with prior lung disease, such as COPD, pneumoconiosis, and bronchiectasis; a dusty environment, such as seen in some mines and farms, also has been identified as a risk factor.[195] The bacillus has become an important cause of systemic disease in patients who have AIDS, approximately 20% to 25% acquiring the infection at some point during the course of their illness.

There is considerable overlap between the radiologic patterns of pulmonary disease caused by nontuberculous mycobacteria and *M. tuberculosis*, precluding confident

Table 5–6. NONTUBERCULOUS (ATYPICAL) MYCOBACTERIAL INFECTION

M. avium-intracellulare and *M. kansasii*
Clinical and radiographic findings resemble tuberculosis
Single or multiple cavities common
Nodular opacities (centrilobular distribution on HRCT)
Unilateral or bilateral
Patchy, predominately upper lobe distribution
HRCT frequently shows extensive bronchiectasis

HRCT, high-resolution computed tomography.

distinction between the two in any particular case (Table 5–6, Fig. 5–44).[170, 199, 200] Nevertheless, certain patterns are seen more commonly in nontuberculous mycobacteria and may be helpful in suggesting the diagnosis in the appropriate clinical setting.[170, 201]

Similar to tuberculosis, a variety of radiologic patterns are seen with nontuberculous mycobacteria. One of the more common, reported in 20% to 60% of patients, consists of single or multiple cavities (Fig. 5–45).[170, 199, 200] Most patients have radiographic evidence of endobronchial spread. In nonimmunocompromised patients, lymph node enlargement and pleural effusion are uncommon.[198] A second radiographic pattern seen in patients who have pulmonary disease caused by *M. avium* complex consists of bilateral small nodular opacities.[204, 205] The nodules usually are well circumscribed, measure less than 1 cm in diameter, and have a centrilobular distribution.[170, 202, 203] They have a tendency for a patchy distribution in all lobes,[170] although they occasionally involve predominantly the upper lobes or middle lobe and lingula.[200, 203, 204] This nodular pattern occurs in 20% to 50% of cases of *M. avium* complex infection in nonimmunocompromised patients and is seen more commonly in women, who account for approximately 80% of such cases.[202, 204] On HRCT, most of these patients have bronchiectasis,[170, 203, 204] usually involving several lobes;[170, 206] occasionally, bronchiectasis involves only the middle lobe and lingular bronchi.[206] Pathologic correlation shows that most of the nodules correspond to foci of granulomatous inflammation in lung parenchyma or peribronchial interstitial tissue.[202]

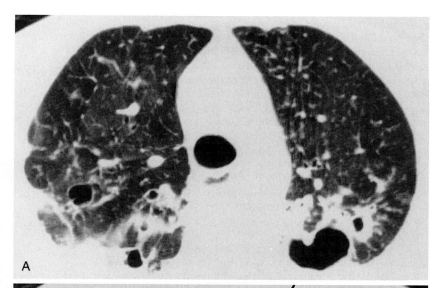

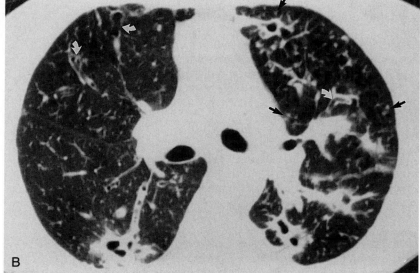

Figure 5–45. Pulmonary *Mycobacterium avium* Complex Infection. HRCT scans *(A* and *B)* show cavities in the upper and lower lobes. There are a few centrilobular nodules *(black arrows)* as well as evidence of bronchiectasis *(white arrows)*. Three consecutive sputum cultures grew *M. avium* complex. The patient was a 66-year-old woman.

The incidence and the pattern of bronchiectasis differ in disease caused by *M. tuberculosis* and *M. avium* complex. In one study in which the HRCT findings were compared in 45 patients who had pulmonary tuberculosis and 32 who had *M. avium* complex, bronchiectasis was identified on HRCT scan in 27% of patients with tuberculosis and 94% of patients with *M. avium* complex.[170] Centrilobular nodules, consolidation, and cavity formation were seen with similar frequency in both infections. When bronchiectasis was present, it involved a mean of 1.8 lobes in patients with tuberculosis and a mean of 4.6 lobes in patients with *M. avium* complex. In patients who had tuberculosis, bronchiectasis most commonly involved the upper lobes, whereas in patients with *M. avium* complex, there was no lobar predominance.

FUNGI AND *ACTINOMYCES*

Fungi can be divided into two major groups according to the pathogenesis of the disease they cause. Some organisms (such as *Histoplasma capsulatum*, *Coccidioides immitis*, and *Blastomyces dermatitidis*) are primary pathogens that most frequently infect healthy individuals. They are found in specific geographic areas—the term *endemic* often is used to describe the infection—and typically dwell in the soil as saprophytes. In appropriate climatic conditions, they germinate and produce spores, which when inhaled by a susceptible host, change form and proliferate. In the individual who has an intact inflammatory response and adequate cell-mediated immunity, such proliferation almost invariably is limited, the resulting disease being subclinical or mild and evidenced only by the development of a positive skin test. In a few apparently normal individuals, however, fulminant primary infection or chronic pulmonary disease, with or without systemic dissemination, can cause significant morbidity and occasionally is fatal. Such complications are much more common and serious in patients who have an underlying immune deficiency, such as AIDS.[207]

A second group of organisms (including *Aspergillus*, *Candida* species, and the species that cause mucormycosis) are opportunistic invaders that chiefly affect immunocompromised hosts or grow in association with underlying pulmonary disease. In contrast to members of the previous group, these organisms can be found throughout the world and usually are ubiquitous in the environment. In addition to saprophytic and invasive infection, some fungi (particularly *Aspergillus* species) can cause disease by inducing an exaggerated hypersensitivity reaction without invading tissue.

Histoplasmosis

Histoplasmosis is an endemic fungal disease, whose clinical and radiographic manifestations are highly variable. Disease is caused by the dimorphic fungus *H. capsulatum*.[1, 210]

Epidemiology

The natural habitat of *H. capsulatum* is soil that contains a high nitrogen content, usually derived from the guano of

Table 5–7. HISTOPLASMOSIS

Histoplasma capsulatum
Central and eastern United States and Canada
Acute disease: radiographic findings
  Usually asymptomatic
  Nonsegmental consolidation
  Hilar lymph node enlargement
  Heavy exposure: multiple nodules 1–4 cm in diameter
Chronic histoplasmosis
  Resembles reactivation tuberculosis
Other manifestations
  Histoplasmoma: may have central or diffuse calcification
  Miliary disease
  Fibrosing mediastinitis
  Broncholithiasis

birds or bats. Areas such as chicken houses, blackbird and pigeon roosts, bat-infested caves or attics, and other sites where bird guano accumulates are the most common sources for outbreaks of infection.[211, 212] Although the organism is of worldwide distribution, most reports of disease have come from North America, particularly the central and eastern portions and notably in the Ohio, Mississippi, and St. Lawrence River valleys, where the organism is considered endemic.[1]

Acute Histoplasmosis

Acute histoplasmosis consists of the abrupt onset of symptoms in a patient who has clinical and laboratory evidence of *H. capsulatum* infection. Symptoms of a flulike

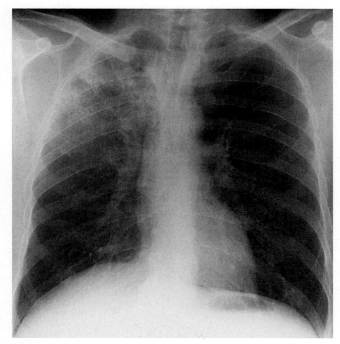

Figure 5–46. Acute Histoplasmosis. A 48-year-old man presented with a 3-week history of right-sided pleuritic chest pain. Posteroanterior chest radiograph shows extensive consolidation in the right upper lobe and small areas of consolidation in the apex of the left lung. Sputum cultures grew *Histoplasma capsulatum*. (Courtesy of Dr. Thomas Hartman, Mayo Clinic, Rochester, MN.)

illness, consisting of fever, headache, chills, and cough, are the most common manifestations.[208]

The chest radiograph is normal in most patients.[213] The most common radiographic findings consist of single or multiple, poorly defined areas of air-space consolidation (Table 5–7).[215] Severe disease is characterized by homogeneous, nonsegmental, parenchymal consolidation simulating acute bacterial air-space pneumonia (Fig. 5–46).[213, 215] In contrast to the latter, the disease tends to clear in one area and appear in another. Hilar lymph node enlargement is common;[213, 215] pleural effusion is rare. After heavy exposure, the radiograph may show widely disseminated, fairly discrete nodular shadows, individual lesions measuring 3 or 4 mm in diameter;[217] such abnormalities may not be apparent for 1 week or more after the onset of symptoms. Hilar lymph node enlargement is present in most cases.[215]

Histoplasmosis also can be manifested by unilateral or bilateral enlargement of hilar or mediastinal lymph nodes in the absence of other radiographic abnormalities.[215] Calcification of lymph nodes is common and may be associated with broncholithiasis (Fig. 5–47);[213] in many such cases, CT scan reveals parabronchial calcification and clarifies the nature of the abnormality.[213, 214]

Histoplasmoma

Histoplasmoma is a relatively common form of pulmonary histoplasmosis that may or may not be associated with a history of previous symptomatic disease.[219, 220] The abnormality typically appears as a sharply defined nodule 0.5 to 3 cm in diameter, in most cases in a lower lobe.[213, 218] Although the lesion may be solitary, smaller satellite lesions often are seen. The nodules may have a central focus of calcification, producing a *target* lesion, or may be diffusely calcified; such calcification frequently is identified on CT scan when it is not apparent on the radiograph (Fig. 5–48).[181, 221] Hilar lymph node calcification is common, although node enlargement is unusual.

Chronic Histoplasmosis

In contrast to most individuals who have acute disease, which clinically and radiographically subsides without treatment in weeks to months, rare cases of histoplasmosis progress and become chronic, either in the lungs or in the mediastinum.

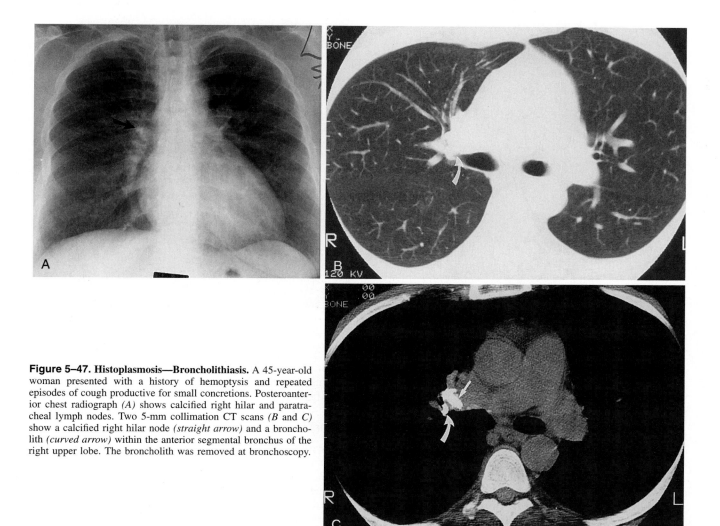

Figure 5–47. Histoplasmosis—Broncholithiasis. A 45-year-old woman presented with a history of hemoptysis and repeated episodes of cough productive for small concretions. Posteroanterior chest radiograph *(A)* shows calcified right hilar and paratracheal lymph nodes. Two 5-mm collimation CT scans *(B and C)* show a calcified right hilar node *(straight arrow)* and a broncholith *(curved arrow)* within the anterior segmental bronchus of the right upper lobe. The broncholith was removed at bronchoscopy.

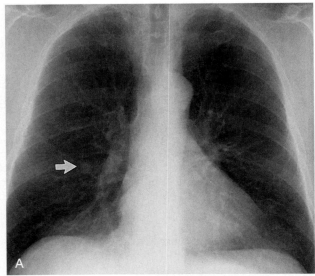

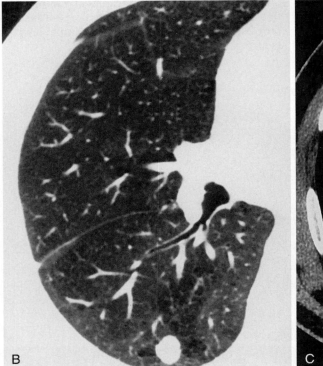

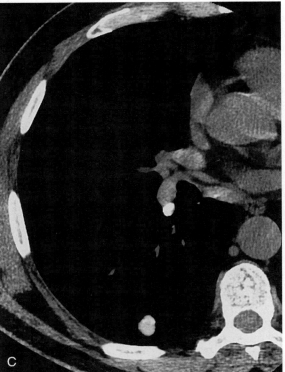

Figure 5–48. Calcified Histoplasmoma. Posteroanterior chest radiograph *(A)* shows a 1.5-cm-diameter nodule in the right lower lobe *(arrow)*; calcification is not apparent. HRCT scans *(B* and *C)* show diffuse calcification of the nodule as well as calcified right hilar and subcarinal nodes. The patient was an asymptomatic 54-year-old man.

Chronic Pulmonary Histoplasmosis

Chronic pulmonary histoplasmosis tends to be associated with cough and expectoration, which in some cases are likely the result of underlying COPD rather than the infection itself. Spillage from infected cavities or bullae may be accompanied by fever.

The radiographic appearance (Fig. 5–49) simulates postprimary tuberculosis,[213, 216] the earliest manifestations consisting of segmental or subsegmental areas of consolidation in the apices of the lungs, frequently outlining areas of centrilobular emphysema. Thick-walled bullae sometimes contain fluid levels; with time, the bullae can disappear completely or can increase gradually in size. In some

patients, there is an increase in the wall thickness of bullae. Serial chest radiographs tend to show progressive loss of volume associated with increased prominence of linear opacities.

Chronic Mediastinal Histoplasmosis

Involvement of the mediastinum by histoplasmosis can result in a variety of clinical and radiologic abnormalities. Sometimes the abnormalities are related to one or more enlarged mediastinal lymph nodes.[222] Rarely an ill-defined, matted mass of necrotic and fibrotic tissue results from direct spread of infection outside the capsule of such nodes or from direct invasion of adjacent pulmonary lesions. Per-

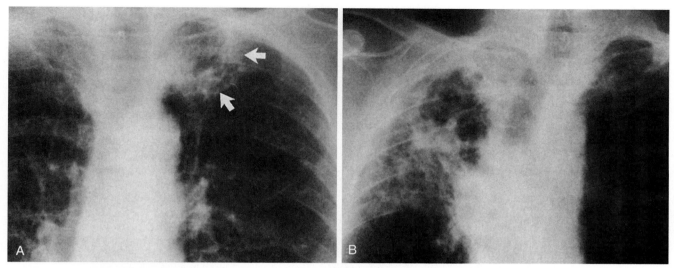

Figure 5–49. Chronic Progressive Histoplasmosis. View of the upper half of the left lung *(A)* reveals a poorly defined, inhomogeneous opacity *(arrows)* containing a central radiolucency representing a cavity. The right lung was clear at that time. Approximately 1 year later *(B)*, the left apical lesion had resolved almost completely, but there was now extensive disease throughout the right upper lobe, associated with considerable loss of volume (note the tracheal shift to the right). The appearance is similar to that of chronic tuberculosis; however, *H. capsulatum* was identified by culture.

haps more frequently (although still rarely), this process is secondary to an exuberant fibrous reaction that has been hypothesized to be caused by chronic immunologic stimulation by histoplasmin antigens similar to that seen in histoplasmomas (fibrosing mediastinitis, *see* Chapter 22).[208, 223]

CT scans of the mediastinum are essential for elucidation of the abnormalities. The most common findings are mediastinal or hilar masses, calcification within the mediastinal mass or associated lymph nodes, superior vena cava obstruction, pulmonary artery narrowing, and bronchial narrowing.[224, 225] The presence of a localized calcified mediastinal soft tissue mass is the most frequent of these abnormalities; in a patient with an appropriate clinical history, this finding strongly suggests a diagnosis of *H. capsulatum*–induced fibrosing mediastinitis and precludes need for biopsy.[224, 225] In patients without calcification or with pro-

gressive radiographic findings, a biopsy specimen should be obtained for a definitive diagnosis.[225]

Disseminated Histoplasmosis

Disseminated histoplasmosis occurs most frequently in infants and young children and in patients who are immunocompromised by conditions such as AIDS or organ transplantation. The radiographic and HRCT findings usually are similar to those of miliary tuberculosis,[184] consisting of 1- to 3-mm-diameter nodules distributed randomly throughout both lungs (Fig. 5–50).

Coccidioidomycosis

Coccidioidomycosis is a highly infectious disease caused by the dimorphic fungus *C. immitis*.[226] It is almost

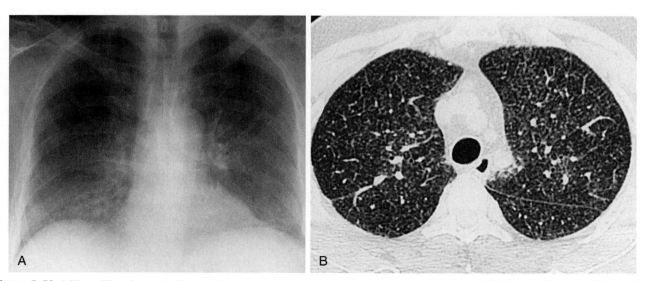

Figure 5–50. Miliary Histoplasmosis. Chest radiograph *(A)* shows fine nodularity throughout both lungs. HRCT scan *(B)* shows diffuse miliary nodules. The patient was a previously healthy man with proven miliary histoplasmosis. (Case courtesy of Dr. Thomas Hartman, Mayo Clinic, Rochester, MN.)

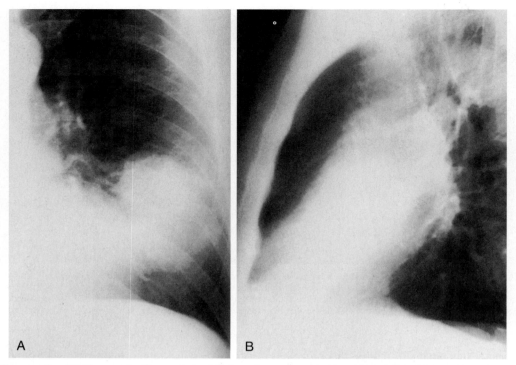

Figure 5–51. Primary Coccidioidomycosis. Views of the left lung from posteroanterior *(A)* and lateral *(B)* radiographs show homogeneous consolidation of much of the lingular segment of the left upper lobe. A faint air bronchogram could be identified on the original radiographs but does not reproduce well. The upper border of the consolidation is sharply circumscribed, resembling a mass. On surgical excision, it proved to be coccidioidomycosis.

exclusively a disease of the Western Hemisphere and is found principally in its endemic areas in the southwestern United States and northern Mexico.[227] In endemic areas, the incidence of infection is high: Approximately 25% of newly arrived individuals develop a positive skin test at the end of 1 year, and 50% develop a positive skin test at the end of 4 years.

Primary Coccidioidomycosis

The frequency with which primary coccidioidomycosis is recognized clinically probably depends on how closely it is looked for as well as on the degree of exposure. Overall, it has been estimated that about 60% to 80% of patients are asymptomatic.[232] When present, symptoms that accompany primary infection often are nonspecific and flulike, consisting of fever, cough (usually nonproductive), chest pain, headache, and (sometimes) a generalized erythematous rash.[233]

The most common radiologic manifestation consists of single or multiple foci of air-space consolidation (Fig. 5–51, Table 5–8).[229] Sometimes the foci of consolidation are transformed into thin-walled cavities that may resolve spontaneously.[230] Small pleural effusions occur in approximately 20% of cases;[228, 231] large effusions are rare. Lymph node enlargement occurs in approximately 20% of cases, seldom in the absence of parenchymal involvement.[228]

Chronic Pulmonary Coccidioidomycosis

In most cases, radiologic changes of chronic pulmonary coccidioidomycosis are found incidentally in asymptomatic

patients.[229] The radiologic manifestations include lung nodules and cavities and, rarely, bronchiectasis, scarring, and calcification.[229]

Radiographically, a nodule develops over approximately 5 to 6 weeks,[231] as a focus of consolidation becomes smaller, denser, and better defined. Occasionally, nodular opacities result from filling in of a cavity.[229] The nodules are 0.5 to 5 cm in diameter and in more than 90% of cases are located in the lung periphery.[229] Although usually single, they occasionally are multiple.[228, 231]

Cavities have been reported to occur in 10% to 15% of patients who have pulmonary disease.[228] They usually are single and located in the upper lobes[209, 235] and may be thin or thick walled (Fig. 5–52); thin-walled (*grape-skin*) cavities have a tendency to change size,[234, 236] possibly reflecting a variable check-valve communication with proximal bronchi. Almost all patients who have nodular coccidi-

Table 5–8. COCCIDIOIDOMYCOSIS

Coccidioides immitis
Southwestern United States and northern Mexico
Primary coccidioidomycosis
    60–80% of patients are asymptomatic
    Single or multiple foci of air-space consolidation
    Lymph node enlargement in 20% of cases
    Small pleural effusion in 20% of cases
Chronic pulmonary coccidioidomycosis
    Usually asymptomatic
    Nodule, usually single, 0.5–5 cm in diameter
    10–15% cavitate, typically thin walled

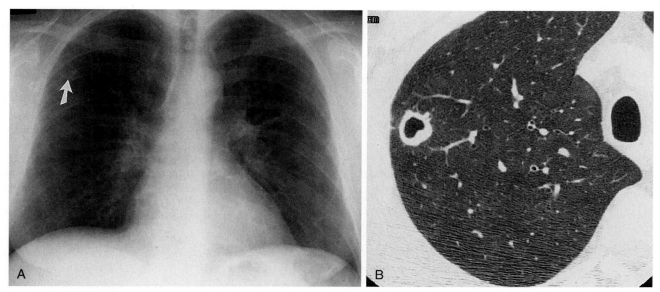

Figure 5–52. Cavitary coccidioidomycosis. Posteroanterior chest radiograph *(A)* in a 44-year-old patient shows a sharply circumscribed, 2 cm in diameter cavitating nodule in the right upper lobe. HRCT *(B)* shows uneven thickness of the wall and smooth outer margins. Coccidioidomycosis was proved by surgical resection.

oidomycosis are asymptomatic, even in the presence of cavitation.

The CT findings of chronic pulmonary coccidioidomycosis were assessed in a retrospective analysis of 18 patients.[238] The abnormalities consisted of solitary nodules measuring 1 to 2 cm in diameter (seen in 17 patients) and two focal areas of air-space opacification (seen in 1 patient). Ten of the nodules had homogeneous attenuation on CT scan, two had central areas of low attenuation resulting from necrosis, two had cavitation, two had foci of calcification, and one had a bubble-like lucency. Three of the nodules were surrounded by halos of ground-glass attenuation, which were shown on histologic examination to represent granulomatous inflammation in two cases and pulmonary hemorrhage in one case.[238]

In fewer than 1% of patients who have pulmonary coccidioidomycosis, the disease is slowly progressive and may mimic reactivation tuberculosis or chronic histoplasmosis.[229, 239] The radiologic findings in these patients consist of upper lobe scarring, multiple nodules, and cavities.[229, 239]

North American Blastomycosis

North American blastomycosis is caused by the dimorphic fungus *B. dermatitidis*.[248] The disease occurs most commonly in the Western Hemisphere, mainly the central and southeastern United States (where endemic areas include the Ohio, Mississippi, and Missouri river valleys [particularly in Wisconsin])[241] and southern Canada (principally Quebec, Ontario, and Manitoba).[242, 243] Although infection in miniepidemics may be associated with flulike symptoms only, it is manifested more commonly by symptoms of acute pneumonia, including the abrupt onset of fever, chills, productive cough, and pleuritic chest pain.[244] Arthralgias and myalgias are common, and erythema nodosum develops occasionally.[240]

The most common radiographic presentation—reported in 25% to 75% of patients—consists of acute air-space consolidation.[246-248] This consolidation may be patchy or confluent and subsegmental, segmental, or nonsegmental (Fig. 5–53). The next most common radiographic presentation—seen in 30% of cases[247]—is a mass, either single or multiple;[247, 249] when solitary, the mass can mimic primary carcinoma.[530] Cavitation occurs in approximately 15% to 20% of cases.[246, 249] Overwhelming infection usually is accompanied by a radiographic pattern of miliary dissemination.[245, 250]

Hilar and mediastinal lymph node enlargement is uncommon, even on CT scan.[251] Pleural effusion has been identified on chest radiographs in 10% to 15% of cases and almost invariably is associated with parenchymal disease.[246, 252]

Cryptococcosis

Cryptococcosis is caused by *Cryptococcus neoformans*, a unimorphic fungus that exists in yeast form in its natural habitat and in animals and humans. The disease is found throughout the world. Although it can occur as pulmonary or disseminated disease in otherwise normal individuals, it is identified most frequently in compromised hosts, particularly patients who have AIDS or lymphoma (especially Hodgkin's disease).[254-256]

The initial lung infection often does not result in symptoms and is recognized infrequently.[253] When disease confined to the lungs causes symptoms, these are usually mild and include cough, scanty mucoid or (rarely) bloody sputum, chest pain, and low-grade fever.[253] The organism has a particular affinity for the central nervous system, a common clinical presentation being meningitis.

The most common radiographic manifestation of pulmonary infection consists of single or multiple nodules, usually subpleural in location and 0.5 to 4 cm in diameter.[257, 258] An alternative presentation is in the form of a localized

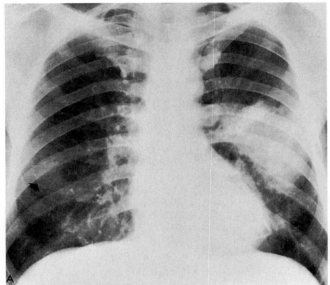

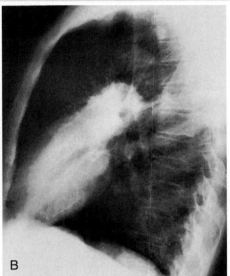

Figure 5–53. North American Blastomycosis. Posteroanterior *(A)* and lateral *(B)* chest radiographs show a large, poorly defined shadow of homogeneous density in the lingula; the consolidation is nonsegmental and shows no evidence of an air bronchogram. The posteroanterior radiograph reveals destruction of the anterior portion of the right fifth rib *(arrow)*. *Blastomyces dermatitidis* was cultured from a 24-hour sputum collection, and from fluid aspirated from the swelling over the right fifth rib.

comorbidity.[260] Similar to other infectious diseases, fulminating cryptococcosis may be associated with adult respiratory distress syndrome.[261]

Pneumocystis carinii

Although *P. carinii* historically has been considered to be a protozoan, morphologic, biochemical, and genetic studies have revealed a much closer relationship with fungi,[262, 263] and it is now considered by most authorities to be classified properly with these organisms.[264] The mode of transmission has not been shown conclusively; however, because of the universal presence of the organism within the lungs, it is presumed to be by inhalation.

Although *P. carinii* infection is common in humans,[265]

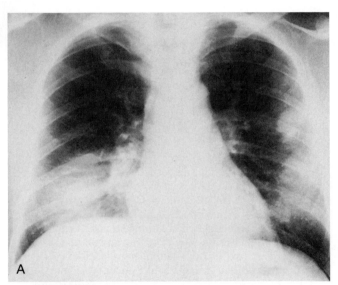

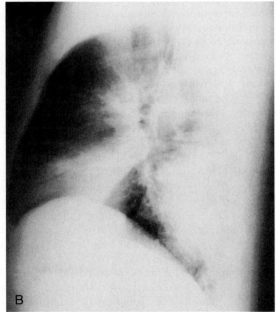

Figure 5–54. Acute Cryptococcal Pneumonia. Posteroanterior *(A)* and lateral *(B)* radiographs show nonsegmental homogeneous consolidation of both lower lobes and the right middle lobe. *Cryptococcus neoformans* was recovered from the sputum.

area of less well-defined air-space consolidation,[257, 258] segmental or nonsegmental in distribution but usually confined to one lobe (Fig. 5–54). Cavitation is uncommon in otherwise healthy individuals but frequently is present in immunocompromised patients (Fig. 5–55).[257, 258] The latter also have a higher incidence of disseminated disease.[257, 259] Such disease, described most commonly in patients with AIDS, can give rise to a miliary pattern or to multiple diffuse, ill-defined opacities.[257, 259] Hilar and mediastinal lymph node enlargement also is relatively frequent in patients who have AIDS.[257, 259]

Pleural effusion is uncommon and usually connotes dissemination of the organism in a patient with underlying

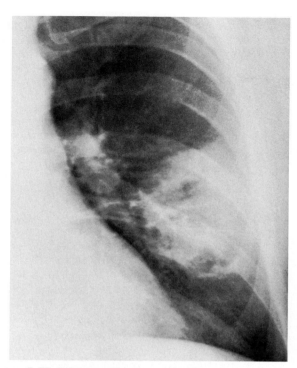

Figure 5–55. Pulmonary Cryptococcosis. View of the left hemithorax from a posteroanterior radiograph shows a well-circumscribed mass situated in the axillary portion of the left lower lobe; its lateral aspect abuts against the visceral pleura. Several irregular areas of radiolucency are present throughout the mass, representing multiple foci of cavitation. The appearance of the mass is characteristic of cryptococcosis, although the cavitation is unusual. *Cryptococcus neoformans* was cultured from the sputum.

it results in clinically significant pneumonia almost uniquely in individuals who have underlying disease. *P. carinii* pneumonia is particularly prevalent and virulent in patients who have AIDS, in whom it has been estimated that at least one episode of pneumonia will occur at some point during the course of the disease in the absence of prophylaxis and antiviral therapy.[266] A second important group at risk is immunosuppressed organ transplant recipients;[267] some investigators have found the risk in this group to be related to the particular type of immunosuppression.[268] In patients who have a malignancy, infection is manifested most often in patients who have lymphoreticular neoplasms (usually associated with concomitant cytotoxic therapy);[269, 270] individuals who have solid tumors (including pulmonary carcinoma) are affected less often.[271] Pneumonia also is seen in patients who have systemic vasculitis or connective tissue disorders (almost invariably in association with corticosteroid and cytotoxic therapy),[271, 272] congenital immunodeficiency diseases, and (rarely) adrenocorticotropic hormone–producing neoplasms.[273, 274]

There are significant differences in the clinical course of patients with and without AIDS. In patients without AIDS, the duration of prodromal symptoms tends to be shorter, often with a relatively acute presentation of fever and hypoxemia.[292, 293] In patients who have AIDS, there often is a prodrome of fever, malaise, cough, and breathlessness, which may be of several weeks' duration before

recognition of the infection. Dyspnea is the most common symptom; in some patients, a dry hacking cough is present.

In the early stage of *P. carinii* pneumonia, a granular pattern or hazy opacity (ground-glass pattern) is apparent, particularly in the perihilar areas (Table 5–9, Fig. 5–56).[276, 277] In more advanced disease, the pattern usually is one of air-space consolidation (although a granular or reticulogranular pattern still may be present at the periphery of the consolidated area).[33] Terminally, the lungs may be massively consolidated, to a point of almost complete airlessness; in some patients, the acute onset and diffuse involvement are characteristic of adult respiratory distress syndrome.[278, 279]

Pneumonia usually is bilateral and most prominent in the lower lobes. Less commonly, it involves the upper lobes predominantly or exclusively. Although this distribution is seen most frequently in patients with AIDS who are receiving prophylactic aerosolized pentamidine,[280, 281] it also may occur in individuals not receiving prophylaxis. Rarely, there is lobar consolidation.[33, 282] An atypical radiographic distribution may be seen in patients whose thorax has been irradiated; in two such cases, lung zones within the irradiation fields were spared apparent *Pneumocystis* involvement, suggesting that the damaged tissue did not support the growth of the organism.[282]

Another uncommon presentation of *P. carinii* pneumonia is as solitary or multiple, nodular opacities;[284, 528] the nodules may be solid or cavitary. Although seen most commonly in patients who have AIDS, such nodules also have been described in patients with lymphoma.[275, 283] A relatively common radiographic manifestation in patients with AIDS is cystic lung disease (*see* Chapter 10). Unusual extrapulmonary radiologic features of *P. carinii* infection include pleural effusion;[285, 286] enlarged noncalcified[286, 287] or calcified[288, 289] hilar and mediastinal lymph nodes; and calcification of the spleen, liver, kidney, adrenal glands, and abdominal lymph nodes.[285, 289]

The predominant CT finding in *P. carinii* pneumonia consists of bilateral areas of ground-glass attenuation. This attenuation may be diffuse or have a distinct mosaic pattern, areas of normal lung intervening between the foci of ground-glass attenuation (Fig. 5–57).[36, 290] Associated thickening of interlobular septa is seen in 20% to 50% of cases,[35, 36] and parenchymal consolidation is seen in approximately 40%.[36] With time, the areas of ground-glass

Table 5–9. *PNEUMOCYSTIS CARINII*

Is currently classified as a fungus
Almost exclusively a pathogen in immunocompromised patients
Most common symptoms: cough and progressive dyspnea
Chest radiograph
    Fine granular, reticulonodular, or ground-glass pattern
    Initially predominately in perihilar regions
    Progresses to diffuse consolidation
    Lymphadenopathy and pleural effusion uncommon
HRCT
    Ground-glass pattern
    Diffuse or geographic distribution
    Consolidation and reticulation may be present
    Cystic changes common in patients who have AIDS

HRCT, high-resolution computed tomography; AIDS, acquired immunodeficiency syndrome.

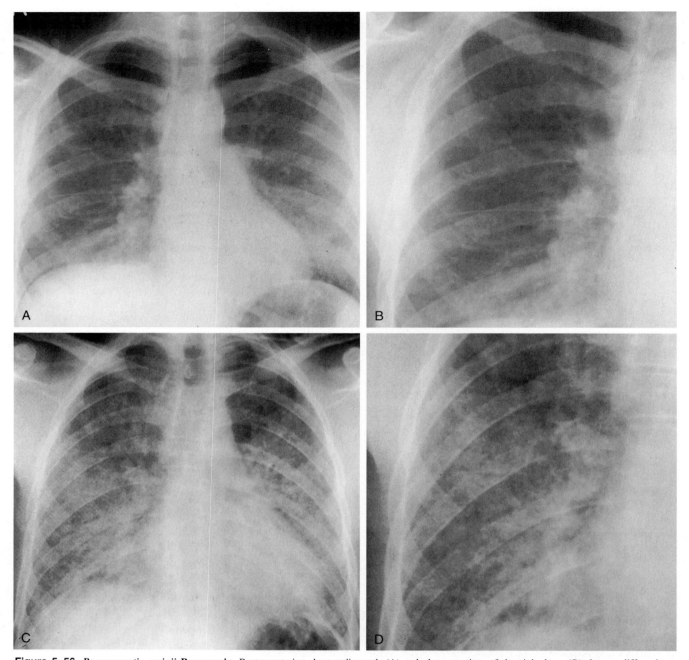

Figure 5–56. *Pneumocystis carinii* **Pneumonia.** Posteroanterior chest radiograph *(A)* and close-up view of the right lung *(B)* show a diffuse hazy increase in lung opacity (ground-glass opacity) throughout both lungs, worse in the lower lobes. The appearance in this clinical setting is suggestive of early *P. carinii* pneumonia. Several days later, the disease had progressed to consolidation *(C* and *D)*. Open-lung biopsy disclosed the classic histopathology of *P. carinii* pneumonia.

attenuation progress to consolidation; eventually, interstitial abnormalities become evident and may predominate.[33] The interstitial findings may consist of thickened interlobular septa or irregular lines of attenuation (Fig. 5–58).[33, 36] Occasionally, patients develop a pattern of diffuse fibrosis[33] or peripheral bronchiectasis and bronchiolectasis.[291]

Candidiasis

Candidiasis is caused by a variety of dimorphic fungi of the *Candida* genus, usually *C. albicans* and, less com-

monly, *C. tropicalis*.[298] The organisms are common human saprophytes, *C. albicans* being found normally in the gastrointestinal tract and mucocutaneous regions and a variety of non-*albicans* species being found on the skin. Their numbers are held in check naturally by saprophytic bacteria. Conditions in which the composition of the normal flora is altered are likely to lead to overgrowth of *Candida* species and an increased risk of infection. Pulmonary infection is relatively uncommon; in one series of 125 pulmonary complications seen in immunocompromised patients, it was the cause in only 6 (5%).[294]

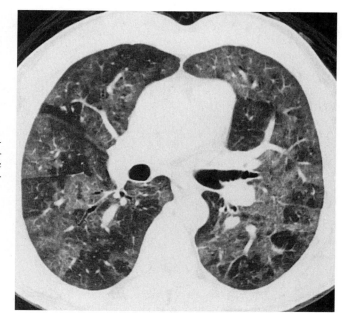

Figure 5–57. *Pneumocystis carinii* **Pneumonia.** HRCT scan shows characteristic appearance consisting of bilateral areas of ground-glass attenuation interspersed with areas of normal-appearing lung causing a mosaic pattern. The patient was a 46-year-old man who had acquired immunodeficiency syndrome.

The symptoms of pulmonary candidiasis are nonspecific and include cough, purulent expectoration, and hemoptysis. Many patients have evidence of involvement of other organs or tissues; such disseminated disease often is a terminal event in debilitated and immunocompromised patients, many of whom are receiving antibiotic, corticosteroid, or other immunosuppressive therapy.

The most common radiographic manifestations consist of unilateral or bilateral areas of segmental or nonsegmental consolidation.[295] Less commonly, the findings consist of a diffuse nodular or miliary pattern (Fig. 5–59).[296, 297] Nodules may range from a few millimeters to 3 cm in diameter.[294] Pleural effusions are seen in approximately 20% of patients.[295]

HRCT findings of *Candida* pneumonia have been reported in a few cases.[299, 300] In one review of nine patients, seven had a bilateral, predominantly nodular pattern, and two had bilateral areas of ground-glass attenuation and consolidation (Fig. 5–60).[299] The nodules were 3 to 30 mm in diameter. Halos of ground-glass attenuation surrounding the nodules were seen in four patients.

Aspergillosis

Although approximately 300 species of *Aspergillus* have been described,[302] only a few have been associated with human disease; the most important is *A. fumigatus.*[303] *Aspergillus* organisms are extremely hardy and ubiquitous in

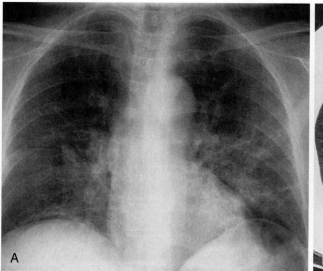

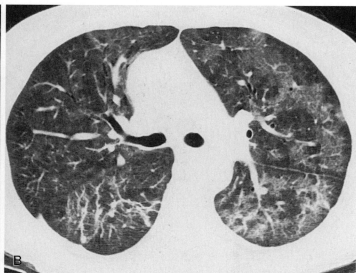

Figure 5–58. *Pneumocystis carinii* **Pneumonia.** Chest radiograph *(A)* shows perihilar consolidation and bilateral irregular linear opacities. HRCT scan *(B)* shows bilateral areas of ground-glass attenuation and irregular linear opacities involving mainly the lower lobes. The patient was a 56-year-old woman who developed *P. carinii* pneumonia after renal transplantation.

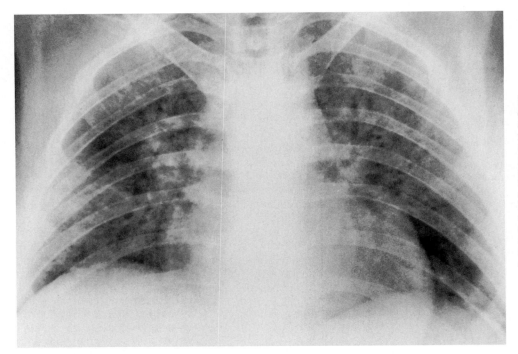

Figure 5–59. Disseminated Candidiasis. This 19-year-old man had acute leukemia, for which he was receiving high doses of antineoplastic drugs and corticosteroids. During this course of therapy, he developed clinical evidence of diffuse pneumonia. This anteroposterior radiograph reveals widespread involvement of both lungs by patchy and confluent areas of air-space consolidation; an air bronchogram is visible in most areas. At necropsy, there was widespread organ involvement by *Candida albicans*.

the environment, having been found in soil, water, and decaying organic material of many types. In most instances, infection is believed to occur by inhalation of airborne conidia from a variety of contaminated areas.

Disease caused by *Aspergillus* species can be manifested in three ways, each with distinctive clinical, radiologic, and pathologic features: (1) *saprophytic infestation*, in which the fungus colonizes airways, cavities (aspergilloma), or necrotic tissue; (2) *allergic disease*, characterized by such entities as allergic bronchopulmonary aspergillosis and extrinsic allergic alveolitis; and (3) *invasive disease*, a form that is usually acute in onset and rapidly fatal and rarely insidious and associated with a relatively good prognosis (Table 5–10). Although these three varieties are not mutu-

ally exclusive—for example, occasional cases of saprophytic or allergic disease progress to invasive aspergillosis—as a rule, crossover does not occur.

Saprophytic Aspergillosis: **Fungus Ball**

A fungus ball (mycetoma, aspergilloma*) is a conglomeration of fungal hyphae admixed with mucus and cellular

---

*Because a variety of fungi other than *Aspergillus* species can produce the complication (*see* farther on), use of the term *aspergilloma* synonymously with fungus ball is, strictly speaking, inappropriate without ancillary immunologic or cultural confirmation; however, because of common usage and because *Aspergillus* organisms are the most frequent causative agents of fungus ball, we and most others use the designation in the absence of definitive proof.

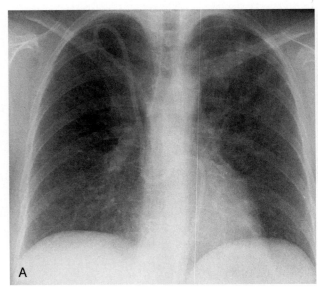

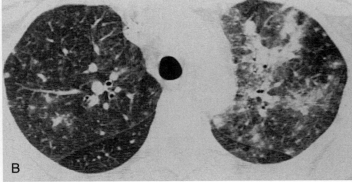

Figure 5–60. *Candida* **Pneumonia.** Posteroanterior chest radiograph *(A)* shows poorly defined areas of consolidation and a few nodular opacities in the upper lobes. HRCT scan *(B)* shows nodules of various sizes, focal areas of consolidation, and ground-glass attenuation. The patient was a 27-year-old woman who developed *Candida* pneumonia after bone marrow transplantation.

Table 5–10. ASPERGILLOSIS

Aspergillus fumigatus
Three distinct clinical and radiologic manifestations
  Saprophytic infestation (aspergilloma)
    Fungus colonizes airways or cavity
    Most commonly previous tuberculosis or sarcoidosis
    Hemoptysis in 50–95% of cases
    Round mass, usually in upper lobe
    Separated from wall by an air space (air crescent sign)
    Moves when patient changes position
  Allergic disease
    Most common form is allergic bronchopulmonary aspergillosis
    Patients almost invariably have asthma
    Mucoid impaction: bifurcating (inverted Y or V) opacities
    Central bronchiectasis
    Predominately upper lobe involvement
  Invasive form
    Most commonly angioinvasive
    Immunocompromised patients
    Most patients have severe neutropenia
    Multiple nodules
    Poorly defined margins on chest radiograph
    Commonly have ground-glass halo on HRCT
    Segmental consolidation

HRCT, high-resolution computed tomography.

debris within a pulmonary cavity or ectatic bronchus. Historically the most common underlying cause was tuberculosis, approximately 25% to 55% of patients having a history of this disease.[304, 305] The second most common underlying condition is sarcoidosis;[304, 306] in one prospective evaluation of 100 patients with this disease, 10 developed an aspergilloma.[318]

Other predisposing conditions associated less often with aspergilloma formation include bronchiectasis of any cause (including cystic fibrosis),[308, 309] chronic fungal cavities,[310, 311] bronchogenic cysts, acute and chronic bacterial abscesses,[312] cavities related to *P. carinii* in patients who have AIDS,[313] cavitary carcinoma,[314] radiation fibrosis,[315] apical fibrobullous changes of rheumatoid disease,[316] ankylosing spondylitis,[317, 318] and pulmonary sequestration.[319]

Common clinical manifestations include cough and expectoration. Hemoptysis has been reported in 50% to 95% of cases.[328–330] The latter varies from relatively minor streaking of the sputum to life-threatening hemorrhage.

Radiographically, a fungus ball consists of a solid, more or less round mass of soft tissue density within a spherical or ovoid cavity, usually in an upper lobe.[321] Typically, the mass is separated from the wall of the cavity by an air space of variable size and shape, resulting in the distinctive air crescent sign (Fig. 5–61). A fluid level is seldom present within the cavity.[322] Occasionally, the mycelial mass grows to fill a cavity completely, effectively obliterating the air space necessary for its radiographic recognition (the abnormality being recognized as a result of hemoptysis or as incidental findings at autopsy). Most cavities are thin walled; in one series, cavities averaged 5.5 by 3.5 cm in diameter.[321] They are often contiguous with a pleural surface, which itself may be thickened.[323] Thickening of the wall of a tuberculous cavity or of the adjacent pleura has been described as an early radiographic sign of *Aspergillus* colonization, antedating the detection of the fungus ball.[324]

The fungus ball usually moves when the patient changes position;[325] however, some are irregular in shape, conforming, for example, to an elongated bronchiectatic cavity, in which case change in the position of the patient may not be accompanied by a concomitant movement of the fungus ball.

Similar to the radiograph, the most characteristic finding of an aspergilloma on CT scan consists of an ovoid or round soft tissue intracavity mass that moves when the patient is turned from the supine to the prone position (*see* Fig. 5–61).[326, 327] Areas of increased attenuation, presumably representing calcium deposits, are relatively common.[326] CT may allow visualization of aspergillomas not apparent on the radiograph[326, 327] as well as multiple aspergillomas (Fig. 5–62). In one review of 25 cases in which abnormalities consistent with an aspergilloma were identified by HRCT scan, irregular fungal strands could be seen between the fungus ball and the surrounding cavity wall in cases in which an air crescent was not visible on the radiograph.[326] CT scan may show fungal fronds situated on the cavity wall that intersect with each other and form an irregular spongelike network that antedates the development of the mature fungus ball (Fig. 5–63).[326]

Allergic Aspergillosis

Hypersensitivity reactions to *Aspergillus* organisms can take three forms: (1) *extrinsic allergic alveolitis*, most likely the result of hypersensitivity to inhaled conidia and usually seen in an occupational setting,[331] such as the production of malt;[332] (2) a *Loeffler-like syndrome*;[304] and (3) allergic bronchopulmonary aspergillosis. The last-named is by far the most common of the three.

The diagnosis of allergic bronchopulmonary aspergillosis can be difficult and depends on the demonstration of several abnormalities;[333] in a particular patient, confidence in diagnosis depends on the number and type of abnormalities that are identified. These abnormalities include (in approximate order of diagnostic importance):

  1. Radiographic or CT manifestations of mucoid impaction or ectasia of proximal bronchi[334, 335]
  2. Asthma (an almost invariable finding in the United States but not in the United Kingdom[336, 337] or some parts of Australia)[338]
  3. Eosinophilia of blood (>1,000/mm³) and sputum (common in adults but often absent in children[336] and not present in every acute attack)[339]
  4. An elevated level of total serum IgE[340]
  5. Characteristic histologic findings on specimens obtained by bronchoscopy[342]
  6. Elevated levels of serum IgE and IgG antibodies to *Aspergillus* (compared with asthmatic patients, who have immediate cutaneous reactivity to *Aspergillus* but do not have allergic bronchopulmonary aspergillosis)[336, 341]
  7. An immediate cutaneous reaction to *Aspergillus* antigen
  8. Precipitating antibodies against *Aspergillus* antigen[343]
  9. Positive sputum culture for *Aspergillus* species[344]
  10. Positive delayed skin reaction to intracutaneous injection of *Aspergillus* antigen

The radiographic findings in allergic bronchopulmonary aspergillosis are identical to those of mucoid impaction

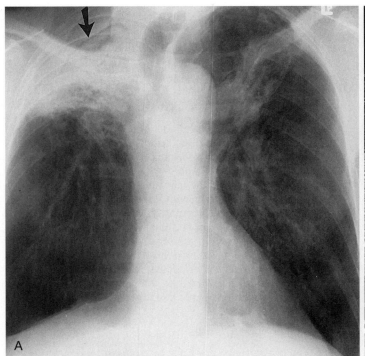

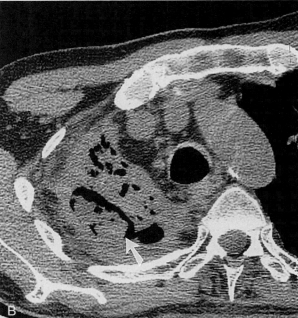

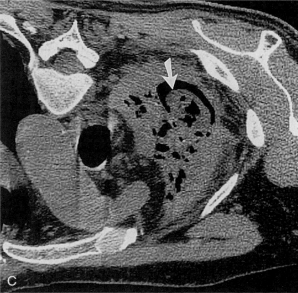

Figure 5–61. Aspergilloma with an Air Crescent Sign and Change in Position. A 65-year-old man with previous tuberculosis presented with hemoptysis. Posteroanterior chest radiograph *(A)* shows extensive scarring in the upper lobes. A large mycetoma in the right upper lobe shows a characteristic crescent of air between the mycetoma and the cavity wall *(arrow)*. Marked pleural thickening surrounds the cavity containing the aspergilloma. HRCT scan with the patient supine *(B)* and prone *(C)* shows change in position of the aspergilloma *(arrows)* despite its large size. Extensive bronchiectasis and marked pleural thickening are seen. *Aspergillus fumigatus* was recovered at bronchoscopy.

(Fig. 5–64).[320, 345] Homogeneous, finger-like shadows of soft tissue density lie in a precise bronchial distribution, usually involving the upper lobes and almost always in the more central segmental bronchi rather than peripheral branches (Fig. 5–65).[320] These bifurcating opacities have been described variously, according to their orientation on the radiograph, as having a *gloved-finger, inverted Y* or *V,* or *cluster-of-grapes* appearance. Although involvement of main and lobar bronchi is uncommon, cases have been described in which an entire lung has collapsed distal to a huge mucous plug.[337, 346, 525] Occasionally, isolated lobar or segmental collapse also occurs, sometimes coincident with clinical exacerbation.[321] The shadows tend to be transient but may persist unchanged for weeks or months or may enlarge.

After expectoration of a mucous plug, residual bronchial

dilation may be evident;[308, 347] when severely dilated, such bronchi may contain a fluid level[334, 348] or an aspergilloma. Occasionally, mucous plugs calcify (*see* Fig. 5–65). Mucoid impaction tends to recur in the same segmental bronchi, suggesting that bronchial damage predisposes to further episodes.[320] Pleural disease is uncommon; however, effusion[349] and spontaneous pneumothorax[350] have been reported.

Similar to radiographs, the CT findings of allergic bronchopulmonary aspergillosis consist principally of mucoid impaction and bronchiectasis, involving predominantly the segmental and subsegmental airways (Fig. 5–66).[335, 351] High attenuation of the mucous plugs, presumably related to the presence of calcium, was evident on HRCT scan in 4 (28%) of 14 patients in one study.[352] Other abnormalities include atelectasis and areas of consolidation.

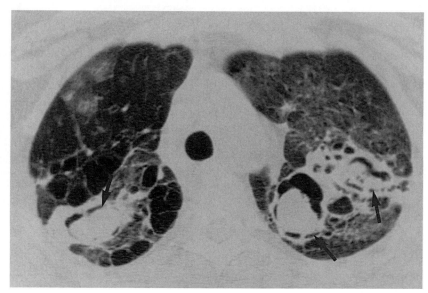

Figure 5–62. Multiple Aspergillomas. CT scan shows several soft tissue masses *(arrows)* within markedly ectatic upper lobe bronchi. Ground-glass opacities and emphysema also can be seen. The patient was a 35-year-old woman who had a 5-year history of sarcoidosis before developing repeated episodes of hemoptysis. (Case courtesy of Dr. Georgeann McGuinness, Department of Radiology, New York University Medical Center, New York, NY.)

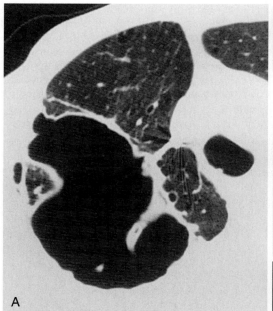

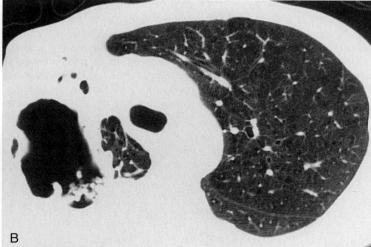

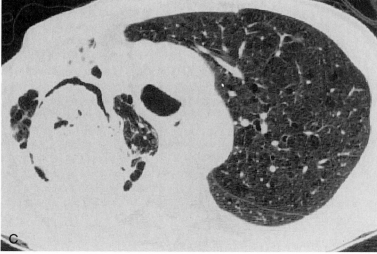

Figure 5–63. Aspergilloma: Development and Growth over Time. A 59-year-old woman with previous right mastectomy and right upper lobectomy presented with cough and weight loss. HRCT scan targeted to the right lung *(A)* showed a large cystic lesion in the superior segment of the right lower lobe. There is evidence of bronchiectasis. No other abnormality was found. All cultures were negative. HRCT scan 18 months later *(B)* shows a small amount of soft tissue in the dependent portion of the cystic lesion. There is increased thickness of the wall of the cyst. The patient also has evidence of extensive bronchiectasis and scarring in the right lung. Four years later, the patient developed hemoptysis. HRCT scan *(C)* shows a large mycetoma within the cavity. *Aspergillus fumigatus* was recovered at bronchoscopy.

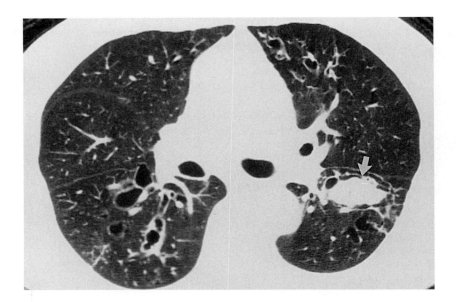

Figure 5–64. Allergic Bronchopulmonary Aspergillosis. HRCT scan shows extensive bronchiectasis involving mainly the central bronchi. Mucoid impaction *(arrow)* is present in an ectatic bronchus within the superior segment of the left lower lobe.

One group of investigators compared the HRCT findings in 44 asthmatic patients who had allergic bronchopulmonary aspergillosis with those of 38 asthmatic patients who did not have the disease.[353] Bronchiectasis was identified on HRCT scan in 42 (95%) of 44 patients who had allergic bronchopulmonary aspergillosis, centrilobular nodules in 41 (93%), and mucoid impaction in 29 (65%). In the asthmatic control group, bronchiectasis was detected in 11 (29%) of 38 patients, centrilobular nodules in 10 (26%), and mucoid impaction in 1 patient. Bronchiectasis usually involved three or more lobes (the lingula was considered a separate lobe) in patients who had allergic bronchopulmonary aspergillosis and only one or two lobes in patients who had asthma alone. Based on the presence of central bronchiectasis involving mainly the upper lobes, two independent observers correctly identified allergic bronchopulmonary aspergillosis as their first-choice diagnosis in 41 (93%) of 44 cases and correctly excluded the diagnosis of allergic bronchopulmonary aspergillosis in 36 (95%) of the asthmatic controls.[353]

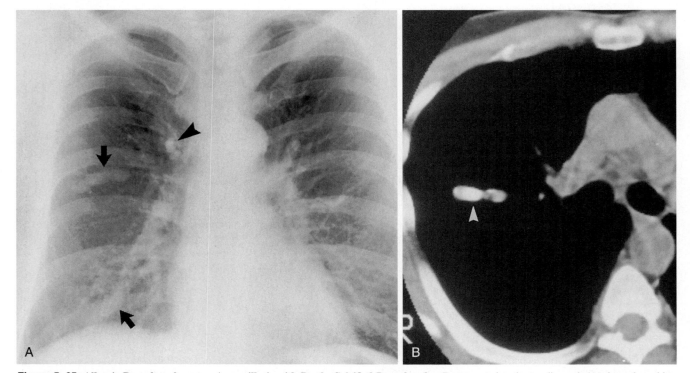

Figure 5–65. Allergic Bronchopulmonary Aspergillosis with Partly Calcified Bronchoceles. Posteroanterior chest radiograph *(A)* shows branching, bandlike opacities in the right lower lobe *(oblique arrow)* and the right upper lobe *(vertical arrow)*; an end-on round opacity *(arrowhead)* is seen in the upper hilum. CT scan *(B)* shows calcific material *(white arrowhead)* within the bronchocele. The patient was a 42-year-old man who had a history of atopic asthma and peripheral blood eosinophilia.

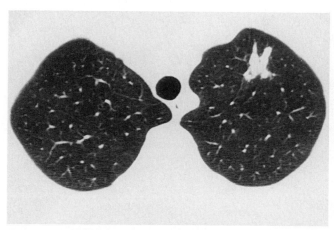

Figure 5–66. Allergic Bronchopulmonary Aspergillosis with Mucoid Impaction. HRCT scan targeted to the left upper lobe shows branching opacities characteristic of mucoid impaction in the left upper lobe. The patient was a 73-year-old woman who had asthma.

Invasive Aspergillosis

Invasive aspergillosis is characterized by extension of *Aspergillus* organisms into viable tissue, usually associated with tissue destruction. The abnormality almost invariably develops in patients whose host defenses are impaired, often as a result of cancer and its therapy.[297] Patients who have acute myelogenous leukemia are particularly susceptible;[356, 357] a significant risk for patients who have chronic myelogenous leukemia has been documented in some studies.[358] A major predisposing factor in these patients is granulocytopenia.[357, 359] Other conditions that are associated with an increased risk of invasive aspergillosis include organ transplantation,[360, 361] viral infection (particularly by influenza virus),[362, 363] renal or hepatic failure,[364, 365] and diabetes.[366] The disease is relatively infrequent in patients who have AIDS,[367] although it can occur, particularly when associated with risk factors such as corticosteroid therapy or neutropenia.[368]

Invasive pulmonary aspergillosis is manifested by four major clinicopathologic forms of disease that are useful to consider separately: (1) acute bronchopneumonia, (2) angioinvasive aspergillosis, (3) acute tracheobronchitis, and (4) chronic necrotizing aspergillosis.[370] The first two comprise most cases; in one review of 84 cases, acute bronchopneumonia and angioinvasive aspergillosis accounted for 30 and 29 cases.[355]

Acute Bronchopneumonia

Patients characteristically present with unremitting fever that responds poorly or not at all to antibiotic therapy; sometimes, there is an initial response, then failure. Dyspnea and tachypnea occur in cases of more extensive disease.

The radiographic pattern is one of patchy or homogeneous air-space consolidation without specific features.[355] In one review of nine patients, the findings included bilateral air-space consolidation in five, unilateral consolidation in one, small ill-defined nodules in two, and a normal chest radiograph in one.[7] The most common findings on CT scan, present also in the patient who had the normal radiograph,

consisted of bilateral, predominantly peribronchial, consolidation (Fig. 5–67). Sometimes the predominant finding on CT scan consists of poorly defined centrilobular nodular opacities measuring 2 to 5 mm in diameter (Fig. 5–68).[7] As might be expected, patients who have CT findings consistent with bronchitis or bronchopneumonia (centrilobular nodules and peribronchial consolidation) are more likely to have diagnostic findings on bronchoalveolar lavage than those who have CT findings consistent with angioinvasive aspergillosis (nodules >1 cm diameter, segmental consolidation); for example, in one study of 21 patients who had proven *Aspergillus* infection, bronchoalveolar lavage yielded fungus in 8 of 10 patients who had CT evidence of bronchiolitis or bronchopneumonia and in only 2 of 11 patients who had angioinvasive disease.[372]

Angioinvasive Aspergillosis

Angioinvasive aspergillosis probably is the most common manifestation of invasive pulmonary aspergillosis. Patients commonly present with fever, dyspnea, nonproductive cough, and pleuritic chest pain.[355]

The radiographic pattern consists of nodules or single or multiple areas of homogeneous consolidation (Fig. 5–69).[297, 371] Cavitation is common[354, 373] and sometimes is manifested by an air crescent partly or completely surrounding a central homogeneous mass (*see* Fig. 5–69).[374] This air crescent sign can develop 1 day to 3 weeks after the appearance of the initial radiographic abnormality.[356, 375] Occasionally, the characteristically patchy consolidation extends to involve an entire lobe, radiographically simulating acute bacterial pneumonia.[377] Pleural involvement is rare but may result in effusion or pneumothorax because of a bronchopleural fistula.[378] Pneumopericardium occurs rarely.[369, 379]

CT scan may show a characteristic finding in early angioinvasive aspergillosis, consisting of a halo of ground-glass attenuation surrounding a soft tissue nodule (Fig. 5–70) (the so-called halo sign).[376] This finding is related to the presence of air-space hemorrhage surrounding the nodule of necrotic lung tissue.[237, 380] With time, these lesions may develop air crescents or progress to frank cavitation (Fig. 5–71).[376] In the appropriate clinical setting, the presence of a soft tissue nodule with a halo sign is highly suggestive of angioinvasive aspergillosis.[376, 380] Vascular obstruction may result in homogeneous subsegmental, segmental, or lobar consolidation due to infarction.[301]

Chronic Necrotizing (Semi-Invasive) Aspergillosis

Chronic necrotizing (semi-invasive) aspergillosis is a rare form of invasive aspergillosis characterized by slowly progressive upper lobe disease that may spread to the contralateral lung, mediastinum, pleural space, or chest wall.[381, 382] Many patients have underlying chronic pulmonary disease, including remote infarction; inactive tuberculosis; COPD; or fibrosis related to previous resectional surgery, radiation therapy, or pneumoconiosis. Although abnormalities of host defense may be apparent, they typically are relatively mild compared with the abnormalities associated with other forms of invasive disease (e.g., diabetes, poor nutrition, connective tissue disorders). A history of intensive immunosuppressive therapy usually is absent;

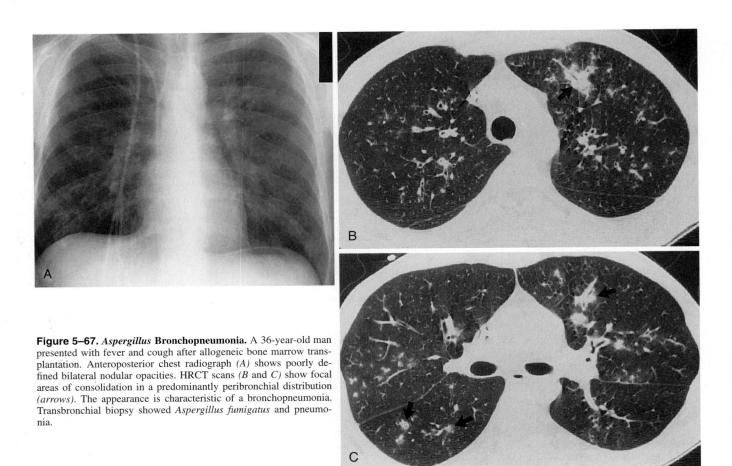

Figure 5–67. *Aspergillus* **Bronchopneumonia.** A 36-year-old man presented with fever and cough after allogeneic bone marrow transplantation. Anteroposterior chest radiograph *(A)* shows poorly defined bilateral nodular opacities. HRCT scans *(B and C)* show focal areas of consolidation in a predominantly peribronchial distribution *(arrows)*. The appearance is characteristic of a bronchopneumonia. Transbronchial biopsy showed *Aspergillus fumigatus* and pneumonia.

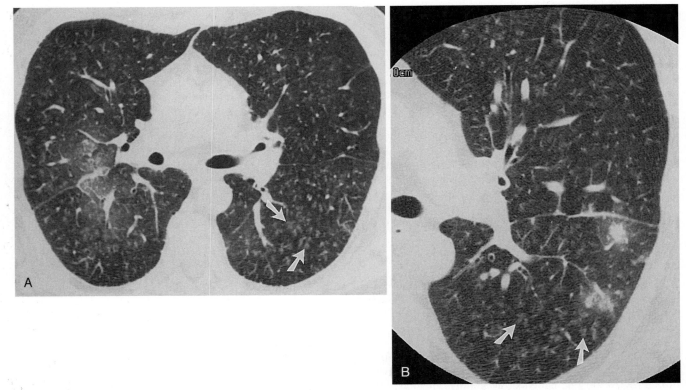

Figure 5–68. *Aspergillus* **Bronchiolitis and Bronchopneumonia.** HRCT scan *(A)* shows localized area of ground-glass attenuation in the right lung and bilateral, poorly defined small nodular opacities. HRCT scan targeted to the left lung *(B)* delineates better the small nodular and branching opacities *(arrows)* and shows them to have a centrilobular distribution characteristic of bronchiolitis. Focal areas of consolidation are visible in the left lower lobe. Open-lung biopsy showed *Aspergillus* bronchiolitis and bronchopneumonia. The patient was a 52-year-old man who had undergone bone marrow transplantation.

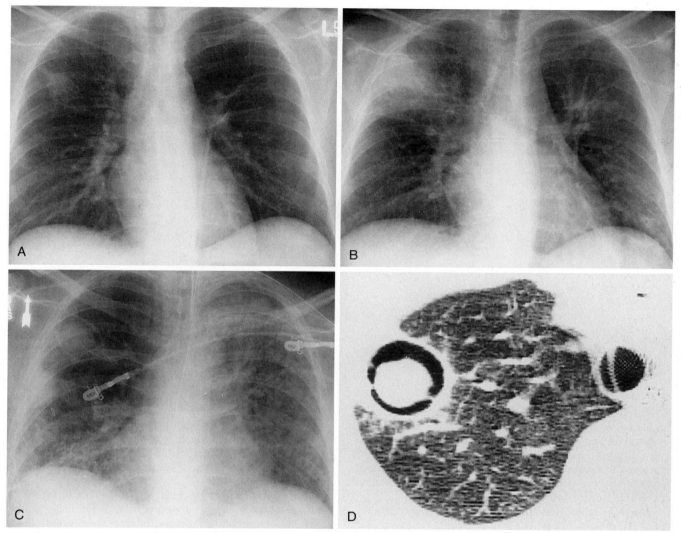

Figure 5–69. Angioinvasive Aspergillosis: Progression of Radiographic Findings. A 23-year-old patient with acute leukemia presented with fever and cough. Anteroposterior chest radiograph *(A)* shows a rounded area of consolidation in the right upper lobe, which 1 week later *(B)* has shown considerable progression. The following day, the patient underwent open-lung biopsy that showed pulmonary hemorrhage but failed to identify any organisms. Anteroposterior chest radiograph 2 weeks after biopsy *(C)* and HRCT scan *(D)* show a smoothly marginated cavity in the right upper lobe containing a soft tissue mass. Repeat biopsy performed under CT guidance confirmed the diagnosis of invasive aspergillosis, the soft tissue mass within the cavity in this case representing necrotic lung (sequestrum).

however, some patients have been taking low doses of corticosteroids.

Radiologic manifestations usually consist of an area of consolidation, a nodule or mass in the upper lobe that develops progressive cavitation over several weeks or months.[327, 383, 384] The cavitation may be associated with an intracavitary soft tissue opacity. Adjacent pleural thickening is common. The process may extend to involve the chest wall and mediastinum.[327] In a review of the radiographic and CT findings in nine patients, the radiologic abnormalities consisted of upper lobe parenchymal consolidation in six and nodules larger than 1 cm in diameter in three.[383] Cavitation was present in four patients, and pleural thickening was present in four patients.[383]

Zygomycosis

Zygomycosis (mucormycosis, phycomycosis) is caused by fungi of the orders Entomophthorales and Mucorales,

which are ubiquitous and worldwide in distribution. The most common radiographic findings consist of unilateral or bilateral air-space consolidation.[385] Lung involvement frequently is segmental and homogeneous, reflecting vascular obstruction.[386–388] The consolidation may be round and rapidly progressive (Fig. 5–72);[389] occasionally, there is lobar expansion.[385] Another common presentation consists of solitary or multiple small or large nodules;[385] in one case, a nodular opacity was found to be a thrombosed vessel subtending a pulmonary infarct.[390] As with angioinvasive aspergillosis, CT scan may show a halo of ground-glass attenuation surrounding the nodule (halo sign).[391]

Actinomycosis

Actinomycosis is caused by members of the family Actinomycetaceae, of which the most important genus is *Actinomyces*. This genus contains several species, including

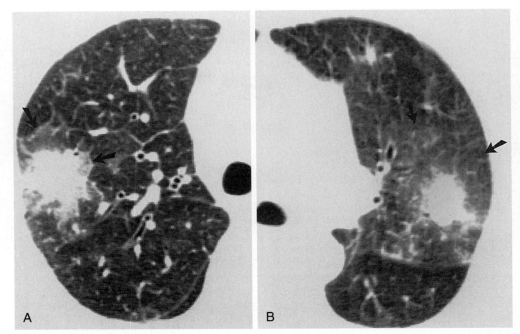

Figure 5–70. Angioinvasive Aspergillosis: CT Halo Sign. HRCT scans of the right upper *(A)* and left upper *(B)* lobes show nodules that are surrounded by a halo of ground-glass attenuation *(arrows)* (halo sign). The patient was a 72-year-old woman with severe neutropenia undergoing chemotherapy for leukemia. Diagnosis was proved by bronchoalveolar lavage.

A. israelii, which is the most important cause of disease in humans. The organism is a normal inhabitant of the human oropharynx and frequently is found in the crypts of surgically excised tonsils[394] and in dental caries and at gingival margins of persons who have poor oral hygiene.[392] In most cases, disease is believed to be acquired by the spread of organisms from these sites.[393]

The initial clinical manifestations of pulmonary involvement are nonproductive cough and low-grade fever. With time, the cough becomes productive of purulent and, in many cases, blood-streaked sputum. As the disease progresses, weight loss, anemia, and finger clubbing may occur.[406] Pleuritic chest pain commonly develops as the infection spreads to the pleura and chest wall.

The typical pattern of acute pulmonary actinomycosis consists of nonsegmental air-space consolidation, commonly in the periphery of the lung and with a predilection for the lower lobes. Once the pneumonia has developed, the course of events depends largely on whether antibiotic therapy is instituted. With appropriate therapy, most cases resolve without complications. If therapy is not instituted, an abscess may develop, and the infection may extend into the pleura and into the chest wall, with abscess formation in these areas. Extension across the interlobar fissures also is common but is not unique to this disease—it also may occur in blastomycosis, cryptococcosis, and tuberculosis.

Although the previous description is perhaps the most common radiographic manifestation of actinomycosis, other abnormalities are frequent. In our experience and that of others, the infection commonly presents radiographically as a mass, sometimes cavitated,[397] that simulates pulmonary carcinoma.[398–400] In patients in whom the pleuropulmonary disease becomes chronic, extensive fibrosis in and about the lung can become a prominent radiographic feature; as a result, there is severe distortion of normal anatomic

structures (Fig. 5–73).[401] Pleural effusion occasionally is the only radiographic manifestation;[402] when an isolated finding or when associated with parenchymal disease, its development almost invariably indicates empyema.[403, 404] Mediastinal and pericardial involvement may occur but are uncommon.[405]

The manifestations of chest wall involvement include a soft tissue mass and rib abnormalities, sometimes without evidence of pulmonary disease.[406] Periosteal proliferation along the ribs may have a peculiar wavy configuration;[397] such involvement of several adjacent ribs in the absence of empyema is suggestive of the disease.[395] Frank rib and, occasionally, vertebral destruction may occur.[397] CT[396, 407] and ultrasonography[408] have been advocated as useful procedures to determine the presence and extent of chest wall involvement.

In one investigation of eight patients, central low attenuation regions were identified in three patients (38%) in the areas of consolidation on CT scan, corresponding to abscess formation pathologically (Fig. 5–74).[396] Pleural thickening was identified on the radiograph in four cases and pleural effusion in three. Pleural thickening localized to the pleura abutting an area of consolidation was seen on CT scan in all patients. Small pleural effusions were identified in five patients (62%); in two patients, the effusion represented an empyema. Invasion through the chest wall was present in only one case; there was no associated rib destruction or periosteal reaction. Hilar or mediastinal lymph node enlargement was seen on CT scan in six cases (75%).

Nocardiosis

Nocardiosis is caused by species of the family Nocardiaceae, of which the most important with respect to human

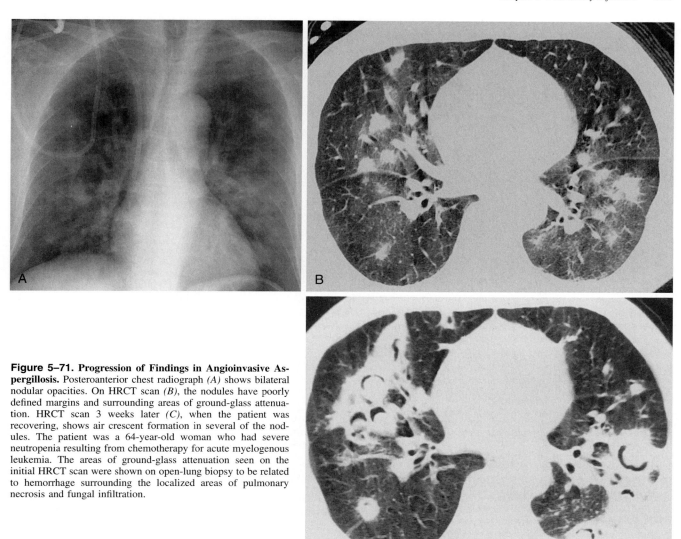

Figure 5–71. Progression of Findings in Angioinvasive Aspergillosis. Posteroanterior chest radiograph *(A)* shows bilateral nodular opacities. On HRCT scan *(B)*, the nodules have poorly defined margins and surrounding areas of ground-glass attenuation. HRCT scan 3 weeks later *(C)*, when the patient was recovering, shows air crescent formation in several of the nodules. The patient was a 64-year-old woman who had severe neutropenia resulting from chemotherapy for acute myelogenous leukemia. The areas of ground-glass attenuation seen on the initial HRCT scan were shown on open-lung biopsy to be related to hemorrhage surrounding the localized areas of pulmonary necrosis and fungal infiltration.

pulmonary disease is *Nocardia asteroides*.[409] The organisms are common inhabitants of soil throughout the world; most cases of pulmonary disease are believed to be acquired by inhalation of material from this source. Cough, purulent sputum, pleural pain, and night sweats are the usual symptoms; hemoptysis occurs occasionally.[429]

Although *Nocardia* formerly was seen almost exclusively as a primary pulmonary pathogen, it now is recognized more frequently as an opportunistic invader in patients who have underlying disease.[409, 411] Patients who have lymphoma,[412, 413] organ transplants,[414, 415] and, for reasons not well understood, alveolar proteinosis appear to be most susceptible.[416] Patients who have systemic lupus erythematosus,[417] who are receiving low-dose methotrexate[418] or corticosteroid therapy,[411] or who have an endogenous source of increased glucocorticoids[419] are vulnerable.[409, 418] It is a relatively uncommon cause of opportunistic infection in AIDS.[410]

The most frequent radiographic abnormality is air-space consolidation, usually homogeneous and nonsegmental[420, 421] but sometimes patchy and inhomogeneous (Fig. 5–75).[422]

In one review of 21 patients, multilobar consolidation was present in most.[423] In contrast to actinomycosis, nocardiosis shows no predilection for the lower lobes.[423] Cavitation is frequent;[422, 423] in one series of 12 cases, it was the most common radiographic manifestation, occurring within a consolidated lobe in three patients and within a solitary mass in four.[424] Similar to actinomycosis, infection may extend into the pleural space and cause effusion or empyema.[423] Evidence of chest wall involvement seldom is seen on the radiograph.[425] Extension to the pericardium or mediastinum occurs occasionally.[423, 426, 427]

CT may be helpful in assessing the extent of disease and as a guide to obtain material for a definitive diagnosis.[427, 428] In one review of the CT findings in five patients, the predominant abnormality consisted of multifocal areas of consolidation.[428] Localized areas of low attenuation with rim enhancement suggestive of abscess formation were present within the areas of consolidation in three patients, and cavitation was present in one patient. Variable sized pulmonary nodules were identified in three patients (Fig. 5–76). Pleural involvement was present in all cases, includ-

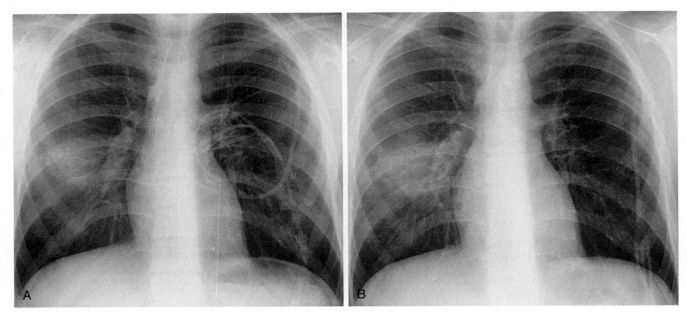

Figure 5–72. Mucormycosis. Posteroanterior *(A)* chest radiograph shows a rounded area of consolidation in the superior segment of the right lower lobe. Follow-up radiograph obtained the next day *(B)* shows considerable increase in size of the consolidation. Because of the patient's severe clinical findings, a right lower lobectomy was performed. Hemorrhagic necrosis with extensive angioinvasive mucormycosis was found. The patient was a 15-year-old boy who had severe neutropenia secondary to chemotherapy for acute leukemia. (Case courtesy of Dr. James Barrie, University of Alberta Hospital, Edmonton, Canada.)

ing pleural effusion in four, empyema in one, and pleural thickening in four. Chest wall extension was identified in three patients.

VIRUSES, *MYCOPLASMA PNEUMONIAE,* AND *CHLAMYDIA PNEUMONIAE*

RNA Viruses

Influenza Virus

Influenza can occur in pandemics, epidemics, or sporadically in individuals or small clusters of patients. Almost all severe epidemics and all pandemics are caused by type A viruses. Although outbreaks caused by type B can occur, they are less frequent, more localized, and more common in schoolchildren than in the general population.[430] Influenza outbreaks tend to occur on an annual basis, typically during the winter in temperate climates; a seasonal association is less clear-cut in tropical areas. Attack rates are highest in schoolchildren; complications and hospitalization are more likely in children and in the elderly (particularly those in nursing homes).

Pneumonia is an uncommon but dreaded complication of influenza infection. Although it may be caused by the virus itself (usually type A and occasionally type B organisms[431, 432]), bacterial superinfection (most often by *S. aureus* and occasionally by *Streptococcus*[529]) is much more frequent. Involvement may be local or general. Local involvement usually is in the form of segmental consolidation that may be homogeneous or patchy and unilateral or bilateral.[433–435] Serial radiographs may show poorly defined, patchy areas of consolidation, 1 to 2 cm in diameter, which become confluent rapidly. In one series, disease was unilateral and bilateral in approximately the same number of cases and widely disseminated in roughly a quarter of the latter cases (Fig. 5–77).[435] Pleural effusion is comparatively rare.[435] Resolution averages about 3 weeks.[435]

Respiratory Syncytial Virus

Respiratory syncytial virus is particularly important as a cause of disease in infants and small children.[436, 439] In a prospective study of respiratory infections in the first 3 years of life, the organism was identified as the cause of disease in 50% of cases.[437] Adult infection usually is mild and limited to the upper respiratory tract, presumably reflecting immunity as a result of childhood infection; however, significant lower respiratory tract involvement can occur, particularly in elderly or chronically ill patients in nursing homes or the hospital[442, 443] and in immunocompromised individuals.[444, 445] Rarely, there is an acute onset of pneumonia with rapid progression to adult respiratory distress syndrome.[446]

A disparity has been noted between the severity of respiratory symptoms and the relative paucity of radiographic findings.[441] In infants, the chest radiograph shows patchy areas of consolidation interspersed with zones of overinflation.[440] In one study of 65 patients, the dominant findings in 60 cases were bronchial wall thickening, peribronchial infiltrates, and perihilar linearity.[438] Patchy sublobular or lobular consolidation was present in 39 cases, whereas more homogeneous consolidation was present in 10; multiple areas of involvement were common. Air-trapping was evident in 41.

Hantaviruses

Hantaviruses are lipid-enveloped RNA viruses that typically cause a symptom complex characterized by fever,

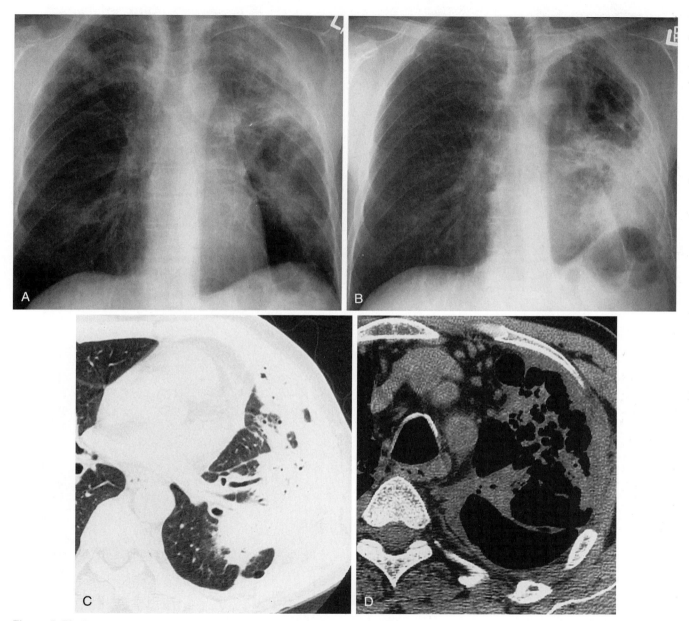

Figure 5–73. Pleuropulmonary Actinomycosis. A 55-year-old alcoholic man presented with a 6-month history of cough, fever, and weight loss. Posteroanterior chest radiograph *(A)* shows bilateral areas of consolidation involving the upper lobes. Cultures, bronchoscopy, and open-lung biopsy failed to yield a definitive diagnosis, and the patient was treated empirically with antibiotics. Posteroanterior chest radiograph performed 4 months later *(B)* shows fibrosis in the left upper lobe and adjacent pleural thickening. Note volume loss of the left lung because of the fibrosis. Consolidation has developed in the lingula and in the left lower lobe. HRCT scan *(C* and *D)* confirms the lingular and left lower lobe consolidation as well as marked pleural thickening, particularly adjacent to the anterolateral aspect of the upper lobe. A small left pleural effusion is evident. Repeat pleural and open-lung biopsy showed *Actinomyces israelii.*

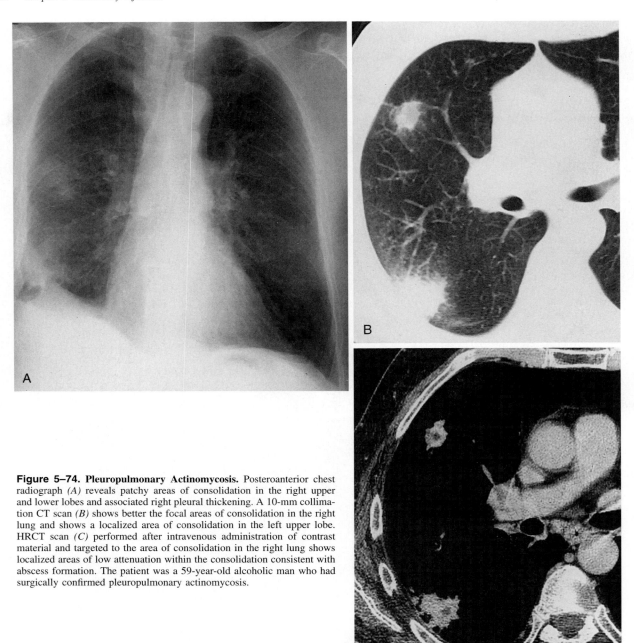

Figure 5–74. Pleuropulmonary Actinomycosis. Posteroanterior chest radiograph *(A)* reveals patchy areas of consolidation in the right upper and lower lobes and associated right pleural thickening. A 10-mm collimation CT scan *(B)* shows better the focal areas of consolidation in the right lung and shows a localized area of consolidation in the left upper lobe. HRCT scan *(C)* performed after intravenous administration of contrast material and targeted to the area of consolidation in the right lung shows localized areas of low attenuation within the consolidation consistent with abscess formation. The patient was a 59-year-old alcoholic man who had surgically confirmed pleuropulmonary actinomycosis.

hypotension, and renal failure and referred to as *hemorrhagic fever with renal syndrome.* In the early 1990s, the Sin Nombre virus was identified as the agent responsible for a frequently more fulminant and clinically severe disease with prominent pulmonary involvement—the hantavirus pulmonary syndrome.[447, 448] The natural reservoir of all hantaviruses is wild rodents, the deer mouse being the most important animal harboring the Sin Nombre variant in the United States.[447] Climatic or other environmental driven changes in the local rodent population are believed to be at least partly responsible for variations in the incidence of disease and the development of local outbreaks. Most cases have been identified in rural areas.

The radiographic findings were described in 16 patients seen during an epidemic in the southwestern United States in 1993.[449] In 13 of the 16 patients, the initial chest radiographs revealed changes indicative of interstitial pulmonary edema, including septal (Kerley B) lines, hilar indistinctness, and peribronchial cuffing (Fig. 5–78). In the three patients who had normal radiographs at presentation, findings consistent with interstitial pulmonary edema developed within 48 hours. Four of 16 patients had radiographic findings consisting predominantly or exclusively of interstitial edema at 48 hours; all 4 patients survived, and their radiographs returned to normal within 5 days after admission. Six of 16 patients had air-space consolidation on the initial chest radiograph; this was perihilar in 3, involved the basal segments in 2, and involved the central upper

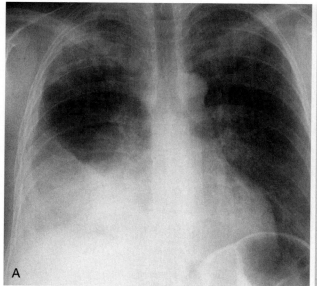

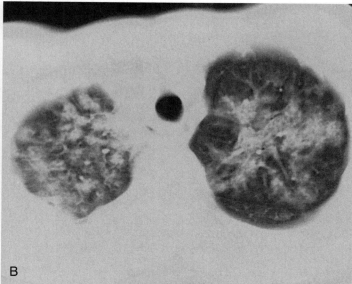

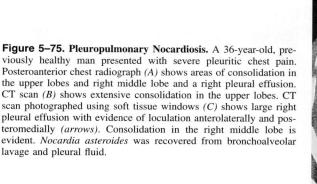

Figure 5–75. Pleuropulmonary Nocardiosis. A 36-year-old, previously healthy man presented with severe pleuritic chest pain. Posteroanterior chest radiograph *(A)* shows areas of consolidation in the upper lobes and right middle lobe and a right pleural effusion. CT scan *(B)* shows extensive consolidation in the upper lobes. CT scan photographed using soft tissue windows *(C)* shows large right pleural effusion with evidence of loculation anterolaterally and posteromedially *(arrows)*. Consolidation in the right middle lobe is evident. *Nocardia asteroides* was recovered from bronchoalveolar lavage and pleural fluid.

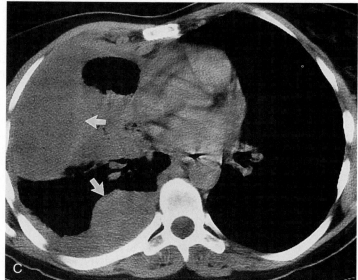

lobe in 1 patient. Within 48 hours after admission, 11 patients developed extensive air-space consolidation. The distribution was bibasilar or perihilar in 10 patients and predominantly peripheral in 1 patient. The time to resolution of the radiographic findings in the nine patients who survived ranged from 5 days to more than 3 weeks. Pleural effusions were present on the initial chest radiographs in two patients and developed within 48 hours in nine other patients. The effusions were small in five patients and large in six patients.

DNA Viruses

Adenovirus

Adenovirus infection forms a small but significant proportion of respiratory disease. In one investigation of more than 18,000 infants and children followed for 10 years, at least 7% of respiratory infections were estimated to be caused by adenovirus.[450] Disease may occur as pharyngitis, pharyngoconjunctivitis, laryngotracheobronchitis, bronchiolitis, pneumonia, or a nonspecific acute respiratory syndrome; there is evidence that the organism may be involved in the pathogeneses of some cases of bronchiectasis.[451]

One of the most extensive reviews of adenoviral pneumonia and its complications in infancy and childhood consisted of a study of 69 patients conducted over a 5-year period.[452] Of the patients, 46 (67%) were North American Indian, Metis, or Inuit, and most were younger than 1 year of age. The most common radiographic findings consisted of diffuse bilateral bronchopneumonia and severe overinflation.

Herpesviruses

Herpes Simplex Type I

Most patients who have herpes simplex virus type I pulmonary or tracheobronchial disease have an underlying predisposing condition, such as severe burns,[454] AIDS, ma-

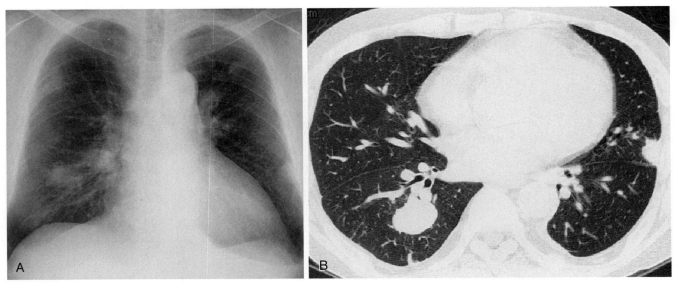

Figure 5–76. *Nocardia* **Pneumonia After Renal Transplantation.** A 41-year-old man on immunosuppressive therapy after renal transplantation presented with fever and cough. Posteroanterior chest radiograph *(A)* shows bilateral nodular opacities. HRCT scan *(B)* shows nodules in lingula and right lower lobe. *Nocardia asteroides* infection was proved by bronchoalveolar lavage.

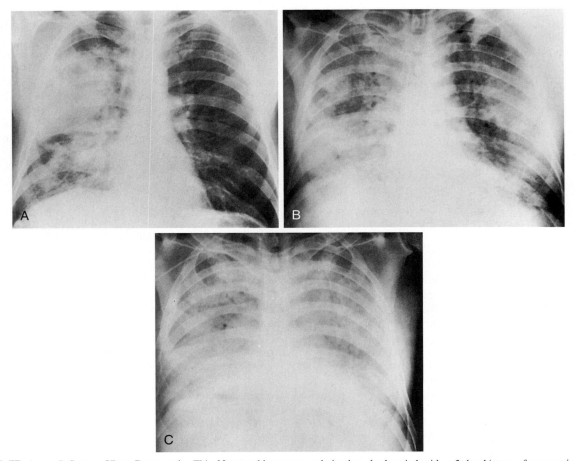

Figure 5–77. Acute Influenza Virus Pneumonia. This 32-year-old man was admitted to the hospital with a 3-day history of progressive dyspnea, cough productive of whitish yellow sputum, right-sided pleuritic chest pain, chills, and fever. Posteroanterior chest radiograph on the day of admission *(A)* shows extensive homogeneous air-space consolidation of the right upper lobe, with patchy shadows of air-space consolidation of the right lower lobe; the left lung is clear. Two days later *(B)*, consolidation of the right lower lobe has become almost uniform, and extension of the air-space disease has occurred throughout the whole of the left lung. Twenty-four hours later *(C)*, both lungs are consolidated almost completely, the only visible air being present within the bronchial tree (a diffuse air bronchogram). Shortly after admission, the patient became comatose and never regained consciousness. Serologic studies revealed a titer of 1:128 (complement-fixation test) for influenza A$_2$. Respiratory syncytial virus and influenza virus were cultured from the blood, from the sputum, and directly from the lung at autopsy.

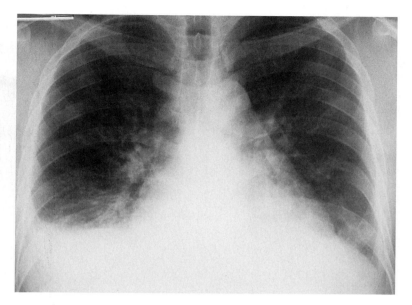

Figure 5–78. Hantavirus Pneumonia. Chest radiograph in a patient with hantavirus pulmonary syndrome shows mild cardiomegaly with prominence of the pulmonary vascular markings and small bilateral pleural effusions. These findings resolved rapidly after renal dialysis. (Case courtesy of Dr. Eun-Young Kang, De rtment of Radiology, Korea University Medical Center, Guro Hospital, Seoul, Korea.)

lignancy, or organ transplants,[453] or have undergone major surgery.[455] The radiographic and CT manifestations usually consist of patchy bilateral subsegmental or segmental areas of consolidation.[455, 456] Additional findings that may be present include lobar areas of consolidation, ground-glass opacities, reticular opacities, and pleural effusions.[455] Occasionally, poorly defined 3- to 20-mm-diameter nodules are seen on radiograph and HRCT scan (Fig. 5–79).[299, 301]

Varicellavirus

Varicellavirus (varicella-zoster virus) infection is seen in two clinical forms: (1) chickenpox (varicella), representing primary and usually disseminated disease in previously uninfected individuals, and (2) zoster (shingles), representing reactivation of latent virus, typically as a unilateral dermatomal skin eruption. Although either form may be associated with pneumonia, most such cases occur in relation to chickenpox.[457]

The overall incidence of varicella-related pneumonia appears to be about 15%,[459, 460] although in adults admitted to the hospital it has been 50%.[461] Most cases occur in very young children or adults.[458] In both groups, pre-existing neoplastic disease—particularly leukemia and lymphoma—and other causes of immunodeficiency are predisposing factors.[462, 463] The incidence and the severity of such pneumonia are significantly greater in pregnant women.[464]

The characteristic radiographic pattern consists of multiple 5- to 10-mm-diameter nodular opacities (Fig. 5–80). Smaller nodular opacities and miliary-like nodules may be seen but are uncommon.[466] The opacities usually are fairly discrete in the lung periphery but tend to coalesce near the hila and in the lung bases.[459] Progression to extensive air-space consolidation can occur rapidly. In a few cases, the changes have been described as transitory, some areas of air-space consolidation clearing, while new areas appear.[465] Occasionally, the nodular opacities mimic pulmonary metastases.[531] Hilar lymph node enlargement occurs but may be difficult to appreciate because of contiguity of the consolidation in the parahilar parenchyma.[459] Pleural effusion is uncommon and never large.[468]

Radiographic clearing usually takes 10 days to several months;[467, 469] however, in one series of 20 patients, chest radiographs of 6 patients showed widespread nodulation considered to represent scarring 6 years after the infection.[465] In one case, fibrosis appeared to increase in extent over a period of 3 to 4 years after the initial infection.[470]

An uncommon manifestation of chickenpox pneumonia consists of tiny widespread foci of calcification throughout both lungs in persons who had chickenpox many years before (typically in adulthood) (Fig. 5–81).[471, 472] The foci of calcification vary in size and number but seldom exceed 2 to 3 mm in diameter; they predominate in the lower half of the lungs. Hilar lymph nodes do not calcify. In one survey of almost 17,000 individuals, 463 (2.7%) had a history of chickenpox as adults;[473] only 8 (1.7%) of these had multifocal calcification.

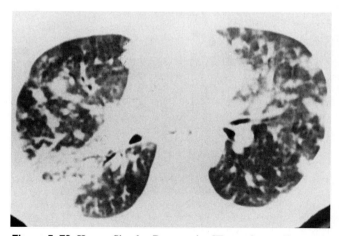

Figure 5–79. Herpes Simplex Pneumonia. CT scan from a 42-year-old immunocompromised woman after bone marrow transplantation shows bilateral nodules 3 to 15 mm in diameter. Focal areas of consolidation in the right lower lobe and lingula also are present. The diagnosis was confirmed at open-lung biopsy.

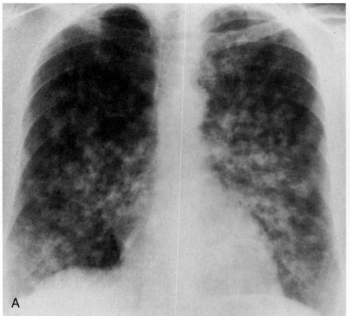

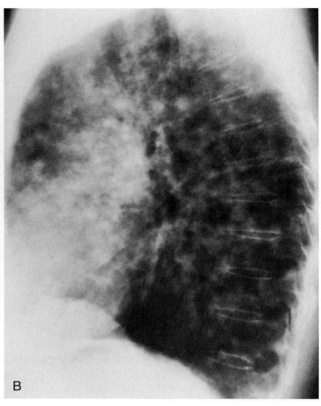

Figure 5–80. Acute Varicella-Zoster Pneumonia. Posteroanterior *(A)* and lateral *(B)* radiographs show multiple, poorly defined nodular opacities and patchy air-space consolidation. The patient was a 42-year-old woman who had non-Hodgkin's lymphoma.

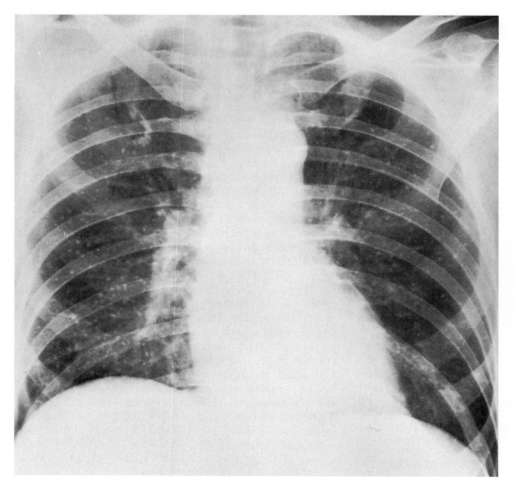

Figure 5–81. Healed Varicella-Zoster (Chickenpox) Pneumonia. Posteroanterior radiograph shows a multitude of tiny calcific shadows 1 to 2 mm in diameter scattered widely and uniformly throughout both lungs. This 42-year-old asymptomatic man had had florid chickenpox 15 years previously; the presence of acute pneumonia was recognized at the time. (Courtesy of Dr. Romeo Ethier, Montreal Neurological Hospital, Montreal, Canada.)

Cytomegalovirus

Acquired CMV infection is common; seropositivity rates vary from 40% to 100% in different adult populations around the world.[474] Higher rates tend to be seen in conditions of lower socioeconomic status.[474] Most affected individuals are asymptomatic, the only sequela of their infection being the presence of latent virus as a potential source of reinfection. As a corollary, CMV is an uncommon cause of community-acquired pneumonia; for example, in one study of 443 patients who had this condition, the pneumonia was caused by CMV in only 4 (0.9%).[475] By contrast, pneumonia and other clinical manifestations of active infection are much more frequent in patients who have underlying disease, particularly immunodeficiency related to organ transplantation (*see* Chapter 11)[476, 477] or AIDS (*see* Chapter 10).

The most common radiographic findings in CMV pneumonia are bilateral linear opacities (reticular pattern), ground-glass opacities, and parenchymal consolidation (Fig. 5–82).[478, 479] Less common manifestations include small nodular opacities, a reticulonodular pattern, and lobar consolidation.[299, 480, 481]

In one investigation of 31 patients who had CMV pneumonia after bone marrow transplantation, radiographic abnormalities consisted of air-space consolidation in 12 (39%), linear opacities (reticular pattern) in 7 (23%), ground-glass opacities in 4 (13%), and a combination of the three patterns in 8 (26%).[479] These abnormalities first were noted 26 to 270 days (median, 96 days) after transplantation, were bilateral in 22 patients and unilateral in 9 patients, and most commonly involved the lower lung zones. Although pleural effusions were present in six patients, they usually could be attributed to other causes, most commonly renal failure. In another study of six patients who had had cardiac transplants, the radiographic findings included diffuse bilateral haze (ground-glass opacities), lobar consolidation with small pleural effusion, and focal subsegmental consolidation.[478]

Findings of CMV pneumonia on CT scan include areas of ground-glass attenuation, parenchymal consolidation, and nodular or reticulonodular opacities.[37, 38, 482] In one investigation of eight patients, seven had a combination of linear opacities and parenchymal consolidation, and one had only consolidation.[482] All abnormalities were bilateral. The consolidation most commonly consisted of poorly marginated opacities that were predominantly peripheral in distribution. Pleural effusion was present in four cases and was bilateral in three. Enlarged hilar or mediastinal nodes were not identified. In a second study of 10 patients, the CT findings included small nodules in 6, consolidation in 4, ground-glass attenuation in 4, and irregular lines in 1 patient (Fig. 5–83).[38] The nodules had a bilateral and symmetric distribution and involved all lung zones. The areas of consolidation were nonsegmental and involved the lower lung zones. Neither nodules nor consolidation showed a tendency toward a peribronchial or subpleural distribution.

Epstein-Barr Virus

Epstein-Barr virus is perhaps best known as the cause of infectious mononucleosis, a syndrome that affects predominantly young adults and consists of pharyngitis; fever; more or less diffuse lymph node enlargement; splenomegaly; and an increase in lymphocytes, often cytologically

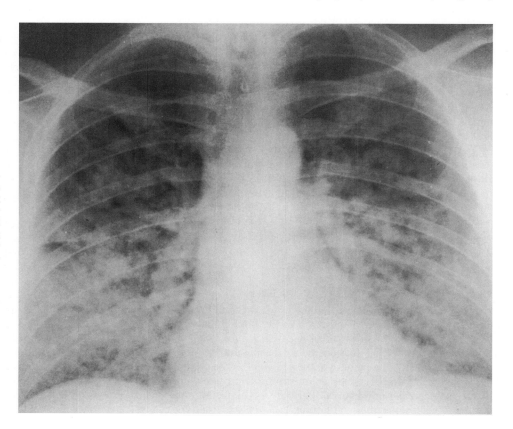

Figure 5–82. Acute Cytomegalovirus Pneumonia in a Renal Transplant Patient. Posteroanterior chest radiograph shows widespread patchy air-space consolidation, more marked in the lower lobes. There is mild left ventricular enlargement. At autopsy several days later, severe cytomegalovirus pneumonia was found.

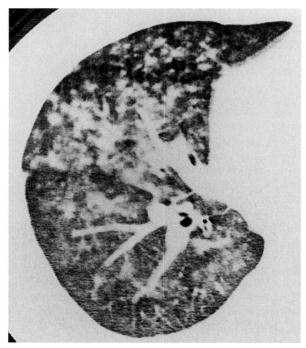

Figure 5–83. Cytomegalovirus Pneumonia. HRCT scan targeted to the right lung shows small nodular opacities 3 to 10 mm in diameter and areas of ground-glass attenuation. Similar abnormalities were evident in the left lung. The patient was a 24-year-old man who had undergone renal transplantation.

atypical, in peripheral blood. Intrathoracic disease is uncommon and is manifested most often by lymph node enlargement (Fig. 5–84), interstitial pneumonitis, or both.[483] In one series of 556 patients, 30 had abnormal physical findings in the chest, and 14 of these patients had radiographic evidence of interstitial pneumonitis.[484] In another series of 59 patients, the radiographic findings were as follows:[485] hilar lymph node enlargement in 8 (13%); a diffuse reticular pattern in 3 (5%), 1 of these patients also showing an air-space pattern; and pleural effusions in 3 (small and bilateral in 2 patients and moderate and unilateral in the other patient).

Epstein-Barr virus has been implicated strongly in the development of several lymphoproliferative disorders. This association has been documented best in Burkitt's lymphoma and in lymphomas complicating systemic immunodeficiency, particularly AIDS, congenital immunodeficiency states, and post-transplant lymphoproliferative disorders (including those of the lung; *see* Chapter 11).[486]

Mycoplasma pneumoniae

Mycoplasma pneumoniae is one of the more common causes of community-acquired pneumonia, accounting for an estimated 10% to 15% of cases in the population as a whole[488, 489] and 50% of cases in specific groups, such as military recruits.[487, 490] Infections occur throughout the year, with a peak during the autumn and early winter. The typical case begins insidiously with fever, nonproductive cough, headache, malaise, and (rarely) chills.[501] Myalgia, arthralgia, and gastrointestinal symptoms usually are mild or

absent. Upper respiratory tract involvement, characterized predominantly by sore throat and symptoms of rhinitis, is present in about 50% of cases.[491]

The radiographic pattern of acute mycoplasmal pneumonia is indistinguishable from that of many viral pneumonias,[28] the manifestations consisting of interstitial or air-space opacities or a combination of both (Fig. 5–85).[492] In the early stages, the interstitial inflammation causes a fine reticular pattern, followed by signs of air-space consolidation in a patchy distribution (Fig. 5–86).[29, 30] In contrast to the nonsegmental distribution of acute bacterial air-space pneumonia (e.g., caused by *S. pneumoniae*), mycoplasmal pneumonia tends to be segmental. In one series of 79 cases, only 2 cases had a radiographic picture that could be confused with bacterial pneumonia; both of these were readily identified clinically and from the leukocyte count as of mycoplasmal or viral origin.[493] Disease is manifested predominantly in the lower lobes: Only 5 of 39 cases in one series had upper lobe involvement.[494]

The main HRCT findings of mycoplasmal pneumonia consist of centrilobular nodular and branching linear opacities in a patchy distribution, thickening of the bronchovascular bundles, and areas of lobular or segmental consolidation (Fig. 5–87).[12, 495] The HRCT findings were compared with the radiographic findings in a retrospective study of 28 patients.[495] The most common abnormality evident on the radiograph was air-space opacification (seen in 24 [85%] patients). On HRCT scan, areas of ground-glass attenuation were seen in 24 (85%) and air-space consolidation in 22 (75%) patients. In 13 (59%) patients, the areas of consolidation had a lobular distribution on HRCT scan. Nodules, usually in a centrilobular distribution, were seen on HRCT scan in 89% of patients and on radiograph in 50%.[495]

Hilar lymph node enlargement is rare in adults[28, 496] but occurs in approximately 30% of children.[497, 498] Pleural effusions occur in approximately 20% of patients but usually are small and unilateral.[31, 499, 500]

Chlamydia pneumoniae

Chlamydia pneumoniae is a common cause of community-acquired pneumonia. In one study of 65 patients presenting to the emergency department with a principal symptom of cough lasting longer than 2 weeks and less than 3 months, 13 (20%) were found to have serologic evidence of recent *C. pneumoniae* infection.[502] The most frequent clinical manifestations are sore throat, nonproductive cough, and fever; hoarseness occurs in some patients.

Radiographic manifestations have been described in one series of 55 adults hospitalized for community-acquired pneumonia.[503] Based on serologic criteria, the patients were categorized as having acute primary (17 patients [31%]) or recurrent (38 patients [69%]) infection. Findings in the first group included air-space consolidation in 11 patients, interstitial infiltrates in 2, combined interstitial and air-space infiltrates in 3, and a normal radiograph in 1 patient. The consolidation was unilateral in 12 patients, lobar in 9, and multifocal in 3. Pleural effusions were present in three patients. Of the 38 patients who had recurrent infection, 11 had air-space consolidation; 14 had interstitial infiltrates; 6 had a combination of air-space and interstitial infiltrates;

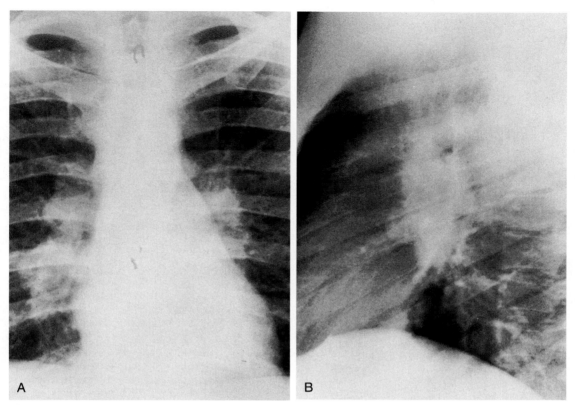

Figure 5–84. Infectious Mononucleosis. This 17-year-old boy presented with history and physical findings compatible with infectious mononucleosis; he had a leukocytosis of 18,000, 50% of which were atypical lymphocytes; serial studies revealed a rising heterophil antibody titer. Views from posteroanterior *(A)* and lateral *(B)* radiographs show marked enlargement of both hila, the lobulated contour being typical of lymph node enlargement. There is no evidence of mediastinal lymphadenopathy or of pulmonary or pleural disease. One month later, chest radiograph was normal.

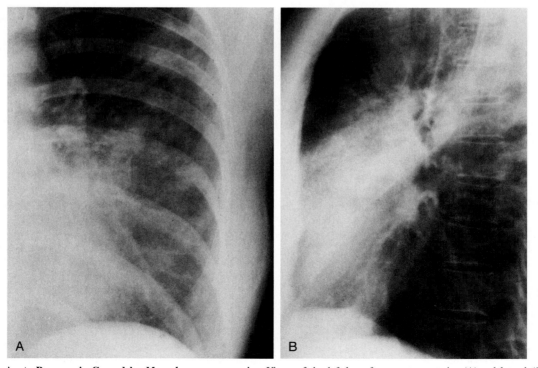

Figure 5–85. Acute Pneumonia Caused by *Mycoplasma pneumoniae.* Views of the left lung from posteroanterior *(A)* and lateral *(B)* radiographs show patchy air-space consolidation in the distribution of the lingular and posterior segments of the left upper lobe. Immunofluorescence microscopy of sputum revealed *M. pneumoniae* organisms.

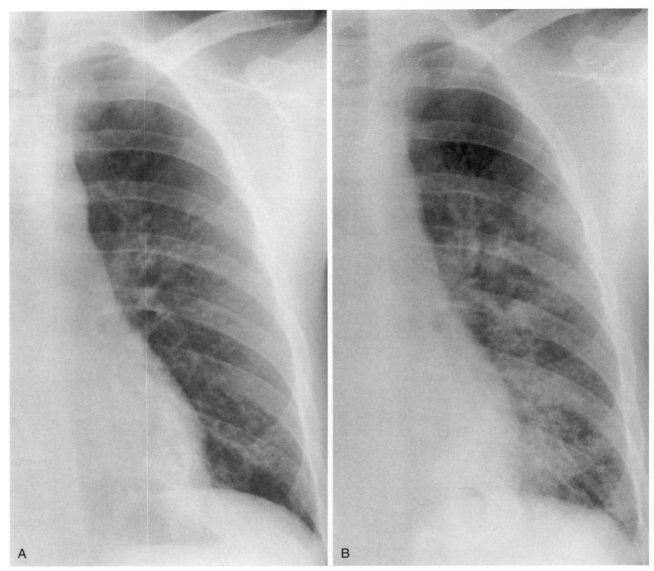

Figure 5–86. Acute Mycoplasmal Pneumonia Showing Sequential Interstitial and Air-Space Features. Detail view *(A)* of the left lung from posteroanterior chest radiograph shows a loss of definition and thickening of the bronchovascular bundles in the left lower lobe. A faint reticulation is suggested in some areas. Several days later *(B)*, after unsuccessful therapy with penicillin, considerable progression of the disease had occurred; patchy air-space opacities now obscure the previous interstitial abnormality. A subsequent chest radiograph showed complete resolution after tetracycline therapy. The patient was a young college student who complained of the acute onset of cough, fever, myalgia, and headache.

and 7 had other findings, including areas of atelectasis, small nodules, and biapical cavitation. Fourteen of the 38 patients had unilateral abnormalities, and 24 patients had bilateral disease. Eleven patients had pleural effusion, typically of small to medium size. In both groups, the radiographic abnormalities tended to progress to bilateral, mixed, interstitial, and air-space infiltrates during the course of infection.

PARASITES

Echinococcus granulosus (Hydatid Disease)

Echinococcus granulosus is the cause of most cases of human hydatid disease and occurs in two varieties, pastoral and sylvatic. These diseases differ in their definitive and

intermediate hosts, their geographic distributions, and to a limited extent their clinical and radiologic features. The *pastoral* variety is the more common of the two and, as the name implies, occurs in rural settings in which sheep, cows, or pigs are the intermediate hosts and dogs the usual definitive hosts. Humans typically acquire the disease by direct contact with infested dogs or by ingestion of contaminated water, food, or soil; humans become accidental intermediate hosts. The disease is particularly common in the sheep-raising regions of southeastern Europe, the Middle East, North Africa, parts of the former Soviet Union, South America (particularly Argentina, Chile, and Uruguay), Australia, and New Zealand. Cases that are seen outside these regions most often occur in immigrants from the endemic areas.

The *sylvatic* variety of echinococcosis has as its defini-

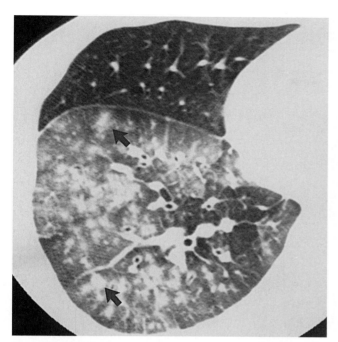

Figure 5–87. *Mycoplasma pneumoniae* **Pneumonia.** HRCT scan at the level of the right lower lobe reveals small nodules *(straight arrows)* in a predominantly centrilobular distribution and areas of ground-glass attenuation. Sharp demarcation between normal and abnormal secondary pulmonary lobules is consistent with lobular pneumonia. (From Reittner P, Müller NL, Heyneman L, et al: Am J Roentgenol 174:37, 2000.)

tive hosts several species of the Canidae family, including the dog, wolf, arctic fox, and coyote. A variety of herbivores, including moose, deer, reindeer, elk, caribou, and bison, serve as intermediate hosts. The disease is seen primarily in Alaska and northern Canada, where it affects mostly native Indians and Inuits.[505]

The mature adult worms, of which there may be thousands, live in the small intestine of the definitive host.

Eggs are passed in the feces onto grazing land or water and are ingested by the intermediate hosts. In these, larvae develop in the duodenum, penetrate its wall, and pass via the portal system to the liver, where most are trapped in hepatic sinusoids; most larvae that escape are trapped in the alveolar capillaries. Most entrapped larvae are killed by the host; the few that survive develop into solitary or multiple cysts that produce brood capsules containing immature worms (protoscolices). The life cycle of the parasite is completed when the definitive host feeds on the remains of an intermediate host that harbors cysts, with subsequent intraintestinal development of adult worms. The effect of the hepatic and pulmonary capillary sieves in containing the larvae is largely responsible for the distribution of disease—approximately 65% to 70% of *E. granulosus* cysts occur in the liver and 15% to 30% in the lungs.

Most intact pulmonary hydatid cysts cause no symptoms; occasionally, an unruptured cyst is associated with nonproductive cough and minimal hemoptysis.[507] When a cyst ruptures, either spontaneously or as a result of secondary infection, there is an abrupt onset of cough, expectoration, and fever; an acute hypersensitivity reaction may develop, with urticaria, pruritus and, in some cases, hypotension.[512]

Radiologically, pulmonary echinococcal cysts characteristically present as solitary, sharply circumscribed, spherical, or oval masses surrounded by normal lung (Fig. 5–88).[508–510] They are multiple in 20% to 30% of patients.[509, 510] Their size ranges from 1 to greater than 20 cm in diameter;[511] the larger cysts usually are seen in the pastoral type of disease, those in the sylvatic variety rarely exceeding 10 cm.[504, 508] Most cysts are located in the lower lobes, more often posteriorly than anteriorly and somewhat more commonly on the right.[506, 512] Although often spherical or oval, cysts sometimes have a bizarre, irregular shape, attributed by some to the fact that they impinge on relatively rigid structures such as bronchovascular bundles as they grow, becoming indented and lobulated.[507, 510] A cyst that is near

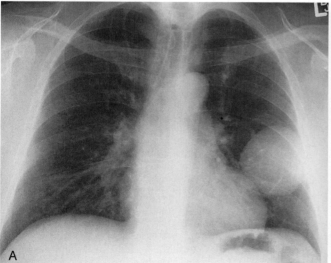
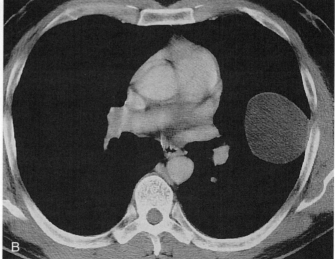

Figure 5–88. Hydatid Cyst: Radiographic and CT Findings. Posteroanterior chest radiograph *(A)* shows a smoothly marginated 6-cm diameter mass in the left lung. CT scan *(B)* shows a cystic lesion containing fluid with attenuation values similar to water (0 HU). The patient was a 51-year-old asymptomatic man who hunted for several years in Northern Canada.

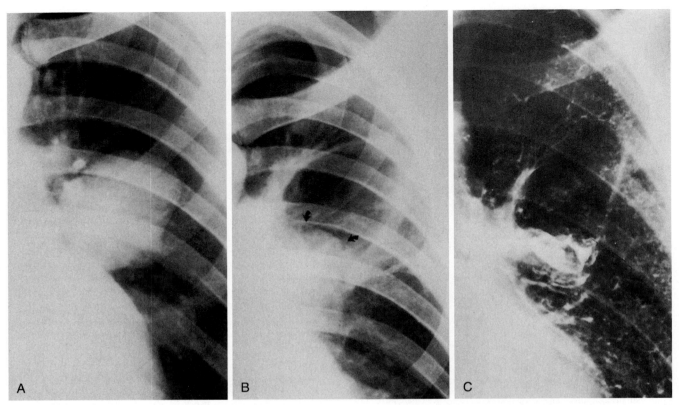

Figure 5–89. Hydatid Cyst with Rupture. Sharply circumscribed homogeneous mass *(A)* visible in the left midlung has a smooth but lobulated contour. Four years later *(B)*, the cyst has expelled all its liquid contents into the tracheobronchial tree and now contains air; an irregular mass present at the bottom of the cyst *(arrows)* represents collapsed membranes. Bronchogram *(C)* shows contrast material within the cyst, outlining the membranes. (Courtesy of Alfred Hospital, Melbourne, Australia.)

the diaphragm, chest wall, or mediastinum also tends to flatten against it, although compression of mediastinal structures may occur.

When communication develops between the cyst and the bronchial tree, air may enter the space between the pericyst and exocyst, producing a thin crescent of air around the periphery of the cyst—the *meniscus* or *crescent sign.*[506, 509] Despite the emphasis that has been placed on this sign in published reports, it was observed in only 5% of 49 patients with the pastoral type of infestation in one study.[506] After the cyst has ruptured into the bronchial tree, its membrane may float on the fluid within the cyst, giving rise to the classic *water-lily sign* or *sign of the camalote* (Fig. 5–89).[509, 513] This sign may be seen in pleural fluid when rupture of the cyst into the pleural space has resulted in hydropneumothorax or pyopneumothorax;[514] in such circumstances, the pneumothorax may be under *tension.*[515] The water-lily sign is rare in the sylvatic form of the disease; in the series cited previously, it was observed in only 1 of 101 patients.[508]

CT scan allows distinction of hydatid cysts from soft tissue nodules by showing a thin-walled, fluid-filled cyst. The fluid has attenuation values close to 0 HU *(see* Fig. 5–88).[516, 517] CT scan can be helpful in identifying pathognomonic features in ruptured or complicated hydatid cysts, such as detached or collapsed endocyst membranes, collapsed daughter cyst membranes, and intact daughter cysts.[516, 518] Cyst rupture may occur without such characteristic signs being evident, however. MR imaging allows

reliable differentiation of the fluid-filled hydatid cysts from solid tumors.[519, 520] The cysts have low signal intensity on T1-weighted MR images and homogeneous high signal intensity on T2-weighted MR images.

References

1. Fraser R, Müller NL, Colman N, et al: Diagnosis of Diseases of the Chest. 4th ed. Philadelphia, WB Saunders, 1999.
2. Macfarlane JT, Miller AC, Roderick-Smith WH, et al: Comparative radiographic features of community acquired Legionnaires disease, pneumococcal pneumonia, mycoplasma pneumonia, and psittacosis. Thorax 39:28, 1984.
3. Wollschlager CM, Khan FA, Khan A: Utility of radiography and clinical features in the diagnosis of community-acquired pneumonia. Clin Chest Med 8:393, 1987.
3a. Shah RM, Gupta S, Angeid-Backman E, O'Donnell J: Pneumococcal pneumonia in patients requiring hospitalization: Effects of bacteremia and HIV seropositivity on radiographic appearance. Am J Roentgenol 175:1533, 2000.
4. Albaum MN, Hill LC, Murphy M, et al: Interobserver reliability of the chest radiograph in community-acquired pneumonia. Chest 110:343, 1996.
5. Goodman LR, Goren RA, Teptick SK: The radiographic evaluation of pulmonary infection. Med Clin North Am 64:553, 1980.
6. Zornoza J, Goldman AM, Wallace S, et al: Radiologic features of gram-negative pneumonias in the neutropenic patient. Am J Roentgenol 127:989, 1976.
7. Logan PM, Primack SL, Miller RR, Müller NL: Invasive aspergillosis of the airways: Radiographic, CT, and pathologic findings. Radiology 193:383, 1994.
8. McGuinness G, Gruden JF, Bhalla M, et al: AIDS-related airway disease. Am J Roentgenol 168:67, 1997.
9. Louria DB, Blumenfeld HL, Ellis JT, et al: Studies on influenza in

the pandemic of 1957–1958: II. Pulmonary complications of influenza. J Clin Invest 38:213, 1959.

10. Wenzel RP, McCormick DP, Beam WE Jr: Parainfluenza pneumonia in adults. JAMA 221:294, 1972.

11. Itoh H, Tokunaga S, Asamoto H, et al: Radiologic-pathologic correlations of small lung nodules with special reference to peribronchiolar nodules. Am J Roentgenol 130:223, 1978.

12. Müller NL, Miller RR: State-of-the-art: Diseases of the bronchioles: CT and histopathologic findings. Radiology 196:3, 1995.

13. Im J-G, Itoh H, Shim Y-S, et al: Pulmonary tuberculosis: CT findings—early active disease and sequential change with antituberculous therapy. Radiology 186:653, 1993.

14. Genereux GP, Stillwell GA: The acute bacterial pneumonias. Semin Roentgenol 15:9, 1980.

15. Collins J, Blankenbaker D, Stern EJ: CT patterns of bronchiolar disease: What is "tree-in-bud"? Am J Roentgenol 171:365, 1998.

16. Fraser RG, Wortzman G: Acute pneumococcal lobar pneumonia: The significance of nonsegmental distribution. J Can Assoc Radiol 10:37, 1959.

17. Barnes DJ, Naraqi S, Igo JD: The diagnostic and prognostic significance of bulging fissures in acute lobar pneumonia. Aust N Z J Med 18:130, 1988.

18. Kaye MG, Fox MJ, Bartlett JG, et al: The clinical spectrum of *Staphylococcus aureus* pulmonary infection. Chest 97:788, 1990.

19. Macfarlane J, Rose D: Radiographic features of staphylococcal pneumonia in adults and children. Thorax 51:539, 1996.

20. Itoh H, Murata K, Konishi J, et al: Diffuse lung disease: Pathologic basis for the high-resolution computed tomography findings. J Thorac Imaging 8:176, 1993.

21. Groskin SA, Panicek DM, Ewing DK, et al: Bacterial lung abscess: A review of the radiographic and clinical features of 50 cases. J Thorac Imaging 6:62, 1991.

22. Hammond JM, Potgieter PD, Hanslo D: The etiology and antimicrobial susceptibility patterns of microorganisms in acute community-acquired lung abscess. Chest 108:937, 1995.

23. Mori T, Ebe T, Takahashi M: Lung abscess: Analysis of 66 cases from 1979 to 1991. Intern Med 32:273, 1993.

24. Penner C, Maycher B, Long R: Pulmonary gangrene: A complication of bacterial pneumonia. Chest 105:567, 1994.

25. Padmanabhan K, Rajgopalan K, Yeo K, et al: Intracavitary mass in a patient with *Klebsiella* pneumonia. Chest 93:187, 1988.

26. Quigley MJ, Fraser RS: Pulmonary pneumatocele: Pathology and pathogenesis. Am J Roentgenol 150:1275, 1988.

27. Feuerstein IM, Archer A, Pluda JM, et al: Thin-walled cavities, cysts, and pneumothorax in *P. carinii* pneumonia: Further observations with histopathologic correlation. Radiology 174:697, 1990.

28. Rosmus HH, Pare JAP, Masson AM, et al: Roentgenographic patterns of acute *Mycoplasma* and viral pneumonitis. J Can Assoc Radiol 19:74, 1968.

29. Borthwick RC, Cameron DC, Philp T: Radiographic patterns of pulmonary involvement in acute mycoplasmal infections. Scand J Respir Dis 59:190, 1978.

30. Cameron DC, Borthwick RN, Philp T: The radiographic patterns of acute mycoplasma pneumonitis. Clin Radiol 28:173, 1977.

31. Putman CE, Curtis AM, Simeone JF, et al: Mycoplasma pneumonia: Clinical and roentgenographic patterns. Am J Roentgenol 124:417, 1975.

32. DeLorenzo LJ, Huang CT, Maguire GP, et al: Roentgenographic patterns of *P. carinii* pneumonia in 104 patients with AIDS. Chest 91:323, 1987.

33. Naidich DP, McGuinness G: Pulmonary manifestations of AIDS: CT and radiographic correlations. Radiol Clin North Am 29:999, 1991.

34. Kuhlman JE: Pneumocystic infections: The radiologist's perspective. Radiology 198:623, 1996.

35. Bergin CJ, Wirth RL, Berry GJ, et al: *Pneumocystis carinii* pneumonia: CT and HRCT observations. J Comput Assist Tomogr 14:756, 1990.

36. Hartman TE, Primack SL, Müller NL, et al: Diagnosis of thoracic complications in AIDS: Accuracy of CT. Am J Roentgenol 162:547, 1994.

37. McGuinness G, Scholes JV, Garay SM, et al: Cytomegalovirus pneumonitis: Spectrum of parenchymal CT findings with pathologic correlation in 21 AIDS patients. Radiology 192:451, 1994.

38. Kang E-Y, Patz EF Jr, Müller NL: Cytomegalovirus pneumonia in transplant patients: CT findings. J Comput Assist Tomogr 20:295, 1996.

39. Gelb AF, Leffler C, Brewin A, et al: Miliary tuberculosis. Am Rev Respir Dis 108:1327, 1973.

40. Kwong JS, Carignan S, Kang EY, et al: Miliary tuberculosis: Diagnostic accuracy of chest radiography. Chest 110:339, 1996.

41. Huang RM, Naidich D, Lubat E, et al: Septic pulmonary emboli: CT radiographic correlation. Am J Roentgenol 153:41, 1989.

42. Kuhlman JE, Fishman EK, Teigen C: Pulmonary septic emboli: Diagnosis with CT. Radiology 174:211, 1990.

43. Biocina B, Sutlic Z, Husedzinovic I, et al: Penetrating cardiothoracic war wounds. Eur J Cardiothorac Surg 11:399, 1997.

44. Pointe HD, Osika E, Montagne JP, et al: Adrenobronchial fistula complicating a neonatal adrenal abscess: Treatment by percutaneous aspiration and antibiotics. Pediatr Radiol 27:184, 1997.

45. O'Brien JD, Ettinger NA: Nephrobronchial fistula and lung abscess resulting from nephrolithiasis and pyelonephritis. Chest 108:1166, 1995.

46. Brooks GF, Butel JS, Ornston LN, et al (eds): Javetz, Melnick, and Adelberg's Medical Microbiology. Norwalk, CT, Appleton & Lange, 1995.

47. Macfarlane J: An overview of community-acquired pneumonia with lessons learned from the British Thoracic Society Study. Semin Respir Infect 9:153, 1994.

48. Porath A, Schlaeffer F, Pick N, et al: Pneumococcal community-acquired pneumonia in 148 hospitalized adult patients. Eur J Clin Microbiol Infect Dis 16:863, 1997.

49. Sankilampi U, Herva E, Haikala R, et al: Epidemiology of invasive *Streptococcus pneumoniae* infections in adults in Finland. Epidemiol Infect 118:7, 1997.

50. Koivula I, Sten M, Mäkelä PH: Risk factors for pneumonia in the elderly. Am J Med 96:313, 1994.

51. Haglung LA, Istre GR, Pickett DA, et al: Invasive pneumococcal disease in central Oklahoma: Emergence of high-level penicillin resistance and multiple antibiotic resistance—Pneumococcus Study Group. J Infect Dis 168:1532, 1993.

52. Leeper KV Jr: Severe community-acquired pneumonia. Semin Respir Infect 11:96, 1996.

53. Bisno AL, Freeman JC: The syndrome of asplenia, pneumococcal sepsis, and disseminated intravascular coagulation. Ann Intern Med 72:389, 1970.

54. Leatherman JW, Iber C, Davies SF: Cavitation in bacteremic pneumococcal pneumonia: Causal role of mixed infection with anaerobic bacteria. Am Rev Respir Dis 129:317, 1984.

55. Hershey CO, Panaro V: Round pneumonia in adults. Arch Intern Med 148:1155, 1988.

56. Lévy M, Dromer F, Brion N, et al: Community-acquired pneumonia: Importance of initial noninvasive bacteriologic and radiographic investigations. Chest 92:43, 1988.

57. Moine P, Vercken JB, Chevret S, et al: Severe community-acquired pneumonia: Etiology, epidemiology, and prognosis factors. Chest 105:1487, 1994.

58. Lippmann ML, Goldberg SK, Walkenstein MD, et al: Bacteremic pneumococcal pneumonia: A community hospital experience. Chest 108:1608, 1995.

59. Brewin A, Arango L, Hadley WK, et al: High-dose penicillin therapy and pneumococcal pneumonia. JAMA 230:409, 1974.

60. Musgrave T, Verghese A: Clinical features of pneumonia in the elderly. Semin Respir Infect 5:269, 1990.

61. Barnes DJ, Naraqi S, Igo JD: The diagnostic and prognostic significance of bulging fissures in acute lobar pneumonia. Aust N Z J Med 18:130, 1988.

62. al-Ujayli B, Nafziger DA, Saravolatz L: Pneumonia due to *Staphylococcus aureus* infection. Clin Chest Med 16:111, 1995.

63. Spencer RC: Predominant pathogens found in the European Prevalence of Infection in Intensive Care Study. Eur J Clin Microbiol Infect Dis 15:281, 1996.

64. Chartrand SA, McCracken GH: Staphylococcal pneumonia in infants and children. Pediatr Infect Dis 1:19, 1982.

65. Dines DE: Diagnostic significance of pneumatocele of the lung. JAMA 204:1169, 1968.

66. Flaherty RA, Keegan JM, Sturdevant HN: Post-pneumonic pulmonary pneumatoceles. Radiology 74:50, 1960.

67. Naraqi S, McDonnell G: Hematogenous staphylococcal pneumonia secondary to soft tissue infection. Chest 79:173, 1981.

68. George DL: Epidemiology of nosocomial pneumonia in intensive care unit patients. Clin Chest Med 16:29, 1995.

69. Rello J, Quintana E, Ausina V, et al: Incidence, etiology, and outcome of nosocomial pneumonia in mechanically ventilated patients. Chest 100:439, 1991.

70. Hospital-acquired pneumonia in adults: Diagnosis, assessment of severity, initial antimicrobial therapy, and preventative strategies. Am J Respir Crit Care Med 153:1711, 1995. [This official statement of the American Thoracic Society was adopted by the ATS Board of Directors, November 1995.]

71. Maloney SA, Jarvis WR: Epidemic nosocomial pneumonia in the intensive care unit. Clin Chest Med 16:209, 1995.

72. Jong GM, Hsiue TR, Chen CR, et al: Rapidly fatal outcome of bacteremic *Klebsiella pneumoniae* pneumonia in alcoholics. Chest 107:214, 1995.

73. Crossley KB, Thurn JR: Nursing home-acquired pneumonia. Semin Respir Infect 4:64, 1989.

74. Pierce AK, Stanford JP: Aerobic gram-negative bacillary pneumonias. Am Rev Respir Dis 110:647, 1974.

75. Schmidt AJ, Stark P: Radiographic findings in *Klebsiella* (Friedlander's) pneumonia: The bulging fissure sign. Semin Respir Infect 13:80, 1998.

76. Holmes RB: Friedlander's pneumonia. Am J Roentgenol 75:728, 1956.

77. Felson B, Rosenberg LS, Hamburger M Jr: Roentgen findings in acute Friedlander's pneumonia. Radiology 53:599, 1949.

78. Moon WK, Im JG, Yeon KM, et al. Complications of *Klebsiella* pneumonia: CT evaluation. J Comput Assist Tomogr 19:176, 1995.

79. Korvick AJ, Hackett AK, Yu VL, et al: *Klebsiella* pneumonia in the modern era: Clinicoradiographic correlations. South Med J 84:200, 1991.

80. Carson MJ, Chadwick DL, Brubaker CA, et al: Thirteen boys with progressive septic granulomatosis. Pediatrics 35:405, 1965.

81. Mundy LM, Auwaerter PG, Oldach D, et al: Community-acquired pneumonia: Impact of immune status. Am J Respir Crit Care Med 152:1309, 1995.

82. Jaffey PB, English PW II, Campbell GA, et al: *Escherichia coli* lobar pneumonia: Fatal infection in a patient with mental retardation. South Med J 89:628, 1996.

83. Tillotson JR, Lerner AM: Pneumonias caused by gram-negative bacilli. Medicine 45:65, 1996.

84. Unger JC, Rose HD, Unger GF: Gram-negative pneumonia. Radiology 107:283, 1973.

85. Dunn M, Wunderink RG: Ventilator-associated pneumonia caused by *Pseudomonas* infection. Clin Chest Med 16:95, 1995.

86. Rello J, Ausina V, Ricart M, et al: Risk factors for infection by *Pseudomonas* in patients with ventilator-associated pneumonia. Intensive Care Med 20:193, 1994.

87. Pennington JE, Reynolds HY, Carbone PP: *Pseudomonas* pneumonia: A retrospective study of 36 cases. Am J Med 55:155, 1973.

88. Winer-Muram HT, Jennings SG, Wunderink RG, et al: Ventilator-associated *Pseudomonas aeruginosa* pneumonia: Radiographic findings. Radiology 195:247, 1995.

89. Joffe N: Roentgenologic aspects of primary *Pseudomonas aeruginosa* pneumonia in mechanically ventilated patients. Am J Roentgenol 107:305, 1969.

90. Iannini PB, Claffey T, Quintiliani R: Bacteremic *Pseudomonas* pneumonia. JAMA 230:558, 1974.

91. McHenry MC, Hawk WA: Bacteremia caused by gram-negative bacilli. Med Clin North Am 58:623, 1974.

92. Tirdel GB, Gibbons GH, Fishman RS: Pneumonia with an enlarged cardiac silhouette. Chest 109:1380, 1996.

93. Wallace RJ Jr, Musher DM, Martin RR: *Haemophilus influenzae* pneumonia in adults. Am J Med 64:87, 1978.

94. Trolfors B, Claesson B, Lagergard T, et al: Incidence, predisposing factors, and manifestations of invasive *Haemophilus influenzae* infections in adults. Eur J Clin Microbiol 3:180, 1984.

95. Johnson SR, Thompson RC, Humphreys H, et al: Clinical features of patients with beta-lactamase-producing *Haemophilus influenzae* isolated from sputum. J Antimicrob Chemother 38:881, 1996.

96. Gillis S, Dann EJ, Berkman N, et al: Fatal *Haemophilus influenzae* septicemia following bronchoscopy in a splenectomized patient. Chest 104:1607, 1993.

97. Falco V, Fernandez de Sevilla T, Alegre J, et al: Bacterial pneumonia in HIV-infected patients: A prospective study of 68 episodes. Eur Respir J 7:235, 1994.

98. Rello J, Rodriguez R, Jubert P, et al: Severe community-acquired pneumonia in the elderly: Epidemiology and prognosis. Study Group for Severe Community-Acquired Pneumonia. Clin Infect Dis 23:723, 1996.

99. Gomez J, Banos V, Ruiz Gomez J, et al: Prospective study of epidemiology and prognostic factors in community-acquired pneumonia. Eur J Clin Microbiol Infect Dis 15:556, 1996.

100. Pearlberg J, Haggar AM, Saravolatz L, et al: *Hemophilus influenzae* pneumonia in the adult: Radiographic appearance with clinical correlation. Radiology 151:23, 1984.

101. Roig J, Domingo C, Morera J: Legionnaires' disease. Chest 105:1817, 1994.

102. Davis GS, Winn WC Jr, Beaty HN: Legionnaires' disease: Infections caused by *Legionella pneumophila* and *Legionella*-like organisms. Clin Chest Med 2:145, 1981.

103. Lieberman D, Porath A, Schlaeffer F, et al: *Legionella* species community-acquired pneumonia—a review of 56 hospitalized adult patients. Chest 109:1243, 1996.

104. Helms CM, Viner JP, Wiesenburger DD, et al: Sporadic legionnaires' disease: Clinical observations on 87 nosocomial and community-acquired cases. Am J Med Sci 288:2, 1984.

105. Kirby BD, Snyder KM, Meyer RD, et al: Legionnaires' disease: Report of sixty-five nosocomially acquired cases and review of the literature. Medicine 59:188, 1980.

106. Moore EH, Webb WR, Gamsu G, et al: Legionnaires' disease in the renal transplant patient: Clinical presentation and radiographic progression. Radiology 153:589, 1984.

107. Prodinger WM, Bonatti H, Allerberger F, et al: *Legionella* pneumonia in transplant recipients: A cluster of cases of eight years' duration. J Hosp Infect 26:191, 1994.

108. Rudin JE, Wing EJ: A comparative study of *Legionella micdadei* and other nosocomial-acquired pneumonia. Chest 86:675, 1984.

109. Dietrich PA, Johnson RD, Fairbank JT, et al: The chest radiograph in legionnaires' disease. Radiology 127:577, 1978.

110. Storch GA, Sagel SS, Baine WB: The chest roentgenogram in sporadic cases of legionnaires' disease. JAMA 245:587, 1981.

111. Kroboth FJ, Yu VL, Reddy SC, et al: Clinicoradiographic correlation with the extent of legionnaires' disease. Am J Roentgenol 141:263, 1983.

112. Pedro-Botet ML, Sabria-Leal M, Haro M, et al: Nosocomial- and community-acquired Legionella pneumonia: Clinical comparative analysis. Eur Respir J 8:1929, 1995.

113. Meyer RD: Legionnaires' disease update: Be prepared for this summer. J Respir Dis 1:12, 1980.

114. Fairbank JT, Mamourian AC, Dietrich PA, et al: The chest radiograph in legionnaires' disease: Further observations. Radiology 147:33, 1983.

115. Fairbank JT, Mamourian AC, Dietrich PA, et al: The chest radiograph in legionnaires' disease. Radiology 147:30, 1983.

116. Meenhorst PL, Mulder JD: The chest x-ray in *Legionella* pneumonia (legionnaires' disease). Eur J Radiol 3:180, 1983.

117. Mirich D, Gray R, Hyland R: Legionella lung cavitation. J Can Assoc Radiol 41:100, 1990.

118. Bali A, Pierry AA, Bernstein A: Spontaneous pneumothorax complicating Legionnaires' disease. Postgrad Med J 57:656, 1981.

119. Carter JB, Wolter RK, Angres G, et al: Nodular legionnaires' disease. Am J Roentgenol 137:612, 1981.

120. Pope TL Jr, Armstrong P, Thompson R, et al: Pittsburgh pneumonia agent: Chest film manifestations. Am J Roentgenol 138:237, 1982.

121. Muder RR, Reddy SC, Yu VL, et al: Pneumonia caused by Pittsburgh pneumonia agent: Radiologic manifestations. Radiology 150:633, 1984.

122. Mehta P, Patel JD, Milder JE: *Legionella micdadei* (Pittsburgh pneumonia agent): Two infections with unusual clinical features. JAMA 249:1620, 1983.

123. Bartlett JG, Gorbach SL, Finegold SM: The bacteriology of aspiration pneumonia. Am J Med 56:202, 1974.

124. Doré P, Robert R, Grollier G, et al: Incidence of anaerobes in ventilator-associated pneumonia with use of a protected specimen brush. Am J Respir Crit Care Med 153:1292, 1996.

125. Marina M, Strong CA, Civen R, et al: Bacteriology of anaerobic pleuropulmonary infections. Clin Infect Dis 16:256, 1993.

126. Bartlett JG: Anaerobic bacterial infections of the lung and pleural space. Clin Infect Dis 16:248, 1993.

127. Brook I, Frazier EH: Aerobic and anaerobic microbiology of empyema: A retrospective review in two military hospitals. Chest 103:1502, 1993.

128. Pollock HM, Hawkins EL, Bonner JR, et al: Diagnosis of bacterial pulmonary infections with quantitative protected-catheter cultures obtained during bronchoscopy. J Clin Microbiol 17:225, 1983.

129. Kato T, Ueemura H, Murakami N, et al: Incidence of anaerobic infections among patients with pulmonary diseases: Japanese experience with transtracheal aspiration and immediate bedside anaerobic inoculation. Clin Infect Dis 23:87, 1996.

130. Bartlett JG, O'Keefe P, Tally FP, et al: Bacteriology of hospital-acquired pneumonia. Arch Intern Med 146:868, 1986.

131. Bartlett JG, Finegold SM: State of the art: Anaerobic infections of the lung and pleural space. Am Rev Respir Dis 110:56, 1974.

132. Abernathy RS: Antibiotic therapy of lung abscess: Effectiveness of penicillin. Dis Chest 53:592, 1968.

133. Gopalakrishna KV, Lerner PI: Primary lung abscess: Analysis of sixty-six cases. Cleve Clin Q 42:3, 1975.

134. Shafron RD, Tate CF Jr: Lung abscess: A five-year evaluation. Dis Chest 53:12, 1968.

135. Gorbach SL, Bartlett JG: Anaerobic infections. N Engl J Med 290:1177, 1974.

136. Landay MJ, Christensen EE, Bynum LJ, et al: Anaerobic pleural and pulmonary infections. Am J Roentgenol 134:233, 1980.

137. Bartlett JG: Anaerobic bacterial pneumonitis. Am Rev Respir Dis 119:19, 1979.

138. Rohlfing BM, White EA, Webb WR, et al: Hilar and mediastinal adenopathy caused by bacterial abscess of the lung. Radiology 128:289, 1978.

139. Rieder HL: Epidemiology of tuberculosis in Europe. Eur Respir J 8(Suppl 20):620s, 1995.

140. Riley RL: Disease transmission and contagion control. Am Rev Respir Dis 125(Suppl):16, 1982.

141. Centers for Disease Control and Prevention: Tuberculosis morbidity: United States, 1996. MMWR Morb Mortal Wkly Rep 46:695, 1997.

142. Leung AN: Pulmonary tuberculosis: The essentials. Radiology 210:307, 1999.

143. Glassroth J, Robbins AG, Snider DE Jr: Tuberculosis in the 1980s. N Engl J Med 302:1441, 1980.

144. Davies BH: Infectivity of tuberculosis. Thorax 35:481, 1980.

145. Stead WW: Pathogenesis of the sporadic case of tuberculosis. N Engl J Med 277:1008, 1967.

146. Stead WW: Pathogenesis of a first episode of chronic pulmonary tuberculosis in man: Recrudescence of residua of the primary infection or exogenous reinfection? Am Rev Respir Dis 95:729, 1967.

147. Small PM, Shafer RW, Hopewell PC, et al: Exogenous reinfection with multi-drug-resistant *Mycobacterium tuberculosis* in patients with advanced HIV infection. N Engl J Med 238:1137, 1993.

148. Nardell E, McInnis B, Thomas B, et al: Exogenous reinfection with tuberculosis in a shelter for the homeless. N Engl J Med 315:1570, 1986.

149. Colice GL: Pulmonary tuberculosis: Is resurgence due to reactivation or new infection? Postgrad Med J 97:35, 1995.

150. Toossi Z, Gogae P, Shiratsuchi H, et al: Enhanced production of TGF-beta by blood monocytes from patients with active tuberculosis and presence of TGF-beta in tuberculous granulomatous lung lesions. J Immunol 154:465, 1995.

151. Weber AL, Bird KT, Janower ML: Primary tuberculosis in childhood with particular emphasis on changes affecting the tracheobronchial tree. Am J Roentgenol 103:123, 1968.

152. Stead WW, Kerby GR, Schlueter DP, et al: The clinical spectrum of primary tuberculosis in adults: Confusion with reinfection in the pathogenesis of chronic tuberculosis. Ann Intern Med 68:731, 1968.

153. Leung AN, Müller NL, Pineda PR, et al: Primary tuberculosis in childhood: Radiographic manifestations. Radiology 182:87, 1992.

154. Choyke PL, Sostman HD, Curtis AM, et al: Adult-onset tuberculosis: Radiology 48:357, 1983.

155. Lee KS, Im JG: CT in adults with tuberculosis of the chest: Characteristic findings and role in management. Am J Roentgenol 164:1361, 1995.

156. Woodring JH, Vandiviere HM, Fried AM, et al: Update: The radiographic features of pulmonary tuberculosis. Am J Roentgenol 146:497, 1986.

157. Im JG, Song KS, Kang HS, et al: Mediastinal tuberculous lymphadenitis: CT manifestations. Radiology 164:115, 1987.

158. Pombo F, Rodriguez E, Mato J, et al: Patterns of contrast enhancement of tuberculous lymph nodes demonstrated by computed tomography. Clin Radiol 46:13, 1992.

159. Pastores SM, Naidich DP, Aranda CP, et al: Intrathoracic adenopathy associated with pulmonary tuberculosis in patients with human immunodeficiency virus infection. Chest 103:1433, 1993.

160. Landy MJ, Rollins NK: Mediastinal histoplasmosis granuloma: Evaluation with CT. Radiology 172:657, 1989.

161. Frostad S: Lymph node perforation through the bronchial tree in children with primary tuberculosis. Acta Tuberc Scand 47(Suppl):104, 1959.

162. Matthews JI, Matarese SL, Carpenter JL: Endobronchial tuberculosis simulating lung cancer. Chest 86:642, 1984.

163. Serviansky B, Schwarz J: Calcified intrathoracic lesions caused by histoplasmosis and tuberculosis. Am J Roentgenol 77:1034, 1957.

164. Alland D, Kalkut GE, Moss AR, et al: Transmission of tuberculosis in New York City: An analysis by DNA fingerprinting and conventional epidemiologic methods. N Engl J Med 330:1710, 1994.

165. Small PM, Hopewell PC, Singh SP, et al: The epidemiology of tuberculosis in San Francisco: A population-based study using conventional and molecular methods. N Engl J Med 330:1703, 1994.

166. Krysl J, Korzeniewska-Kosela M, Müller NL, et al: Radiologic features of pulmonary tuberculosis: An assessment of 188 cases. Can Assoc Radiol J 45:101, 1994.

167. Lee KS, Hwang JW, Chung MP, et al: Utility of CT in the evaluation of pulmonary tuberculosis in patients without AIDS. Chest 110:977, 1996.

168. Adler H: Phthisiogenetic studies by means of tomography in cases of localized pulmonary tuberculosis in adults. Acta Tuberc Scand 47(Suppl):13, 1959.

169. Im JG, Itoh H, Han MC: CT of pulmonary tuberculosis. Semin Ultrasound CT MRI 16:420, 1995.

170. Primack SL, Logan PM, Hartman TE, et al: Pulmonary tuberculosis and *Mycobacterium avium-intracellulare*: A comparison of CT findings. Radiology 194:413, 1995.

171. Lee KS, Song KS, Lim TH, et al: Adult-onset pulmonary tuberculosis: Findings on chest radiographs and CT scans. Am J Roentgenol 160:753, 1993.

172. Penner C, Roberts D, Kunimoto D, et al: Tuberculosis as a primary cause of respiratory failure requiring mechanical ventilation. Am J Respir Crit Care Med 151:867, 1995.

173. Hatipoglu ON, Osma E, Manisali M, et al: High resolution computed tomographic findings in pulmonary tuberculosis. Thorax 51:397, 1996.

174. Poey C, Verhaegen F, Giron J, et al: High-resolution chest CT in tuberculosis: Evolutive patterns and signs of activity. J Comput Assist Tomogr 21:601, 1997.

175. Cohen JR, Amorosa JK, Smith PR: The air-fluid level in cavitary pulmonary tuberculosis. Radiology 127:315, 1978.

176. Sochocky S: Tuberculoma of the lung. Am Rev Tuberc 78:403, 1958.

177. Bleyer JM, Marks JH: Tuberculomas and hamartomas of the lung: Comparative study of 66 proved cases. Am J Roentgenol 77:1013, 1957.

178. Winer-Muram HT, Rubin SA: Thoracic complications of tuberculosis. J Thorac Imaging 5:46, 1990.

179. Zwirewich CV, Vedal S, Miller RR, et al: Solitary pulmonary nodule: High-resolution CT and radiologic-pathologic correlation. Radiology 179:469, 1991.

180. Swensen SJ, Brown LR, Colby TV, et al: Pulmonary nodules: CT evaluation of enhancement with iodinated contrast material. Radiology 194:393, 1995.

181. Siegelman SS, Khouri NF, Leo FP, et al: Solitary pulmonary nodules: CT assessment. Radiology 160:307, 1986.

182. Optican RJ, Ost A, Ravin CE: High-resolution computed tomography in the diagnosis of miliary tuberculosis. Chest 102:941, 1992.

183. Oh YW, Kim YH, Lee NJ, et al: High-resolution CT appearance of miliary tuberculosis. J Comput Assist Tomogr 18:862, 1994.

184. McGuinness G, Naidich DP, Jagirdar J, et al: High resolution CT findings in miliary lung disease. J Comput Assist Tomogr 16:384, 1992.

185. Eykyn S, Davidson C: Rigors in tuberculosis. Postgrad Med J 69:724, 1993.

186. Holmes P, Faulks L: Presentation of pulmonary tuberculosis. Aust N Z J Med 11:651, 1981.

187. Farer LS, Lowell LM, Meador MP: Extrapulmonary tuberculosis in the United States. Am J Epidemiol 109:205, 1979.

188. Small PM, Schecter GF, Goodman PC, et al: Treatment of tuberculo-

sis in patients with advanced human immunodeficiency virus infection. N Engl J Med 324:289, 1991.

189. Hong SH, Im J-G, Lee JS, et al: High-resolution CT findings of miliary tuberculosis. J Comput Assist Tomogr 22:220, 1998.

190. Weaver P, Lifeso RM: The radiological diagnosis of tuberculosis of the adult spine. Skeletal Radiol 12:178, 1984.

191. Maritz NGJ, De Villiers JFK, Van Castricum OQS: Computed tomography in tuberculosis of the spine. Comp Radiol 6:1, 1982.

192. Whelan MA, Naidich DP, Post JD, et al: Computed tomography of spinal tuberculosis. J Comput Assist Tomogr 7:25, 1983.

193. Coppola J, Müller NL, Connell DG: Computed tomography of musculoskeletal tuberculosis. J Can Assoc Radiol 38:199, 1987.

194. de Roos A, van Persijn van Meerten EL, Bloem JL, et al: MRI of tuberculous spondylitis. Am J Roentgenol 147:79, 1986.

195. Wolinsky E: Nontuberculous mycobacteria and associated disease. Am Rev Respir Dis 119:107, 1979.

196. Tortoli E, Piersimoni C, Kirschner P, et al: Characterization of mycobacterial isolates phylogenetically related to, but different from, *Mycobacterium simiae*. J Clin Microbiol 35:697, 1997.

197. Liu F, Andrews D, Wright DN: *Mycobacterium thermoresistiblie* infection in an immunocompromised host. J Clin Microbiol 1:546, 1984.

198. Christensen EE, Dietz GW, Ahn CH, et al: Pulmonary manifestations of *Mycobacterium intracellulare*. Am J Roentgenol 133:59, 1979.

199. Albelda SM, Kern JA, Marinelli DL, et al: Expanding spectrum of pulmonary disease caused by nontuberculous mycobacteria. Radiology 157:289, 1985.

200. Woodring JH, Mac Vandiviere H, Melvin IG: Roentgenographic features of pulmonary disease caused by atypical mycobacteria. South Med J 80:1488, 1987.

201. Evans AJ, Crisp AJ, Hubbard RB, et al: Pulmonary *Mycobacterium kansasii* infection: Comparison of radiological appearances with pulmonary tuberculosis. Thorax 51:1243, 1996.

202. Moore EH: Atypical mycobacterial infection in the lung: CT appearance. Radiology 187:777, 1993.

203. Lynch DA, Simone PM, Fox MA, et al: CT features of pulmonary *Mycobacterium avium* complex infection. J Comput Assist Tomogr 19:353, 1995.

204. Miller WT Jr: Spectrum of pulmonary nontuberculous mycobacterial infection. Radiology 191:343, 1994.

205. Prince DS, Peterson DD, Steiner RM, et al: Infection with *Mycobacterium avium* complex in patients without predisposing conditions. N Engl J Med 321:863, 1989.

206. Hartman TE, Swensen SJ, Williams DE: *Mycobacterium avium-intracellulare* complex: Evaluation with CT. Radiology 187:23, 1993.

207. Stansell JD: Pulmonary fungal infections in HIV-infected persons. Semin Respir Infect 8:116, 1993.

208. Goodwin RA, Loyd JE, Des Prez RM: Histoplasmosis in normal hosts. Medicine 60:231, 1981.

209. Goodwin RA Jr, Owens FT, Snell JD, et al: Chronic pulmonary histoplasmosis. Medicine 55:413, 1976.

210. Bradsher RW: Histoplasmosis and blastomycosis. Clin Infect Dis 22(Suppl 2):S102, 1996.

211. Taylor ML, Granados J, Toriello C: Biological and sociocultural approaches of histoplasmosis in the state of Guerrero, Mexico. Mycoses 39:375, 1996.

212. Stobierski MG, Hospedales CJ, Hall WN, et al: Outbreak of histoplasmosis among employees in a paper factory—Michigan, 1993. J Clin Microbiol 34:1220, 1996.

213. Gurney JW, Conces DJ Jr: Pulmonary histoplasmosis. Radiology 199:297, 1996.

214. Conces DJ, Tarver RD, Vix VA: Broncholithiasis: CT features in 15 patients. Am J Roentgenol 157:249, 1991.

215. Conces DJ Jr: Histoplasmosis. Semin Roentgenol 1:14, 1996.

216. Wheat LJ, Wass J, Norton J, et al: Cavitary histoplasmosis occurring during two large urban outbreaks: Analysis of clinical, epidemiologic, roentgenographic, and laboratory features. Medicine 63:201, 1984.

217. Furcolow ML, Grayston JT: Occurrence of histoplasmosis in epidemics: Etiologic studies. Am Rev Tuberc 68:307, 1953.

218. Connell JV Jr, Muhm JR: Radiographic manifestations of pulmonary histoplasmosis: A 10-year review. Radiology 121:281, 1976.

219. Prager RL, Burney DP, Waterhouse G, et al: Pulmonary, mediastinal, and cardiac presentations of histoplasmosis. Ann Thorac Surg 30:385, 1980.

220. Straus SE, Jacobson ES: The spectrum of histoplasmosis in a general hospital: A review of 55 cases diagnosed at Barnes Hospital between 1966 and 1977. Am J Med Sci 279:147, 1980.

221. Zerhouni EA, Stitik FP, Siegelman SS, et al: CT of the pulmonary nodule: A cooperative study. Radiology 160:319, 1986.

222. Savides TJ, Gress FG, Wheat LJ, et al: Dysphagia due to mediastinal granulomas: Diagnosis with endoscopic ultrasonography. Gastroenterology 109:366, 1995.

223. Mathisen DJ, Grillo HC: Clinical manifestation of mediastinal fibrosis and histoplasmosis. Ann Thorac Surg 54:1053, 1992.

224. Weinstein JB, Aronberg DJ, Sagel SS: CT of fibrosing mediastinitis: Findings and their utility. Am J Roentgenol 141:247, 1983.

225. Sherrick AD, Brown LR, Harms GF, et al: The radiographic findings of fibrosing mediastinitis. Chest 106:484, 1994.

226. Stevens DA: Coccidioidomycosis. N Engl J Med 332:1077, 1995.

227. Ajello L: Coccidioidomycosis and histoplasmosis: A review of their epidemiology and geographical distribution. Mycopathol Mycol Appl 45:221, 1971.

228. Greendyke WH, Resnick DL, Harvey WC: The varied roentgen manifestations of primary coccidioidomycosis. Am J Roentgenol 109:491, 1970.

229. Batra P, Batra RS: Thoracic coccidioidomycosis. Semin Roentgenol 1:28, 1996.

230. Klein EW, Griffin JP: Coccidioidomycosis (diagnosis outside the Sonoran Zone): The roentgen features of acute multiple pulmonary cavities. Am J Roentgenol 94:653, 1965.

231. Batra P: Pulmonary coccidioidomycosis. J Thorac Imaging 7:29, 1992.

232. Cantanzaro A: Pulmonary coccidioidomycosis. Med Clin North Am 64:461, 1980.

233. Bayer AS, Yoshikawa TT, Galpin JE: Unusual syndromes of coccidioidomycosis—diagnostic and therapeutic considerations. Medicine 55:131, 1976.

234. Schwarz J, Baum GL: Coccidioidomycosis. Semin Roentgenol 5:29, 1970.

235. Winn WA: A long-term study of 300 patients with cavitary-abscess lesions of the lung of coccidioidal origin: An analytical study with special reference to treatment. Dis Chest 54(Suppl I):268, 1968.

236. Spivey CG Jr, Jones FL, Bopp RK: Cavitary coccidioidomycosis: Experience in a tuberculosis hospital outside the endemic area. Dis Chest 56:13, 1969.

237. Primack SL, Hartman TE, Lee KS, et al: Pulmonary nodules and the CT halo sign. Radiology 190:513, 1994.

238. Kim K-I, Leung AN, Flint JDA, Müller NL: Chronic pulmonary coccidioidomycosis: Computed tomographic and pathologic findings in 18 patients. Can Assoc Radiol J 49:401, 1998.

239. Bayer AS, Yoshikawa TT, Guze LB: Chronic progressive coccidioidal pneumonitis: Report of six cases with clinical, roentgenographic, serologic, and therapeutic features. Arch Intern Med 139:536, 1979.

240. Sarosi GA, Davies SF: Blastomycosis. Am Rev Respir Dis 120:911, 1979.

241. Furcolow ML, Chick EW, Busey JP, et al: Prevalence and incidence studies of human and canine blastomycosis: I. Cases in the United States, 1885–1968. Am Rev Respir Dis 102:60, 1970.

242. Kane J, Righter J, Krajden S, et al: Blastomycosis: A new endemic focus in Canada. Can Med Assoc J 129:728, 1983.

243. St. Germain G, Murray G, Duperval R: Blastomycosis in Quebec (1981–90): Report of 23 cases and review of published cases from Quebec. Can J Infect Dis 4:89, 1993.

244. Klein BS, Vergeront JM, Weeks RJ, et al: Isolation of *Blastomyces dermatitidis* in soil associated with a large outbreak of blastomycosis in Wisconsin. N Engl J Med 314:529, 1986.

245. Stelling CB, Woodring JH, Rehm SR, et al: Miliary pulmonary blastomycosis. Radiology 150:7, 1984.

246. Sheflin JR, Campbell JA, Thompson GP: Pulmonary blastomycosis: Findings on chest radiographs in 63 patients. Am J Roentgenol 154:1177, 1990.

247. Brown LR, Swensen SJ, Van Scoy RE, et al: Roentgenologic features of pulmonary blastomycosis. Mayo Clin Proc 66:29, 1991.

248. Kuzo RS, Goodman LR: Blastomycosis. Semin Roentgenol 1:45, 1996.

249. Halvorsen RA, Duncan JD, Merten DF, et al: Pulmonary blastomycosis: Radiologic manifestations. Radiology 150:1, 1984.

250. Griffith JE, Campbell GD: Acute miliary blastomycosis presenting as fulminating respiratory failure. Chest 75:630, 1979.

251. Winer-Muram HT, Beals DH, Cole Jr FH: Blastomycosis of the lung: CT features. Radiology 182:829, 1992.

252. Kinasewitz GT, Penn RL, George RB: The spectrum and significance of pleural disease in blastomycosis. Chest 86:580, 1984.

253. Rozenbaum R, Goncalves AJ: Clinical epidemiological study of 171 cases of cryptococcosis. Clin Infect Dis 18:369, 1994.

254. McDonnell JM, Hutchins GM: Pulmonary cryptococcosis. Hum Pathol 16:121, 1985.

255. Kerkering TM, Duma RJ, Shadomy S: The evolution of pulmonary cryptococcosis: Clinical implications from a study of 41 patients with and without compromising host factors. Ann Intern Med 94:611, 1981.

256. Zuger A, Louie E, Holzman RS, et al: Cryptococcal disease in patients with the acquired immunodeficiency syndrome: Diagnostic features and outcome of treatment. Ann Intern Med 104:234, 1986.

257. Patz EF Jr, Goodman PC: Pulmonary cryptococcosis. J Thorac Imaging 7:51, 1992.

258. Woodring JH, Ciporkin G, Lee C, et al: Pulmonary cryptococcosis. Semin Roentgenol 1:67, 1996.

259. Miller WT Jr, Edelman JM, Miller WT: Cryptococcal pulmonary infection in patients with AIDS: Radiographic appearance. Radiology 175:725, 1990.

260. Young EJ, Hirsh DD, Fainstein V, et al: Pleural effusions due to *Cryptococcus neoformans*: A review of the literature and report of two cases with cryptococcal antigen determinations. Am Rev Respir 121:743, 1980.

261. Perla EN, Maayan S, Miller SN, et al: Disseminated cryptococcosis presenting as the adult respiratory distress syndrome. N Y State J Med 85:704, 1985.

262. Edman JC, Kovacs JA, Masur H, et al: Ribosomal RNA sequence shows *Pneumocystis carinii* to be a member of the fungi. Nature 33:519, 1988.

263. Bedrossian CWM: Ultrastructure of *Pneumocystis carinii*: A review of internal and surface characteristics. Semin Diagn Pathol 6:212, 1989.

264. Smulian AG, Walzer PD: The biology of *Pneumocystis carinii*. Crit Rev Microbiol 18:191, 1992.

265. Lundgren B, Lebech M, Lind K, et al: Antibody response to a major human *Pneumocystis carinii* surface antigen in patients without evidence of immunosuppression and in patients with suspected atypical pneumonia. Eur J Clin Microbiol Infect Dis 12:105, 1993.

266. Kovacs JA: Diagnosis, treatment and prevention of *Pneumocystis carinii* pneumonia in HIV-infection patients. AIDS Updates 2:1, 1989.

267. Ballardie FW, Winearis CG, Cohen J, et al: *Pneumocystis carinii* pneumonia in renal transplant recipients: Clinical and radiographic features, diagnosis and complications of treatment. QJM 57:729, 1985.

268. Lufft V, Kliem V, Behrend M, et al: Incidence of *Pneumocystis carinii* pneumonia after renal transplantation: Impact of immunosuppression. Transplantation 62:421, 1996.

269. Varthalitis I, Aoun M, Daneau D, et al: *Pneumocystis carinii* pneumonia in patients with cancer: An increasing incidence. Cancer 71:481, 1993.

270. van der Lelie J, Venema D, Kuijper EJ, et al: *Pneumocystis carinii* pneumonia in HIV-negative patients with haematologic disease. Infection 25:78, 1997.

271. Fossieck BE, Spagnolo SV: *Pneumocystis carinii* pneumonitis in patients with lung cancer. Chest 78:721, 1980.

272. Godeau B, Coutant-Perronne V, Le Thi Huong D, et al: *Pneumocystis carinii* pneumonia in the course of connective tissue disease: Report of 34 cases. J Rheumatol 21:246, 1994.

273. Natale RB, Yagoda A, Brown A, et al: Combined *Pneumocystis carinii* and *Nocardia asteroides* pneumonitis in a patient with an ACTH-producing carcinoid. Cancer 47:2933, 1981.

274. Fulkerson WJ, Newman JH: Endogenous Cushing's syndrome complicated by *Pneumocystis carinii* pneumonia. Am Rev Respir Dis 129:188, 1984.

275. Hartz JW, Geisinger KR, Scharyj M, et al: Granulomatous pneumocystosis presenting as a solitary pulmonary nodule. Arch Pathol Lab Med 109:466, 1985.

276. Peters SG, Prakash UB: *Pneumocystis carinii* pneumonia: Review of 53 cases. Am J Med 82:73, 1987.

277. Cohen BA, Pomeranz S, Rabinowitz JG, et al: Pulmonary complications of AIDS: Radiologic features. Am J Roentgenol 143:115, 1984.

278. Suffredini AF, Tobin MJ, Wajszczuk CP, et al: Acute respiratory failure due to *Pneumocystis carinii* pneumonia: Clinical, radiographic, and pathologic course. Crit Care Med 13:237, 1985.

279. Maxfield RA, Sorkin IB, Faxxini EP, et al: Respiratory failure in patients with acquired immunodeficiency syndrome and *Pneumocystis carinii* pneumonia. Crit Care Med 14:443, 1986.

280. Chaffey MH, Klein JS, Gamsu G, et al: Radiographic distribution of *Pneumocystis carinii* pneumonia in patients with AIDS treated with prophylactic inhaled pentamidine. Radiology 175:715, 1990.

281. Milligan SA, Stulbarg MS, Gamsu G, et al: *Pneumocystis carinii* pneumonia radiographically simulating tuberculosis. Am Rev Respir Dis 132:1124, 1985.

282. Forrest JV: Radiographic findings in *Pneumocystis carinii* pneumonia. Radiology 103:539, 1972.

283. Cross AS, Steigbigel RT: *Pneumocystis carinii* pneumonia presenting as localized nodular densities. N Engl J Med 291:831, 1974.

284. Barrio JL, Suarez M, Rodriguez JL, et al: *Pneumocystis carinii* pneumonia presenting as cavitating and noncavitating solitary pulmonary nodules in patients with the acquired immunodeficiency syndrome. Am Rev Respir Dis 134:1094, 1986.

285. Lubat E, Megibow AJ, Balthazar EJ, et al: Extrapulmonary *Pneumocystis carinii* infection in AIDS: CT findings. Radiology 174:157, 1990.

286. Eagar GM, Friedland JA, Sagel SS: Tumefactive *Pneumocystis carinii* infection in AIDS: Report of three cases. Am J Roentgenol 160:1197, 1993.

287. Mayor B, Schnyder P, Giron J, et al: Mediastinal and hilar lymphadenopathy due to *Pneumocystis carinii* infection in AIDS patients: CT features. J Comp Assist Tomogr 18:408, 1994.

288. Groskin SA, Massi AF, Randall PA: Calcified hilar and mediastinal lymph nodes in an AIDS patient with *Pneumocystis carinii* infection. Radiology 175:345, 1990.

289. Radin DR, Baker EL, Klatt EC, et al: Visceral and nodal calcification in patients with AIDS-related *Pneumocystis carinii* infection. Am J Roentgenol 154:27, 1990.

290. Kuhlman JE, Kavuru M, Fishman ED, et al: *Pneumocystis carinii* pneumonia: Spectrum of parenchymal CT findings. Radiology 175:711, 1990.

291. McGuinness G, Naidich DP, Garcy SM, et al: AIDS associated bronchiectasis: CT features. J Comput Assist Tomogr 17:260, 1993.

292. Kovacs JA, Hiemenz JW, Macher AM, et al: *Pneumocystis carinii* pneumonia: A comparison between patients with the acquired immunodeficiency syndrome and patients with other immunodeficiencies. Ann Intern Med 100:663, 1984.

293. Sterling RP, Bradley BB, Khalil KG, et al: Comparison of biopsy-proven *Pneumocystis carinii* pneumonia in acquired immune deficiency syndrome patients and renal allograft recipients. Ann Thorac Surg 38:494, 1984.

294. Logan PM, Primack SL, Staples C, et al: Acute lung disease in the immunocompromised host: Diagnostic accuracy of the chest radiograph. Chest 108:1283, 1995.

295. Buff SJ, McLelland R, Gallis HA, et al: *Candida albicans* pneumonia: Radiographic appearance. Am J Roentgenol 138:645, 1982.

296. Ramirez G, Shuster M, Kozub W, et al: Fatal acute *C. albicans* bronchopneumonia: Report of a case. JAMA 199:340, 1967.

297. Pagani JJ, Libshitz HI: Opportunistic fungal pneumonia in cancer patients. Am J Roentgenol 137:1033, 1981.

298. Samuels BI, Bodey GP, Libshitz HI: Imaging in candidiasis. Semin Roentgenol 31:76, 1996.

299. Janzen DL, Padley SPG, Adler BD, et al: Acute pulmonary complications in immunocompromised non-AIDS patients: Comparison of diagnostic accuracy of CT and chest radiography. Clin Radiol 47:159, 1993.

300. Primack SL, Müller NL: High-resolution computed tomography in acute diffuse lung disease in the immunocompromised patient. Radiol Clin North Am 32:731, 1994.

301. Brown MJ, Miller RR, Müller NL: Acute lung disease in the immunocompromised host: CT and pathologic examination findings. Radiology 190:247, 1994.

302. Bardana EJ Jr: The clinical spectrum of aspergillosis: Part 1. Epidemiology, pathogenicity, infection in animals and immunology of *Aspergillus*. CRC Crit Rev Clin Lab Sci 13:21, 1981.

303. Young RC, Jennings A, Bennett J: Species identification of invasive aspergillosis in man. Am J Clin Pathol 58:554, 1972.

304. Bardana EJ Jr: The clinical spectrum of aspergillosis: Part 2. Classi-

fication and description of saprophytic, allergic, and invasive variants of human disease. CRC Crit Rev Clin Lab Sci 13:85, 1981.

305. Chatzimichalis A, Massard G, Kessler R, et al: Bronchopulmonary aspergilloma: A reappraisal. Ann Thorac Surg 65:927, 1998.

306. Battaglini JW, Murray GF, Keagy BA, et al: Surgical management of symptomatic pulmonary aspergilloma. Ann Thorac Surg 39:512, 1985.

307. Wollschlager C, Khan F: Aspergillomas complicating sarcoidosis: A prospective study in 100 patients. Chest 86:585, 1984.

308. Campbell MJ, Clayton YM: Bronchopulmonary aspergillosis: A correlation of the clinical and laboratory findings in 272 patients investigated for bronchopulmonary aspergillosis. Am Rev Respir Dis 89:186, 1964.

309. Maguire CP, Hayes JP, Hayes M, et al: Three cases of pulmonary aspergilloma in adult patients with cystic fibrosis. Thorax 50:805, 1995.

310. Sarosi GA, Silberfarb PM, Saliba NA, et al: Aspergillomas occurring in blastomycotic cavities. Am Rev Respir Dis 104:581, 1971.

311. Rosenheim SH, Schwarz J: Cavitary pulmonary cryptococcosis complicated by aspergilloma. Am Rev Respir Dis 111:549, 1975.

312. Fahey PJ, Utell MJ, Hyde RW: Spontaneous lysis of mycetomas after acute cavitating lung disease. Am Rev Respir Dis 123:336, 1981.

313. Addrizzo-Harris DJ, Harkin TJ, McGuinness G, et al: Pulmonary aspergilloma and AIDS: A comparison of HIV-infected and HIV-negative individuals. Chest 111:612, 1997.

314. McGregor DH, Papasian CJ, Pierce PD: Aspergilloma within cavitating pulmonary adenocarcinoma. Am J Clin Pathol 91:100, 1989.

315. Ward MJ, Davies D: Pulmonary aspergilloma after radiation therapy. Br J Dis Chest 76:361, 1982.

316. Petrie JP, Caughey DE: Bilateral apical fibrobullous disease complicated by bilateral *Aspergillus* mycetomata in rheumatoid arthritis. N Z Med J 96:7, 1983.

317. Krohn J, Halvorsen JH: Aspergilloma of the lung in ankylosing spondylitis. Scand J Respir Dis 63(Suppl):131, 1968.

318. Aslam PA, Eastridge CE, Hughes FA Jr: Aspergillosis of the lung—an eighteen-year experience. Chest 49:28, 1971.

319. Freixinet J, de Cos J, Rodriguez de Castro F, et al: Colonisation with *Aspergillus* of an intralobar pulmonary sequestration. Thorax 50:810, 1995.

320. Henderson AH: Allergic aspergillosis: Review of 32 cases. Thorax 23:501, 1968.

321. Goldberg B: Radiological appearances in pulmonary aspergillosis. Clin Radiol 13:106, 1962.

322. Levin EJ: Pulmonary intracavitary fungus ball. Radiology 66:9, 1956.

323. Libshitz HI, Atkinson GW, Israel HL: Pleural thickening as a manifestation of *Aspergillus* superinfection. Am J Roentgenol 120:883, 1974.

324. Le Hegarat R, Vie A, Allain YM, et al: L'épaississement des parois, signe précoce et peu connu dans l'aspergillome pulmonaire. [Thickening of the walls, early and little known sign of pulmonary aspergilloma.] J Radiol Electrol Med Nucl 47:535, 1966.

325. Irwin A: Radiology of the aspergilloma. Clin Radiol 18:432, 1967.

326. Roberts CM, Citron KM, Strickland B: Intrathoracic aspergilloma: Role of CT in diagnosis and treatment. Radiology 165:123, 1987.

327. Gefter WB: The spectrum of pulmonary aspergillosis. J Thorac Imaging 7:56, 1992.

328. Pennington JE: *Aspergillus* lung disease. Med Clin North Am 64:475, 1980.

329. Freundlich IM, Israel HL: Pulmonary aspergillosis. Clin Radiol 24:248, 1973.

330. Faulkner SL, Vernon R, Brown PP, et al: Hemoptysis and pulmonary aspergilloma: Operative versus nonoperative treatment. Ann Thorac Surg 25:389, 1978.

331. Hinojosa M, Fraj J, De la Hoz B, et al: Hypersensitivity pneumonitis in workers exposed to esparto grass (*Stipa tenacissima*) fibers. J Allergy Clin Immunol 98:985, 1996.

332. Channell S, Blyth W, Lloyd M, et al: Allergic alveolitis in maltworkers: A clinical, mycological, and immunological study. QJM 38:351, 1969.

333. Rosenberg M, Patterson R, Mintzer R: Clinical and immunologic criteria for the diagnosis of allergic bronchopulmonary aspergillosis. Ann Intern Med 86:405, 1977.

334. Mintzer RA, Rogers LF, Kruglik GD, et al: The spectrum of radio-

logic findings in allergic bronchopulmonary aspergillosis. Radiology 127:301, 1978.

335. Angus RM, Davies M-L, Cowman MD, et al: Computed tomographic scanning of the lung in patients with allergic bronchopulmonary aspergillosis and in asthmatic patients with a positive skin test to *Aspergillus fumigatus*. Thorax 49:586, 1994.

336. Ricketti AJ, Greenberger PA, Mintzer RA, et al: Allergic bronchopulmonary aspergillosis. Chest 86:773, 1984.

337. Berkin KE, Vernon DRH, Kerr JW: Lung collapse caused by allergic bronchopulmonary aspergillosis in nonasthmatic patients. BMJ 285:552, 1982.

338. Glancy JJ, Elder JL, McAleer R: Allergic bronchopulmonary fungal disease without clinical asthma. Thorax 36:345, 1981.

339. Breslin AB, Jenkins CR: Experience with allergic bronchopulmonary aspergillosis: Some unusual features. Clin Allergy 14:21, 1984.

340. Imbeau SA, Nichols D, Flaherty D, et al: Relationships between prednisone therapy, disease activity, and the total serum IgE in allergic bronchopulmonary aspergillosis. J Allergy Clin Immunol 62:91, 1978.

341. Malo J-L, Longbottom J, Mitchell J, et al: Studies in chronic allergic bronchopulmonary aspergillosis: 3. Immunological findings. Thorax 32:269, 1977.

342. Aubry M-C, Fraser R: The role of bronchial biopsy and washing in the diagnosis of allergic bronchopulmonary aspergillosis. Mod Pathol 11:607, 1998.

343. Longbottom JJ, Pepys J: Pulmonary aspergillosis: Diagnostic immunological significance of antigens and C-substance in *Aspergillus fumigatus*. J Pathol Bacteriol 88:141, 1964.

344. Safirstein BH: Aspergilloma consequent to allergic bronchopulmonary aspergillosis. Am Rev Respir Dis 108:940, 1973.

345. Urschel HC, Paulson DL, Shaw RR: Mucoid impaction of the bronchi. Ann Thorac Surg 2:1, 1966.

346. Lipinski JK, Weisbrod GL, Sanders DE: Unusual manifestations of pulmonary aspergillosis. J Can Assoc Radiol 29:216, 1978.

347. Pepys J, Riddell RW, Citron KM, et al: Clinical and immunologic significance of *Aspergillus fumigatus* in the sputum. Am Rev Respir Dis 80:167, 1959.

348. Fisher MR, Mendelson EB, Mintzer RA: Allergic bronchopulmonary aspergillosis: A pictorial essay. Radiographics 4:445, 1984.

349. Murphy D, Lane DJ: Pleural effusion in allergic bronchopulmonary aspergillosis: 2 case reports. Br J Dis Chest 75:91, 1981.

350. Ricketti AJ, Greenberger PA, Glassroth J: Spontaneous pneumothorax in allergic bronchopulmonary aspergillosis. Arch Intern Med 144:151, 1984.

351. Neeld DA, Goodman LR, Gurney JW, et al: Computerized tomography in the evaluation of allergic bronchopulmonary aspergillosis. Am Rev Respir Dis 142:1200, 1990.

352. Logan PM, Müller NL: High-attenuation mucous plugging in allergic bronchopulmonary aspergillosis. Can Assoc Radiol J 47:374, 1996.

353. Ward S, Heyneman L, Lee MJ, et al: Accuracy of CT in the diagnosis of allergic bronchopulmonary aspergillosis in asthmatic patients. Am J Roentgenol 173:937, 1999.

354. Meyer RD, Young LS, Armstrong D, et al: Aspergillosis complicating neoplastic disease. Am J Med 54:6, 1973.

355. Young RC, Bennett JE, Vogel CL, et al: Aspergillosis: The spectrum of the disease in 98 patients. Medicine 49:147, 1970.

356. Kuhlman JE, Fishman EK, Burch PA, et al: Invasive pulmonary aspergillosis in acute leukemia: The contribution of CT to early diagnosis and aggressive management. Chest 92:95, 1987.

357. Robertson MJ, Larson RA: Recurrent fungal pneumonias in patients with acute nonlymphocytic leukemia undergoing multiple courses of intensive chemotherapy. Am J Med 84:233, 1988.

358. Klimowski LL, Rotstein C, Cummings KM: Incidence of nosocomial aspergillosis in patients with leukemia over a twenty-year period. Infect Control Hosp Epidemiol 10:299, 1989.

359. Gerson SL, Talbot GH, Hurwitz S, et al: Prolonged granulocytopenia: The major risk factor for invasive pulmonary aspergillosis in patients with acute leukemia. Ann Intern Med 100:345, 1984.

360. Weiland D, Ferguson RM, Peterson PK, et al: Aspergillosis in 25 renal transplant patients: Epidemiology, clinical presentation, diagnosis and management. Ann Surg 198:622, 1983.

361. Yeldandi V, Laghi F, McCabe MA, et al: Aspergillus and lung transplantation. J Heart Lung Transplant 14:883, 1995.

362. Horn CR, Wood NC, Hughes JA: Invasive aspergillosis following post-influenzal pneumonia. Br J Dis Chest 77:407, 1983.

363. Lewis M, Kallenbach J, Ruff P, et al: Invasive pulmonary aspergillosis complicating influenza A pneumonia in a previously healthy patient. Chest 87:691, 1985.

364. Park GR, Drummond GB, Lamb D, et al: Disseminated aspergillosis occurring in patients with respiratory, renal and hepatic failure. Lancet 2:179, 1982.

365. Walsh TJ, Hamilton SR: Disseminated aspergillosis complicating hepatic failure. Arch Intern Med 143:1189, 1983.

366. Pizzani JN, Knapp A: Diabetic ketoacidosis and invasive aspergillosis. Lung 159:43, 1981.

367. Denning DW, Follansbee SE, Scolaro M, et al: Pulmonary aspergillosis in the acquired immunodeficiency syndrome. N Engl J Med 324:654, 1991.

368. Keating JJ, Rogers T, Petrou M, et al: Management of pulmonary aspergillosis in AIDS: An emerging clinical problem. J Clin Pathol 47:805, 1994.

369. Müller NL, Miller RR, Ostrow DN, et al: Tension pneumopericardium: An unusual manifestation of invasive pulmonary aspergillosis. Am J Roentgenol 148:678, 1987.

370. Fraser RS: Pulmonary aspergillosis: Pathologic and pathogenetic features. *In* Rosen PP, Fechner RE (eds): Pathology Annual Part 1. Vol 28. Norwalk, CT, Appleton & Lange, 1993, p 231.

371. Herbert PA, Bayer AS: Fungal pneumonia: Part 4. Invasive pulmonary aspergillosis. Chest 80:220, 1981.

372. Brown MJ, Worthy SA, Flint JDA, Müller NL: Invasive aspergillosis in the immunocompromised host: Utility of computed tomography and bronchoalveolar lavage. Clin Radiol 53:255, 1997.

373. Kirshenbaum JM, Lorell BH, Schoen FJ, et al: Angioinvasive pulmonary aspergillosis: Presentation as massive pulmonary saddle embolism in an immunocompromised patient. J Am Coll Cardiol 6:486, 1985.

374. Curtis AM, Smith GJW, Ravin CE: Air crescent sign of invasive aspergillosis. Radiology 133:17, 1979.

375. Albeda SM, Talbot GH, Gerson SL, et al: Pulmonary cavitation and massive hemoptysis in invasive pulmonary aspergillosis: Influence of bone marrow recovery in patients with acute leukemia. Am Rev Respir Dis 131:115, 1985.

376. Kuhlman JE, Fishman EK, Siegelman SS: Invasive pulmonary aspergillosis in acute leukemia: Characteristic findings on CT, the CT halo sign, and the role of CT in early diagnosis. Radiology 157:611, 1985.

377. Young RC, Vogel CL, Devita VT: *Aspergillus* lobar pneumonia. JAMA 208:1156, 1969.

378. Albelda SM, Gefter WB, Epstein DM, et al: Bronchopleural fistula complicating invasive pulmonary aspergillosis. Am Rev Respir Dis 126:163, 1982.

379. van Ede AE, Meis JF, Koot RA, et al: Pneumopericardium complicating invasive pulmonary aspergillosis: Case report and review. Infection 22:102, 1994.

380. Hruban RH, Meziane MA, Zerhouni EA, et al: Radiologic-pathologic correlations of the CT halo sign in invasive pulmonary aspergillosis. J Comput Assist Tomogr 11:534, 1987.

381. Binder RE, Faling LJ, Pugatch RD, et al: Chronic necrotizing pulmonary aspergillosis: A discrete clinical entity. Medicine 61:109, 1982.

382. Gefter WB, Weingrad TR, Epstein DM, et al: "Semi-invasive" pulmonary aspergillosis: A new look at the spectrum of *Aspergillus* infections of the lung. Radiology 140:313, 1981.

383. Franquet T, Müller NL, Giménez A, et al: Semiinvasive pulmonary aspergillosis in chronic obstructive pulmonary disease: Radiologic and pathologic findings in nine patients. Am J Roentgenol 174:51, 2000.

384. Kim SY, Lee KS, Han J, et al: Semiinvasive pulmonary aspergillosis: CT and pathologic findings in six patients. Am J Roentgenol 174:795, 2000.

385. McAdams HP, Rosado de Christenson M, Strollo DC, et al: Pulmonary mucormycosis: Radiologic findings in 32 cases. Am J Roentgenol 168:1541, 1997.

386. McBride RA, Corson JM, Dammin GJ: Mcuormycosis: Two cases of disseminated disease with cultural identification of rhizopus: Review of literature. Am J Med 28:832, 1960.

387. Donner MW, McAfee JG: Roentgenographic manifestations of diabetes mellitus. Am J Med Sci 239:622, 1960.

388. Gabriele OF: Mucormycosis. Am J Roentgenol 83:227, 1960.

389. Rubin SA, Chaljub G, Winer-Muram HT, et al: Pulmonary zygomycosis: A radiographic and clinical spectrum. J Thorac Imaging 7:85, 1992.

390. Gale AM, Kleitsch WP: Solitary pulmonary nodule due to phycomycosis (mucormycosis). Chest 62:752, 1972.

391. Jamadar DA, Kazerooni EA, Daly BD, et al: Pulmonary zygomycosis: CT appearance. J Comput Assist Tomogr 19:733, 1995.

392. Suzuki JB, Delisle AL: Pulmonary actinomycosis of periodontal origin. J Periodontol 55:581, 1984.

393. Apotheloz C, Regamey C: Disseminated infection due to *Actinomyces meyeri*: Case report and review. Clin Infect Dis 22:621, 1996.

394. Brown JR: Human actinomycosis: A study of 181 subjects. Hum Pathol 4:319, 1973.

395. Bates M, Cruickshank G: Thoracic actinomycosis. Thorax 12:99, 1957.

396. Kwong JS, Müller NL, Godwin JD, et al: Thoracic actinomycosis: CT findings in eight patients. Radiology 183:189, 1992.

397. Flynn MW, Felson B: The roentgen manifestations of thoracic actinomycosis. Am J Roentgenol 110:707, 1970.

398. Eiben C, Indihar FJ, Hunter SW: Thoracic actinomycosis mimicking the pancoast syndrome. Minn Med 66:541, 1983.

399. Balikian JP, Cheng TH, Costello P, et al: Pulmonary actinomycosis: A report of three cases. Radiology 128:613, 1978.

400. Hsieh MJ, Liu HP, Chang JP, et al: Thoracic actinomycosis. Chest 104:366, 1993.

401. Schwarz J, Baum GL: Actinomycosis. Semin Roentgenol 5:58, 1970.

402. Coodley EL, Yoshinaka R: Pleural effusion as the major manifestation of actinomycosis. Chest 106:1615, 1994.

403. Harrison RN, Thomas DJB: Acute actinomycotic empyema. Thorax 34:406, 1979.

404. Merdler C, Greif J, Burke M, et al: Primary actinomycotic empyema. South Med J 76:411, 1983.

405. Morgan DE, Nath H, Sanders C, et al: Mediastinal actinomycosis. Am J Roentgenol 155:735, 1990.

406. Harvey JC, Cantrell JR, Fisher AM: Actinomycosis: Its recognition and treatment. Ann Intern Med 46:868, 1957.

407. Webb WR, Sagel SS: Actinomycosis involving the chest wall: CT findings. Am J Roentgenol 139:1007, 1982.

408. Dershaw DD: Actinomycosis of the chest wall: Ultrasound findings in empyema necessitans. Chest 86:779, 1984.

409. Georghiou PR, Blacklock ZM: Infection with *Nocardia* species in Queensland: A review of 102 clinical isolates. Med J Aust 156:692, 1992.

410. Coker RJ, Bignardi G, Horner P, et al: *Nocardia* infection in AIDS: A clinical and microbiological challenge. J Clin Pathol 45:821, 1992.

411. Menendez R, Cordero PJ, Santos M, et al: Pulmonary infection with *Nocardia* species: A report of 10 cases and review. Eur Respir J 10:1542, 1997.

412. Young LS, Armstrong D, Blevins A, et al: *Nocardia asteroides* infection complicating neoplastic disease. Am J Med 501:356, 1971.

413. Pinkhas J, Oliver I, De Vries A, et al: Pulmonary nocardiosis complicating malignant lymphoma successfully treated with chemotherapy. Chest 63:367, 1973.

414. Krick JA, Stinson EB, Remington JS: *Nocardia* infection in heart transplant patients. Ann Intern Med 82:18, 1975.

415. Bach MC, Sahyoun A, Adler JL, et al: Influence of rejection therapy on fungal and nocardial infections in renal transplant recipients. Lancet 1:80, 1973.

416. Andriole VT, Ballas M, Wilson GL: The association of nocardiosis and pulmonary alveolar proteinosis: A case study. Ann Intern Med 60:266, 1964.

417. Mok CC, Yuen KY, Lau CS: Nocardiosis in systemic lupus erythematosus. Semin Arthritis Rheum 26:675, 1997.

418. Presant CA, Wiernik PH, Serpick AA: Factors affecting survival in nocardiosis. Am Rev Respir Dis 108:1444, 1973.

419. Pesce CM, Quaglia AC: *Nocardia* lung infection with hematogenous spread in a woman with adrenal cortical hyperfunction. Eur J Respir Dis 65:613, 1984.

420. Hathaway BM, Mason KN: Nocardiosis: A study of fourteen cases. Am J Med 32:903, 1962.

421. Weed LA, Anderson HA, Good CA, et al: Nocardiosis: Clinical, bacteriologic and pathological aspects. N Engl J Med 253:1137, 1955.

422. Raich RA, Casey F, Hall WH: Pulmonary and cutaneous nocardiosis: The significance of the laboratory isolation of *Nocardia*. Am Rev Respir Dis 83:505, 1961.

423. Feigin DS: Nocardiosis of the lung: Chest radiographic findings in 21 cases. Radiology 159:9, 1986.

424. Grossman CB, Bragg DG, Armstrong D: Roentgen manifestations of pulmonary nocardiosis. Radiology 96:325, 1970.

425. Neu HC, Silva M, Hazen E, et al: Necrotizing nocardial pneumonitis. Ann Intern Med 66:274, 1967.

426. Balikian JP, Herman PG, Kopit S: Pulmonary nocardiosis. Radiology 126:569, 1978.

427. Raby N, Forbes G, Williams R: *Nocardia* infection in patients with liver transplants or chronic liver disease: Radiologic findings. Radiology 174:713, 1990.

428. Yoon HK, Im J-G, Ahn JM, et al: Pulmonary nocardiosis: CT findings. J Comput Assist Tomogr 19:52, 1995.

429. Van Kralingen KW, Hekker TA, Bril H, et al: Haemoptysis and an abnormal x-ray after prolonged treatment in the ICU. Eur Respir J 7:419, 1994.

430. Hobson D: Acute respiratory virus infections. BMJ 2:229, 1973.

431. Nolan TF Jr, Goodman RA, Hinman AR, et al: Morbidity and mortality associated with influenza B in the United States, 1979–1980: A report from the Centers for Disease Control. J Infect Dis 142:360, 1980.

432. Glezen WP: Viral pneumonia as a cause and result of hospitalization. J Infect Dis 147:765, 1983.

433. Soto PJ, Broun GO, Wyatt JP: Asian influenzal pneumonitis: A structural and virologic analysis. Am J Med 27:18, 1959.

434. Fry J: Influenza A (Asian) 1957: Clinical and epidemiological features in a general practice. BMJ 1:259, 1959.

435. Galloway RW, Miller RS: Lung changes in the recent influenza epidemic. Br J Radiol 32:28, 1959.

436. Glezen WP, Denny FW: Epidemiology of acute lower respiratory disease in children. N Engl J Med 288:498, 1973.

437. Taussig LM, Wright AL, Morgan WJ, et al: The Tucson Children's Respiratory Study: I. Design and implementation of a prospective study of acute and chronic respiratory illness in children. Am J Epidemiol 129:1219, 1989.

438. Osborne D: Radiologic appearance of viral disease of the lower respiratory tract in infants and children. Am J Roentgenol 130:29, 1978.

439. Downham MAPS, Gardner PS, McQuillin J, et al: Role of respiratory viruses in childhood mortality. BMJ 1:235, 1975.

440. Sterner G, Wolontis S, Bloth B, et al: Respiratory syncytial virus—an outbreak of acute respiratory illnesses in a home for infants. Acta Paediatr Scand 55:273, 1966.

441. Forbes JA, Bennett NMcK, Gray NJ: Epidemic bronchiolitis caused by a respiratory syncytial virus: Clinical aspects. Med J Aust 2:933, 1961.

442. Sorvillo FJ, Huie SF, Strassburg MA, et al: An outbreak of respiratory syncytial virus pneumonia in a nursing home for the elderly. J Infect 9:252, 1984.

443. Morales F, Calder MA, Inglis JM, et al: A study of respiratory infections in the elderly to assess the role of respiratory syncytial virus. J Infect 7:236, 1983.

444. Parham DM, Bozeman P, Killian C, et al: Cytologic diagnosis of respiratory syncytial virus infection in a bronchoalveolar lavage specimen from a bone marrow transplant recipient. Am J Clin Pathol 99:588, 1993.

445. van Dissel JT, Zijlmans JM, Kroes AC, et al: Respiratory syncytial virus, a rare cause of severe pneumonia following bone marrow transplantation. Ann Hematol 71:253, 1995.

446. Zaroukian MH, Kashyap GH, Wentworth BB: Case report: Respiratory syncytial virus infection: A cause of respiratory distress syndrome and pneumonia in adults. Am J Med Sci 295:218, 1988.

447. Butler JC, Peters CJ: Hantaviruses and hantavirus pulmonary syndrome. Clin Infect Dis 19:387, 1994.

448. Khan AS, Khabbaz RF, Armstrong LR, et al: Hantavirus pulmonary syndrome: The first 100 US cases. J Infect Dis 173:1297, 1996.

449. Ketai LH, Williamson MR, Telepak RJ, et al: Hantavirus pulmonary syndrome: Radiographic findings in 16 patients. Radiology 191:665, 1994.

450. Brandt CD, Kim HW, Vargosko AJ, et al: Infections in 18,000 infants and children in a controlled study of respiratory tract disease: I. Adenovirus pathogenicity in relation to serologic type and illness syndrome. Am J Epidemiol 90:484, 1969.

451. Bateman ED, Hayashi S, Kuwano K, et al: Latent adenoviral infection in follicular bronchiectasis. Am J Respir Crit Care Med 151:170, 1995.

452. Gold R, Wilt JC, Adhikari PK, et al: Adenoviral pneumonia and its complications in infancy and childhood. J Can Assoc Radiol 20:218, 1969.

453. Schullere D, Spessert C, Fraser VJ, et al: Herpes simplex virus from respiratory tract secretions: Epidemiology, clinical characteristics, and outcome in immunocompromised and nonimmunocompromised hosts. Am J Med 94:29, 1993.

454. Nash G, Foley FD: Herpetic infection of the middle and lower respiratory tract. Am J Clin Pathol 54:857, 1970.

455. Aquino SL, Dunagan DP, Chiles C, et al: Herpes simplex virus 1 pneumonia: Patterns on CT scans and conventional chest radiographs. J Comput Assist Tomogr 22:795, 1998.

456. Graham BS, Snell JD Jr: Herpes simplex virus infection in the adult lower respiratory tract. Medicine 62:384, 1983.

457. Pek S, Gikas PW: Pneumonia due to herpes zoster: Report of a case and review of the literature. Ann Intern Med 62:350, 1965.

458. Weller TH: Varicella and herpes zoster: Changing concepts of the natural history, control, and importance of a not-so-benign virus (first of two parts). N Engl J Med 309:1434, 1983.

459. Triebwasser JH, Harris RE, Bryant RE, et al: Varicella pneumonia in adults: A report of seven cases and a review of literature. Medicine 46:409, 1967.

460. Weber DM, Pellecchia JA: Varicella pneumonia: Study of prevalence in adult men. JAMA 192:572, 1965.

461. Mermelstein RH, Freireich AW: Varicella pneumonia. Ann Intern Med 55:456, 1961.

462. Jura E, Chadwick EG, Josephs SH, et al: Varicella-zoster virus infections in children infected with human immunodeficiency virus. Pediatr Infect J 8:586, 1989.

463. Locksley RM, Flournoy N, Sullivan KM, et al: Infection with varicella-zoster virus after marrow transplantation. J Infect Dis 152:1172, 1985.

464. Esmonde TF, Herdman G, Anderson G: Chickenpox pneumonia: An association with pregnancy. Thorax 44:812, 1989.

465. Sargent EN, Carson MJ, Reilly ED: Roentgenographic manifestations of varicella pneumonia with postmortem correlation. Am J Roentgenol 98:305, 1966.

466. Southard ME: Roentgen findings in chickenpox pneumonia: Review of the literature and report of five cases. Am J Roentgenol 76:533, 1956.

467. Tan DYM, Kaufman SA, Levene G: Primary chickenpox pneumonia. Am J Roentgenol 76:527, 1956.

468. Charles RE, Katz RL, Ordonez NG, et al: Varicella-zoster infection with pleural involvement: A cytologic and ultrastructural study of a case. Am J Clin Pathol 85:522, 1986.

469. Kriss N: Chickenpox pneumonia: A case report. Radiology 66:727, 1956.

470. Raider L: Calcification in chickenpox pneumonia. Chest 60:504, 1971.

471. Abrahams EW, Evans C, Knyvett AF, et al: Varicella pneumonia: A possible cause of subsequent pulmonary calcification. Med J Aust 2:781, 1964.

472. Knyvett AF, Stringer RE, Abrahams EW: The radiology of chickenpox lung. J Coll Radiol Australas 9:134, 1965.

473. Brunton FJ, Moore ME: A survey of pulmonary calcification following adult chicken-pox. Br J Radiol 42:256, 1969.

474. Ho M: Epidemiology of CMV infections. Rev Infect Dis 12:S701, 1990.

475. Marrie TJ, Janigan DT, Haldane EV, et al: Does CMV play a role in community-acquired pneumonia? Clin Invest Med 8:286, 1985.

476. Ettinger NA, Bailey TC, Trulock EP, et al: Cytomegalovirus infection and pneumonitis: Impact after isolated lung transplantation. Am Rev Respir Dis 147:1017, 1993.

477. Meyers JD, Flournoy N, Thomas ED: Nonbacterial pneumonia after allogeneic marrow transplantation: A review of ten years' experience. Rev Infect Dis 4:1119, 1982.

478. Austin JHM, Schulman LL, Mastrobattista JD: Pulmonary infection after cardiac transplantation: Clinical and radiologic correlations. Radiology 172:259, 1989.

479. Olliff JFC, Williams MP: Radiological appearances of cytomegalovirus infections. Clin Radiol 40:463, 1989.

480. Schulman LL: Cytomegalovirus pneumonitis and lobar consolidation. Chest 91:558, 1987.

481. Moore EH, Webb WR, Amend WJC: Pulmonary infections in renal transplantation patients treated with cyclosporine. Radiology 167:97, 1988.

482. Aafedt BC, Halvorsen RA, Tylen U, et al: Cytomegalovirus pneumonia: Computed tomography findings. J Can Assoc Radiol 41:276, 1990.

483. Hoagland RJ: The clinical manifestations of infectious mononucleosis: A report of two hundred cases. Am J Med Sci 240:21, 1960.

484. Wechsler HF, Rosenblum AH, Sills CT: Infectious mononucleosis: Report of an epidemic in an army post. Ann Intern Med 25:113, 1946.

485. Lander P, Palayew MJ: Infectious mononucleosis—a review of chest roentgenographic manifestations. J Can Assoc Radiol 25:303, 1974.

486. Cohen JI: Epstein-Barr virus lymphoproliferative disease associated with acquired immunodeficiency. Medicine 70:137, 1991.

487. Levine DP, Lerner AM: The clinical spectrum of *Mycoplasma pneumoniae* infections. Med Clin North Am 62:961, 1978.

488. Ortqvist A, Jedlung A, Grillner I, et al: Etiology, outcome and prognostic factors in community-acquired pneumonia requiring hospitalization. Eur Respir J 3:1105, 1990.

489. Almirall J, Morato I, Riera F, et al: Incidence of community-acquired pneumonia and *Chlamydia pneumoniae* infection: A prospective multicentre study. Eur Respir J 6:14, 1993.

490. Amundson DE, Weiss PJ: Pneumonia in military recruits. Milit Med 159:629, 1994.

491. Purcell RH, Chanock RM: Role of mycoplasmas in human respiratory disease. Med Clin North Am 51:791, 1967.

492. Brolin I, Wernstedt L: Radiographic appearance of mycoplasmal pneumonia. Scand J Respir Dis 59:179, 1978.

493. Alexander ER, Foy JM, Kenny GE, et al: Pneumonia due to *Mycoplasma pneumoniae*: Its incidence in the membership of a cooperative medical group. N Engl J Med 275:131, 1966.

494. Grayston JT, Alexander ER, Kenny GE, et al: *Mycoplasma pneumoniae* infections: Clinical and epidemiologic studies. JAMA 191:369, 1965.

495. Reittner P, Müller NL, Heyneman L, et al: *Mycoplasma pneumoniae* pneumonia: Radiographic and high-resolution CT features in 28 patients. Am J Roentgenol 174:37, 2000.

496. Izumikawa K, Hara K: Clinical features of mycoplasmal pneumonia in adults. Yale J Biol Med 56:505, 1983.

497. Thombs DD: Cold agglutinin-positive pneumonia: A review of thirty cases in children. Ohio State Med J 63:1171, 1967.

498. Nitu Y: *M. pneumoniae* respiratory diseases: Clinical features—children. Yale J Biol Med 56:493, 1983.

499. Lambert HP: *Mycoplasma pneumoniae* infections. J Clin Pathol 21(Suppl 2):52, 1968.

500. Dean NL: Mycoplasma pneumonias in the community hospital: The "unusual" manifestations become common. Clin Chest Med 2:121, 1981.

501. Ali NJ, Sillis M, Andrews BE, et al: The clinical spectrum and diagnosis of *Mycoplasma pneumoniae* infection. QJM 58:241, 1986.

502. Wright SW, Edwards KM, Decker MD, et al: Prevalence of positive serology for acute *Chlamydia pneumoniae* infection in emergency department patients with persistent cough. Acad Emerg Med 4:179, 1997.

503. McConnell CT, Plouffe JF, File TM, et al, CBPIS Study Group: Radiographic appearance of *Chlamydia pneumoniae* (TWAR Strain) respiratory infections. Radiology 192:819, 1994.

504. Bhatia G: *Echinococcus*. Semin Respir Infect 12:171, 1997.

505. Moore RD, Urschel JD, Fraser RE, et al: Cystic hydatid lung disease in northwest Canada. Can J Surg 37:20, 1994.

506. McPhail JL, Arora TS: Intrathoracic hydatid disease. Dis Chest 52:772, 1967.

507. Sadrieh M, Dutz W, Navabpoor MS: Review of 150 cases of hydatid cyst of the lung. Dis Chest 52:662, 1967.

508. Wilson JF, Diddams AC, Rausch RL: Cystic hydatid disease in Alaska: A review of 101 autochthonous cases of *Echinococcus granulosus* infection. Am Rev Respir Dis 98:1, 1968.

509. Bloomfield JA: Protean radiological manifestations of hydatid infestation. Aust Radiol 10:330, 1966.

510. McElvaney G, Müller NL, Pitman RG, et al: Clinical-radiologic-pathologic conference: A family with lung nodules discovered by radiographic survey. J Can Assoc Radiol 39:17, 1988.

511. Halezeroglu S, Celik M, Uysal A, et al: Giant hydatid cysts of the lung. J Thorac Cardiovasc Surg 113:712, 1997.

512. Ozdemir IA, Kalaycioglu E: Surgical treatment and complications of thoracic hydatid disease: Report of 61 cases. Eur J Respir Dis 64:217, 1983.

513. Ozer Z, Cetin M, Kahraman C: Pleural involvement by hydatid cysts of the lung. Thorac Cardiovasc Surg 33:103, 1985.

514. Rakower J, Milwidsky H: Hydatid pleural disease. Am Rev Respir Dis 90:623, 1964.

515. Bakir F, Al-Omeri MM: Echinococcal tension pneumothorax. Thorax 24:547, 1969.

516. Saksouk FA, Fahl MH, Rizk GK: Computed tomography of pulmonary hydatid disease. J Comput Assist Tomogr 10:226, 1986.

517. von Sinner WN: Radiographic, CT, and MRI spectrum of hydatid disease of the chest: Pictorial essay. Eur Radiol 3:62, 1993.

518. von Sinner WN: New diagnostic signs in hydatid disease: Radiography, ultrasound, CT and MRI correlated to pathology. Eur J Radiol 12:150, 1991.

519. von Sinner WN, Rifai A, teStrake L, et al: Magnetic resonance imaging of thoracic hydatid disease: Correlation with clinical findings, radiography, ultrasonography, CT, and pathology. Acta Radiol 31:59, 1990.

520. von Sinner WN, Linjawi T, Al Watban J: Mediastinal hydatid disease: Report of three cases. J Can Assoc Radiol 41:79, 1990.

521. Marrie TJ: Pneumococcal pneumonia: Epidemiology and clinical features. Semin Respir Infect 14:227, 1999.

522. Ruiz M, Santiago E, Marcos MA, et al: Etiology of community-acquired pneumonia. Am J Respir Crit Care Med 160:397, 1999.

523. George DL, Falk PS, Wunderink RG, et al: Epidemiology of ventilator-acquired pneumonia based on protected bronchoscopic sampling. Am J Respir Crit Care Med 158:1839, 1998.

524. van Rie A, Warren R, Richardson M, et al: Exogenous reinfection as cause of recurrent tuberculosis after curative treatment. N Engl J Med 341:1174, 1999.

525. Ellis RH: Total collapse of the lung in aspergillosis. Thorax 20:118, 1965.

526. Kroboth FJ, Yu VL, Reddy SC, et al: Clinicoradiographic correlations with the extent of legionnaires' disease. Am J Roentgenol 141:263, 1983.

527. Hoffmann L, Neumann P, Naegele E, et al: Tuberculous round foci of the lungs from the viewpoint of tuberculosis care and chest surgery [German]. Beitr Klin Tuberk 124:558, 1962.

528. Bleiweiss IJ, Jagirdar JS, Klein MJ, et al: Granulomatous *Pneumocystis carinii* pneumonia in three patients with the acquired immune deficiency syndrome. Chest 94:580, 1988.

529. Schwarzmann SW, Adler JL, Sullivan RJ, et al: Bacterial pneumonia during the Hong Kong influenza epidemic of 1968-1969: Experience in a city-county hospital. Arch Intern Med 127:519, 1971.

530. Nash G: Necrotizing tracheobronchitis and bronchopneumonia consistent with herpetic infection. Hum Pathol 3:283, 1972.

531. Kushihashi T, Munechika H, Motoya H, et al: CT and MR findings in tuberculous mediastinitis. J Comput Assist Tomogr 19:379, 1995.

CHAPTER 6

Pulmonary Neoplasms

PULMONARY CARCINOMA

In this text, the term *pulmonary carcinoma* is used to refer to neoplasms that arise from the surface epithelium of the airways and alveoli. Such neoplasms consist of four main histologic types: squamous cell carcinoma, small cell carcinoma, adenocarcinoma, and large cell carcinoma. Although these tumors commonly are referred to as *bronchogenic carcinoma*, we prefer to use the designation *pulmonary carcinoma* in recognition of the fact that most adenocarcinomas probably arise from bronchiolar or alveolar epithelial cells.

Pulmonary carcinoma is one of the most important human neoplasms, not only because of its frequency, but also because of its dismal prognosis. It is the most common cause of cancer-related death in men and women in North America and worldwide.[2] In 1997, pulmonary carcinoma was responsible for an estimated 170,000 deaths in the United States,[4] accounting for more than one third of all cancer deaths in men and close to one quarter in women.[2] Overall, only about 10% to 15% of patients survive 5 years or longer.[15] In general hospitals, the incidence of unresectability of non–small cell carcinoma is 80% to 85%.[174a, 175]

The most important causative agent of pulmonary carcinoma is tobacco smoke. Although the attributable proportion of tumors caused by this agent varies with smoking prevalence and intensity in any given population,[3] it has been estimated that approximately 85% of all tumors in North America and Europe are the result of cigarette consumption.[3, 5] An increased risk for development of pulmonary carcinoma is present in individuals who have had exposure to inorganic substances such as asbestos,[6] arsenic,[7] and nickel[8] or to radiation in mines;[9] in patients who have undergone radiotherapy;[10, 11] and in patients who have diffuse interstitial pulmonary fibrosis.[12, 13]

Pathologic Characteristics
Adenocarcinoma

Although pulmonary adenocarcinoma is divided into several histologic subtypes in the World Health Organization classification,[1] the distinctiveness of the subgroups is open to question, and from a practical point of view, the neoplasm is considered best in two major groups—bronchioloalveolar carcinoma (sometimes subdivided into mucinous and nonmucinous variants[22]) and nonbronchioloalveolar carcinoma. The distinction between the two lies in their pattern of growth: In bronchioloalveolar carcinoma, tumor cells grow on the alveolar surface with minimal or no invasion of the underlying interstitial tissue; as a result, the overall architecture of the underlying lung parenchyma still can be recognized.

Adenocarcinoma is the most common histologic type of pulmonary carcinoma, comprising about 30% to 35% of all cases. Approximately 50% of tumors present as a nodule or mass located in the periphery of the lung, 15% present as a hilar or perihilar mass, and 35% present as a combination of parenchymal mass and hilar or mediastinal lymphadenopathy.[28]

Squamous Cell Carcinoma

Although formerly the most common subtype of pulmonary carcinoma, squamous cell carcinoma has decreased in relative incidence in many areas since the 1960s and now generally is believed to be second to adenocarcinoma in overall frequency, comprising approximately 25% to 30% of all pulmonary carcinomas. The tumor originates most frequently in a segmental or lobar bronchus and characteristically grows into the airway lumen, causing atelectasis and obstructive pneumonitis in the distal lung.[16, 17] In one review of 98 patients who had squamous cell carcinoma, 43% had such complications.[28]

Small Cell Carcinoma

Small cell carcinoma comprises about 15% to 20% of all pulmonary carcinomas. It typically arises in association with proximal airways, particularly lobar and main bronchi;[18, 19] occasional tumors (<5%) appear to originate in the lung periphery without any obvious association with an airway.[20, 21] In the early stage, centrally located tumors tend to be poorly delimited and spread in the submucosa and peribronchovascular connective tissue. Endobronchial growth is seen much less frequently than in squamous cell carcinoma; when airway obstruction occurs, it is usually as a result of airway compression by the expanding tumor rather than by intraluminal growth. Invasion of small blood vessels and lymphatics is present in most tumors at an early stage, and regional bronchopulmonary and hilar lymph nodes almost invariably are enlarged at the time of diagnosis as a result of metastatic or invasive carcinoma.

Large Cell Carcinoma

A diagnosis of large cell carcinoma is applied to tumors that do not possess the typical appearance of small cell carcinoma and that have no evidence by light microscopy of either squamous or glandular differentiation. If these criteria are adhered to, large cell carcinoma comprises about 10% to 15% of all pulmonary carcinomas. Although they may have a variety of gross pathologic features, most tumors present as large peripheral masses.[23]

Clinical Manifestations

Symptoms of pulmonary carcinoma can be the result of local bronchopulmonary disease (e.g., cough and hemoptysis), extension of tumor to adjacent structures (particularly the chest wall and mediastinum), distant metastases (especially to bone, liver, and brain), nonspecific constitutional effects (fatigue, anorexia, and weight loss), and immunologic reactions to or hormone secretion by the tumor (paraneoplastic syndromes). About 10% of patients are asymptomatic when first seen, the diagnosis being suspected initially from an abnormal chest radiograph.

Tumors of the thoracic inlet almost invariably result in symptoms and signs related to local invasion (Pancoast tumor). Important structures within the superior thoracic inlet are (from front to back) the subclavian and jugular veins, the phrenic and vagus nerves, the subclavian and common carotid arteries, the recurrent laryngeal nerve, the eighth cervical and first thoracic nerves, the sympathetic chain and stellate ganglion, and the first four ribs and upper vertebrae. A Pancoast tumor may involve one or several of these structures and result in a variety of signs and symptoms, including pain and weakness of the shoulder and arm, swelling of the arm, and Horner's syndrome.[116]

Constitutional symptoms, such as malaise, weakness, lassitude, fever, and weight loss, are common. In addition to these relatively nonspecific constitutional manifestations, some patients—particularly those who have small cell carcinoma—have symptoms and signs not directly related to neoplastic infiltration itself.[117] These paraneoplastic syndromes are said to occur in 10% of patients[119] and may be seen in the absence of symptoms related to intrathoracic disease.[121] The disorders are mediated by hormones or peptides secreted by the tumor or by antitumor antibodies that cross-react with normal tissues.[118] Such paraneoplastic syndromes include hypertrophic osteoarthropathy, myopathy, peripheral neuropathy, a variety of central nervous system syndromes (e.g., subacute cerebellar degeneration), a Cushing's-like syndrome, hypercalcemia, and inappropriate secretion of antidiuretic hormone.[117, 119]

Hypertrophic osteoarthropathy is an important manifestation of pulmonary disease, carcinoma being the most common cause. It has been found in about 3% of patients who have pulmonary carcinoma.[120] It is distinctly uncommon in patients who have small cell carcinoma,[122] and its presence should suggest the diagnosis of non–small cell tumor.[120] The main symptom is deep-seated, burning pain in distal parts of the extremities. Clubbing of the fingers and toes and edema, warmth, and tenderness of the hands, wrists, feet, and lower legs usually are evident. Radiography reveals subperiosteal new bone formation, chiefly of the distal bones of the extremities. Because radionuclide bone scanning is a sensitive detector of new bone formation, it may offer a more complete appreciation of the extent of the abnormality than is possible by radiography alone.

Radiologic Manifestations

The radiographic manifestations of pulmonary carcinoma are related to its size and its anatomic location, particularly with respect to its relationship to an airway.

Table 6–1. PULMONARY CARCINOMA: RADIOLOGIC MANIFESTATIONS

Obstructive pneumonitis and atelectasis
    May involve a segment, a lobe, or the entire lung
    Most commonly squamous or small cell carcinoma
Lung nodule or mass
    Most commonly adenocarcinoma or squamous cell carcinoma
    Usually has spiculated or lobulated margins
    Enhances more than 15 HU following administration of intravenous
        contrast
Apical mass (Pancoast tumor)
    Usually adenocarcinoma or squamous cell carcinoma
Cavitated mass
    Most commonly squamous cell carcinoma
Nodule or mass associated with lymphadenopathy
    Any cell type
Unilateral hilar or mediastinal lymphadenopathy alone
    Most commonly small cell carcinoma

The earliest finding often is not the lesion itself but the obstructive pneumonitis or atelectasis that the tumor engenders (Table 6–1).

Anatomic Location

Pulmonary carcinoma occurs with a relative frequency of 3:2 in the right versus the left lung[24, 25] and the upper versus the lower lobe.[25, 26] Although squamous cell and small cell carcinomas may occur centrally or peripherally, there is clear-cut predominance of both tumors in the former location.[27, 28] In approximately 50% of cases, adenocarcinoma presents as an isolated peripheral lesion; in the other 50%, it occurs as a peripheral lesion associated with hilar lymphadenopathy or as a central tumor.[28, 29] Of tumors that arise in the conducting airways, most are situated in relation to segmental and lobar bronchi.[16, 18] Carcinoma arising in the trachea is rare, amounting to less than 1% of cases.[30] Approximately 4% of carcinomas arise in the extreme apex of the upper lobes (Pancoast tumors).[28]

Obstructive Pneumonitis

Radiographic findings secondary to airway obstruction are present in approximately 40% of patients at the time of presentation.[28] The most frequent are related to a combination of pathologic changes that includes atelectasis, bronchiectasis with mucous plugging, and consolidation. The atelectasis most often is segmental or lobar (Fig. 6–1); occasionally an entire lung is affected (Fig. 6–2). Because airway obstruction usually is complete, air cannot pass distally, and an air bronchogram is absent; this sign is virtually pathognomonic of an endobronchial obstructing lesion and is of utmost importance in diagnosis. Bronchi distal to the obstruction usually are dilated and filled with mucus or pus. Occasionally a tumor is identified as a focal convexity, whereas the interlobar fissure distally is concave as a result of atelectasis, an S-shaped configuration known as *Golden's S sign* (*see* Fig. 6–1).[32]

When an obstructing tumor is not apparent on radiograph, it usually can be seen on dynamic or spiral computed tomography (CT) after intravenous administration of a bolus of contrast material or on magnetic resonance (MR) imaging.[34, 35] For example, in one retrospective study of 50 patients who had segmental or lobar atelectasis, pulmonary carcinomas causing bronchial obstruction were identified correctly in 24 of 27 (89%) patients on chest radiograph and in all 27 cases on CT scan.[33] Optimal visualization of the tumor in these cases requires the use of an intravenous bolus of contrast material and dynamic or spiral CT (*see* Fig. 6–1);[34, 36] using these techniques, the tumor enhances only slightly, whereas the atelectatic lung shows considerable enhancement.

Distinction of carcinoma from post–obstructive atelectasis can be made on T2-weighted spin-echo MR images (Fig. 6–3)[34, 37] or on T1-weighted MR images after intravenous administration of gadolinium.[38, 39] The results of studies comparing MR imaging with CT have been variable; in two series, MR imaging was considered to be superior

Table 6–2. CLINICAL AND RADIOLOGIC CRITERIA IN THE DIFFERENTIATION OF BENIGN AND MALIGNANT SOLITARY PULMONARY NODULES

	Benign	Malignant
Clinical		
Age	<35 yr; exception is hamartoma	>35 yr
Symptoms	Absent	Present
Past history and functional inquiry	High incidence of granuloma in area; exposure to tuberculosis; nonsmoker	Diagnosis of primary lesion elsewhere; smoker; exposure to carcinogens
Radiographic		
Size	Small (<2 cm in diameter)	Large (>2 cm in diameter)
Location	No predilection except for tuberculosis (upper lobes)	Predominantly upper lobes except for lung metastases
Contour	Margins smooth	Margins spiculated
Calcification	Almost pathognomonic of a benign lesion if laminated, diffuse, or central	Rare, may be eccentric (engulfed granuloma)
Satellite lesions	More common	Less common
Serial studies showing no change over 2 yr	Almost diagnostic of benign lesion	Most unlikely
Doubling time	<30 or >490 days	Between these extremes
Computed Tomography		
Calcification	Diffuse or central	Absent or eccentric
Fat	Virtually diagnostic of hamartoma	Absent
Bubble-like lucencies	Uncommon	Common, particularly in adenocarcinomas
Enhancement with intravenous contrast material	<15 HU	>15 HU

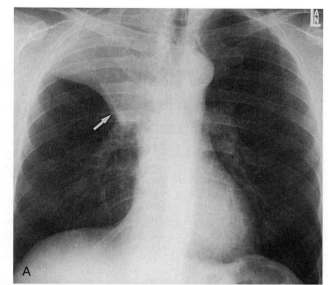

Figure 6–1. Lobar Atelectasis Resulting from Pulmonary Carcinoma. Anteroposterior chest radiograph *(A)* in a 67-year-old man shows atelectasis and obstructive pneumonitis of the right upper lobe. The focal convexity in the hilar region *(arrow)*, which indicates the location of the tumor, and the concave appearance of the interlobar fissure distally as a result of atelectasis give a configuration that resembles an S (Golden's S sign). Contrast-enhanced CT scan *(B)* shows the central tumor *(straight arrows)* and the atelectatic right upper lobe *(open arrows)*. Biopsy showed squamous cell carcinoma.

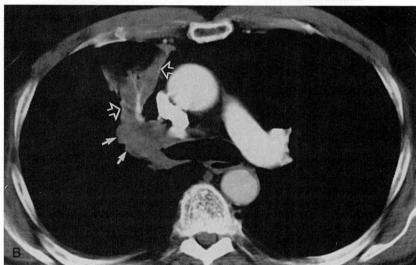

to CT in the distinction of tumor from post–obstructive atelectasis changes,[38, 39] whereas in one study it was considered inferior.[34]

Solitary Pulmonary Nodule

There is a wide variation in the criteria for designating a radiologic opacity a solitary nodule, with resultant differences in radiologic features and prognostic implications. The shape usually is described as round or oval. Although in the past the size was accepted to vary from 1 to 6 cm in diameter,[40, 41] it is more customary today to restrict the maximum diameter to 3 cm,[42, 43] with larger lesions being identified as masses.

Approximately 60% of solitary nodules are benign, and 40% are malignant.[43] Using clinical and radiographic findings (Table 6–2), the distinction between benign and malignant lesions often can be established with a reasonable degree of confidence, helping to make a decision as to whether surgical intervention is warranted. Experience has shown that it is best to divide solitary nodules into two broad categories for the purposes of differential diagnosis:

(1) lesions that are clearly benign, as determined by rigidly defined radiologic signs,[47, 50] and (2) lesions of indeterminate nature, comprising all other lesions. The *benign/indeterminate* categorization replaces the more traditional *benign/malignant* distinction. The main reason for this separation is that the criteria of benignity are more certain than are the radiologic signs of malignancy. The four signs of greatest value in assessing a solitary pulmonary nodule are size, calcification, character of the tumor-lung interface, and doubling time.

Size

Based on the data in the literature, the likelihood ratio for malignancy of solitary nodules has been estimated to be 0.52 for nodules less than 1 cm in diameter, 0.74 for nodules 1.1 to 2 cm, 3.7 for nodules 2.1 to 3 cm, and 5.2 for nodules greater than 3 cm.[51] When interpreting these figures, it is important to remember that the likelihood of carcinoma is influenced strongly by other factors, such as age and smoking history.

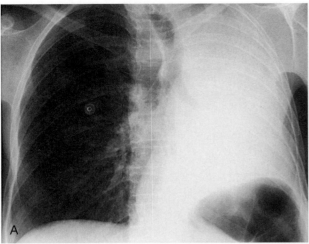

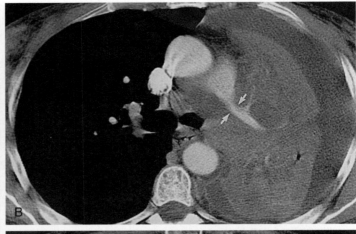

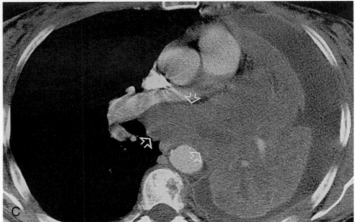

Figure 6–2. Atelectasis and Obstructive Pneumonitis of the Left Lung. Posteroanterior chest radiograph *(A)* shows consolidation and atelectasis of the left lung, mediastinal displacement to the left, and overinflation of the right lung. The marked elevation of the left hemidiaphragm in this patient was the result of phrenic nerve involvement by tumor. Contrast-enhanced CT scan *(B)* at the level of the proximal left main bronchus shows tumor infiltration into the mediastinum and encasement of the left pulmonary artery *(arrows)*. Obstructive pneumonitis and atelectasis of the left lung and a left pleural effusion also are evident. CT scan at the more caudad level *(C)* shows extensive tumor infiltration of the mediastinum *(open arrows)* with complete obstruction of the left bronchus. The diagnosis of small cell carcinoma was proved by bronchial biopsy.

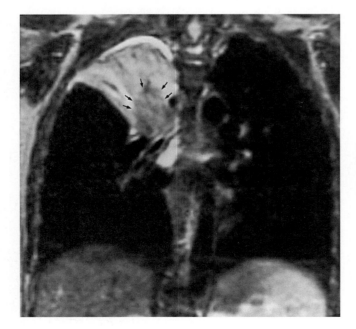

Figure 6–3. Obstructive Pneumonitis and Atelectasis. Coronal spin-echo T2-weighted MR image (TR/TE, 2,400/120) shows right upper lobe atelectasis and obstructive pneumonitis. The obstructing pulmonary carcinoma *(arrows)* has a relatively low signal intensity compared with the consolidated lung. The diagnosis of adenocarcinoma was proved surgically.

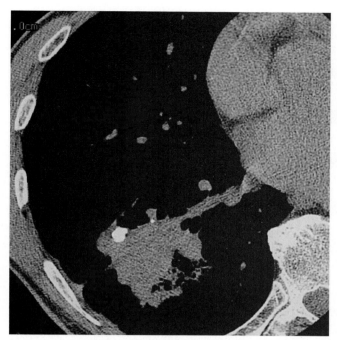

Figure 6–4. Calcification in Pulmonary Carcinoma. HRCT scan in a 75-year-old man shows a 4-cm-diameter tumor in the right lower lobe. Focal areas of eccentric calcification are present. At right lower lobectomy, the tumor was shown to be a bronchioloalveolar carcinoma that had engulfed adjacent calcified granulomas.

Calcification

The presence or absence of calcium is the most important feature that distinguishes benign from malignant nodules.[46, 50] The presence of diffuse, laminated, or central calcification is almost certain evidence of benignity, with only rare tumors with these features proving to be malignant.[46, 47] The presence of an eccentric calcific opacity in a nodule or mass occasionally represents incorporation of a calcified granuloma within the substance of a carcinoma (Fig. 6–4). Although calcification can be seen on thin-section CT (1- to 3-mm collimation scans) in about 5% to 10% of pulmonary carcinomas,[53, 54] it usually affects tumors greater than 3 cm in diameter; for example, in one study of 39 calcified tumors, only 6 (15%) were smaller than this.[54] The calcification within the pulmonary carcinomas was mild and had not been identified on the original chest radiograph in any instance.

The author of a review in 1994 identified 11 studies in which CT densitometry had been used to evaluate pulmonary nodules.[56] The authors of these studies used either the presence of attenuation values with a threshold of 164 to 200 HU to identify the presence of calcification or an internal reference phantom standardized to a given attenuation value (which ranged from 185 to 264 HU in different series). Of 504 nodules denser than the reference, 490 (97%) were benign, and 14 (3%) were malignant. Of 1,109 nodules less dense than the reference, 782 (71%) were malignant, and 327 (29%) were benign. In most of these cases, the calcification identified on CT scan was not apparent on conventional radiographs.

Optimal assessment on CT scan requires the use of a series of thin sections (1- to 3-mm collimation) through the nodule. In one study of 62 benign nodules, calcification was identified on thin-section CT scan in 36% of tumors compared with only 12% on conventional CT scan.[55] Foci of calcification that are visible on thin-section CT usually have attenuation values of 400 HU or higher.[52, 57] In the absence of such foci, attenuation values of 200 HU or higher can be considered to represent calcification.[52, 57]

Character of the Nodule-Lung Interface

Pulmonary carcinomas commonly have an irregular spiculated interface (Fig. 6–5). In one study of 283 tumors, 184 (65%) had focal or diffuse spiculation of their margins, 91 (32%) had smooth but lobulated margins, and 8 (3%) had smooth nonlobulated margins.[46] In a review of the literature published in 1993, it was concluded that the likelihood ratio for malignancy of a nodule that has irregular or spiculated margins is 5.54; the corresponding figures for lobulated and smoothly marginated nodules are 0.74 and 0.30.[51] Radiologic-pathologic correlation has shown that spiculation may reflect the presence of fibrosis in the surrounding parenchyma, direct infiltration of carcinoma into the adjacent parenchyma, or localized lymphangitic spread.[58]

The *tail sign* (pleural tag) consists of a linear opacity that extends from a peripheral nodule or mass to the visceral pleura. The tag can represent a strand of fibrous tissue that extends from the nodule to the visceral pleura[58, 59] or can result from inward retraction and apposition of a thickened visceral pleura. As the visceral pleura invaginates, a

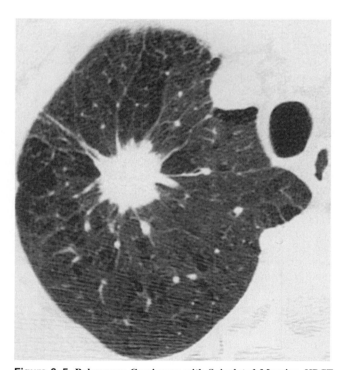

Figure 6–5. Pulmonary Carcinoma with Spiculated Margins. HRCT scan in a 62-year-old man shows a 2.5-cm-diameter nodule in the right upper lobe. The nodule has multiple spicules radiating from the lesion into the surrounding parenchyma (corona radiata). The diagnosis of adenocarcinoma was proved at surgery.

small quantity of extrapleural fat is drawn into the area, creating the opacity.[60] Pleural tags have been reported on thin-section CT scan in 60% to 80% of peripheral pulmonary carcinomas.[58, 62] Although they are associated most commonly with adenocarcinoma,[58, 63] they may be seen with other histologic subtypes;[58, 64] they also may be identified in pulmonary metastases[64, 65] and granulomas.[64, 65] As a result of the latter observation, the sign is of limited value in the differential diagnosis of benign from malignant lesions.[64, 65]

Doubling Time

Use of doubling time* in estimating growth rate may be valuable in differentiating benign from malignant nodules in individual patients. The process requires at least two serial chest radiographs showing a roughly spherical lesion whose diameter can be averaged from measurements in at least two planes.[70]

In a study of 218 pulmonary nodules (177 malignant and 41 benign), virtually all nodules whose doubling time was 7 days or less were benign;[71] similarly, nodules whose volume doubles in 465 days or more almost always were benign. A pulmonary nodule whose rate of growth falls between these limits must be considered malignant. Perhaps the most useful application of the growth rate principle in assessing solitary nodules is in patients older than 40 years of age, in whom the incidence of malignancy increases markedly. In one study of individuals in this age group, almost every solitary nodule whose doubling time was less than 37 days was benign;[71] of 72 malignant nodules, the slowest growing nodules doubled their volume in 200 days. Other investigators have quoted only slightly different figures.[72, 73]

The doubling time provides a more accurate assessment of the nature of a solitary nodule than does simple increase in size. Because benign lesions such as hamartoma and histoplasmoma also may grow slowly,[74, 75] increase in size by itself should not be the sole consideration governing the therapeutic approach to a pulmonary nodule. Absence of growth over a 2-year period is a fairly reliable indicator of benignity.[71, 76] The validity of a 2-year stability as an indicator of benignity has been questioned, however.[78] Small changes in size may be difficult to appreciate on the chest radiograph; for example, a 5-mm-diameter nodule increases to only 6 mm diameter after one doubling and to only 8 mm diameter after two doublings. Occasional carcinomas have been found to have apparent stability for a period of 2 or more years.[77] Despite these observations, we believe that a 2-year stability can be considered a reasonably reliable criterion for benignity. Patients who have such nodules should continue to be followed, however.[78]

Air Bronchogram

On thin-section CT scan, air bronchograms and air bronchiolograms are seen more commonly in pulmonary carci-

---

*Doubling refers to volume, not diameter. Assuming a nodule to be spherical, its diameter must be multiplied by 1.25 to obtain the diameter of a sphere whose volume is double (e.g., the volume of a nodule 2 cm in diameter is doubled by the time its diameter reaches 2.5 cm). A doubling of diameter represents an eightfold increase in volume.

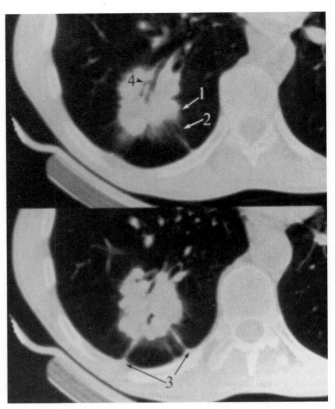

Figure 6–6. Air Bronchogram in Bronchioloalveolar Carcinoma. CT scans through a right lower lobe mass show several signs that strongly favor malignancy: marginal nodulation *(1)*, fine spiculations *(2)*, and pleural retraction *(3)*. Air bronchogram *(4)* with narrowed, amputated airways suggests a diagnosis of bronchioloalveolar carcinoma, which was established after surgical excision. The patient was a 55-year-old woman.

nomas than in benign nodules (Fig. 6–6).[58, 61] For example, in one review of 132 patients, air bronchograms were identified on thin-section CT scan in 33 (29%) of 115 pulmonary carcinomas and in only 1 (6%) of 17 benign nodules.[66] The patent airways frequently are tortuous and ectatic.[66] When cut in cross-section, they are seen as focal air collections, usually measuring 5 mm or less in diameter, a finding commonly referred to as *bubble-like lucency* or *pseudocavitation* (Fig. 6–7).[68, 69]

As might be expected, bubble-like lucencies are particularly common in bronchioloalveolar carcinoma; in one review of the findings in 30 patients who had this tumor, they were seen in 18 (60%).[67] In another study, bubble-like lucencies were seen within solitary nodules on thin-section CT scan in 21 of 85 malignant nodules (25%) and in only 1 (9%) of 11 benign nodules;[58] they were present in 7 (55%) of 13 bronchioloalveolar carcinomas, 9 (31%) of 28 nonbronchioloalveolar adenocarcinomas, and approximately 10% of squamous carcinomas and large cell carcinomas.

Nodule Enhancement

Computed Tomography

The potential usefulness of measuring nodule enhancement on thin-section CT scan as a means of distinguishing

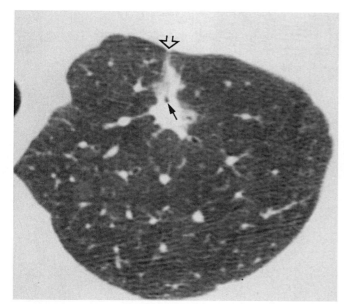

Figure 6–7. Bubble-Like Lucency in Bronchioloalveolar Carcinoma. View of the left upper lobe from HRCT scan in a 49-year-old woman shows a 2-cm-diameter, spiculated nodule. A small localized area of air density (bubble-like lucency) *(straight arrow)* is present within the nodule. A pleural tag also is present *(open arrow)*. The diagnosis of bronchioloalveolar carcinoma was confirmed at surgery. Correlation of HRCT scan with the excised specimen showed that the bubble-like lucency represented a bronchus surrounded by tumor.

between benign and malignant nodules has been investigated by several groups.[42, 44, 79] In one prospective study of 107 patients using an enhancement of at least 20 HU as a marker for malignancy, the authors found a 98% sensitivity and a 73% specificity for the diagnosis of carcinoma (Fig. 6–8).[79] Eight nodules had enhancement measuring 16 to 24 HU; four of these were malignant, and four were benign, leading the authors to define this range as indeterminate.[79] The value of contrast enhancement was confirmed in a prospective multicenter study of 356 nodules (185 benign, 171 malignant).[80] Using 15 HU as a threshold for a positive

test result, the sensitivity was 98% and the specificity was 58% in excluding malignancy.

The results of these studies indicate that lack of enhancement or enhancement of less than 15 HU after intravenous administration of contrast material is virtually diagnostic of a benign lesion. The greatest value of nodule enhancement studies is in providing support for conservative follow-up of noncalcified lesions that are considered likely to be benign. Because of the number of false-positive examinations, the presence of contrast enhancement is less helpful in diagnosis.

Although the results of these studies are encouraging, they are applicable only to nodules measuring 6 to 30 mm in diameter that have homogeneous attenuation. The technique requires meticulous attention to detail. CT scans are obtained using 3-mm collimation, preferentially using spiral technique and reconstruction at 1- to 2-mm intervals. The attenuation is measured in the section closest to the center of the nodule using a region of interest of approximately 60% of the diameter of the nodule. After initial measurement of nodule attenuation on unenhanced scans, iodinated intravenous contrast material is injected for a total dose of 420 mg of iodine per kilogram at a concentration of 300 mg per ml (100 ml for a 70-kg subject) at a rate of 2 ml/sec. Images are obtained at 1-, 2-, 3-, and 4-minute intervals, and attenuation values are measured using identical technique as in the precontrast scan.[79, 80]

Positron Emission Tomography

Several groups of investigators have assessed the potential use of positron emission tomography (PET) after intravenous administration of 2-(fluorine-18)-fluoro-2-deoxy-D-glucose (^{18}FDG)* in the assessment of lung nodules (Fig. 6–9).[81, 82, 84] A review of the studies published before 1999 indicated that FDG-PET imaging had a sensitivity of 96%

---

*^{18}FDG is a glucose analogue labeled with a positron emitter, ^{18}F; it is transported through the cell membrane and phosphorylated through normal glycolytic pathways, after which it is not metabolized further and remains within the cell.

Figure 6–8. Nodule Enhancement in Pulmonary Carcinoma. View of the right lung from a 3-mm collimation spiral CT scan shows a 1.2-cm-diameter, noncalcified nodule *(arrow)* in the right middle lobe. CT scan performed at the same level 2 minutes after intravenous administration of contrast material shows marked enhancement of the nodule. The attenuation increased from 10 HU before intravenous contrast administration to 53 HU after contrast administration. At right middle lobectomy, the nodule was an adenocarcinoma.

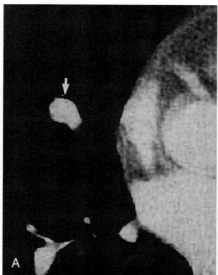
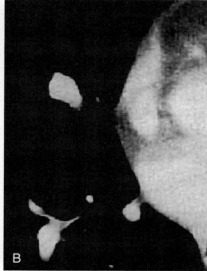

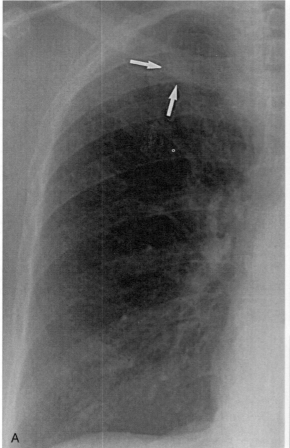

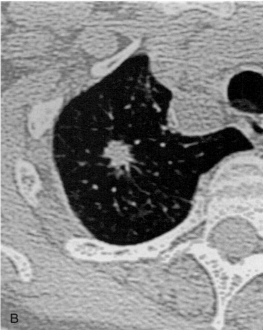

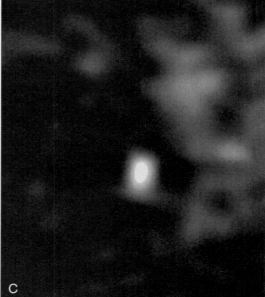

Figure 6–9. Positron Emission Tomography (PET). View from posteroanterior chest radiograph *(A)* shows a poorly defined nodular opacity in the right upper lobe *(arrows)*. Thin-section CT scan *(B)* confirms the presence of an 8-mm-diameter nodule with spiculated margins. PET image *(C)* shows increased activity of the lung nodule. The diagnosis of stage I right upper lobe adenocarcinoma was confirmed at surgery. (Case courtesy of Dr. Ned Patz, Duke University Medical Center, Durham, NC.)

and specificity of 88% in the assessment of nodules 10 mm or larger.[83] Because the probability of malignancy is low (<5%) in patients with negative FDG-PET scans, these patients can be followed radiologically.[83] False-negative FDG-PET studies can occur in patients with carcinoid tumors, bronchioloalveolar carcinomas, and pulmonary carcinomas measuring less than 10 mm in diameter.[83, 84] False-positive scans can occur with infectious or inflammatory conditions, such as tuberculosis, histoplasmosis, and rheumatoid nodules.[83, 84] The main disadvantages of the technique are limited availability and high cost.

Solitary Pulmonary Mass

As discussed previously, the division of solitary opacities within the lung into two categories, nodules (measuring ≦3 cm in diameter) and masses (measuring >3 cm in diameter) serves only one useful purpose—a mass is much more likely than is a nodule to be malignant. Calcification in a mass does not exclude malignancy as it does in the case of a solitary nodule. For example, in one study of 353 carcinomas, 20 (6%) had calcification evident on CT scan;[53] 17 of the 20 containing calcification (85%) were greater than 3 cm in diameter. In another study, the mean diameter of 39 carcinomas that had calcification on CT was 6.2 cm;[54] 33 tumors (85%) were greater than 3 cm in diameter. The calcification in these large tumors may be punctate, chunky, or amorphous in appearance and central, peripheral, or diffuse in distribution (Fig. 6–10).[54] It may be related to psammoma bodies, dystrophic calcification, or incorporation of a focus of prior granulomatous in-

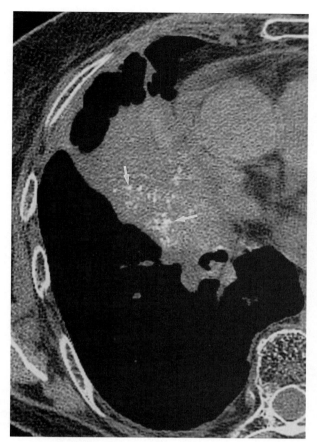

Figure 6–10. Calcifications in Pulmonary Carcinoma. HRCT scan in a 70-year-old woman shows large mass in the right middle lobe containing numerous small, speckled areas of calcification *(arrows)*. The diagnosis of adenocarcinoma was made by bronchial biopsy.

flammation or calcified bronchial cartilage within the tumor.[54, 85]

Cavitation

The incidence of cavitation in pulmonary carcinoma is about 10%.[31] Although the complication can occur in tumors of any size, most are greater than 3 cm in diameter.[45] The most common histologic type is squamous cell carcinoma; in a review of the radiographic findings in 600 carcinomas, cavitation was seen in 22% of 263 squamous cell carcinomas, 6% of 97 large cell carcinomas, 2% of 126 adenocarcinomas, and none of 114 small cell carcinomas.[31] Most cavities have an irregular inner surface as a result of variably sized nodules of neoplastic tissue projecting into the cavity and of the patchy nature of the necrosis (Fig. 6–11). The cavities may be central or eccentric and 1 to 10 cm in diameter.

Air-Space (Pneumonic) Pattern

The air-space pattern of disease is restricted almost entirely to bronchioloalveolar carcinoma (Fig. 6–12). The changes may be local or disseminated widely, the former predominating in 60% to 90% of reported series.[69, 87] Some patients in whom the disease appears to be local when first

seen have deposits elsewhere in the lungs that can be seen on CT scan.[88] In others, increase in size of the initial tumor is associated with widespread dissemination on radiographs. Radiographic air-space abnormalities range from a hazy increase in density (ground-glass pattern) to dense consolidation and may be seen as an isolated finding or in conjunction with single or multiple nodules.[87, 89]

On CT scan, this pattern corresponds to areas of ground-glass opacity or consolidation, reflecting the characteristic nondestructive growth of carcinoma on alveolar septa, the presence of secretions in adjacent air spaces, or both. The abnormalities can be focal, measuring less than 1 cm to several centimeters in diameter (Fig. 6–13); patchy; or nonsegmental;[68, 69] lobar consolidation may occur and be associated with volume loss or lobar expansion.[69, 86] In one study of 42 patients who had bronchioloalveolar carcinoma, 16 (40%) presented with a solitary nodule or mass, 10 (24%) presented with lobar consolidation, 13 (30%) presented with multilobar consolidation, and 3 (7%) presented with diffuse nodules.[90]

Air bronchograms or bronchiolograms and bubble-like lucencies are seen in 50% to 80% of cases.[58, 67] After intravenous administration of contrast material, clear distinction of pulmonary vessels from the relatively low attenuation of the surrounding parenchyma often is present, a finding known as the *CT angiogram sign*.[92] Although this sign was described first in bronchioloalveolar carcinoma, it also can be seen in a variety of other conditions, including obstructive pneumonitis, lymphoma, lipid pneumonia, bacterial pneumonia, infarction, and edema.[91, 93] The sign can be considered suggestive of bronchioloalveolar carcinoma

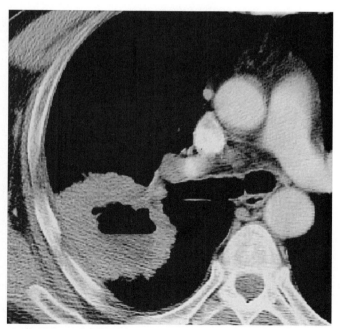

Figure 6–11. Cavitary Pulmonary Carcinoma. View of the right lung from contrast-enhanced CT scan in a 56-year-old man shows a 5-cm-diameter, cavitating mass in the right upper lobe. The cavity has thick walls and a nodular inner contour characteristic of carcinoma. Also noted are an air-fluid level within the tumor and right hilar lymphadenopathy. The diagnosis of cavitating squamous cell carcinoma was proved at surgery.

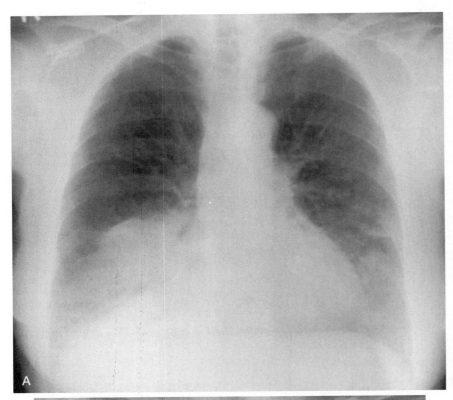

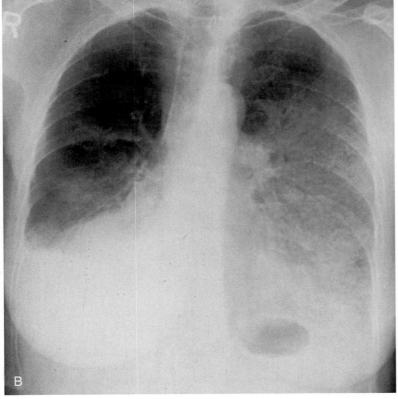

Figure 6–12. Progressive Multicentric Bronchioloalveolar Carcinoma. Posteroanterior chest radiograph *(A)* shows bilateral air-space opacities involving the middle lobe and parts of both lower lobes. One year later, posteroanterior chest radiograph *(B)* shows more extensive consolidation throughout all areas, including both upper lobes. The patient was a 56-year-old woman who died of her disease shortly thereafter; at autopsy, all parts of both lungs were involved with diffuse bronchioloalveolar carcinoma.

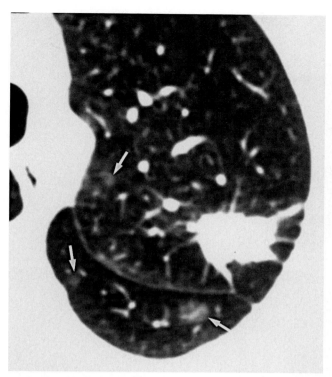

Figure 6–13. Bronchioloalveolar Carcinoma. View of the left lung from HRCT scan in a 68-year-old man shows a 3-cm-diameter, spiculated nodule in the left upper lobe. There are small focal areas of ground-glass attenuation *(arrows)*. At surgery, the latter areas and the dominant nodule were shown to represent multicentric bronchioloalveolar carcinoma.

only if the mean attenuation of the consolidated lung is less than that of the chest wall musculature.[93]

Hilar Enlargement

Unilateral hilar enlargement may be the earliest radiographic manifestation of pulmonary carcinoma.[28] It may represent a primary carcinoma that has arisen in a main or lobar bronchus or, more commonly, enlarged bronchopulmonary or hilar lymph nodes that are the site of direct invasion or metastasis from a small primary lesion in the adjacent bronchus or peripheral parenchyma. The pattern is particularly characteristic of small cell carcinoma.

Mediastinal Involvement

The mediastinum can be involved by metastases to lymph nodes or, less commonly, by direct invasion from a contiguous neoplasm in the lung parenchyma. In a review of the radiographic presentation in 345 patients who had pulmonary carcinoma, a mediastinal mass or mediastinal lymph node enlargement was seen in 53 of 86 (62%) small cell carcinomas, 45 of 125 (36%) adenocarcinomas, 7 of 22 (32%) large cell carcinomas, and 25 of 98 (26%) squamous carcinomas.[28] Although uncommon, enlargement of mediastinal lymph nodes may be the main or sole abnormality seen radiographically,[14] in which case it usually indicates the presence of small cell carcinoma.[27, 28] The chief radiographic sign is mediastinal widening, usually with an undulating or lobulated contour (Fig. 6–14).

Apical Pulmonary Neoplasms

Approximately 5% of pulmonary carcinomas arise in the apex of the lung. The term *Pancoast syndrome* can be applied to any situation in which such a neoplasm is accompanied by shoulder or arm pain. In an investigation of 345 patients who had newly diagnosed pulmonary carcinoma, 12 (3.5%) had an apical mass, including 5 of 125 (4%) adenocarcinomas, 4 of 98 (4%) squamous cell carcinomas, and 3 of 86 (3%) small cell carcinomas.[28] In another study of 27 patients who had apical tumors, 21 were adenocarcinomas, 5 were squamous cell carcinomas, 1 was a small cell carcinoma, and 1 was a large cell carcinoma.[94] In other series, however, adenocarcinoma was only slightly more common than squamous cell carcinoma[95–98] or less common than squamous cell carcinoma.[97]

Several workers have shown that MR imaging is superior to CT in the assessment of these tumors.[94, 102, 105] The procedure allows direct coronal, sagittal, and oblique imaging that yields excellent anatomic detail of the thoracic inlet and brachial plexus (Fig. 6–15). It also provides better soft tissue differentiation than CT, allowing superior depiction of chest wall invasion, which is visualized as disruption of the normal extrapleural fat.

Pleural Involvement

There is considerable variation in the reported prevalence of pleural effusion in pulmonary carcinoma. It was observed in 4% of 600 patients in one study,[31] 15% of 417 patients in a second study,[14] and 23% of 331 patients in a third study.[28] The complication does not denote invasion by neoplastic cells; serous effusion sometimes occurs as a result of lymphatic obstruction or atelectasis.[103]

Chest Wall Involvement

The presence of rib destruction or an obvious chest wall mass on CT scan allows reliable diagnosis of chest wall invasion;[99, 101, 104] however, these findings have a low sensitivity, being present in only 20% to 40% of patients who have this complication.[99, 100] Other findings, such as the presence of obtuse angles between the mass and chest wall, greater than 3 cm contact between mass and chest wall, and focal pleural thickening, are not reliable indicators.[99, 101] A review of the studies published before 1999 indicates that when these signs are included, the reported sensitivity of CT for detecting chest wall invasion ranges from 38% to 87%, and the specificity ranges from 40% to 90%.[104]

Although MR imaging has been shown to be superior to CT in the assessment of chest wall invasion in apical tumors,[94, 105] its value in the detection of lateral chest wall invasion is controversial. In one study of 13 patients, MR imaging had a negative predictive value of 100%, correctly depicting the lack of chest wall invasion in 9 patients.[106] In this study, the procedure allowed accurate diagnosis of the presence or absence of chest wall invasion in nine patients in whom the CT findings were equivocal. In the report of the Radiology Diagnostic Oncology Group trial, however, which included 23 patients who had surgical and pathologic correlation, CT and MR imaging were equivalent in the assessment of chest wall invasion.[107] The earliest finding

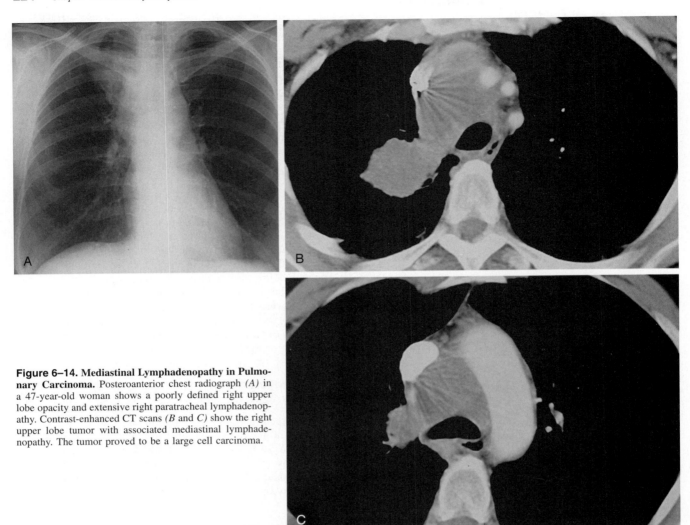

Figure 6–14. Mediastinal Lymphadenopathy in Pulmonary Carcinoma. Posteroanterior chest radiograph *(A)* in a 47-year-old woman shows a poorly defined right upper lobe opacity and extensive right paratracheal lymphadenopathy. Contrast-enhanced CT scans *(B and C)* show the right upper lobe tumor with associated mediastinal lymphadenopathy. The tumor proved to be a large cell carcinoma.

of chest wall invasion on MR imaging is disruption of the normal extrapleural fat by soft tissue, which has moderate signal intensity on T1-weighted spin-echo images and high signal intensity on T2-weighted images (*see* Fig. 6–15).[109] Inflammatory and neoplastic tissue have similar signal characteristics.[108, 110]

Disruption of the pleural surface and extension into the chest wall by pulmonary carcinoma can be assessed well by ultrasonography.[111, 112] In one study of 120 patients, the procedure allowed correct identification of chest wall infiltration in all of 19 patients who had invasion proved at surgery (sensitivity 100%) and absence of chest wall invasion in 99 of 101 patients (specificity 98%).[112]

Bone Involvement

The skeleton may be involved in pulmonary carcinoma by direct extension to the ribs or vertebrae (Fig. 6–16) or by metastasis to these or other sites (Fig. 6–17). Rib or vertebral destruction sometimes is visible on the chest radiograph but is depicted best on CT scan. The incidence of bone metastases at the time of death has been reported to be 10% to 40%.[113, 114] Although they are predominantly osteolytic, purely osteoblastic lesions may occur.

Staging

Schemes for Staging

The most widely used scheme for staging non–small cell carcinoma of the lung is the TNM classification. A variety of alterations in this scheme have been made to group better patients with similar prognosis and treatment options. The most recent revision was approved by the American Joint Committee on Cancer (AJCC) and the Union Internationale Contre le Cancer (UICC) in 1997.[123] An accompanying article outlines refinements made in regional lymph node classification.[124] Specific properties of each of the T, N, and M subtypes as defined by this revision are shown in Table 6–3. The various combinations of T, N, and M that define different stages are depicted in Table 6–4.

Patients who have small cell carcinoma frequently are staged in a simpler fashion into two categories: (1) *limited* disease, defined as carcinoma confined to a tolerable radiation port (depending on the investigators, this has included regional mediastinal and supraclavicular lymph nodes as well as pleural effusion), and (2) *extensive* disease, in which carcinoma has extended beyond these limits.[15, 127]

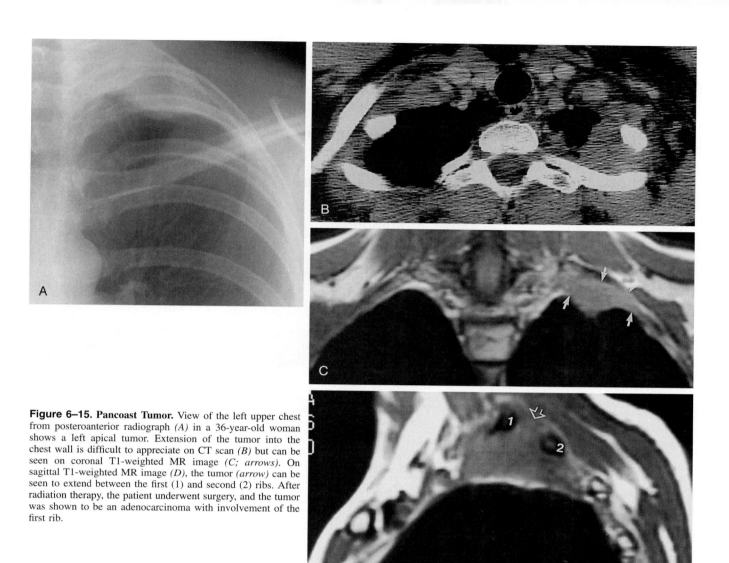

Figure 6–15. Pancoast Tumor. View of the left upper chest from posteroanterior radiograph *(A)* in a 36-year-old woman shows a left apical tumor. Extension of the tumor into the chest wall is difficult to appreciate on CT scan *(B)* but can be seen on coronal T1-weighted MR image *(C; arrows)*. On sagittal T1-weighted MR image *(D)*, the tumor *(arrow)* can be seen to extend between the first *(1)* and second *(2)* ribs. After radiation therapy, the patient underwent surgery, and the tumor was shown to be an adenocarcinoma with involvement of the first rib.

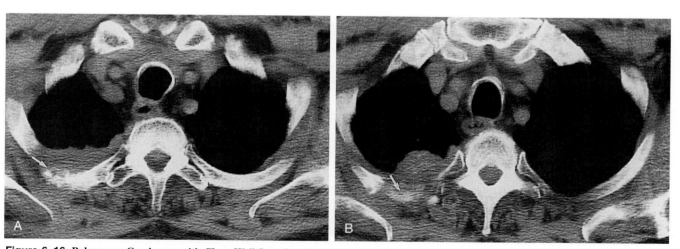

Figure 6–16. Pulmonary Carcinoma with Chest Wall Invasion. CT scans *(A and B)* in a 67-year-old man show a right apical tumor with evidence of chest wall invasion, as shown by the partial destruction of the right posterior third rib *(arrows)*. The tumor was resected together with the right second, third, and fourth ribs and shown to be a squamous cell carcinoma.

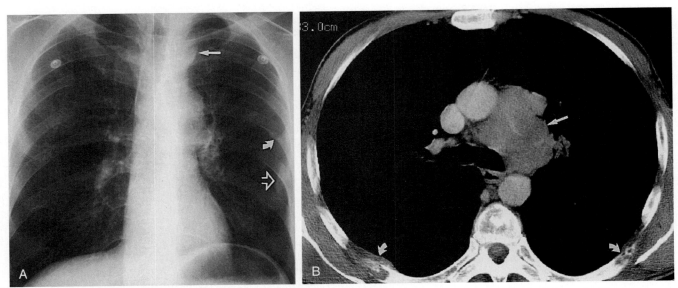

Figure 6–17. Metastatic Pulmonary Carcinoma. A 37-year-old man presented with a 1-month history of weight loss and chest pain. Chest radiograph *(A)* shows localized convexity in the left upper mediastinum *(straight arrow)*, focal irregularity of the left posterior sixth rib *(curved arrow)*, and an extrapleural sign associated with the anterolateral left fifth rib *(open arrow)*. Contrast-enhanced CT scan *(B)* shows extensive mediastinal lymphadenopathy *(straight arrow)* and lytic rib lesions *(curved arrows)*. The diagnosis was metastatic small cell carcinoma.

Table 6–3. TNM DESCRIPTORS

Primary Tumor (T)

TX   Primary tumor cannot be assessed or tumor proved by the presence of malignant cells in sputum or bronchial washings but not visualized by imaging or bronchoscopy

T0   No evidence of primary tumor

Tis   Carcinoma in situ

T1   Tumor ≤3 cm in greatest dimension, surrounded by lung or visceral pleura, without bronchoscopic evidence of invasion more proximal than the lobar bronchus* (i.e., not in the main bronchus)

T2   Tumor with any of the following features of size or extent
More than 3 cm in greatest dimension
Involves main bronchus, ≥2 cm distal to the carina
Invades the visceral pleura
Associated with atelectasis or obstructive pneumonitis that extends to the hilar region but does not involve the entire lung

T3   Tumor of any size that directly invades any of the following: chest wall (including superior sulcus tumors), diaphragm, mediastinal pleura, parietal pericardium; or tumor in the main bronchus <2 cm distal to the carina but without involvement of the carina; or associated atelectasis or obstructive pneumonitis of the entire lung

T4   Tumor of any size that invades any of the following: mediastinum, heart, great vessels, trachea, esophagus, vertebral body, carina; or tumor with a malignant pleural or pericardial effusion,† or with a satellite tumor nodule or nodules within the ipsilateral primary-tumor lobe of the lung

Regional Lymph Nodes (N)

NX   Regional lymph nodes cannot be assessed

N0   No regional lymph node metastasis

N1   Metastasis to ipsilateral peribronchial and/or ipsilateral hilar lymph nodes and intrapulmonary nodes involved by direct extension of the primary tumor

N2   Metastasis to an ipsilateral mediastinal and/or subcarinal lymph node or nodes

N3   Metastasis to contralateral mediastinal, contralateral hilar, ipsilateral or contralateral scalene, or supraclavicular lymph node or nodes

Distant Metastasis (M)

MX   Presence of distant metastasis cannot be assessed

M0   No distant metastasis

M1   Distant metastasis present‡

---

*The uncommon superficial tumor of any size with its invasive component limited to the bronchial wall, which may extend proximal to the main bronchus, is also classified T1.

†Most pleural effusions associated with lung cancer are due to tumor. There are a few patients, however, in whom multiple cytopathologic examinations of pleural fluid show no tumor. In these cases, the fluid is nonbloody and is not an exudate. When these elements and clinical judgment dictate that the effusion is not related to the tumor, the effusion should be excluded as a staging element, and the patient's disease should be staged T1, T2, or T3. Pericardial effusion is classified according to the same rules.

‡A separate metastatic tumor nodule or nodules in the ipsilateral nonprimary tumor lobe or lobes of the lung are also classified M1.

Adapted from Mountain CF: Revisions in the international system for staging lung cancer. Chest 111:1710, 1997.

Table 6–4. STAGE GROUPING: TNM SUBSETS*

Stage	TNM Subset
0	Carcinoma in situ
1A	T1N0M0
1B	T2N0M0
IIA	T1N1M0
IIB	T2N1M0
	T3N0M0
IIIA	T3N1M0
	T1N2M0
	T2N2M0
	T3N2M0
IIIB	T4N0M0
	T4N1M0
	T4N2M0
	T1N3M0
	T2N3M0
	T3N3M0
	T4N3M0
IV	Any T Any N M1

*Staging is not relevant for occult carcinoma, designated TXN0M0.

From Mountain CF: Revisions in the international system for staging lung cancer. Chest 111:1710, 1997.

Methods of Staging

A variety of techniques can be used to investigate T, N, and M parameters to determine the appropriate tumor stage.

T (Primary Tumor)

Radiography. Of the criteria that define the T categories in the TNM classification, most already have been established during the initial diagnostic workup. For example, chest radiographs would have revealed the size of the lesion in patients in whom it is circumscribed and the degree of associated atelectasis or obstructive pneumonitis in the presence of airway obstruction in patients in whom it is not. In the latter situation, bronchoscopy would have documented the proximal extent of the neoplasm. The chest radiograph would have established the presence or absence of pleural effusion, the exception being the situation in which atelectasis or obstructive pneumonitis of a lower lobe obscures its presence.

In some cases, extrapulmonary spread may be evident without the results of special investigations. For example, direct extension of a neoplasm into the chest wall may be established by radiographic evidence of destruction of ribs or vertebrae or clinical evidence of a palpable mass. Evidence of invasion of the mediastinum may be suggested by marked elevation of a hemidiaphragm (related to phrenic nerve paralysis) or by clinical signs of superior vena cava syndrome or laryngeal paralysis. Paramediastinal tumors sometimes displace or narrow the tracheal air column, providing convincing radiographic evidence of mediastinal invasion. In the absence of signs such as these, the chest radiograph generally is unreliable in detecting invasion of the chest wall, diaphragm, or mediastinum, and it is necessary to resort to CT or MR imaging for such evaluation.[47, 107]

Computed Tomography. CT can detect reliably invasion of the mediastinum, provided that major mediastinal vessels or bronchi are surrounded by tumor (Fig. 6–18).[130] A tumor that abuts but does not obviously invade the mediastinum cannot be considered as invasive, however, even when associated with obliteration of the fat plane between the mediastinum and the tumor mass.[47] CT criteria suggesting that a tumor abutting the mediastinum is likely to be resectable (albeit possibly minimally invasive) include (1) less than 3 cm contact between the tumor and the adjacent mediastinum, (2) less than 90 degrees circumferential contact between the tumor and the aorta, and (3) the presence of fat between the tumor and the adjacent mediastinal structures.[129] Carcinomas that involve the tracheal carina or that surround, encase, or abut more than 180 degrees of the aorta, main or proximal portion of the right or left pulmonary arteries, or esophagus are likely to be extensively invasive and unresectable.[47, 130]

The detection of a T4 status is considered one of the main indications for use of CT in the staging of pulmonary carcinoma.[131] For example, in one study of 275 patients, CT scans showed surgically unresectable tumors (T4) in 34 patients (12%).[47] In another prospective study of 250 patients, only 2 patients underwent thoracotomy and were

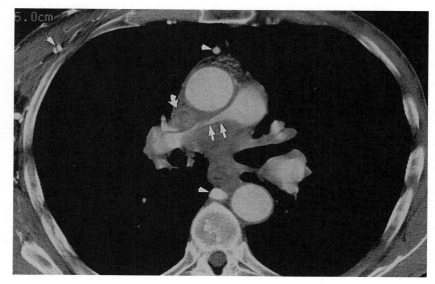

Figure 6–18. Unresectable Pulmonary Carcinoma. Contrast-enhanced CT scan shows extensive mediastinal involvement by tumor with encasement of the right pulmonary artery *(straight arrows)* and obstruction of the superior vena cava *(curved arrow)*. Note collateral venous circulation in the chest wall and mediastinum *(arrowheads)*. The diagnosis was biopsy-proven large cell carcinoma.

found to have T4 disease undetected by CT scan.[107] Although tumors that abut the mediastinum for less than 3 cm generally are resectable and tumors that encase major mediastinal vessels or bronchi are unresectable, there are no reliable criteria to predict resectability of tumors that abut the mediastinum for more than 3 cm but are not associated with major mediastinal extension (Fig. 6–19).[132, 133]

Magnetic Resonance Imaging. MR imaging is superior to CT in the demonstration of the pericardium, cardiac chambers, and mediastinal vessels with the added advantage of not requiring intravenous contrast material.[134, 135] Disruption of the normal 2- to 3-mm low signal intensity of the pericardium is suggestive of pericardial infiltration, although this does not preclude complete surgical resection (Fig. 6–20). Coronal images are particularly helpful in the assessment of tumor extension into the subcarinal region, aortopulmonary window and superior vena cava.[107, 109, 134] Disadvantages of MR imaging include lower spatial resolution and artifacts as a result of respiratory motion.

The merit of MR imaging over CT in the overall assessment of mediastinal invasion is controversial. In two studies, MR imaging was found to be slightly more accurate than CT in the diagnosis of mediastinal invasion.[39, 107] In one of these studies (which involved 170 patients who had non–small cell carcinoma [including 30 patients who had T3 or T4 tumors]), MR imaging allowed better delineation of mediastinal and superior sulcus invasion; however, there was no significant difference in the overall diagnostic accu-

racy between CT and MR imaging.[107] The sensitivity of CT and MR imaging was 63% and 56%, and the specificity was 84% and 80%, for distinguishing T3 and T4 tumors from less extensive pulmonary carcinomas. Similar to CT, the main limitation of MR imaging is the inability to distinguish tumor invasion of mediastinal fat from inflammatory changes.[38, 135]

N (Lymph Nodes)

Radiography. Hilar (N1), ipsilateral (N2) or contralateral (N3) mediastinal lymph node metastases often are present at the time of initial diagnosis of pulmonary carcinoma. The following represent the most widely accepted criteria for radiologic assessment.

1. Lymph nodes should be classified according to a standardized lymph node map. The one adopted by the AJCC and the UICC in 1997 (Fig. 6–21 and Table 6–5) is the preferred scheme at present.[124] Guides to the AJCC-UICC nodal map classification on CT have been published based on the demonstration of enlarged nodes on contrast-enhanced spiral CT.[125, 126]

2. The most reliable and practical measurement of lymph node size on CT is its short-axis diameter (i.e., the shortest diameter on the cross-sectional image); this parameter correlates better than the long-axis diameter with the node volume and is less influenced by the spatial orientation of the node.[136] Although some authors have

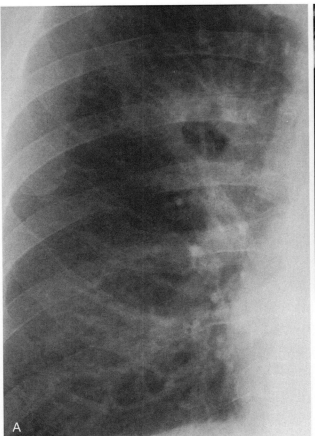

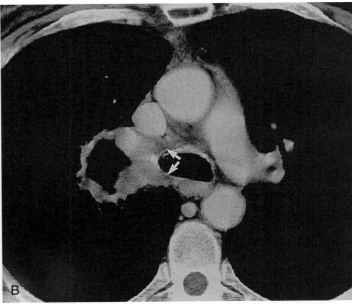

Figure 6–19. Resectable (T3) Pulmonary Carcinoma. View of the right lung from anteroposterior chest radiograph *(A)* shows a 4-cm-diameter, cavitating mass in the right upper lobe. Contrast-enhanced CT scan *(B)* shows the mass as well as soft tissue extension anterior and posterior *(arrows)* to the right main bronchus. The diagnosis of squamous cell carcinoma was confirmed at bronchoscopy. The patient was a 60-year-old man who presented with hemoptysis. The tumor (stage IIIa) was resected completely at pneumonectomy.

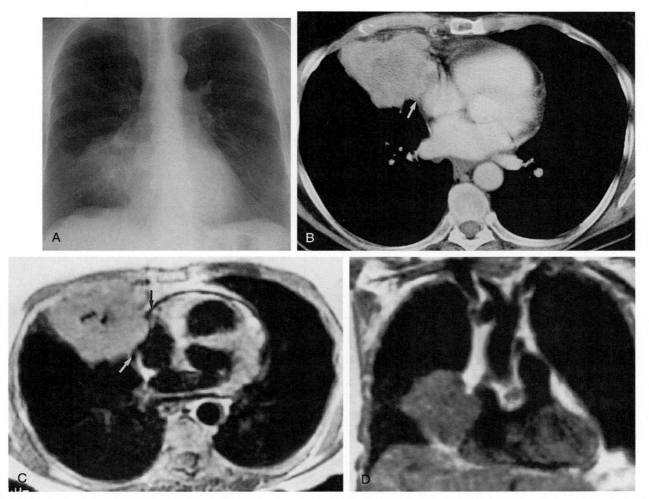

Figure 6–20. Resectable (T3) Pulmonary Carcinoma. Posteroanterior chest radiograph *(A)* in a 62-year-old woman shows a large right middle lobe tumor abutting the heart. Contrast-enhanced CT scan *(B)* shows focal thickening of the pericardium *(arrow)* and focal mediastinal invasion. The extent of mediastinal invasion cannot be assessed reliably on the CT image. Transverse, cardiac-gated, spin-echo MR image *(C)* shows better the pericardium *(arrows)* and the focal extension of tumor as well as focal compression of the right atrium. Coronal MR image *(D)* shows better the relationship of the tumor with the right atrium. Neither the CT nor the MR images allow definite diagnosis or exclusion of invasion of the right atrium. At surgery, this was shown to be a resectable (T3) squamous cell carcinoma with focal pericardial invasion, which compressed the right atrium but did not involve the right atrial wall (stage IIb pulmonary carcinoma).

suggested the use of various nodal size criteria specific for each mediastinal nodal station,[137, 138] for practical reasons we and others consider a diameter greater than 10 mm in short axis as abnormal regardless of nodal station.[56, 108]

3. Factors that facilitate visualization of mediastinal lymph nodes include the presence of mediastinal fat, use of intravenous contrast material, and thinner CT sections. Intravenous contrast material is particularly helpful in the distinction of the truncus anterior from a right paratracheal lymph node and in the assessment of the aortopulmonary window region, where the superior aspect of the main or left pulmonary artery may be misinterpreted as an enlarged lymph node on scans performed without intravenous contrast material. Despite these advantages, we believe that intravenous contrast material is not required routinely for the assessment of mediastinal nodes when using spiral CT technique and 5- to 7-mm collimation scans. In a study of 79 patients, 5-mm collimation scans without the use of intravenous contrast material allowed identification of more nodes than 10-mm-thick sections with intravenous contrast material.[139] In another study of 96 patients who had nonenhanced and contrast-enhanced spiral CT, the staging of mediastinal lymph nodes changed in only 1 patient: from N3 on noncontrast CT to N1 on contrast-enhanced CT.[140] At mediastinoscopy, this patient was found to have N2 disease.

Although intravenous contrast material is not required for the evaluation of mediastinal lymph nodes, assessment of hilar lymph nodes requires the use of intravenous injection of contrast material and dynamic incremental[141] or spiral CT (Fig. 6–22).[142, 143] Intravenous contrast material is recommended in patients in whom hilar lymph node enlargement is suspected on the radiograph.

Although there is no question that CT is superior to chest radiography in the detection of mediastinal lymph node metastases (Fig. 6–23), the specificity for the diagnosis is slightly less.[144, 145] For example, in one study of

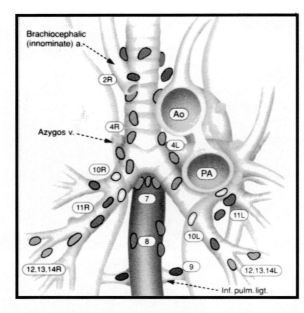

Superior Mediastinal Nodes

- ● **1** Highest Mediastinal
- ● **2** Upper Paratracheal
- ● **3** Pre-vascular and Retrotracheal
- ● **4** Lower Paratracheal (including Azygos Nodes)

N_2 = single digit, ipsilateral
N_3 = single digit, contralateral or supraclavicular

Aortic Nodes

- ● **5** Subaortic (A-P window)
- ● **6** Para-aortic (ascending aorta or phrenic)

Inferior Mediastinal Nodes

- ● **7** Subcarinal
- ● **8** Paraesophageal (below carina)
- ● **9** Pulmonary Ligament

N_1 Nodes

- ○ **10** Hilar
- ● **11** Interlobar
- ○ **12** Lobar
- ○ **13** Segmental
- ○ **14** Subsegmental

Figure 6–21. Regional Lymph Node Stations for Lung Cancer Staging. (From Mountain CF, Dresler CM: Chest 111:1719, 1997.)

418 patients, the sensitivity and specificity of the chest radiograph for the detection of mediastinal lymph node metastases were 40% and 99%; for the same group, CT had a sensitivity and a specificity of 84%.[145] In another investigation of 170 patients, the sensitivity and specificity of the radiograph were 9% and 92%, whereas the corresponding figures for CT were 52% and 69%.[144] Appreciation of mediastinal lymph node enlargement on radiography almost invariably indicates the presence of metastatic carcinoma.

As the results of the previous studies suggest, there has been considerable variability in the reported sensitivity and specificity of CT in the assessment of mediastinal nodal metastases; although several groups have shown a sensitivity greater than 85%,[146, 147] others have reported values of 40% to 70%.[144, 148] This variability is related to several factors, including different size criteria for abnormal lymph nodes, different patient populations studied, use of a per-patient versus a per-nodal station analysis, interobserver variability, and differences in the diagnostic gold standard.

Although there is considerable variability in the reported CT accuracy in the diagnosis of mediastinal lymph node metastases, the authors of a meta-analysis of 42 studies published between 1980 and 1988 concluded that the sensitivity was 83% and the specificity was 81% on a per-patient basis.[149] These figures are similar to those of a prospective multicenter Canadian Lung Oncology Group study of mediastinal nodal metastases, in which CT was found to have a sensitivity of 78% and a specificity of 69%.[150] The results of the latter study showed that CT

Table 6–5. LYMPH NODE MAP DEFINITIONS

Nodal Station	Anatomic Landmarks
N2 nodes—all N2 nodes lie within the mediastinal pleural envelope	
1 Highest mediastinal nodes	Nodes lying above a horizontal line at the upper rim of the brachiocephalic (left innominate) vein where it ascends to the left, crossing in front of the trachea at its midline.
2 Upper paratracheal nodes	Nodes lying above a horizontal line drawn tangential to the upper margin of the aortic arch and below the inferior boundary of No. 1 nodes.
3 Prevascular and retrotracheal nodes	Prevascular and retrotracheal nodes may be designated 3A and 3P; midline nodes are considered to be ipsilateral.
4 Lower paratracheal nodes	The lower paratracheal nodes on the right lie to the right of the midline of the trachea between a horizontal line drawn tangential to the upper margin of the aortic arch and a line extending across the right main bronchus at the upper margin of the upper lobe bronchus and contained within the mediastinal pleural envelope; the lower paratracheal nodes on the left lie to the left of the midline of the trachea between a horizontal line drawn tangential to the upper margin of the aortic arch and a line extending across the left main bronchus at the level of the upper margin of the left upper lobe bronchus, medial to the ligamentum arteriosum and contained within the mediastinal pleural envelope.
	Researchers may wish to designate the lower paratracheal nodes as No. 4s (superior) and No. 4i (inferior) subsets for study purposes. The No. 4s nodes may be defined by a horizontal line extending across the trachea and drawn tangential to the cephalic border of the azygos vein. The No. 4i nodes may be defined by the lower boundary of No. 4s and the lower boundary of No. 4, as described above.
5 Subaortic nodes (aortopulmonary window)	Subaortic nodes are lateral to the ligamentum arteriosum or the aorta or left pulmonary artery and proximal to the first branch of the left pulmonary artery and lie within the mediastinal pleural envelope.
6 Para-aortic nodes (ascending aorta or phrenic)	Nodes lying anterior and lateral to the ascending aorta and the aortic arch or the innominate artery, beneath a line tangential to the upper margin of the aortic arch.
7 Subcarinal nodes	Nodes lying caudal to the carina of the trachea but not associated with the lower lobe bronchi or arteries within the lung.
8 Paraesophageal nodes (below carina)	Nodes lying adjacent to the wall of the esophagus and to the right or left of the midline, excluding subcarinal nodes.
9 Pulmonary ligament nodes	Nodes lying within the pulmonary ligament, including those in the posterior wall and lower part of the inferior pulmonary vein.
N1 nodes—all N1 nodes lie distal to the mediastinal pleural reflection and within the visceral pleura	
10 Hilar nodes	Proximal lobar nodes, distal to the mediastinal pleural reflection and the nodes adjacent to the bronchus intermedius on the right; radiographically, the hilar shadow may be created by enlargement of both hilar and interlobar nodes.
11 Interlobar nodes	Nodes lying between the lobar bronchi.
12 Lobar nodes	Nodes adjacent to the distal lobar bronchi.
13 Segmental nodes	Nodes adjacent to the segmental bronchi.
14 Subsegmental nodes	Nodes around the subsegmental bronchi.

From Mountain CF, Dresler CM: Regional lymph node classification for lung cancer staging. Chest 111:1720, 1997.

was more cost-effective than mediastinoscopy and that CT rather than mediastinoscopy should be performed in all patients who are suspected to have pulmonary carcinoma. Patients who are still considered to have normal-sized nodes may proceed directly to thoracotomy.[150] Because of the relative lack of specificity of enlarged nodes detected by CT alone, biopsy usually is required to confirm the presence of metastases.

Positive nodes missed on CT scan are less likely to be associated with extracapsular spread of tumor than nodes larger than 1 cm in diameter.[151, 152] Patients who have metastasis to normal-sized nodes are more likely to have negative results at mediastinoscopy and to have the affected nodes discovered only at subsequent thoracotomy. There is evidence that patients who have microscopic metastases discovered at the time of thoracotomy have an improved survival rate if the primary tumor and the involved mediastinal nodes are resected.[151]

Magnetic Resonance Imaging. Similar to CT, MR imaging relies on size criteria to determine nodal abnormalities and is comparable to CT in the assessment of mediastinal nodal metastasis.[107, 153]

Positron Emission Tomography. Although CT and MR imaging rely on the anatomic assessment of lymph nodes, PET relies on a biochemical difference between normal and neoplastic cells. Mediastinal nodes containing carcinoma have been shown to have increased uptake and accumulation of FDG (Fig. 6–24). Several groups have shown that PET is superior to CT in the assessment of mediastinal nodal metastases.[154–156] In one study of 99 patients, the sensitivity and specificity for the diagnosis of N2 disease were 83% and 94% for PET compared with 63% and 73% for CT.[155] In another investigation of 100 patients, mediastinal lymph nodes were staged correctly in 85% of cases with PET compared with 58% with CT.[157] The authors of a meta-analysis of 14 studies published between

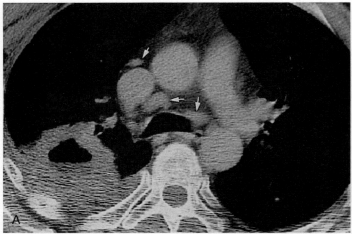

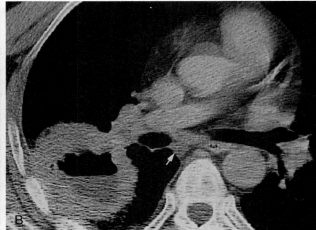

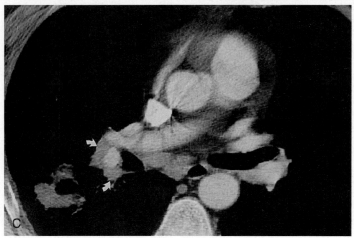

Figure 6–22. Value of Contrast Enhancement. CT scans performed without intravenous contrast material *(A and B)* show 5-cm-diameter, cavitated tumor in the right lung. Mediastinal nodes *(arrows)* can be identified without the use of intravenous contrast material as soft tissue opacities surrounded by fat. The CT scan at the level of the right hilum *(B)* does not allow adequate assessment of hilar and interlobar nodes. After intravenous administration of contrast material *(C)*, the enlarged right hilar nodes *(curved arrows)* can be distinguished readily from the interlobar pulmonary artery. The patient was a 56-year-old man who had surgically proven squamous carcinoma with involvement of the right interlobar (10) lymph nodes. The mediastinal nodes did not contain carcinoma.

1990 and 1998 concluded that the sensitivity of PET for the detection of mediastinal nodal metastases is 79% and the specificity is 91%.[158] By comparison, meta-analysis of 29 studies using CT published during the same period showed a sensitivity of 60% and a specificity of 77%.[158] The sensitivity of PET in the meta-analysis of the studies published in the 1990s is similar to the previously mentioned meta-analysis of CT studies performed in the 1980s,[149] whereas that of CT is substantially lower.

M (Distant Metastases)

The most widely used techniques to investigate patients who have possible extrathoracic metastases are CT (to show metastases to the adrenal glands and liver), MR imaging (to assess the brain and adrenals), and radionuclide scans (to identify skeletal metastases). The use of these techniques should be considered in the context of the clinical picture. In patients who have non–small cell carcinoma, brain MR imaging and radionuclide scanning of bone generally are indicated only if there is clinical or laboratory evidence of metastatic disease. Such evidence includes not only organ-specific signs and symptoms (liver enlargement, bone pain), but also nonspecific symptoms of anorexia, weight loss, and fatigue. In one study of 309 patients who had non–small cell carcinoma in an early

stage (T1 or T2, N0 or N1), routine bone, brain, and liver scans or bone scan and abdominal and brain CT were done before anticipated surgery.[159] Only 1 of the 472 studies (0.2%) revealed an unexpected metastasis; all other metastatic disease detected was associated with clinical signs and symptoms or abnormal biochemical profiles.

In a 1995 meta-analysis of 25 studies that addressed the issue of the appropriateness of preoperative evaluation of metastatic disease, the authors concluded that a negative clinical evaluation had a high negative predictive value (consistently exceeding 90%) for finding occult metastases by bone scan and CT evaluation of the brain and abdomen.[115] These values were more impressive (>97%) when an expanded clinical evaluation, which included consideration of constitutional symptoms, was used. Although some investigators have reported occult brain metastases in asymptomatic individuals, especially those who have adenocarcinoma,[160, 161] such findings must be balanced against the low cost-effectiveness of the procedure. In the meta-analysis cited previously, the prevalence of brain metastases was only 5% in asymptomatic patients. Because gadolinium-enhanced MR imaging is more sensitive than CT in the detection of such metastases, it is possible that the prevalence is higher than that suggested by the CT data.

Routine contrast-enhanced CT through the liver for the staging of lung cancer rarely changes tumor stage and is

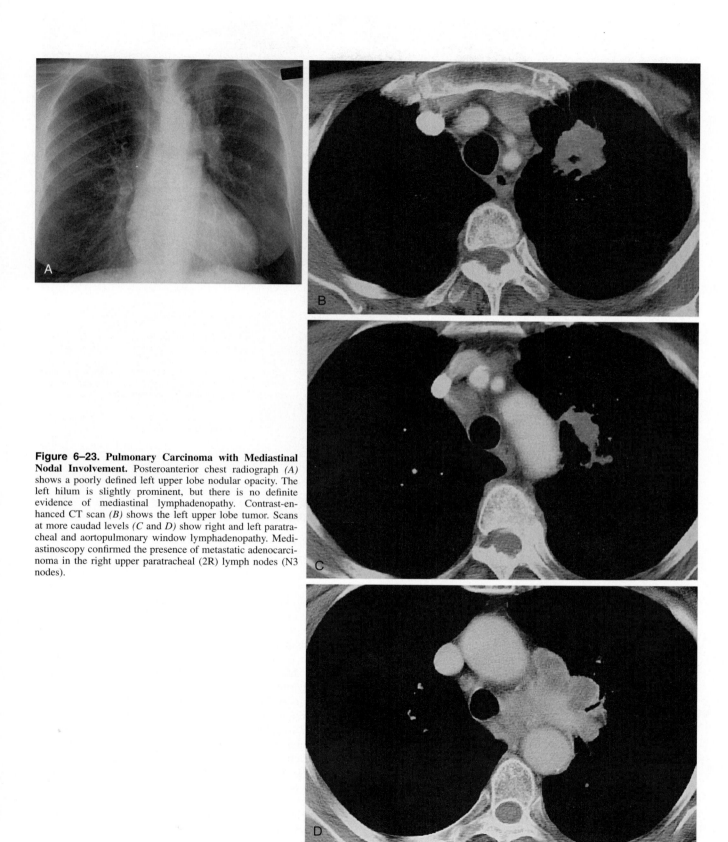

Figure 6–23. Pulmonary Carcinoma with Mediastinal Nodal Involvement. Posteroanterior chest radiograph *(A)* shows a poorly defined left upper lobe nodular opacity. The left hilum is slightly prominent, but there is no definite evidence of mediastinal lymphadenopathy. Contrast-enhanced CT scan *(B)* shows the left upper lobe tumor. Scans at more caudad levels *(C* and *D)* show right and left paratracheal and aortopulmonary window lymphadenopathy. Mediastinoscopy confirmed the presence of metastatic adenocarcinoma in the right upper paratracheal (2R) lymph nodes (N3 nodes).

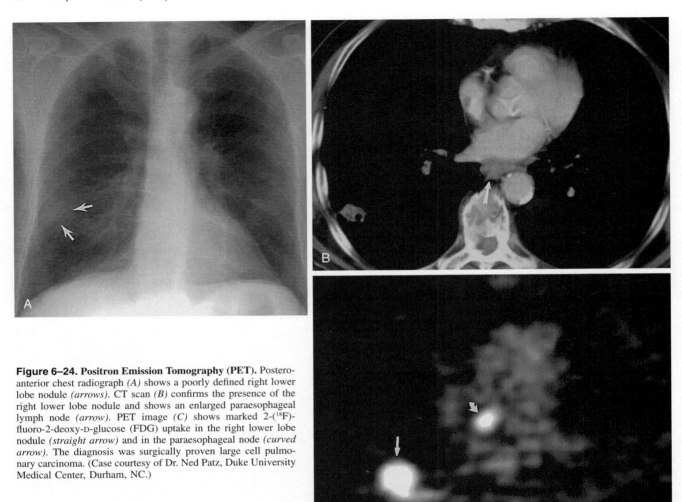

Figure 6–24. Positron Emission Tomography (PET). Posteroanterior chest radiograph *(A)* shows a poorly defined right lower lobe nodule *(arrows)*. CT scan *(B)* confirms the presence of the right lower lobe nodule and shows an enlarged paraesophageal lymph node *(arrow)*. PET image *(C)* shows marked 2-(^{18}F)-fluoro-2-deoxy-D-glucose (FDG) uptake in the right lower lobe nodule *(straight arrow)* and in the paraesophageal node *(curved arrow)*. The diagnosis was surgically proven large cell pulmonary carcinoma. (Case courtesy of Dr. Ned Patz, Duke University Medical Center, Durham, NC.)

not warranted.[104, 115] Because the adrenal glands are common sites for metastatic pulmonary carcinoma and because of the ease of examination, however, most radiologists extend the chest CT scan to include the adrenal glands in patients who have a pulmonary tumor.[47, 140, 162] In one study of 110 patients who had pulmonary carcinoma (cell type not specified), adrenal masses were identified in 11 (10%);[128] in 5 patients, the adrenal glands were the only site of metastasis.

The other main differential diagnosis of an adrenal mass in a patient who has pulmonary carcinoma is a nonfunctioning adenoma. The most helpful diagnostic features on CT scan for distinguishing between a metastasis and an adenoma are tumor size and attenuation value. Lesions 1 cm or less in diameter are more likely to be adenomas, whereas lesions 3 cm or larger usually are metastases (Fig. 6–25). A more reliable distinction is obtained by measuring the attenuation of the mass on an unenhanced CT scan: Adrenal adenomas typically have homogeneous low attenuation, whereas metastases have high attenuation values. As might be expected, the sensitivity and specificity of CT are influenced by the density threshold (attenuation value) used for distinguishing benign from malignant lesions. One group of investigators analyzed the results derived from 10 studies that included a total of 272 benign and 223 malignant adrenal tumors.[163] The sensitivity for detecting the former lesions was 47% at a threshold of 2 HU and 88% at a threshold of 20 HU; the specificity was 100% at a threshold of 2 HU and 84% at a threshold of 20 HU. Although total reliance on attenuation values for distinguishing benign from malignant lesions is unwise, a threshold value of 10 HU generally is accepted as reliable,[164] provided that the mass has homogeneous attenuation and smooth margins. Unenhanced CT with a 10H threshold has a sensitivity of 73% and a specificity of 96% in the diagnosis of adrenal adenoma.[165] Based on the data in the literature prior to 2000, one group of investigators has shown that unenhanced CT with a 10H threshold is currently the most cost-effective method for distinguishing adrenal adenoma from metastasis in patients with newly diagnosed pulmonary carcinoma.[166]

Several groups have assessed the diagnostic accuracy of MR imaging in the detection of adrenal metastases and in their distinction from adenomas. The results of the initial studies showed considerable overlap between the MR signal characteristics of malignant and benign lesions on conventional spin-echo and gradient recalled echo images.[167, 168] The ability to distinguish metastases from adenomas has

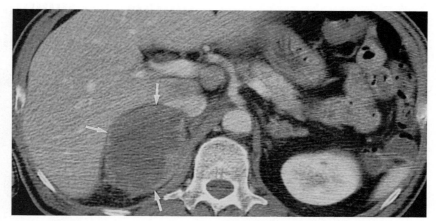

Figure 6–25. Adrenal Metastasis. Contrast-enhanced CT scan in a 69-year-old man shows a 6-cm-diameter, inhomogeneous right adrenal mass *(arrows)*. The diagnosis of metastatic adenocarcinoma was established by ultrasound-guided biopsy. The primary tumor was a 2-cm-diameter left upper lobe pulmonary carcinoma.

improved considerably with the introduction of more sophisticated MR techniques, such as fat saturation, chemical shift, and dynamic gadolinium-enhanced MR imaging.[170–172] On spin-echo MR images performed using fat saturation technique, adrenal adenomas have a characteristic hyperintense rim;[169] in one study of 48 patients, this sign was seen in 26 of 28 (92%) adenomas and in only 1 of 20 (5%) metastases.[169] One group of investigators correlated the MR findings with histologic results in 114 patients with 134 adrenal masses.[172] Chemical shift and dynamic gadolinium-enhanced MR imaging had a sensitivity of 91% and a specificity of 94% in distinguishing benign and malignant adrenal masses.[172]

Preliminary results suggest that FDG-PET imaging can characterize metabolically adrenal masses and allow distinction of adrenal metastases from benign lesions.[173, 174] Whole-body PET imaging has the advantage over other imaging modalities of showing not only adrenal metastases, but also other metastases that may not be apparent on CT, MR imaging, or bone scintigraphy.[157] In one investigation of 100 patients with newly diagnosed pulmonary carcinoma, PET correctly indicated the M status in 40 (91%) of 44 patients with metastatic disease compared with 35 (80%) with conventional imaging.[157] PET and CT correctly identified all six adrenal metastases (sensitivity 100%), but PET had a specificity and positive predictive value of 100% compared with 93% and 46% for CT. PET correctly identified 11 (91%) of 12 patients with bone metastases compared with 6 (50%) identified on scintigraphy; both modalities had a specificity of 92%.[157]

MISCELLANEOUS NEOPLASMS AND NON-NEOPLASTIC TUMORS

Neuroendocrine Neoplasms

Pulmonary neuroendocrine neoplasms show ultrastructural and immunohistochemical features similar to the neuroendocrine cells normally present in small numbers within the tracheobronchial epithelium. The prime example of neuroendocrine neoplasm is the carcinoid tumor. Although some authors also classify small cell carcinoma with neuroendocrine tumors, we prefer to consider it separately because of its closer clinical and epidemiologic association with the other more common forms of pulmonary carcinoma.

Carcinoid Tumor

Pulmonary carcinoid tumor is a low-grade malignant neoplasm believed to be derived from surface or glandular epithelium of the conducting or transitional airways. It is uncommon, accounting for only about 0.5% to 2.5% of all pulmonary neoplasms.[176, 177] It is slightly more common in women than in men; the average age at presentation is 45 years.[179] On the basis of pathologic features, tumors can be divided into typical and atypical types, the latter representing about 10% to 20% of tumors.[178, 179]

Clinical manifestations include cough, expectoration, fever, and chest pain; hemoptysis occurs in 30% to 50% of cases.[180, 195] Some patients have symptoms simulating asthma.[183] Although carcinoid tumors typically contain one or more immunoreactive neuroendocrine products, clinical signs and symptoms related to their presence are uncommon. Carcinoid syndrome is present in fewer than 1% of patients, almost exclusively in patients who have liver metastases.[179] Uncommonly a small tumor is associated with paraneoplastic clinical manifestations, usually Cushing's syndrome.[196]

Radiologic manifestations depend largely on the location of the tumor (Table 6–6). Because 80% to 85% are located in lobar or segmental bronchi, evidence of airway obstruction is the most common radiographic finding. In most cases, the obstruction is complete, with peripheral atelectasis and obstructive pneumonitis. The characteristic radiographic pattern consists of homogeneous increase in density confined precisely to a lobe or to one or more segments, usually with considerable loss of volume (Fig.

Table 6–6. CARCINOID TUMOR

Accounts for 0.5%–2.5% of pulmonary neoplasms
Slightly more common in women
Average age 45 yr
Common symptoms: cough and hemoptysis
80%–85% are central
    Segmental or lobar atelectasis or obstructive pneumonitis
    Endobronchial mass on CT
    Calcification apparent on CT in 40% of cases
15%–20% are peripheral
    Solitary nodule
    Usually homogeneous attenuation and smooth margins
    Calcification apparent on CT in 10%–15% of cases

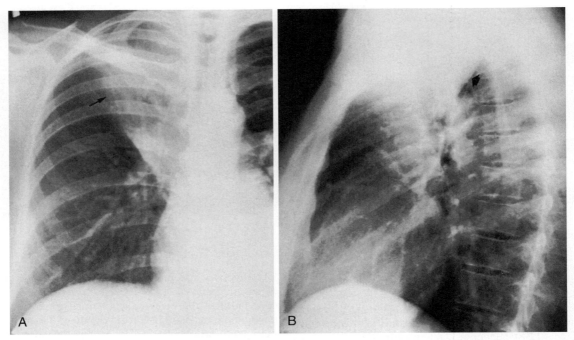

Figure 6–26. Carcinoid Tumor. Views of the right hemithorax from posteroanterior *(A)* and lateral *(B)* radiographs show a roughly triangular shadow of homogeneous density occupying the superomedial portion of the right lung. The inferolateral border of the shadow is formed by the upwardly displaced minor fissure *(arrow in A)* and the posterior border of the anteriorly displaced major fissure *(arrow in B)*. This shadow represents combined consolidation and atelectasis of the right upper lobe resulting from an endobronchial carcinoid tumor. The patient was a 30-year-old woman.

6–26). Segmental atelectasis and pneumonitis may show periodic exacerbations and remissions, presumably reflecting intermittent relief of the obstruction. Recurrent infections distal to the neoplasm can result in bronchiectasis and lung abscesses. Occasionally, retention of mucus in airways distal to the tumor results in mucoid impaction unaccompanied by atelectasis.

When the carcinoid tumor only partially occludes a bronchus, the reduction in ventilation of affected parenchyma can result in hypoxic vasoconstriction and reduction in volume; the oligemia can constitute a subtle but highly suggestive sign of the presence of an endobronchial lesion and should lead to a recommendation for bronchoscopy (Fig. 6–27).[181] This phenomenon has been reported in cases in which carcinoid tumors arising in main bronchi caused expiratory air-trapping and marked reduction in perfusion of whole lungs.[182, 183]

Peripheral carcinoid tumors appear radiologically as solitary nodules. They usually are homogeneous in density, sharply defined, round or oval, and slightly lobulated.[184, 194] Most measure 1 to 3 cm in diameter,[177, 193] although they may grow to 10 cm.[184, 186]

Despite the fairly common demonstration of bone within carcinoid tumors pathologically, ossification seldom is visible on the chest radiograph;[187, 188] in one review of 72 patients, it was documented in only 3 (4%).[189] The abnormality can be identified on CT scan in approximately 30% of cases.[185, 190] Ossification is more common in central than in peripheral tumors: In two studies, it was identified in 3 of 5 (60%)[185] and 7 of 18 (39%)[190] central carcinoids and in only 1 of 7 (14%) and 1 of 13 (8%) peripheral tumors. The pattern of calcification is variable and may include

small or large; smooth or irregular; and central, eccentric, or peripheral foci.[185, 190]

Atypical carcinoid tumors tend to be larger than typical tumors (Fig. 6–28), sometimes attaining a huge size.[191] They are associated more commonly with hilar and mediastinal lymph node enlargement.[192, 193]

Neoplasms of Tracheobronchial Glands

Neoplasms of tracheobronchial glands account for 0.1% to 0.2% of all tracheobronchial tumors;[197, 198] most are adenoid cystic or mucoepidermoid carcinoma; other varieties are exceptionally rare. Clinical manifestations include cough, dyspnea, hoarseness, wheezing, and hemoptysis.

Adenoid Cystic Carcinoma

Approximately 80% of lower respiratory tract adenoid cystic carcinomas arise in the trachea and main bronchi (about equal frequency in each location);[200, 201] approximately 10% to 15% develop in the lung periphery.[202] Although the tumor forms an extremely small proportion of neoplasms arising in the bronchi, its relative incidence in the trachea is much higher, where, with squamous cell carcinoma, it comprises most primary tumors.[197, 198]

The conventional radiographic features of adenoid cystic carcinoma consist of an endotracheal or endobronchial lobulated, polypoid or smooth, hemispheric mass that encroaches on the airway lumen to a variable degree (Fig. 6–29).[203, 204] CT is superior to chest radiography in showing the presence of tracheal tumors and is particularly helpful in assessing the presence of extraluminal extent and mediastinal invasion (*see* Fig. 6–29).[199, 205]

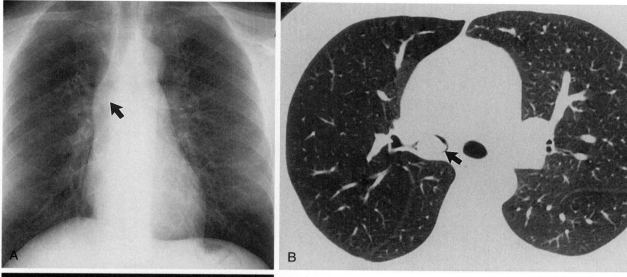

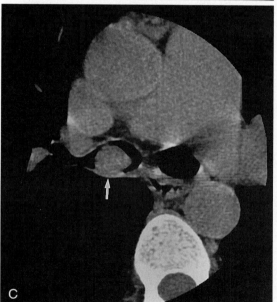

Figure 6–27. Central Carcinoid Tumor—Partial Airway Obstruction with Hypoxic Vasoconstriction. Posteroanterior chest radiograph (A) in a 48-year-old woman shows a tumor in the right main bronchus (arrow). The right lung is slightly smaller than the left and shows decreased vascularity. HRCT scan (B) confirms the presence of intraluminal tumor in the right main bronchus (arrow); decreased vascularity and decreased attenuation of the right lung in comparison to the left are evident, presumably as a result of reflex vasoconstriction. Soft tissue windows (C) show focal thickening of the posterior wall of the right main bronchus (arrow); there is no evidence of extrabronchial extension. The diagnosis of typical carcinoid tumor was made at bronchoscopy and confirmed at surgery.

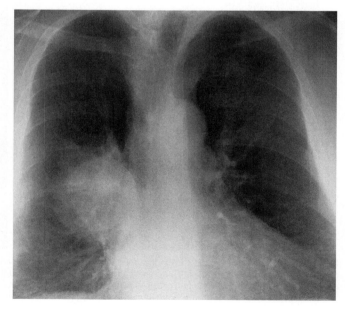

Figure 6–28. Atypical Carcinoid Tumor. Chest radiograph in a 64-year-old man shows a 6-cm-diameter mass in the right lower lobe. At surgery, the patient also had right hilar lymph node metastases.

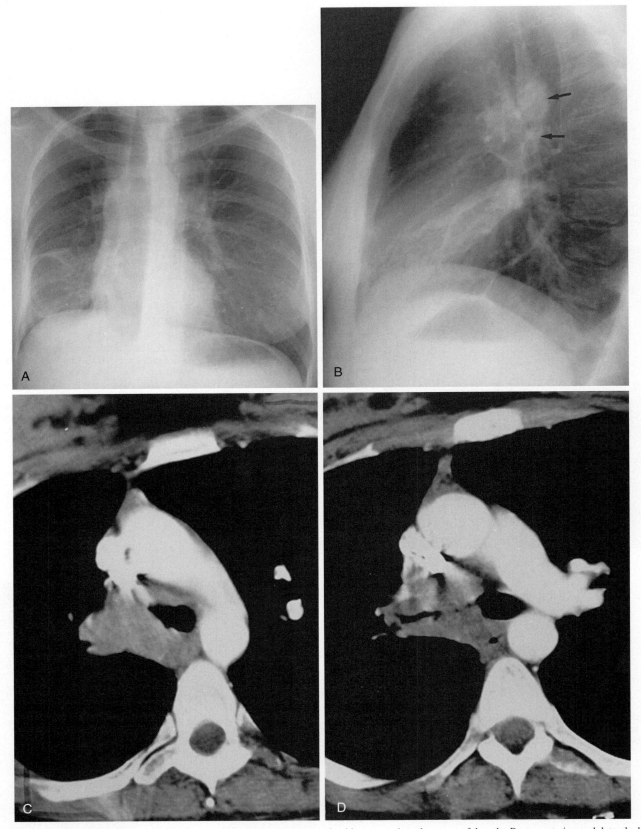

Figure 6–29. Adenoid Cystic Carcinoma. A 27-year-old man presented with progressive shortness of breath. Posteroanterior and lateral chest radiographs *(A* and *B)* show areas of atelectasis in the right lower and middle lobes. Lateral radiograph also shows thickening of the posterior wall of the distal trachea and right bronchus *(arrows)*. Contrast-enhanced CT scans *(C* and *D)* show circumferential tumor at the level of the tracheal carina and right main and right upper lobe bronchi with associated narrowing of the lumen. Focal extension into the left main bronchus is evident.

Mucoepidermoid Carcinoma

After adenoid cystic carcinoma, mucoepidermoid carcinoma probably is the most common form of tracheobronchial gland neoplasm;[206, 208] despite this, only 7 cases (2 tracheal and 5 bronchial) were identified in one series during the same period as were 4,250 primary pulmonary carcinomas (a proportion of only 0.16%).[318]

The radiologic appearance depends on tumor location, size, and presence or absence of obstructive pneumonitis. The radiographic findings consist of a solitary nodule or mass, lobar or segmental consolidation or atelectasis, or a central mass with associated obstructive pneumonitis or atelectasis.[206, 207] On CT scan, the tumors usually are smoothly oval or lobulated in shape.[207] Punctate calcification within the tumor is evident on CT scan in 50% of cases.[207] Occasionally the tumors may involve the trachea rather than the bronchi and present as a polypoid intraluminal nodule on radiograph and CT scan.[205]

Tracheobronchial Papillomas

Multiple Papillomas

Squamous papillomatosis of the respiratory tract is an uncommon abnormality that usually is seen in the larynx of children 18 months to 3 years old.[209] There is convincing evidence from immunohistochemical, ultrastructural, and molecular biologic studies that most, if not all, cases are caused by human papillomavirus.[211, 212] Although most papillomas are limited to the larynx, involvement of the lower respiratory tract occurs occasionally. The average time between the appearance of lesions in the larynx and the detection of bronchopulmonary disease is 10 years.[210] Clinically the diagnosis should be suspected in any patient who has a history of laryngeal papillomas and who develops cough, hemoptysis, asthma-like symptoms, recurrent pneumonia, or atelectasis.

Tracheal and bronchial papillomas may be identified on radiograph and CT scan as small nodules projecting into the lumen of the airway.[204] On CT scan, the presence of numerous papillomas may be manifested as diffuse nodular thickening of the trachea.[214] The papillomas may lead to bronchial obstruction, resulting in atelectasis, obstructive pneumonitis, and bronchiectasis.[215, 216] Involvement of distal airways and parenchyma can result in multiple, sharply circumscribed nodules.[216, 217] These nodules tend to be located in the perihilar lung parenchyma and are most numerous in the posterior half of the thorax.[216] The nodules may grow to several centimeters in diameter, at which point they frequently become cavitated and have walls measuring 2 to 3 mm in thickness (Fig. 6–30).[204, 216] Fluid levels sometimes can be identified.[216] Many of these cavities are related to papillomatosis; however, they may be caused by a complicating necrotic squamous cell carcinoma[213] or an abscess secondary to obstructive pneumonitis.[218]

Solitary Papilloma

Solitary papillomas of the tracheobronchial tree are less common than the multiple form. They almost invariably occur in adults, often middle-aged or older, and usually in men.[219, 220] The radiologic manifestations depend on the size and location of the papilloma. Many lesions that occur in the trachea or main bronchi measure less than 1 cm in diameter and are not detected on chest radiograph.[199] When radiologic and CT findings are evident, they usually consist of a polypoid mass projecting into the airway lumen.[204, 205] Partial bronchial obstruction may result in reflex vasocon-

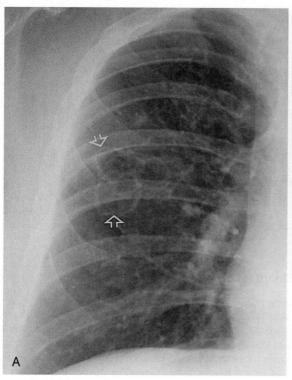

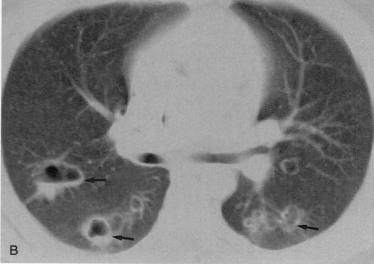

Figure 6–30. Tracheobronchial Papillomatosis. View of the right lung from posteroanterior chest radiograph *(A)* reveals several thin-walled cavities *(arrows).* Similar findings were present in the left lung. CT scan *(B)* shows bilateral thin-walled cavities, several of which contain air-fluid levels *(arrows).* The patient was a 31-year-old woman with long-standing tracheobronchial papillomatosis. (Case courtesy of Dr. Jim Barrie, University of Alberta Hospital, Edmonton, Alberta.)

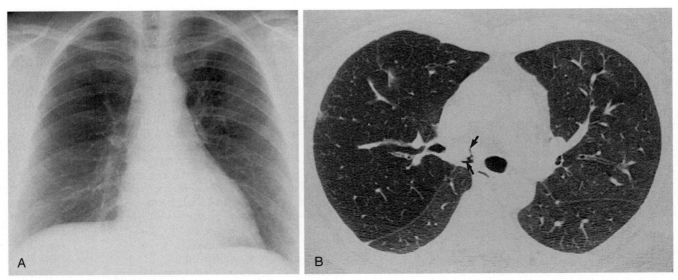

Figure 6–31. Endobronchial Papilloma. Posteroanterior chest radiograph *(A)* in a 51-year-old woman shows a subtle decrease in vascularity and hyperlucency of the right upper lobe, features that are easier to appreciate on HRCT scan *(B)*. HRCT scan also shows a soft tissue tumor *(arrows)* within the right main bronchus. The patient presented with a history of progressive wheezing and had been diagnosed as having asthma. The diagnosis of endobronchial papilloma was confirmed by bronchoscopic biopsy and resection.

striction leading to decreased perfusion and hyperlucency of the affected lung or lobe (Fig. 6–31). Complete obstruction is manifested by atelectasis and obstructive pneumonitis.

Hamartoma

A hamartoma is a tumor-like malformation composed of tissues that normally are present in the organ in which the tumor occurs, but in which the tissue elements, although mature, are disorganized. In the lung, the term traditionally has been used to refer to a parenchymal tumor that is lobulated in contour and consists predominantly of cartilage and adipose tissue; similar tumors occur occasionally in endobronchial and, exceptionally, in endotracheal[222] locations. Despite the widespread use of the term *hamartoma*, the belief that these lesions represent true developmental malformations has been questioned,[221, 223] and it is now generally believed that they are regarded better as benign neoplasms, probably derived from a bronchial wall mesenchymal cell.

Hamartomas are uncommon pulmonary tumors (Table 6–7). In one study of 2,958 solitary lung tumors, 5.7% were found to be hamartomas.[48] Most hamartomas are discovered in adulthood, with a peak incidence in the 50s.[224] Most do not cause symptoms.

The radiologic manifestations typically consist of a well-circumscribed, smoothly marginated solitary nodule without lobar predilection (Fig. 6–32).[48] Most are smaller than 4 cm in diameter.[48, 224] Although calcification has been identified pathologically in 15% of tumors in some series,[226] it is visible on chest radiograph in less than 10% of cases.[227] The radiographic pattern of calcification may resemble popcorn; although virtually diagnostic, this appearance is relatively uncommon. As indicated previously, serial radiography may reveal slow or (exceptionally) rapid growth,[225] increasing the difficulty in differentiation from pulmonary carcinoma. Cavitation (*cystic hamartoma*) is extremely rare.[228, 229]

CT findings were reported in a study of 31 proven and 16 presumed tumors.[49] CT was performed using thin sections (2-mm collimation); the criteria permitting a diagnosis of hamartoma included a smoothly contoured nodule 2.5 cm or less in diameter and focal collections of fat (CT numbers between −40 and −120 HU in at least eight voxels) or fat alternating with areas of calcification (CT numbers >175 HU) (*see* Fig. 6–32). Of the 47 tumors, 17 showed no discernible calcium or fat (the diagnosis was made by other means), 2 showed diffuse calcification, 18 showed areas of fat, and 10 showed foci of calcium and fat; 28 (60%) of the 47 hamartomas were diagnosed correctly by CT without the necessity of a more invasive procedure. Occasionally, hamartomas show focal areas of calcification without evidence of fat (Fig. 6–33).

Non-Neoplastic Tumors

Plasma cell granuloma and *fibrous histiocytoma* are terms that refer to a group of pulmonary tumors characterized histologically by a mixture of fibroblasts, histiocytes, lymphocytes, and plasma cells. Because the proportion of these cells varies considerably from tumor to tumor, a variety of terms has been employed to describe them, and

Table 6–7. HAMARTOMA

Accounts for 6% of solitary nodules
Peak incidence: 50–60 yr
Asymptomatic
Well-defined nodule, smooth margins
Usually measures less than 4 cm in diameter
60% show foci of fat on 1–2 mm collimation CT
25% show foci of calcification on thin-section CT
Popcorn-like calcification seldom evident on radiograph

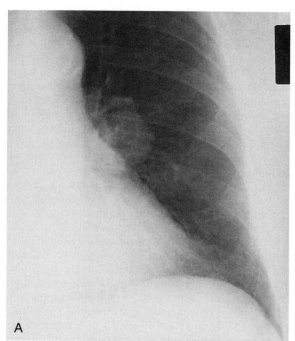

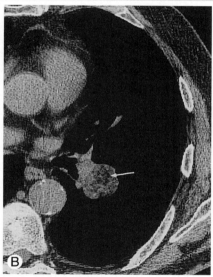

Figure 6–32. Pulmonary Hamartoma. View of the left lung from posteroanterior chest radiograph *(A)* shows a 3-cm-diameter nodule adjacent to the left hilum. HRCT scan *(B)* performed through the center of the nodule shows focal areas of fat *(arrows)*. This CT appearance is diagnostic of pulmonary hamartoma.

a dual concept of their pathogenesis was considered at one time. There is, however, considerable histologic overlap between the two forms of tumor—tumors composed predominantly of fibroblasts containing focal areas characteristic of plasma cell granuloma, and vice versa.[230] As a result, it is now widely believed that these tumors represent a single entity with a variable histologic appearance and that they should all be designated *inflammatory pseudotumor*[232] or *inflammatory myofibroblastic tumor.*[233] In one review of 181 cases, there was an age range of 1 to 72 years and no sex predominance;[236] however, a high proportion occur in children and adolescents, and they have been considered

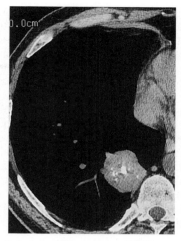

Figure 6–33. Pulmonary Hamartoma. HRCT scan shows a 4-cm-diameter tumor in the right lower lobe; several foci of calcification are evident. The diagnosis of hamartoma was proved at surgery. The patient was an asymptomatic 52-year-old man.

the most common primary pulmonary tumor in this age group.[231]

Radiologic manifestations consist of a solitary pulmonary nodule or a homogeneous area of consolidation that can mimic a primary or metastatic neoplasm (Fig. 6–34).[234, 235] Calcification is present occasionally,[235] and cavitation rarely is present.[231] Endobronchial tumors can cause obstructive pneumonitis. In a review of 60 patients who had inflammatory pseudotumors from the Armed Forces Institute of Pathology, 52 (87%) were found to have solitary peripheral nodules or masses; 3 (5%), multiple nodules; 2, mediastinal masses; and 1 each, an endotracheal or

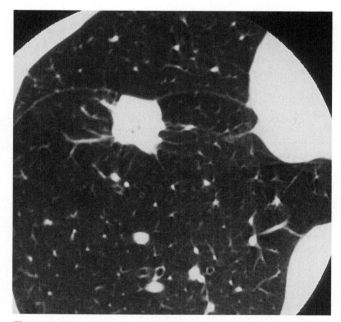

Figure 6–34. Inflammatory Pseudotumor. HRCT scan shows a lobulated, spiculated soft tissue lesion in the right lower lobe. Small areas of low attenuation consistent with air (bubble lucencies) are evident within the lesion. Histologic assessment of the resected specimen showed an inflammatory pseudotumor. The patient was asymptomatic.

endobronchial tumor and with a sharply defined circumscribed pleural mass.[237] Tumors were larger than 3 cm in diameter in 31 patients. Secondary airway luminal involvement by a parenchymal lesion was identified in six patients and lobar atelectasis in five. Hilar or mediastinal lymph node enlargement and pleural effusion occurred in a few cases.

On CT scan, the lesions had smooth or lobulated margins; homogeneous or heterogeneous attenuation; and either no enhancement or homogeneous, heterogeneous, or peripheral rim enhancement after intravenous administration of contrast medium.[237] Heterogeneous signal intensity was evident on T1-weighted MR images and high signal intensity on T2-weighted images; the endotracheal tumor showed heterogeneous enhancement on MR imaging after administration of gadolinium.

PULMONARY METASTASES

The entire output of the right side of the heart as well as virtually all lymphatic fluid produced by body tissues flows through the pulmonary vascular system. Secondary neoplastic involvement of the lungs is common, with the incidence of pulmonary metastases ranging from 30% to almost 55% in various series.[238–240]

Depending on the predominant location of tumor, pulmonary metastases can be considered under four headings: (1) parenchymal nodules, (2) interstitial thickening (lymphangitic spread of tumor), (3) pulmonary hypertension and infarction (tumor emboli), and (4) airway obstruction (endobronchial tumor) (Table 6–8).

Parenchymal Nodules

The most common manifestation of neoplastic metastases to the lungs consists of one or more nodules within the parenchyma. These nodules usually are derived from small tumor emboli that lodge in peripheral pulmonary arteries or arterioles and subsequently extend into the adjacent lung tissue. Nodules are multiple in most cases and tend to be most numerous in the basal portions of the lungs, reflecting

---

Table 6–8. PULMONARY METASTASES: PATTERNS OF PRESENTATION

Parenchymal Nodules
  Most common presentation
  Usually multiple: any extrathoracic primary
  Single nodule: carcinoma (Ca) of colon or kidneys and osteosarcoma
  Cavitation: Ca of head and neck or cervix
  Lower lobe and peripheral predominance
  Spiral CT is most reliable imaging method for detection
Lymphangitic Carcinomatosis
  Common primaries: Ca of lungs, breast, stomach, and pancreas
    Thickening of interlobular septa
    Thickening of peribronchovascular interstitium
    Thickening may be smooth or nodular
    Usually bilateral except in pulmonary carcinoma
    Lymphadenopathy in 30% of patients
    Pleural effusion in 30% of patients
Pulmonary Hypertension and Infarction: Rare
Endobronchial or Endotracheal Metastases: Uncommon
  Usually Ca of breast, colorectum, kidneys, or melanoma
  Partial or complete airway obstruction

---

the effect of gravity on blood flow.[246, 247] They range in size from barely visible to huge growths that occupy virtually the entire volume of a lung. Although most often discrete, individual deposits may enlarge and become confluent, resulting in multinodular masses. When multiple, the nodules usually are of varying size; less often, they are approximately equal, suggesting a single shower of tumor emboli. Rarely, nodular deposits are so numerous and of such minute size as to suggest the diagnosis of miliary tuberculosis radiographically and pathologically.[248]

CT has a considerably greater sensitivity than chest radiography for the identification of pulmonary metastases.[250, 252] The sensitivity is influenced by the technique employed. Using conventional CT with contiguous 10-mm collimation scans, sensitivity is approximately 70%;[252] however, detection of nodules is improved significantly with the use of spiral CT,[254] particularly by using 3- to 5-mm collimation and performing overlapping reconstructions.[255] The sensitivity of spiral CT in the detection of pulmonary nodules in patients with extrathoracic malignancies was assessed in a study of 13 patients who had a total of 90 surgically proven pulmonary nodules.[256] Spiral CT was performed using a slice thickness of 5 mm and reconstruction intervals of 3 mm and 5 mm. The sensitivity was 95% for nodules equal or greater than 6 mm in diameter and 69% for nodules smaller than 6 mm. For lesions smaller than 10 mm in diameter, sensitivity was better using a reconstruction interval of 3 mm rather than of 5 mm.[256] Detection can be improved further by cine viewing of spiral CT scans on a workstation as compared with static film-based images.[257] Despite this increased sensitivity, CT does not allow detection of all metastatic nodules and small lesions; in particular, nodules less than 3 mm in diameter frequently are missed.[258, 259]

Although CT is highly sensitive in the detection of pulmonary metastases, it is not specific; many of the nodules identified represent granulomas or pulmonary lymphoid nodules.[252, 253] In one study of 91 patients with known extrathoracic malignancy, of whom 31 underwent resection, 27 (87%) were found to have primary or metastatic disease, and 4 were found to have benign lesions.[249] Because many false-positive diagnoses with CT are related to granulomas, the specificity of CT is greater in areas in which tuberculosis and fungal disease are less common. In two studies from the United Kingdom, where fungal granulomas are virtually nonexistent, 94% of 200 nodules[260] and 98% of 100 nodules[261] were metastases.

The presence of pulmonary metastases can be assessed using MR imaging.[262, 263] In an early study using spin-echo MR imaging at 0.35 T, small nodules adjacent to vessels often were missed on CT scan but could be identified with MR imaging.[262] Nodules near the diaphragm frequently were missed because of respiratory motion. In an investigation of 11 patients, the results of MR imaging performed at 0.5 T were compared with those of CT and chest radiography.[263] MR imaging and CT allowed detection of at least one metastatic nodule in all cases compared with 64% of cases on chest radiography. MR imaging was as sensitive as CT in the detection of individual nodules. Of the various MR sequences used, the short inversion time inversion-recovery (STIR) sequences had the highest sensitivity for the detection of individual nodules. Although no false-positive interpretations were seen on CT, 13 were made on MR imaging; these were most common in the lower lobes, presumably as a result of diaphragmatic motion. Although these studies suggest a potential role for MR imaging in the assessment of pulmonary metastases, we consider that its current shortcomings outweigh its benefits and recommend CT as the imaging modality of choice.

When pulmonary parenchymal nodules are multiple, the probability that they represent metastases is increased; conversely, although a solitary nodule can be a metastasis, the possibility that it represents a primary carcinoma is increased. From a diagnostic viewpoint, neoplastic parenchymal nodules can be discussed under the headings *solitary* and *multiple*.

Solitary Nodules

Metastatic neoplasms that present as solitary parenchymal nodules comprise a distinct group that must be differentiated from any other cause of a solitary nodule in the lungs (Fig. 6–35). They are relatively uncommon, account-

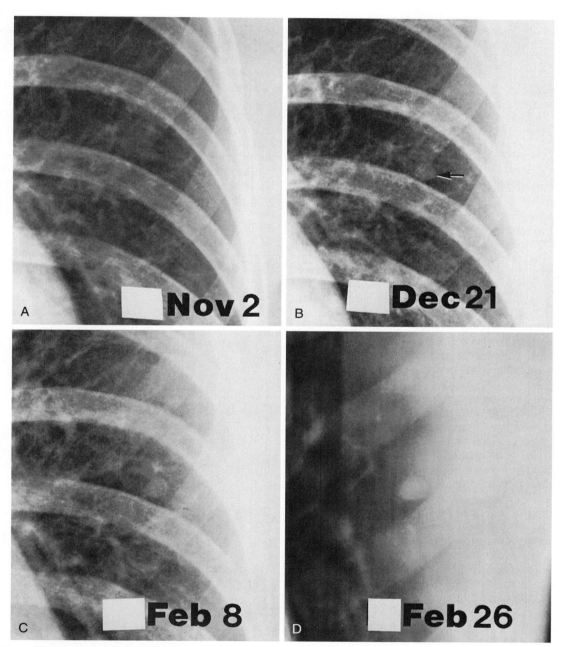

Figure 6–35. Solitary Metastasis from Wilms' Tumor. Detail views of left midlung zone from four sequential radiographs, covering a span of almost 4 months. In the first radiograph *(A)*, an abnormality cannot be identified, even in retrospect. Slightly less than 2 months later *(B)*, a tiny nodule measuring 6 mm in diameter had appeared *(arrow)*. Two months later *(C and D)*, the nodule had increased to 8 mm in diameter, representing a doubling in volume. This 19-year-old man had had a left nephrectomy many years previously for Wilms' tumor; subsequently the upper lobe of the right lung and the right lobe of the liver had been resected for metastatic disease. The nodule shown on these radiographs appeared 1 year after the lobectomy and partial hepatectomy. On resection, it proved to be metastatic Wilms' tumor.

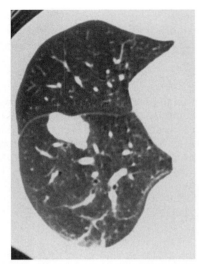

Figure 6–36. Lobulated Metastasis. CT scan shows a 3-cm-diameter nodule with a lobulated contour within the right lower lobe. At thoracotomy, this was proved to be metastatic adenocarcinoma, the primary site being the colon.

ing for only about 2% to 10% of cases of solitary pulmonary nodules.[46, 47] In one study of 634 patients who had solitary nodules on CT scan, 72 of the lesions (11%) were proved to represent metastases from an extrathoracic neoplasm;[46] 71 of the 72 nodules measured 0.5 to 3 cm in diameter. In another investigation of 275 patients who had CT findings interpreted as consistent with pulmonary carcinoma, 6 (2%) proved to have metastatic disease.[47] Most of these solitary metastatic lesions occur in patients aged 45 years and older.[46] Certain primary neoplasms are more likely than others to produce solitary metastases, including carcinoma of the colon (particularly of the rectosigmoid area), kidney, testicle, and breast; sarcomas (particularly those originating in bone); and malignant melanoma.[41, 264]

On high-resolution computed tomography (HRCT) scan, approximately 50% of metastatic nodules have smooth margins, and 50% have irregular margins.[58, 265] They may be round or oval or have a lobulated contour (Fig. 6–36). Irregular margins with spiculation may result from a desmoplastic reaction or tumor infiltration within the adjacent bronchovascular connective tissue or lymphatics (lymphangitic spread).[58, 265]

Identification of a concomitant primary neoplasm elsewhere or a history of prior neoplasia does not indicate that a solitary nodule in the lung is metastatic.[252] In one investigation of 50 patients previously treated for a malignancy and without evidence of metastases elsewhere, 18 had single intrathoracic lesions that proved to be unrelated pulmonary or mediastinal tumors;[266] 9 others had benign pulmonary lesions. In another series of 54 patients with known colonic carcinoma and a solitary pulmonary nodule, only 25 lesions were found to be metastases.[267]

In patients who have an extrathoracic malignancy and a solitary nodule on radiograph or CT scan, additional nodules frequently are identified at surgery.[251, 252] For example, in one study of 84 patients with known extrathoracic malignancy, a solitary nodule was seen in 65 lungs on chest radiography;[252] in 21 (32%) of these, more than one nodule was found on CT scan. In 9 of the remaining 44 lungs (20%) in which only one nodule was shown on CT scan, additional nodules were found at surgery. In the other 35 (80%), only one nodule was found at surgery.

The distinction between a new primary and a metastasis has important prognostic and therapeutic implications, particularly with the increasing use of pulmonary metastatectomy.[268, 269] Although there is debate about the efficacy of this procedure, review of the literature suggests that it is likely to be beneficial in selected patients with certain neoplasms.[269a] With few exceptions, there are no criteria by which a solitary metastasis can be distinguished definitively from a primary pulmonary carcinoma on the chest radiograph or CT scan (Fig. 6–37).[46, 47] Despite this lack of criteria, certain features are associated with an increased probability of one or the other.[270] The nature of the primary extrapulmonary tumor is important: A solitary nodule in a patient who has a high-grade sarcoma or deeply invasive melanoma is much more likely to be a metastasis than a new primary. Such a nodule in a patient who has a squamous cell carcinoma of the oropharyngeal region is possibly a primary pulmonary carcinoma. The time interval between the initial tumor and the appearance of the pulmonary lesion is important, although not independent of tumor type. An interval greater than 5 years in a patient who has

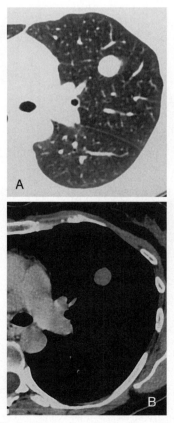

Figure 6–37. Single Metastasis—CT Findings. CT scans *(A and B)* show a smoothly marginated, noncalcified nodule in the left upper lobe; the appearance is indistinguishable from that of a noncalcified granuloma. At thoracotomy, this was proved to be a single metastatic leiomyosarcoma. The primary site subsequently was determined to be the lower extremity.

a history of osteosarcoma is almost certain to be associated with a new pulmonary primary; however, in carcinomas originating in the breast or kidney, in which metastases can occur many years after the original tumor is identified, this conclusion is less likely to be correct. Older age and a history of cigarette smoking increase the likelihood that the tumor is primary in the lung.

When a solitary pulmonary nodule is identified in a patient who does not have a history of cancer, some physicians put the patient through a battery of radiologic and other diagnostic procedures in an attempt to identify or exclude a primary nonpulmonary malignancy. Because most such searches are fruitless,[271, 272] however, we believe that search for an extrapulmonary primary in the presence of a solitary pulmonary nodule should be limited to cases in which there is specific organ dysfunction.

Multiple Nodules

The radiographic pattern of multiple pulmonary nodules varies from diffuse micronodular shadows resembling miliary disease to large, well-defined *cannonball* masses (Fig. 6–38). In the former situation, the lesions may be of uniform size, indicating a simultaneous origin in one shower of emboli, or may differ, suggesting embolic events of different ages. Although most individual shadows usually are defined fairly sharply, some may be indistinct; when these shadows reach 5 to 6 mm in diameter, they can simulate air-space disease.[273]

On CT scan, nodular metastases are seen most commonly in the outer third of the lungs, particularly the subpleural regions of the lower zones.[158, 251] Although metastases less than 2 cm in diameter frequently are round and have smooth margins (Fig. 6–39), they may have various shapes; larger nodules frequently are lobulated and have irregular margins.[274, 275] Irregular margins appear to be particularly common in metastatic adenocarcinoma.[265] Occasionally a halo of ground-glass attenuation can be seen to surround the nodules, a finding that is most common in highly vascular or hemorrhagic tumors, such as angiosarcoma.[276]

Although intravascular tumor emboli can be seen histopathologically in many patients who have nodular metastases, they tend to occur in arterioles or small arteries and usually are not seen on CT scan.[265] Rarely, they can be identified as nodular or beaded thickening of the peripheral pulmonary arteries (Fig. 6–40).[277] Although this appearance may suggest the diagnosis of metastasis, a similar appearance has been reported in a patient who had perivascular granulomatous inflammation caused by *Histoplasma capsulatum*.[278] It has been suggested that pulmonary vessels often can be seen leading directly to the pulmonary metastasis (the *feeding vessel* sign).[279, 280] Although this finding is seen with metastatic tumors, it is uncommon. In one analysis of the HRCT and pathologic findings of 190 nodules, including radiographs and stereomicroscopy of autopsy specimens, only 21 (11%) were found to be related closely to a vessel (more specifically, the centrilobular bronchovascular bundle).[281] A total of 130 (68%) nodules were located between the centrilobular bronchovascular bundle and the perilobular structures, and 39 (21%) were in the periphery of the secondary pulmonary lobule. The vessels supplying the metastatic nodule could not be visualized on HRCT scan.[281]

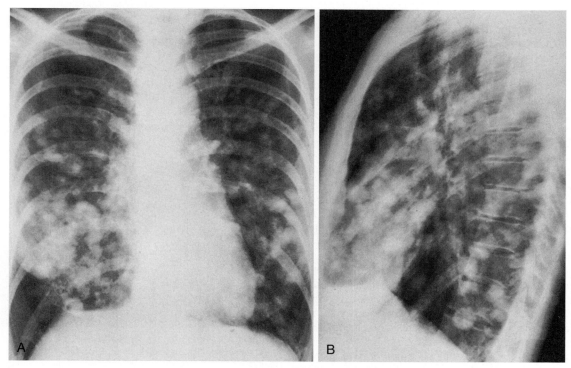

Figure 6–38. Metastatic Adenoid Cystic Carcinoma of the Left Submaxillary Gland—Multiple Parenchymal Nodules. Posteroanterior *(A)* and lateral *(B)* radiographs reveal multiple nodules of homogeneous density ranging in size from 5 mm to 2 cm, distributed widely through both lungs. The apices and bases are relatively less affected than the midzones. There is no evidence of cavitation.

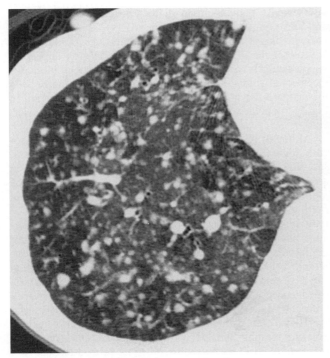

Figure 6–39. Metastatic Carcinoma—CT Appearance. CT scan shows numerous, smoothly marginated nodules 2 to 10 mm in diameter in the right lower lobe. The patient was a 70-year-old woman with metastatic adenocarcinoma of unknown primary.

Cavitation of nodular metastases is not as common as in primary lung carcinoma;[282, 283] in one report, it was identified in 4% of metastatic deposits and 9% of primary neoplasms.[283] Similar to primary pulmonary tumors, the complication occurs most often in squamous cell carcinoma and is more common in the upper than the lower lobes. The site of the primary neoplasm is most frequently in the head and neck in men (Fig. 6–41) and the cervix in women.[283, 284] Although uncommon, cavitation also can occur in metastatic adenocarcinoma, particularly in lesions originating in the large bowel,[283, 285] and in metastatic sarcoma, particularly osteogenic; excavation of the latter may account for the relatively high incidence of concomitant pneumothorax in this tumor (*see* farther on).

Calcification of metastatic lesions is rare and almost invariably indicates that the primary neoplasm is osteogenic sarcoma, chondrosarcoma, or synovial sarcoma (Fig. 6–42).[286] If small, such metastases can mimic benign lesions; in one patient who had metastatic synovial sarcoma, one nodule simulated a hamartoma, and two others simulated granulomas.[286] Calcification can develop at the site of pulmonary metastases that have vanished after successful chemotherapy.[287] This chemotherapeutic effect can be manifested as persistent nodules that, on histologic examination, show only necrosis and fibrosis without residual viable neoplastic tissue.[288, 289] Metastatic testicular neoplasms are particularly prone to this outcome.[316, 317]

The occurrence of spontaneous pneumothorax in association with metastatic disease to the lungs should suggest sarcoma as the primary neoplasm. Although a variety of tumors have been reported,[290] the incidence is especially

high in osteogenic sarcoma;[290] in one study of 552 cases of this tumor, pneumothorax developed in 5% who had pulmonary metastases.[291] It has been suggested that the complication is more frequent in patients undergoing chemotherapy.[292] It may occur before radiographic visibility of metastases.[290]

Interstitial Thickening (Lymphangitic Carcinomatosis)

Interstitial thickening is frequent. In one study of 174 cases of metastatic pulmonary disease, it was seen in 97 (55%); in more than half the cases, it was the predominant mode of spread.[244] In another investigation of 222 consecutive autopsies of patients who had solid tumors, the abnormality was found in 78 (35%).[293] Although virtually any metastatic neoplasm can show lymphangitic spread, they most commonly originate in the breast, stomach, pancreas, and prostate;[242, 243] in addition, it is common for primary pulmonary carcinoma, particularly small cell carcinoma and adenocarcinoma, to spread by this route.

Pathologically, lymphangitic spread varies from a slight accentuation of the interlobular septa and peribronchovascular connective tissue to obvious thickening (5 to 10 mm) of these structures (Fig. 6–43). Associated pleural involvement is common.

The characteristic radiographic pattern consists of coarsened bronchovascular markings of irregular contour, sometimes indistinctly defined, simulating interstitial pulmonary edema. Although the pattern is uniform throughout both

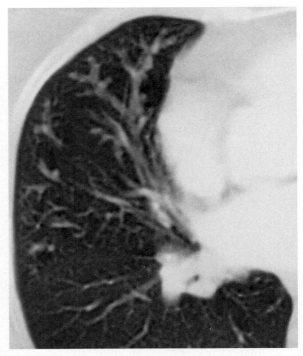

Figure 6–40. Intravascular Tumor Emboli. Detail view of the right lung shows nodular thickening of the pulmonary arteries in the right middle lobe. The appearance is characteristic of intravascular tumor emboli. The patient had proven metastatic carcinoma of the breast. (Courtesy of Drs. Lynn Broderick and Robert Tarver, Indiana University Medical Center, Indianapolis, IN.)

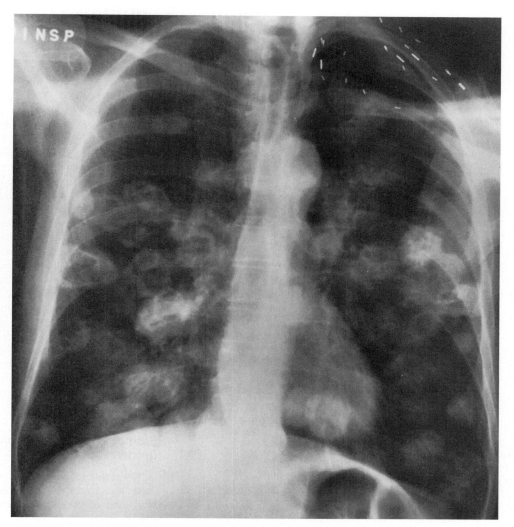

Figure 6–41. Cavitation in Metastatic Carcinoma. Posteroanterior radiograph reveals multiple nodules throughout both lungs ranging from 5 mm to 3 cm in diameter. Most of the nodules are cavitated. For an unknown reason, such thin-walled cavities tend to occur in metastases from primary neoplasms arising in the head and neck, at least in men (in women, the primary neoplasm tends to be in the genital tract). In this patient, the primary carcinoma was in the pharynx. (The surgical clips over the left supraclavicular region are from a previous radical neck dissection.)

lungs in most patients, it tends to be more obvious in the lower zones. Septal lines (Kerley B lines) commonly are present (Fig. 6–44).[242, 298] The linear accentuation sometimes is associated with a nodular component, resulting

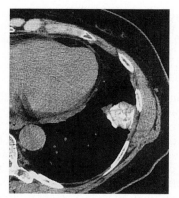

Figure 6–42. Calcified Metastatic Osteosarcoma. A 71-year-old woman with previously resected primary osteosarcoma of the femur developed two new pulmonary nodules. CT scan shows a 2.5-cm-diameter lobulated nodule in the left lower lobe. It is extensively calcified. CT scan 6 months previously had been normal.

from intraparenchymal extension of tumor, creating a coarse reticulonodular pattern. Although often bilateral, the abnormality may be confined to one lung or one lobe, as was the case in 28 of 100 patients in one series;[294] 21 of the 28 patients had a primary pulmonary carcinoma. Hilar and mediastinal lymph node enlargement is seen radiographically in 20% to 40% of patients and pleural effusion in 30% to 50%.[242, 295] Although characteristic, these findings lack specificity and sensitivity for the diagnosis. In one study, an accurate diagnosis of lymphangitic carcinomatosis was suggested on chest radiograph in only 20 of 87 (23%) patients.[296] The chest radiograph is normal in 30% to 50% of patients who have pathologically proven lymphangitic carcinomatosis.[242, 296, 297]

Lymphangitic carcinomatosis also has a characteristic HRCT appearance, consisting of smooth or nodular thickening of the interlobular septa and peribronchovascular interstitium with preservation of normal lung architecture (Fig. 6–45).[295, 298] The thickened interlobular septa may be seen as peripheral lines extending to the pleural surface or centrally as polygonal arcades, frequently with a nodular or beaded appearance.[295, 299] This nodular thickening is highly suggestive of the diagnosis and is not seen in pulmonary edema or interstitial fibrosis.[299] Lymphangitic carcino-

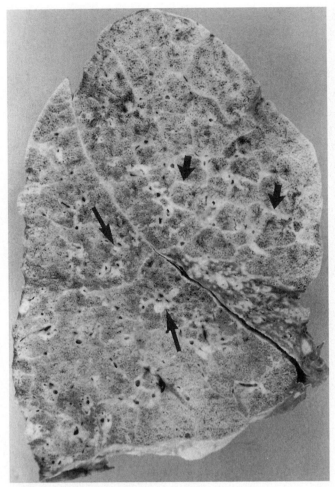

Figure 6–43. Lymphangitic Spread—Carcinoma of the Breast. Section of left lung shows extensive infiltration of interlobular septa *(short arrows)* and peribronchovascular tissue *(long arrows)* by breast carcinoma.

matosis may be associated with interstitial edema, in which case the thickened interlobular septa may have a smooth appearance. Thickening of interlobular septa of adjacent lobules leads to an appearance of polygonal arcades.[298] Characteristically the arcades are associated with a prominent central dot, representing thickening of the interstitium along the centrilobular bronchovascular bundles.[295, 298] Tumor and edema in the pleural interstitial tissue leads to smooth or nodular thickening of the interlobar fissures. Discrete nodules separate from the interlobular septa also may be seen but are relatively uncommon.[295] Pleural effusion is seen on CT scan in approximately 30% of cases, and hilar or mediastinal lymph node enlargement is seen in approximately 40%.[295]

At the time of diagnosis, the HRCT findings of lymphangitic carcinomatosis are unilateral or markedly asymmetric in 50% of cases (Fig. 6–46).[295, 300] As indicated previously, such unilateral disease is particularly common in patients who have pulmonary carcinoma. In some, the abnormalities involve predominantly the peripheral lung, leading to prominent thickening of the interlobular septa; in others, the abnormalities involve predominantly the central bronchovascular bundles.[300]

Disease may be appreciated on HRCT scan in patients who have normal or nonspecific radiographic findings.[298, 301] For example, in one study of 12 patients with pathologically proven lymphangitic carcinomatosis, 3 (25%) had normal chest radiographs and characteristic abnormalities on HRCT scan.[298] The diagnostic accuracy of CT was compared with that of chest radiography in another study of 118 consecutive patients who had various chronic diffuse infiltrative lung diseases.[301] The CT and radiographic findings were assessed independently by three observers without knowledge of clinical or pathologic data. Of 18 patients who had lymphangitic carcinomatosis, a confident diagnosis was made on the chest radiograph in 20%; this interpretation was correct in 64% of readings. By contrast, a confident diagnosis of lymphangitic carcinomatosis was suggested on CT scan in 54% of readings, the interpretation being correct in 93% of cases.

The relative value of clinical, chest radiograph, and CT findings in making a specific diagnosis of chronic diffuse infiltrative lung diseases was assessed in another investigation of 208 consecutive patients, of whom 13 had pathologically proven lymphangitic carcinomatosis.[302] A confident diagnosis was made based on a combination of clinical and radiographic findings in 54% of patients (the assessment being correct in 92%) and on a combination of clinical, radiographic, and CT findings in 92% (correct in all instances).[302] A confident diagnosis was not made on clinical grounds alone in any case.

Pulmonary Hypertension and Infarction (Intravascular Emboli)

Intravascular metastatic neoplasm is common in the lungs at autopsy; for example, in one study of 366 patients who died of choriocarcinoma or carcinoma of the breast, kidney, liver, or stomach, 95 (26%) showed tumor within the pulmonary arterial tree.[241] The complication is seen most often with adenocarcinoma,[245, 291] especially of the breast or stomach; an unusually high frequency is seen in hepatocellular carcinoma, out of proportion to the incidence of the neoplasm.[241, 291]

Most often, tumor is identified only histologically. Medium-sized to small-sized muscular arteries and arterioles usually are affected; rarely, alveolar septal capillaries are involved.[303, 304] As indicated previously, concomitant lymphangitic carcinomatosis is common, either focally or widespread.[293, 305] Occasionally, grossly visible emboli can be identified in segmental or larger arteries.[245, 306] Such tumor emboli can result in infarction[241, 307] or sudden death.[308, 309]

Although intravascular tumor emboli usually are accompanied by radiographic evidence of another pattern of pulmonary involvement (most often lymphangitic carcinomatosis), they may be the sole manifestation of metastatic pulmonary disease. In such cases, the chest radiograph may be normal[310] or may show dilation of central pulmonary arteries and the right ventricle, reflecting pulmonary hypertension. As indicated previously, emboli rarely are identified on CT scan as nodular or beaded thickening of the pulmonary arteries *(see* Fig. 6–40).[277] The propensity for tumor emboli to obstruct arterioles can result in an abnormal radionuclide perfusion lung scan characterized by mis-

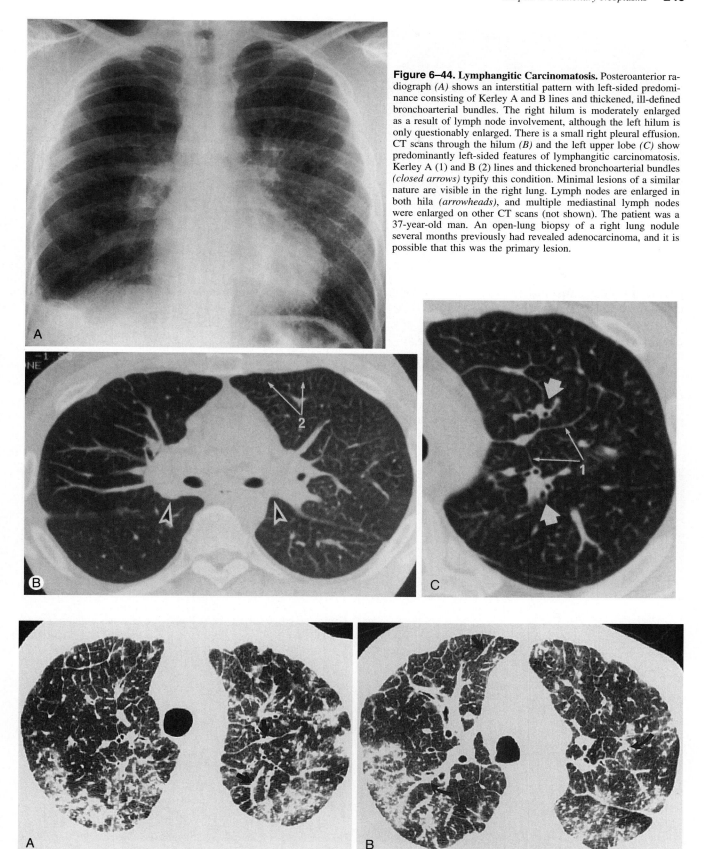

Figure 6–44. Lymphangitic Carcinomatosis. Posteroanterior radiograph *(A)* shows an interstitial pattern with left-sided predominance consisting of Kerley A and B lines and thickened, ill-defined bronchoarterial bundles. The right hilum is moderately enlarged as a result of lymph node involvement, although the left hilum is only questionably enlarged. There is a small right pleural effusion. CT scans through the hilum *(B)* and the left upper lobe *(C)* show predominantly left-sided features of lymphangitic carcinomatosis. Kerley A (1) and B (2) lines and thickened bronchoarterial bundles *(closed arrows)* typify this condition. Minimal lesions of a similar nature are visible in the right lung. Lymph nodes are enlarged in both hila *(arrowheads)*, and multiple mediastinal lymph nodes were enlarged on other CT scans (not shown). The patient was a 37-year-old man. An open-lung biopsy of a right lung nodule several months previously had revealed adenocarcinoma, and it is possible that this was the primary lesion.

Figure 6–45. Lymphangitic Carcinomatosis. HRCT scans *(A and B)* show smooth and nodular *(straight arrow)* thickening of the interlobular septa and nodular thickening along the bronchovascular bundles *(curved arrows)*. The patient was a dyspneic 72-year-old man who had lymphangitic carcinomatosis secondary to poorly differentiated adenocarcinoma of the rectum.

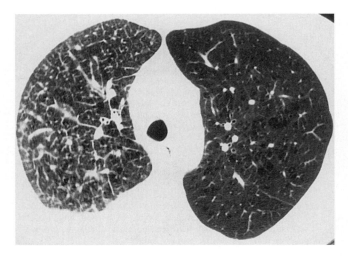

Figure 6–46. Asymmetric Lymphangitic Carcinomatosis. HRCT scan shows interlobular septal thickening throughout the right upper lobe. A small right pleural effusion also is present. The left lung shows only a few thickened interlobular septa and evidence of emphysema. The patient was a 67-year-old woman who had lymphangitic carcinomatosis proved by a transbronchial biopsy. (From Leung AN, Staples CA, Müller NL: Am J Roentgenol 157:693, 1991.)

matching ventilation-perfusion defects that are virtually indistinguishable from thromboembolic disease.[311]

Airway Obstruction (Bronchial and Tracheal Metastasis)

Endobronchial metastases usually are secondary to carcinoma of the breast, colorectum, and kidney or to melanoma.[312–314] Most cases are incidental findings seen by the pathologist at autopsy; when seen by the bronchoscopist during endoscopy, they usually are of such small size

and limited extent that they do not manifest themselves radiographically. When present, the usual radiologic findings are those of bronchial obstruction, either partial (causing oligemia and expiratory air-trapping) or complete (with atelectasis and obstructive pneumonitis).

Hematogenous metastases to the trachea are rare. Similar to endobronchial metastases, the most common primary sites are kidney, breast, colon, and melanoma.[205, 315] Occasionally a metastasis is detected as a polypoid soft tissue mass on the chest radiograph or CT scan (Fig. 6–47).[199]

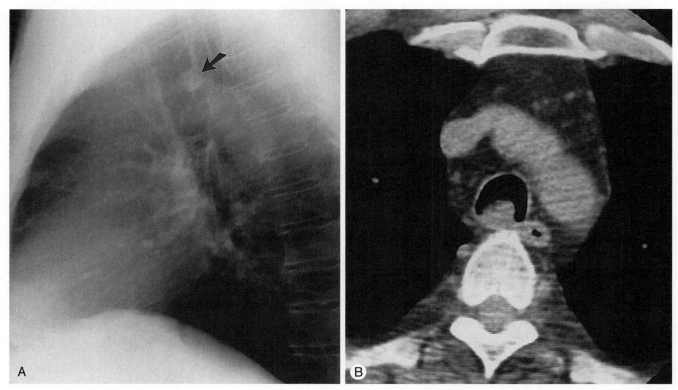

Figure 6–47. Endotracheal Metastasis. Lateral chest radiograph *(A)* shows a 1.5-cm-diameter focal soft tissue opacity abutting the posterior wall of the trachea *(arrow)*. CT scan *(B)* confirms the presence of the endotracheal tumor. The diagnosis of metastatic melanoma was confirmed by bronchoscopy. The patient was a 56-year-old man with a known history of melanoma. (From Kwong JS, Adler BD, Padley SPG, et al: Am J Roentgenol 161:519, 1993.)

References

1. Travis WD, Colby TV, Corrin B, et al, and Collaborators from 14 Countries: World Health Organization Pathology Panel: World Health Organization Histological Typing of Lung and Pleural Tumors: International Histological Classification of Tumors. 3rd ed. Berlin, Springer-Verlag, 1999.
2. Travis WD, Lubin J, Ries L, et al: United States lung carcinoma incidence trends—declining for most histologic types among males, increasing among females. Cancer 77:2464, 1996.
3. Beckett WS: Epidemiology and etiology of lung cancer. Clin Chest Med 14:1, 1993.
4. American Thoracic Society/European Respiratory Society: Pretreatment evaluation of nonsmall-cell lung cancer. Am J Respir Crit Care Med 156:320, 1997.
5. Bartecchi CE, MacKenzie TD, Schrier RW: The human costs of tobacco use. N Engl J Med 907:330, 1994.
6. McDonald JC, Liddell FDK, Dufresne A, et al: The 1891–1920 birth cohort of Quebec chrysotile miners and millers: Mortality 1976–88. Br J Ind Med 50:1073, 1993.
7. Järup L, Pershagen G: Arsenic exposure, smoking, and lung cancer in smelter workers: A case-control study. Am J Epidemiol 134:545, 1991.
8. Chovil A, Sutherland B, Halliday M: Respiratory cancer in a cohort of nickel sinter plant workers. Br J Ind Med 38:327, 1981.
9. Sevc J, Tomasek L, Kunz E, et al: A survey of the Czechoslovak follow-up of lung cancer mortality in uranium miners. Health Phys 64:355, 1993.
10. Oliphant L, McFadden RG: Lung cancer following therapy for Hodgkin's disease. Can Med Assoc J 132:533, 1985.
11. Wiernik PH, Sklarin NT, Dutcher JP, et al: Adjuvant radiotherapy for breast cancer as a risk factor for the development of lung cancer. Med Oncol 11:121, 1994.
12. Lee HJ, Im JG, Ahn JM, et al: Lung cancer in patients with idiopathic pulmonary fibrosis: CT findings. J Comput Assist Tomogr 20:979, 1996.
13. Hubbard R, Venn A, Lewis S, et al: Lung cancer and cryptogenic fibrosing alveolitis. Am J Respir Crit Care Med 161:5, 2000.
14. Cohen S, Hossain SA: Primary carcinoma of the lung: A review of 417 histologically proved cases. Dis Chest 49:67, 1966.
15. Filderman AE, Matthay RA: Bronchogenic carcinoma. In Bone RC, Dantzker DR,George RB, et al (eds): Pulmonary and Critical Care Medicine. St. Louis, Mosby, 1997.
16. Lisa JR, Trinidad S, Rosenblatt MB: Site of origin, histogenesis, and cytostructure of bronchogenic carcinoma. Am J Clin Pathol 44:375, 1965.
17. Melamed MR, Zaman MB, Flehinger BJ, et al: Radiologically occult in situ and incipient invasive epidermoid lung cancer: Detection by sputum cytology in a survey of asymptomatic cigarette smokers. Am J Surg Pathol 1:5, 1977.
18. Carter D: Small-cell carcinoma of the lung. Am J Surg Pathol 7:787, 1983.
19. Yesner R: Small cell tumors of the lung. Am J Surg Pathol 7:775, 1983.
20. Kriesman H, Wolkove N, Quoix E: Small cell lung cancer presenting as a solitary pulmonary nodule. Chest 101:225, 1992.
21. Gephardt GN, Grady KJ, Ahmad M, et al: Peripheral small cell undifferentiated carcinoma of the lung: Clinicopathologic features of 17 cases. Cancer 61:1002, 1988.
22. Manning JT Jr, Spjut HJ, Tschen JA: Bronchioloalveolar carcinoma: The significance of two histopathologic types. Cancer 54:525, 1984.
23. Horie A, Ohta M: Ultrasound features of large cell carcinoma of the lung with reference to the prognosis of patients. Hum Pathol 12:423, 1981.
24. Garland LH: Bronchial carcinomas: Lobar distribution of lesions in 250 cases. Calif Med 94:7, 1961.
25. Macfarlane JCW, Doughty BJ, Crosbie WA: Carcinoma of the lung: An analysis of 362 cases diagnosed and treated in one year. Br J Dis Chest 56:57, 1962.
26. Byers TE, Vena JE, Rzepka TF: Predilection of lung cancer for the upper lobes: An epidemiologic inquiry. J Natl Cancer Inst 72:1271, 1984.
27. Chute CG, Greenberg ER, Baron J, et al: Presenting conditions of 1539 population-based lung cancer patients by cell type and stage in New Hampshire and Vermont. Cancer 56:2107, 1985.
28. Quinn D, Gianlupi A, Broste S: The changing radiographic presentation of bronchogenic carcinoma with reference to cell types. Chest 110:1474, 1996.
29. Woodring JH, Stelling CB: Adenocarcinoma of the lung: A tumor with changing pleomorphic character. Am J Roentgenol 140:657, 1983.
30. Ranke EJ, Presley SS, Holinger PH: Tracheogenic carcinoma. JAMA 182:519, 1962.
31. Byrd RB, Carr DT, Miller WE, et al: Radiographic abnormalities in carcinoma of the lung as relation to histological cell type. Thorax 24:573, 1969.
32. Golden R: The effect of bronchostenosis upon the roentgen-ray shadows in carcinoma of the bronchus. Am J Roentgenol 13:21, 1925.
33. Woodring JH: Determining the cause of pulmonary atelectasis: A comparison of plain radiography and CT. Am J Roentgenol 150:757, 1988.
34. Tobler J, Levitt RG, Glazer HS, et al: Differentiation of proximal bronchogenic carcinoma from post-obstructive lobar collapse by magnetic resonance imaging: Comparison with computed tomography. Invest Radiol 22:538, 1987.
35. Molina PL, Hiken JN, Glazer HS: Imaging evaluation of obstructive atelectasis. J Thorac Imaging 11:176, 1996.
36. Onitsuka H, Tsukuda M, Araki A, et al: Differentiation of central lung tumor from postobstructive lobar collapse by rapid sequence computed tomography. J Thorac Imaging 6:28, 1991.
37. Herold CJ, Kuhlman JE, Zerhouni EA: Pulmonary atelectasis: Signal patterns with MR imaging. Radiology 178:715, 1991.
38. Stiglbauer R, Schurawitzki H, Klepetko W: Contrast-enhanced MRI for the staging of bronchogenic carcinoma: Comparison with CT and histopathologic staging-preliminary results. Clin Radiol 44:293, 1991.
39. Kameda K, Adachi S, Kono M: Detection of T-factor in lung cancer using magnetic resonance imaging and computed tomography. J Thorac Imaging 3:73, 1988.
40. Edwards WM, Cox RS Jr, Garland LH: The solitary nodule (coin lesion) of the lung: An analysis of 52 consecutive cases treated by thoracotomy and a study of preoperative diagnostic accuracy. Am J Roentgenol 88:1020, 1962.
41. Steele JD: The solitary pulmonary nodule: Report of a cooperative study of resected asymptomatic solitary pulmonary nodules in males. J Thorac Cardiovasc Surg 46:21, 1963.
42. Swensen SJ, Morin RL, Schueler BA, et al: Solitary pulmonary nodule: CT evaluation of enhancement with iodinated contrast material—a preliminary report. Radiology 182:343, 1992.
43. Erasmus JJ, Connolly JE, McAdams HP, et al: Solitary pulmonary nodules: Part I. Morphologic evaluation for differentiation of benign and malignant lesions. Radiographics 20:43, 2000.
44. Yamashita K, Matsunobe S, Tsuda T: Intratumoral necrosis of lung carcinoma: A potential pitfall in incremental dynamic computed tomography analysis of solitary nodules? J Thorac Imaging 12:181, 1997.
45. Mack MJ, Hazebrigg SR, Landreneau RJ, et al: Thoracoscopy for the diagnosis of the indeterminate solitary pulmonary nodule. Ann Thorac Surg 56:825, 1993.
46. Siegelman SS, Khouri NF, Leo FP, et al: Solitary pulmonary nodules: CT assessment. Radiology 160:307, 1986.
47. Primack SL, Lee KS, Logan PM, et al: Bronchogenic carcinoma: Utility of CT in the evaluation of patients with suspected lesions. Radiology 193:795, 1994.
48. Bateson EM: An analysis of 155 solitary lung lesions illustrating the differential diagnosis of mixed tumours of the lung. Clin Radiol 16:51, 1965.
49. Siegelman SS, Khouri NF, Scott WW, et al: Pulmonary hamartoma: CT findings. Radiology 160:313, 1986.
50. Cummings SR, Lillington GA, Richard RJ: Managing solitary pulmonary nodules: The choice of strategy is a "close call." Am Rev Respir Dis 134:453, 1986.
51. Gurney JW: Determining the likelihood of malignancy in solitary pulmonary nodules with Bayesian analysis: Part I. Theory. Radiology 186:405, 1993.
52. Webb WR: Radiologic evaluation of the solitary pulmonary nodule. Am J Roentgenol 154:701, 1990.
53. Mahoney MC, Shipley RT, Corcoran HL, et al: CT demonstration of calcification in carcinoma of the lung. Am J Roentgenol 154:255, 1990.

54. Grewal RG, Austin JHM: CT demonstration of calcification in carcinoma of the lung. J Comput Assist Tomogr 18:867, 1994.
55. Khan A, Herman PG, Vorwerk P, et al: Solitary pulmonary nodules: Comparison of classification with standard, thin-section, and reference phantom CT. Radiology 179:477, 1991.
56. Colice GL: Chest CT for known or suspected lung cancer. Chest 106:1538, 1994.
57. Im J-G, Gamsu G, Birnberg FA, et al: CT densitometry of pulmonary nodules in a frozen human thorax. Am J Roentgenol 150:61, 1988.
58. Zwirewich CV, Vedal S, Miller RR, Müller NL: Solitary pulmonary nodule: High-resolution CT and radiologic-pathologic correlation. Radiology 179:469, 1991.
59. Shapiro R, Wilson GL, Yesner R, et al: A useful roentgen sign in the diagnosis of localized bronchioloalveolar carcinoma. Am J Roentgenol 114:516, 1972.
60. Sone S, Sakai F, Takashima S, et al: Factors affecting the radiologic appearance of peripheral bronchogenic carcinomas. J Thorac Imaging 12:159, 1997.
61. Kuriyama K, Tateishi R, Doi O, et al: Prevalence of air bronchograms in small peripheral carcinomas of the lung on thin-section CT: Comparison with benign tumors. Am J Roentgenol 156:921, 1991.
62. Kuriyama K, Tateishi R, Doi O, et al: CT-pathologic correlation in small peripheral lung cancers. AJR 149:1129, 1987.
63. Schraufnagel DE, Peloquin A, Paré JAP, et al: Differentiating bronchioloalveolar carcinoma from adenocarcinoma. Am Rev Respir Dis 125:74, 1982.
64. Webb WR: The pleural tail sign. Radiology 127:309, 1978.
65. Hill CA: "Tail" signs associated with pulmonary lesions: Critical reappraisal. Am J Roentgenol 139:311, 1982.
66. Kui M, Templeton PA, White CS, et al: Evaluation of the air bronchogram sign on CT in solitary pulmonary lesions. J Comput Assist Tomogr 20:983, 1996.
67. Kuhlman JE, Fishman EK, Kuhajda FP, et al: Solitary bronchioloalveolar carcinoma: CT criteria. Radiology 167:379, 1988.
68. Adler B, Padley S, Miller RR, et al: High-resolution CT of bronchioloalveolar carcinoma. Am J Roentgenol 159:275, 1992.
69. Lee KS, Kim Y, Han J, et al: Bronchioloalveolar carcinoma: Clinical, histopathologic, and radiologic findings. Radiographics 17:1345, 1997.
70. Garland LH: The rate of growth and natural duration of primary bronchial cancer. Am J Roentgenol 96:604, 1966.
71. Nathan MH, Collins VP, Adams RA: Differentiation of benign and malignant pulmonary nodules by growth rate. Radiology 79:221, 1962.
72. Weiss W, Boucot KR, Cooper DA: The survival of men with measurable proved lung cancer in relation to growth rate. Am J Roentgenol 98:404, 1966.
73. Garland LH, Coulson W, Wollin E: The rate of growth and apparent duration of untreated primary bronchial carcinoma. Cancer 16:694, 1963.
74. Jensen JG, Schiodt T: Growth conditions of hamartoma of the lung: A study based on 22 cases operated on after radiographic observation for from one to 18 years. Thorax 13:233, 1958.
75. Weisel W, Glicklich M, Landis FB: Pulmonary hamartoma, an enlarging neoplasm. Arch Surg 71:128, 1955.
76. Good CA, Wilson TW: The solitary circumscribed pulmonary nodule: Study of seven hundred five cases encountered roentgenologically in a period of three- and one-half years. JAMA 166:210, 1958.
77. Bennett DE, Sasser WF, Ferguson TB: Adenocarcinoma of the lung in men. Cancer 23:431, 1969.
78. Yankelevitz DF, Henschke CI: Does 2-year stability imply that pulmonary nodules are benign? Am J Roentgenol 168:325, 1997.
79. Swensen SJ, Brown LR, Colby TV, et al: Lung nodule enhancement at CT: Prospective findings. Radiology 201:447, 1996.
80. Swensen SJ, Viggiano RW, Midthun DE, et al: Lung nodule enhancement at CT: Multicenter study. Radiology 214:73, 2000.
81. Patz EF, Lowe VJ, Hoffman JM, et al: Focal pulmonary abnormalities: Evaluation with F-18 fluorodeoxyglucose PET scanning. Radiology 188:487, 1993.
82. Scott WJ, Schwabe JL, Gupta NC, et al: Positron emission tomography of lung tumours and mediastinal lymph nodes using [^{18}F] fluorodeoxyglucose. Ann Thorac Surg 58:698, 1994.
83. Erasmus JJ, McAdams HP, Patz EF Jr: Non-small cell lung cancer: FDG-PET imaging. J Thorac Imaging 14:247, 1999.
84. Lowe VJ, Fletcher JW, Gobar L, et al: Prospective investigation of PET in lung nodules (PIOPILN). J Clin Oncol 16:1075, 1998.
85. Nakata H, Hirakata K, Watanabe H, et al: Lung cancer associated with punctate calcification: CT and histological correlation. Radiat Med 15:91, 1997.
86. Huang D, Weisbrod GL, Chamberlain DW: Unusual radiologic presentations of bronchioloalveolar carcinoma. J Can Assoc Radiol 37:94, 1986.
87. Hill CA: Bronchioloalveolar carcinoma: A review. Radiology 150:15, 1984.
88. Zwirewich CV, Miller RR, Müller NL: Multicentric adenocarcinoma of the lung: CT-pathologic correlation. Radiology 176:185, 1990.
89. Gaeta M, Caruso R, Barone M, et al: Ground-glass attenuation in nodular bronchioloalveolar carcinoma: CT patterns and prognostic value. J Comput Assist Tomogr 22:215, 1998.
90. Trigaux JP, Genevois PA, Goncette L, et al: Bronchioloalveolar carcinoma: Computed tomography findings. Eur Respir J 9:9, 1996.
91. Aquino SL, Chiles C, Halford P: Distinction of consolidative bronchioloalveolar carcinoma from pneumonia: Do CT criteria work? Am J Roentgenol 171:359, 1998.
92. Im JG, Han MC, Yu EJ, et al: Lobar bronchioloalveolar carcinoma: "Angiogram sign" on CT scans. Radiology 176:749, 1990.
93. Maldonado RL: The CT angiogram sign. Radiology 210:323, 1999.
94. Heelan RT, Demas BE, Caravelli JF, et al: Superior sulcus tumors: CT and MR imaging. Radiology 170:637, 1989.
95. Stanford W, Barnes RP, Tucker AR: Influence of staging in superior sulcus (Pancoast) tumors of the lung. Ann Thorac Surg 29:406, 1980.
96. Anderson TM, Moy PM, Holmes EC, et al: Factors affecting survival in superior sulcus tumors. J Clin Oncol 4:1598, 1986.
97. Attar S, Krasna MJ, Sonett JR, et al: Superior sulcus (Pancoast) tumor: Experience with 105 patients. Ann Thorac Surg 66:193, 1998.
98. Shahian DM, Neptune WB, Ellis FH Jr: Pancoast tumors: Improved survival with preoperative and postoperative radiotherapy. Ann Thorac Surg 43:32, 1987.
99. Scott IR, Müller NL, Miller RR, et al: Resectable stage III lung cancer: CT, surgical, and pathologic correlation. Radiology 166:75, 1988.
100. Pennes DR, Glazer GM, Wimbish KJ, et al: Chest wall invasion by lung cancer: Limitations of CT evaluation. Am J Roentgenol 144:507, 1985.
101. Pearlberg JL, Sandler MA, Beute GH, et al: Limitations of CT in evaluation of neoplasms involving chest wall. J Comput Assist Tomogr 11:290, 1987.
102. Takasugi J, Rapoport S, Shaw C: Superior sulcus tumors: The role of imaging. J Thorac Imaging 4:41, 1989.
103. Sahn S: Pleural effusion in lung cancer. Clin Chest Med 14:189, 1993.
104. Quint LE, Francis IR: Radiologic staging of lung cancer. J Thorac Imaging 14:235, 1999.
105. McLoud TC, Filon RB, Edelman RR, et al: MR imaging of superior sulcus carcinoma. J Comput Assist Tomogr 13:233, 1989.
106. Haggar AM, Pearlberg JL, Froelich JW, et al: Chest-wall invasion by carcinoma of the lung: Detection by MR imaging. Am J Roentgenol 148:1075, 1987.
107. Webb WR, Gatsonis C, Zerhouni EA, et al: CT and MR imaging in staging non-small cell bronchogenic carcinoma: Report of the radiologic diagnostic oncology group. Radiology 178:705, 1991.
108. Quint LE, Francis IR, Wahl RL, et al: Preoperative staging of non-small-cell carcinoma of the lung: Imaging methods. Am J Roentgenol 164:1349, 1995.
109. Gefter WB: Magnetic resonance imaging in the evaluation of lung cancer. Semin Roentgenol 25:73, 1990.
110. Webb WR, Sostman HD: MR imaging of thoracic disease: Clinical uses. Radiology 182:621, 1992.
111. Sugana Y, Kobayashi H, Kitamura S, et al: Ultrasonographic evaluation of pleural and chest wall invasion of lung cancer. Chest 94:1271, 1988.
112. Susuki N, Saitoh T, Kitamura S: Tumor invasion of the chest wall in lung cancer: Diagnosis with US. Radiology 187:39, 1993.
113. Lamay P, Anthoine D, Rebeix G, et al: Ostéoses et myéloses cancéreuses d'origine bronchique. [Metastatic lesions of bone and bone marrow in bronchogenic carcinoma.] Rev Tuberc 29:401, 1965.
114. Clain A: Secondary malignant disease of bone. Br J Cancer 19:15, 1965.
115. Silvestri GA, Littenberg B, Colice GL: The clinical evaluation for detecting metastatic lung cancer: A meta-analysis. Am J Respir Crit Care Med 152:225, 1995.

116. Hepper NGG, Herskovic T, Witten DM, et al: Thoracic inlet tumors. Ann Intern Med 64:979, 1966.

117. Marchioli CC, Graziano SL: Paraneoplastic syndromes associated with small cell lung cancer. Chest Surg Clin N Am 7:65, 1997.

118. Eisen T, Hickish T, Smith IE, et al: Small-cell lung cancer. Lancet 345:1285, 1995.

119. Patel AM, Davila DG, Peters SG: Paraneoplastic syndrome associated with lung cancer. Mayo Clin Proc 68:278, 1993.

120. Rassam JW, Anderson G: Incidence of paramalignant disorders in bronchogenic carcinoma. Thorax 30:86, 1975.

121. Pate JW, Campbell RE, Hughes FA: Unsuspected bronchogenic carcinoma. Dis Chest 37:56, 1960.

122. Fujishita T, Mizushima Y, Yoshida Y, et al: A case of small cell carcinoma of the lung associated with hypertrophic pulmonary osteoarthropathy. Tumori 82:259, 1996.

123. Mountain CF: Revisions in the International System for Staging Lung Cancer. Chest 111:1710, 1997.

124. Mountain CF, Dresler CM: Regional lymph node classification for lung cancer staging. Chest 111:1718, 1997.

125. Cymbalista M, Waysberg A, Zacharias C, et al: CT demonstration of the 1996 AJCC-UICC regional lymph node classification for lung cancer staging. Radiographics 19:899, 1999.

126. Ko JP, Drucker EA, Shepard J-AO, et al: CT depiction of regional nodal stations for lung cancer staging. Am J Roentgenol 174:775, 2000.

127. Abrams J, Doyle LA, Aisner J: Staging prognostic factors, and special considerations in small cell lung cancer. Semin Oncol 15:261, 1988.

128. Ekholm S, Albrechtsson U, Kugelberg J, et al: Computed tomography in preoperative stating of bronchogenic carcinoma. CT 4:763, 1980.

129. Glazer HS, Kaiser LR, Anderson DJ, et al: Indeterminate mediastinal invasion in bronchogenic carcinoma: CT evaluation. Radiology 173:37, 1989.

130. Gay SB, Black WB, Armstrong P, et al: Chest CT of unresectable lung cancer. Radiographics 8:735, 1988.

131. Epstein DM, Stephenson LW, Gefter WB, et al: Value of CT in the preoperative assessment of lung cancer: A survey of thoracic surgeons. Radiology 161:423, 1986.

132. Herman SJ, Winton TL, Weisbrod GL, et al: Mediastinal invasion by bronchogenic carcinoma: CT signs. Radiology 190:841, 1994.

133. White PG, Adams H, Crane MD, et al: Preoperative staging of carcinoma of the bronchus: Can computed tomographic scanning reliably identify stage III tumors? Thorax 49:951, 1994.

134. Weinreb JC, Naidich DP: Thoracic magnetic resonance imaging. Clin Chest Med 12:33, 1991.

135. Mayr B, Lenhard M, Fink U, et al: Preoperative evaluation of bronchogenic carcinoma: Value of MR in T- and N-staging. Eur J Radiol 14:245, 1992.

136. Quint LE, Glazer GM, Orringer MB, et al: Mediastinal lymph node detection and sizing at CT and autopsy. Am J Roentgenol 147:469, 1986.

137. Buy JN, Ghossain MA, Poirson F, et al: Computed tomography of mediastinal lymph nodes in nonsmall cell lung cancer: A new approach based on the lymphatic pathway of tumor spread. J Comput Assist Tomogr 12:545, 1988.

138. Ikezoe J, Kadowaki K, Morimoto S, et al: Mediastinal lymph node metastases from non-small cell bronchogenic carcinoma: Reevaluation with CT. J Comput Assist Tomogr 14:340, 1990.

139. Haramati LB, Cartagena AM, Austin JHM: CT evaluation of mediastinal lymphadenopathy: Non-contrast 5 mm vs. post-contrast 10 mm sections. J Comput Assist Tomogr 19:375, 1995.

140. Patz EF Jr, Erasmus JJ, McAdams HP, et al: Lung cancer staging and management: Comparison of contrast-enhanced and nonenhanced helical CT of the thorax. Radiology 212:56, 1999.

141. Glazer GM, Francis IR, Gebarski K, et al: Dynamic incremental computed tomography in evaluation of the pulmonary hila. J Comput Assist Tomogr 7:59, 1983.

142. Remy-Jardin M, Duyck P, Remy J, et al: Hilar lymph nodes: Identification with spiral CT and histologic correlation. Radiology 196:387, 1995.

143. Shimoyama K, Murata K, Takahashi M, et al: Pulmonary hilar lymph node metastases from lung cancer: Evaluation based on morphology at thin-section, incremental, dynamic CT. Radiology 203:187, 1997.

144. McKenna RJ Jr, Libshitz HI, Mountain CE, et al: Roentgenographic evaluation of mediastinal nodes for preoperative assessment in lung cancer. Chest 88:206, 1985.

145. Lewis JW, Pearlberg JL, Beaute GH, et al: Can computed tomography of the chest stage lung cancer? Yes and no. Ann Thorac Surg 49:591, 1990.

146. Daly BD, Pugatch RD, Gale ME, et al: Computed tomography, an effective technique for mediastinal staging in lung cancer. J Thorac Cardiovasc Surg 88:486, 1984.

147. Glazer GM, Orringer MB, Gross BH, et al: The mediastinum in non-small cell lung cancer: CT-surgical correlation. Am J Roentgenol 142:1101, 1984.

148. McLoud TC, Bourgouin PM, Greenberg RW, et al: Bronchogenic carcinoma: Analysis of staging in the mediastinum with CT by correlative lymph node mapping and sampling. Radiology 182:319, 1992.

149. Dales RA, Stark RM, Raman S: Computed tomography to stage lung cancer: Approaching a controversy using meta-analysis. Am Rev Respir Dis 141:1096, 1990.

150. Guyatt DH, Cook DJ, Walter S: The Canadian Lung Oncology Group. Investigation for mediastinal disease in patients with apparently operable lung cancer. Ann Thorac Surg 60:1382, 1995.

151. Pearson FG, DeLarue NC, Ilves R, et al: Significance of positive superior mediastinal nodes identified at mediastinoscopy in patients with resectable cancer of the lung. J Thorac Cardiovasc Surg 83:11, 1982.

152. Gross BH, Glazer GM, Orringer MB, et al: Bronchogenic carcinoma metastatic to normal-sized lymph nodes: Frequency and significance. Radiology 166:71, 1988.

153. Poon PY, Bronskill MJ, Henkelman RM, et al: Mediastinal lymph node metastases from bronchogenic carcinoma: Detection with MR imaging and CT. Radiology 162:651, 1987.

154. Patz EF, Lowe VJ, Goodman PC, et al: Thoracic nodal staging with PET imaging with 18FDG in patients with bronchogenic carcinoma. Chest 108:1617, 1995.

155. Valk PE, Pounds TR, Hopkins DM, et al: Staging non-small cell lung cancer by whole-body positron emission tomographic imaging. Ann Thorac Surg 60:1573, 1995.

156. Vansteenkiste JF, Stroobants SG, De Leyn PR, et al: Mediastinal lymph node staging with FDG-PET scan in patients with potentially operable non-small cell lung cancer: A prospective analysis of 50 cases. Chest 112:1480, 1997.

157. Marom EM, McAdams HP, Erasmus JJ, et al: Staging non-small cell lung cancer with whole-body PET. Radiology 212:803, 1999.

158. Dwamena BA, Sonnad SS, Angobaldo JO, et al: Metastases from non-small cell lung cancer: Mediastinal staging in the 1990s—meta-analytic comparison of PET and CT. Radiology 213:530, 1999.

159. Ichinose Y, Hara N, Ohta M, et al: Preoperative examination to detect distant metastasis is not advocated for asymptomatic patients with stages 1 and 2 non-small cell lung cancer—preoperative examination for lung cancer. Chest 96:1104, 1989.

160. Ferrigno D, Buccheri G: Cranial computed tomography as a part of the initial staging procedures for patients with nonsmall-cell lung cancer. Chest 106:1025, 1994.

161. Mintz BJ, Tuhrim S, Alexander S, et al: Intracranial metastases in the initial staging of bronchogenic carcinoma. Chest 86:849, 1984.

162. Webb WR, Golden JA: Imaging strategies in the staging of lung cancer. Clin Chest Med 12:133, 1991.

163. Boland GWL, Lee MJ, Gazelle GS, et al: Characterization of adrenal masses using unenhanced CT: An analysis of the CT literature. Am J Roentgenol 171:201, 1998.

164. Macari M, Rofsy NM, Naidich DP, et al: Non-small cell lung carcinoma: Usefulness of unenhanced helical CT of the adrenal glands in the unmonitored environment. Radiology 209:807, 1998.

165. van Erkel AR, van Gils APG, Lequin M, et al: CT and MR distinction of adenomas and nonadenomas of the adrenal glands. J Comput Assist Tomogr 18:432, 1994.

166. Remer EM, Obuchowski N, Ellis JD, et al: Adrenal mass evaluation in patients with lung carcinoma: A cost-effectiveness analysis. Am J Roentgenol 174:1033, 2000.

167. Reinig JW, Doppman JL, Dwyer AJ, et al: Adrenal masses differentiated by MR. Radiology 158:81, 1986.

168. Reinig JW, Stutley JE, Leonhardt CM, et al: Differentiation of adrenal masses with MR imaging: Comparison of techniques. Radiology 192:41, 1994.

169. Ichikawa T, Ohtomo K, Uchiyama G, et al: Adrenal adenomas: Characteristic hyperintense rim sign on fat-saturated spin-echo MR images. Radiology 193:247, 1994.
170. Korobkin M, Lombardi TJ, Aisen AM, et al: Characterization of adrenal masses with chemical shift and gadolinium-enhanced MR imaging. Radiology 197:411, 1995.
171. Schwartz LH, Panicek DM, Koutcher JA, et al: Adrenal masses in patients with malignancy: Prospective comparison of echo-planar, fast spin-echo, and chemical shift MR imaging. Radiology 197:421, 1995.
172. Heinz-Peer G, Hönigschnabl S, Schneider B, et al: Characterization of adrenal masses using MR imaging with histopathologic correlation. Am J Roentgenol 173:15, 1999.
173. Erasmus JJ, Patz EF Jr, McAdams HP, et al: Evaluation of adrenal masses in patients with bronchogenic carcinoma using F-18 fluorodeoxyglucose positron emission tomography. Am J Roentgenol 168:1357, 1997.
174. Maurea S, Mainolfi C, Bazzicalupo L, et al: Imaging of adrenal tumors using FDG PET: Comparison of benign and malignant lesions. Am J Roentgenol 173:25, 1999.
174a. Malmberg R, Bergman B, Branehog I, et al: Lung cancer in West Sweden 1976–1985: A study of trends and survival with special reference to surgical treatment. Acta Oncol 35:185, 1996.
175. Wada H, Tanaka F, Yanagihara K, et al: Time trends and survival after operations for primary lung cancer from 1976 through 1990. J Thorac Cardiovasc Surg 112:349, 1996.
176. Paladugu RR, Benfield JR, Pak HY, et al: Bronchopulmonary Kulchitzky cell carcinomas: A new classification scheme for typical and atypical carcinoids. Cancer 55:1303, 1985.
177. Harpole DH Jr, Feldman JM, Buchanan S, et al: Bronchial carcinoid tumors: A retrospective analysis of 126 patients. Ann Thorac Surg 54:50, 1992.
178. Arrigoni MG, Woolner LB, Bernatz PE: Atypical carcinoid tumors of the lung. J Cardiovasc Thorac Surg 64:413, 1972.
179. Rosado de Christenson ML, Abbott GF, Kirejczyk WM, et al: Thoracic carcinoids: Radiologic-pathologic correlation. Radiographics 19:707, 1999.
180. Hurt R, Bates M: Carcinoid tumours of the bronchus: A 33 year experience. Thorax 39:617, 1984.
181. Chaudhuri TK, Chaudhuri TK, Schapiro RL, et al: Abnormal lung perfusion in a patient with bronchial adenoma. Chest 62:110, 1972.
182. McGuinnis EJ, Lull RJ: Bronchial adenoma causing unilateral absence of pulmonary perfusion. Radiology 120:367, 1976.
183. Wynn SR, O'Connell EJ, Frigas E, et al: Exercise-induced "asthma" as a presentation of bronchial carcinoid. Ann Allergy 57:139, 1986.
184. Nessi R, Ricci PB, Ricci SB, et al: Bronchial carcinoid tumors: Radiologic observations in 49 cases. J Thorac Imaging 6:47, 1991.
185. Magid D, Siegelman SS, Eggleston JC, et al: Pulmonary carcinoid tumors: CT assessment. J Comput Assist Tomogr 13:244, 1989.
186. Markel SF, Abell MR, Haight C, et al: Neoplasms of bronchus commonly designated as adenomas. Cancer 17:590, 1964.
187. Troupin R: Ossifying bronchial carcinoid: A case report. Am J Roentgenol 104:808, 1968.
188. Heimburger IL, Kilman JW, Battersby JS: Peripheral bronchial adenomas. J Thorac Cardiovasc Surg 52:542, 1966.
189. Lawson RM, Ramanathan L, Hurley G, et al: Bronchial adenoma: Review of an 18-year experience at the Brompton Hospital. Thorax 31:245, 1976.
190. Zwiebel BR, Austin JHM, Grimes MM: Bronchial carcinoid tumors: Assessment with CT of location and intratumoral calcification in 31 patients. Radiology 179:483, 1991.
191. Sheppard BB, Follette DM, Meyers FJ: Giant carcinoid tumor of the lung. Ann Thorac Surg 63:851, 1997.
192. Choplin RH, Kawamoto DH, Dyer RB, et al: Atypical carcinoid of the lung: Radiographic features. Am J Roentgenol 146:665, 1986.
193. Forster BB, Müller NL, Miller RR, et al: Neuroendocrine carcinomas of the lung: Clinical, radiologic, and pathologic correlation. Radiology 170:441, 1989.
194. Müller NL, Miller RR: Neuroendocrine carcinomas of the lung. Semin Roentgenol 25:96, 1990.
195. Todd TR, Cooper JD, Weissberg D, et al: Bronchial carcinoid tumors: 20 years' experience. J Thorac Cardiovasc Surg 79:532, 1980.
196. DeStephano DB, Lloyd RV, Schteingart DE: Cushing's syndrome produced by a bronchial carcinoid tumor: Case studies. Hum Pathol 15:890, 1984.

197. Gelder CM, Hetzel MR: Primary tracheal tumours: A national survey. Thorax 48:688, 1993.
198. Howard DJ, Haribhakti VV: Primary tumours of the trachea: Analysis of clinical features and treatment results. J Laryngol Otol 108:230, 1994.
199. Kwong JS, Adler BD, Padley SPG, et al: Diagnosis of diseases of the trachea and main bronchi: Chest radiography versus CT. Am J Roentgenol 161:519, 1993.
200. Reid JD: Adenoid cystic carcinoma (cylindroma) of the bronchial tree. Cancer 5:685, 1952.
201. Enterline HT, Schoenberg HW: Carcinoma (cylindromatous type) of trachea and bronchi and bronchial adenoma: A comparative study. Cancer 7:663, 1954.
202. Gallagher CG, Stark R, Teskey J, et al: Atypical manifestations of pulmonary adenoid cystic carcinoma. Br J Dis Chest 80:396, 1986.
203. Cleveland RH, Nice CM, Ziskind J: Primary adenoid cystic carcinoma (cylindroma) of the trachea. Radiology 122:597, 1977.
204. McCarthy MJ, Rosado de Christenson ML: Tumors of the trachea. J Thorac Imaging 10:180, 1995.
205. Kwong JS, Müller NL, Miller RR: Diseases of the trachea and main-stem bronchi: Correlation of CT with pathologic findings. Radiographics 12:645, 1992.
206. Yousem SA, Hochholzer L: Mucoepidermoid tumors of the lung. Cancer 60:1346, 1987.
207. Kim TS, Lee KS, Han J, et al: Mucoepidermoid carcinoma of the tracheobronchial tree: Radiographic and CT findings in 12 patients. Radiology 212:643, 1999.
208. Heitmiller RF, Mathisen DJ, Ferry JA, et al: Mucoepidermoid lung tumors. Ann Thorac Surg 47:394, 1989.
209. Multiple papillomas of the larynx in children (editorial). Lancet 1:367, 1981.
210. Smith L, Gooding CA: Pulmonary involvement in laryngeal papillomatosis. Pediatr Radiol 2:161, 1974.
211. Hartley C, Hamilton J, Birzgalis AR, et al: Recurrent respiratory papillomatosis—the Manchester experience, 1974–1992. J Laryngol Otol 108:226, 1994.
212. Tachezy R, Hamsikova E, Valvoda J, et al: Antibody response to a synthetic peptide derived from the human papillomavirus type 6/11 L2 protein in recurrent respiratory papillomatosis: Correlation between Southern blot hybridization, polymerase chain reaction, and serology. J Med Virol 42:52, 1994.
213. Brach BB, Klein RC, Matthews AJ, et al: Papillomatosis of the respiratory tract: Upper airway obstruction and carcinoma. Arch Otolaryngol 104:413, 1978.
214. Takasugi JE, Godwin JD: The airway. Semin Roentgenol 26:175, 1991.
215. Kramer SS, Wehunt WD, Stocker JT, et al: Pulmonary manifestations of juvenile laryngotracheal papillomatosis. Am J Roentgenol 144:687, 1985.
216. Rosenbaum HD, Alavi SM, Bryant LR: Pulmonary parenchymal spread of juvenile laryngeal papillomatosis. Radiology 90:654, 1968.
217. Laubscher FA: Solitary squamous cell papilloma of bronchial origin. Am J Clin Pathol 52:599, 1969.
218. Drennan JM, Douglas AC: Solitary papilloma of a bronchus. J Clin Pathol 18:401, 1965.
219. Maxwell RJ, Gibbons JR, O'Hara MD: Solitary squamous papilloma of the bronchus. Thorax 40:68, 1985.
220. Zimmermann A, Lang HR, Muhlberger F, et al: Papilloma of the bronchus. Respiration 39:286, 1980.
221. Tomashefski JF Jr: Benign endobronchial mesenchymal tumors: Their relationship to parenchymal pulmonary hamartomas. Am J Surg Pathol 6:531, 1982.
222. Suzuki N, Ohno S, Ishii Y, et al: Peripheral intrapulmonary hamartoma accompanied by a similar endotracheal lesion. Chest 106:1291, 1994.
223. Van Den Bosch JMM, Wagenaar SS, Corrin B, et al: Mesenchymoma of the lung (so called hamartoma): A review of 154 parenchymal and endobronchial cases. Thorax 42:790, 1987.
224. Bateson EM, Abbott EK: Mixed tumors of the lung, or hamartochondromas: A review of the radiological appearances of cases published in the literature and a report of fifteen new cases. Clin Radiol 11:232, 1960.
225. Sagel SS, Ablow RC: Hamartoma: On occasion a rapidly growing tumor of the lung. Radiology 91:971, 1968.
226. Gjevre JA, Myers JL, Prakash UBS: Pulmonary hamartomas. Mayo Clin Proc 71:14, 1996.

227. Poirer TJ, Van Ordstrand HS: Pulmonary chondromatous hamartomas: Report of seventeen cases and review of the literature. Chest 59:50, 1971.
228. Doppman J, Wilson G: Cystic pulmonary hamartoma. Br J Radiol 38:629, 1965.
229. Demos TC, Armin A, Chandrasekhar AJ, et al: Cystic hamartoma of the lung. J Can Assoc Radiol 34:149, 1983.
230. Spencer H: The pulmonary plasma cell/histiocytoma complex. Histopathology 8:903, 1984.
231. Bahadori M, Liebow AA: Plasma cell granulomas of the lung. Cancer 31:191, 1973.
232. Matsubara O, Tan-Liu NS, Kenney RM, et al: Inflammatory pseudotumors of the lung: Progression from organizing pneumonia to fibrous histiocytoma or to plasma cell granuloma in 32 cases. Hum Pathol 19:807, 1988.
233. Pettinato G, Manivel JC, DeRosa N, et al: Inflammatory myofibroblastic tumor (plasma cell granuloma): Clinicopathologic study of 20 cases with immunohistochemical and ultrastructural observations. Am J Clin Pathol 94:538, 1990.
234. Schwartz EE, Katz SM, Mandell GA: Postinflammatory pseudotumors of the lung: Fibrous histiocytoma and related lesions. Radiology 136:609, 1980.
235. McCall IH, Woo-Ming M: The radiological appearances of plasma cell granuloma of the lung. Clin Radiol 29:145, 1978.
236. Berardi RS, Lee SS, Chen HP, et al: Inflammatory pseudotumors of the lung. Surg Gynecol Obstet 156:89, 1983.
237. Agrons GA, Rosado de Christenson ML, Kirejczyk WM, et al: Pulmonary inflammatory pseudotumor: Radiologic features. Radiology 206:511, 1998.
238. Woodard PK, Dehdashti F, Putman CE: Radiologic diagnosis of extrathoracic metastases to the lung. Oncology 12:431, 1998.
239. Putnam JB Jr, Roth JA: Surgical treatment for pulmonary metastases from sarcoma. Hematol Oncol Clin North Am 9:869, 1995.
240. Johnson RM, Lindskog GE: 100 cases of tumor metastatic to the lung and mediastinum. JAMA 202:94, 1967.
241. Winterbauer RH, Elfenbein IB, Ball WC Jr: Incidence and clinical significance of tumor embolization to the lungs. Am J Med 45:271, 1968.
242. Janower ML, Blennerhassett JB: Lymphangitic spread of metastatic cancer to the lung: A radiologic-pathologic classification. Radiology 101:267, 1971.
243. Harold JT: Lymphangitis carcinomatosa of the lungs. QJM 83:353, 1952.
244. Hagerstrand I, Fichera G: The small lymph vessels of the lungs in lymphangiosis carcinomatosa. Acta Pathol Microbiol Scand 65:505, 1965.
245. Gonzalez-Vitale JC, Garcia-Bunuel R: Pulmonary tumor emboli and cor pulmonale in primary carcinoma of the lung. Cancer 38:2105, 1976.
246. Crow J, Slavin G, Kreel L: Pulmonary metastasis: A pathologic and radiologic study. Cancer 47:2595, 1981.
247. Hirakata K, Nakata H, Nakagawa T: CT of pulmonary metastases with pathological correlation. Semin Ultrasound CT MRI 16:379, 1995.
248. Burton RM: A case of chorion-epithelioma with pulmonary complications. Tubercle 44:487, 1963.
249. Muhm JR, Brown LR, Crowe JR, et al: Comparison of whole lung tomography for detecting pulmonary nodules. Am J Roentgenol 131:981, 1978.
250. Gross BH, Glazer GM, Bookstein FL: Multiple pulmonary nodules detected by computed tomography: Diagnostic implications. J Comput Assist Tomogr 9:880, 1985.
251. Davis SD: CT evaluation for pulmonary metastases in patients with extrathoracic malignancy. Radiology 180:1, 1991.
252. Peuchot M, Libshitz HI: Pulmonary metastatic disease: Radiologic-surgical correlation. Radiology 164:719, 1987.
253. Yokomise H, Mizuno H, Ike O, et al: Importance of intrapulmonary lymph nodes in the differential diagnosis of small pulmonary shadows. Chest 113:703, 1998.
254. Remy-Jardin M, Remy J, Giraud F, et al: Pulmonary nodules: Detection with thick-section spiral CT versus conventional CT. Radiology 187:513, 1993.
255. Buckley JA, Scott WW, Siegelman SS, et al: Pulmonary nodules: Effect of increased data sampling on detection with spiral CT and confidence in diagnosis. Radiology 196:395, 1995.
256. Diederich S, Semik M, Lentschig MG, et al: Helical CT of pulmonary nodules in patients with extrathoracic malignancy: CT-surgical correlation. Am J Roentgenol 172:353, 1999.
257. Tillich M, Kammerhuber F, Reittner P, et al: Detection of pulmonary nodules with helical CT: Comparison of cine and film-based viewing. Am J Roentgenol 169:1611, 1997.
258. Schaner EG, Chang AE, Doppman JL, et al: Comparison of computed and conventional whole lung tomography in detecting pulmonary nodules: A prospective radiologic-pathologic study. Am J Roentgenol 131:51, 1978.
259. Chang AE, Schaner EG, Conkle DM, et al: Evaluation of computed tomography in the detection of pulmonary metastases: A prospective study. Cancer 43:913, 1979.
260. Williams MP, Husband JE, Heron CW: Intrathoracic manifestations of metastatic testicular seminoma: A comparison of chest radiographic and CT findings. Am J Roentgenol 149:473, 1987.
261. Edwards SE, Kelsey-Fry I: Prevalence of nodules on computed tomography of patients without known malignant disease. Br J Radiol 55:715, 1982.
262. Müller NL, Gamsu G, Webb WR: Pulmonary nodules: Detection using magnetic resonance and computed tomography. Radiology 155:687, 1985.
263. Feuerstein IM, Jicha DL, Pass HI, et al: Pulmonary metastases: MR imaging with surgical correlation—a prospective study. Radiology 182:123, 1992.
264. Clagett OT, Woolner LB: Surgical treatment of solitary metastatic pulmonary lesion. Med Clin North Am 48:939, 1964.
265. Hirakata K, Nakata H, Haratake J: Appearance of pulmonary metastases on high-resolution CT scans: Comparison with histopathologic findings from autopsy specimens. Am J Roentgenol 161:37, 1993.
266. Adkins PC, Wesselhoeft CW Jr, Newman W, et al: Thoracotomy on the patient with previous malignancy: Metastasis or new primary? J Thorac Cardiovasc Surg 56:351, 1968.
267. Cahan WG, Castro El B, Hajdu SI: The significance of a solitary lung shadow in patients with colon carcinoma. Cancer 33:414, 1974.
268. Girard P, Baldeyrou P, Le Chevalier T, et al: Surgical resection of pulmonary metastases: Up to what number? Am J Respir Crit Care Med 149:469, 1994.
269. Heij HA, Vos A, de Kraker J, et al: Prognostic factors in surgery for pulmonary metastases in children. Surgery 115:687, 1994.
269a. Matthay RA, Arroliga AC: Resection of pulmonary metastases. Am Rev Respir Dis 148:1691, 1993.
270. Askin FB: Something old? Something new? Second primary or pulmonary metastasis in the patient with known extrathoracic carcinoma. Am J Clin Pathol 100:4, 1993.
271. Nystrom JS, Weiner JM, Wolf RM, et al: Identifying the primary site in metastatic cancer of unknown origin. JAMA 241:381, 1979.
272. Steckel RJ, Kagan AR: Diagnostic persistence in working up metastatic cancer with an unknown primary site. Radiology 134:367, 1980.
273. Ziskind MM, Weill H, Payzant AR: The recognition and significance of acinus-filling processes of the lungs. Am Rev Respir Dis 87:551, 1963.
274. Friedmann G, Bohndorf K, Kruger J: Radiology of pulmonary metastases: Comparison of imaging techniques with operative findings. Thorac Cardiovasc Surg 34:120, 1986.
275. Shirakusa T, Tsutsui M, Motonaga R, et al: Resection of metastatic lung tumor: The evaluation of histologic appearance in the lung. Am Surg 54:655, 1988.
276. Primack SL, Hartman TE, Lee KS, et al: Pulmonary nodules and the CT halo sign. Radiology 190:513, 1994.
277. Shepard JO, Moore EH, Templeton PA, et al: Pulmonary intravascular tumor emboli: Dilated and beaded peripheral pulmonary arteries at CT. Radiology 187:797, 1993.
278. Kaste SC, Winer-Muram HT, Jenkins III JJ: Pulmonary nodules with a linear and beaded appearance: A nonspecific finding. Radiology 195:874, 1995.
279. Meziane MA, Hruban RH, Zerhouni EA, et al: High-resolution CT of the lung parenchyma with pathologic correlation. Radiographics 8:27, 1988.
280. Milne ENC, Zerhouni EA: Blood supply of pulmonary metastases. J Thorac Imaging 2:15, 1987.
281. Murata K, Takahashi M, Mori M, et al: Pulmonary metastatic nodules: CT-pathologic correlation. Radiology 182:331, 1992.
282. LeMay M, Piro AJ: Cavitary pulmonary metastases. Ann Intern Med 62:59, 1965.

283. Dodd GD, Boyle JJ: Excavating pulmonary metastases. Am J Roentgenol 85:277, 1961.

284. Don C, Gray DG: Cavitating secondary carcinoma of the lung. J Can Assoc Radiol 18:310, 1967.

285. Chaudhuri MR: Cavitary pulmonary metastases. Thorax 25:375, 1970.

286. Zollikofer C, Castaneda-Zuniga W, Stenlund R, et al: Lung metastases from synovial sarcoma simulating granulomas. Am J Roentgenol 135:161, 1980.

287. Cockshott WP, de V Hendrickse JP: Pulmonary calcification at the site of trophoblastic metastases. Br J Radiol 42:17, 1969.

288. Vogelzang NJ, Stenlund R: Residual pulmonary nodules after combination chemotherapy of testicular cancer. Radiology 146:195, 1983.

289. Libshitz HI, Jing B-S, Wallace S, et al: Sterilized metastases: A diagnostic and therapeutic dilemma. Am J Roentgenol 140:15, 1983.

290. Dines DE, Cortese DA, Brennan MD, et al: Malignant pulmonary neoplasms predisposing to spontaneous pneumothorax. Mayo Clin Proc 48:541, 1973.

291. Kane RD, Hawkins HK, Miller JA, et al: Microscopic pulmonary tumor emboli associated with dyspnea. Cancer 36:1473, 1975.

292. Smevik B, Olbjorn K: The risk of spontaneous pneumothorax in patients with osteogenic sarcoma and testicular cancer. Cancer 49:1734, 1982.

293. Soares FA, Pinto PFE, Magnani GA, et al: Pulmonary tumor embolism to arterial vessels and carcinomatous lymphangitis: A comparative clinicopathological study. Arch Pathol Lab Med 117:827, 1993.

294. Youngberg AS: Unilateral diffuse lung opacity. Radiology 123:277, 1977.

295. Munk PL, Müller NL, Miller RR, et al: Pulmonary lymphangitic carcinomatosis: CT and pathologic findings. Radiology 166:705, 1988.

296. Goldsmith SH, Bailey HD, Callahan EL, et al: Pulmonary metastases from breast carcinoma. Arch Surg 94:483, 1967.

297. Sadoff L, Grossman J, Weiner N: Lymphangitic pulmonary metastasis secondary to breast cancer with normal chest x-rays and abnormal perfusion lung scans. Oncology 31:164, 1975.

298. Stein MG, Mayo J, Müller NL, et al: Pulmonary lymphangitic spread of carcinoma: Appearance on CT scans. Radiology 162:371, 1987.

299. Ren H, Hruban RH, Kuhlman JE, et al: Computed tomography of inflation-fixed lungs: The beaded septum sign of pulmonary metastases. J Comput Assist Tomogr 13:411, 1989.

300. Johkoh T, Ikezoe J, Tomiyama N, et al: CT findings in lymphangitic carcinomatosis of the lung: Correlation with histologic findings and pulmonary function tests. Am J Roentgenol 158:1217, 1992.

301. Mathieson JR, Mayo JR, Staples CA, et al: Chronic diffuse infiltrative lung disease: Comparison of diagnostic accuracy of CT and chest radiography. Radiology 171:111, 1989.

302. Grenier P, Chevret S, Beigelman C, et al: Chronic diffuse infiltrative lung disease: Determination of the diagnostic value of clinical data, chest radiography, and CT with bayesian analysis. Radiology 191:383, 1994.

303. Soares FA, Magnani LGA, Mello de Oliveira JA: Pulmonary tumor embolism to alveolar septal capillaries: A prospective study of 12 cases. Arch Pathol Lab Med 115:127, 1991.

304. Soares FA, Magnani LGA, Mello de Oliveira JA: Pulmonary tumor embolism to alveolar septal capillaries: An unusual cause of sudden cor pulmonale. Arch Pathol Lab Med 116:187, 1992.

305. Chakeres DW, Spiegel PK: Fatal pulmonary hypertension secondary to intravascular metastatic tumor emboli. Am J Roentgenol 139:997, 1982.

306. Bagshawe KD, Noble MIM: Cardiorespiratory aspects of trophoblastic tumours. QJM 35:39, 1966.

307. Kang CH, Choi J-A, Kim HR, et al: Lung metastases manifesting as pulmonary infarction by mucin and tumor embolization: Radiographic, high-resolution CT, and pathologic findings. J Comput Assist Tomogr 23:644, 1999.

308. Parker KM, Embry JH: Sudden death due to tricuspid valve myxoma with massive pulmonary embolism in a 15-month old male. J Forensic Sci 42:524, 1997.

309. Dada MA, Van Velden DJ: Sudden death caused by testicular germ cell tumour. Med Sci Law 35:357, 1995.

310. Altemus LR, Lee RE: Carcinomatosis of the lung with pulmonary hypertension: Pathoradiologic spectrum. Arch Intern Med 119:32, 1967.

311. Bates SC, Tranum BL: Perfusion lung scan: An aid in detection of lymphangitic carcinomatosis. Cancer 50:232, 1982.

312. Jariwalla AG, Seaton A, McCormack RJM, et al: Intrabronchial metastases from renal carcinoma with recurrent tumour expectoration. Thorax 36:179, 1981.

313. Albertini RE, Ekberg NL: Endobronchial metastasis in breast cancer. Thorax 35:435, 1980.

314. Sutton FD Jr, Vestal RE, Creagh CE: Varied presentations of metastatic pulmonary melanoma. Chest 65:415, 1974.

315. Morency G, Chalaoui J, Samson SJ: Malignant neoplasms of the trachea. J Can Assoc Radiol 40:198, 1989.

316. Madden M, Goldstraw P, Corrin B: Effect of chemotherapy on the histological appearances of testicular teratoma metastatic to the lung: Correlation with patient survival. J Clin Pathol 37:1212, 1984.

317. Moran CA, Travis WD, Carter D, et al: Metastatic mature teratoma in lung following testicular embryonal carcinoma and teratocarcinoma. Arch Pathol Lab Med 117:641, 1993.

318. Leonardi HK, Jung-Legg Y, Legg MA, et al: Tracheobronchial mucoepidermoid carcinoma: Clinicopathological features and results of treatment. J Thorac Cardiovasc Surg 76:431, 1978.

CHAPTER 7

Lymphoproliferative Disorders and Leukemia

PULMONARY LYMPHOID HYPERPLASIA

Focal Lymphoid Hyperplasia

Focal lymphoid hyperplasia (nodular lymphoid hyperplasia, pseudolymphoma) is an uncommon abnormality characterized pathologically by a localized proliferation of lymphocytes, plasma cells, and histiocytes, most or all of which are cytologically benign.[5] The fundamental nature of the abnormality has been debated. Originally, it was considered to be a reactive (hyperplastic) lesion to an unknown stimulus that simulated lymphoma histologically (hence the term *pseudolymphoma*). On the basis of the results of immunohistochemical and molecular studies performed in the 1980s and 1990s, however, it now is apparent that many of the lesions are low-grade lymphomas. Despite the availability of modern diagnostic techniques, the distinction between a benign and a malignant tumor still is difficult in some cases.

The most frequent radiologic manifestations consist of a solitary nodule or a focal area of consolidation usually limited to one lobe (Fig. 7–1, Table 7–1).[6, 7] The tumors usually measure 2 to 5 cm in diameter,[5] although masses

and areas of consolidation measuring 10 cm in diameter have been described.[8] Virtually all lesions contain air bronchograms.[7] Less common manifestations include multiple nodules or multiple areas of consolidation and cavitation.[7] There is no associated lymphadenopathy; its presence or the presence of pleural effusion should suggest a diagnosis of lymphoma.[6]

Diffuse Lymphoid Hyperplasia

Two varieties of diffuse pulmonary lymphoid hyperplasia have been described according to anatomic location. The first affects predominantly the parenchymal interstitium (lymphoid or lymphocytic interstitial pneumonia) and the second affects predominantly the interstitium adjacent to conducting airways (follicular bronchitis and bronchiolitis).[9] Although the two traditionally have been considered as separate entities, it has been argued that they represent a spectrum of reactive histologic change to a variety of stimuli.[9] Similar to focal lymphoid hyperplasia, the distinction of the diffuse process from lymphoma is difficult in some cases (particularly for lymphocytic interstitial pneumonia).

Table 7–1. LYMPHOID HYPERPLASIA: CHARACTERISTIC RADIOLOGIC FINDINGS

Focal Lymphoid Hyperplasia (Pseudolymphoma)

Solitary nodule
Focal area of consolidation

Diffuse Lymphoid Hyperplasia

Lymphocytic interstitial pneumonia
  Chest radiograph
    Reticulonodular pattern
  HRCT
    Ground-glass pattern
    Poorly defined centrilobular nodules
    Multiple cysts in 70% of cases
Follicular bronchitis and bronchiolitis
  Chest radiograph
    Reticulonodular pattern
  HRCT
    Centrilobular nodules
    Peribronchovascular nodules
    Subpleural nodules

HRCT, high-resolution computed tomography.

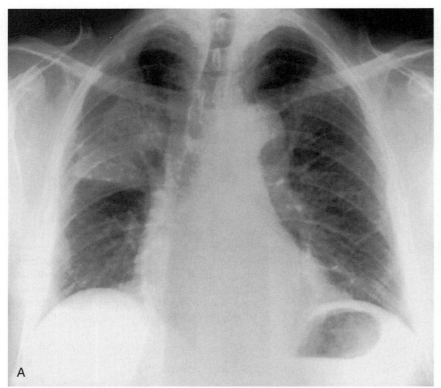

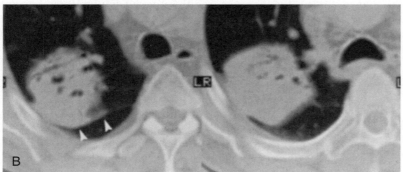

Figure 7–1. Focal Lymphoid Hyperplasia. Posteroanterior chest radiograph *(A)* shows an area of air-space consolidation in the posterior segment of the right upper lobe. The right hilum and mediastinum are normal. Sequential 10-mm collimation CT scans through the posterior segmental lesion *(B)* reveal a nodular area of consolidation that abuts the major fissure *(arrowheads)* and contains an air bronchogram. Pathologic analysis of the resected lobe disclosed features of lymphoid hyperplasia. The patient was a 57-year-old man.

Lymphocytic Interstitial Pneumonia

Lymphocytic interstitial pneumonia is probably the more common of the two abnormalities of diffuse lymphoid hyperplasia. Affected patients usually have underlying disease, most often rheumatoid disease, Sjögren's syndrome, or acquired immunodeficiency syndrome (AIDS). With the exception of AIDS, in which affected patients typically are children, most patients are adults (mean age, about 50 years).[11, 12] Pathologically the abnormality is characterized by a more or less diffuse interstitial infiltrate of mononuclear cells, in the typical case, predominantly lymphocytes;[11] plasma cells occasionally are prominent.[12, 13] Interstitial fibrosis also is present in some cases and can become severe enough to result in a honeycomb appearance.[10, 14]

The most frequently reported radiographic findings consist of a reticular or reticulonodular pattern involving mainly the lower lung zones (*see* Table 7–1).[11, 15] In some cases, branching and linear opacities consistent with interlobular septal thickening have been described in the lung periphery;[14] however, such thickening is more suggestive of

lymphoma than lymphocytic interstitial pneumonia. Other radiographic patterns include bilateral areas of ground-glass opacity[16] or consolidation (Fig. 7–2).[17] A nodular pattern also may occur,[15] most commonly in patients who have AIDS.[6, 18] Hilar and mediastinal lymph node enlargement has been described in patients who have AIDS and lymphocytic interstitial pneumonia,[18, 19] but this finding seldom is present in patients without AIDS.[6, 17, 20] Pleural effusion is rare.

The most common abnormalities on high-resolution computed tomography (HRCT) scan consist of bilateral areas of ground-glass attenuation (*see* Fig. 7–2) and poorly defined centrilobular nodules; other common findings include subpleural nodules, thickening of the bronchovascular bundles, and cysts (Fig. 7–3).[16, 21, 22] In one investigation of HRCT findings in 22 patients, all were found to have areas of ground-glass attenuation and poorly defined centrilobular nodules; 19 (86%), subpleural nodules; 19 (86%), thickening of the bronchovascular bundles; 18 (82%), mild interlobular septal thickening; and 15 (68%), cystic air spaces.[22] In another investigation of 17 patients with

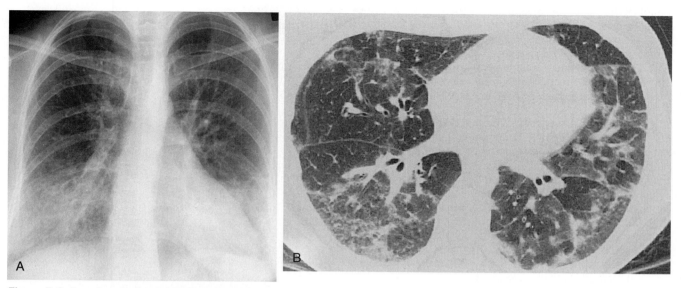

Figure 7–2. Lymphocytic Interstitial Pneumonia. Posteroanterior chest radiograph *(A)* in a 26-year-old woman with rheumatoid arthritis shows bilateral areas of ground-glass opacity and consolidation involving the lower lung zones. HRCT scan *(B)* shows extensive bilateral areas of ground-glass attenuation and focal areas of consolidation. The diagnosis of lymphoid interstitial pneumonia was proved at video-assisted thoracoscopic biopsy.

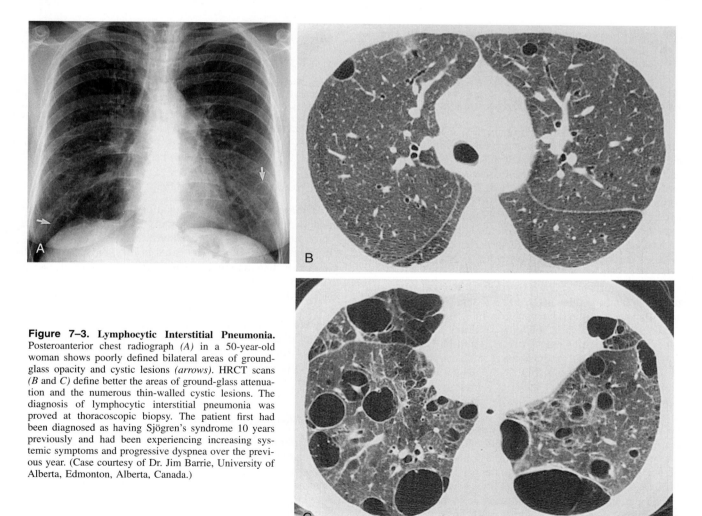

Figure 7–3. Lymphocytic Interstitial Pneumonia. Posteroanterior chest radiograph *(A)* in a 50-year-old woman shows poorly defined bilateral areas of ground-glass opacity and cystic lesions *(arrows).* HRCT scans *(B and C)* define better the areas of ground-glass attenuation and the numerous thin-walled cystic lesions. The diagnosis of lymphocytic interstitial pneumonia was proved at thoracoscopic biopsy. The patient first had been diagnosed as having Sjögren's syndrome 10 years previously and had been experiencing increasing systemic symptoms and progressive dyspnea over the previous year. (Case courtesy of Dr. Jim Barrie, University of Alberta, Edmonton, Alberta, Canada.)

lymphocytic interstitial pneumonia, ground-glass opacities were seen in 13 (76%); cysts, in 14 (82%); and nodules, in 12 (71%).[23] The nodules in lymphocytic interstitial pneumonia usually measure less than 10 mm in diameter.[22, 23] Although lymph node enlargement seldom is evident on chest radiograph, mediastinal lymphadenopathy has been reported in approximately two thirds of the patients on HRCT scan.[22]

One group of investigators compared HRCT findings in 17 patients with lymphocytic interstitial pneumonia and 44 patients with malignant lymphoma of the lung.[23] The most helpful findings in distinguishing lymphocytic interstitial pneumonia from lymphoma were the presence of cysts in lymphocytic interstitial pneumonia and the presence of large nodules (11 to 30 mm in diameter), consolidation, and pleural effusion in lymphoma. Of patients with lymphocytic interstitial pneumonia, 82% had cysts, 18% had consolidation, 6% had large nodules, and none had pleural effusion. Of patients with pulmonary lymphoma, 2% had cysts, 66% had air-space consolidation, 41% had large nodules, and 25% had pleural effusion.[23]

The natural history of lymphocytic interstitial pneumonia is variable. In some individuals, there is progression of disease within the lung, sometimes associated with fibrosis and an evolution similar to that of idiopathic pulmonary fibrosis. Honeycombing is seen occasionally on HRCT scan in such patients.[22] In other individuals, the disease evolves into clear-cut lymphoma.[24, 25]

Follicular Bronchitis and Bronchiolitis

Follicular bronchitis and bronchiolitis are characterized histologically by a mononuclear cell infiltrate (predominantly lymphocytes, with lesser numbers of plasma cells and histiocytes) in the interstitial tissue adjacent to bronchi and bronchioles. As the name suggests, germinal center formation is common, resulting in a distinctly nodular appearance to the abnormality.[26] Similar to lymphocytic interstitial pneumonia, many patients have a history of an underlying immunodeficiency disorder or connective tissue disease, particularly Sjögren's syndrome or rheumatoid arthritis.[26]

Chest radiograph characteristically shows a diffuse reticular or reticulonodular pattern (*see* Table 7–1).[26, 27] HRCT scan shows small nodular opacities in a peribronchovascular centrilobular and subpleural distribution.[28, 29] In most cases, these opacities measure 1 to 3 mm in diameter (Fig. 7–4), although focal nodular cases of consolidation 1 cm in diameter may be seen (Fig. 7–5).[29]

In one investigation of the HRCT findings in 12 patients who had biopsy-proven follicular bronchiolitis, the predominant abnormalities consisted of nodules and areas of ground-glass attenuation.[29] The nodules had a centrilobular distribution in all 12 patients; additional peribronchial nodules were present in 5 (42%) patients, and subpleural nodules were present in 3 (25%) patients. The nodules were diffuse but involved mainly the lower lung zones. Nine (75%) patients had patchy bilateral areas of ground-glass attenuation. Additional findings seen in a few patients included mild interlobular septal thickening, bronchial wall thickening, and peribronchial consolidation.

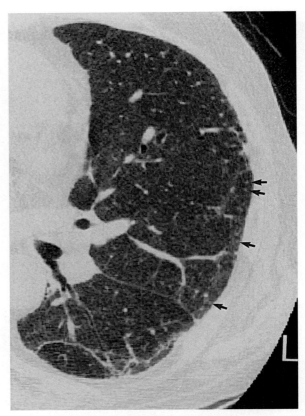

Figure 7–4. Follicular Bronchiolitis. View of the left lung from HRCT scan shows centrilobular subpleural nodules measuring 1 to 3 mm in diameter *(arrows)*. Evidence of mild fibrosis with irregular linear opacities and thickening of interlobular septa, particularly in the left lower lobe, is noted. The patient was a 64-year-old man who had progressive systemic sclerosis.

NON-HODGKIN'S LYMPHOMA

The most frequent manifestation of thoracic involvement in non-Hodgkin's lymphoma is mediastinal or hilar lymph node enlargement, a feature that was evident radiographically in 36% of 1,269 cases in one study.[30] Although pulmonary parenchymal disease is less common, it also is evident in many patients. The latter form of the disease can be considered conveniently in two groups: (1) patients in whom lymphoma apparently is limited to the lungs with or without mediastinal lymph node involvement at the time of diagnosis (*primary* pulmonary lymphoma) and (2) patients in whom concomitant or previous extrathoracic lymphoma is evident as well (*secondary* pulmonary lymphoma).

Mediastinal Lymphoma

Lymphoma involving the mediastinum may be part of a generalized process or may occur exclusively or predominantly at this site; in the latter situation, the tumor is sometimes known as *primary mediastinal lymphoma*. Although virtually any histologic type of lymphoma may be identified,[142] the two most common forms are lymphoblastic and diffuse large cell. The former tends to occur mainly in children and adolescents and the latter in young to

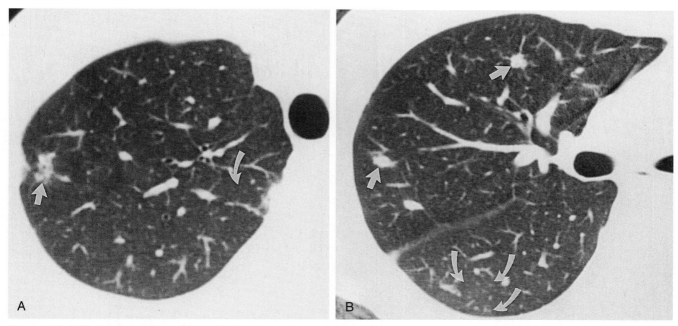

Figure 7–5. Follicular Bronchitis and Bronchiolitis. Views of the right lung near the apex *(A)* and at the level of the bronchus intermedius *(B)* from HRCT scan show focal nodular infiltrates surrounding bronchi *(straight arrows)* and a few small centrilobular nodular opacities *(curved arrows)* resulting from follicular bronchiolitis. The patient was a 24-year-old woman who had rheumatoid arthritis.

middle-aged adults.[67, 68] The radiologic manifestations of these two forms are similar and are described together.

Radiologically the most commonly involved lymph nodes are those in the anterior mediastinal and paratracheal regions.[54, 55] In one investigation of 181 consecutive patients who had no previous treatment, involvement of these groups was apparent radiographically in 24% and on computed tomography (CT) scan in 34% (Table 7–2).[55] Other nodal stations that may be involved include, in decreasing order of frequency, the subcarinal, hilar, internal mammary, pericardial, and posterior mediastinal regions.[55] In 40% of cases, lymphadenopathy involves a single nodal group;[54] when multiple groups are affected, involvement may be noncontiguous. The enlarged nodes may have homogeneous soft tissue attenuation (Fig. 7–6) or, less commonly, a central area of decreased attenuation and rim enhancement. The nodes may encase major vessels and lead to obstruction of the superior vena cava (Fig. 7–7). Irradiation or chemotherapy (or both) can result in a rapid resolution of disease. After treatment, particularly radiotherapy, dystrophic calcification may occur, most commonly within lymph nodes in the anterior mediastinum.[69] Rarely, nodal calcification is present at the time of initial diagnosis.[44]

The contribution of CT to the initial staging of patients

who have non-Hodgkin's lymphoma was assessed in a study of 181 consecutive individuals.[55] Intrathoracic abnormalities were seen in 45%. Prevascular and paratracheal lymph node enlargement was the most common abnormality, being present in approximately 75% of patients who had intrathoracic disease. (As might be expected, lymphadenopathy was seen more commonly on CT than on radiography; CT was particularly helpful in the detection of subcarinal and pericardial node enlargement.) Pulmonary parenchymal involvement was evident on CT scan in 24 patients (13%); in approximately one third of these, the abnormalities were not evident on radiography. The most common findings in the lung parenchyma included nodules, masses, and focal areas of air-space consolidation; less commonly, direct parenchymal infiltration from adjacent mediastinal lymph nodes was evident (Fig. 7–8).[55] Pleural effusion was seen on CT scan in 36 (20%) patients; focal soft tissue pleural masses, in 9 (5%); and chest wall involvement, in 9. Overall the findings on routine chest CT scan increased the stage in 16 patients (9%) but did not influence therapy.

Magnetic resonance (MR) imaging shows the same anatomic features as CT. Lymphoma usually has a homogeneous appearance on MR imaging, the signal intensity being slightly greater than muscle on T1-weighted and T2-weighted images.[70] Although MR imaging enables greater soft tissue contrast than CT, it seldom is used in the initial assessment of patients who have lymphoma. MR imaging may be helpful, however, in patients who are allergic to intravenous contrast agents or who have superior vena cava syndrome or in the assessment of pericardial or chest wall invasion. In one study of 57 patients who had biopsy-proven non-Hodgkin's lymphoma or Hodgkin's disease, chest wall involvement was evident on MR imaging in 20 and on CT in 7,[71] and pleural disease was seen on MR

Table 7–2. NON-HODGKIN'S LYMPHOMA: CHARACTERISTIC RADIOLOGIC FINDINGS

Intrathoracic disease present in one third of patients
Mediastinal lymph node enlargement most common finding
Most frequently involves anterior mediastinal nodes
Involves several nodal stations in 60% of patients
Enlarged nodes may be in noncontiguous stations
Nodes may calcify after radiotherapy
Concomitant parenchymal involvement in 10%

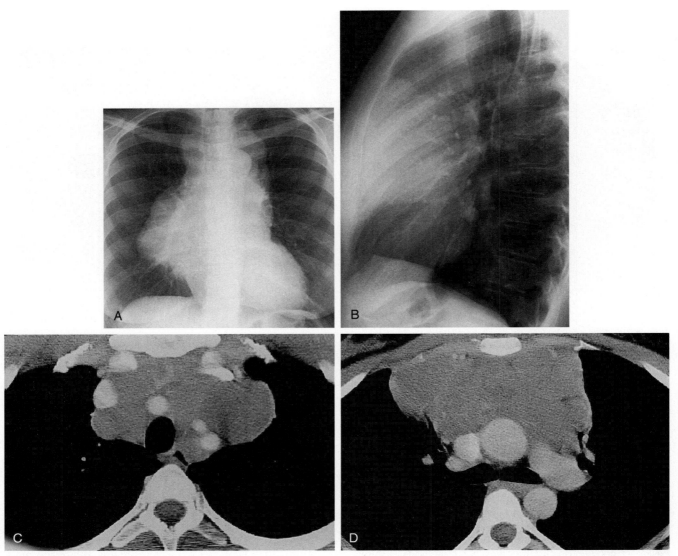

Figure 7–6. Mediastinal B-Cell Lymphoma. Posteroanterior *(A)* and lateral *(B)* chest radiographs reveal a large, lobulated anterior mediastinal mass. Note the absence of hilar lymphadenopathy, the interlobar arteries being seen clearly through the soft tissue masses (*hilum overlay* sign). Contrast-enhanced spiral CT scans *(C and D)* show diffuse enlargement of the anterior mediastinal and paratracheal lymph nodes with obliteration of the fat planes between the nodes. Despite the extensive lymphadenopathy, there is no evidence of compression of the vascular structures. Mediastinoscopy revealed diffuse large cell lymphoma. The patient was a 31-year-old woman.

imaging in 14 patients and on CT in 5. Of the 15 patients in the study who had chest wall disease and were treated with radiation therapy, 3 (20%) had the portals changed because of the MR imaging findings.[71]

Gallium 67 scintigraphy is inferior to CT in the initial assessment of patients who have lymphoma. The procedure has an important role, however, in the evaluation of patients who have a residual tumor mass after treatment, uptake being present in lymphoma but not in necrotic and fibrotic tissue.[72–74] Preliminary results suggest that 2-(^{18}F)-fluoro-2-deoxy-D-glucose (FDG) positron emission tomography (PET) may be superior to CT in showing nodal involvement in non-Hodgkin's lymphoma and Hodgkin's disease.[75] FDG is a glucose analogue that is metabolized in proportion to the glycolytic metabolic rate, which is elevated in tumors;[76] uptake of the substance in non-Hodgkin's

lymphoma has been shown to correlate with tumor grade (and consequently prognosis).[77–79]

Primary Pulmonary Lymphoma

The criteria for accepting a lymphoma as originating in the lung are variable. Perhaps the most widely accepted criteria are those of Saltzstein,[1] who considered a lesion to be primary if it affected the lung (with or without involvement of hilar and mediastinal lymph nodes) and showed no evidence of extrathoracic disease for at least 3 months after the initial diagnosis. Such neoplasms are uncommon: In one study of 1,269 cases of lymphoma, only 0.34% were deemed to have a pulmonary origin.[30] Although virtually any histologic type of lymphoma can arise in the lung, the most common are classified as low-grade B-cell

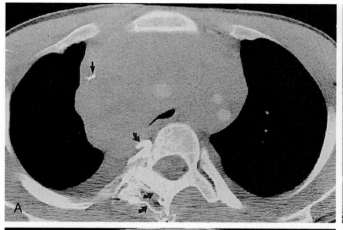

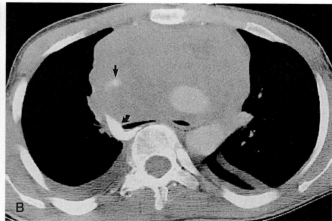

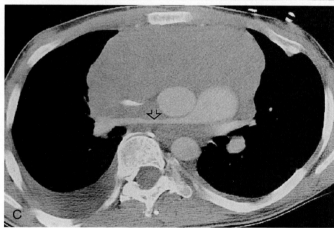

Figure 7–7. Mediastinal Lymphoblastic T-Cell Lymphoma with Superior Vena Cava Obstruction. Contrast-enhanced CT scan through the upper chest *(A)* shows diffuse soft tissue infiltration of the mediastinum resulting in marked compression and deformity of the trachea. Intravenous contrast material can be seen within an encased, markedly narrowed right brachiocephalic vein *(straight arrow)* and within collateral veins *(curved arrows)*. Small bilateral pleural effusions are noted. CT scan at the level of the main bronchi *(B)* reveals encasement of the superior vena cava *(straight arrow)* and prominent collateral circulation through the azygos vein *(curved arrow)*. CT scan at the level of the bronchus intermedius *(C)* shows narrowing and elongation of the right pulmonary artery *(open arrow)*. The patient was an 18-year-old man who presented with progressive shortness of breath and clinical findings of superior vena cava obstruction.

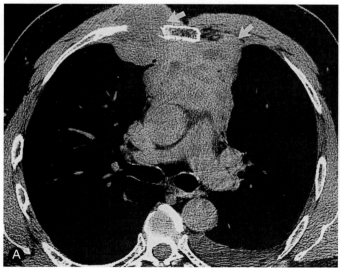

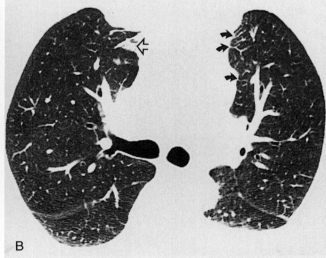

Figure 7–8. B-Cell Lymphoma with Chest Wall and Pulmonary Invasion. CT scan *(A)* in a 51-year-old man shows inhomogeneous enlargement of the anterior mediastinal nodes with direct extension into the chest wall *(arrows)*. A small left pleural effusion is evident. Lung windows *(B)* show thickening of interlobular septa *(curved arrows)* adjacent to the enlarged mediastinal lymph nodes consistent with direct extension of lymphoma into the lungs. The focal area of consolidation in the right lung *(open arrow)* is presumed to represent secondary lymphoma.

lymphoma (MALToma) and angiocentric immunoproliferative lesion (lymphomatoid granulomatosis).

Low-Grade B-Cell Lymphoma

It now is believed widely that many extranodal lymphomas, including those that arise in the lung, are derived from mucosa-associated lymphoid tissue (MALT); hence the term *MALToma* that sometimes is used to describe the tumors.[5, 32, 33] In the lung, the tumors are believed to arise from marginal zone cells that are present in normal or hyperplastic bronchus–associated lymphoid tissue.[32] This form of lymphoma is the most frequent to involve the lungs primarily, accounting for 60% to 90% of cases.[2, 31] Most tumors occur in adults, with a mean age at diagnosis of about 55 to 60 years.[3, 4] Men and women are affected equally.

The most common radiologic manifestation consists of nodules or nodular areas of consolidation (Table 7–3).[143–145] The nodules range from 2 mm to 8 cm in diameter and may be single or, more commonly, multiple.[144, 145] The nodules or areas of consolidation are usually centered on the airways.[144] Air bronchograms are visible on radiography or CT in 50% to 100% of cases (Fig. 7–9).[35, 144] The areas of consolidation may range from a small subsegmental region to an entire lobe and be single or multiple (Fig. 7–10).[3, 36, 37] CT may depict multifocal or bilateral abnormalities in patients with a single parenchymal finding on chest radiography.[144] Less common abnormalities seen on CT include peribronchovascular interstitial thickening, septal lines, and ground-glass opacities.[143, 144] The parenchymal abnormalities typically show an indolent course with slow growth over months or years.[35, 38] Pleural effusion is present in 10% to 20% of cases, usually in association with evidence of parenchymal involvement.[3, 35, 145] Lymph node enlargement is evident radiographically in fewer than 5% of cases at presentation,[2] and on CT in as many as 10% of cases.[143]

On CT scan, the bronchi within affected lung parenchyma frequently are dilated[144] but may occasionally appear stretched and slightly narrowed.[36] Rarely, airway involvement is manifested by bronchial wall thickening and marked narrowing of the bronchial lumen.[39]

As the name suggests, patients who have primary pulmonary low-grade B-cell lymphoma generally have an excellent prognosis.[3, 40] For example, in one study of 43

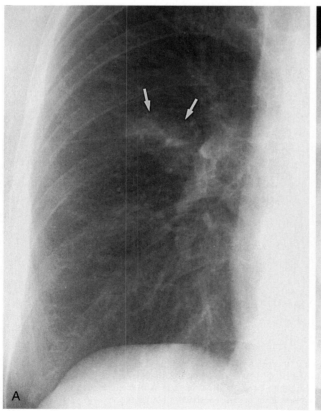
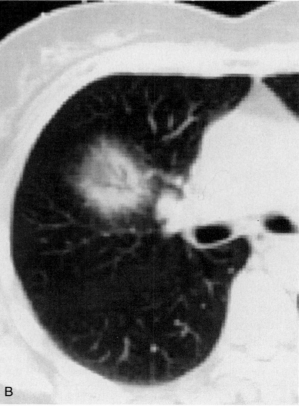

Figure 7–9. Primary Pulmonary Low-Grade B-Cell Lymphoma (MALToma). Close-up views of the right lung from posteroanterior chest radiograph *(A)* and conventional CT scan *(B)* show a 3-cm area of consolidation in the right upper lobe *(arrows).* An air bronchogram is visible on the CT scan. The diagnosis of low-grade B-cell lymphoma was proved at surgery. The patient was a 68-year-old woman.

esis) refers to a group

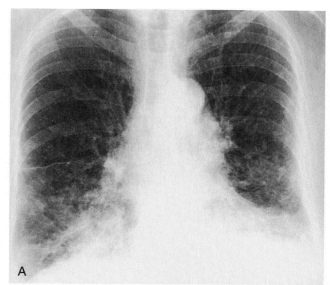

Figure 7–10. Primary Pulmonary Low-Grade B-Cell Lymphoma. Posteroanterior chest radiograph *(A)* shows poorly defined nodular opacities throughout both lungs and areas of consolidation in the lower lung zones. Small bilateral pleural effusions are seen. Magnified views of the right lung from HRCT scans *(B and C)* show nodular thickening of the interlobar fissures *(straight arrows)* and bronchovascular bundles *(curved arrows)*. Also present are a focal area of consolidation *(open arrow)* with air bronchograms in the right middle lobe and a small right pleural effusion. Similar findings were present in the left lung. The patient was a 73-year-old woman who presented with a 6-month history of dry cough and progressive shortness of breath.

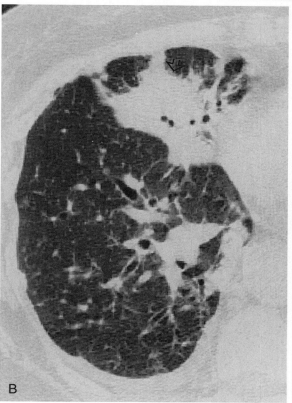

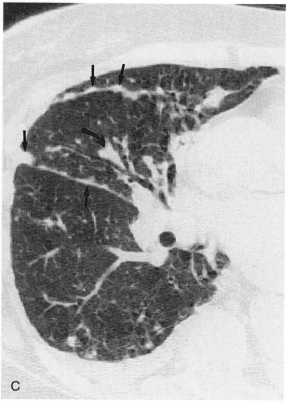

patients, the overall 5-year survival was 84%, a value equivalent to that of the appropriate unaffected (control) population.[31] Despite this finding, patients who had systemic symptoms (fever, night sweats, or weight loss) had a significantly poorer prognosis, the 5-year survival being only about 55%.

Angiocentric Immunoproliferative Lesion (Lymphomatoid Granulomatosis)

The term *angiocentric immunoproliferative lesion* (angioimmunoproliferative lesion, lymphomatoid granulomato-

sis) refers to a group of abnormalities characterized histologically by a lymphoid infiltrate that is polymorphic (i.e., composed of several cell types), has a variable degree of cytologic atypia, and shows prominent vascular infiltration. Tumors vary from those that are composed predominantly of benign-appearing cells (grade I) to those that are frankly malignant (grade III). The neoplastic cells may express either T-cell or B-cell phenotype. Patients who have grade II or III lesions tend to have involvement of extrathoracic tissues, particularly the skin and central nervous system.

The most common radiologic manifestation (present in 70% to 80% of patients) is one of multiple nodules or

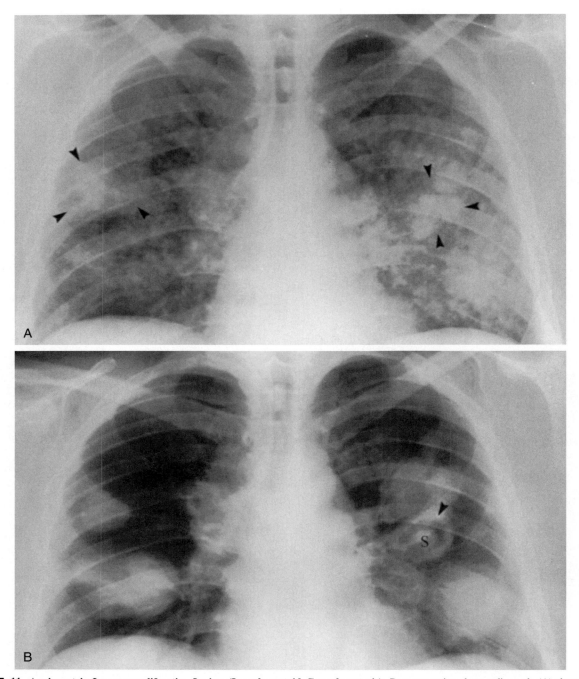

Figure 7–11. Angiocentric Immunoproliferative Lesion (Lymphomatoid Granulomatosis). Posteroanterior chest radiograph *(A)* shows bilateral confluent and isolated nodular opacities; some of the larger opacities *(arrowheads)* possess features of air-space consolidation. Bilateral hilar lymph node enlargement is present, and the aortopulmonary window is prominent, suggesting mediastinal node involvement. Two months later, a repeat chest radiograph *(B)* shows that the diffuse disease has resolved but has been replaced by large cavitary and noncavitary nodules. One cavitary lesion on the left *(arrowhead)* contains a central loose body (S) that could represent infarcted tissue or a blood clot. Several of the nodules relate to the more confluent areas of consolidation identified in the first radiograph *(A)*. Open-lung biopsy revealed infarcts caused by involvement of peripheral vessels by lymphomatoid granulomatosis. The patient was a 52-year-old man.

masses 0.5 to 8 cm in diameter.[48, 49, 51] In some patients, the initial abnormality consists of poorly defined opacities, which then progress over many weeks to form nodules or masses. The nodules frequently have ill-defined margins and show a tendency to coalesce (Fig. 7–11);[49] although they may be diffuse throughout both lungs, they tend to be most numerous in the lower lung zones.[46, 49] Cavitation is

present in 30% to 40% of patients.[46, 48, 49] Neither the nodules nor the masses contain air bronchograms.[49]

Other radiologic findings include areas of consolidation (described in 50% of patients)[48] and a reticulonodular pattern (in approximately 20%).[48, 49] Pleural effusions are present in 10% to 25% of patients.[48–50] Hilar lymph node enlargement is uncommon, being seen in only 14 of 284

(5%) patients reported in four studies.[47–49, 52] Rapid progression of any of the parenchymal abnormalities may be seen.

High-Grade Lymphoma

Most cases of primary high-grade pulmonary lymphoma are of B-cell type; occasional cases of anaplastic (Ki-1) lymphoma[41] or peripheral T-cell[42, 43] lymphoma have been reported. Some tumors appear to be derived from the low-grade B-cell lymphoma described previously.[5] Others occur in patients who have organ transplants (post-transplant lymphoproliferative disorder; *see* Chapter 11).

Radiologic manifestations are nonspecific and include localized opacities with or without air bronchograms, bilateral consolidation, and a diffuse reticulonodular pattern.[44] Occasionally, the pattern progresses from a localized opacity to extensive bilateral consolidation within a few weeks of initial presentation;[45] associated respiratory failure is common.

Secondary Pulmonary Lymphoma

Pleuropulmonary involvement with lymphoma in patients known to have disease outside of the thorax is much more common than the primary condition; for example, in one series of 1,269 cases, the pleura was affected in 21% and the lungs in 29%.[30] In another review of 651 patients, 54 (8%) had histologically documented pulmonary involvement.[53] Similar to carcinoma, such disease can develop by direct spread from involved mediastinal or hilar lymph nodes or by intravascular dissemination (metastasis).

Pulmonary involvement is apparent radiographically at presentation in approximately 5% to 10% of patients who have non-Hodgkin's lymphoma.[54, 55] The typical pattern consists of solitary or multiple nodules or masses 0.5 to 8 cm in diameter.[54, 55] They usually are most frequent in the lower lobes (Fig. 7–12).[56, 57] The nodules are round, ovoid, or polyhedral in shape and usually possess poorly defined margins, sometimes with linear strands extending into adjacent lung parenchyma. In cases of untreated lymphoma, the masses tend to coalesce, producing an opacity identical

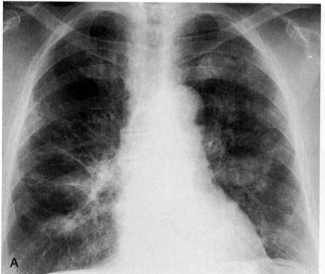
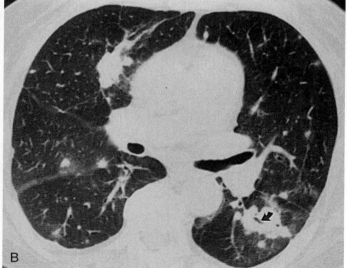
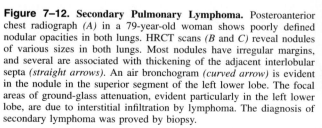
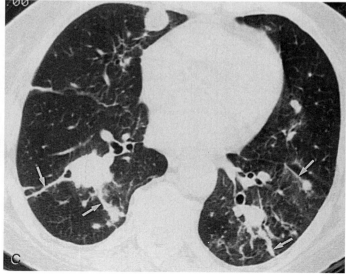

Figure 7–12. Secondary Pulmonary Lymphoma. Posteroanterior chest radiograph *(A)* in a 79-year-old woman shows poorly defined nodular opacities in both lungs. HRCT scans *(B and C)* reveal nodules of various sizes in both lungs. Most nodules have irregular margins, and several are associated with thickening of the adjacent interlobular septa *(straight arrows)*. An air bronchogram *(curved arrow)* is evident in the nodule in the superior segment of the left lower lobe. The focal areas of ground-glass attenuation, evident particularly in the left lower lobe, are due to interstitial infiltration by lymphoma. The diagnosis of secondary lymphoma was proved by biopsy.

to and indistinguishable from that of primary pulmonary lymphoma.[56] Cavitation occurs rarely.[54, 58, 59] In one series of patients who had large cell lymphoma, cystlike lesions situated within or contiguous to masses were observed in 17 patients;[1] in 8 patients, the cystic changes resembled cavitation radiographically.

In contrast to primary pulmonary lymphoma, the secondary variety tends to affect the larger airways (in most cases probably reflecting extension from bronchopulmonary lymph nodes) and may result in atelectasis and obstructive pneumonitis.[60, 61] A diffuse reticulonodular pattern with thickening of the interlobar septa resembling lymphangitic carcinomatosis sometimes occurs.[34, 56, 62] Less common findings include ground-glass opacities or air-space consolidation, particularly in patients who have recurrent disease.[34, 63]

Pleural involvement can be manifested in several ways. Effusion alone is uncommon;[64] however, it develops in association with parenchymal lymphoma at some point in the course of the disease in many patients (24 of 54 in one investigation[53]). Pleural thickening may be seen radiologically at presentation or during recurrence (occasionally as the only site).[65] The appearance may consist of plaquelike areas, focal nodules, masses, or, less commonly, diffuse thickening.[65, 66]

PLASMA CELL NEOPLASMS

Multiple Myeloma

Multiple myeloma is characterized pathologically by a proliferation of plasma cells with varying degrees of atypia.[81, 82] Thoracic involvement is common: In one review of 958 patients, evidence of skeletal or pleuropulmonary disease was found at some time during the course of the disorder in 443 (46%);[80] radiographic abnormalities were present in 25% at the time of diagnosis.

The usual radiographic appearance consists of one or more well-defined, osteolytic lesions; diffuse osteoporosis; fracture; or a combination of lesions. An involved rib may show focal expansion. Extension and proliferation of tumor cells outside the ribs in the adjacent chest wall result in a typical radiologic appearance of a smooth homogeneous soft tissue mass protruding into the thorax and compressing the lung (Fig. 7–13). Such tumor masses can grow to a large size, sometimes almost completely opacifying the hemithorax.[83] The association of an osteolytic lesion in a rib with a soft tissue mass protruding into the thorax should suggest the diagnosis strongly;[91] however, this combination also can occur with metastatic carcinoma, with other primary chest wall diseases (such as osteomyelitis), and with lesions originating in the lung (such as pulmonary carcinoma and fungal infections).

Infiltration of the lungs or pleura by neoplastic cells is much less common than infiltration of the skeleton. Pleural effusion caused by malignant infiltration has been reported rarely;[84, 85] for reasons that are unclear, this appears to occur more often on the left side. Pleural thickening and nodularity sometimes are evident in addition to the effusion.[86]

Plasmacytoma

A plasmacytoma is a more or less well-defined neoplastic proliferation of plasma cells in the absence of a general-

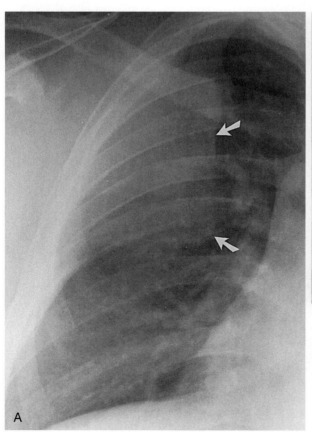

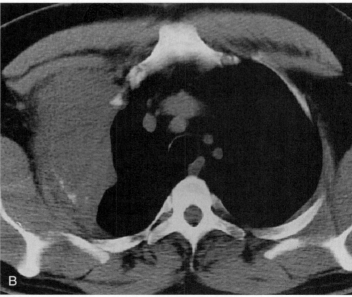

Figure 7–13. Multiple Myeloma. View of the right chest from posteroanterior radiograph *(A)* shows destruction of the anterior aspect of the right second rib associated with a soft tissue mass *(arrows)*. CT scan *(B)* confirms the rib destruction and shows tumor extending into the chest wall.

ized plasma cell dyscrasia. As such, it excludes the far more common situation in which a localized plasma cell tumor is a manifestation of multiple myeloma. These tumors can consist of an expansile osteolytic lesion of bone or a visceral or soft tissue mass; the latter often is termed *extramedullary plasmacytoma*. Most such tumors are located in the upper respiratory tract, particularly the pharynx; in one large review of 272 cases, only 13 (4.7%) tumors were situated in the lungs or trachea.[87] In a literature review in 1992, only 19 well-documented examples were described in the lower respiratory tract.[88]

HODGKIN'S DISEASE

Intrathoracic involvement in Hodgkin's disease is common and occurs most often in the form of lymph node enlargement. In one series of 659 patients, mediastinal lymph node enlargement was present in 405 (61%) and hilar lymph node enlargement in 193 (29%) at the time of diagnosis.[89] Evidence of pleuropulmonary involvement is present at the time of diagnosis in 10% to 15% of patients[54, 89] and at some time during the course of the disease in 15% to 40%.[115] Most cases are of the nodular sclerosis subtype; in the review of 89 patients who had lung involvement cited previously, 77 (17%) of these patients were from the 460 patients who had nodular sclerosis, whereas only 6 (4%) occurred in the 146 patients who had the mixed cellularity subtype.[89]

Intrathoracic involvement usually is associated with evidence of Hodgkin's disease elsewhere in the body; for example, in one series of 1,470 consecutive patients, only 44 (3%) were found to have purely intrathoracic disease after appropriate clinical and pathologic staging.[90] Primary pulmonary Hodgkin's disease (unassociated with clinical or radiologic evidence of disease in lymph nodes or other tissues) is more uncommon:[90, 115] In a study of 155 cases of Hodgkin's disease from Yale University between 1980 and 1987, only one such case was identified; a review of the literature published at the same time documented only 60 additional reports.[115]

The incidence of various intrathoracic abnormalities identifiable on plain chest radiographs was assessed in a study of 300 consecutive patients who had untreated Hodgkin's disease and non-Hodgkin's lymphoma.[54] Hodgkin's disease was found to be associated with a higher incidence of intrathoracic disease at presentation (67% compared with 43%), manifested predominantly by bulky anterior mediastinal lymph node enlargement. In this study, lung involvement was more common in Hodgkin's disease (approximately 12% versus 4%) and always was accompanied by mediastinal or hilar lymph node enlargement or both.

Mediastinal Lymph Node Enlargement

Mediastinal lymph node enlargement is seen on the initial chest radiograph in 60% to 75% of patients (Fig. 7–14).[54, 89, 91] Involvement of the anterior mediastinal and paratracheal lymph nodes is four times more common in Hodgkin's disease than in non-Hodgkin's lymphoma, being evident at presentation on chest radiograph in 90% and on CT scan in 98% of patients who have intrathoracic disease (Table 7–4).[54, 91] Disease most commonly involves the ante-

Table 7–4. HODGKIN'S DISEASE: CHARACTERISTIC RADIOLOGIC FINDINGS

Intrathoracic disease present in 60% of patients
Mediastinal lymph node enlargement most common finding
Almost always involves anterior mediastinal nodes
Also involves contiguous nodal groups in 90% of patients
Nodes may calcify after radiotherapy
Concomitant parenchymal involvement in 10% of cases
Pleural involvement in 10%–15% of cases

rior mediastinal nodes followed in decreasing frequency by paratracheal, hilar, subcarinal, internal mammary, pericardiophrenic, and posterior mediastinal (Fig. 7–15).[54, 91] Infiltration of contiguous groups of lymph nodes occurs in approximately 90% of patients.[92, 93]

Dystrophic calcification develops in involved lymph nodes in some cases after mediastinal radiation (Fig. 7–16).[69, 100] Although some investigators consider the complication to be unrelated to the degree of radiation,[99] others link it with relatively high doses.[100] The time interval between irradiation and the appearance of calcification may be 1 to 9 years.

Similar to carcinoma, Hodgkin's disease can extend beyond affected lymph nodes into mediastinal interstitial tissue and invade such structures as the esophagus, superior vena cava, and pericardium. Corresponding radiologic manifestations, such as pericardial effusion, may be seen.[98, 101] An exception is diaphragmatic paralysis secondary to invasion of the phrenic nerve; in contrast to pulmonary carcinoma, Hodgkin's disease rarely results in this complication.[98, 101, 102] Involvement of the anterior mediastinal and internal mammary nodes may be associated with invasion of the sternum or the parasternal tissue[94–96] unilaterally or bilaterally.[97] The results of one study suggest that MR imaging may be superior to CT in the detection of chest wall involvement, either by showing extension not apparent on CT or by identifying additional sites of chest wall disease.[71]

Pleuropulmonary Disease

Involvement of peribronchovascular tissue by Hodgkin's disease is manifested radiographically by a coarse reticulonodular and linear pattern that extends outward from the hila (Fig. 7–17). Lymphoid tissue at the bifurcation of bronchi and vessels also can be affected,[98, 102] and involvement of the interlobular septa can result in Kerley lines.[102] Consolidation of lung parenchyma remote from the mediastinum is common (Fig. 7–18).[98]

Pleural or subpleural nodules or plaques are seen on CT in 30% of patients at some time in the course of the disease.[65] The size of such nodules ranges widely and may vary with time; individual foci may coalesce to form a large homogeneous nonsegmental mass,[98] sometimes involving a whole lobe.[98, 104] This type of parenchymal consolidation is unassociated with loss of volume (Fig. 7–19); its borders can be shaggy and ill-defined or sharply margined. Because the airways are unaffected, an air bronchogram may be visible. Such masses can undergo necrosis and form a cavity that may be thin or thick walled; in many cases,

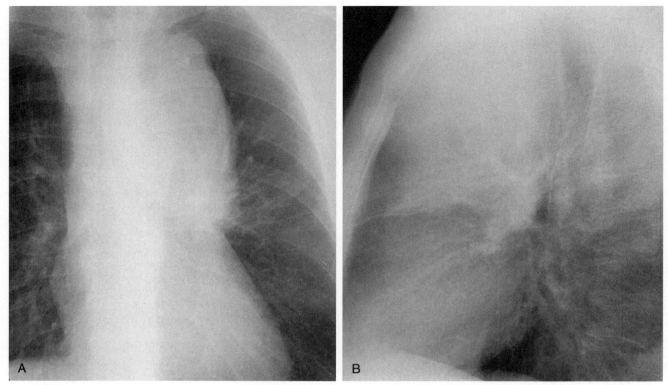

Figure 7–14. Hodgkin's Disease. Close-up view of the mediastinum from posteroanterior chest radiograph *(A)* reveals asymmetric widening of the mediastinum with a lobulated contour consistent with extensive anterior mediastinal lymph node enlargement. Increased soft tissue opacity in the region of the superior vena cava is consistent with paratracheal lymph node enlargement. Lateral view *(B)* confirms the presence of extensive anterior mediastinal lymphadenopathy. The patient was a 57-year-old man with Hodgkin's disease proved by biopsy of the enlarged paratracheal lymph nodes.

they are multiple and are situated in the lower lobes.[105–107] In one patient, cavitated nodules were recurrent.[108]

Rarely, there is a generalized miliary or reticulonodular pattern,[103] in which case differentiation from lymphangitic spread of carcinoma or sarcoidosis may be difficult or impossible without biopsy.[104, 109] Bronchial occlusion almost always is caused by tumor within the airway lumen or wall[60, 110–112] and can result in lobar or segmental atelectasis and obstructive pneumonitis. In one study of six patients, atelectasis was caused by an endobronchial lesion in four; in three, this was the principal initial pulmonary manifestation.[60]

Pleural effusion is seen at presentation in approximately 10% of patients[54, 91] and eventually develops in approximately 30%, most often in association with other intrathoracic manifestations of the disease.[98] The fluid can be serous, chylous, pseudochylous,[113] or (rarely) serosanguineous. The incidence of pneumothorax is increased in patients who have Hodgkin's disease; in one study of 1,977 patients who had lymphoma, the complication was 10 times higher than expected, most patients being younger than 30 years of age.[114] Treatment with radiotherapy, lung involvement, radiation fibrosis, and infection appear to be risk factors.

The radiographic findings of primary pulmonary Hodgkin's disease consist of single or multiple nodules or masses or focal areas of consolidation.[115] The masses may cavitate. Similar findings have been described on CT scan.[116]

Chest Wall and Other Skeletal Involvement

Approximately 15% of patients who have Hodgkin's disease manifest bone involvement radiographically.[117] The thoracic skeleton usually[96, 102, 113] but not invariably[104] is affected by direct extension of tumor from the mediastinum or lungs. In such cases, destruction of ribs, vertebrae, or the sternum typically results in focal lytic areas. By contrast, vertebral involvement other than by direct extension often is purely osteoblastic (ivory vertebra) (Fig. 7–20). Involvement of the nonthoracic skeleton (most commonly the spine or pelvis) usually results in mixed lytic and blastic lesions.[117]

Follow-Up

Therapy usually is followed by slow involution of enlarged mediastinal lymph nodes. In one study, 86% of patients who had Stage 1 or 2 disease and mediastinal nodal involvement had a normal-appearing chest radiograph 11 months after treatment.[118] By contrast, in another investigation of 57 patients, residual abnormalities were evident on the chest radiograph in 50 (88%);[25] at a median follow-up of 48 months, 24 of the 57 patients (42%) still had abnormalities. In this study, the presence of residual mediastinal abnormalities did not by itself indicate persistent active disease or an increased risk of relapse.[119] The significance of residual mediastinal masses on chest radiographs was assessed further in a study of 110 patients

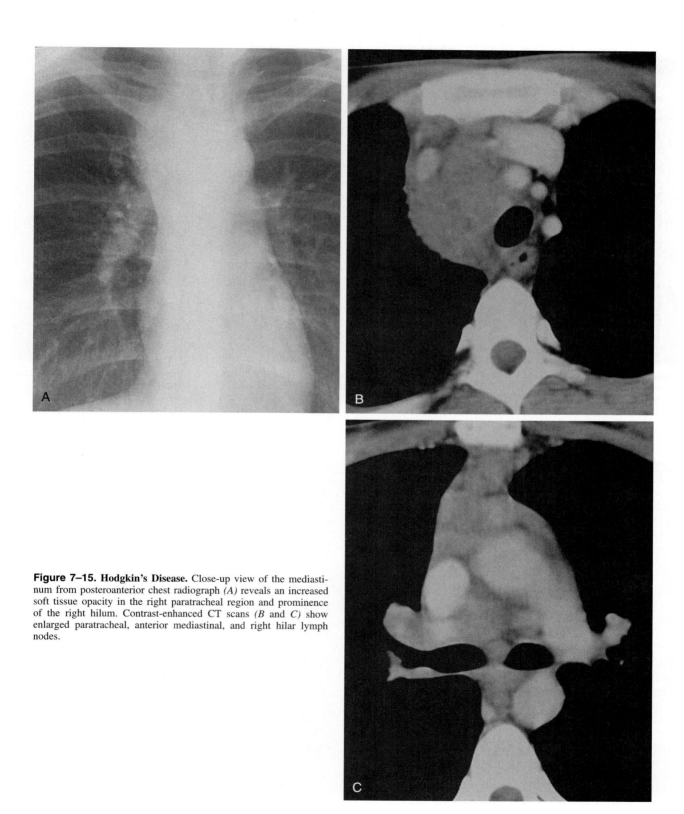

Figure 7–15. Hodgkin's Disease. Close-up view of the mediastinum from posteroanterior chest radiograph *(A)* reveals an increased soft tissue opacity in the right paratracheal region and prominence of the right hilum. Contrast-enhanced CT scans *(B* and *C)* show enlarged paratracheal, anterior mediastinal, and right hilar lymph nodes.

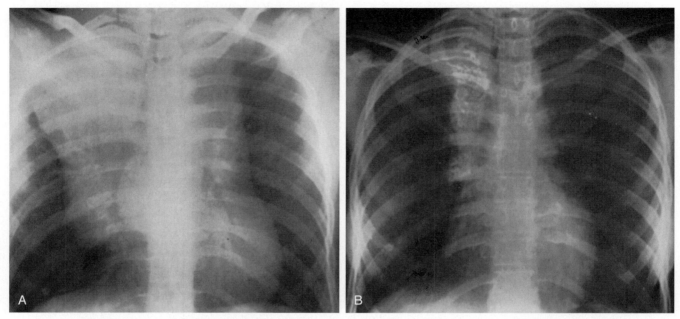

Figure 7–16. Calcification of Mediastinal Lymph Nodes After Irradiation for Hodgkin's Disease. Marked enlargement of anterior mediastinal nodes *(A)* largely had disappeared 3 years later *(B)*, but the nodes had undergone extensive calcification. The patient was a teenage girl.

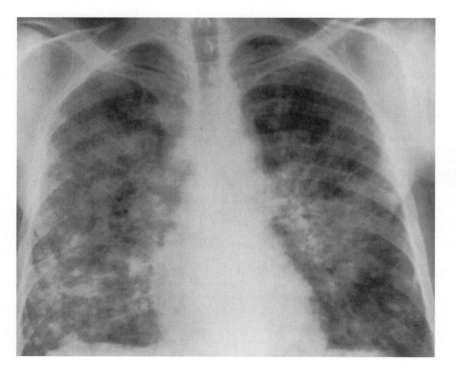

Figure 7–17. Mixed Interstitial Air-Space Pattern of Pulmonary Involvement in Hodgkin's Disease. Posteroanterior chest radiograph shows bilateral patchy air-space opacities throughout both lungs, worse on the right. The bronchovascular bundles are thickened, and septal lines are present in upper and lower lobes. Mediastinal and hilar nodes are enlarged.

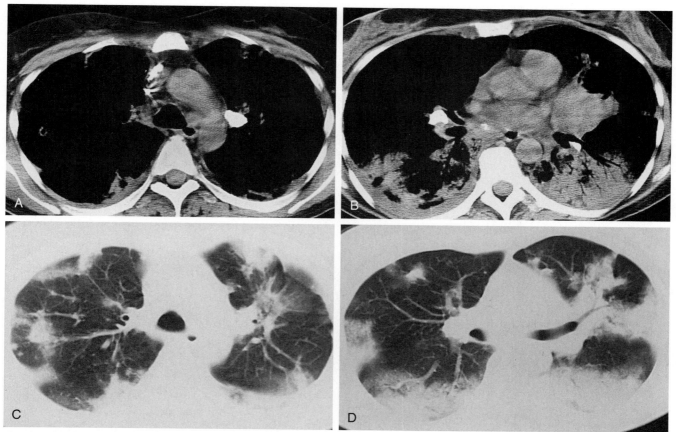

Figure 7–18. Parenchymal Consolidation in Hodgkin's Disease. Conventional CT scans *(A* and *B)* in a 45-year-old woman with previously treated Hodgkin's disease show calcified mediastinal and hilar lymph nodes and enlarged subcarinal and left hilar lymph nodes. Lung windows *(C* and *D)* reveal peribronchial and peripheral areas of consolidation. Surgical lung biopsy demonstrated Hodgkin's disease.

treated for advanced Hodgkin's disease with chemotherapy, radiation therapy, or both.[120] The relapse rate was not influenced by the rapidity of resolution of the radiographic findings and was similar in patients who had normal radiographs and patients who had residual radiographic abnormalities 1 year after treatment. These studies indicate that residual abnormalities on chest radiograph or on CT scan may represent only nonviable or fibrotic tissue.[120, 121] The differentiation of residual tumor from necrotic tumor or fibrotic tissue usually can be made with gallium 67 scintigraphy.[122, 123]

Because its low water content leads to a short T2, fibrous tissue also can be distinguished readily from tumor on MR imaging. The study reveals a heterogeneous pattern immediately after treatment, which subsequently progresses to the low signal intensity on T2-weighted images that is characteristic of scar tissue.[124] Radiation-induced inflammatory changes also may result in increased signal intensity on T2-weighted images.

LEUKEMIA

Thoracic involvement is common at autopsy in patients who have leukemia of all types. Mediastinal and hilar lymph node infiltration is the most frequent finding, particularly in acute lymphoblastic leukemia and chronic lymphocytic leukemia. Pleuropulmonary infiltration is evi-

dent histologically in 20% to 40% of patients.[126, 127] The likelihood that clinical and radiographic abnormalities are related to pleuropulmonary leukemic infiltration alone is low, however;[128–130] most abnormalities are caused by infection, hemorrhage, drug reactions, or heart failure.[131–133]

The most common radiologic intrathoracic manifestations of leukemia are mediastinal and hilar lymph node enlargement (Fig. 7–21).[135, 140] CT may show a focal mediastinal mass or infiltration of mediastinal fat.[135] Other findings include cardiac enlargement as a result of a focal pericardial mass or pericardial effusion, pleural effusions, pleural masses, and pulmonary opacities.[135]

Pulmonary disease in patients who have leukemia most often is caused by disease other than leukemic cell infiltration. For example, in one series of 21 patients who had abnormal chest radiographs, all of whom were considered during life to have leukemic infiltration of the lungs, only 2 had such a finding at autopsy.[125] The most common pulmonary abnormality is localized or diffuse air-space consolidation, caused almost invariably by pneumonia, edema, or hemorrhage.[125, 134, 139] In an autopsy review of 60 patients who died from acute or chronic myelogenous or lymphocytic leukemia,[131] radiographically demonstrable disease was related to hemorrhage in 74%, infection in 67%, edema or congestion in 57%, and leukemic infiltration in 26%; only 5% were radiographically normal.

Pulmonary disease associated with involvement by leu-

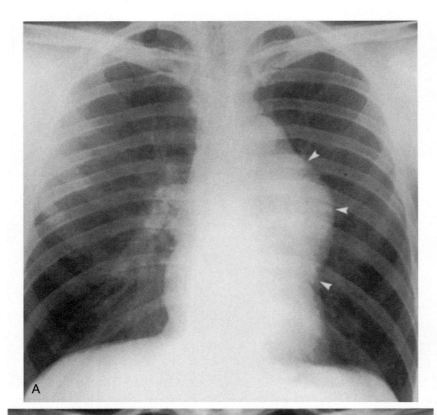

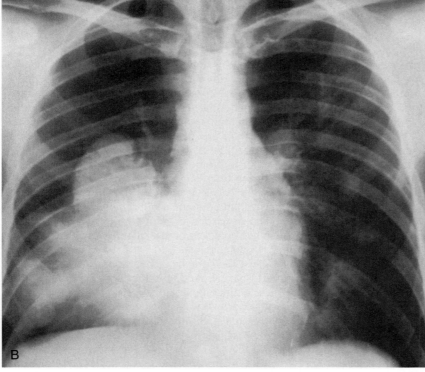

Figure 7–19. Parenchymal Consolidation in Hodgkin's Disease. Posteroanterior chest radiograph *(A)* reveals a smoothly contoured left anterior mediastinal mass *(arrowheads)* caused by Hodgkin's involvement of lymph nodes. Five years later, posteroanterior radiograph *(B)* shows regression of the mediastinal lesion, but in the interim massive consolidation of the right middle and lower lobes caused by direct spread of Hodgkin's disease from hilar and mediastinal nodes had developed. In the left lung, poorly defined opacities characteristic of subpleural parenchymal consolidation have developed at a distance from the hilum and mediastinum.

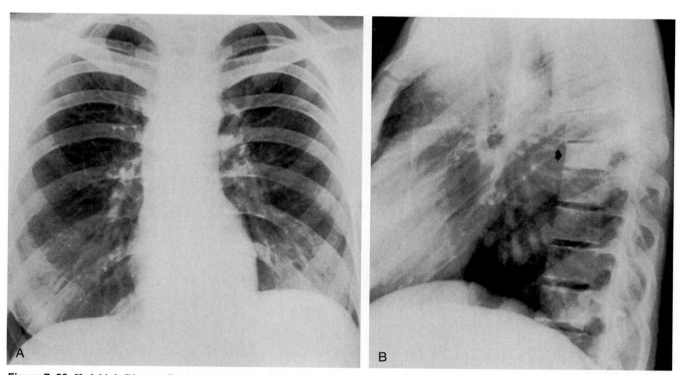

Figure 7–20. Hodgkin's Disease: Combined Splenomegaly and Bone Involvement. Posteroanterior *(A)* and lateral *(B)* radiographs of this 26-year-old woman show elevation of the left hemidiaphragm as a result of a markedly enlarged spleen. The lungs are clear, and there is no evidence of hilar or mediastinal node enlargement. In lateral projection, the 7th thoracic vertebral body *(arrow)* can be seen to be slightly compressed and to be uniformly dense *(ivory vertebra)*; the 11th thoracic vertebral body is sclerotic in its posterior portion. This combination of changes is highly suggestive of the diagnosis of Hodgkin's disease. Some months later, this patient developed massive consolidation of the right lung from Hodgkin's disease.

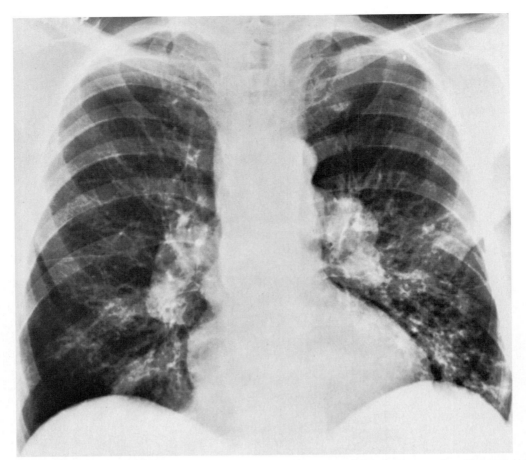

Figure 7–21. Hilar Lymph Node Enlargement in Chronic Lymphocytic Leukemia. Posteroanterior chest radiograph reveals markedly enlarged lymph nodes in both hila and (probably) slight enlargement of the nodes in the paratracheal chain bilaterally. There is no evidence of significant pulmonary or pleural disease (the minor parenchymal changes in the left lower lobe represent resolving bronchopneumonia). The patient was a 65-year-old man who had chronic lymphocytic leukemia.

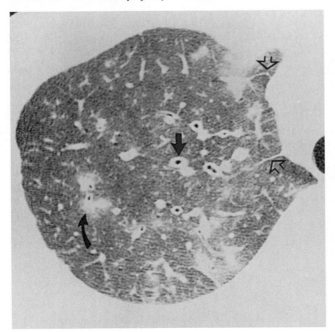

Figure 7–22. Chronic Myelogenous Leukemia. HRCT scan targeted to the right upper lobe in a 51-year-old patient with chronic myelogenous leukemia shows thickening of the bronchovascular bundles *(curved arrow)* and interlobular septa *(open arrows)*. Poorly defined peribronchial nodules *(straight arrow)*, ground-glass attenuation, and regions of peripheral consolidation also are present. (From Heyneman L, et al: Am J Roentgenol 174:517, 2000.)

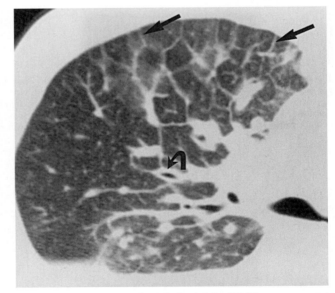

Figure 7–23. Acute Lymphocytic Leukemia. HRCT scan targeted to the right upper lobe in a 27-year-old patient with acute lymphocytic leukemia shows predominantly smooth thickening of the interlobular septa *(straight arrows)* and the bronchovascular bundles *(curved arrow)*. Right hilar lymphadenopathy and a right pleural effusion also are present. (From Heyneman L, et al: Am J Roentgenol 174:517, 2000.)

kemic cells usually results in diffuse bilateral reticulation or linearity that resembles interstitial edema or lymphangitic carcinomatosis. Less common radiographic manifestations include air-space consolidation and nodules.[136, 137, 141] The HRCT findings of pulmonary leukemic infiltrates were reviewed in 10 patients who had histopathologically proven disease and no other concomitant pulmonary complications.[138] The predominant abnormalities consisted of interlobular septal thickening, seen in all patients, and thickening of the bronchovascular bundles, seen in nine patients (Fig. 7–22). The septal thickening was smooth in six patients and nodular in four (Fig. 7–23). Nodules measuring 5 to 10 mm in diameter were present in eight patients. Less common findings included focal areas of ground-glass attenuation or consolidation.[138]

References

1. Saltzstein SL: Pulmonary malignant lymphomas and pseudolymphomas: Classification, therapy, and prognosis. Cancer 16:928, 1963.
2. Koss MN, Hochholzer L, Nichols PW, et al: Primary non-Hodgkin's lymphoma and pseudolymphoma of lung: A study of 161 patients. Hum Pathol 14:1024, 1983.
3. Turner RR, Colby TV, Doggett RS: Well-differentiated lymphocytic lymphoma. Cancer 54:2088, 1984.
4. Kennedy JL, Nathwani BN, Burke JS, et al: Pulmonary lymphomas and other pulmonary lymphoid lesions: A clinicopathologic and immunologic study of 64 patients. Cancer 56:539, 1985.
5. Koss MN: Pulmonary lymphoid disorders. Semin Diagn Pathol 12:158, 1995.
6. Bragg DG, Chor PJ, Murray KA, et al: Lymphoproliferative disorders of the lung: Histopathology, clinical manifestations, and imaging features. Am J Roentgenol 163:273, 1994.
7. Holland EA, Ghahremani GG, Fry WA, et al: Evolution of pulmonary pseudolymphomas: Clinical and radiologic manifestations. J Thorac Imaging 6:74, 1991.
8. Hutchinson WB, Friedenberg MJ, Saltzstein SL: Primary pulmonary pseudolymphoma. Radiology 82:48, 1964.
9. Nicholson AG, Wotherspoon AC, Diss TC, et al: Reactive pulmonary lymphoid disorders. Histopathology 26:405, 1995.
10. Strimlan CV, Rosenow EC, Weiland LH, et al: Lymphocytic interstitial pneumonitis. Ann Intern Med 88:616, 1978.
11. Koss MN, Hochholzer L, Langloss JM, et al: Lymphoid interstitial pneumonia: Clinicopathological and immunopathological findings in 18 cases. Pathology 19:178, 1987.
12. Greenberg SD, Haley MD, Jenkins DE, et al: Lymphoplasmacytic pneumonia with accompanying dysproteinemia. Arch Pathol 96:73, 1973.
13. Moran TJ, Totten RS: Lymphoid interstitial pneumonia with dysproteinemia: Report of two cases with plasma cell predominance. Am J Clin Pathol 54:747, 1970.
14. Liebow AA, Carrington CB: The interstitial pneumonias. *In* Simon M, Potchen EJ, Le May M (eds): Frontiers of Pulmonary Radiology. New York, Grune & Stratton, 1969, p 102.
15. Julsrud PR, Brown LR, Li CY, et al: Pulmonary processes of mature-appearing lymphocytes: Pseudolymphoma, well-differentiated lymphocytic lymphoma, and lymphocytic interstitial pneumonia. Radiology 127:289, 1978.
16. Ichikawa Y, Kinoshita M, Koga T, et al: Lung cyst formation in lymphocytic interstitial pneumonia: CT features. J Comput Assist Tomogr 18:745, 1994.
17. Feigin DS, Siegelman SS, Theros EG, et al: Nonmalignant lymphoid disorders of the chest. Am J Roentgenol 129:221, 1977.
18. McGuinness G, Scholes JV, Jagirdar JS, et al: Unusual lymphoproliferative disorders in nine adults with HIV or AIDS: CT and pathologic findings. Radiology 197:59, 1995.
19. Oldham SAA, Castillo M, Jacobson FL, et al: HIV-associated lymphocytic interstitial pneumonia: Radiologic manifestations and pathologic correlation. Radiology 170:83, 1989.
20. Torii K, Ogawa K, Kawabata Y, et al: Lymphoid interstitial pneumonia as a pulmonary lesion of idiopathic plasmacytic lymphadenopathy with hyperimmunoglobulinemia. Intern Med 33:237, 1994.
21. Carignan S, Staples CA, Müller NL: Intrathoracic lymphoproliferative disorders in the immunocompromised patient: CT findings. Radiology 197:53, 1995.
22. Johkoh T, Müller NL, Pickford HA, et al: Lymphocytic interstitial pneumonia: Thin-section CT findings in 22 patients. Radiology 212:567, 1999.
23. Honda O, Johkoh T, Ichikado K, et al: Differential diagnosis of lymphocytic interstitial pneumonia and malignant lymphoma on high-resolution CT. Am J Roentgenol 173:71, 1999.
24. Banerjee D, Ahmad D: Malignant lymphoma complicating lymphocytic interstitial pneumonia: A monoclonal B-cell neoplasm arising in a polyclonal lymphoproliferative disorder. Hum Pathol 13:780, 1982.
25. Schuurman H-J, Gooszen HC, Tan IWN, et al: Low-grade lymphoma of immature T-cell phenotype in a case of lymphocytic interstitial pneumonia and Sjögren's syndrome. Histopathology 11:1193, 1987.
26. Yousem SA, Colby TV, Carrington CB: Follicular bronchitis/bronchiolitis. Hum Pathol 16:700, 1985.
27. Fortoul TI, Cano-Valle F, Oliva E, et al: Follicular bronchiolitis in association with connective tissue diseases. Lung 163:305, 1985.
28. Kinoshita M, Higashi T, Tanaka C, et al: Follicular bronchiolitis associated with rheumatoid arthritis. Intern Med 31:674, 1992.
29. Howling SJ, Hansell DM, Wells AU, et al: Follicular bronchiolitis: Thin-section CT and histologic findings. Radiology 212:637, 1999.
30. Rosenberg SA, Diamond HD, Jaslowitz B, et al: Lymphosarcoma: A review of 1269 cases. Medicine 40:31, 1961.
31. Li G, Hansmann M-L, Zwingers T, et al: Primary lymphomas of the lung: Morphological, immunohistochemical and clinical features. Histopathology 16:519, 1990.
32. Harris NL: Low-grade B-cell lymphoma of mucosa-associated lymphoid tissue and monocytoid B-cell lymphoma: Related entities that are distinct from other low-grade B-cell lymphomas. Arch Pathol Lab Med 117:771, 1993.
33. Koss M, Zeren EH: Low-grade B-cell lymphomas of lung and lymphomatoid granulomatosis. Pathology 4:125, 1996.
34. Lee KS, Kim Y, Primack SL: Imaging of pulmonary lymphomas. Am J Roentgenol 168:339, 1997.
35. Cordier JF, Chailleux E, Lauque D, et al: Primary pulmonary lymphomas: A clinical study of 70 cases in nonimmunocompromised patients. Chest 103:201, 1993.
36. Bozanko CMM, Korobkin M, Fantone JC, et al: Lobar primary pulmonary lymphoma: CT findings. J Comput Assist Tomogr 15:679, 1991.
37. O'Donnell PG, Jackson SA, Tung KT, et al: Radiological appearances of lymphomas arising from mucosa-associated lymphoid tissue (MALT) in the lung. Clin Radiol 53:258, 1998.
38. Au V, Leung AN: Radiologic manifestations of lymphoma in the thorax. Am J Roentgenol 168:93, 1997.
39. Gollub MJ, Castellino RA: Diffuse endobronchial non-Hodgkin's lymphoma: CT demonstration. Am J Roentgenol 164:1093, 1995.
40. Tamura A, Komatsu H, Yanai N, et al: Primary pulmonary lymphoma: Relationship between clinical features and pathologic findings in 24 cases. The Japan National Chest Hospital Study Group for Lung Cancer. Jpn J Clin Oncol 25:140, 1995.
41. Close PM, Macrae MB, Hammond JM, et al: Anaplastic large-cell Ki-1 lymphoma: Pulmonary presentation mimicking miliary tuberculosis. Am J Clin Pathol 99:631, 1993.
42. Cheng AL, Su IJ, Chen YC, et al: Characteristic clinicopathologic features of Epstein-Barr virus-associated peripheral T-cell lymphoma. Cancer 72:909, 1993.
43. Harrison NK, Twelves C, Addis BJ: Peripheral T-cell lymphoma presenting with angioedema and diffuse pulmonary infiltrates. Am Rev Respir Dis 138:976, 1988.
44. Lautin EM, Rosenblatt M, Friedman AC, et al: Calcification in non-Hodgkin lymphoma occurring before therapy: Identification on plain films and CT. Am J Roentgenol 155:739, 1990.
45. Eliasson AH, Rajagopal KR, Dow NS: Respiratory failure in rapidly progressing pulmonary lymphoma. Am Rev Respir Dis 141:231, 1990.
46. Liebow AA, Carrington CRB, Friedman PJ: Lymphomatoid granulomatosis. Hum Pathol 3:457, 1972.
47. Katzenstein A-LA, Carrington CB, Liebow AA: Lymphomatoid granulomatosis. Cancer 43:360, 1979.
48. Wechsler RJ, Steiner RM, Israel HL, et al: Chest radiograph in lymphomatoid granulomatosis: Comparison with Wegener granulomatosis. Am J Roentgenol 142:79, 1984.

49. Prénovault JMN, Weisbrod GL, Herman SJ: Lymphomatoid granulomatosis: A review of 12 cases. J Can Assoc Radiol 39:263, 1988.
50. Pisani RJ, De Remee RA: Clinical implications of the histopathologic diagnosis of pulmonary lymphomatoid granulomatosis. Mayo Clin Proc 65:151, 1990.
51. Donnelly TJ, Tuder RM, Vendegna TR: A 48-year-old woman with peripheral neuropathy, hypercalcemia, and pulmonary infiltrates. Chest 114:1205, 1998.
52. Fauci AS, Haynes BF, Costa J, et al: Lymphomatoid granulomatosis: Prospective clinical and therapeutic experience over 10 years. N Engl J Med 306:68, 1982.
53. Mentzer SJ, Reilly JJ, Skarin AT, et al: Patterns of lung involvement by malignant lymphoma. Surgery 113:507, 1993.
54. Filly R, Blank N, Castellino RA: Radiographic distribution of intrathoracic disease in previously untreated patients with Hodgkin's disease and non-Hodgkin's lymphoma. Radiology 120:277, 1976.
55. Castellino RA, Hilton S, O'Brien JP, et al: Non-Hodgkin lymphoma: Contribution of chest CT in the initial staging evaluation. Radiology 199:129, 1996.
56. Robbins LL: The roentgenological appearance of parenchymal involvement of the lungs by malignant lymphoma. Cancer 6:80, 1953.
57. Lewis ER, Caskey CI, Fishman EK: Lymphoma of the lung: CT findings in 31 patients. Am J Roentgenol 156:711, 1991.
58. Van Schoor J, Joos G, Pauwels R: Non-Hodgkin's lymphoma presenting as multiple cavitating pulmonary nodules. Eur Respir J 6:1229, 1993.
59. Jackson SA, Tung KT, Mead GM: Multiple cavitating pulmonary lesions in non-Hodgkin's lymphoma. Clin Radiol 49:883, 1994.
60. Samuels ML, Howe CD, Dodd GD, et al: Endobronchial malignant lymphoma: Report of five cases in adults. Am J Roentgenol 85:87, 1961.
61. Havard CWH, Nichols JB, Stanfield AG: Primary lymphosarcoma of the lung. Thorax 17:190, 1962.
62. Goldstein J, Burns JC: Lymphoma of lung masquerading as sarcoidosis. Tubercle 42:507, 1961.
63. Brown MJ, Miller RR, Müller NL: Acute lung disease in the immunocompromised host: CT and pathologic examination findings. Radiology 190:247, 1994.
64. Celikoglu F, Teirstein AS, Krellenstein DJ, et al: Pleural effusion in non-Hodgkin's lymphoma. Chest 101:1357, 1992.
65. Shuman LS, Libshitz HI: Solid pleural manifestations of lymphoma. Am J Roentgenol 142:269, 1984.
66. Leung AN, Müller NL, Miller RR: CT in differential diagnosis of diffuse pleural disease. Am J Roentgenol 154:487, 1990.
67. Waldron JA Jr, Dohring EJ, Farber LR: Primary large cell lymphomas of the mediastinum: An analysis of 20 cases. Semin Diagn Pathol 2:281, 1985.
68. Perrone T, Frizzera G, Rosai J: Mediastinal diffuse large-cell lymphoma with sclerosis: A clinicopathologic study of 60 cases. Am J Surg Pathol 10:176, 1986.
69. Fishman EK, Kuhlman JE, Jones RJ: CT of lymphoma: Spectrum of disease. Radiographics 11:647, 1991.
70. Negendank WG, Al-Katib AM, Karanes C, et al: Lymphomas: MR imaging contrast characteristics with clinical-pathologic correlations. Radiology 177:209, 1990.
71. Carlsen SE, Bergin CJ, Hoppe RT: MR imaging to detect chest wall and pleural involvement in patients with lymphoma: Effect on radiation therapy planning. Am J Roentgenol 160:1191, 1993.
72. Israel O, Front D, Lam M, et al: Gallium 67 imaging in monitoring lymphoma response to treatment. Cancer 61:2439, 1988.
73. Front D, Israel O, Epelbaum R, et al: Ga-67 SPECT before and after treatment of lymphoma. Radiology 175:515, 1990.
74. Front D, Bar-Shalom R, Epelbaum R, et al: Early detection of lymphoma recurrence with gallium-67 scintigraphy. J Nucl Med 34:2101, 1993.
75. Moog F, Bangerter M, Diederichs CG, et al: Lymphoma: Role of whole-body 2-deoxy-2-[F-18]-fluoro-D-glucose (FDG) PET in nodal staging. Radiology 203:795, 1997.
76. Som P, Atkins HL, Bandophadhyah D: A fluorinated glucose analog, 2-fluoro-2-deoxy-D-glucose (F-18). J Nucl Med 21:670, 1980.
77. Rodriguez M, Rehn S, Ahlström H, et al: Predicting malignancy grade with PET in non-Hodgkin's lymphoma. J Nucl Med 36:1790, 1995.
78. Lapela M, Leskinen S, Minn H, et al: Increased glucose metabolism in untreated non-Hodgkin's lymphoma: A study with positron emission tomography and fluorine-18 fluorodeoxyglucose. Blood 9:3522, 1995.
79. Okada J, Yoshikawa K, Imazeki K, et al: The use of FDG-PET in the detection and management of malignant lymphoma: Correlation of uptake with prognosis. J Nucl Med 32:686, 1991.
80. Kintzer JS, Rosenow EC, Kyle RA: Thoracic and pulmonary abnormalities in multiple myeloma. Arch Intern Med 138:727, 1978.
81. Garewal H, Durie BG: Aggressive phase of multiple myeloma with pulmonary plasma cell infiltrates. JAMA 248:1875, 1982.
82. Gilchrist D, Chan CK, LaRoye GJ, et al: Bronchial mucosal infiltration and unilateral lung collapse: An unusual complication of multiple myeloma. Am J Med 85:74, 1988.
83. Kinare SG, Parulkar GB, Panday SR, et al: Extensive ossification in a pulmonary plasmacytoma. Thorax 20:206, 1965.
84. Kwan WC, Lam SC, Klimo P: Kappa light-chain myeloma with pleural involvement. Chest 86:494, 1984.
85. Witt DH, Zalusky R, Castella A, et al: Light chain myeloma with meningeal and pleural involvement. Am J Med 80:1213, 1986.
86. Moulopoulos LA, Granfield CAJ, Dimopoulos MA, et al: Extraosseous multiple myeloma: Imaging features. Am J Roentgenol 161:1083, 1993.
87. Wiltshaw E: The natural history of extramedullary plasmacytoma and its relation to solitary myeloma of bone and myelomatosis. Medicine 55:217, 1976.
88. Joseph G, Pandit M, Korfhage L: Primary pulmonry plasmacytoma. Cancer 71:721, 1993.
89. Colby TV, Hoppe RT, Warnke RA: Hodgkin's disease: A clinicopathologic study of 659 cases. Cancer 49:1848, 1981.
90. Johnson DW, Hoppe RT, Cox RS, et al: Hodgkin's disease limited to intrathoracic sites. Cancer 52:8, 1983.
91. Castellino RA, Blank N, Hoppe RT, et al: Hodgkin disease: Contributions of chest CT in the initial staging evaluation. Radiology 160:603, 1996.
92. Cobby M, Whipp E, Bullimore J, et al: CT appearances of relapse of lymphoma in the lung. Clin Radiol 41:232, 1990.
93. Rosenberg SA, Kaplan HS: Evidence for an orderly progression in the spread of Hodgkin's disease. Cancer Res 26:1225, 1966.
94. Cropp AJ, DiMarco AF, Lankerani M: False-positive transbronchial needle aspiration in bronchogenic carcinoma. Chest 85:696, 1984.
95. Leading article: Outlook in Hodgkin's disease. BMJ 2:328, 1967.
96. Goldman JM: Parasternal chest wall involvement in Hodgkin's disease. Chest 59:133, 1971.
97. Press GA, Glazer HS, Wasserman TH, et al: Thoracic wall involvement by Hodgkin disease and non-Hodgkin lymphoma: CT evaluation. Radiology 157:195, 1985.
98. Fisher AHM, Kendall B, Van Leuven BD: Hodgkin's disease: A radiological survey. Clin Radiol 13:115, 1962.
99. Wyman SM, Weber AL: Calcification in intrathoracic nodes in Hodgkin's disease. Radiology 93:1021, 1969.
100. Brereton HD, Johnson RE: Calcification in mediastinal lymph nodes after radiation therapy of Hodgkin's disease. Radiology 112:705, 1974.
101. Whitcomb ME, Schwartz MI, Keller AR, et al: Hodgkin's disease of the lung. Am Rev Respir Dis 106:79, 1972.
102. Martin JJ: The Nisbet Symposium: Hodgkin's disease: Radiological aspects of the disease. Australas Radiol 11:206, 1967.
103. Sheinmel A, Roswit B, Lawrence LR: Hodgkin's disease of the lung: Roentgen appearance and therapeutic management. Radiology 54:165, 1950.
104. Ellman P, Bowdler AJ: Pulmonary manifestations of Hodgkin's disease. Br J Dis Chest 54:59, 1960.
105. Dhingra HK, Flance IJ: Cavitary primary pulmonary Hodgkin's diseae presenting as pruritus. Chest 58:71, 1970.
106. Simon G: Intra-thoracic Hodgkin's disease: Part I. Less common intra-thoracic manifestations of Hodgkin's disease. Br J Radiol 40:926, 1967.
107. Madewell JE, Daroca PJ, Reed JC: Pulmonary parenchymal Hodgkin's disease: RPC from the AFIP. Radiology 117:555, 1975.
108. Shahar J, Angelillo VA, Katz D, et al: Recurrent cavitary nodules secondary to Hodgkin's disease. Chest 91:273, 1987.
109. Holeshi S: Unusual x-ray appearances in Hodgkin's disease. Proc R Soc Med 48:1049, 1955.
110. Seward CW, Safdar SH: Endobronchial Hodgkin's disease presenting as a primary pulmonary lesion. Chest 62:649, 1972.

111. Vaughan BF: Endobronchial Hodgkin's disease. Br J Radiol 31:45, 1958.
112. Renzi G, Lesage R: Endobronchial Hodgkin's disease and broncho-esophageal fistula. Chest 61:696, 1972.
113. Strickland B: Intra-thoracic Hodgkin's disease: Part II. Peripheral manifestations of Hodgkin's disease in the chest. Br J Radiol 40:930, 1967.
114. Yellin A, Benfield JR: Pneumothorax associated with lymphoma. Am Rev Respir Dis 134:590, 1986.
115. Radin AI: Primary pulmonary Hodgkin's disease. Cancer 65:550, 1990.
116. Cartier Y, Johkoh T, Honda O, et al: Primary pulmonary Hodgkin's disease: CT findings in three patients. Clin Radiol 54:182, 1999.
117. Beachley MC, Lau BP, King ER: Bone involvement in Hodgkin's disease. Am J Roentgenol 114:559, 1972.
118. North LB, Fuller LM, Sullivan-Halley JA, et al: Regression of mediastinal Hodgkin disease after therapy: Evaluation of time interval. Radiology 164:599, 1987.
119. Jochelson M, Mauch P, Balikian J, et al: The significance of the residual mediastinal mass in treated Hodgkin's disease. J Clin Oncol 3:637, 1985.
120. Radford JA, Cowan RA, Flanagan M, et al: The significance of residual mediastinal abnormality on the chest radiograph following the treatment of Hodgkin's disease. J Clin Oncol 6:940, 1988.
121. Canellos GP: Residual mass in lymphoma may not be residual disease (editorial). J Clin Oncol 6:931, 1988.
122. Wylie BR, Southee AE, Joshua DE, et al: Gallium scanning in the management of mediastinal Hodgkin's disease. Eur J Haematol 42:344, 1989.
123. Kramer EL, Divgi CR: Pulmonary applications of nuclear medicine. Clin Chest Med 12:55, 1991.
124. Nyman RS, Rehn SM, Glimelius BLG, et al: Residual mediastinal masses in Hodgkin disease: Prediction of size with MR imaging. Radiology 170:435, 1989.
125. Green RA, Nichlos NJ: Pulmonary involvement in leukemia. Am Rev Respir Dis 80:883, 1959.
126. Doran HM, Sheppard MN, Collins PW, et al: Pathology of the lung in leukaemia and lymphoma: A study of 87 autopsies. Histopathology 18:211, 1991.
127. Rollins SD, Colby TV: Lung biopsy in chronic lymphocytic leukemia. Arch Pathol Lab Med 112:607, 1988.
128. March WL Jr, Bylund DJ, Heath VC, et al: Osteoarticular and pulmonary manifestations of acute leukemia: Case report and review of the literature. Cancer 57:385, 1986.
129. Rossi GA, Balbi B, Risso M, et al: Acute myelomonocytic leukemia: Demonstration of pulmonary involvement by bronchoalveolar lavage. Chest 87:259, 1985.
130. Hildebrand FL Jr, Rosenow EC 3rd, Habermann TM, et al: Pulmonary complications of leukemia. Chest 98:1233, 1990.
131. Maile CW, Moore AV, Ulreich S, et al: Chest radiographic-pathologic correlation in adult leukemia patients. Invest Radiol 18:495, 1983.
132. Suzumiya J, Marutsuka K, Nabeshima K, et al: Autopsy findings in 47 cases of adult T-cell leukemia/lymphoma in Miyazaki prefecture, Japan. Leuk Lymphoma 11:281, 1993.
133. Tenholder MF, Hooper RG: Pulmonary infiltrates in leukemia. Chest 78:468, 1980.
134. Bell CM, Stewart TE: Acute respiratory distress syndrome associated with tumour lysis syndrome in acute leukemia. Can Respir J 4:48, 1997.
135. Takasugi JE, Godwin JD, Marglin SI, et al: Intrathoracic granulocytic sarcomas. J Thorac Imaging 11:223, 1996.
136. Sueyoshi E, Uetani M, Hayashi K, et al: Adult T-cell leukemia with multiple pulmonary nodules due to leukemic cell infiltration. Am J Roentgenol 167:540, 1996.
137. Kovalski R, Hansen-Flaschen J, Lodato RF, et al: Localized leukemic pulmonary infiltrates: Diagnosis by bronchoscopy and resolution with therapy. Chest 97:674, 1990.
138. Heyneman LE, Johkoh T, Ward S, et al: Pulmonary leukemic infiltrates: High-resolution CT findings in 10 patients. Am J Roentgenol 174:517, 2000.
139. Blank N, Castellino RA, Shah V: Radiographic aspects of pulmonary infection in patients with altered immunity. Radiol Clin North Am 11:175, 1973.
140. Klatte EC, Yardley J, Smith EB, et al: The pulmonary manifestations and complications of leukemia. Am J Roentgenol 89:598, 1963.
141. Jenkins PF, Ward MJ, Davies P, et al: Non-Hodgkin's lymphoma, chronic lymphatic leukaemia and the lung. Br J Dis Chest 75:22, 1981.
142. Suster S, Moran CA: Pleomorphic large cell lymphomas of the mediastinum. Am J Surg Pathol 20:224, 1996.
143. McCulloch GL, Sinnatamby R, Stewart S, et al: High-resolution computed tomographic appearance of MALToma of the lung. Eur Radiol 8:1669, 1998.
144. Wislez M, Cadranel J, Antoine M, et al: Lymphoma of pulmonary mucosa–associated lymphoid tissue: CT scan findings and pathological correlations. Eur Resp J 14:423, 1999.
145. Knisely BL, Mastey LA, Mergo PJ, et al: Pulmonary mucosa–associated lymphoid tissue lymphoma: CT and pathologic findings. Am J Roentgenol 172:1321, 1999.

CHAPTER 8

Immunologic Lung Disease

CONNECTIVE TISSUE DISEASES

The autoimmune connective tissue diseases comprise a group of disorders whose common denominator is damage to components of connective tissue at a variety of sites in the body. Specific diseases include systemic lupus erythematosus (SLE), rheumatoid disease, progressive systemic sclerosis (PSS), dermatomyositis and polymyositis, ankylosing spondylitis, Sjögren's syndrome, mixed connective tissue disease (MCTD), and relapsing polychondritis.

Systemic Lupus Erythematosus

SLE is a multisystem autoimmune disorder for which several classifications of diagnostic criteria have been proposed (Table 8–1).[2] Patients are considered to have the disease if four criteria are met sequentially or simultaneously during any period of observation. The mean age at diagnosis is approximately 40 years.[5] The prevalence is 10 times greater in women than in men.[5]

Overall, about 50% to 60% of patients with SLE have pleuropulmonary involvement at some time during its course.[3] In a series of 1,000 European patients studied prospectively, 3% had clinically evident lung involvement and 17% had pleural involvement at the time of onset of

Table 8–1. CLINICAL FEATURES OF CLASSIC SYSTEMIC LUPUS ERYTHEMATOSUS

Rash	Serositis
Discoid lupus	Renal disorder
Photosensitivity	Neurologic disorder
Oral ulcers	Hematologic disorder
Arthritis	Immunologic disorder

From Panush RS, Greer JM, Morshedian KK: What is lupus? What is not lupus? Rheum Dis Clin North Am 19:223, 1993.

disease;[4] over the period of observation, a further 7% developed lung disease and 36% developed pleural disease. The pleuropulmonary manifestations of SLE are summarized in Table 8–2. The radiologic manifestations of drug-induced SLE are no different from those of the idiopathic form.[27]

Because of its high sensitivity, the screening test used most commonly in patients suspected of having SLE is a search for antinuclear antibodies (ANA). The test has relatively poor specificity, however, and may be positive in a variety of other connective tissue disorders as well as in otherwise normal individuals.[156]

Radiologic Manifestations

Radiologic abnormalities may be seen in the lungs, pleura, and heart, alone or in combination. In one investigation of 275 patients, 46% had normal chest radiographs, 35% had pleural effusion or thickening, 13% had pulmonary abnormalities, and 37% had cardiomegaly or pericardial effusion.[9] As is evident from these figures, pleural effusion is the most common thoracic manifestation.[10] Pleural effusion is frequently bilateral; although usually small (Fig. 8–1), it may be massive. The effusions may resolve completely[14] or result in mild residual pleural thickening.[9]

Radiographic abnormalities in the lungs usually are nonspecific and commonly consist of poorly defined patchy areas of parenchymal consolidation involving mainly the lung bases.[13] In most patients—70% in some series[13]—these areas are the result of infection; occasionally, they represent bronchiolitis obliterans organizing pneumonia (BOOP).[15]

Acute lupus pneumonitis is an uncommon manifestation of SLE characterized by fever, dyspnea, hypoxemia, and patchy unilateral or bilateral areas of consolidation (Fig. 8–2)[10, 11] in the absence of infection. Its incidence is estimated to be 1% to 4%.[12] Pathologic findings are variable; some cases show diffuse alveolar damage (intra-alveolar proteinaceous exudate, hyaline membranes, and an interstitial mononuclear inflammatory infiltrate),[6] and others show capillaritis and alveolar hemorrhage.[8] The triad of anemia, air-space consolidation, and hemoptysis should suggest the diagnosis of alveolar hemorrhage. The manifestation is

Table 8–2. PLEUROPULMONARY DISEASE IN SYSTEMIC LUPUS ERYTHEMATOSUS

Pleural disease
  Pleuritis with and without effusion
Parenchymal disease
  Acute lupus pneumonitis
  Bronchiolitis obliterans organizing pneumonia (BOOP)
  Interstitial pneumonitis and fibrosis
  Pulmonary hemorrhage
Vascular disease
  Pulmonary artery thrombosis
  Pulmonary thromboembolism
  Pulmonary hypertension
Airway disease
  Obliterative bronchiolitis
  Upper airway disease
Neuromuscular disease
  Diaphragmatic dysfunction

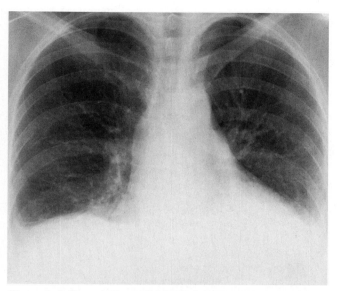

Figure 8–1. Systemic Lupus Erythematosus. Posteroanterior chest radiograph shows small pleural effusions and decreased lung volumes. Mild enlargement of the cardiopericardial silhouette was shown at echocardiography to be due to a pericardial effusion. This constellation of findings is characteristic of systemic lupus erythematosus. The patient was a 30-year-old woman.

rare; it occurred in only 1.6% of patients in one series[28] and was responsible for 3.7% of 510 hospitalizations for complications of SLE in another series.[29]

Alveolar hemorrhage is manifested radiologically by bilateral, patchy, ill-defined areas of consolidation involving mainly the lower lung zones.[13] In patients who have severe hemorrhage, radiographs may show extensive bilateral areas of ground-glass opacity or multifocal or confluent areas of consolidation (Fig. 8–3).[14, 16] It has been suggested that magnetic resonance (MR) imaging may show characteristic findings in these cases, consisting of intermediate signal intensity on proton density spin-echo images and low signal on T2-weighted images.[17]

Radiographic evidence of interstitial fibrosis is seen in a small percentage of patients who have SLE (Fig. 8–4): It was reported in 3 of 28 patients in one series[18] and 1 of 44 patients in a second series[19] and was not evident in any of 270 patients in a third series.[9] In another investigation of the incidence of abnormalities in an outpatient SLE clinic over a 1-year period, diffuse interstitial lung disease was found in 18 patients (approximately 3% of those studied).[20]

Horizontal line shadows are seen relatively commonly in patients who have SLE. They usually are present in the lung bases, sometimes are migratory, and probably are attributable to subsegmental atelectasis. Cavitary pulmonary nodules are rare; in one study of six patients who had SLE or MCTD and this abnormality,[21] the lesion proved to be the result of infection or infarction in five. Although local parenchymal changes may be fairly extensive without producing symptoms,[22] it is likely that the converse more often is the case—many patients complain of dyspnea and have considerable impairment of pulmonary function without manifesting parenchymal abnormalities on radiograph. In some of these patients, sequential radiographs show progressive loss of lung volume with elevation of the

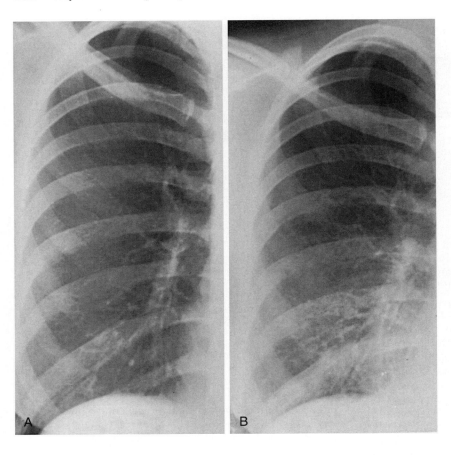

Figure 8–2. Acute Lupus Pneumonitis. Detail view of the right lung from posteroanterior radiograph *(A)* is normal. Two days later, after the onset of dyspnea and cough in this patient who had systemic lupus erythematosus *(B)*, the right lung shows increased opacity and poorly defined lung markings in the mid and lower portions of the chest. Similar features were identified in the left lung (not shown). There is no recruitment of upper zone vessels to suggest that pulmonary venous hypertension was a cause for the pulmonary abnormality. The changes are consistent with acute noncardiac pulmonary edema.

hemidiaphragms.[7] This *shrinking lung* syndrome generally is considered to be the result of diaphragmatic weakness.[23, 30]

The presence and extent of parenchymal abnormalities in patients who have SLE frequently are underestimated on chest radiograph.[24–26] In a prospective study in 48 patients who had serologically confirmed disease but no prior clinical evidence of pulmonary involvement, chest radiographs showed evidence of fibrosis in 3 (6%) patients and no abnormalities in 45 patients (94%).[24] Of the 45 patients who had normal radiographs, 17 (38%) had abnormal findings on high-resolution computed tomography (HRCT). The most common findings were interlobular septal thickening (33% of patients), intralobular interstitial thickening (33%), small rounded areas of consolidation (22%), and areas of ground-glass attenuation (13%). The abnormalities

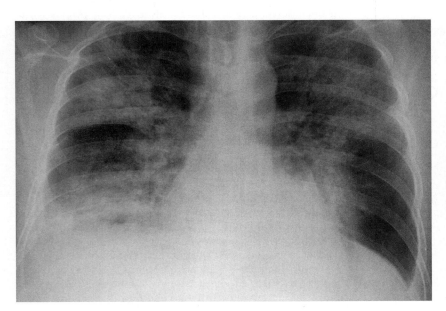

Figure 8–3. Diffuse Pulmonary Hemorrhage in Systemic Lupus Erythematosus. Posteroanterior chest radiograph shows extensive bilateral areas of consolidation with relative sparing of the peripheral lung regions. Small bilateral pleural effusions also are evident. The patient was a 24-year-old man with systemic lupus erythematosus who presented with hemoptysis. The pulmonary opacities resolved within 72 hours.

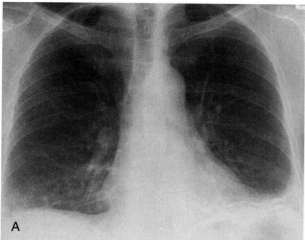

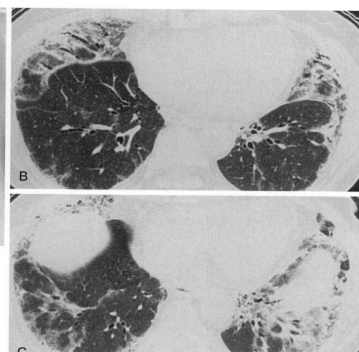

Figure 8–4. Systemic Lupus Erythematosus: Pulmonary Fibrosis. Posteroanterior chest radiograph *(A)* shows irregular linear opacities in the lower lung zones. HRCT scans *(B* and *C)* show parenchymal abnormalities involving mainly the right middle lobe, lingula, and left lower lobes. The findings consist of areas of ground-glass attenuation as well as irregular linear opacities, distortion of lung architecture, and bronchial dilation indicative of fibrosis. The patient was a 53-year-old woman who had long-standing systemic lupus erythematosus.

occurred mainly in the lower lobes in 14 patients and in the middle lobes in 3; the fibrosis involved mainly the subpleural lung regions and had an appearance similar to that of interstitial fibrosis seen in other connective tissue disorders. The duration of SLE clinically in this group of patients was 8 to 52 months.

In another prospective study, 34 patients who had SLE were assessed using chest radiography, HRCT, and pulmonary function tests.[25] The plain chest radiograph was abnormal in 8 patients (24%), pulmonary function abnormalities were present in 14 patients (41%), and HRCT abnormalities were identified in 24 patients (70%). The authors reported that 11 patients (32%) had definite evidence of interstitial lung disease on HRCT, which was mild in 5 patients and moderately advanced in 6 patients. Nine of the 11 patients who had evidence of interstitial lung disease on HRCT scan were asymptomatic, 7 had normal chest radiographs, and 4 had normal pulmonary function tests. Airway disease—defined as bronchial dilation or bronchial wall thickening—was observed in 12 patients (9 of whom had never smoked cigarettes).

As might be expected, the prevalence of parenchymal abnormalities is highest in patients who have long-standing SLE and chronic respiratory symptoms. In one study of 10 patients who had a mean duration of SLE of 7.5 years and who had respiratory symptoms for a mean of 2.5 years, all patients had abnormal pulmonary function tests and HRCT scans (4 had normal chest radiographs).[26] The most common abnormalities on HRCT scan were areas of ground-glass attenuation (seen in eight patients), honeycombing (seen in seven patients), and pleural thickening (seen in eight patients). Two patients had airway abnormalities, consisting of bronchial dilation in one and centrilobular nodular and branching linear opacities (*tree-in-bud* appearance) in the other.

Cardiovascular changes frequently occur in association with pulmonary and pleural manifestations. An increase in the size of the cardiac silhouette generally is the result of pericardial effusion, which usually is relatively small but may be massive.[9] Cardiomegaly and pulmonary edema may be caused by primary lupus myocardiopathy.

Rheumatoid Disease

The frequency with which rheumatoid arthritis is associated with extra-articular manifestations—76% of cases in one series of 127 patients[31]—justifies the concept of rheumatoid disease as a systemic process. In contrast to the female sex predominance characteristic of rheumatoid arthritis (female-to-male, 2:1 or 3:1[32]), extra-articular manifestations of rheumatoid disease are more common in men. The pleuropulmonary manifestations of rheumatoid disease are listed in Table 8–3.

Similar to other connective tissue diseases, serologic abnormalities are common in rheumatoid disease and presumably reflect an underlying derangement of immunologic function. The presence of rheumatoid factor (anti-IgG immunoglobulin) is the most common abnormality.

Parenchymal Disease

Diffuse Interstitial Pneumonitis and Fibrosis

Interstitial pneumonitis associated with rheumatoid disease is most frequent in seropositive men between 50 and 60 years of age.[34] The most common symptom is dyspnea on effort,[43] sometimes associated with cough and pleuritic pain. Finger clubbing may be present. This condition is similar pathologically to interstitial pneumonitis that occurs in relation to a variety of other connective tissue diseases.

Table 8–3. PLEUROPULMONARY MANIFESTATIONS OF RHEUMATOID DISEASE

Parenchymal disease
    Interstitial pneumonitis and fibrosis
    Upper lobe fibrobullous disease
    Bronchiolitis obliterans with organizing pneumonia (BOOP)
    Rheumatoid nodule
    Caplan's syndrome
Airway disease
    Obliterative bronchiolitis
    Follicular bronchiolitis
    Bronchiectasis
    Upper airway disease
Pleural disease
    Pleural effusion
    Pneumothorax
Vascular disease
    Pulmonary hypertension
    Pulmonary arteritis
    Hyperviscosity syndrome
Secondary abnormalities
    Drug reactions
    Infection
    Malignancy
Miscellaneous conditions

The prevalence of radiographic evidence of pulmonary fibrosis in patients who have rheumatoid disease ranges from about 2% to 10% in different series.[37, 38] Perhaps the most representative data come from a study in which the chest radiographs of 309 patients who had rheumatoid disease were compared with those of sex-matched and age-matched controls;[39] in this study, a reticulonodular pattern consistent with fibrosis was seen in 4.5% of patients who had rheumatoid disease as compared with 0.3% of controls.

The pattern and distribution of fibrosis on chest radiograph and HRCT scan are indistinguishable from those of idiopathic pulmonary fibrosis.[14, 40, 41] In the early stage, the radiographic appearance consists of irregular linear opacities causing a fine reticular or reticulonodular pattern involving mainly the lower lung zones (Fig. 8–5).[10, 14] With progression of disease, the reticular or reticulonodular pattern becomes more coarse and diffuse, and honeycombing may be seen.[10]

HRCT may show evidence of fibrosis in patients with normal chest radiographs.[42] Similar to the radiograph, the predominant abnormality on HRCT scan consists of a reticular pattern caused by a combination of intralobular linear opacities and irregular thickening of interlobular septa (*see* Fig. 8–5).[36, 40] They are present mainly in the subpleural parenchyma and the lower lung zones.[45] Although irregular linear opacities representing fibrosis can be seen on HRCT scan at any level, honeycombing usually is most marked near the diaphragm.[36, 40]

In one review of the HRCT findings in 77 patients, 8 (10%) were found to have features of pulmonary fibrosis (small irregular linear opacities with associated architectural distortion and honeycombing).[36] Seven patients also had areas of ground-glass attenuation, and five patients had pleural thickening or effusion. Honeycombing was seen exclusively in the peripheral lung in five patients and involved the central and peripheral lung in three. Follow-up of four patients over a 4-year period showed progression of honeycombing from the peripheral to the central parts of both lungs and from the bases toward the apices.[36] In three patients, the areas of ground-glass attenuation were replaced by honeycombing.

Upper Lobe Fibrobullous Disease

Although rare, the number of reports of fibrosis confined to the upper lobes and associated with bullae or cavities is sufficient to justify inclusion of this form of parenchymal abnormality as a separate manifestation of rheumatoid disease.[44, 45] The pathogenic basis of this unusual variety is unclear. Chest radiographs show patchy upper lobe fibrosis and cystic spaces consistent with either cavities or bullae, the pattern closely resembling that seen in patients who have advanced ankylosing spondylitis.[44]

Bronchiolitis Obliterans with Organizing Pneumonia

BOOP has been documented uncommonly in patients who have rheumatoid disease.[75, 76] The radiologic findings are identical to those of idiopathic BOOP and consist mainly of air-space consolidation that usually is bilateral and patchy in distribution.[10] In approximately 60% of patients, the consolidation involves mainly the peripheral or peribronchial lung regions.[10]

Rheumatoid Nodules

The rheumatoid nodule represents a relatively rare cause of solitary or multiple nodules in the lungs. It has been estimated that nodules can be detected radiographically in approximately 2 per 1,000 patients who have rheumatoid disease.[50] As might be expected, rheumatoid nodules are seen more commonly with computed tomography (CT), being observed in 3 of 77 patients in one series.[36] Typically, rheumatoid nodules present as well-circumscribed masses, usually multiple, 5 mm to 7 cm in diameter, commonly situated in the periphery of the lung next to the pleura (Fig. 8–6).[36, 47] The nodules may be numerous, resembling metastases, and may wax and wane in concert with subcutaneous nodules and in proportion to the activity of underlying arthritis.[51, 52] Cavitation is common, the walls being thick and having a smooth inner lining. During remission of arthritis, the cavities may become thin walled and disappear gradually, and during exacerbations, they may refill and become opacified.[46] Pleural effusion[46, 53] and spontaneous pneumothorax[46, 51] may coexist. Unless the latter complication supervenes, patients usually have no pulmonary symptoms related to the nodules.

Caplan's Syndrome

Caplan's syndrome was described first in coal miners in South Wales and is characterized radiographically by single or multiple, well-defined, spherical pulmonary opacities 0.5 to 5.0 cm in diameter occurring in inorganic dust–exposed individuals who have rheumatoid disease.[54] In contrast with the slow development of progressive massive fibrosis in coal workers' pneumoconiosis, these lesions usually develop rapidly and tend to appear in crops. In many cases, the background of simple pneumoconiosis is slight or absent.[55] Since the original description of the disease in coal workers, it has been recognized that the lesions also may be associated with exposure to silica or silicates in a variety of industries.[56]

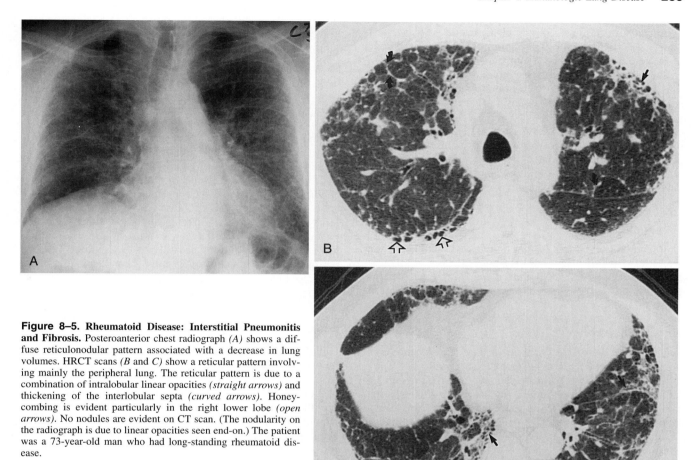

Figure 8–5. Rheumatoid Disease: Interstitial Pneumonitis and Fibrosis. Posteroanterior chest radiograph *(A)* shows a diffuse reticulonodular pattern associated with a decrease in lung volumes. HRCT scans *(B* and *C)* show a reticular pattern involving mainly the peripheral lung. The reticular pattern is due to a combination of intralobular linear opacities *(straight arrows)* and thickening of the interlobular septa *(curved arrows).* Honeycombing is evident particularly in the right lower lobe *(open arrows).* No nodules are evident on CT scan. (The nodularity on the radiograph is due to linear opacities seen end-on.) The patient was a 73-year-old man who had long-standing rheumatoid disease.

Radiographically, there is little to distinguish the nodular lesions of Caplan's syndrome from rheumatoid nodules unassociated with pneumoconiosis. As indicated previously, the nodules tend to develop rapidly and appear in crops. They may increase in number, remain unchanged, or calcify; cavitation may occur and may be followed by fibrosis or disappearance of the lesion.[54, 57]

Pleural Disease

Pleuritis and Pleural Effusion

Pleural abnormalities probably are the most common thoracic manifestation of rheumatoid disease.[1] In autopsy series, the reported prevalence of pathologically evident pleural disease is 38% to 73%;[61] the most common finding

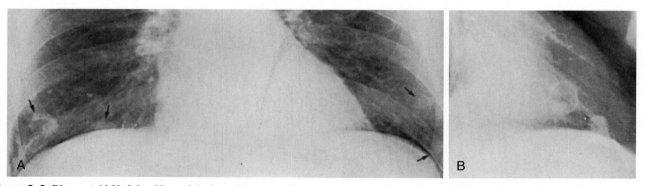

Figure 8–6. Rheumatoid Nodules. View of the lower lung zones from posteroanterior chest radiograph *(A)* in a 41-year-old man with 1-year history of rheumatoid arthritis shows two well-circumscribed nodules in the base of the right lung and at least two nodules in the left base *(arrows)*; the more lateral of the two lesions on the right has cavitated. A thoracotomy was performed, and three nodules were removed from the right middle and lower lobes; characteristic histologic features of rheumatoid nodules were seen. Six years later, oblique radiograph of the lower portion of the left lung *(B)* reveals two nodules, one of which presents as a ring shadow and the other as a nodule of homogeneous density.

is mild pleural fibrosis. Pleural effusions occur in approximately 5% of patients.[61] They may result in no symptoms or be associated with chest pain, fever, or dyspnea.[61]

Pleural effusions usually are small and unilateral[60, 61] but may be bilateral or large.[62, 63] Although they usually resolve over weeks or months, they may recur or persist for many months or years (Fig. 8–7).[64] One third of patients have concurrent parenchymal lung involvement, either interstitial fibrosis or rheumatoid nodules.[61] Similar to diffuse pulmonary interstitial fibrosis, pleural effusion associated with rheumatoid disease is much more likely to occur in patients who have subcutaneous nodules than in those who do not.[58, 59]

Pneumothorax

Pneumothorax is an uncommon complication of rheumatoid disease. It often is associated with rupture of rheumatoid nodules into the pleural space;[65] in some patients, pneumothorax is associated with advanced interstitial fibrosis.

Airway Disease

Clinically significant airway disease is uncommon in nonsmoking patients who have rheumatoid arthritis.[33] Nevertheless, about 15% of such patients have been found to have at least some functional evidence of air-flow obstruction.[49, 66] Airway abnormalities seen with increased prevalence in patients who have rheumatoid disease include obliterative bronchiolitis, follicular bronchitis/bronchiolitis, and bronchiectasis.

Obliterative Bronchiolitis

Obliterative bronchiolitis is seen with increased prevalence in patients who have rheumatoid disease.[67, 68] At the time the complication is recognized, many patients have been receiving penicillamine;[70, 71] rarely a history of gold therapy is elicited.[69, 72] The clinical symptoms usually consist of dry cough and rapidly progressive dyspnea.[61]

The chest radiograph usually is normal or shows only hyperinflation.[67, 73] In one investigation of the HRCT findings in four patients, all of whom had a clinical diagnosis of obliterative bronchiolitis and were receiving penicillamine, abnormalities consisted of a mosaic perfusion pattern with areas of lung showing decreased attenuation and vascularity and other areas showing increased attenuation and vascularity;[74] bronchiectasis, mainly at a subsegmental level, was noted. In another study of two patients, mosaic perfusion and bronchiectasis were found;[73] in addition, expiratory CT showed focal areas of air-trapping consistent with small airway obstruction (Fig. 8–8).

Follicular Bronchitis/Bronchiolitis

Follicular bronchitis/bronchiolitis is a relatively uncommon histologic manifestation of pulmonary rheumatoid disease. Pathologically, this condition is characterized by the presence of abundant lymphoid tissue, frequently with prominent germinal centers, situated in the walls of bronchioles and, to some extent, bronchi.[77] The most common symptoms consist of cough and sputum production and progressive shortness of breath.[48, 77]

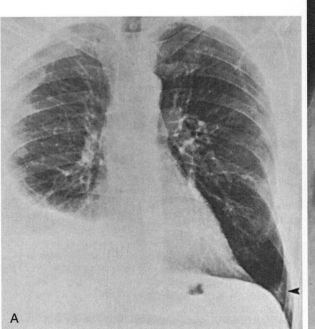
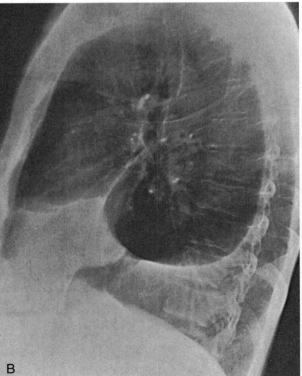

Figure 8–7. Rheumatoid Pleural Effusion. Posteroanterior *(A)* and lateral *(B)* radiographs reveal a moderate accumulation of fluid in the right pleural space. Apart from the solitary nodular opacity in the left costophrenic angle *(arrow)*, the nature of which was not established, the lungs are clear. The effusion showed little change in quantity during several months of observation. The patient was a 54-year-old man who had rheumatoid arthritis.

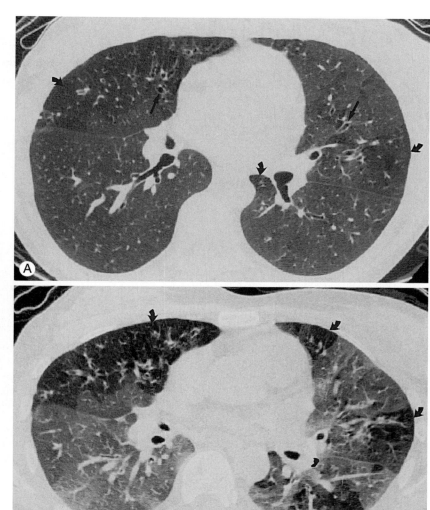

Figure 8–8. Rheumatoid Disease: Obliterative Bronchiolitis. HRCT scan performed at end inspiration *(A)* shows bronchiectasis in the right middle lobe and lingula *(straight arrows)*. Note the areas of decreased attenuation and vascularity in the middle lobe, lingula, and left lower lobe *(curved arrows)* with slight increase in vascularity in normal lung, a pattern known as *mosaic perfusion.* Another scan performed at maximal expiration *(B)* shows areas of air-trapping *(arrows)*. There is marked decrease in vascularity in the areas of air-trapping. The patient was a 30-year-old woman who had rheumatoid disease and a clinical diagnosis of obliterative bronchiolitis. She was not receiving penicillamine.

Chest radiograph characteristically shows a diffuse reticulonodular pattern.[48, 77] HRCT scan shows nodules, mainly in a centrilobular, subpleural, and peribronchial distribution;[36, 48, 307] these usually are small but may measure 1 cm or more in diameter (Fig. 8–9). Other findings include bronchial wall thickening, centrilobular branching linear opacities, and ground-glass opacities.[307] In a review of the CT findings in 12 patients with follicular bronchiolitis, small centrilobular nodules were present in all 12 patients and peribronchial nodules in 5.[307] Nodules larger than 10 mm in diameter were seen in only one patient. Areas of ground-glass attenuation were present in 9 patients (75%), bronchial dilatation in 4, and bronchial wall thickening in 4.

Bronchiectasis

An association between rheumatoid arthritis and bronchiectasis has been shown by several groups of investigators.[78–80] The bronchiectasis may precede the development of arthritis but usually follows it.[80, 81] Most patients have no symptoms related to the bronchiectasis.[61]

In one investigation of 20 lifelong nonsmoking patients who had normal chest radiographs and who underwent HRCT scanning of the chest, 5 were found unexpectedly to have bronchiectasis.[82] In another series, patients who had rheumatoid arthritis and interstitial lung disease on chest radiograph were compared with a control group of patients who had rheumatoid disease and no evidence of interstitial lung disease on HRCT scan.[83] Bronchiectasis was seen in six of the patients who had interstitial lung disease; although this was likely traction bronchiectasis in four patients, in two patients it was thought to be the predominant finding. Four of the patients who had normal chest radiographs had bronchiectasis on HRCT scans. In a third series of 84 unselected patients who had rheumatoid arthritis, bronchiectasis and bronchiolectasis were the most common abnormalities, being observed in 30% (Fig. 8–10);[36] only a few of these patients (7 of 23) had evidence of honeycombing or other distortion of lung architecture.

Pulmonary Hypertension and Vasculitis

Pulmonary arterial hypertension in rheumatoid disease occurs most frequently in association with diffuse intersti-

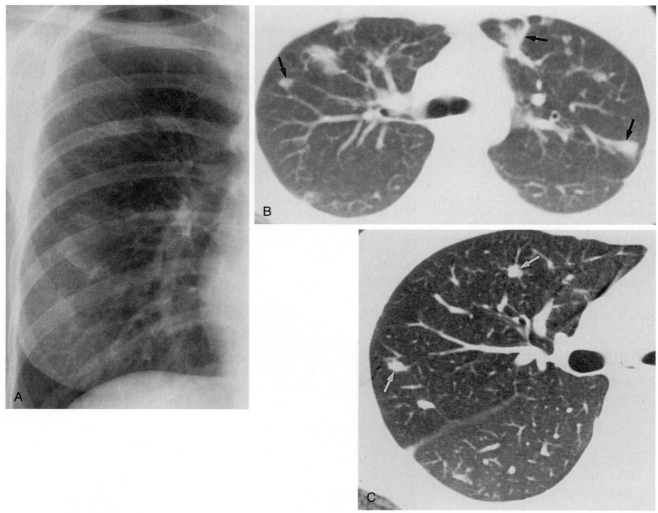

Figure 8–9. Rheumatoid Disease: Follicular Bronchiolitis. View of the right lung from posteroanterior chest radiograph *(A)* shows ill-defined nodular opacities. A similar pattern was present in the left lung. Conventional 10-mm collimation CT scan *(B)* shows focal nodular areas of consolidation in both lungs, located in a predominantly peribronchovascular distribution *(arrows)*. HRCT scan targeted to the right lung *(C)* shows sharply defined peribronchovascular nodular infiltrates in the right upper lobe *(arrows)*. The patient was a 24-year-old woman who had rheumatoid disease and biopsy-proven follicular bronchiolitis.

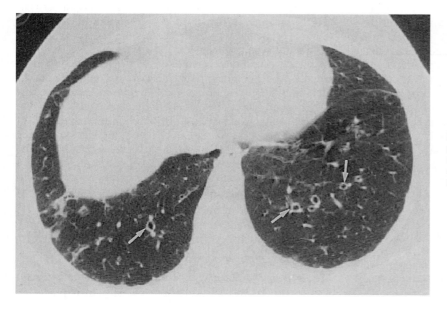

Figure 8–10. Rheumatoid Disease: Bronchiectasis. HRCT scan in a 54-year-old woman with long-standing rheumatoid disease and chronic symptoms of nonproductive cough shows bronchiectasis in both lower lobes *(arrows)*.

tial fibrosis,[84] in which case its pathogenesis and pathologic characteristics are the same as those associated with fibrosis of other causes.[84] Rarely, hypertension develops in the absence of parenchymal disease;[85] in this situation, it often is associated with Raynaud's phenomenon.[35] Pulmonary vasculitis and hemorrhage rarely are seen in rheumatoid arthritis.[61]

Progressive Systemic Sclerosis

PSS (scleroderma) is a generalized disorder characterized by inflammatory, fibrotic, and degenerative changes of connective tissue, often accompanied by vasculopathy. It is an uncommon condition, with an estimated incidence of only 12 cases per 1 million population per year.[86] Most patients are in their thirties to fifties. There is a female predominance of approximately 3:1.[87] The thoracic manifestations of the disease are summarized in Table 8–4.

Pulmonary complications are the most common cause of death in patients who have PSS, the most frequent manifestation being fibrosis, which occurs in about 80% of cases.[88] The main pulmonary symptom is dyspnea on exertion, which is present in approximately 60% of patients who have PSS.[88]

Pulmonary arterial hypertension has been reported in 6% to 60% of patients with PSS, the prevalence being influenced by the diagnostic method used to establish its presence and by the population being studied.[88] It usually is secondary to severe interstitial fibrosis but occasionally occurs in its absence.[88, 94]

Radiologic Manifestations

The systemic nature of PSS often can be appreciated on chest radiograph, which may show abnormalities of the lungs, pleura, esophagus, and chest wall.

Lungs

Evidence of interstitial fibrosis has been reported to be present on chest radiographs in 25% to 65% of patients

Table 8–4. THORACIC MANIFESTATIONS OF PROGRESSIVE SYSTEMIC SCLEROSIS

Parenchymal disease
    Interstitial pneumonitis and fibrosis
    Bronchiolitis obliterans organizing pneumonia
Airway disease
    Follicular bronchiolitis
Pleural abnormalities
    Pleural thickening
    Pleural effusion
Vascular disease
    Pulmonary hypertension
Secondary abnormalities
    Aspiration pneumonia
    Mediastinal lymph node enlargement
    Malignancy
Miscellaneous abnormalities
    Thickened inelastic skin
    Esophageal dilation
    Air esophagogram
    Sclerosis of cardiac muscle
    Erosion of superior cortex of ribs

who have PSS.[88, 92] The initial radiographic abnormalities may be subtle and typically consist of fine reticulation;[88] as the disease progresses, the reticulation tends to become coarser and easier to detect as it extends from the bases to involve the lower two thirds of the lungs (Fig. 8–11).[88] Similar to idiopathic pulmonary fibrosis and rheumatoid disease, there is a tendency for predominant involvement of the lower lung zones, with little or no evidence of upper zone abnormality, at least in the initial stages of the disease.[92]

HRCT frequently shows evidence of interstitial pneumonitis and fibrosis in patients who have normal or questionable radiographic findings.[92, 95] For example, in one prospective study of 23 patients, a definitive reticular pattern consistent with fibrosis was seen on chest radiograph in 9 (39%), and minimal or equivocal findings were seen in 6 (26%); by contrast, evidence of fibrosis was seen on HRCT scan in 21 patients (91%).[92] Only nine patients (39%) had dyspnea at rest or on exercise. In a second study of 18 patients who had PSS and dyspnea or restrictive lung disease as determined by pulmonary function tests, 10 (59%) had evidence of fibrosis on chest radiograph as compared with 15 (88%) on HRCT scan.[96]

The HRCT findings include parenchymal and subpleural micronodules, intralobular linear opacities giving a reticular pattern, subpleural lines, areas of ground-glass attenuation, and honeycombing (*see* Fig. 8–11).[90, 92] The abnormalities involve mainly the lower lobes and are located predominantly in peripheral and posterior regions.[90] Because of this distribution, CT scans should be performed with the patient prone to detect mild abnormalities and to avoid confusing early disease with gravity-induced dependent density.[90] When the chest radiograph is normal or equivocal, nodules measuring 2 to 3 mm in diameter are seen commonly on CT scan, reflecting the presence of follicular bronchiolitis.[90]

The pattern of abnormality on HRCT scan has been shown to reflect the relative proportions of fibrosis and inflammation. In one study of 12 patients, comparison was made between CT findings and open-lung biopsy specimens obtained from 20 different lobes.[97] In 13 of the lobes, HRCT showed a predominant reticular pattern; in the other 7 lobes, there was an equivalent extent of reticulation and areas of ground-glass attenuation. On histologic examination, the predominant reticular pattern was associated with a predominantly fibrotic appearance in 12 of 13 lobes; in the lobes that had an equivalent extent of reticulation and areas of ground-glass attenuation, there was an inflammatory appearance in 4 and a fibrotic appearance in 3 lobes. CT allowed correct discrimination between inflammatory and fibrotic histologic findings in 16 (80%) of 20 biopsy specimens. In another investigation, short-term functional improvement after therapy with corticosteroids was observed in three of seven patients who had an equivalent extent of ground-glass attenuation and reticulation and in none of six patients who had predominant reticulation.[98] Despite this apparent therapeutic benefit, in a follow-up of 66 patients who had interstitial pneumonitis and fibrosis associated with PSS, the CT appearances were not predictive of 4-year survival.[98]

Patients who have interstitial pneumonitis and fibrosis associated with PSS frequently have mediastinal lymph

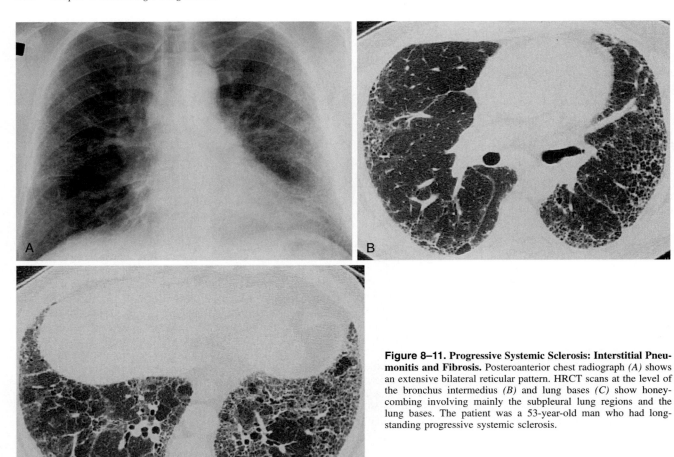

Figure 8–11. Progressive Systemic Sclerosis: Interstitial Pneumonitis and Fibrosis. Posteroanterior chest radiograph *(A)* shows an extensive bilateral reticular pattern. HRCT scans at the level of the bronchus intermedius *(B)* and lung bases *(C)* show honeycombing involving mainly the subpleural lung regions and the lung bases. The patient was a 53-year-old man who had long-standing progressive systemic sclerosis.

node enlargement on CT scan (defined as a short-axis diameter >10 mm). In one series of 53 patients, mediastinal lymphadenopathy was not seen in any of the patients who had normal parenchyma on CT scan but was present in 23% of patients who had mild parenchymal disease and in 42% of the patients who had honeycombing.[90] In another study of 25 patients who had PSS and diffuse interstitial lung disease, mediastinal lymph node enlargement was present in 15 (60%).[99] The likelihood of lymphadenopathy appears to be related to the presence of parenchymal abnormalities rather than the specific pattern of disease seen on HRCT scan. In a review of the CT findings in 73 patients, lymph node enlargement was identified in 35 (48%).[100] Lymph node enlargement was present in 70% of patients who had parenchymal abnormalities regardless of whether the pattern consisted of areas of ground-glass attenuation, a linear pattern, or honeycombing. Only 6 (17%) of the 35 patients who had normal lung parenchyma on CT scan had lymph node enlargement. When considering pulmonary abnormalities, the lung disease might be secondary; for example, esophageal dysmotility may lead to aspiration pneumonia.[22]

Pleura

Radiographic evidence of pleural effusion or thickening is less common in PSS than in other connective tissue diseases, being seen in approximately 10% to 15% of patients.[101] Pleural thickening is seen more commonly on CT scan: In one series of 55 patients evaluated with HRCT, diffuse pleural thickening was seen in one third, all of whom had pulmonary abnormalities.[90] Pneumothorax is rare.[92]

Esophagus

The esophagus is reported to be involved clinically and radiologically in about 50% of patients who have PSS;[102] however, it is likely that the true frequency is greater because patients who have minimal involvement unaccompanied by dysphagia are unlikely to be referred for radiologic examination.[89] For example, in one study of 36 patients who underwent manometric or barium examination of the esophagus, 33 manifested abnormal esophageal motility.[91] Although most patients who have radiographic evidence of esophageal involvement complain of dysphagia, this is not invariable.[89]

The atrophy and atony of the esophagus that result in aperistalsis can lead to dilation, which may be manifested on plain radiographs as an air esophagogram (Fig. 8–12). The presence or absence of esophageal aperistalsis can be assessed better by fluoroscopic study and barium swallow, however—preferably with the patient in the horizontal po-

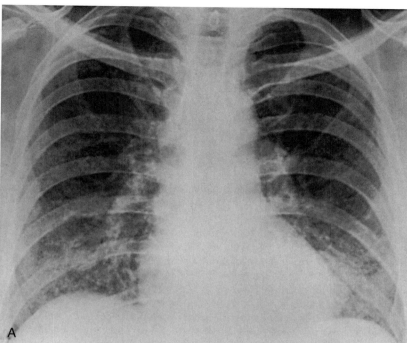

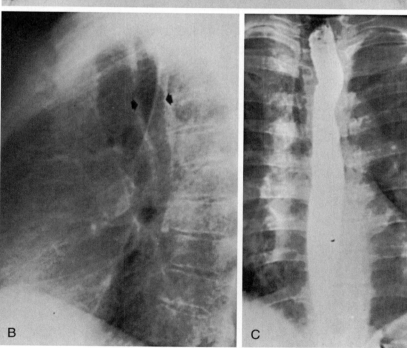

Figure 8–12. Esophageal Distention in Progressive Systemic Sclerosis. Posteroanterior *(A)* and lateral *(B)* radiographs of the chest reveal a fine reticular pattern throughout both lungs; the reticulation is more prominent in the bases. In lateral projection, an abnormal accumulation of gas behind the trachea *(arrows)* represents an air-distended esophagus. Chest radiograph after ingestion of barium *(C)* shows uniform dilation of the esophagus: Fluoroscopic examination revealed aperistalsis. The patient was a 53-year-old man who had progressive systemic sclerosis.

sition because the motility disturbance often is not evident in the erect position. The presence of a substantial amount of gas in the esophagus on a lateral radiograph of the chest is a useful sign of PSS, especially if it is unassociated with an air-fluid level and if gas is present in the gastric fundus.[103] The latter two qualifications are important because an esophageal air-fluid level and a gasless stomach are characteristic features of achalasia, the chief differential diagnostic possibility. The association of an air-containing esophagus with the lung changes described previously is virtually pathognomonic of PSS.[104]

Chest Wall

Erosion of the cortex of the superior aspects of the ribs in the posterior axillary line (superior rib notching) has been reported in approximately 15% of patients who have PSS.[93] The abnormality is not specific because it also may be observed in rheumatoid disease, SLE, and Sjögren's syndrome. Its pathogenesis is unknown.

Dermatomyositis and Polymyositis

The terms *dermatomyositis* and *polymyositis* refer to a group of disorders characterized by weakness and some-

Table 8–5. THORACIC MANIFESTATIONS OF DERMATOMYOSITIS/POLYMYOSITIS

Parenchymal disease
    Interstitial pneumonitis and fibrosis
    Bronchiolitis obliterans organizing pneumonia (BOOP)
Vascular disease
    Pulmonary hypertension
Muscular involvement
    Small lung volumes
    Elevation of diaphragm
Secondary abnormalities
    Aspiration pneumonia
Miscellaneous abnormalities
    Coexistent malignancy

times pain in the proximal limb muscles and (occasionally) in the muscles of the neck. About 50% of patients have dermatomyositis, which is distinguished from polymyositis by a characteristic heliotrope skin rash and erythema or purpura on the extensor surfaces of the extremity joints.[105] About 80% of patients who have dermatomyositis and polymyositis and interstitial lung disease have antibodies directed against the aminoacyl-tRNA synthetases, such as anti-Jo-1.[111] In these cases, malignancy usually is not present.[110]

The disease is worldwide in distribution and occurs twice as often in women as in men. It shows two peak age incidences, the first in ages 1 to 10 and the second in the forties and fifties.[106]

The thorax is affected commonly at some point in the disease, generally in one or more of three forms: (1) hypoventilation and respiratory failure as a result of direct involvement of the respiratory muscles, (2) interstitial pneumonitis indistinguishable from that seen in other connective tissue diseases, and (3) aspiration pneumonia secondary to pharyngeal muscle weakness. The thoracic manifestations are summarized in Table 8–5. The most common clinical presentation in patients who have thoracic involvement is progressive dyspnea with or without cough.[108] Less often, the patient presents with acute symptoms as a result of diffuse alveolar damage or BOOP.[108]

Radiologic Manifestations

The reported frequency of parenchymal abnormalities evident on chest radiograph is 0 to 9%.[109, 113] The most representative figure is probably that derived from a Mayo Clinic study in which 213 patients had the diagnosis established by a combination of muscle biopsy, electromyography, and detection of enzyme abnormalities; in this investigation, only 10 patients (5%) showed radiographic evidence of interstitial pulmonary disease.[107]

The radiographic findings of interstitial fibrosis in patients who have dermatomyositis and polymyositis are indistinguishable from those of idiopathic pulmonary fibrosis and consist of a symmetric, predominantly basal, reticular or reticulonodular pattern.[107, 114] This pattern can become diffuse over time and progress to honeycombing.[114] Some patients develop relatively acute abnormalities over a 2- to 3-week period.[107, 115] In these individuals, chest radiograph usually shows bilateral areas of consolidation superimposed on a reticulonodular pattern, an abnormality related to diffuse alveolar damage[112, 115] or BOOP.[112, 115] On HRCT scan, the consolidation may have a predominantly peribronchoarterial or subpleural distribution (Fig. 8–13).[116, 117] Less

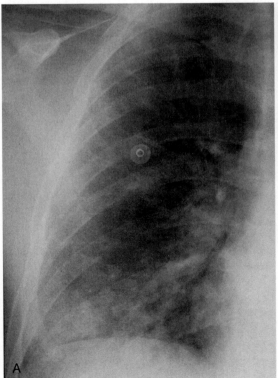

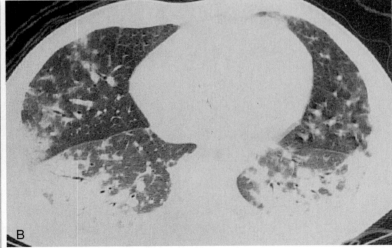

Figure 8–13. Polymyositis: Bronchiolitis Obliterans Organizing Pneumonia. View of the right lung from posteroanterior chest radiograph *(A)* shows areas of consolidation. Similar findings were present in the left lung. HRCT scan through the lower lung zones *(B)* shows that the consolidation involves mainly the peripheral lung regions. The patient was a 27-year-old man who presented with fever, cough, progressive shortness of breath, and muscle weakness. The diagnoses of bronchiolitis obliterans organizing pneumonia and polymyositis were proved by biopsy.

commonly, BOOP may present with bilateral interstitial or nodular opacities.[112]

In one investigation, the authors reviewed the findings in 25 patients who underwent HRCT examination because of abnormal chest radiographs or pulmonary function test results.[117] Of 25 patients, 23 had parenchymal abnormalities on HRCT scan, including linear opacities (92%), ground-glass attenuation (92%), air-space consolidation (52%), small nodules (28%), and honeycombing (16%).[117] The linear opacities involved mainly the peripheral portions of the middle and lower lung zones, similar to the distribution of interstitial pneumonitis and fibrosis in other connective tissue diseases. In most cases, the consolidation involved the middle and lower lung zones and was shown histologically to represent BOOP; in two cases, it was diffuse and was shown at autopsy to be related to diffuse alveolar damage.[117] In another study of 19 patients, all had bilateral areas of ground-glass attenuation and patchy areas of consolidation involving mainly the lower lung zones;[118] a predominantly subpleural distribution was present in 16 patients (84%).

Other common findings included interlobular septal thickening, subpleural lines, and irregular peribronchoarterial thickening. Bronchial or bronchiolar dilation (traction bronchiectasis or bronchiolectasis) was seen in seven patients; none had honeycombing. HRCT scans performed during mean follow-up of 2 years after treatment with corticosteroids, immunosuppressive agents, or both showed marked improvement in all but one patient.

When polymyositis involves the respiratory muscles, particularly the diaphragm, diaphragmatic elevation and small lung volumes are apparent, often in conjunction with basal linear opacities.[119] When pharyngeal muscle paralysis is present, unilateral or bilateral segmental pneumonia may result from aspiration of food and oral secretions; such aspiration pneumonia has been reported in 15% to 20% of patients.[115]

Sjögren's Syndrome

Sjögren's syndrome is a chronic autoimmune inflammatory disease characterized by the clinical triad of dry eyes (keratoconjunctivitis sicca), dry mouth (xerostomia), and arthritis.[120] Although this syndrome may be seen in the absence of other connective tissue disease (primary Sjögren's syndrome), this is uncommon; for example, in one study of 171 patients, rheumatoid arthritis or another connective tissue disorder coexisted in 100 (59%) patients.[121] Sjögren's syndrome affects 0.1% of the general population and is more common in women (female-to-male ratio 9:1).[120] Patients who have Sjögren's syndrome frequently have pleuropulmonary abnormalities. Some of these abnormalities are related to other connective tissue diseases, whereas others probably are specific for the syndrome (Table 8–6).

Radiologic Manifestations

The frequency of abnormalities on chest radiograph varies considerably in different series. In one study of 42 patients, 14 (33%) showed a reticulonodular pattern,[123] whereas in another review of 343 patients, pulmonary

Table 8–6. THORACIC MANIFESTATIONS OF SJÖGREN'S SYNDROME

Parenchymal disease
  Interstitial pneumonitis and fibrosis
  Lymphocytic interstitial pneumonia
  Bronchiolitis obliterans organizing pneumonia (BOOP)
  Lymphoma
  Amyloidosis
Airway disease
  Follicular bronchiolitis
Vascular disease
  Pulmonary hypertension
Pleural disease
  Pleuritis with or without effusion

involvement was shown in 31 (9%).[124] In a third study of 171 patients, only 3 (1.7%) showed radiographic abnormalities consistent with fibrosis.[122]

The reticulonodular pattern usually has a basal predominance.[125] Lung biopsy in a few patients has shown that this pattern may be caused by lymphocytic interstitial pneumonia, interstitial fibrosis, or, less commonly, lymphoma.[125, 126] HRCT findings were assessed in a prospective study of 50 patients in whom the onset of Sjögren's syndrome had occurred a mean of 12 years (range, 2 to 37 years) before the scans;[127] 37 (74%) of the 50 patients had no respiratory symptoms at the time of HRCT scan. Abnormalities were detected in 17 (34%) patients on HRCT scan compared with 7 (14%) patients on chest radiographs. The most common findings consisted of bronchiolectasis and poorly defined centrilobular nodular or branching linear opacities (seen in 11 patients), areas of ground-glass attenuation (seen in 7 patients), and honeycombing (seen in 4 patients). Honeycombing was bilateral and present almost exclusively in the periphery of the lower lobes.

A characteristic pattern of extensive areas of ground-glass attenuation with scattered thin-walled cysts has been reported in patients who have lymphocytic interstitial pneumonitis (Fig. 8–14).[128, 131] Similar findings have been described in lymphocytic interstitial pneumonia not associated with Sjögren's syndrome.[128, 132] An open-lung biopsy specimen in one patient showed interstitial and peribronchiolar lymphoplasmacytic infiltrates associated with overinflation of the secondary pulmonary lobule.[129] Other common findings include poorly defined centrilobular nodules, subpleural nodules, and thickening of the bronchovascular bundles and interlobular septa.[131] In one series, HRCT findings consisted of thin-walled cysts 2 to 15 mm in diameter and multiple irregular, solid soft tissue nodules, most of which were adjacent to the cysts.[130] The soft tissue nodules were shown histologically to represent pulmonary nodular amyloidosis.

Mixed Connective Tissue Disease

Many patients who have connective tissue disease show features of more than one specific entity, in which case they commonly are referred to as having *overlap syndromes* or *unclassified (undifferentiated) connective tissue disease.*[134, 135] One form of such overlap disease consists of a symptom complex with features of SLE, PSS, and polymyositis.[137] Patients who have this abnormality (MCTD) typically have

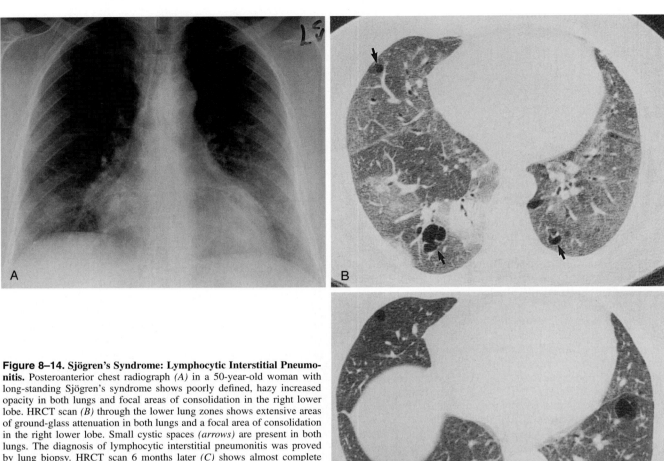

Figure 8–14. Sjögren's Syndrome: Lymphocytic Interstitial Pneumonitis. Posteroanterior chest radiograph *(A)* in a 50-year-old woman with long-standing Sjögren's syndrome shows poorly defined, hazy increased opacity in both lungs and focal areas of consolidation in the right lower lobe. HRCT scan *(B)* through the lower lung zones shows extensive areas of ground-glass attenuation in both lungs and a focal area of consolidation in the right lower lobe. Small cystic spaces *(arrows)* are present in both lungs. The diagnosis of lymphocytic interstitial pneumonitis was proved by lung biopsy. HRCT scan 6 months later *(C)* shows almost complete resolution of the parenchymal opacities. The cysts have become more conspicuous, however. They presumably are related to partial obstruction of small airways. The patient was a lifelong nonsmoker.

high serum titers of antibody to extractable nuclear antigen (anti-nRNP Ab).[136]

As might be expected, the radiologic manifestations of MCTD include those seen in SLE, PSS, and polymyositis.[138] The frequency of pulmonary abnormalities varies considerably in different series. For example, in a retrospective study of 81 patients from the Mayo Clinic, an interstitial pattern was seen on chest radiograph in 19%;[139] careful prospective study of 34 patients in another investigation showed interstitial infiltrates in 85%.[134] The infiltrates consisted of irregular linear opacities having a reticular pattern and involving mainly the lung bases.[142] With progression of disease, the fibrosis gradually extends superiorly; in the late stage, honeycombing may be identified.[134, 138] HRCT corroborates the radiographic findings and shows a predominantly subpleural distribution of fibrosis, similar to that seen in the interstitial fibrosis associated with other connective tissue diseases.[138] Other radiographic abnormalities include areas of parenchymal consolidation that may be related to aspiration pneumonia[138] or diffuse pulmonary hemorrhage.[140, 261]

Pleural effusion has been reported in 5% of patients.[139] Pericardial effusion and evidence of congestive heart failure secondary to myocarditis also may be seen.[138]

Relapsing Polychondritis

Relapsing polychondritis is characterized principally by inflammation and destruction of cartilage in a variety of sites throughout the body; disease of the eye, ear, and systemic vessels also is seen occasionally. The condition is uncommon: By 1991, slightly more than 600 cases had been reported in the world literature.[142] There is no sex predominance, and the disease occurs at all ages, with a peak incidence between 40 and 60 years.[141]

The most common clinical manifestations consist of pain, erythema, and swelling of one or both external ears.[143] Polyarthritis, often migratory, is seen in 50% to 80% of patients.[143] Respiratory symptoms as a result of involvement of the glottis, trachea, or proximal bronchi include dyspnea, cough, stridor, and wheezing.[143]

Radiologic Manifestations

The most common radiographic manifestation in the chest is tracheal stenosis.[144] Less often, there is narrowing of the major[144, 145] or segmental bronchi.[146] The tracheal narrowing usually measures only a few centimeters in length,[147] although diffuse stenosis may occur.[148] Thickening of the tracheal or bronchial wall can be seen on CT scan, in association with narrowing of the lumen (Fig. 8–15).[149, 150] Occasionally, bronchiectasis is evident, presumably secondary to recurrent pneumonia.[146] The extent and degree of tracheal and bronchial stenosis is assessed best using spiral CT with thin collimation (3 mm) and multiplanar or three-dimensional reconstructions.[151, 152] Dynamic collapse of the airways can be visualized using dynamic imaging with multidetector spiral CT.[152a]

Pulmonary Involvement in Inflammatory Bowel Disease

Although idiopathic inflammatory bowel disease (Crohn's disease and ulcerative colitis) generally is not considered to be in the spectrum of the connective tissue diseases, it may be immunologically mediated and is included in this section. Clinically apparent respiratory involvement in these disorders is rare. Most of the descriptions of an association between pleuroparenchymal disease and inflammatory bowel disease are culled from individual case reports; these reports were summarized and 33 new patients were described in a 1993 review.[153]

Airway complications probably are the most common manifestations, especially in patients who have ulcerative colitis.[153] Chronic bronchitis and bronchiectasis have been seen in many such patients in the absence of a smoking history;[154, 155] ulcerative tracheobronchitis (Fig. 8–16),[157]

BOOP,[158, 159] obliterative bronchiolitis,[160] granulomatous bronchiolitis,[305] and diffuse panbronchiolitis[161] have been described. Subglottic stenosis has been a manifestation of ulcerative colitis and Crohn's disease.

Radiographic and HRCT findings were described in seven patients with ulcerative colitis who presented with cough and recurrent respiratory infections.[162] Chest radiographs were normal in two patients and showed evidence of bronchial wall thickening in three and bronchiectasis in two. HRCT findings included bronchiectasis in six patients and centrilobular nodularity suggestive of peripheral airway disease in four. Three patients had narrowing of the major bronchi, in one case associated with narrowing of the distal trachea. Bronchial biopsy in six patients showed acute and chronic inflammation of the mucosa and submucosa associated with peribronchial fibrosis.

VASCULITIS

This section includes a variety of conditions whose sole or predominant histologic feature is inflammation of pulmonary vessels; discussion is limited to disorders in which the inflammatory reaction is directed primarily against the vessel wall and is of proven or presumed immunologic origin. Such disease occurs in several well-characterized clinicopathologic entities, such as Wegener's granulomatosis, Churg-Strauss syndrome, microscopic polyangiitis, Takayasu's arteritis, and Behçet's disease. Other conditions in which systemic vasculitis is prominent but in which the nature of associated pulmonary disease is poorly defined (such as polyarteritis nodosa) also are discussed.

Wegener's Granulomatosis

Wegener's granulomatosis is a multisystem disease with variable clinical expression that, in its full-blown state, is

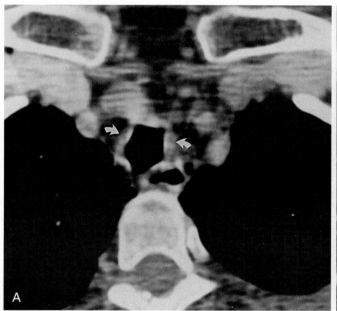
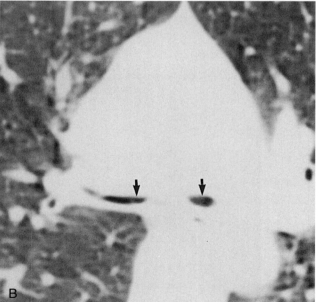

Figure 8–15. Relapsing Polychondritis. HRCT scan *(A)* shows mild circumferential thickening of the tracheal wall *(arrows)*. Scan at the level of the main bronchi photographed at lung windows *(B)* shows narrowing of the lumen of the right and the left main bronchi *(arrows)*. The patient was a 51-year-old woman who presented with a 6-month history of sore throat, hoarseness, and dry cough. The diagnosis was proved by tracheal biopsy. (From Müller NL, et al: Can Assoc Radiol J 40:213, 1989.)

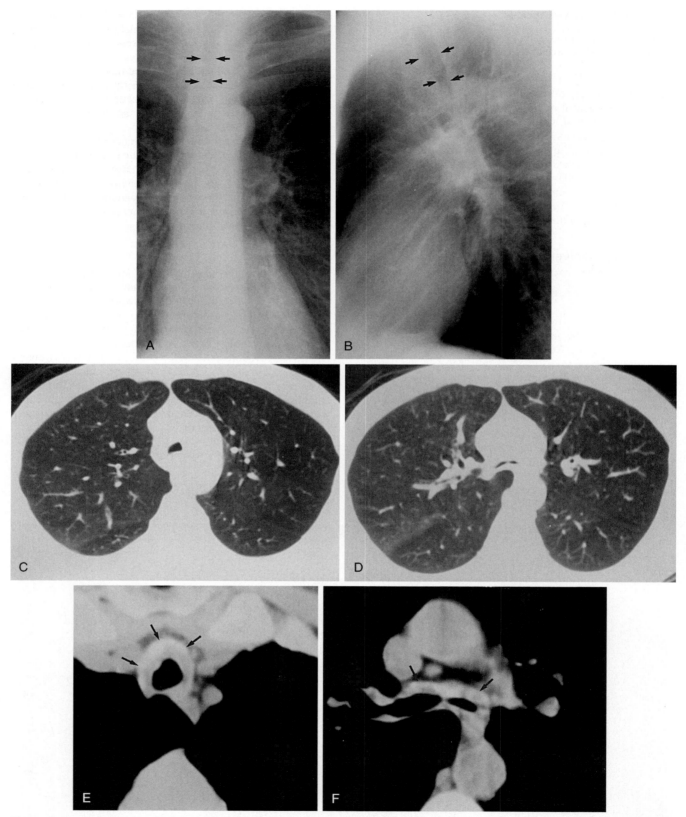

Figure 8–16. Ulcerative Tracheobronchitis Associated with Ulcerative Colitis. A 50-year-old man who had ulcerative colitis presented with progressive shortness of breath and stridor. Views from posteroanterior *(A)* and lateral *(B)* chest radiographs show diffuse narrowing of the tracheal lumen *(arrows)*. The degree of tracheal narrowing and the presence of bilateral bronchial narrowing are seen better on CT scans photographed on lung windows *(C and D)*. Soft tissue windows show marked thickening of the wall of the trachea *(E)* and the right and left main bronchi *(F; arrows)*. The diagnosis of ulcerative tracheobronchitis was proved by biopsy.

Table 8–7. THORACIC MANIFESTATIONS OF WEGENER'S GRANULOMATOSIS

Parenchymal abnormalities
    Multiple nodules, approximately 50% cavitate
    Air-space consolidation
    Ground-glass attenuation
Airway abnormalities
    Tracheal or bronchial wall thickening
    Tracheal or bronchial stenosis
Pleural abnormalities
    Pleural effusion in about 10% of cases
    Rarely pleural thickening or pneumothorax
Lymph node enlargement
    Hilar or mediastinal lymph node enlargement in about 5% of cases

characterized pathologically by necrotizing granulomatous inflammation of the upper and lower respiratory tracts, glomerulonephritis, and necrotizing vasculitis of the lungs and a variety of other organs and tissues. It is a rare disease; in the United States, the prevalence has been estimated to be about 3 per 100,000.[165] The disease typically affects adults in their thirties to fifties, the mean age in three large series being 46, 41, and 56 years.[165–167]

The onset may be acute (and its course fulminating)[188] but more commonly is insidious. Although the disease may be associated initially with such nonspecific symptoms as fever, general malaise, weight loss, and fatigue, most patients present with complaints referable to the nose, paranasal sinuses, ear, or chest.[166]

Thoracic symptoms consist most often of cough, hemoptysis, dyspnea, and pleuritic pain.[166, 167] Cough, usually nonproductive, is the most frequent, occurring in 60 of 77 patients with pulmonary disease in one review.[167] Hemoptysis is seen in about 30% to 40% of these patients; occasionally, it is massive, the clinical presentation mimicking Goodpasture's syndrome.[168] Dyspnea occurs particularly with alveolar hemorrhage and, occasionally, as a result of tracheal involvement.[189, 190]

The upper respiratory tract is affected at the onset of disease in about 50% to 75% of patients and at some time during its course in almost all patients.[166] The most common manifestations are those related to sinusitis and nasal ulceration. The latter may be associated with destruction of bone and cartilage and significant nasal deformity. Manifestations of otitis, including pain and hearing loss, also are common. Although manifestations of renal disease occur in 75% to 85% of patients at some time in the course of the disease,[166] only rarely are they the presenting clinical features.[192]

The diagnosis and management of Wegener's granulomatosis have been aided by the ability to measure serum antineutrophil cytoplasmic antibodies (ANCA) levels. Some investigators have found c-ANCA in approximately 85% to 90% of patients who have disseminated Wegener's granulomatosis[193, 194] and in about 75% of those who have limited disease.[195]

Radiologic Manifestations

In an analysis of the findings in 158 patients with Wegener's granulomatosis who were referred to the U.S. National Institutes of Health (NIH), pulmonary parenchymal abnormalities were identified on the initial chest radiograph in 45% and eventually developed in 85% (Table 8–7).[166] The typical abnormality consists of nodules ranging in size from a few millimeters to 10 cm in diameter (Fig. 8–17);[167, 170] rarely, there is a reticulonodular interstitial pattern.[172] In 80% to 95% of cases, the nodules are fewer than 10.[170, 171] The nodules are bilateral in approximately 75% of cases[167] and usually are distributed widely, with no predilection for any lung zone.[167] With progression of disease, the nodules tend to increase in size and in number.[167] Calcification is rare.[169, 173] Cavitation occurs eventually in approximately 50% of cases.[167, 175] The cavities usually are thick walled and tend to have an irregular, shaggy inner lining;[167, 175] less commonly, they are thin walled[169, 175] or contain an air-fluid level (Fig. 8–18). The cavities may become large, sometimes involving a whole lobe.[173] Rarely, individual pulmonary opacities, with or without cavitation, decrease in size or disappear before therapy.[174]

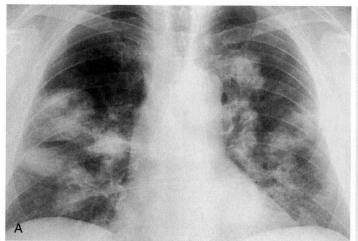

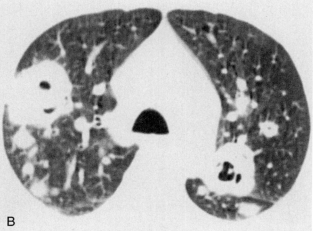

A   B

Figure 8–17. Wegener's Granulomatosis. Posteroanterior chest radiograph *(A)* and CT scan at the level of the upper lobes *(B)* show multiple bilateral nodules a few millimeters to 5 cm in diameter. The larger nodules are cavitated. The patient was a 54-year-old man; open-lung biopsy showed features typical of Wegener's granulomatosis.

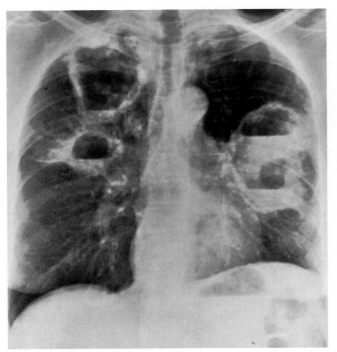

Figure 8–18. Wegener's Granulomatosis—Cavitation. Posteroanterior chest radiograph in a 55-year-old woman shows multiple, large, thick-walled cavities with air-fluid levels. The left upper lung zone is oligemic, suggesting the possibility of compromise of the left upper lobe bronchus and resulting hypoxic vasoconstriction.

CT may show nodules that are not apparent on radiography and is superior in showing the presence of cavitation;[169, 177] cavitation is evident on CT scan in most nodules that measure more than 2 cm.[171] As on radiography, the nodules tend to have a random distribution;[171, 176] occasion-

ally, they are predominantly or exclusively subpleural in location[176] or have a peribronchovascular distribution.[175, 178]

Acute air-space consolidation or ground-glass opacities secondary to pulmonary hemorrhage (Fig. 8–19) is the second most common radiographic finding in Wegener's granulomatosis and may occur with or without the presence of nodules.[167, 175] The areas of consolidation are variable in appearance, some being dense and localized,[167] some involving a whole lobe,[179] and some being bilateral and patchy or confluent.[175] In one review of the radiographic findings in 77 patients who had pulmonary Wegener's granulomatosis, nodules were identified on the radiograph in 69% and areas of consolidation in 53%;[167] 49% of nodules and 17% of areas of consolidation had evidence of cavitation. Diffuse bilateral areas of ground-glass opacity or consolidation were seen in 8% of cases. On CT scan, the areas of consolidation may be random in distribution; sometimes they appear as peripheral wedge-shaped lesions abutting the pleura, mimicking pulmonary infarcts,[178] or have a peribronchoarterial distribution (Fig. 8–20).[175, 180] Calcification within areas of consolidation is rare.[167] Less common parenchymal abnormalities evident on CT scan include interlobular septal thickening, centrilobular interstitial thickening, and parenchymal bands.[177]

Tracheobronchial involvement occurs in about 15% of patients during the course of the disease.[133, 166] Bronchial wall involvement may result in airway narrowing and lead to segmental, lobar, or total lung atelectasis.[167, 173] The bronchial abnormalities themselves or those affecting the trachea seldom are visible on radiograph.[170, 181] In one study of 51 patients who underwent bronchoscopy, 30 (59%) had tracheal or endobronchial disease, including subglottic stenosis, ulcerating tracheobronchitis, and tracheal or bronchial stenosis;[181] in none of these patients were these abnormalities evident on the radiograph. By contrast, tracheal and bronchial wall thickening and luminal narrowing usu-

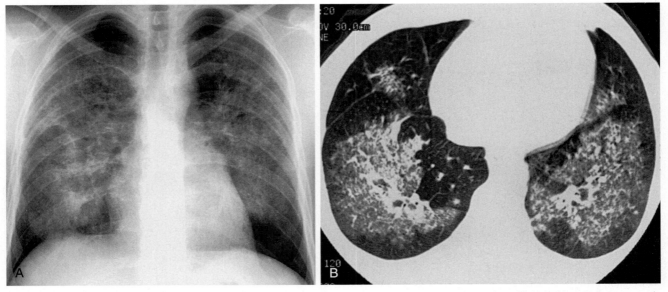

Figure 8–19. Wegener's Granulomatosis—Air-Space Hemorrhage. Posteroanterior chest radiograph *(A)* in a 20-year-old man shows extensive bilateral areas of consolidation with relative sparing of the lung apices and lung bases. Several irregular linear opacities suggestive of fibrosis are evident. HRCT scan *(B)* shows bilateral areas of ground-glass attenuation and consolidation with relative sparing of the subpleural lung regions. A few small nodular opacities and irregular linear opacities are evident. The patient had recurrent pulmonary hemorrhage.

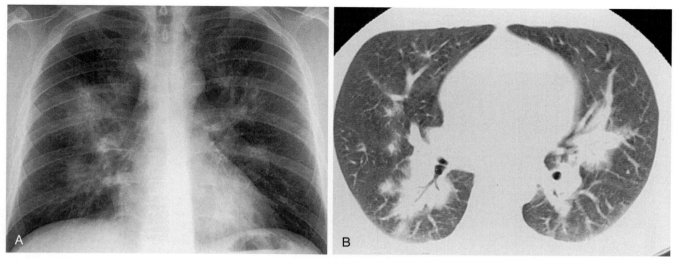

Figure 8–20. Wegener's Granulomatosis. Posteroanterior chest radiograph *(A)* in a 39-year-old man shows patchy bilateral areas of consolidation involving mainly the perihilar regions. CT scan *(B)* shows peribronchial distribution of the areas of consolidation. The diagnosis of Wegener's granulomatosis was proved by lung biopsy. (Case courtesy of Dr. Andrew Mason, St. Paul's Hospital, Vancouver, Canada.)

ally can be detected on CT scan.[176, 179] Of tracheal lesions on CT scan, 90% are located in the subglottic region.[191] Common findings include circumferential wall thickening, stenosis, and mucosal irregularity.[191] The tracheal rings may be abnormally thickened and calcified.[182] Rarely, tracheal[183] or esophageal[184] involvement leads to a tracheoesophageal fistula.

Pleural effusions may be unilateral or bilateral and small or large. Pleural effusions have been reported in 3% and 55% of patients in different series,[175, 176, 184] the best estimate of frequency probably being about 10%.[167] Rarely, there is unilateral or bilateral pleural thickening,[173] pneumothorax,[185] hydropneumothorax,[175] or pyopneumothorax.[186]

Hilar or mediastinal lymph node enlargement, or both, has been reported on radiography or CT in 2% to 15% of cases.[167, 175] The hilar lymph node enlargement may be unilateral or bilateral. Occasionally, enlarged mediastinal nodes compress the trachea or bronchi.[187]

Churg-Strauss Syndrome

Churg-Strauss syndrome is a clinicopathologic entity characterized clinically by asthma, fever, and eosinophilia and pathologically by necrotizing vasculitis and extravascular granulomatous inflammation.[196] The condition is rare. The annual incidence in the Norfolk region of England has been estimated to be 2.4 per 1 million (approximately 30% that of Wegener's granulomatosis and the same as that of microscopic polyangiitis).[164]

Patients typically have a history of allergic phenomena—most often nasal polyposis, sinusitis, or asthma—that precedes the other components of the disease by months or years. Pulmonary manifestations that develop during the vasculitic phase of disease include cough and (rarely) hemoptysis.

Extrapulmonary involvement is seen most often in the skin, gastrointestinal tract, and nervous system. Skin rash is one of the most common clinical features. In one review of 90 patients, skin rash was seen in 36 (40%);[204] in 5

patients, it was the initial manifestation of disease. The most common findings reported in this review were purpura and petechiae on the lower extremities and cutaneous nodules and papules on the elbows. Gastrointestinal disease occurs in 35% to 60% of patients,[202] manifested most often by pain and less frequently by diarrhea or bleeding. Neurologic involvement most often takes the form of a peripheral neuropathy, usually mononeuritis multiplex.[203]

Radiologic Manifestations

Chest radiograph is abnormal in approximately 70% of patients (Table 8–8).[197] In most, the abnormalities consist of transient, patchy nonsegmental areas of consolidation without predilection for any lung zone.[197, 198] In 40%, these changes precede the development of clinical evidence of systemic vasculitis.[197] The areas of consolidation may be symmetric and have a nonsegmental distribution similar to that observed in chronic eosinophilic pneumonia (Fig. 8–21).[197, 198] A diffuse interstitial, reticular, or reticulonodular pattern and miliary nodules also may occur but are uncommon.[197, 198] Occasionally the abnormalities consist of bilateral small and large nodular opacities that may become confluent; in contrast to Wegener's granulomatosis, cavitation is rare.[197, 199] Unilateral or bilateral pleural effusions occur in approximately 30% of patients.[197] Hilar lymph node enlargement has been observed occasionally.[197]

Table 8–8. THORACIC MANIFESTATIONS OF CHURG-STRAUSS SYNDROME

Parenchymal abnormalities
   Patchy bilateral air-space consolidation: most common finding
   Small or large nodular opacities
   Reticular or reticulonodular pattern: uncommon
Pleural abnormalities
   Pleural effusion in 30% of patients
Lymph node enlargement
   Hilar or mediastinal lymph node enlargement: uncommon

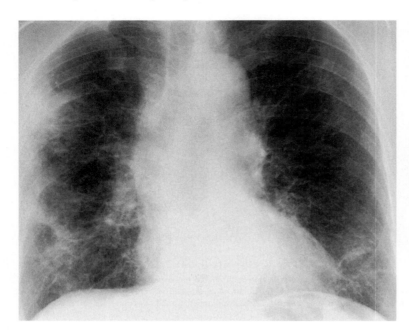

Figure 8–21. Churg-Strauss Syndrome. Posteroanterior chest radiograph in a 71-year-old woman shows patchy bilateral areas of consolidation in a predominantly subpleural distribution. The diagnosis of Churg-Strauss syndrome was proved by open-lung biopsy.

In one review of the HRCT findings at the time of diagnosis in 17 patients, the most common abnormality (seen in approximately 60%) consisted of areas of ground-glass attenuation or consolidation in a patchy or a predominant peripheral distribution (Fig. 8–22);[200] 2 patients also had small centrilobular nodules. In another two patients, the predominant abnormality consisted of multiple nodules measuring 0.5 to 3.5 cm in diameter, several of which were cavitated. One patient had interlobular septal thickening related to interstitial pulmonary edema secondary to cardiac involvement, two patients had bronchial wall thickening or dilation (findings commonly seen in patients who have asthma), and two patients had normal examinations. Small unilateral or bilateral pleural effusions were identified in two patients.

A single case has been reported in which HRCT showed enlarged peripheral pulmonary arteries, some of which had an irregular, stellate configuration that correlated with the presence of vasculitis histologically.[201]

Microscopic Polyangiitis

In the past, primary vasculitis of systemic arteries sometimes was considered as a single entity, termed *polyarteritis nodosa*. Now it is believed widely that such vasculitis is better considered as two disease processes, one involving only medium-size or small arteries and termed *classic polyarteritis nodosa* and the other characterized by inflammation of arterioles, venules, and capillaries (including those of the glomeruli) and referred to as *microscopic polyangiitis*.[163] Because classic polyarteritis nodosa is much less common than microscopic polyangiitis[163, 205] and because its involvement of the pulmonary circulation is almost nonexistent,[174] the following discussion is limited to microscopic polyarteritis.

Depending on the extent and nature of renal, pulmonary, and systemic vascular involvement, clinical findings of microscopic polyarteritis can be variable. Renal disease is the most common and important manifestation and is present at the onset of disease in most patients. Pulmonary involvement develops in about 15% to 30% of patients and is characterized principally by hemoptysis;[202] cough, chest pain, and shortness of breath may be present.[206] Men are affected somewhat more commonly than women are, and the average age of onset is about 50 years.[202] Antineutrophil cytoplasmic antibodies (usually p-ANCAs) are present in most patients.[202]

The radiographic features consist of patchy, bilateral airspace opacities caused by alveolar hemorrhage.[207, 208] Pleural effusion has been reported in approximately 15% of cases and pulmonary edema in 6%.[208]

Takayasu's Arteritis

Takayasu's arteritis is an uncommon condition affecting principally the aorta and its major branches; approximately

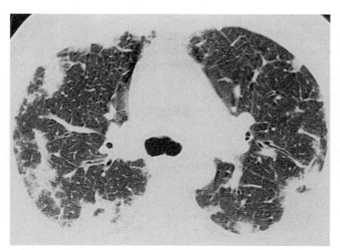

Figure 8–22. Churg-Strauss Syndrome. HRCT scan in a 52-year-old man shows bilateral areas of consolidation in a predominantly subpleural distribution. The diagnosis was proved by open-lung biopsy.

300 cases had been reported by 1996.[209] The abnormality has been classified into several types, depending on the specific sites involved.[210] Although vasculitis usually is confined to the systemic circulation, pulmonary artery involvement is found in many cases; in one review of 76 autopsies, the main pulmonary artery was found to be affected in 34 cases and the intrapulmonary arterial branches in 21.[211] Angiographic studies have shown a wide variation in the incidence of pulmonary involvement (15% to 85% of patients).[212–214]

The disease has a marked predilection for women (approximately 90% to 95% of cases[215]) and usually has its onset between 10 and 40 years of age. Most reports have originated in Southeast Asia; however, it has been suggested that the disease might be underdiagnosed in Europe and North America.[216]

Radiologic Manifestations

The most common radiographic abnormalities involve the aorta and consist of contour irregularities (reported in 10% to 73% of patients) and calcification (reported in 10% to 25% of patients).[214, 217] These findings are uncommon in normal premenopausal women, and their presence should alert the physician to the diagnosis.[214] In one review of 49 patients, abnormalities were detected on chest radiograph in 67%;[214] the most common abnormalities consisted of a wavy or scalloped contour of the descending thoracic aorta (45%) (Fig. 8–23), ectasia of the aortic arch (18%), calcification of the wall of the aorta at the level of its arch or

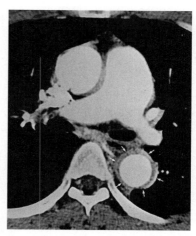

Figure 8–24. Takayasu's Arteritis. Contrast-enhanced CT scan in a 32-year-old woman shows circumferential thickening of the wall of the descending thoracic aorta *(arrows)*, a characteristic finding in Takayasu's arteritis. (Case courtesy of Dr. Jung-Gi Im, Department of Radiology, Seoul National University Hospital, Seoul, Korea.)

descending portion (18%) and cardiomegaly (16%).[214] Less common abnormalities include dilation of the ascending aorta, aneurysms of the descending aorta, oligemia distal to obstructed pulmonary arteries, and pulmonary edema.[214, 217]

In one retrospective CT analysis of pulmonary parenchymal abnormalities in 25 patients, localized areas of low attenuation and decreased vascularity were identified in 11 (44%);[218] these were shown to correspond to areas of decreased vascularity distal to pulmonary arteritis on pulmonary angiography and to perfusion defects on 99m-macroaggregated albumin perfusion scintigraphy. The findings were seen better on HRCT scan than on conventional CT scan. Other abnormalities seen on CT scan included localized subpleural irregular linear opacities (in 48% of patients) and localized areas of pleural thickening (in 36% of patients).

Aortic and pulmonary artery abnormalities in Takayasu's arteritis may be assessed using contrast-enhanced spiral CT or MR imaging (Fig. 8–24).[219–221] In one prospective study of 12 patients and 10 healthy adults involving CT angiography, precontrast images revealed high attenuation of the aortic wall in 10 patients and mural calcification of the aorta in 9.[219] Arterial-phase images showed circumferential thickening of 1 to 4 mm of the aortic wall in all patients and enhancement in five patients; delayed-phase CT images obtained 20 to 40 minutes after intravenous injection showed circumferential enhancement of the aortic wall in eight patients. (The wall of the aorta in the 10 healthy adults was <1 mm or was imperceptible, showed no calcification, and could not be visualized on the precontrast and delayed images). In two patients, the pulmonary trunk and right and left main pulmonary arteries showed variable wall thickening with early and delayed enhancement.

Thickening and enhancement of the vessel wall may also be seen on contrast-enhanced MR imaging.[308] In one investigation of 26 patients with Takayasu's arteritis, the presence of enhancement of thickened aortic wall on MR imaging correlated with clinical and laboratory findings of disease activity.[308]

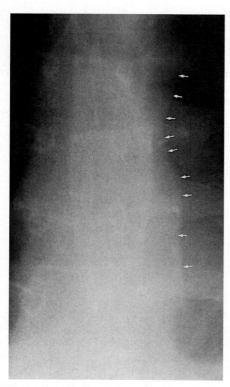

Figure 8–23. Takayasu's Arteritis. Close-up view of the mediastinum from posteroanterior chest radiograph in a 21-year-old woman shows a wavy contour of the descending thoracic aorta *(arrows)*. The diagnosis was confirmed at aortography.

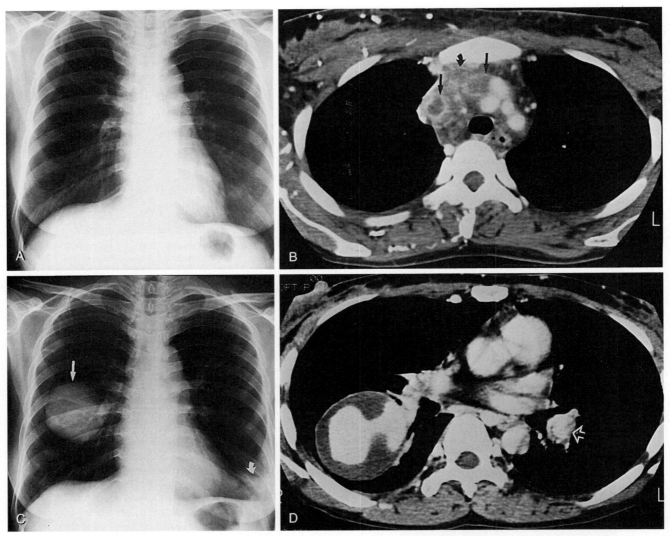

Figure 8–25. Behçet's Disease. Posteroanterior chest radiograph *(A)* in a 37-year-old woman with Behçet's disease shows widening of the right upper mediastinum. Contrast-enhanced CT scan *(B)* shows thrombosis of the right and left brachiocephalic veins *(straight arrows)* and increased attenuation of the mediastinal fat *(curved arrow)*, a finding that is suggestive of edema. Collateral veins are visible in the mediastinum and chest wall. Posteroanterior chest radiograph obtained 6 months later *(C)* shows a round, well-defined mass in the right lower lobe *(straight arrow)* and localized consolidation in the left lower lobe *(curved arrow)*. The upper mediastinum appears normal. Contrast-enhanced CT scan *(D)* obtained at the same time as the posteroanterior chest radiograph *(C)* shows a large aneurysm of the right pulmonary artery with enhancement of the patent lumen and a circumferential thrombus. Note dilated left descending pulmonary artery *(arrowhead)*. (A to D from Ahn JM, Im JG, Ryoo JW, et al: Radiology 194:199, 1995. Case courtesy of Dr. Jung-Gi Im, Department of Radiology, Seoul National University Hospital, Seoul, Korea.)

Several investigators have assessed the incidence and patterns of pulmonary artery involvement after conventional or digital pulmonary angiography.[212, 214, 222] As mentioned previously, the incidence of pulmonary involvement in the various series ranged from 15% to 86% of patients. The high incidence in some of the studies probably reflects a selection bias because pulmonary angiography was not performed routinely.[214] Based on findings on CT[218] and MR imaging,[220] we believe that pulmonary artery involvement probably occurs in about 50% to 70% of cases. The frequency of such involvement shows a positive correlation with the degree of brachiocephalic vessel disease but not with extent or severity of aortic disease.[220] Rarely, pulmonary artery disease is the initial manifestation of Takayasu's arteritis.[223] The most common abnormalities consist of stenosis or occlusion of segmental or subsegmental branches, usually of an upper lobe; less often, abnormalities involve the middle lobe, lingula, or lower lobe segmental or subsegmental vessels. The abnormalities tend to progress over time.[220] Scintigraphy may show decreased perfusion distal to narrowed or occluded pulmonary arteries.[214]

Behçet's Disease

Behçet's disease is an uncommon disorder characterized by exacerbations and remissions of uveitis and oral and genital ulcers. Other findings include skin lesions (particularly erythema nodosum); arthritis; thrombophlebitis; neurologic syndromes; and, less frequently, colitis, epididymitis, orchitis, and systemic arterial thrombosis and aneurysms.[227] Men are affected more often than women; the age of onset is usually between 20 and 30 years. The incidence is highest in the Middle East and Japan.[225]

Pulmonary involvement is infrequent. In one retrospective autopsy review of 170 patients, pulmonary thrombosis was identified only once.[225] In another review of 72 patients, 7 were found to have evidence of pulmonary vascular involvement.[226] Such pulmonary disease usually is manifested several years after the onset of systemic disease.[237] Clinical findings include dyspnea, cough, chest pain, and hemoptysis.[226] Hemoptysis is the most common and serious, sometimes being massive and leading to death.[237, 238]

Radiologic Manifestations

Pulmonary arterial disease usually is related to thrombosis or aneurysm formation. Aneurysms are manifested radiographically by round perihilar opacities or the rapid development of unilateral hilar enlargement.[229, 230] The aneurysms may be single or multiple, unilateral or bilateral, and usually measure 1 to 3 cm in diameter.[229, 230] Although they may have sharply defined margins, the latter more commonly are defined poorly as a result of surrounding hemorrhage.[229] The presence, size, and location of the aneurysms can be assessed with CT, MR imaging, or angiography (Fig. 8–25);[229, 230, 232] CT and MR imaging may show thrombosed aneurysms, which are not seen at angiography.[229, 233] When considering pulmonary angiography in patients who have Behçet's disease, insertion of a venous catheter may lead to venous thrombosis or to propagation of an existing thrombus,[228, 229] complications that may result in significant deterioration in the patient's state.[226, 237]

Thrombotic occlusion of the pulmonary vasculature most commonly involves the right interlobar artery followed in decreasing order by lobar and segmental arteries.[233] Such occlusion may result in localized areas of consolidation as a result of infarction (rarely associated with cavitation),[231] areas of oligemia,[231] and areas of atelectasis.[229] Lung scintigraphy shows ventilation-perfusion mismatch or a combination of matched and mismatched perfusion defects.[234, 306] Pulmonary hemorrhage as a result of vasculitis or pulmonary artery rupture can result in focal, multifocal, or diffuse air-space consolidation.[229, 237]

Thrombosis of the superior vena cava may be manifested by mediastinal widening on the chest radiograph (*see* Fig. 8–25).[230] CT scans in five patients who had such widening showed it to be secondary to thrombosis or narrowing of the superior vena cava leading to collateral circulation and mediastinal edema.[230] Occasionally, mediastinal widening may result from aortic aneurysm formation.[229]

Unilateral or bilateral pleural effusions may occur, usually as a result of pulmonary infarction.[224, 231] Rarely the effusion represents hemothorax secondary to rupture of a pulmonary artery,[235] chylothorax secondary to thrombosis of the superior vena cava and brachiocephalic vein,[236] or vasculitis of the pleura itself.[229] A case of hydropneumothorax secondary to rupture of a cavitated infarct into the pleural space has been described.[231]

Necrotizing Sarcoid Granulomatosis

Necrotizing sarcoid granulomatosis is a rare disorder that usually is recognized only after histologic examination of excised lung tissue. It first was defined pathologically as a mass of confluent granulomas associated with a variable amount of necrosis and prominent, focally destructive vasculitis.[239] About 100 cases had been reported by 1996.[240] Most patients are middle-aged adults: The average age of onset reported in three studies was 49 years.[241–243] The condition has a distinct female predominance.[241, 244] Patients may be asymptomatic or present with cough, fever, sweats, malaise, dyspnea, hemoptysis, or pleuritic pain.[244]

The fundamental nature of the condition is uncertain. Because non-necrotizing vasculitis is common in otherwise classic sarcoidosis[245] and because occasional cases of necrotizing sarcoid granulomatosis have been associated with granulomatous inflammation in hilar lymph nodes and other extrapulmonary sites,[241, 246] it has been suggested that the condition might be a variant of sarcoidosis, possibly representing the histologic counterpart of the nodular form of the disease observed radiologically.[247]

The radiologic pattern in most patients is that of multiple well-defined nodules (Fig. 8–26).[242, 248] Most commonly, the nodules are 5 to 10 mm in diameter; however, a miliary

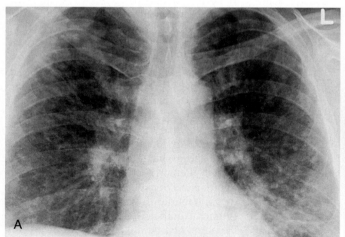
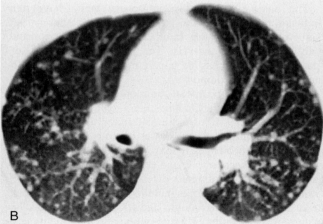

Figure 8–26. Necrotizing Sarcoid Granulomatosis. View of the chest from posteroanterior radiograph *(A)* in a 41-year-old man shows numerous bilateral small nodular opacities. Conventional CT scan *(B)* shows that most of the nodules are associated closely with pulmonary vessels. Subpleural nodules are evident. The diagnosis of necrotizing sarcoid granulomatosis was proved by open-lung biopsy.

pattern and nodules 4 cm in diameter may be seen.[242, 248] On HRCT scan, the nodules have a predominantly peribronchoarterial and subpleural distribution, similar to that of sarcoidosis.[249] The nodules may increase in size and number over time or, occasionally, resolve;[242] cavitation occurs rarely.[241]

Other radiologic manifestations include a solitary nodule or mass,[242, 249] bilateral areas of consolidation, and, less commonly, a bilateral interstitial reticular pattern.[242, 249] On HRCT scan, the areas of consolidation may have a predominantly peribronchoarterial or subpleural distribution.[249, 250] Hilar lymph node enlargement was not a feature in the original report of 11 cases[239] but was noted in 1 of 13 patients in one series[241] and in 6 of 12 patients in another.[242] Pleural effusion may occur[241] but is uncommon.

Goodpasture's Syndrome and Idiopathic Pulmonary Hemorrhage

Goodpasture's syndrome and idiopathic pulmonary hemorrhage are characterized by repeated episodes of pulmonary hemorrhage, iron-deficiency anemia, and acute or chronic pulmonary insufficiency. Goodpasture's syndrome includes renal disease in addition to the pulmonary manifestations. It is distinguished from other pulmonary-renal syndromes associated with diffuse alveolar hemorrhage and glomerulonephritis by the presence of an anti–basement membrane antibody in the circulation.

Idiopathic pulmonary hemorrhage occurs most commonly in children, usually younger than 10 years old (although cases developing during adulthood or extending from childhood to adulthood are well described).[253, 254] In the younger age group, the disease shows no sex predominance;[251] in adults, it occurs twice as often in men as in women. By contrast, Goodpasture's syndrome is primarily a disease of young adults older than age 16,[255, 256] although elderly people also can be affected.[255, 257] It occurs twice as commonly in men as in women.[257]

Clinical Manifestations

The onset of idiopathic pulmonary hemorrhage may be insidious, with anemia, pallor, weakness, lethargy, and (sometimes) a dry cough. In other cases, the onset is acute, with fever and hemoptysis. The typical changes of air-space hemorrhage may be apparent radiographically without a history of hemoptysis.[271a]

Hemoptysis is the most common presenting symptom of patients who have Goodpasture's syndrome, occurring in about 80% to 95% of those affected.[257] Although it may be life-threatening, it is seldom as copious as in idiopathic pulmonary hemorrhage. It may occur early or late in the course of the disease[251, 269] and typically precedes the clinical manifestations of renal disease by several months.[257] Other presenting symptoms include dyspnea, fatigue, weakness, lassitude, pallor, cough, and (occasionally) frank hematuria.[256] Circulating or tissue-bound anti–basement membrane antibodies can be identified by enzyme-linked immunosorbent assay or immunofluorescent examination.[272]

Radiologic Manifestations

The radiologic manifestations of Goodpasture's syndrome and idiopathic pulmonary hemorrhage are identical and depend in large measure on the number of hemorrhagic episodes that have occurred. In the early stages of the disease, the radiographic pattern is one of patchy areas of air-space consolidation scattered fairly evenly throughout the lungs (Fig. 8–27). An air bronchogram usually is identifiable in areas of major consolidation. At this stage, the appearance simulates pulmonary edema. Opacities usually are widespread but may be more prominent in the perihilar areas and in the mid and lower lung zones. The apices and costophrenic angles almost invariably are spared;[258] should they show evidence of consolidation, superimposed pneumonia is likely.[259] Although parenchymal involvement usually is bilateral, it is commonly asymmetric and occasionally may be unilateral.[259] Less common radiographic findings include ground-glass opacities and migratory areas of consolidation.[260, 261] The chest radiograph may be normal; in one review of 25 patients who had Goodpasture's syndrome, normal findings were documented in 7 of 39 (18%) episodes.[259]

The CT manifestations of acute pulmonary hemorrhage consist of areas of ground-glass attenuation or consolidation; these may be patchy or diffuse[261, 262] but tend to involve mainly the dependent lung regions.[263] CT may show parenchymal abnormalities in patients who have normal or questionable radiographic findings.[261]

Serial radiographs obtained over the several days after an acute episode of pulmonary hemorrhage usually reveal a highly predictable progressive change in pattern (*see* Fig. 8–27): The fluffy deposits characteristic of air-space consolidation disappear within 2 to 3 days and are replaced by a reticulonodular pattern whose distribution is identical to that of the air-space disease.[267] In one study of six patients, HRCT performed during this resolving phase showed poorly defined 1- to 3-mm-diameter centrilobular nodules in all patients, patchy areas of ground-glass attenuation in four, and interlobular septal thickening in four.[262] This reticular pattern diminishes gradually during the next several days, and the appearance of the chest radiograph usually returns to normal about 10 to 12 days after the original episode.[261]

With repeated episodes of hemorrhage, increasing amounts of hemosiderin are deposited within the interstitial tissue and are associated with progressive fibrosis. In most cases, chest radiograph shows only partial clearing after each hemorrhagic episode, revealing persistence of a fine reticulonodular pattern indicative of the irreversible interstitial disease.[268, 269] HRCT at this stage shows 1- to 3-mm-diameter centrilobular nodules throughout the lung parenchyma (Fig. 8–28);[264, 265] interlobular septal thickening also may be seen.[266] Once these changes have developed, new episodes of pulmonary hemorrhage usually result in the typical pattern of air-space consolidation being superimposed on the diffuse interstitial disease.[251, 270] Rarely, acute episodes occur without significant variation in the radiologic pattern.[252] Uncommonly, pulmonary hypertension and chronic cor pulmonale develop as a result of diffuse pulmonary fibrosis.[251]

Pleural effusion is rare, and its presence usually indi-

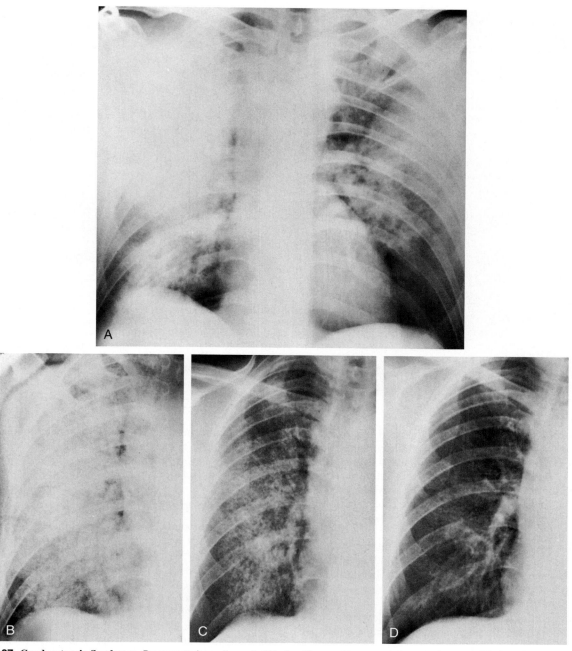

Figure 8–27. Goodpasture's Syndrome. Posteroanterior radiograph *(A)* of a 49-year-old man reveals extensive consolidation of both lungs. A well-defined air bronchogram is visualized. Three days later *(B)*, the pattern was somewhat more granular, and 10 days after the initial episode *(C)*, the pattern has become distinctly reticular. Six days later *(D)*, only a fine reticular pattern remains in an anatomic distribution identical to the original involvement. The sequence of changes illustrated by this patient with Goodpasture's syndrome is typical of massive pulmonary hemorrhage.

cates cardiac decompensation or superimposed pneumonia.[258] Hilar and, rarely, paratracheal lymph node enlargement has been described in idiopathic pulmonary hemorrhage.[268, 271]

EOSINOPHILIC LUNG DISEASE

The term *eosinophilic lung disease* encompasses a group of diverse disorders characterized pathologically by the accumulation of abundant eosinophils in alveolar air spaces and interstitial tissue. Peripheral blood eosinophilia is fre-

quently prominent. The disorders can be classified into groups with and without defined causes (Table 8–9); disorders of unknown origin are defined and distinguished from one another largely by their clinical features.

Idiopathic Eosinophilic Lung Disease

Simple Pulmonary Eosinophilia

Simple pulmonary eosinophilia (Loeffler's syndrome) is characterized by transient, nonsegmental areas of parenchy-

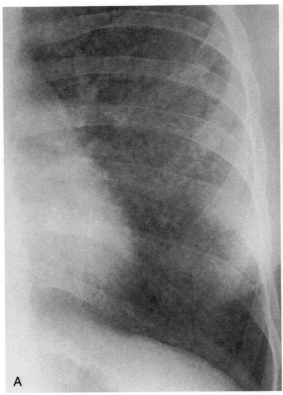

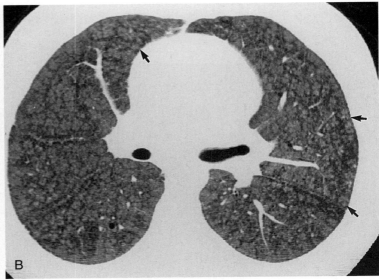

Figure 8–28. Idiopathic Pulmonary Hemorrhage. View of the left lung from posteroanterior chest radiograph in a 22-year-old woman *(A)* reveals numerous poorly defined, small nodular opacities. HRCT scan *(B)* shows the centrilobular distribution of the poorly defined nodular opacities *(arrows)*. The patient had a history of recurrent pulmonary hemorrhage since the age of 4 years. The nodular opacities had remained unchanged over the previous 3 years.

mal consolidation on chest radiographs and blood eosinophilia. Some authors would include in this syndrome conditions that occur in association with many causative agents, particularly parasites;[274] however, it seems more reasonable to confine the use of the term to cases in which the cause is unknown (one third of cases[275]), while categorizing cases with known causes as specific forms of eosinophilic lung disease.

Patients typically have few or no symptoms, the diagnosis often being suspected initially by the finding of characteristic opacities on chest radiograph. A background of asthma and atopy is common.[278] A total white cell count of more than 20,000 per mm³ is common; an increase in eosinophils is responsible for most of the elevation.

The radiographic findings characteristically consist of

Table 8–9. EOSINOPHILIC LUNG DISEASE

Classification	Disease or Specific Agent
Idiopathic eosinophilic lung disease	Simple pulmonary eosinophilia (Loeffler's syndrome)
	Acute eosinophilic pneumonia
	Chronic eosinophilic pneumonia
	Hypereosinophilic syndrome
Eosinophilic lung disease of specific cause	
Drugs	Nonsteroidal anti-inflammatory agents, penicillin, sulfonamides
Parasites	Ascariasis, strongyloidiasis, tropical eosinophilia
Fungi	Allergic bronchopulmonary aspergillosis
Connective tissue disease and vasculitides	Churg-Strauss syndrome, rheumatoid disease

transitory and migratory areas of parenchymal consolidation. These are nonsegmental, may be single or multiple, and usually have ill-defined margins (Fig. 8–29).[273, 276] The areas of consolidation often are peripheral.[273]

Acute Eosinophilic Pneumonia

Acute eosinophilic pneumonia is an acute febrile illness associated with hypoxemic respiratory failure.[279, 280] Patients typically present with breathlessness, myalgia, and pleuritic chest pain. Peripheral eosinophilia usually is absent, although a marked elevation of bronchoalveolar lavage eosinophils is characteristic and is helpful in establishing diagnosis.[279, 280]

Radiographically and on CT scan, the findings are similar to those of pulmonary edema. The earliest radiographic manifestation consists of reticular opacities, frequently with Kerley B lines.[273] These opacities progress rapidly over a few hours or days to bilateral interstitial and air-space opacities involving mainly the lower lung zones (Fig. 8–30).[273, 281] Small bilateral pleural effusions are seen at some point in the course of the disease in most patients.[282] CT scans show bilateral areas of ground-glass attenuation, smooth interlobular septal thickening, small pleural effusions, and, occasionally, localized areas of consolidation or small nodules (*see* Fig. 8–30).[282, 283] In contrast to chronic eosinophilic pneumonia, a peripheral distribution is seldom seen.[273, 281]

Chronic Eosinophilic Pneumonia

The chronicity, severity of symptoms, and (at times) radiologic appearance distinguish chronic eosinophilic

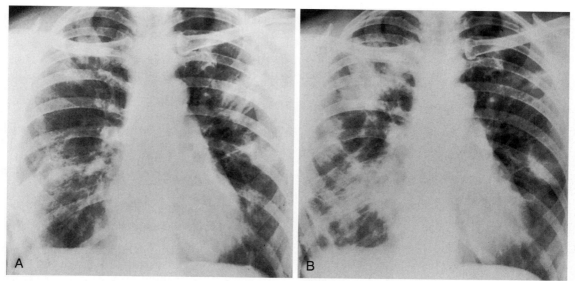

Figure 8–29. Simple Pulmonary Eosinophilia. Posteroanterior chest radiograph *(A)* in a 61-year-old woman shows bilateral areas of consolidation occupying no precise segmental distribution; in particular, there is a broad shadow of increased density along the lower axillary zone of the right lung. At this time, her total white cell count was 11,000 per ml with 1,700 (15%) eosinophils. One week later *(B)*, the anatomic distribution of the areas of consolidation had changed considerably, being more extensive in the right upper and both lower lobes and less extensive in the left upper lobe; at this time, the total white cell count was 14,000 per ml with 20% eosinophils. A diagnosis of simple pulmonary eosinophilia was made; treatment resulted in prompt remission of symptoms and complete resolution of the radiographic abnormalities.

pneumonia from simple pulmonary eosinophilia. Atopy is present in about 50% of patients, asthma being the most common manifestation;[277] most patients are otherwise well before the onset of symptoms. Disease usually is manifested by high fever, malaise, weight loss, cough, and dyspnea;[277] hemoptysis, chest pain, and myalgia occur rarely.[273] The onset of symptoms may be insidious; patients are ill for an average of 7.7 months before diagnosis.[284]

The radiographic pattern consists of bilateral, nonsegmental homogeneous consolidation in the lung periphery

(Fig. 8–31).[284] This pattern has led some observers to apply the designation *reversed pulmonary edema pattern* because of its confinement to the lung periphery in contrast to the perihilar or central distribution of pulmonary edema.[285] Compared with the transitory and migratory character of the areas of consolidation in simple eosinophilic pneumonia, the lesions of chronic eosinophilic pneumonia tend to persist unchanged for many days or weeks unless corticosteroid therapy is instituted.

Although the reversed pulmonary edema pattern of con-

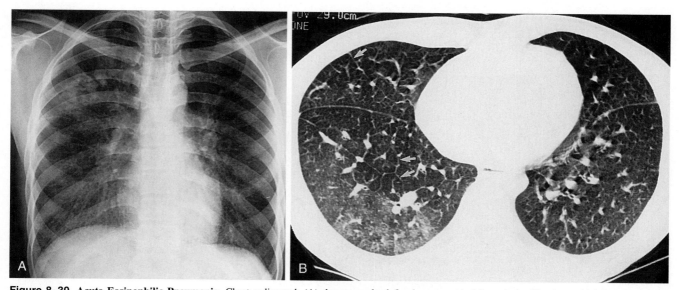

Figure 8–30. Acute Eosinophilic Pneumonia. Chest radiograph *(A)* shows poorly defined asymmetric bilateral opacification, which is most marked in the right upper lobe. HRCT scan performed 2 days later *(B)* shows asymmetric bilateral areas of ground-glass attenuation. Mild interlobular septal thickening *(arrows)* is evident in the right lung. Transbronchial biopsy showed numerous eosinophils and mononuclear cells in the alveolar spaces and alveolar walls. The patient was a 25-year-old man. (From Cheon JE, et al: Am J Roentgenol 167:1195, 1996. Courtesy of Dr. Kyung Soo Lee, Samsung Medical Center, Seoul, South Korea.)

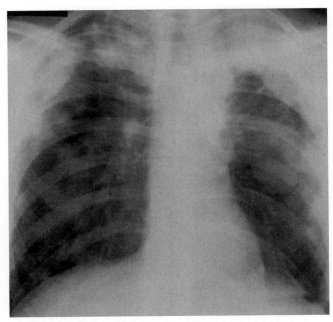

Figure 8–31. Chronic Eosinophilic Pneumonia. Posteroanterior chest radiograph reveals bilateral air-space consolidation, predominantly upper lobe in distribution; the peripheral (cortical) distribution is highly characteristic of the disease. The patient was a middle-aged woman who presented with wheezing, cough, nocturnal fever, and blood eosinophilia.

findings included evidence of cavitation in 5 of 119 cases, pleural effusion in 2, a nodular pattern in 3, and atelectasis in 2.

In contrast to radiographs, the peripheral distribution of the consolidation can be identified in virtually all cases on CT scans (Fig. 8–32).[286] In one study of 17 patients, a peripheral distribution of consolidation was evident on radiograph in 11 patients and on CT scan in 16.[287] Ground-glass attenuation may be seen, usually in association with areas of consolidation but occasionally as an isolated finding.[287] Mediastinal lymph node enlargement has been reported in a few cases on CT scans[286, 288] and rarely on radiographs.[288]

Hypereosinophilic Syndrome

Hypereosinophilic syndrome consists of prolonged blood eosinophilia associated with tissue infiltration by eosinophils and multiorgan disease. An underlying cause may or may not be evident. Three criteria have been established for the diagnosis of idiopathic disease:[289] (1) persistent eosinophilia of 1,500 per mm^3 for at least 6 months or death before 6 months in individuals who have appropriate signs and symptoms; (2) lack of evidence for parasitic, allergic, or other recognized cause of eosinophilia; and (3) signs and symptoms of organ involvement unexplained by other pathology.

Symptoms are nonspecific, and the diagnosis often is considered only when leukocytosis and eosinophilia are detected. The major cause of morbidity and mortality is cardiac disease; the supportive structures of the atrioventricular valves are particularly prone to fibrosis, resulting in mitral and occasionally tricuspid insufficiency.[319]

Initially, chest radiographs may reveal transient hazy opacities or areas of consolidation (Fig. 8–33) that can

solidation is characteristic of chronic eosinophilic pneumonia, particularly if it involves mainly the upper lobes, it is not a universal finding. In one review of the radiographic manifestations of 119 patients described in the literature by 1988, consolidation was found to involve mainly the outer two thirds of the lungs in 74 (62%) patients and was limited to the lung periphery in 30 (25%) patients.[284] Uncommon

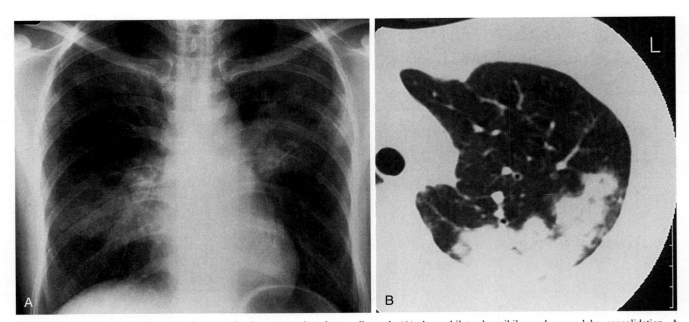

Figure 8–32. Chronic Eosinophilic Pneumonia. Posteroanterior chest radiograph *(A)* shows bilateral perihilar and upper lobe consolidation. A peripheral predominance is not readily apparent on the radiograph. Conventional 10-mm collimation CT scan targeted to the left upper lobe *(B)* shows the peripheral distribution of the consolidation. The patient was a 42-year-old woman. (Case courtesy of Dr. Hiroshi Niimi, Department of Radiology, St. Marianna University School of Medicine, Yokohama, Japan.)

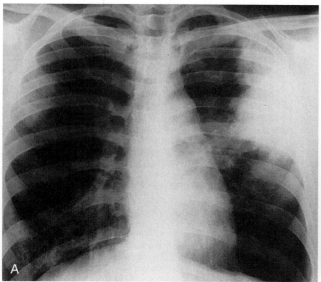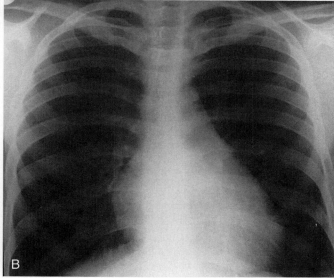

Figure 8–33. Hypereosinophilic Syndrome. Posteroanterior chest radiograph *(A)* shows asymmetric bilateral areas of consolidation involving predominantly the peripheral regions of the upper lobes. The patient was a 20-year-old man who recently had developed asthma and had marked eosinophilia. The parenchymal abnormalities resolved after treatment with corticosteroids. The patient subsequently developed myocarditis, however. A follow-up chest radiograph *(B)* shows mild enlargement of the cardiac silhouette. The lungs are clear. (Case courtesy of Dr. Christopher Flower, Addenbrooke's Hospital, Cambridge, England.)

resolve spontaneously. Sometimes, these are associated with bronchospasm. An interstitial pattern also has been described, presumably caused by perivascular eosinophilic infiltration or fibrosis.[289, 290] The HRCT manifestations include focal areas of ground-glass attenuation or a few nodules surrounded by a halo of ground-glass attenuation.[294] Cardiac decompensation eventually is manifested by cardiomegaly, pulmonary edema, and pleural effusion.[291] Occasionally, pleural effusions are seen in patients who do not have heart failure, possibly as a result of pulmonary emboli.[292] Spontaneous pneumothorax has been reported.[293]

Eosinophilic Lung Disease of Specific Etiology

Drugs

Drugs are an important cause of eosinophilic lung disease.[273] It is important to consider the reaction in any patient who presents with air-space consolidation or interstitial changes and blood or bronchoalveolar lavage eosinophilia and has a history of drug exposure by any route. Reactions range from those similar to simple pulmonary eosinophilia to those imitating acute eosinophilic pneumonia. Implicated drugs include antibiotics,[295–297] nonsteroidal anti-inflammatory agents,[298, 299] drugs used for inflammatory bowel disease,[300, 301] and inhaled illicit drugs such as cocaine[302, 303] and heroin.[304]

Parasitic Infestation

Parasites are common causes of eosinophilic lung infiltration and peripheral blood eosinophilia in developing countries. With increasing immigration to developed countries from these areas and with increasing foreign travel, however, physicians should be familiar with the manifestations of these infections. All infestations are caused by

metazoans, most from roundworms such as *Ascaris lumbricoides*, *Strongyloides stercoralis*, and *Wuchereria bancrofti*.

Fungal Infection

The major fungal disease associated with pulmonary eosinophilia is allergic bronchopulmonary aspergillosis (*see* Chapter 5); uncommonly a variety of other mycotic organisms cause a similar hypersensitivity reaction.

References

1. Wiedemann HP, Matthay RA: Pulmonary manifestations of the collagen vascular diseases. Clin Chest Med 10:677, 1989.
2. Panush RS, Greer JM, Morshedian KK: What is lupus? What is not lupus? Rheum Dis Clin North Am 19:223, 1993.
3. Quismorio FP: Clinical and pathologic features of lung involvement in systemic lupus erythematosus. Semin Respir Med 9:297, 1988.
4. Cervera R, Khamashta MA, Font J, et al: Systemic lupus erythematosus: Clinical and immunologic patterns of disease expression in a cohort of 1,000 patients. Medicine (Baltimore) 72:113, 1993.
5. Hopkinson ND, Doherty M, Powell RJ: Clinical features and race-specific incidence/prevalence rates of systemic lupus erythematosus in a geographically complete cohort of patients. Ann Rheum Dis 53:675, 1994.
6. Matthay RA, Schwartz MI, Petty TL, et al: Pulmonary manifestations of systemic lupus erythematosus: Review of twelve cases of acute lupus pneumonitis. Medicine (Baltimore) 54:397, 1975.
7. Hoffbrand BI, Beck ER: "Unexplained" dyspnoea and shrinking lungs in systemic lupus erythematosus. BMJ 1:1273, 1965.
8. Myers JL, Katzenstein AA: Microangiitis in lupus-induced pulmonary hemorrhage. Am J Clin Pathol 85:552, 1986.
9. Bulgrin JG, Dubois EL, Jacobson G: Chest roentgenographic changes in systemic lupus erythematosus. Radiology 74:42, 1960.
10. Primack SL, Müller NL: Radiologic manifestations of the systemic autoimmune diseases. Clin Chest Med 19:573, 1998.
11. Murin S, Wiedemann HP, Matthay RA: Pulmonary manifestations of systemic lupus erythematosus. Clin Chest Med 19:641, 1998.
12. Orens JB, Martinez FJ, Lynch JP III: Pleuropulmonary manifestations of systemic lupus erythematosus. Rheum Dis Clin North Am 20:159, 1994.

13. Wiedemann HP, Matthay RA: Pulmonary manifestations of systemic lupus erythematosus. J Thorac Imaging 7:1, 1992.

14. Gamsu G: Radiographic manifestations of thoracic involvement by collagen vascular diseases. J Thorac Imaging 7:1, 1992.

15. Gammon RB, Bridges TA, Al-Nezir H, et al: Bronchiolitis obliterans organizing pneumonia associated with systemic lupus erythematosus. Chest 102:1171, 1992.

16. Onomura K, Nakata H, Tanaka Y, et al: Pulmonary hemorrhage in patients with systemic lupus erythematosus. J Thorac Imaging 6:57, 1991.

17. Hsu BY, Edwards DK, Drambert MA: Pulmonary hemorrhage complicating systemic lupus erythematosus: Role of MR imaging in diagnosis. Am J Roentgenol 158:519, 1992.

18. Huang CT, Hennigar GR, Lyons HA: Pulmonary dysfunction in systemic lupus erythematosus. N Engl J Med 272:288, 1965.

19. Gross M, Esterly JR, Earle RH: Pulmonary alterations in systemic lupus erythematosus. Am Rev Respir Dis 105:572, 1972.

20. Eisenberg H, Dubois EL, Sherwin RP, et al: Diffuse interstitial lung disease in systemic lupus erythematosus. Ann Intern Med 79:37, 1973.

21. Webb WR, Gamsu G: Cavitary pulmonary nodules with systemic lupus erythematosus: Differential diagnosis. Am J Roentgenol 136:27, 1981.

22. Divertie MB: Lung involvement in the connective-tissue disorders. Med Clin North Am 48:1015, 1964.

23. Thompson PJ, Dhillon DP, Ledingham J, et al: Shrinking lungs, diaphragmatic dysfunction, and systemic lupus erythematosus. Am Rev Respir Dis 132:926, 1985.

24. Bankier AA, Kiener HP, Wiesmayr MN, et al: Discrete lung involvement in systemic lupus erythematosus: CT assessment. Radiology 196:835, 1995.

25. Fenlon HM, Doran M, Sant SM, et al: High-resolution chest CT in systemic lupus erythematosus. Am J Roentgenol 166:301, 1996.

26. Ooi GC, Ngan H, Peh WCG, et al: Systemic lupus erythematosus patients with respiratory symptoms: The value of HRCT. Clin Radiol 52:775, 1997.

27. Auerback RC, Snyder NE, Bragg DG: The chest roentgenographic manifestations of pronestyl-induced lupus erythematosus. Radiology 109:287, 1973.

28. Abud-Mendoza C, Diaz-Jouanen E, Alarcon-Sergovia D: Fatal pulmonary hemorrhage in systemic lupus erythematosus: Occurrence without hemoptysis. J Rheumatol 12:558, 1985.

29. Zamora MR, Warner ML, Tuder R, et al: Diffuse alveolar hemorrhage and systemic lupus erythematosus: Clinical presentation, histology, survival, and outcome. Medicine (Baltimore) 76:192, 1997.

30. Wilcox PG, Stein HB, Clarke SD, et al: Phrenic nerve function in patients with diaphragmatic weakness and systemic lupus erythematosus. Chest 93:352, 1988.

31. Gordon DA, Stein JL, Broder I: The extra-articular features of rheumatoid arthritis: A systemic analysis of 127 cases. Am J Med 54:445, 1973.

32. Kohler PF, Vaughan J: The autoimmune diseases. JAMA 248:2646, 1982.

33. Baydur A, Mongan ES: Thoracic manifestations in rheumatoid arthritis. Semin Respir Med 9:305, 1988.

34. Anaya JM, Diethelm L, Oritz LA, et al: Pulmonary involvement in rheumatoid arthritis. Semin Arthritis Rheum 24:242, 1995.

35. Walker WC, Wright V: Pulmonary lesions and rheumatoid arthritis. Medicine (Baltimore) 47:501, 1968.

36. Remy-Jardin M, Remy J, Cortet B, et al: Lung changes in rheumatoid arthritis: CT findings. Radiology 193:375, 1994.

37. Walker WC, Wright V: Rheumatoid pleuritis. Ann Rheum Dis 26:467, 1967.

38. Frank ST, Weg JG, Harkleroad LE, et al: Pulmonary dysfunction in rheumatoid disease. Chest 63:27, 1973.

39. Jurik AG, Davidsen D, Graudal H: Prevalence of pulmonary involvement in rheumatoid arthritis and its relationship to some characteristics of the patients—a radiological and clinical study. Scand J Rheumatol 11:217, 1982.

40. Staples CA, Müller NL, Vedal S, et al: Usual interstitial pneumonia: Correlation of CT with clinical, functional, and radiologic findings. Radiology 162:377, 1987.

41. Akira M, Sakatani M, Hara H: Thin-section CT findings in rheumatoid arthritis-associated lung disease: CT patterns and their courses. J Comput Assist Tomogr 23:941, 1999.

42. Fujii M, Adachi S, Shimizu T, et al: Interstitial lung disease in rheumatoid arthritis: Assessment with high-resolution computed tomography. J Thorac Imaging 8:54, 1993.

43. Brannan HM, Good CA, Divertie MB, et al: Pulmonary disease associated with rheumatoid arthritis. JAMA 189:914, 1964.

44. Strohl KP, Feldman NT, Ingram RH Jr: Apical fibrobullous disease with rheumatoid arthritis. Chest 75:739, 1979.

45. McCann BG, Hart GJ, Stokes TC, et al: Obliterative bronchiolitis and upper-zone pulmonary consolidation in rheumatoid arthritis. Thorax 38:73, 1983.

46. Burrows FGO: Pulmonary nodules in rheumatoid disease: A report of two cases. Br J Radiol 40:256, 1967.

47. Sienewicz DJ, Martin JR, Moore S, et al: Rheumatoid nodules in the lung. J Can Assoc Radiol 13:73, 1962.

48. Hayakawa H, Sato A, Imokawa S, et al: Bronchiolar disease in rheumatoid arthritis. Am J Respir Crit Care Med 154:1531, 1996.

49. Perez T, Remy-Jardin M, Cortet B: Airways involvement in rheumatoid arthritis: Clinical, functional, and HRCT findings. Am J Respir Crit Care Med 157:1658, 1998.

50. Shannon TM, Gale ME: Noncardiac manifestations of rheumatoid arthritis in the thorax. J Thorac Imaging 7:19, 1992.

51. Portner MM, Gracie WA Jr: Rheumatoid lung disease with cavitary nodules, pneumothorax, and eosinophilia. N Engl J Med 275:697, 1966.

52. Morgan WKC, Wolfel DA: The lungs and pleura in rheumatoid arthritis. Am J Roentgenol 98:334, 1966.

53. Stengel BF, Watson RA, Darling RJ: Pulmonary rheumatoid nodule with cavitation and chronic lipid effusion. JAMA 198:1263, 1966.

54. Caplan A: Certain unusual radiological appearances in the chest of coal miners suffering from rheumatoid arthritis. Thorax 8:29, 1953.

55. Constantinidis K: Pneumoconiosis and rheumatoid arthritis: Caplan's syndrome. Br J Clin Pract 31:25, 1977.

56. Chatgidakis CB, Theron CP: Rheumatoid pneumoconiosis (Caplan's syndrome): A discussion of the disease and a report of a case in a European Witwatersrand gold miner. Arch Environ Health 2:397, 1961.

57. Ramirez R-J, Lopez-Majano V, Schultz G: Caplan's syndrome: A clinicopathologic study. Am J Med 37:643, 1964.

58. Mays EE: Rheumatoid pleuritis: Observations in eight cases and suggestions for making the diagnosis in patients without the "typical findings." Dis Chest 53:202, 1968.

59. Campbell GD, Ferrington E: Rheumatoid pleuritis with effusion. Dis Chest 53:521, 1968.

60. Martel W, Abell MR, Mikkelsne WM, et al: Pulmonary and pleural lesions in rheumatoid disease. Radiology 90:641, 1968.

61. Tanoue LT: Pulmonary manifestations of rheumatoid arthritis. Clin Chest Med 19:667, 1998.

62. Brennan SR, Daly JJ: Large pleural effusions in rheumatoid arthritis. Br J Dis Chest 73:133, 1979.

63. Pritkin JD, Jensen WA, Yenokida GG, et al: Respiratory failure due to a massive rheumatoid effusion. J Rheumatol 17:673, 1990.

64. Faurschou P, Francis D, Faarup P: Thoracoscopic, histologic, and clinical findings in nine cases of rheumatoid pleural effusions. Thorax 40:371, 1985.

65. Adelman HM, Dupont EL, Flannery MT, et al: Case report: Recurrent pneumothorax in a patient with rheumatoid arthritis. Am J Med Sci 308:171, 1994.

66. Vergnenegre A, Pugnere N, Antonini MT, et al: Airway obstruction and rheumatoid arthritis. Eur Respir J 10:1072, 1997.

67. Geddes DM, Corrin B, Brewerton DA, et al: Progressive airway obliteration in adults and its association with rheumatoid disease. QJM 46:427, 1977.

68. Begin R, Masse S, Cantin A, et al: Airway disease in a subset of nonsmoking rheumatoid patients: Characterization of the disease and evidence for an autoimmune pathogenesis. Am J Med 72:743, 1982.

69. Lahdensuo A, Mattila J, Vilppula A: Bronchiolitis in rheumatoid arthritis. Chest 85:705, 1984.

70. Murphy KC, Atkins CJ, Offer RC, et al: Obliterative bronchiolitis in two rheumatoid arthritis patients treated with penicillamine. Arthritis Rheum 24:557, 1981.

71. Stein HC, Patternson AC, Offer RC, et al: Adverse effects of D-penicillamine in rheumatoid arthritis. Ann Intern Med 92:24, 1980.

72. Holness L, Tenenbaum J, Cooter NBE, et al: Fatal bronchiolitis obliterans associated with chrysotherapy. Ann Rheum Dis 42:593, 1983.

73. Aquino SL, Webb RW, Golden J: Bronchiolitis obliterans associated with rheumatoid arthritis: Findings on HRCT and dynamic expiratory CT. J Comput Assist Tomogr 18:555, 1994.

74. Padley SPG, Adler BD, Hansell DM, et al: Bronchiolitis obliterans: High-resolution CT findings and correlation with pulmonary function tests. Clin Radiol 47:236, 1993.

75. Rees JH, Woodhead MA, Sheppard MN, et al: Rheumatoid arthritis and cryptogenic organising pneumonitis. Respir Med 85:243, 1991.

76. van Thiel RJ, van der Burg S, Groote AD, et al: Bronchiolitis obliterans organizing pneumonia and rheumatoid arthritis. Eur Respir J 4:905, 1991.

77. Yousem SA, Colby TV, Carrington CB: Follicular bronchitis/bronchiolitis. Hum Pathol 16:700, 1985.

78. Bamji A, Cooke N: Rheumatoid arthritis and chronic bronchial suppuration. Scand J Rheum 14:15, 1985.

79. Solanki T, Neville E: Bronchiectasis and rheumatoid disease: Is there an association? Br J Rheumatol 31:691, 1992.

80. Despaux J, Polio JC, Toussirot E, et al: Rheumatoid arthritis and bronchiectasis: A retrospective study of 14 cases. Rev Rhum Engl Ed 63:801, 1996.

81. McMahon MJ, Swinson DR, Shettar S, et al: Bronchiectasis and rheumatoid arthritis: A clinical study. Ann Rheum Dis 52:776, 1993.

82. Hassan WU, Keaney NP, Holland CD, et al: High-resolution computed tomography of the lung in lifelong non-smoking patients with rheumatoid arthritis. Ann Rheum Dis 54:308, 1995.

83. McDonagh J, Greaves M, Wright AR, et al: High-resolution computed tomography of the lungs in patients with rheumatoid arthritis and interstitial lung disease. Br J Rheumatol 33:118, 1994.

84. Heath D, Gillund TD, Kay JM, et al: Pulmonary vascular disease in honeycomb lung. J Pathol Bacteriol 95:423, 1968.

85. Kay JM, Banik S: Unexplained pulmonary hypertension with pulmonary arteritis in rheumatoid disease. Br J Dis Chest 71:63, 1977.

86. Maddison PJ, Stephens C, Briggs D, et al: Connective tissue disease and autoantibodies in the kindreds of 63 patients with systemic sclerosis. Medicine (Baltimore) 72:103, 1993.

87. Medsger TA Jr, Masi AT: Epidemiology of systemic sclerosis (scleroderma). Ann Intern Med 74:714, 1971.

88. Minai OA, Dweik RA, Arroliga AC: Manifestations of scleroderma pulmonary disease. Clin Chest Med 19:713, 1998.

89. Bianchi FA, Bistue AR, Wendt VE, et al: Analysis of twenty-seven cases of progressive systemic sclerosis (including two with combined systemic lupus erythematosus) and a review of the literature. J Chron Dis 19:953, 1966.

90. Remy-Jardin M, Remy J, Wallaert B, et al: Pulmonary involvement in progressive systemic sclerosis: Sequential evaluation with CT, pulmonary function tests, and bronchoalveolar lavage. Radiology 188:499, 1993.

91. Taormina VJ, Miller WT, Gefter WB, et al: Progressive systemic sclerosis subgroups: Variable pulmonary features. Am J Roentgenol 137:277, 1981.

92. Schurawitzki H, Stiglbauer R, Graninger W, et al: Interstitial lung disease in progressive systemic sclerosis: High-resolution CT versus radiography. Radiology 176:755, 1990.

93. Arroliga AC, Podell DN, Matthay RA: Pulmonary manifestations of scleroderma. J Thorac Imaging 7:30, 1992.

94. Ungerer RG, Tashkin DP, Furst D, et al: Prevalence and clinical correlates of pulmonary arterial hypertension in progressive systemic sclerosis. Am J Med 75:65, 1983.

95. Harrison NK, Glanville AR, Strickland B, et al: Pulmonary involvement in systemic sclerosis: The detection of early changes in thin section CT scan, bronchoalveolar lavage and TC-DTPA clearance. Respir Med 83:403, 1989.

96. Warrick JH, Bhalla M, Schabel SI, et al: High-resolution computed tomography in early scleroderma lung disease. J Rheumatol 18:1520, 1991.

97. Wells AU, Hansell DM, Corrin B, et al: High-resolution computed tomography as a predictor of lung histology in systemic sclerosis. Thorax 47:508, 1992.

98. Wells AU, Hansell DM, Rubens MB, et al: The predictive value of appearances on thin-section computed tomography in fibrosing alveolitis. Am Rev Respir Dis 148:1076, 1993.

99. Bhalla M, Silver RM, Shepard JAO, et al: Chest CT in patients with scleroderma: Prevalence of asymptomatic esophageal dilatation and mediastinal lymphadenopathy. Am J Roentgenol 161:269, 1993.

100. Wechsler RJ, Steiner RM, Spirn PW, et al: The relationship of thoracic lymphadenopathy to pulmonary interstitial disease in diffuse and limited systemic sclerosis: CT findings. Am J Roentgenol 167:101, 1996.

101. McCarthy DS, Baragar FD, Dhingra S, et al: The lung in systemic sclerosis (scleroderma): A review and new information. Semin Arthritis Rheum 17:271, 1988.

102. Farmer RG, Gifford RW Jr, Hines EA Jr: Prognostic significance of Raynaud's phenomenon and other clinical characteristics of systemic scleroderma: A study of 271 cases. Circulation 21:1088, 1960.

103. Martinez LO: Air in the esophagus as a sign of scleroderma (differential diagnosis with some other entities). J Can Assoc Radiol 25:234, 1974.

104. Dinsmore RE, Goodman D, Dreyfuss JR: The air esophagram: A sign of scleroderma involving the esophagus. Radiology 87:348, 1966.

105. Tanimoto K, Nakano K, Kano S, et al: Classification criteria for polymyositis and dermatomyositis. J Rheumatol 22:668, 1995.

106. Bohan A, Peter JB: Polymyositis and dermatomyositis: I. N Engl J Med 292:344, 1975.

107. Frazier AR, Miller RD: Interstitial pneumonitis in association with polymyositis and dermatomyositis. Chest 65:403, 1974.

108. Schwarz MI: The lung in polymyositis. Clin Chest Med 19:701, 1998.

109. Salmeron G, Greenberg SD, Lidsky MD: Polymyositis and diffuse interstitial lung disease: A review of the pulmonary histopathologic findings. Arch Intern Med 141:1005, 1981.

110. Plotz PH, Rider LG, Targoff IN, et al: Myositis: Immunologic contributions to understanding cause, pathogenesis, and therapy. Ann Intern Med 122:715, 1995.

111. Grau JM, Miro O, Pedrol E, et al: Interstitial lung disease related to dermatomyositis: Comparative study with patients without lung involvement. J Rheumatol 23:1921, 1996.

112. Tazelaar HD, Viggiano RW, Pickersgill J, et al: Interstitial lung disease in polymyositis and dermatomyositis: Clinical features and prognosis as correlated with histologic findings. Am Rev Respir Dis 141:727, 1990.

113. Bohan A, Peter JB, Bowman RL, et al: A computer-assisted analysis of 153 patients with polymyositis and dermatomyositis. Medicine (Baltimore) 56:255, 1977.

114. Schwarz MI, Matthay RA, Sahn SA, et al: Interstitial lung disease in polymyositis and dermatomyositis: Analysis of six cases and review of the literature. Medicine (Baltimore) 55:89, 1976.

115. Schwarz MI: Pulmonary and cardiac manifestations of polymyositis-dermatomyositis. J Thorac Imaging 7:46, 1992.

116. Müller NL, Miller RR: Diseases of the bronchioles: CT and histopathologic findings. Radiology 196:3, 1995.

117. Ikezoe J, Johkoh T, Nohno N, et al: High-resolution CT findings of lung disease in patients with polymyositis and dermatomyositis. J Thorac Imaging 11:250, 1996.

118. Mino M, Noma S, Taguchi Y, et al: Pulmonary involvement in polymyositis and dermatomyositis: Sequential evaluation with CT. Am J Roentgenol 169:83, 1997.

119. Schiavi EA, Roncoroni AJ, Puy RJM: Isolated bilateral diaphragmatic paresis with interstitial lung disease: An unusual presentation of dermatomyositis. Am Rev Respir Dis 129:337, 1984.

120. Cain HC, Noble PW, Matthay RA: Pulmonary manifestations of Sjögren's syndrome. Clin Chest Med 19:687, 1998.

121. Whaley K, Williamson J, Chisholm DK, et al: Sjögren's syndrome: I. Sicca components. QJM 42:279, 1973.

122. Whaley K, Webb J, McEvoy BA, et al: Sjögren's syndrome: II. Clinical associations and immunological phenomena. QJM 42:513, 1973.

123. Silbiger ML, Peterson CC Jr: Sjögren's syndrome: Its roentgenographic features. Am J Roentgenol 100:554, 1967.

124. Strimlan CV, Rosenow EC III, Divertie MB, et al: Pulmonary manifestations of Sjögren's syndrome. Chest 70:354, 1976.

125. Tanoue LT: Pulmonary involvement in collagen vascular disease: A review of the pulmonary manifestations of the Marfan syndrome, ankylosing spondylitis, Sjögren's syndrome, and relapsing polychondritis. J Thorac Imaging 7:62, 1992.

126. Kadota JI, Kusano S, Kawakami K, et al: Usual interstitial pneumonia associated with primary Sjögren's syndrome. Chest 180:1756, 1995.

127. Franquet T, Giménez A, Monill JM, et al: Primary Sjögren's syndrome and associated lung disease: CT findings in 50 patients. Am J Roentgenol 169:655, 1997.

128. Carignan S, Staples CA, Müller NL: Intrathoracic lymphoprolifera-tive disorders in the immunocompromised patient: CT findings. Radiology 197:53, 1995.

129. Meyer CA, Pina JS, Taillon D, et al: Inspiratory and expiratory high-resolution CT findings in a patient with Sjögren's syndrome and cystic lung disease. Am J Roentgenol 168:101, 1997.

130. Desai SR, Nicholson AG, Stewart S, et al: Benign pulmonary lymphocytic infiltration and amyloidosis: Computed tomographic and pathologic features in three cases. J Thorac Imaging 12:215, 1997.

131. Johkoh T, Müller NL, Pickford HA, et al: Lymphocytic interstitial pneumonia: Thin-section CT findings in 22 patients. Radiology 212:567, 1999.

132. Ichikawa Y, Kinoshita M, Koga T, et al: Lung cyst formation in lymphocytic interstitial pneumonia: CT features. J Comput Assist Tomogr 18:745, 1994.

133. Kelly C, Gardiner P, Pal B, et al: Lung function in primary Sjögren's syndrome: A cross sectional and longitudinal study. Thorax 46:180, 1991.

134. Sullivan WD, Hurst DJ, Harman CE, et al: A prospective evaluation emphasizing pulmonary involvement in patients with connective tissue disease. Medicine (Baltimore) 63:92, 1984.

135. Danieli MG, Fraticelli P, Salvi A, et al: Undifferentiated connective tissue disease: Natural history and evolution into definite CTD assessed in 84 patients initially diagnosed as early UCTD. Clin Rheumatol 17:195, 1998.

136. Lazaro MA, Maldonado Cocco JA, Catoggio LJ, et al: Clinical and serologic characteristics of patients with overlap syndrome: Is mixed connective tissue disease a distinct clinical entity? Medicine (Balti-more) 68:58, 1989.

137. Sharp GC, Irvin WS, Tan EM, et al: Mixed connective tissue disease: Apparently distinct rheumatoid disease syndrome associated with a specific antibody to an extractable nuclear antigen (ENA). Am J Med 52:148, 1972.

138. Prakash UBS: Lungs in mixed connective tissue disease. J Thorac Imaging 7:55, 1992.

139. Prakash UBS, Luthra HS, Divertie MB: Intrathoracic manifestations in mixed connective tissue disease. Mayo Clin Proc 60:813, 1985.

140. Germain MJ, Davidman M: Pulmonary hemorrhage and acute renal failure in a patient with mixed connective tissue disease. Am J Kidney Dis 3:420, 1984.

141. McAdam LP, O'Hanlan MA, Bluestone R, et al: Relapsing poly-chondritis: Prospective study of 23 patients and a review of the literature. Medicine (Baltimore) 55:193, 1976.

142. Eng J, Sabanathan S: Airway complications in relapsing polychon-dritis. Ann Thorac Surg 51:686, 1991.

143. Lee-Chiong TL Jr: Pulmonary manifestations of ankylosing spondy-litis and relapsing polychondritis. Clin Chest Med 19:747, 1998.

144. Dolan DL, Lemmon GB Jr, Teitelbaum SL: Relapsing polychon-dritis: Analytical literature review and studies on pathogenesis. Am J Med 41:285, 1966.

145. Crockford MP, Kerr IH: Relapsing polychondritis. Clin Radiol 39:386, 1988.

146. Davis SD, Berkmen YM, King T: Peripheral bronchial involvement in relapsing polychondritis: Demonstration by thin-section CT. Am J Roentgenol 153:953, 1989.

147. Kilman WJ: Narrowing of the airway in relapsing polychondritis. Radiology 126:373, 1978.

148. Choplin RH, Wehunt WD, Theros EG: Diffuse lesions of the trachea. Semin Roentgenol 18:38, 1983.

149. Müller NL, Miller RR, Ostrow DN, et al: Clinico-radiologic-patho-logic conference: Diffuse thickening of the tracheal wall. Can Assoc Radiol J 40:213, 1989.

150. Im JG, Chung JW, Han SK, et al: CT manifestations of tracheobron-chial involvement in relapsing polychondritis. J Comput Assist To-mogr 12:792, 1988.

151. Quint LE, Whyte RI, Kazerooni EA, et al: Stenosis of the central airways: Evaluation by helical CT with multiplanar reconstructions. Radiology 194:871, 1995.

152. Remy-Jardin M, Remy J, Artaud D, et al: Volume rendering of the tracheobronchial tree: Clinical evaluation of bronchographic images. Radiology 208:761, 1998.

152a. Gilkeson RC, Ciancibello LM, Hejal RB, et al: Tracheobronchoma-lacia: Dynamic airway evaluation with multidetector CT. Am J Roentgenol 176:205, 2001.

153. Camus P, Piard F, Ashcroft T, et al: The lung in inflammatory bowel disease. Medicine (Baltimore) 72:151, 1993.

154. Spira A, Grossman R, Balter M: Large airway disease associated with inflammatory bowel disease. Chest 113:1723, 1998.

155. Eaton TE, Lambie N, Wells AU: Bronchiectasis following colectomy for Crohn's disease. Thorax 53:529, 1998.

156. Tam EM, Feltkamp TE, Smolen JS, et al: Range of antinuclear antibodies in "healthy" individuals. Arthritis Rheum 40:1601, 1997.

157. Vasishta S, Wood JB, McGinty F: Ulcerative tracheobronchitis years after colectomy for ulcerative colitis. Chest 106:1279, 1994.

158. Swinburn CR, Jackson GJ, Cobden I, et al: Bronchiolitis obliterans organising pneumonia in a patient with ulcerative colitis. Thorax 43:735, 1988.

159. Matsumoto K, Hirano T, Kondo Y, et al: A case of bronchiolitis obliterans organizing pneumonia associated with ulcerative colitis. Jpn J Thorac Dis 31:245, 1993.

160. Wilcox P, Miller R, Miller G, et al: Airway involvement in ulcerative colitis. Chest 92:18, 1987.

161. Desai SJ, Gephardt GN, Stoller JK: Diffuse panbronchiolitis preced-ing ulcerative colitis. Chest 95:1342, 1989.

162. Garg K, Lynch DA, Newell JD II: Inflammatory airways disease in ulcerative colitis: CT and high-resolution CT features. J Thorac Imaging 8:159, 1993.

163. Jennette JC, Falk RJ, Andrassy K, et al: Nomenclature of systemic vasculitides. Proposal of an International Consensus Conference. Arthritis Rheum 37:1287, 1994.

164. Watts RA, Carruthers DM, Scott DG: Epidemiology of systemic vasculitis: Changing incidence or definition? Semin Arthritis Rheum 25:28, 1995.

165. Cotch MF, Hoffman GS, Yerg DE, et al: The epidemiology of Wegener's granulomatosis: Estimates of the five-year period preva-lence, annual mortality, and geographic disease distribution from population-based data sources. Arthritis Rheum 39:87, 1996.

166. Hoffman GS, Kerr GS, Leavitt RS, et al: Wegener granulomatosis: An analysis of 158 patients. Ann Intern Med 116:488, 1992.

167. Cordier JF, Valeyre D, Guillevin L, et al: Pulmonary Wegener's granulomatosis: A clinical and imaging study of 77 cases. Chest 97:906, 1990.

168. Stokes TC, McCann BG, Rees RT, et al: Acute fulminating intrapul-monary haemorrhage in Wegener's granulomatosis. Thorax 37:315, 1982.

169. Frazier AA, Rosado de Christenson ML, Galvin JR, et al: Pulmonary angiitis and granulomatosis: Radiologic-pathologic correlation. Ra-diographics 18:687, 1998.

170. Aberle DR, Gamsu G, Lynch D: Thoracic manifestations of Wegener granulomatosis: Diagnosis and course. Radiology 174:703, 1990.

171. Weir IH, Müller NL, Chiles C, et al: Wegener's granulomatosis: Findings from computed tomography of the chest in 10 patients. Can Assoc Radiol J 43:31, 1992.

172. Wechsler RJ, Steiner RM, Israel HL: Chest radiography in lymphomatoid granulomatosis: Comparison with Wegener granulo-matosis. Am J Roentgenol 142:679, 1984.

173. Maguire R, Fauci AS, Doppman JL, et al: Unusual radiographic features of Wegener's granulomatosis. Am J Roentgenol 130:233, 1978.

174. Hunninghake GW, Fauci AS: Pulmonary involvement in the colla-gen vascular diseases. Am Rev Respir Dis 119:471, 1979.

175. Papiris SA, Manoussakis MN, Drosos AA, et al: Imaging of thoracic Wegener's granulomatosis: The computed tomographic appearance. Am J Med 93:529, 1992.

176. Maskell GF, Lockwood CM, Flower CDR: Computed tomography of the lung in Wegener's granulomatosis. Clin Radiol 48:377, 1993.

177. Reuter M, Schnabel A, Wesner F, et al: Pulmonary Wegener's granulomatosis: Correlation between high-resolution CT findings and clinical scoring of disease activity. Chest 114:500, 1998.

178. Kuhlman JE, Hruban RH, Fishman ER: Wegener granulomatosis: CT features of parenchymal lung disease. J Comput Assist Tomogr 15:948, 1991.

179. Gohel VK, Dalinka MK, Israel HL, et al: The radiological manifes-tations of Wegener's granulomatosis. Br J Radiol 46:427, 1973.

180. Foo SS, Weisbrod GL, Herman SJ, et al: Wegener granulomatosis presenting on CT with atypical bronchovasocentric distribution. J Comput Assist Tomogr 14:1004, 1990.

181. Daum TE, Specks U, Colby TV, et al: Tracheobronchial involvement in Wegener's granulomatosis. Am J Respir Crit Care Med 151:522, 1995.

182. Baker SB, Robinson DR: Unusual renal manifestations of Wegener's granulomatosis: Report of two cases. Am J Med 64:883, 1978.

183. Conces DJ Jr, Kesler KA, Datzman M, et al: Tracheoesophageal

fistula due to Wegener's granulomatosis. J Thorac Imaging 10:126, 1995.

184. Pinching AJ, Lockwood CM, Pussell BA, et al: Wegener's granulomatosis: Observations on 18 patients with severe renal disease. QJM 52:435, 1983.

185. Jaspan T, Davison AM, Walker WC: Spontaneous pneumothorax in Wegener's granulomatosis. Thorax 37:774, 1982.

186. Wolffenbuttel BH, Weber RF, Kho GS: Pyopneumothorax: A rare complication of Wegener's granulomatosis. Eur J Respir Dis 67:223, 1985.

187. Cohen MI, Gore RM, August CZ, et al: Tracheal and bronchial stenosis associated with mediastinal adenopathy in Wegener granulomatosis: CT findings. J Comput Assist Tomogr 8:327, 1984.

188. Kjellstrand CM, Simmons RL, Uranga VM, et al: Acute fulminant Wegener granulomatosis: Therapy with immunosuppression, hemodialysis, and renal transplantation. Arch Intern Med 134:40, 1974.

189. Arauz JC, Fonseca R: Wegener's granulomatosis appearing initially in the trachea. Ann Otorhinol Laryngol 91:593, 1982.

190. Hellmann D, Laing T, Petri M, et al: Wegener's granulomatosis: Isolated involvement of the trachea and larynx. Ann Rheum Dis 46:628, 1987.

191. Screaton NJ, Sivosothy P, Flower CDR, et al: Tracheal involvement in Wegener's granulomatosis: Evaluation using spiral CT. Clin Radiol 53:809, 1998.

192. Woodworth TG, Abuelo JG, Austin HA III, et al: Severe glomerulonephritis with late emergence of classic Wegener's granulomatosis: Report of 4 cases and review of the literature. Medicine 66:181, 1987.

193. Egner W, Chapel HM: Titration of antibodies against neutrophil cytoplasmic antigens is useful in monitoring disease activity in systemic vasculitides. Clin Exp Immunol 82:244, 1990.

194. Weber MFA, Andrassy K, Pullig O, et al: Antineutrophil cytoplasmic antibodies and antiglomerular basement membrane antibodies in Goodpasture's syndrome and in Wegener's granulomatosis. J Am Soc Nephrol 2:1227, 1992.

195. Kallenberg CGM, Mulder AHL, Cohen Tervaert JW: Anti-neutrophil cytoplasmic antibodies: A still growing class of autoantibodies in inflammatory disorders. Am J Med 93:675, 1992.

196. Churg J, Strauss L: Allergic granulomatosis, allergic angiitis, and periarteritis nodosa. Am J Pathol 27:277, 1951.

197. Lanham JG, Elkon KB, Pusey CD, et al: Systemic vasculitis with asthma and eosinophilia: A clinical approach to the Churg-Strauss syndrome. Medicine 63:65, 1984.

198. Chumbley LC, Harrison EG, DeRemee RA: Allergic granulomatosis and angiitis (Churg-Strauss syndrome): Report and analysis of 30 cases. Mayo Clin Proc 52:477, 1977.

199. Degesys GE, Mintzer RA, Vrla RF: Allergic granulomatosis: Churg-Strauss syndrome. Am J Roentgenol 135:1281, 1980.

200. Worthy SA, Müller NL, Hansell DM, et al: Churg-Strauss syndrome: The spectrum of pulmonary CT findings in 17 patients. Am J Roentgenol 170:297, 1998.

201. Buschman DL, James AW Jr, Talmadge EK: Churg-Strauss pulmonary vasculitis: High-resolution computed tomography scanning and pathologic findings. Am Rev Respir Dis 142:458, 1990.

202. Lhote F, Guillevin L: Polyarteritis nodosa, microscopic polyangiitis, and Churg-Strauss syndrome: Clinical aspects and treatment. Rheum Dis Clin North Am 21:911, 1995.

203. Sehgal M, Swanson JW, DeRemee RA, et al: Neurologic manifestations of Churg-Strauss syndrome. Mayo Clin Proc 70:337, 1995.

204. Davis MD, Baoud MS, McEvoy MT, et al: Cutaneous manifestations of Churg-Strauss syndrome: A clinicopathologic correlation. J Am Acad Dermatol 37:199, 1997.

205. Watts RA, Joliffe VA, Carruthers DM, et al: Effect of classification on the incidence of PAN and microscopic polyangiitis. Arthritis Rheum 39:1208, 1997.

206. Mark EJ, Ramirez JR: Pulmonary capillaritis and hemorrhage in patients with systemic vasculitis. Arch Pathol Lab Med 109:413, 1985.

207. Lewis EJ, Schur PH, Busch GJ, et al: Immunopathologic features of a patient with glomerulonephritis and pulmonary hemorrhage. Am J Med 54:507, 1973.

208. Haworth SJ, Savage COS, Carr D, et al: Pulmonary hemorrhage complicating Wegener's granulomatosis and microscopic polyarteritis. BMJ 290:1175, 1985.

209. Dabague J, Reyes PA: Takayasu arteritis in Mexico: A 38-year clinical perspective through literature review. Int J Cardiol 54:S103, 1996.

210. Hata A, Noda M, Moriwaki R, et al: Angiographic findings of Takayasu arteritis: New classification. Int J Cardiol 54:S155, 1996.

211. Nasu T: Takayasu's truncoarteritis in Japan: A statistical observation of 76 autopsy cases. Pathol Microbiol 43:140, 1975.

212. Sharma S, Kamalakar T, Rajani M, et al: The incidence and patterns of pulmonary artery involvement in Takayasu's arteritis. Clin Radiol 42:177, 1990.

213. Neng-shu H, Fan L, En-hui W, et al: Pulmonary artery involvement in aorto-arteritis: An analysis of DSA. Chin Med J 103:666, 1990.

214. Yamato M, Lecky JW, Hiramatsu K, et al: Takayasu arteritis: Radiographic and angiographic findings in 59 patients. Radiology 161:329, 1986.

215. Kerr GS, Hallahan CW, Giordano J, et al: Takayasu arteritis. Ann Intern Med 120:919, 1994.

216. Sharma BK, Siveski-Iliskovic N, Singal PK: Takayasu arteritis may be underdiagnosed in North America. Can J Cardiol 11:311, 1995.

217. Hachiya J: Current concept of Takayasu's arteritis. Semin Roentgenol 5:245, 1970.

218. Takahashi K, Honda M, Furuse M, et al: CT findings of pulmonary parenchyma in Takayasu arteritis. J Comput Assist Tomogr 20:742, 1996.

219. Park JH, Chung JW, Im JG, et al: Takayasu arteritis: Evaluation of mural changes in the aorta and pulmonary artery with CT angiography. Radiology 196:89, 1995.

220. Yamada I, Numano F, Suzuki S: Takayasu arteritis: Evaluation with MR imaging. Radiology 188:89, 1993.

221. Matsunaga N, Hayashi K, Sakamoto I, et al: Takayasu arteritis: Protean radiologic manifestations and diagnosis. Radiographics 17:579, 1997.

222. Yamada I, Shibuya H, Matsubara O, et al: Pulmonary artery disease in Takayasu's arteritis: Angiographic findings. Am J Roentgenol 159:263, 1992.

223. Hayashi K, Nagasaki M, Matsunaga N, et al: Initial pulmonary artery involvement in Takayasu arteritis. Radiology 159:401, 1986.

224. Hayashi K, Sakamoto I, Matsunaga N: Pulmonary arterial lesions in Takayasu arteritis: Relationship of inflammatory activity to scintigraphic findings and sequential changes. Ann Nucl Med 10:219, 1996,

225. Lakhanpal S, Tani K, Lie JT, et al: Pathologic features of Behçet's syndrome: A review of Japanese autopsy registry data. Hum Pathol 16:790, 1985.

226. Raz I, Okon E, Chajek-Shaul T: Pulmonary manifestations in Behçet's syndrome. Chest 95:585, 1989.

227. Herreman G, Beaufils H, Godeau P, et al: Behçet's syndrome and renal involvement: A histological and immunofluorescent study of 11 renal biopsies. Am J Med Sci 284:10, 1982.

228. Efthimiou J, Johnston C, Spiro SG, et al: Pulmonary disease in Behçet's syndrome. QJM 58:259, 1986.

229. Tunaci A, Berkmen YM, Gökmen E: Thoracic involvement in Behçet's disease: Pathologic, clinical, and imaging features. Am J Roentgenol 164:51, 1995.

230. Ahn JM, Im JG, Ryoo JW, et al: Thoracic manifestations of Behçet syndrome: Radiographic and CT findings in nine patients. Radiology 194:199, 1995.

231. Grenier P, Bletry O, Cornud F, et al: Pulmonary involvement in Behçet disease. Am J Roentgenol 137:565, 1981.

232. Puckette TC, Jolles H, Proto AV: Magnetic resonance imaging confirmation of pulmonary artery aneurysm in Behçet's disease. J Thorac Imaging 9:172, 1994.

233. Numan F, Islak C, Berkmen T, et al: Behçet disease: Pulmonary arterial involvement in 15 cases. Radiology 192:465, 1994.

234. Winer-Muram HT, Headley AS, Menke P, et al: Radiologic manifestations of thoracic vascular Behçet's disease in African-American men. J Thorac Imaging 9:176, 1994.

235. Davies JD: Behçet's syndrome with hemoptysis and pulmonary lesions. J Pathol 109:351, 1973.

236. Çöplü L, Emri S, Selçuk ZT, et al: Life threatening chylous pleural and pericardial effusion in a patient with Behçet's syndrome. Thorax 47:64, 1992.

237. Erkan F, Cavdar T: Pulmonary vasculitis in Behçet's disease. Am Rev Respir Dis 146:232, 1992.

238. Reza MJ, Dermanes DJ: Behçet's disease: A case with hemoptysis, pseudotumor cerebri, and arteritis. J Rheumatol 5:320, 1978.

239. Liebow AA: Pulmonary angiitis and granulomatosis. Am Rev Respir Dis 108:1, 1973.

240. Le Gall F, Loeuillet L, Delaval P, et al: Necrotizing sarcoid granulomatosis with and without extrapulmonary involvement. Pathol Res Pract 192:306, 1996.

241. Koss MN, Hochholzer L, Feigin DS, et al: Necrotizing sarcoid-like granulomatosis: Clinical, pathologic, and immunopathologic findings. Hum Pathol 11:510, 1980.

242. Churg A, Carrington CB, Gupta R: Necrotizing sarcoid granulomatosis. Chest 76:706, 1979.

243. Saldana MJ: Necrotizing sarcoid granulomatosis: Clinicopathologic observations in 24 patients (abstract). Lab Invest 38:364, 1978.

244. Chittock DR, Joseph MG, Paterson NA, et al: Necrotizing sarcoid granulomatosis with pleural involvement: Clinical and radiographic features. Chest 106:672, 1994.

245. Rosen Y, Moon S, Huang C-T, et al: Granulomatous pulmonary angiitis in sarcoidosis. Arch Pathol Lab Med 101:170, 1977.

246. Dykhuizen RS, Smith CC, Kennedy MM, et al: Necrotizing sarcoid granulomatosis with extrapulmonary involvement. Eur Respir J 10:245, 1997.

247. Fisher MR, Christ ML, Bernstein JR: Necrotizing sarcoid-like granulomatosis radiologic-pathologic correlation. J Can Assoc Radiol 35:313, 1984.

248. Stephen JG, Braimbridge MV, Corrin B, et al: Necrotizing "sarcoidal" angiitis and granulomatosis of the lung. Thorax 31:356, 1976.

249. Niimi H, Hartman TE, Müller NL: Necrotizing sarcoid granulomatosis: Computed tomography and pathologic findings. J Comput Assist Tomogr 19:920, 1995.

250. Adlakha A, Kang E, Adlkha K, et al: Nonproductive cough dyspnea, malaise, and night sweats in a 47-year-old woman. Chest 109:1385, 1996.

251. Soergel H, Sommers SC: Idiopathic pulmonary hemosiderosis and related syndromes. Am J Med 32:499, 1962.

252. Boyd DHA: Idiopathic pulmonary hemosiderosis in adults and adolescents. Br J Dis Chest 53:41, 1959.

253. Rezkalla MA, Simmons JL: Idiopathic pulmonary hemosiderosis and alveolar hemorrhage syndrome: Case report and review of the literature. S D J Med 48:79, 1995.

254. Pacheco A, Casanova C, Fogue L, et al: Long-term clinical follow-up of adult idiopathic pulmonary hemosiderosis and celiac disease. Chest 99:1525, 1991.

255. Proskey AJ, Weatherbee L, Easterling RE, et al: Goodpasture's syndrome: A report of five cases and review of the literature. Am J Med 48:162, 1970.

256. Teague CA, Doak PB, Simpson IJ, et al: Goodpasture's syndrome: An analysis of 29 cases. Kidney Int 13:492, 1978.

257. Kelly PT, Haponik EF: Goodpasture syndrome: Molecular and clinical advances. Medicine 73:171, 1994.

258. Slonim L: Goodpasture's syndrome and its radiological features. Australas Radiol 13:164, 1969.

259. Bowley NB, Steiner RE, Chin WS: The chest x-ray in antiglomerular basement membrane antibody disease (Goodpasture's syndrome). Clin Radiol 30:419, 1979.

260. Albelda SM, Gefter WB, Epstein DM, et al: Diffuse pulmonary hemorrhage: A review and classification. Radiology 154:289, 1985.

261. Müller NL, Miller RR: Diffuse pulmonary hemorrhage. Radiol Clin North Am 29:965, 1991.

262. Chea FK, Sheppard MN, Hansell DM: Computed tomography of diffuse pulmonary hemorrhage with pathologic correlation. Clin Radiol 48:89, 1993.

263. Niimi A, Amitani R, Kurasawa T, et al: Two cases of idiopathic pulmonary hemosiderosis: Analysis of chest CT findings. Nippon Kyobu Shikkan Gakkai Zasshi 30:1749, 1992.

264. Seely JM, Effmann EL, Müller NL: High-resolution CT in pediatric lung disease: Imaging findings. Am J Roentgenol 168:1269, 1997.

265. Engeler CE: High-resolution CT of airspace nodules in idiopathic pulmonary hemosiderosis. Eur Radiol 5:663, 1995.

266. Lynch DA, Brasch RC, Hardy KA, et al: Pediatric pulmonary disease: Assessment with high-resolution ultrafast CT. Radiology 176:243, 1990.

267. Theros EG, Reeder MM, Eckert JF: An exercise in radiologic-pathologic correlation. Radiology 90:784, 1968.

268. Bruwer AJ, Kennedy RLJ, Edwards JE: Recurrent pulmonary hemorrhage with hemosiderosis: So-called idiopathic pulmonary hemosiderosis. Am J Roentgenol 76:98, 1956.

269. Sybers RG, Sybers JL, Dickie HA, et al: Roentgenographic aspects of hemorrhagic pulmonary-renal disease (Goodpasture's syndrome). Am J Roentgenol 94:674, 1965.

270. Brannan HM, McCaughey WTE, Good CA: The roentgenographic appearance of pulmonary hemorrhage associated with glomerulonephritis. Am J Roentgenol 90:83, 1963.

271. Case Records of the Massachusetts General Hospital. N Engl J Med 319:227, 1988.

271a. Aledort LM, Lord GP: Idiopathic pulmonary hemosiderosis: Severe anemia without hemoptysis—one year follow-up of pulmonary function. Arch Intern Med 120:220, 1967.

272. van Drop R, Daha MR, Muizert Y, et al: A rapid ELISA for measurement of anti-glomerular basement membrane antibodies using microwaves. J Clin Lab Immunol 40:135, 1993.

273. Allen JN, Davis WB: Eosinophilic lung diseases. Am J Respir Crit Care Med 150:1423, 1994.

274. Löffler W: Zur differential-diagnose der lungeninfiltrierungan: II. Über flüchtige succedan-infiltrate (mit eosinophilie). Beitr Klin Tuberk 79:368, 1932.

275. Ford RM: Transient pulmonary eosinophilia and asthma: A review of 20 cases occurring in 5,702 asthma sufferers. Am Rev Respir Dis 93:797, 1966.

276. Citro LA, Gordon ME, Miller WT: Eosinophilic lung disease (or how to slice P.I.E.). Am J Roentgenol Rad Ther Nucl Med 117:787, 1973.

277. Carrington CB, Addington WW, Goff AM, et al: Chronic eosinophilic pneumonia. N Engl J Med 280:787, 1969.

278. Chapman BJ, Capewell S, Gibson R, et al: Pulmonary eosinophilia with and without allergic bronchopulmonary aspergillosis. Thorax 44:919, 1989.

279. Allen JN, Pacht ER, Gadek JE, et al: Acute eosinophilic pneumonia as a reversible cause of noninfectious respiratory failure. N Engl J Med 321:569, 1989.

280. Badesch DB, King TE Jr, Schwarz MI: Acute eosinophilic pneumonia: A hypersensitivity phenomenon? Am Rev Respir Dis 139:249, 1989.

281. Hayakawa H, Sato A, Toyoshima M, et al: A clinical study of idiopathic eosinophilic pneumonia. Chest 105:1462, 1994.

282. Cheon JE, Lee KS, Jung GS, et al: Acute eosinophilic pneumonia: Radiographic and CT findings in six patients. Am J Roentgenol 167:1195, 1996.

283. King MA, Pope-Harman AL, Allen JN, et al: Acute eosinophilic pneumonia: Radiologic and clinical features. Radiology 203:715, 1997.

284. Jederlinic PJ, Sicilian L, Gaensler EA: Chronic eosinophilic pneumonia: A report of 19 cases and a review of the literature. Medicine 67:154, 1988.

285. Gaensler EA, Carrington CB: Peripheral opacities in chronic eosinophilic pneumonia: The photographic negative of pulmonary edema. Am J Roentgenol 128:1, 1977.

286. Mayo JR, Müller NL, Road J, et al: Chronic eosinophilic pneumonia: CT findings in six cases. Am J Roentgenol 153:727, 1989.

287. Ebara H, Ikezoe J, Johkoh T, et al: Chronic eosinophilic pneumonia: Evolution of chest radiograms and CT features. J Comput Assist Tomogr 18:737, 1994.

288. Zaki I, Wears R, Parnell A, et al: Case report: Mediastinal lymphadenopathy in eosinophilic pneumonia. Clin Radiol 48:61, 1993.

289. Fauci AS, Harley JB, Roberts WC, et al: The idiopathic hypereosinophilic syndrome. Ann Intern Med 97:78, 1982.

290. Hill R, Wang NS, Berry G: Hypereosinophilic syndrome with pulmonary vascular involvement. Angiology 35:238, 1984.

291. Epstein DM, Taormina V, Gefter WB, et al: The hypereosinophilic syndrome. Radiology 140:59, 1981.

292. Chusid MJ, Dale DC, West BC, et al: The hypereosinophilic syndrome: Analysis of fourteen cases with review of the literature. Medicine 54:1, 1975.

293. Geltner D, Friedman G, Naparstek E, et al: Acute lymphoblastic leukemia: Its occurrence with "hypereosinophilic syndrome" and bilateral spontaneous pneumothorax. Arch Intern Med 138:292, 1978.

294. Kang E-Y, Shim JJ, Kim JS, et al: Pulmonary involvement of idiopathic hypereosinophilic syndrome: CT findings in five patients. J Comput Assist Tomogr 21:612, 1997.

295. Reichlin S, Loveless MH, Kane EG: Loeffler's syndrome following penicillin therapy. Ann Intern Med 38:113, 1953.

296. Fiengenberg DS, Weiss H, Kirshman H: Migratory pneumonia with eosinophilia associated with sulfonamide administration. Arch Intern Med 120:85, 1967.

297. Ho D, Tashkin DP, Bein ME, et al: Pulmonary infiltrates with eosinophilia associated with tetracycline. Chest 76:33, 1979.

298. Goodwin SD, Glenny RW: Nonsteroidal anti-inflammatory drug-associated pulmonary infiltrates with eosinophilia: Review of the literature and Food and Drug Administration adverse drug reaction reports. Arch Intern Med 152:1521, 1992.

299. Khahil H, Molinary E, Stoller JK: Diclofenax (Voltaren)-induced eosinophilic pneumonitis. Arch Intern Med 153:1649, 1993.

300. Yamakado S, Yoshida Y, Yamada T, et al: Pulmonary infiltration and eosinophilia associated with sulfasalazine therapy or ulcerative colitis: A case report and review of literature. Intern Med 31:108, 1992.

301. Panayiotou BN: Pulmonary infiltrates and eosinophilia associated with sulphasalazine administration. Aust N Z J Med 21:348, 1991.

302. Oh PI, Balter MS: Cocaine induced eosinophilic lung disease. Thorax 47:478, 1992.

303. Nadeem S, Nasir N, Israel RH: Löffler's syndrome secondary to crack cocaine. Chest 105:1599, 1994.

304. Brander PE, Tukiainen P: Acute eosinophilic pneumonia in a heroin smoker. Eur Respir J 6:750, 1993.

305. Vandenplas O, Casel S, Delos M, et al: Granulomatous bronchiolitis associated with Crohn's disease. Am J Respir Crit Care Med 158:1676, 1998.

306. Erkan F, Cavdar R: Pulmonary vasculitis in Behçet's disease. Am Rev Respir Dis 146:232, 1992.

307. Howling SJ, Hansell DM, Wells AU, et al: Follicular bronchiolitis: Thin-section CT and histologic findings. Radiology 121:637, 1999.

308. Choe YH, Han BK, Koh EM, et al: Takayasu's arteritis: Assessment of disease activity with contract-enhanced MR imaging. Am J Roentgenol 175:505, 2000.

CHAPTER 9

Chronic Interstitial Lung Diseases

SARCOIDOSIS

Sarcoidosis is a relatively common disease that is difficult to characterize precisely. In 1991, members of the World Association of Sarcoidosis and Other Granulomatous Disorders proposed that it should be defined descriptively.[1, 2] Although their definition is cumbersome, it encompasses most of the important features of the disease and emphasizes the fact that the criteria for diagnosis are based on a combination of clinical, radiologic, and laboratory findings. According to the World Association:[1]

[Sarcoidosis is a] multisystem disorder of unknown cause(s). It most commonly affects young and middle-aged adults and frequently presents with bilateral hilar lymphadenopathy, pulmonary infiltration (sic), and ocular and skin lesions. Liver, spleen, lymph nodes, salivary glands, heart, nervous system, muscles, bone and other organs may also be involved. The diagnosis is established when clinico-radiological findings are supported by histologic evidence of non-caseating epithelioid cell granulomas. Granulomas of known causes and local sarcoid reactions must be excluded.

Frequently observed immunologic features are depression of cutaneous delayed-type hypersensitivity and increased helper cell (CD4)–to–suppressor cell (CD8) ratio

at the site of involvement. Circulating immune complexes along with other signs of B-cell hyperactivity also may be detectable. Other markers of the disease include elevated levels of serum angiotensin converting enzyme, increased uptake of radioactive gallium, abnormal calcium metabolism, and abnormal fluorescein angiography. The Kveim-Siltzbach test, when appropriate cell suspensions are available, may be of diagnostic help.

The course and prognosis may correlate with the mode of the onset and the extent of the disease. An acute onset with erythema nodosum or asymptomatic bilateral hilar lymphadenopathy usually heralds a self-limiting course, whereas an insidious onset, especially with multiple extrapulmonary lesions, may be followed by relentless, progressive fibrosis of the lungs and other organs. Corticosteroids relieve symptoms, suppress the formation of granulomas, and normalize the serum angiotensin converting enzyme levels and the gallium uptake.

As this description indicates, sarcoidosis is a systemic disease with a variety of clinical and radiologic features that are associated histologically with granulomatous inflammation. Because other diseases, such as tuberculosis or fungal infection, hypersensitivity pneumonitis, and lymphoma, can simulate the histologic or radiologic features of the disease,[3] the diagnosis is always one of exclusion. The disease is more common in temperate than in tropical climates.[4] In the United States, a reasonable estimate of the prevalence of a radiographic pattern consistent with the diagnosis is about 10 per 100,000 examinations.[4] African Americans, especially women, have a particularly high prevalence.[9]

Although the disease may occur at any age, it is recognized most commonly in patients between the ages of 20 and 40 years.[4, 6] In one review of 1,254 patients, 50% were in this age group;[6] only 2% were younger than age 10 years, and only 4% were older than 60. Overall mortality has been estimated at 1% to 5%.[208]

Pathologic Characteristics

The pathologic hallmark of sarcoidosis is the granuloma, which is identical to that caused by many well-defined etiologic agents—a more or less well-circumscribed collection of epithelioid histiocytes sometimes associated with multinucleated giant cells. Pulmonary involvement characteristically is most prominent in the peribronchovascular, interlobular septal, and pleural interstitial tissue (Fig. 9–1). In the early stages, granulomas typically are discrete and

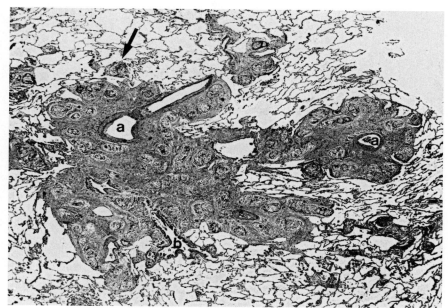

Figure 9–1. Pulmonary Sarcoidosis. Low magnification view of lung parenchyma shows numerous granulomas associated with a moderate amount of collagen; granulomas and fibrous tissue are located predominantly in the interstitium adjacent to pulmonary arteries (a) and bronchioles (b). Only an occasional granuloma appears to be located within parenchymal interstitium *(arrow)*. (×15.)

histologically *active*; as the disease progresses, granulomas often become confluent and associated with fibrosis, resulting in more or less diffuse interstitial thickening. The parenchymal interstitium may be affected, although invariably much less so than that in peribronchovascular, septal, and pleural locations. Granulomatous inflammation and fibrosis also can be seen in the bronchial mucosa,[10] sometimes to such an extent as to cause airway stenosis.[11]

Clinical Manifestations

Symptoms occur in approximately 50% of affected individuals.[4] These symptoms often develop insidiously and frequently are associated with multisystem involvement. Constitutional symptoms, including weight loss, fatigue, weakness, and malaise, are common. Fever occurs in about 15% to 20% of patients.[6] An acute onset of symptoms, usually including erythema nodosum, is particularly common in Scandinavian women; a third of Scandinavian women have presented in this fashion.[7] A predilection for erythema nodosum has been reported in Irish women in London and in Puerto Ricans in New York City.[98] Löfgren's syndrome (erythema nodosum or periarticular ankle inflammation with unilateral or bilateral hilar or right paratracheal lymph node enlargement) usually is self-limited.[209]

Symptoms of pulmonary involvement develop in about one third of patients[5] and include dry cough and shortness of breath.[3, 5] Such symptoms tend to be mild even in patients who have extensive parenchymal abnormalities on the chest radiograph or computed tomography (CT) scan.

Radiologic Manifestations

The radiographic changes in thoracic sarcoidosis can be classified usefully for descriptive purposes into four groups or stages:[12]

Stage 0—no demonstrable abnormality
Stage 1—hilar and mediastinal lymph node enlargement unassociated with pulmonary abnormality
Stage 2—hilar and mediastinal lymph node enlargement associated with pulmonary abnormality
Stage 3—diffuse pulmonary disease unassociated with lymph node enlargement

The main utility of this staging system is in predicting outcome. In one survey of 3,676 patients from nine countries, 8% were found to have normal chest radiographs at presentation;[13] 51% had Stage 1 disease, 29% had Stage 2 disease, and 12% had Stage 3 disease. On follow-up, 65% of patients who had Stage 1 disease showed resolution of the radiographic findings compared with 49% of patients who had Stage 2 disease and 20% of patients who had Stage 3 disease.

Lymph Node Enlargement Without Pulmonary Abnormality

On chest radiograph, lymph node enlargement without parenchymal disease is seen at presentation in approximately 50% of patients.[13, 17] The combination of bilateral hilar and right paratracheal lymph node enlargement is a characteristic and common manifestation (Fig. 9–2);[15] the former is present in more than 95% of patients and the latter in about 70% with intrathoracic lymph node enlargement.[14, 18] Other common sites of lymphadenopathy evident on radiograph include the aortopulmonary window (approximately 50% of cases) and subcarinal region (20% of cases).[14, 15] Anterior mediastinal lymph node enlargement seldom is prominent but can be identified on the radiograph in approximately 15% of cases.[14] Enlargement of posterior mediastinal nodes is uncommon in our experience, although the incidence in reported series varies greatly (e.g., in only 1 of 62 patients in one series[18] and in 6 [20%] of 30 patients in another).[19]

Hilar lymph node enlargement usually is bilateral and symmetric. Unilateral enlargement is uncommon, being reported in only 3% to 5% of proven cases.[20, 21] Occasionally, hilar and mediastinal node enlargement is sufficient to

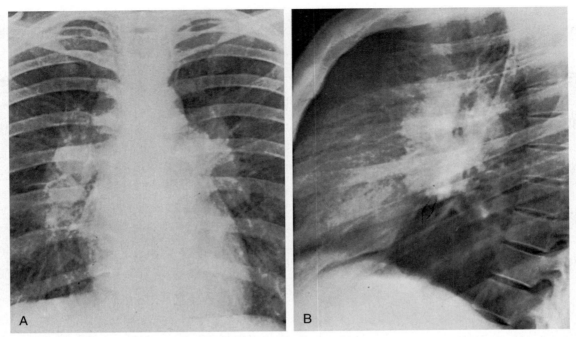

Figure 9–2. Sarcoidosis: Lymph Node Involvement Alone. Posteroanterior *(A)* and lateral *(B)* radiographs of a 32-year-old asymptomatic woman show marked enlargement of both hila, the lobulated contour being typical of lymph node enlargement. Nodes are enlarged in the right paratracheal and aortopulmonary regions. The lungs are clear.

compress the adjacent bronchi. Such compression may lead to lobar atelectasis, most commonly involving the middle lobe.[16] Rarely, enlarged nodes cause narrowing of a central pulmonary artery, particularly the truncus anterior, and lead to decreased pulmonary perfusion.[16] Similarly, a few cases of superior vena caval syndrome or obstruction of the innominate vein by massively enlarged lymph nodes have been reported.[16]

Calcification of hilar lymph nodes is apparent radiographically in approximately 5% of patients at presentation.[20] In some cases, the calcification resembles the eggshell calcification of silicosis.[20] (Sarcoidosis is considered to be the most common cause of circumferential or eggshell calcification in patients not exposed to silica.[24]) Nodal calcification is usually a late manifestation. In one study of 111 patients followed for 10 years or more, calcification of mediastinal lymph nodes was detected radiographically in more than 20%.[25]

Paratracheal node enlargement seldom occurs without concomitant enlargement of hilar nodes.[26] This bilaterally symmetric hilar and paratracheal lymph node enlargement contrasts sharply with the node enlargement of primary tuberculosis, which tends to be unilateral.[27] The contrast is more evident with lymphoma. In Hodgkin's disease, enlargement tends to occur predominantly in the anterior mediastinal and paratracheal groups; when it involves the hilar nodes, it is predominantly unilateral and asymmetric. As indicated previously, although anterior mediastinal lymph node enlargement may occur in sarcoidosis, it is seldom a prominent feature, and it is characteristically associated with paratracheal and symmetric bilateral hilar lymphadenopathy.

The prevalence of lymph node enlargement and its distribution as described previously refer to the findings on

the chest radiograph. As might be expected, hilar and mediastinal lymphadenopathy is seen more commonly on CT scan than on radiograph.[28, 29] The mediastinal disease can be seen to involve more nodal stations on CT scans than on radiograph (Fig. 9–3).[28, 29] CT may show enlarged nodes in sites other than the hila and mediastinum, including internal mammary, axillary, and infradiaphragmatic regions.[31, 32] Calcification of hilar and mediastinal lymph nodes is seen more commonly on CT scans than on radiographs (Fig. 9–4).[33, 34] In one study of 18 patients, this finding was identified on CT at presentation in 4 (22%) patients and on follow-up scans performed 4 to 49 months later in 8 (44%) patients.[33] The calcification usually is focal and most commonly involves the mediastinal and hilar nodes.[14] The diameter of the calcified nodes usually is greater than 10 mm.[14]

Stages 0 and 1 refer only to *radiographically* evident disease and not to disease determined by pathologic or physiologic examination. Similar to other interstitial diseases, the lungs can be involved by sarcoidosis in the absence of a demonstrable abnormality on chest radiograph.[36, 37] The chest radiograph is normal (Stage 0) in about 10% of patients who have biopsy-proven pulmonary sarcoidosis.[13, 35] Similarly, in a study of 21 consecutive patients with Stage 1 disease who underwent open-lung biopsy, typical sarcoid granulomas were present in the lung parenchyma in all;[37] however, the extent of granulomatous inflammation and fibrosis was significantly less than that seen in open-lung biopsy specimens of patients who had radiographic evidence of diffuse lung involvement. The authors of the last study also cited six articles from the literature in which the results of lung biopsy of patients with Stage 1 disease were reported: Lung tissue containing granulomas was obtained in 50% to 100% of cases.[37] As

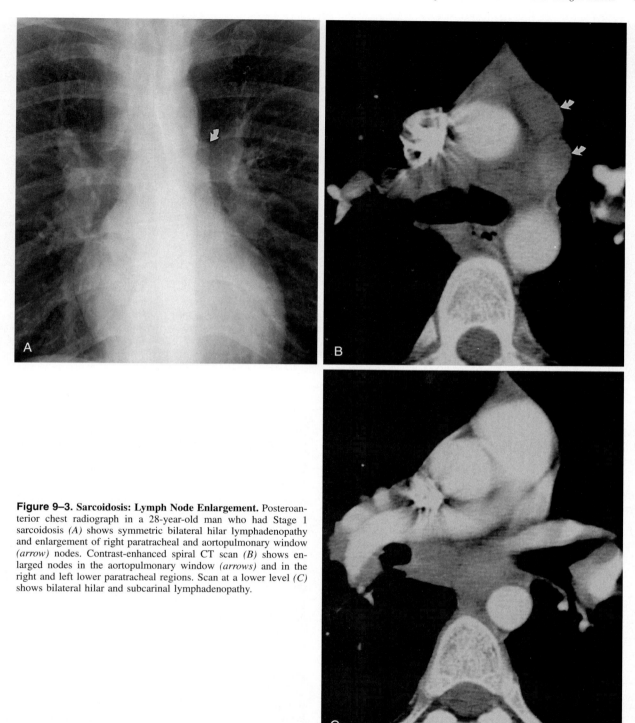

Figure 9–3. Sarcoidosis: Lymph Node Enlargement. Posteroanterior chest radiograph in a 28-year-old man who had Stage 1 sarcoidosis *(A)* shows symmetric bilateral hilar lymphadenopathy and enlargement of right paratracheal and aortopulmonary window *(arrow)* nodes. Contrast-enhanced spiral CT scan *(B)* shows enlarged nodes in the aortopulmonary window *(arrows)* and in the right and left lower paratracheal regions. Scan at a lower level *(C)* shows bilateral hilar and subcarinal lymphadenopathy.

might be expected, parenchymal abnormalities were seen more commonly on high-resolution computed tomography (HRCT) scan than on radiograph.[28] In one study of 44 patients, mild parenchymal abnormalities were detected on HRCT scan in all six patients who had radiographic Stage 1 disease.[38]

Of patients who have Stage 1 sarcoidosis, 65% to 80% eventually show complete radiographic resolution.[13, 39] In one study of 308 patients, normal chest radiographs were observed in 44% after 1 year of follow-up and in 82% after 5 years.[39] Occasionally, enlarged hilar and mediastinal nodes regress to normal size only to undergo enlargement again at a later date.[40, 41] By contrast, hilar and paratracheal node enlargement can persist unchanged for many years.[42, 43] In one study of 12 patients who had chronic hilar and mediastinal lymph node enlargement, 7 patients remained asymptomatic for a mean period of 16 years despite persistent node enlargement, 2 patients had disfiguring facial

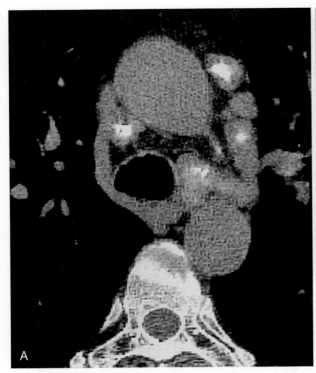

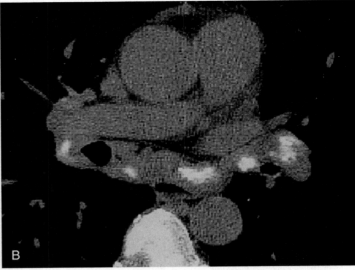

Figure 9–4. Sarcoidosis: Calcified Lymph Nodes. HRCT scan *(A)* in a 59-year-old man with long-standing Stage 2 sarcoidosis shows calcified aortopulmonary window and paratracheal lymph nodes. A scan at a lower level *(B)* shows calcified bilateral hilar and subcarinal lymph nodes.

sarcoidosis for which corticosteroid therapy was administered for 18 and 27 years, and 3 patients developed diffuse pulmonary disease after 10 years of stable node enlargement.[44]

Diffuse Pulmonary Disease with or Without Lymph Node Enlargement

Parenchymal disease is seen on chest radiograph at presentation in approximately 40% of patients who have sarcoidosis and occurs at some time during the course of the disease in 50% to 65% of patients (Table 9–1).[13, 39, 45] At presentation, the pulmonary disease is associated with lymph node enlargement (Stage 2) in approximately 30% of patients; the remaining 10% have no evidence of lymph

Table 9–1. SARCOIDOSIS: RADIOLOGIC MANIFESTATIONS

Bilateral hilar and paratracheal lymph node enlargement	
Without parenchymal abnormalities	50% of patients
With parenchymal disease	30% of patients
Normal chest radiograph	10% of patients
Parenchymal abnormalities without lymphadenopathy	10% of patients
Characteristic parenchymal abnormalities	
Chest radiograph	
Nodular, reticulonodular, or reticular pattern	
Bilateral, symmetric	
Predominantly upper lung zones	
Predominantly central lung regions	
HRCT	
Thickening of peribronchovascular interstitium	
Peribronchovascular nodules in central lung regions	
Subpleural nodules including interlobar fissures	

HRCT, high-resolution computed tomography.

node enlargement (Stage 3).[13, 39] In one 15-year follow-up study of 308 patients, 9% who had Stage 1 disease at presentation progressed to Stage 2, and an additional 2% progressed to Stage 3 apparently without passing through Stage 2.[39] In approximately 70% of 128 patients who had Stage 2 disease at presentation, the radiographic findings returned to normal, in 5% they remained at Stage 2, and in 25% they progressed to Stage 3.

The parenchymal abnormalities in sarcoidosis typically are bilateral and symmetric; although they may be diffuse, in 50% to 80% of patients they involve mainly the upper lung zones.[46, 47] Occasionally, disease is asymmetric, either during the stage of development or resolution;[43] sometimes, it is unilateral.[50] The most frequent patterns are nodular and reticulonodular; less commonly, a reticular pattern, air-space consolidation, or ground-glass opacities predominate.[51, 52] The pattern and extent of parenchymal abnormalities are depicted better on HRCT scan than on radiograph.[51, 54]

Nodular Pattern. A nodular pattern is present on chest radiograph in 30% to 60% of patients (Fig. 9–5).[52, 54] The nodules usually have irregular margins and involve mainly the middle and upper lung zones. Nodules are variable in size and frequently range from 1 to 10 mm in diameter, although most measure less than 3 mm.

On HRCT scan, nodules are seen at presentation in 90% to 100% of patients who have parenchymal abnormalities.[28, 38] They are most numerous along the bronchoarterial and pleural interstitium and adjacent to the interlobar fissures (Fig. 9–6).[28, 38] Extensive nodular thickening of the bronchoarterial interstitium involving mainly the middle and upper lung zones is a characteristic feature of the disease.[46, 56] Nodules commonly are seen along the interlobular septa and centrilobular structures.[28, 55] Correlation of

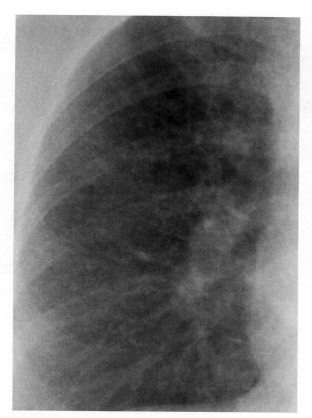

Figure 9–5. Sarcoidosis: Nodular Pattern. View of the right lung from posteroanterior chest radiograph shows numerous nodules measuring approximately 3 mm in diameter, most abundant in the middle and upper lung zones. Similar findings were present in the left lung. The patient was a 37-year-old woman who had Stage 2 sarcoidosis.

HRCT with pathologic findings has shown that the nodules represent a conglomeration of granulomas.[28, 57]

Uncommonly, nodules are diffuse throughout the lung parenchyma; in one study of 150 patients, a diffuse miliary pattern was observed in 2.[22] Rarely, profuse micronodular calcification results in an appearance similar to alveolar microlithiasis.[23] Nodules may appear as dense, round, sharply marginated opacities greater than 1 cm in diameter simulating metastatic cancer.[58, 59] This pattern was observed in 3 of 150 patients in one study;[45] all were African American. Rarely, nodules of this type are solitary.[60, 61] Although nodules greater than 1 cm in diameter are seldom the only finding in pulmonary sarcoidosis, large nodules frequently are seen in association with smaller nodular opacities. Nodules greater than 1 cm in diameter associated with smaller nodules were observed on HRCT scan in 33% of 159 patients in one study;[47] three of the larger nodules were cavitated.

Reticulonodular Pattern. A reticulonodular pattern is present in 25% to 50% of patients who have radiographically evident parenchymal abnormalities (Fig. 9–7).[51, 52] The pattern may result from a combination of nodules and thickening of the interlobular septa or a combination of nodules and intralobular linear opacities.

Reticular Pattern. A reticular pattern is seen in 15% to 20% of patients (Fig. 9–8).[51, 52] This pattern may result from thickening of interlobular septa, intralobular linear opacities, traction bronchiectasis, or, less commonly, honeycombing. On HRCT scan, smooth or nodular thickening of interlobular septa has been described in 20% to 90% of patients, and nonseptal irregular lines have been described in 20% to 70% (Fig. 9–9).[28, 47, 55] The interlobular septal thickening is seldom extensive and, similar to the nodular opacities, tends to involve mainly the central regions of the middle and upper lung zones. Irregular linear opacities usually are associated with distortion of the architecture of the secondary pulmonary lobules, indicating the presence of fibrosis; however, they occasionally are reversible.[28, 54] Fibrosis also leads to dilation and distortion of bronchi (traction bronchiectasis), predominantly in the parahilar regions of the upper lung zones, and to honeycombing (Fig. 9–10).[48] The latter usually involves the subpleural lung regions of the middle and upper lung zones.[48] Occasionally the fibrosis has a predominantly lower lung zone distribution similar to that seen in idiopathic pulmonary fibrosis.[49]

Air-Space Consolidation. Parenchymal consolidation is the predominant finding on chest radiograph in 10% to 20% of patients who have sarcoidosis (Fig. 9–11).[28, 45] The consolidation typically has a bilateral and symmetric distribution, involving mainly the middle and upper lung zones. The appearance may resemble pulmonary edema.[12, 15] Occasionally, it has a lobar distribution;[47] rarely, it has a peripheral distribution resembling chronic eosinophilic pneumonia.[63] In patients in whom the disease is confined largely to the upper lung zones, the pattern may mimic postprimary tuberculosis; in one series of 616 patients, this was identified in 54 (9%).[64]

On HRCT scan, the areas of consolidation may be peribronchial (*see* Fig. 9–11) or, less commonly, peripheral in distribution.[65] Air bronchograms can be seen in most cases.[65] In one review of the HRCT findings in 10 patients, additional findings of small nodules, thickening of the bronchoarterial interstitium, and interlobular septa were present in all;[65] the areas of consolidation involved mainly the upper lung zones in 4 patients, the lower lung zones in 1 patient, and all lung zones in 5 patients. The extent of consolidation and of nodules on HRCT scan correlates with disease activity as assessed by gallium scintigraphy and serum angiotensin–converting enzyme levels.[66] Occasionally the areas of consolidation have a ringlike appearance with a central area of normal lung, a finding referred to as a *fairy ring* appearance.[67]

Ground-Glass Opacities. Hazy areas of increased opacity without obscuration of the vascular markings (ground-glass opacities) seldom are seen on radiograph but commonly are present on HRCT scan (Fig. 9–12). In one review of chest radiographs from 1,652 patients, only 10 (0.6%) showed diffuse ground-glass abnormalities; all had associated hilar or mediastinal lymph node enlargement.[68] By contrast, areas of ground-glass attenuation have been reported on HRCT scan in 20% to 60% of patients.[47, 57, 62] In most of these cases, the ground-glass attenuation is a secondary feature seen in association with small nodules; rarely, it is the predominant abnormality.[57, 69] Correlation of HRCT and pathologic findings has shown the pattern to be related to the presence of interstitial granulomatous inflammation;[57, 70] occasionally, it is the result of microscopic foci of fibrosis in the parenchyma.[69]

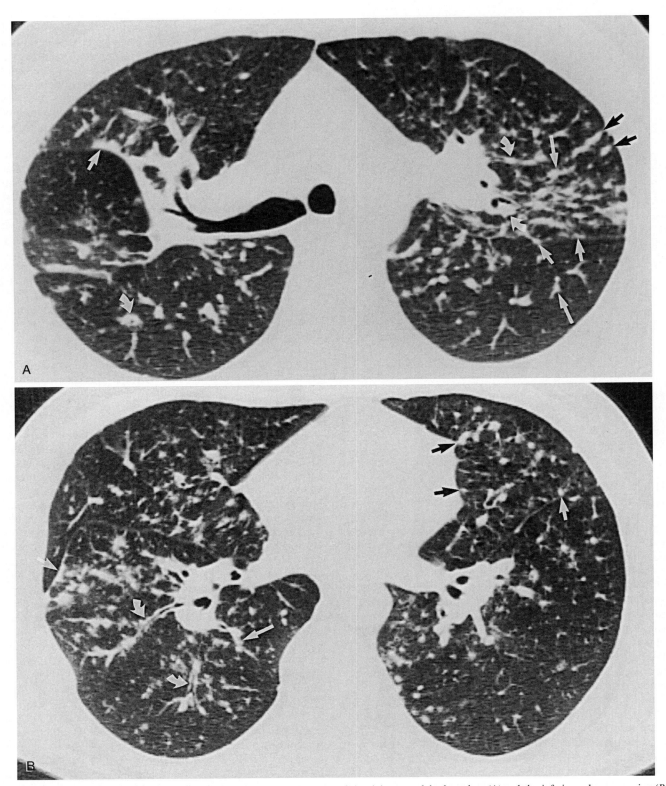

Figure 9–6. Sarcoidosis: HRCT Appearance. HRCT scans at the level of the right upper lobe bronchus *(A)* and the inferior pulmonary veins *(B)* show multiple small nodules. These nodules are located mainly along the bronchi *(curved white arrows)*, pulmonary vessels *(long straight white arrows)*, subpleural lung regions, and interlobar fissures *(short straight white arrows)*. Nodular thickening of interlobular septa is evident *(black arrows)*. The patient was a 37-year-old man who had Stage 2 sarcoidosis.

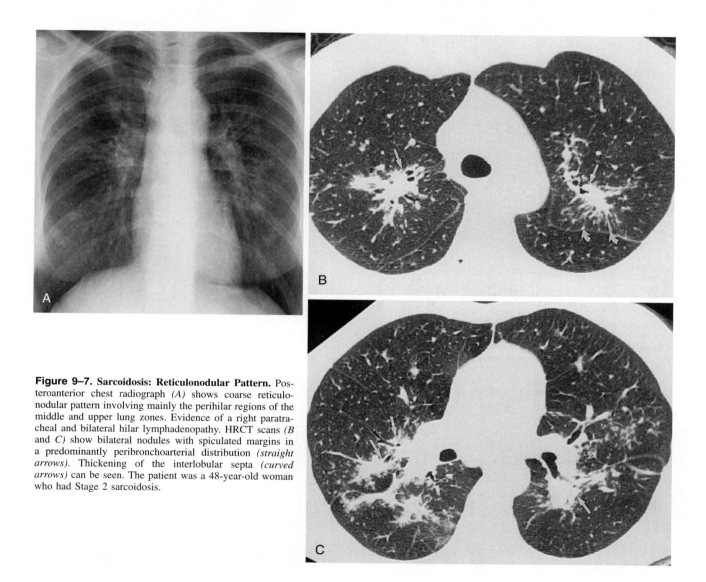

Figure 9–7. Sarcoidosis: Reticulonodular Pattern. Posteroanterior chest radiograph *(A)* shows coarse reticulonodular pattern involving mainly the perihilar regions of the middle and upper lung zones. Evidence of a right paratracheal and bilateral hilar lymphadenopathy. HRCT scans *(B and C)* show bilateral nodules with spiculated margins in a predominantly peribronchoarterial distribution *(straight arrows)*. Thickening of the interlobular septa *(curved arrows)* can be seen. The patient was a 48-year-old woman who had Stage 2 sarcoidosis.

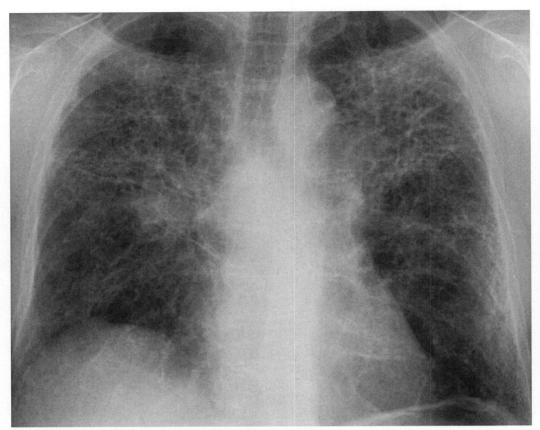

Figure 9–8. Sarcoidosis: Reticular Pattern Associated with Fibrosis. Posteroanterior chest radiograph in a 67-year-old woman with sarcoidosis shows a coarse reticular pattern involving mainly the perihilar regions of the middle and upper lung zones.

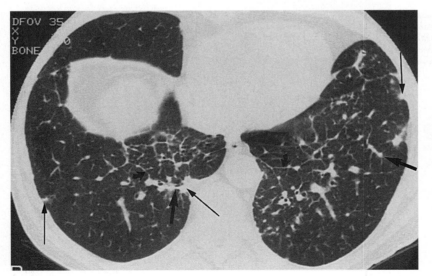

Figure 9–9. Sarcoidosis: Interlobular Septal Thickening. HRCT scan through the lower lung zones shows smooth *(curved arrows)* and nodular *(short straight arrows)* thickening of the interlobular septa. Subpleural nodules *(long thin arrows)* are evident.

Figure 9–10. Sarcoidosis: Pulmonary Fibrosis.
HRCT scan at the level of the aortic arch in a 36-year-old man who had sarcoidosis shows fibrosis involving mainly the peribronchoarterial interstitium. The fibrosis is associated with distortion of lung architecture and posterior displacement of the ectatic upper lobe bronchi. Note thickening of interlobular septa *(straight arrows)*, a few residual centrilobular nodules *(curved arrows)*, and focal areas of ground-glass attenuation *(open arrows)*.

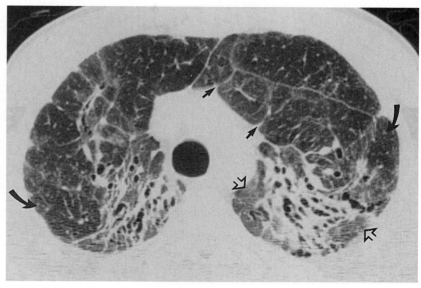

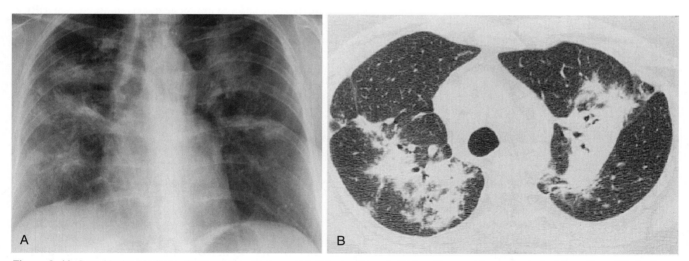

Figure 9–11. Sarcoidosis: Air-Space Consolidation. Posteroanterior chest radiograph *(A)* in a 39-year-old woman who had Stage 2 sarcoidosis shows patchy bilateral areas of consolidation. Air bronchograms can be seen, particularly on the right side. The consolidation involves mainly the perihilar regions of the middle and upper lung zones. HRCT scan *(B)* shows peribronchial distribution of the areas of consolidation and clearly defined air bronchograms.

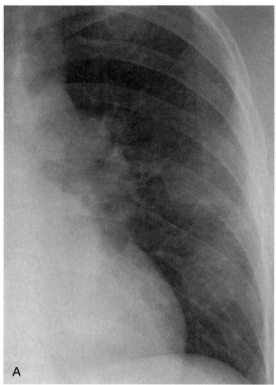

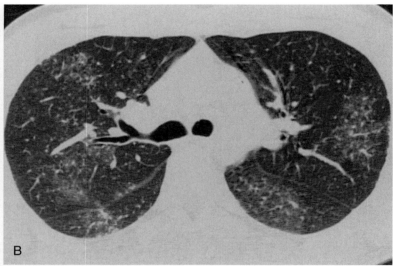

Figure 9–12. Sarcoidosis: Ground-Glass Attenuation. Close-up view of the left lung from posteroanterior chest radiograph *(A)* and HRCT scan *(B)* show patchy areas of ground-glass attenuation containing a few poorly defined nodules. The patient was a 32-year-old man who had Stage 2 sarcoidosis. The diagnosis was proved by transbronchial biopsy.

When pulmonary disease and lymph node enlargement coexist, their radiologic appearance is no different from that of separate involvement. The two manifestations may differ greatly, however, in their temporal relationship in different patients. Diffuse pulmonary disease usually appears when hilar node enlargement is present, although the latter may be regressing. Node enlargement may disappear and be replaced by diffuse pulmonary involvement, either concurrently or several years later, or it may remain and diffuse pulmonary involvement may be superimposed on it.

Fibrosis. As indicated previously, radiologic abnormalities resolve in approximately 50% to 70% of patients who have Stage 2 disease and 20% to 40% of patients who have Stage 3 disease.[13, 39] Many patients who have persistent radiographic abnormalities improve clinically;[71] approximately 20% develop radiologic changes indicative of pulmonary fibrosis.[8, 15] There are no radiographic criteria that allow distinction of reversible from irreversible disease.[15] On HRCT scan, nodules, consolidation, ground-glass attenuation, and interlobular septal thickening may resolve, remain stable, or progress on follow-up.[33, 72] Irregular linear opacities most commonly are irreversible but occasionally resolve.[33, 72] Irreversible abnormalities indicative of fibrosis on HRCT scan include architectural distortion, traction bronchiectasis, and honeycombing.[33, 72] Except for the demonstration of irreversible abnormalities in pulmonary fibrosis, HRCT is not helpful in predicting outcome because there is no difference in the pattern or extent of parenchymal abnormalities in patients who have persistent or progressive disease and patients who improve on follow-up.[55]

The fibrosis in sarcoidosis typically involves mainly the upper lung zones (Fig. 9–13).[12, 15] It usually is associated with superior retraction of the hila, bulla formation, traction bronchiectasis, and compensatory overinflation of the lower lobes *(see* Fig. 9–8).[73] When fibrosis and compensatory overinflation are severe, changes indicative of pulmonary hypertension and cor pulmonale may be seen. On HRCT scan, the fibrosis has a characteristic peribronchovascular distribution radiating from the hila to the upper lobes *(see* Fig. 9–10).[33, 38] Additional findings include irregular lines of attenuation with associated architectural distortion, central conglomeration of ectatic bronchi (Fig. 9–14), conglomerate masses, and, in approximately 40% of cases, subpleural honeycombing.[48] Radiologic differentiation of conglomerate masses of fibrosis in sarcoidosis from those in silicosis can be made readily by the presence of air bronchograms in the former.[48]

Other Radiologic Manifestations

Cavitation. Cavitation is a rare manifestation of sarcoidosis.[47] In one series of 1,254 patients in which the thorax was involved in 94%, cavitation was present in only 8 (0.6%).[6] The abnormality more commonly is apparent on HRCT scan than on radiograph; in one review of 159 patients, cavitated nodules were seen in 3.[47] The cavities tend to be thin walled and are seen in association with other parenchymal abnormalities.[74, 77] They may resolve spontaneously[75] or be complicated by superimposed infection or fungus ball formation.[29, 76, 77] The latter complication occurs in approximately 40% of cystic lesions in sarcoidosis; although most often located in foci of bronchiectasis, they may be seen in bullae or cavities of uncertain origin (Fig. 9–15).[53, 77]

Atelectasis and Air-Trapping. Atelectasis is a rare manifestation of pulmonary sarcoidosis, being observed in

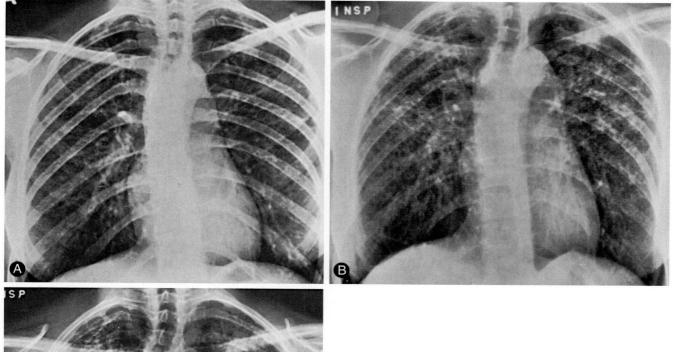

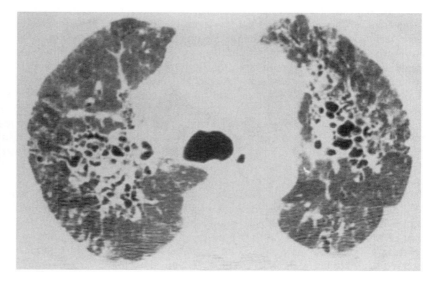

Figure 9–13. Sarcoidosis: Progressive Pulmonary Fibrosis. Initial chest radiograph *(A)* of this 37-year-old woman shows a coarse reticular pattern throughout both lungs with definite upper zonal predominance. There is no evidence of hilar or mediastinal lymph node enlargement. Open-lung biopsy showed non-necrotizing granulomas consistent with sarcoidosis. Three years later *(B)*, the reticulation had become more marked, and there had occurred an upward displacement and flaring of lower zone vessels, indicating the fibrotic nature of the upper zone disease. This was more evident 1 year later *(C)*. Despite the fibrotic nature of the disease, there was no overall reduction in lung volume, chiefly because of overinflation of lower zone parenchyma.

Figure 9–14. Sarcoidosis: Pulmonary Fibrosis. HRCT scan at the level of the tracheal carina shows central conglomeration of ectatic bronchi (traction bronchiectasis) and subpleural nodules. The patient was a 60-year-old man who had Stage 3 sarcoidosis.

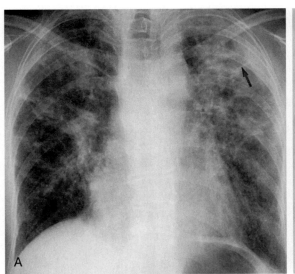
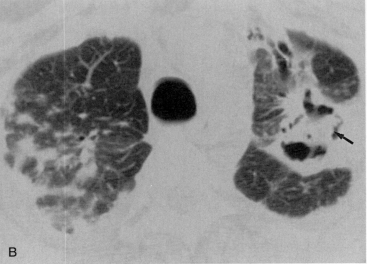

Figure 9–15. Sarcoidosis: Fungus Ball Formation. Posteroanterior chest radiograph *(A)* in a 61-year-old woman who had long-standing sarcoidosis shows a coarse reticulonodular pattern in the upper lobes associated with superior retraction of the hila (indicative of pulmonary fibrosis). A cavity *(arrow)* is seen in the left upper lobe. CT scan *(B)* shows a fungus ball *(arrow)* within the cavity. The patient presented with a history of weight loss and recurrent episodes of blood-streaked sputum.

only 1 of 150 cases in one series,[45] in 1 of 198 cases in another,[20] and in 3 of 300 cases in a third.[78] The atelectasis may be caused by extrinsic compression of bronchi by enlarged lymph nodes, by bronchial mucosal inflammation and fibrosis, or, perhaps most commonly, by a combination of the two.[16, 81] Occasionally, enlarged nodes compress and narrow major bronchi without causing atelectasis.[82] Endobronchial involvement and nodal compression can cause regional alveolar hypoventilation and resultant hypoxic vasoconstriction and local oligemia. Although sarcoidosis rarely causes large airway obstruction, evidence of small airway disease is commonly seen, particularly on HRCT.[79, 83, 212] The findings consist of localized areas of decreased attenuation and oligemia on inspiratory scans and air-trapping on expiratory scans. The areas of decreased attenuation and air-trapping usually have a lobular distribution.[49] In one investigation of 45 patients, localized areas of air-trapping consistent with small airway disease were present on expiratory HRCT scans in 40 patients. Occasionally, the air-trapping on expiratory HRCT may involve subsegmental or segmental regions of lung.[79, 213] Rarely, sarcoidosis presents as emphysema with severe air-flow obstruction.[80] The emphysema presumably results from endoluminal lesions within bronchi and bronchioles leading to peripheral air-trapping and alveolar distention and rupture.[80]

Pleural Disease. Tabulation of the findings of several studies involving 3,146 patients revealed a prevalence of pleural effusion of 2.4%.[16] Approximately one third of pleural effusions are bilateral. In one study of 227 patients in which evidence of pleural involvement specifically was sought, effusion was found in 15 (7%).[84] All of the patients who had effusion manifested moderately advanced pulmonary sarcoidosis; non-necrotizing granulomas were identified on pleural biopsy in 7 of the 15 cases. Pleural effusion tended to clear in 4 to 8 weeks but in some cases progressed to chronic pleural thickening. Given the rarity

with which sarcoidosis causes pleural effusion, its presence should raise the possibility of complicating tuberculosis,[85] coincidental pneumonia, or heart failure.[6, 43]

Pleural thickening and fibrothorax are much more common in sarcoidosis than has been emphasized in the literature, having been identified often at thoracotomy and autopsy.[16] In the study cited previously, the abnormality was identified in 8 (3%) of 227 patients.[84] Such thickening can occur independently of effusion and may be unilateral or bilateral.[84, 86] Affected patients usually are asymptomatic but may have progressive dyspnea.[86] Rarely, sarcoidosis presents as a discrete pleural mass.[87]

Spontaneous pneumothorax has been estimated to occur in 1% to 2% of patients.[88, 89] Bullae tend to develop in the upper lobes in advanced fibrotic disease, and they have been said to rupture in approximately 5% of cases.[88] It is probable, however, that in the absence of bullae, pneumothorax represents a coincidental occurrence and is of the same etiology as that which occurs spontaneously in a susceptible young male population. Bilateral pneumothorax occurs rarely.[82, 90]

Skeletal Disease. Radiographic evidence of bone involvement is seen in approximately 3% of patients,[16] usually in the setting of long-standing disease. The short tubular bones of the hands and feet are affected most commonly.[16, 91] Findings include cystic lesions, punched-out cortical lesions, or a lacelike trabecular pattern. Rapid progression may lead to pathologic fractures.[16] Rarely, combined osteolytic and osteoblastic changes have been described in the vertebral bodies, sternum, or ribs.[16, 92] In one study of 25 untreated patients who had chronic sarcoidosis, 14 had evidence of vertebral osteoporosis.[93]

Cardiovascular Disease. Although abnormalities of the heart, pericardium, and pulmonary vasculature are seen commonly on histologic examination, they are usually of insufficient severity to cause radiographic manifestations. Radiographically evident enlargement of the cardiac silhouette may be the result of congestive cardiomyopathy, valvular disease, pericardial effusion, and left ventricular aneurysm.[94–96] Such cardiac abnormalities may occur in patients with or without lymph node enlargement or evidence of pulmonary disease.[95] Pulmonary hypertension and cor pulmonale, caused by a combination of obliteration of the pulmonary vascular bed and hypoxic vasoconstriction, tend to occur in the late stage of the disease but can develop earlier.[82] Obstruction of major pulmonary arteries and veins and the superior vena cava by enlarged lymph nodes is rare.[82]

Abdominal Manifestations. Abdominal lymph node enlargement, hepatomegaly, and splenomegaly are common radiologic findings.[32, 97] In one investigation of 59 patients, abdominal CT scans showed extensive lymph node enlargement in 6 (10%), hepatomegaly in 5 (8%), and splenomegaly in 4 (6%) patients.[32] Nodules were seen in the spleen in eight patients (15%) and in the liver in three (5%). In another review of 46 patients, lymph node enlargement was present in 20 (43%), splenomegaly or low attenuation lesions in 24 (52%), and hepatomegaly or low attenuation liver lesions in 7 (15%).[97]

Gallium 67 Scanning

Gallium 67 scintigraphy has been used for many years to detect sites of inflammation or neoplasia in the lungs and elsewhere.[99] The results of many (albeit not all[100]) investigations suggest that the correlation between the percentage of lymphocytes found in bronchoalveolar lavage fluid and gallium 67 scintiscans is good.[101, 102] The sensitivity of gallium 67 scintigraphy in detecting inflammatory lesions in general has been estimated to range from 80% to more than 90%. This test has been used on occasion to detect the presence of pulmonary disease in patients who have Stages 0 and 1 disease.[103, 104]

IDIOPATHIC INTERSTITIAL PNEUMONIAS

The interstitial pneumonias are a heterogeneous group of inflammatory diseases that have been referred to by a variety of terms,[106, 125] the earliest of which were based on their histologic patterns.[105] These terms included *usual interstitial pneumonia*, characterized by variable thickening of alveolar interstitium by fibrous tissue and mononuclear inflammatory cells; *desquamative interstitial pneumonia*, in which there is a striking accumulation of macrophages in the alveolar air spaces associated with relatively mild but uniform interstitial thickening; *lymphoid interstitial pneumonia*, in which there is marked infiltration of parenchymal interstitium by lymphocytes, plasma cells, or both; and *giant cell interstitial pneumonia*, consisting of an interstitial infiltrate of mononuclear inflammatory cells associated with large numbers of multinucleated giant cells in the interstitium and adjacent air spaces.

Some of these histologic patterns can be regarded as a tissue reaction to several causative agents rather than as a manifestation of a specific disease. The pattern of giant cell interstitial pneumonia can be seen with infection by several viruses and with exposure to hard metal dust, whereas lymphoid interstitial pneumonia can be seen in patients who have autoimmune disease, such as Sjögren's

Table 9–2. IDIOPATHIC INTERSTITIAL PNEUMONIAS: CHARACTERISTIC HISTOLOGIC FINDINGS

Usual interstitial pneumonia
    Heterogeneous pattern with foci of normal lung, active inflammation, and end-stage fibrosis
Desquamative interstitial pneumonia
    Homogeneous pattern with predominance of intra-alveolar macrophages
Nonspecific interstitial pneumonia
    Homogeneous pattern with predominance of interstitial mononuclear cell infiltrate
Acute interstitial pneumonia
    Diffuse alveolar damage, pulmonary edema, hyaline membranes

syndrome, or who have acquired immunodeficiency syndrome (AIDS). The other patterns are associated less clearly with specific causative agents and often have been refered to as *idiopathic pulmonary fibrosis* or *cryptogenic fibrosing alveolitis*.[106, 125] Although several classifications of such idiopathic conditions have been proposed,[105, 106, 125] we favor a division into four subtypes: usual interstitial pneumonia, desquamative interstitial pneumonia, nonspecific interstitial pneumonia, and acute interstitial pneumonia (Table 9–2). The grouping of these four forms of idiopathic interstitial pneumonia under the single term *idiopathic pulmonary fibrosis* is unfortunate because the various entities have different clinical, radiologic, and histologic manifestations and different prognoses.[125] The international consensus statement published in 2000 recommended that the designation *idiopathic pulmonary fibrosis* be limited to disease that has a pattern of usual interstitial pneumonia on histologic examination.[152] As its name implies, idiopathic pulmonary fibrosis is unassociated with other conditions known to be associated with interstitial pneumonitis and fibrosis, such as connective tissue disease, hypersensitivity pneumonitis, exposure to occupational inorganic dusts (pneumoconiosis), or drug intake.[152]

Idiopathic Pulmonary Fibrosis

Pathologic Characteristics

As indicated, idiopathic pulmonary fibrosis is characterized histologically by a variable degree of interstitial disease, with areas of normal and markedly diseased lung being present in different regions of the same lobe as well as in a single lobule. In early disease, alveolar septa are thickened slightly by an infiltrate of inflammatory cells; lymphocytes usually are the most numerous. In more advanced disease, the interstitial thickening is greater and usually is associated with some degree of fibrosis. In the most severely affected areas, interstitial thickening is so marked that alveoli are reduced to small slits or are obliterated completely; at this stage, fibrous tissue usually is more abundant than the inflammatory cell infiltrate. Such fibrosis often is associated with dilation of transitional airways (traction bronchiolectasis), representing the histologic counterpart of grossly evident honeycomb lung.

Grossly the early stage of idiopathic pulmonary fibrosis consists of only a slight coarseness of the normal parenchyma, typically most severe in the subpleural regions and

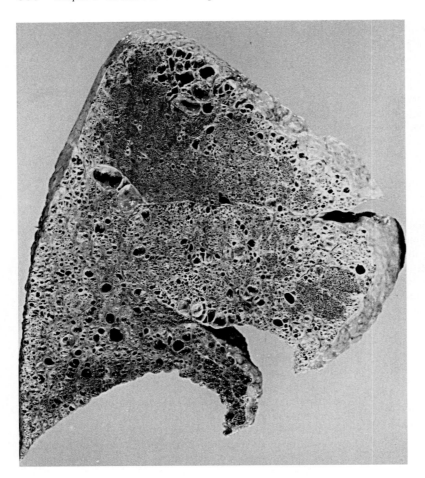

Figure 9–16. Idiopathic Pulmonary Fibrosis: Advanced Stage. Sagittal section of a right lung shows advanced interstitial fibrosis with extensive *honeycomb* change. There is relative sparing of the central portion of the upper lobe.

in the basal and posterior portions of the lower lobes. As disease progresses, clear-cut areas of fibrosis alternating with small cystic spaces 1 to 2 mm in diameter become evident. Eventually, large portions of a lobe can be affected, resulting in numerous 5- to 10-mm cystic spaces separated by a variable amount of firm fibrous tissue (*honeycomb lung*) (Fig. 9–16). These changes usually are most prominent in the lower lobes, particularly the subpleural regions; the central portion of all the lobes is relatively spared.

Abnormalities of the large airways, of which bronchiectasis is the most common, also can be seen in idiopathic pulmonary fibrosis; in one autopsy study of 12 patients who had advanced disease, this complication was identified in 9.[110] The observation that the ectasia is confined largely to areas of pronounced interstitial fibrosis suggests that its cause is retraction of the adjacent fibrous tissue (traction bronchiectasis).

Clinical Manifestations

Most patients are between 50 and 70 years old. Symptoms include progressive dyspnea over several months, nonproductive cough, weight loss, and fatigue.[109] Clubbing is common,[142] and its presence can antedate symptoms and other signs of pulmonary disease.[143] In most patients, deterioration is gradual and inexorable with increasing shortness of breath often accompanied by the development of cor pulmonale. Most patients succumb to respiratory failure, frequently precipitated by infection;[146] about 20% die from cardiac disease.[145] The overall mean survival is less than 5 years.[147, 148]

Radiologic Manifestations

Radiographic Findings

The most common radiographic finding, described in approximately 80% of patients who have biopsy-proven disease, consists of bilateral irregular linear opacities causing a reticular pattern (Table 9–3, Fig. 9–17).[111–113] Although these opacities may be diffuse throughout both lungs, in 50% to 80% of cases they involve predominantly or exclusively the lower lung zones;[112, 113] in 60%, a pre-

Table 9–3. IDIOPATHIC PULMONARY FIBROSIS: CHARACTERISTIC CLINICAL AND RADIOLOGIC MANIFESTATIONS

Patients between 50 and 70 years old
Progressive dyspnea, dry cough over several months
Clubbing and crackles on physical examination
Irregular linear opacities (reticular pattern) on radiograph
Bilateral, symmetric distribution
Lower lobe predominance
Progressive loss in lung volume
Reticulation and honeycombing on HRCT
Predominantly subpleural and basal distribution on HRCT

HRCT, high-resolution computed tomography.

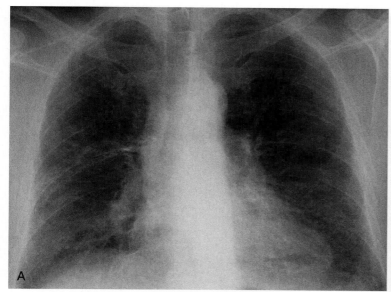

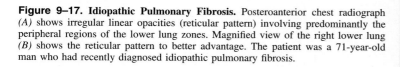

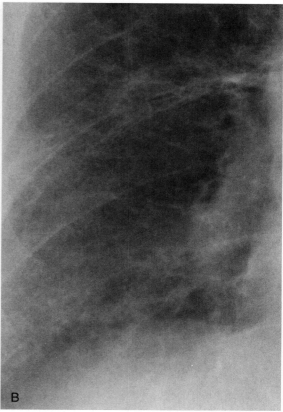

Figure 9–17. Idiopathic Pulmonary Fibrosis. Posteroanterior chest radiograph *(A)* shows irregular linear opacities (reticular pattern) involving predominantly the peripheral regions of the lower lung zones. Magnified view of the right lower lung *(B)* shows the reticular pattern to better advantage. The patient was a 71-year-old man who had recently diagnosed idiopathic pulmonary fibrosis.

dominant peripheral distribution is apparent.[54] Cystic changes related to honeycombing can be identified in 30% to 70% of patients.[46, 115] Basal areas of ground-glass opacity are present in approximately 30% of patients and diffuse ground-glass opacity in 10% to 15%.[111, 114] Less common abnormalities include small nodular opacities (seen in approximately 10% of patients) and a combination of irregular linear and nodular opacities (reticulonodular pattern [seen in 20%]).[112]

In patients who have mild disease, the findings usually consist of symmetric, basal, small- to medium-size, irregular linear shadows (reticular pattern).[111, 116] As the disease progresses, the abnormalities become more diffuse and assume a coarser reticular or reticulonodular pattern associated with progressive loss of volume. *End-stage* disease is characterized by the presence of cysts measuring 0.5–1 cm in diameter.[115, 116] Radiographic evidence of pleural disease is uncommon; in one study of 95 patients, effusions were observed in 4%, pneumothorax in 7%, and diffuse pleural thickening in 6%.[117]

Decreased lung volumes are evident radiographically at presentation in 50% to 60% of cases.[44, 111] We have been impressed by the striking loss of lung volume apparent on serial radiograph studies over a period of several years and consider that a diffuse or predominantly basal reticular pattern accompanied by progressive elevation of the diaphragm—signs that occur much less frequently in other forms of diffuse interstitial fibrosis—strongly suggests the diagnosis of either idiopathic pulmonary fibrosis or progressive systemic sclerosis.[118]

The accuracy of chest radiography in the diagnosis of idiopathic pulmonary fibrosis has been assessed in several studies.[46, 54, 120] In one investigation of 118 consecutive patients who had various chronic interstitial or air-space diseases, radiographs were reviewed independently by three observers without knowledge of clinical or pathologic data.[46] A confident diagnosis of idiopathic pulmonary fibrosis was made on the basis of the radiographic findings in 30% of cases; this diagnosis was correct in 87% of cases. In another study of 86 patients who had various chronic interstitial lung diseases (of which 24 were idiopathic pulmonary fibrosis) and 14 control subjects, a correct diagnosis of idiopathic pulmonary fibrosis was suggested as a first-choice diagnosis in 17 of 24 (69%).[120] The diagnostic value of chest radiography when combined with clinical information was evaluated in another study of 208 patients who had various chronic interstitial lung diseases;[54] the diagnosis of idiopathic pulmonary fibrosis was made with a high degree of confidence in 47% of patients who had idiopathic pulmonary fibrosis based on clinical data alone and in 79% of patients based on a combination of clinical and radiographic findings. Although these studies confirm that the radiographic findings of idiopathic pulmonary fibrosis often are sufficient to suggest the diagnosis, the chest radiograph is normal in about 10% to 15% of patients.[111, 121]

Computed Tomography Findings

Idiopathic pulmonary fibrosis is characterized on CT scan by the presence of fine or coarse, irregular lines of attenuation (reticular pattern) involving predominantly the subpleural lung regions and the lower lung zones (Fig. 9–18).[122, 125] A patchy distribution is apparent in most cases,

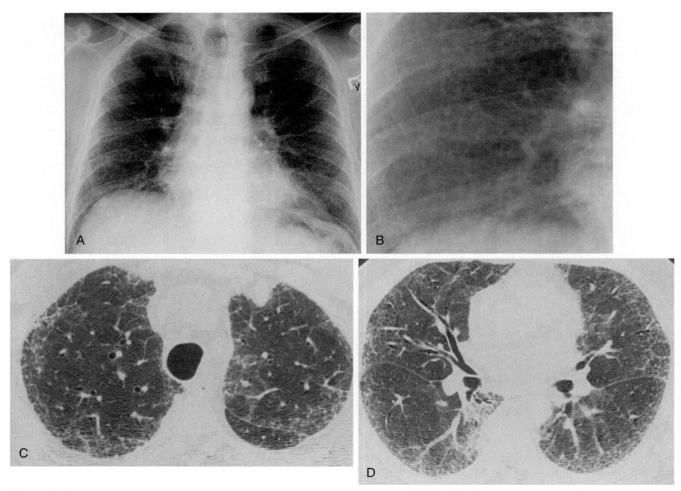

Figure 9–18. Idiopathic Pulmonary Fibrosis. Posteroanterior chest radiograph *(A)* shows a fine bilateral reticular pattern and associated loss of lung volume. The reticular pattern is appreciated better on the magnified view of the right lower lung *(B)*. HRCT scan through the lung apices *(C)* shows irregular lines of attenuation involving predominantly the subpleural lung regions. HRCT scan at the level of the right middle lobe bronchus *(D)* shows more extensive parenchymal involvement. The predominant subpleural distribution is still apparent, however. The reticular pattern on CT scan is due to irregular thickening of interlobular septa and the presence of intralobular lines. Areas of ground-glass attenuation are present also involving mainly the subpleural lung regions. The patient was a 66-year-old man.

with areas that have a reticular pattern intermingled with areas of normal lung (Fig. 9–19).[122, 125] The irregular lines of attenuation usually are associated with irregular pleural, vascular, and bronchial interfaces; evidence of architectural distortion; and dilation of bronchi and bronchioles (traction bronchiectasis and bronchiolectasis).[123, 125] Air-containing cysts measuring 2 to 20 mm in diameter (honeycombing) are seen in 80% to 90% of patients at presentation (*see* Fig. 9–19).[115, 126] These findings are appreciated much better on HRCT scans than on conventional 7- to 10-mm collimation scans.[122]

A crescentic, predominantly subpleural distribution of the reticular pattern of fibrosis is evident on HRCT scan in about 80% to 95% of patients.[119, 122, 155] In about 70% of patients, the fibrosis is most severe in the lower lung zones; in about 20%, all zones are involved to a similar degree; and in 10%, mainly the upper lung zones are affected.[46, 127] Serial HRCT scans show an increase in the extent of the reticular pattern and evidence of honeycombing in virtually all cases (Fig. 9–20).[126, 128] The progression of honeycombing is significantly faster in patients who have exten-

sive areas of ground-glass attenuation on HRCT scan or marked disease activity on open-lung biopsy specimens.[128] Cystic spaces related to honeycombing have been shown to decrease in size on HRCT scans performed after forced expiration.[132, 133] Rarely, fine linear or small nodular foci of calcification are seen within areas of fibrosis as a result of ossification.[134] The subpleural predominance of reticulation or honeycombing is the most characteristic feature of idiopathic pulmonary fibrosis on HRCT scan; lack of this feature should suggest an alternative diagnosis.

Areas of ground-glass attenuation have been described on HRCT scan in 65% to 100% of patients (Fig. 9–21).[48, 123, 129] These areas usually reflect the presence of active inflammation and potentially treatable disease.[69, 130, 135] In one study of 12 patients in whom the presence of ground-glass attenuation on CT scans was compared with pathologic measures of disease activity, 7 patients were categorized histologically as having mild disease activity and 5 patients were categorized as having moderate to marked activity;[135] CT scans showed areas of ground-glass attenuation in all 5 patients who had marked disease activity

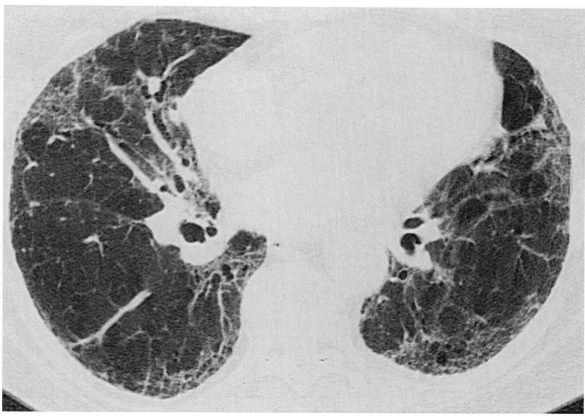

Figure 9–19. Idiopathic Pulmonary Fibrosis. HRCT scan shows a characteristic variegated pattern of idiopathic pulmonary fibrosis, the findings consisting of areas with irregular lines, areas with honeycombing, and areas of ground-glass attenuation intermingled with areas of normal lung. The parenchymal abnormalities have a patchy but predominantly subpleural distribution. The patient was an 80-year-old woman.

Figure 9–20. Idiopathic Pulmonary Fibrosis with Traction Bronchiectasis. HRCT scan shows bilateral honeycombing involving predominantly the subpleural lung regions. Bronchial dilation (traction bronchiectasis) *(arrows)* is evident within the areas of fibrosis, particularly in the right lower lobe. The patient was an 81-year-old man.

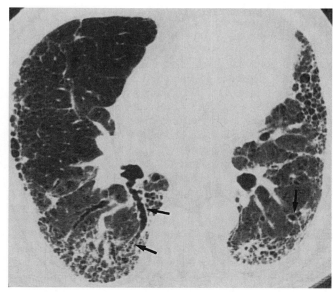

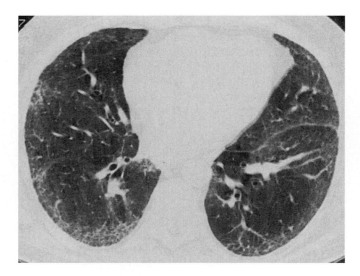

Figure 9–21. Idiopathic Pulmonary Fibrosis with Ground-Glass Attenuation. HRCT scan shows bilateral areas of ground-glass attenuation in a patchy distribution. Also noted are irregular thickening of interlobular septa and intralobular lines giving a fine reticular pattern, particularly in the subpleural regions of the lower lobes. Lung biopsy showed usual interstitial pneumonia with predominant inflammation and relatively mild fibrosis. The patient was a 61-year-old man.

(sensitivity, 100%) and 2 of 7 patients who had mild activity (specificity, 70%).[135] In another investigation of 14 patients, 12 (86%) with idiopathic pulmonary fibrosis who had areas of ground-glass attenuation on HRCT scan had marked inflammation on biopsy.[69]

Mediastinal lymph node enlargement is evident on CT in 70% to 90% of patients.[136, 137] The enlargement is usually mild, with nodes measuring 10 to 15 mm in short-axis diameter and involving only one or two nodal stations (most commonly the right lower paratracheal region).[136] As a result, the node enlargement typically is not apparent on radiograph. There is evidence that the prevalence of lymph node enlargement is lower in patients receiving corticosteroid therapy. In one investigation, enlarged mediastinal nodes were seen on HRCT scan in 3 of 22 (14%) patients who had received oral corticosteroids 2 months before the date of the CT examination and in 23 of 32 (71%) patients who had not taken corticosteroids for at least 6 months before the HRCT scan.[138]

The diagnostic accuracy of HRCT in the diagnosis of idiopathic pulmonary fibrosis has been assessed in several studies.[46, 54, 139] In one study, the accuracy of CT was compared with that of chest radiography in the prediction of specific diagnoses in 34 patients who had idiopathic pulmonary fibrosis and 84 patients who had other chronic interstitial diseases.[119] The radiographs and CT scans were assessed independently by three observers without knowledge of clinical or pathologic data. A confident diagnosis of idiopathic pulmonary fibrosis was made on CT scan in 73% of patients; this diagnosis was correct 95% of the time. By comparison, a confident diagnosis was made in only 30% of chest radiographs (the diagnosis being correct in 87% of cases).

In another study of 41 patients who had idiopathic pulmonary fibrosis and 45 who had various other diffuse lung diseases, two independent observers correctly and confidently discriminated between the two groups with an accuracy of 88% on HRCT and 76% on chest radiography.[139] The false-negative rate for idiopathic pulmonary fibrosis decreased from 29% on chest radiography to 11% on HRCT, and the false-positive rate decreased from 19% to 13%.[139] In a third investigation of 85 patients (including 18 who had idiopathic pulmonary fibrosis and who underwent biopsy), CT scan images were reviewed by two radiologists who reached a decision by consensus.[141] The correct diagnosis of idiopathic pulmonary fibrosis was made as a first-choice diagnosis in 16 of 18 (89%) patients; the diagnosis was correct in all 12 patients in whom a first-choice diagnosis of idiopathic pulmonary fibrosis was made with a high degree of confidence. The accuracy of a confident diagnosis of idiopathic pulmonary fibrosis made on HRCT by an experienced chest radiologist is approximately 95%. The accuracy of interpretation by less experienced observers is substantially lower.[47, 140]

The diagnostic accuracy based on the HRCT findings increases with severity of disease. In one study, the scans of 61 consecutive patients who had end-stage lung disease (defined by the presence of honeycombing, extensive cystic changes, or conglomerate fibrosis) were assessed independently by two observers without knowledge of clinical or pathologic data;[211] a correct first-choice diagnosis of idiopathic pulmonary fibrosis was made in 23 of the 26 cases (88%); when the observers were confident in their first-choice diagnosis (based on the presence of predominantly subpleural and lower lung zone honeycombing), they made a correct diagnosis in all cases. (The diagnosis of idiopathic pulmonary fibrosis in these patients was established by biopsy specimens taken from relatively uninvolved areas or before the development of end-stage disease.)

Conditions that commonly have similar parenchymal abnormalities as idiopathic pulmonary fibrosis are progressive systemic sclerosis, rheumatoid arthritis, and asbestosis.[150–152] Asbestosis can be recognized readily on HRCT scan by the presence of pleural plaques. A reticular pattern and honeycombing also are commonly seen in chronic hypersensitivity pneumonitis. The distinction from idiopathic pulmonary fibrosis usually can be made readily on HRCT scan by the presence of centrilobular nodules and the relative sparing of the lung bases in patients with hypersensitivity pneumonitis.[153]

HRCT has been shown to be much more sensitive than chest radiography in the detection of early or mild interstitial lung disease.[121, 152, 154] Rarely, patients with normal idiopathic pulmonary fibrosis can have a normal HRCT scan, however.[121, 152]

Desquamative Interstitial Pneumonia

The cause and pathogenesis of desquamative interstitial pneumonia are unknown. The histologic pattern has been seen in association with nitrofurantoin therapy,[156] leukemia,[157] and a variety of inhaled particulates.[158–160] Desquamative interstitial pneumonia also bears some resemblance to smoking-related respiratory bronchiolitis (*see* Chapter 15).[161] Because about 90% of patients who have desquamative interstitial pneumonia are smokers,[111, 165] and because there is considerable overlap between the histologic findings of desquamative interstitial pneumonia and those of respiratory bronchiolitis–interstitial lung disease, it has been suggested that the term *desquamative interstitial pneumonia* be replaced by respiratory bronchiolitis–interstitial lung disease.[106] Histologically, respiratory bronchiolitis–interstitial lung disease has a predominantly bronchiolocentric distribution, however, whereas desquamative interstitial pneumonia is diffuse. Although respiratory bronchiolitis–interstitial lung disease and desquamative interstitial pneumonia may represent different parts of the spectrum of the same disease process, we consider them to be separate entities.

In contrast to the variable histologic appearance characteristic of idiopathic pulmonary fibrosis, the pattern of desquamative interstitial pneumonia is distinctly uniform, with all portions of lung on a tissue section appearing more or less similar. The alveolar interstitium usually is mildly to moderately thickened by an infiltrate of mononuclear inflammatory cells (predominantly lymphocytes) and a small amount of collagen. Alveolar air spaces characteristically are filled with numerous alveolar macrophages.

Desquamative interstitial pneumonia is uncommon, accounting for approximately 5% of cases of interstitial pneumonitis of unknown etiology.[108, 175] Most patients are between 30 and 50 years old. The most common clinical manifestation is dyspnea on exertion.[167] Rarely, disease is discovered after the performance of a routine chest radiograph.[167] Cough has been reported in about half of patients; fever, diaphoresis, weight loss, weakness, myalgia, chest pain, and fatigue are seen in a few patients.

The characteristic radiographic pattern consists of symmetric bilateral ground-glass opacification, which can be diffuse but usually involves mainly the lower lung zones (Table 9–4, Fig. 9–22).[153, 162] In patients who have fibrosis, irregular linear opacities can be seen predominantly in the lower lung zones.[111, 163] Hilar lymph node enlargement has been reported in a few cases;[162, 164] pleural effusion is rare.[155] The chest radiograph has been reported to be normal in 3% to 22% of patients who have biopsy-proven disease.[111, 120, 163]

The predominant abnormality on HRCT scan is the presence of bilateral areas of ground-glass attenuation.[165, 166] In one review of 22 patients, this ground-glass attenuation involved the mid and lower lung zones in all patients and the upper lung zones in 18 (82%) patients.[165] The distribution was predominantly peripheral in 13 patients (59%), patchy and bilateral in 5 (23%), and diffuse in 4 (18%). Irregular lines of attenuation (reticular pattern) suggestive

Table 9–4. DESQUAMATIVE INTERSTITIAL PNEUMONIA: CHARACTERISTIC CLINICAL AND RADIOLOGIC MANIFESTATIONS

Patients between 30 and 50 years old
90% of patients are smokers
Progressive dyspnea, dry cough over several months
Ground-glass opacities on chest radiograph
Bilateral symmetric distributon
Lower lobe predominance
Mild if any reticulation on radiograph
Ground-glass attenuation on HRCT
Predominantly basal distribution
Mild if any reticulation on HRCT
Minimal if any honeycombing

HRCT, high-resolution computed tomography.

of fibrosis were seen in 11 patients (50%), and cystic changes (honeycombing) were seen in 7 (32%). The fibrosis was most marked in the lower lung zones in 11 patients, mid lung zones in 1 patient, and upper lung zones in 1 patient. Mild honeycombing was seen in 7 of the 22 patients and was present almost exclusively in the lung bases. In a second investigation of eight patients, all showed areas of ground-glass attenuation involving the mid and lower lung zones, predominantly in the lung periphery;[166] less common findings included a mild reticular pattern in five patients, architectural distortion in three, and traction bronchiectasis in one. Although small cystic changes were seen in areas with ground-glass attenuation, these were considered to represent traction bronchiolectasis rather than areas of honeycombing.

The natural history of areas of ground-glass attenuation was assessed in a follow-up study of 11 patients.[129] On initial CT scans, all 11 patients had areas of ground-glass attenuation involving approximately 50% of the lung parenchyma, 5 patients had irregular linear opacities involving approximately 5% of the lung parenchyma, and 1 patient had mild honeycombing. Follow-up HRCT scans performed after a median interval of 10 months and after treatment (predominantly corticosteroids alone) showed a decrease in the extent of parenchymal abnormalities in six patients, no change in three, and a slight increase in the extent of abnormalities in two. The improvement on the follow-up CT scan was related to a decrease in the extent of areas of ground-glass attenuation (Fig. 9–23). The two patients who had progression of disease showed an increase in the extent of irregular lines or the development of mild honeycombing.[129] In another follow-up investigation of eight patients, all showed initial decrease in extent of ground-glass attenuation with treatment; however, the extent of ground-glass attenuation subsequently increased in three patients despite treatment.[166]

Nonspecific Interstitial Pneumonia

Nonspecific interstitial pneumonia is a form of interstitial lung disease that resembles idiopathic pulmonary fibrosis clinically but that appears to be associated with a significantly different course and outcome.[168, 210] The abnormality differs pathologically from idiopathic pulmonary fibrosis by its uniform appearance: Idiopathic pulmo-

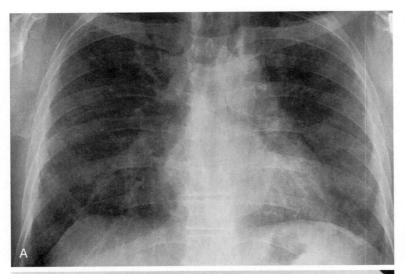

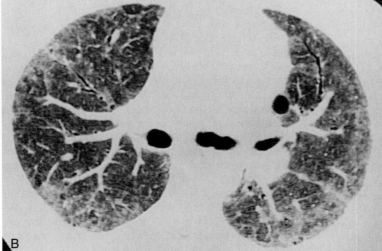

Figure 9–22. Desquamative Interstitial Pneumonia. Anteroposterior chest radiograph *(A)* shows ground-glass opacification throughout all lung zones. HRCT scan *(B)* shows extensive bilateral ground-glass attenuation most marked in the subpleural lung regions. Incidental note is made of a bulla adjacent to the left heart border.

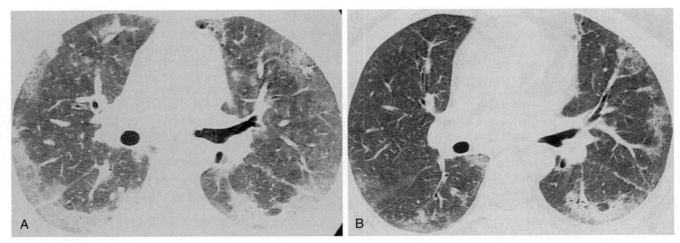

Figure 9–23. Desquamative Interstitial Pneumonia: Improvement on Follow-Up. HRCT scan at presentation *(A)* shows extensive bilateral areas of ground-glass attenuation involving predominantly the subpleural lung regions. A few irregular linear opacities are present in the subpleural regions and are consistent with mild fibrosis. HRCT scan 18 months later *(B)* shows marked improvement in the areas of ground-glass attenuation. Mild residual fibrosis is present, particularly in the subpleural regions of the left lung. (Courtesy of Dr. Georgeann McGuinness, Department of Radiology, New York University Medical Center, New York.)

nary fibrosis typically shows a combination of active inflammation and fibrogenesis associated with changes of more long-standing injury, such as mature fibrous tissue and cyst formation, whereas nonspecific interstitial pneumonia is characterized by an appearance that suggests a single initiating event.

This form of interstitial lung disease accounts for about 5% to 15% of patients who historically were included in series of patients believed to have idiopathic pulmonary fibrosis.[144, 175] Symptoms are similar to those associated with idiopathic pulmonary fibrosis but often are less severe and considerably more indolent in progression. Some patients have been reported to have influenza-like symptoms associated with mild dyspnea.[176] In one study of 15 such patients, the mean duration of symptoms before diagnosis was 18 months.[210] Most patients are between 40 and 70 years old.[106]

The term *nonspecific interstitial pneumonia* initially was proposed as a diagnosis of exclusion for pathologic specimens that did not have the typical findings of usual interstitial pneumonia, desquamative interstitial pneumonia, acute interstitial pneumonia, or bronchiolitis obliterans organizing pneumonia.[168] Nonspecific interstitial pneumonia encompasses a wide range of histologic features with varying degrees of interstitial inflammation and fibrosis.[168, 169]

The most common radiographic manifestations consist of areas of ground-glass opacification or consolidation involving mainly the mid and lower lung zones (Table 9–5, Fig. 9–24).[170] Other abnormalities include a reticular pattern[168] and a combination of interstitial and air-space patterns.[168, 170, 173]

Table 9–5. NONSPECIFIC INTERSTITIAL PNEUMONIA: CHARACTERISTIC CLINICAL AND RADIOLOGIC MANIFESTATIONS

Patients between 40 and 70 years old
Progressive dyspnea, dry cough over several months
Ground-glass opacities, reticulation or consolidation on chest radiograph
Bilateral, symmetric distribution
Lower lobe predominance
HRCT pattern variable. Most common finding: bilateral ground-glass attenuation. Other findings: consolidation and reticulation
Other finding:
Distribution can be peribronchovascular, random, or, less commonly, predominantly subpleural

HRCT, high-resolution computed tomography.

The HRCT manifestations are heterogeneous and often mimic those of desquamative interstitial pneumonia, bronchiolitis obliterans organizing pneumonia, or usual interstitial pneumonia.[171, 174] The most common manifestations consist of bilateral symmetric areas of ground-glass attenuation with or without areas of consolidation.[170–172] The ground-glass opacities can have a subpleural distribution, can have a random distribution, or can be diffuse.[172] The areas of consolidation may have a predominantly peribronchial or subpleural distribution.[171, 172, 174] Other common abnormalities include irregular linear opacities, thickening of the bronchovascular bundles, and bronchial dilation.[172, 174] Irregular linear opacities are seen in 40% to 80% of patients.[151, 171] They tend to involve mainly the subpleural lung regions and lower lung zones. Honeycombing has been reported in 0 to 30% of cases.[151, 171]

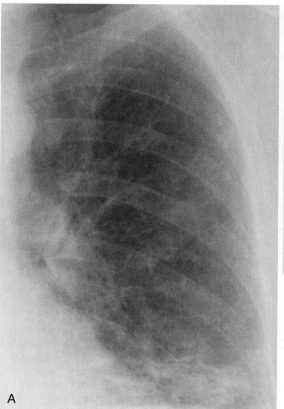

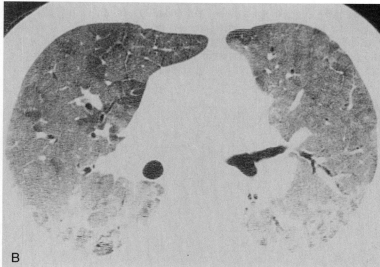

Figure 9–24. Nonspecific Interstitial Pneumonia. View of the left lung from posteroanterior chest radiograph *(A)* shows diffuse ground-glass opacification of the left lung and focal areas of consolidation and irregular linear opacities in the left lower lung zone. Similar findings were present in the right lung. HRCT scan *(B)* shows extensive bilateral areas of ground-glass attenuation. Small focal areas of consolidation are present in the dependent lung regions. The patient was a 44-year-old man who had biopsy-proven nonspecific interstitial pneumonitis.

The heterogeneous appearance of nonspecific interstitial pneumonia on HRCT is not surprising given the initial definition of nonspecific interstitial pneumonia as a pathologic diagnosis of exclusion for patients who do not have histologic features characteristic of usual interstitial pneumonia, desquamative interstitial pneumonia, acute interstitial pneumonia, or bronchiolitis obliterans organizing pneumonia.[168, 171, 174] The heterogeneous appearance also raises the possibility that nonspecific interstitial pneumonia, as currently defined, may represent more than one disease entity.

Survival of patients who have nonspecific interstitial pneumonia is substantially better than that of patients who have idiopathic pulmonary fibrosis.[108, 144, 177, 210] In one study, almost 80% of 14 patients who had nonspecific interstitial pneumonia were alive 10 years after diagnosis compared with less than 10% of 63 patients who had idiopathic pulmonary fibrosis.[144] In another investigation of 48 patients considered to have nonspecific interstitial pneumonia, only 5 (11%) had died in the follow-up period, and almost 50% recovered completely, figures much better than those for idiopathic pulmonary fibrosis.[168]

Acute Interstitial Pneumonia

In 1935, Hamman and Rich[178] described an acute (fulminating) variety of interstitial pulmonary disease characterized by rapid progression of signs and symptoms leading to death in less than 1 year. Review of the histologic descriptions of some of their patients and more recent studies of patients who had similar clinical disease have shown the underlying pathologic abnormality to be diffuse alveolar damage.[179–181] About 25% to 30% of patients have an exudative pattern (air-space proteinaceous exudate, interstitial edema and mild inflammation, and hyaline membranes), and the remaining patients have a proliferative (fibroblastic) pattern. Presumably because of the latter appearance, the abnormality was termed *diffuse interstitial*

fibrosis by Hamman and Rich;[178] subsequent authors have preferred the designation *acute interstitial pneumonia*.[179, 180] A more appropriate clinical description might be adult respiratory distress syndrome.

The cause and pathogenesis of acute interstitial pneumonia are unclear. This abnormality may represent simply a particularly severe form of idiopathic pulmonary fibrosis; this hypothesis is supported by the observation that some patients who have otherwise typical idiopathic pulmonary fibrosis undergo a phase of rapidly progressive disease characterized radiologically by adult respiratory distress syndrome and pathologically by diffuse alveolar damage. Despite these arguments, we believe that the features of most cases of *de novo* acute interstitial pneumonitis are so different from those of the usual case of idiopathic pulmonary fibrosis that they should be considered separately.

Patients usually present with dyspnea, which is rapidly progressive over a period of weeks. Most patients are between 40 and 70 years old. Some patients complain of an influenza-like illness and fever.[149]

The radiologic manifestations are similar to those of adult respiratory distress syndrome.[180, 182] The main finding on the chest radiograph is bilateral air-space consolidation (Table 9–6, Fig. 9–25).[182] In one study of nine patients, this finding was present in all;[182] it was diffuse in five, involved mainly the upper lung zones in two, and involved mainly the lower lung zones in two. The HRCT findings consist of extensive bilateral areas of ground-glass attenuation, architectural distortion, traction bronchiectasis, and focal areas of air-space consolidation.[174, 182, 214] In a review of the HRCT findings in 36 patients, ground-glass opacities, architectural distortion, and traction bronchiectasis were seen in all cases and air-space consolidation in 33 patients (92%).[214] The presence of traction bronchiectasis correlates with disease duration.[214] It usually reflects the proliferative or fibrotic phase of acute interstitial pneumonia.[215] Other common manifestations include intralobular linear opacities, interlobular septal thickening, and thick-

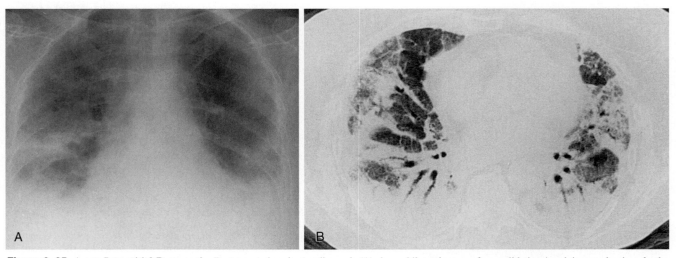

Figure 9–25. Acute Interstitial Pneumonia. Posteroanterior chest radiograph *(A)* shows bilateral areas of consolidation involving predominantly the lower lung zones. CT scan *(B)* shows areas of consolidation with air bronchograms in the dependent portions of the lower lobes and areas of ground-glass attenuation in the middle lobe and lingula. The patient was an 83-year-old woman in whom the diagnosis of acute interstitial pneumonitis was proved at autopsy. (From Primack SL, Hartman TE, Ikezoe J, et al: Acute interstitial pneumonia. Radiographic and CT findings in nine patients. Radiology 188:817, 1993.)

Table 9–6. ACUTE INTERSTITIAL PNEUMONIA: CHARACTERISTIC CLINICAL AND RADIOLOGIC MANIFESTATIONS

Patients between 40 and 70 years old
Rapidly progressive dyspnea over days or weeks
Extensive bilateral air-space consolidation
Symmetric distribution
Ground-glass attenuation and consolidation on HRCT
Architectural distortion, traction bronchiectasis
Intralobular linear opacities
Radiologic findings similar to ARDS

HRCT, high-resolution computed tomography; ARDS, adult respiratory distress syndrome.

ening of the bronchovascular bundles.[214] An anteroposterior gradient in the ground-glass attenuation or consolidation with considerable increase in attenuation in the dependent lung regions (*see* Fig. 9–25) is present in approximately 25% of patients.[214]

LANGERHANS' CELL HISTIOCYTOSIS

Langerhans' cell histiocytosis (Langerhans' cell granulomatosis, eosinophilic granuloma, histiocytosis X) is an uncommon disease characterized pathologically by a proliferation of specialized histiocytes known as *Langerhans' cells*.[183] There is a strong association of pulmonary disease (pulmonary Langerhans' cell histiocytosis) with cigarette smoking;[187] 100% of patients in some series were current smokers.[188]

Grossly, the lungs in the early or active stage of pulmonary Langerhans' cell histiocytosis show multiple nodules, mostly measuring 1 to 10 mm in diameter. With time, the relatively discrete nodular lesions become confluent, resulting in irregularly shaped areas of fibrosis containing cysts of variable size. In long-standing disease, the appearance is similar to that of advanced idiopathic pulmonary fibrosis, with the presence of bands of fibrous tissue and multiple cysts of variable size (Fig. 9–26). The major distinguishing features between the two are that pulmonary Langerhans' cell histiocytosis tends to be more severe in the upper lobes and to affect peripheral and central regions more evenly.[185, 186]

Abnormalities in the early stage of disease are located predominantly in the interstitial connective tissue of small membranous and proximal respiratory bronchioles and consist mainly of a cellular infiltrate.[188] In more advanced disease, this infiltrate typically extends into the adjacent alveolar interstitium, and the central portion of the lesion undergoes fibrosis, resulting in a characteristic stellate shape. For reasons that are unclear, some affected bronchioles appear to dilate, resulting in the cysts seen in gross specimens and radiologic images. It also is possible that some cysts originate by cavitation of the cellular nodules. In advanced disease, the lung may consist almost entirely of fibrous tissue and cystic spaces, with only scattered Langerhans' cells and few or no eosinophils.

Pulmonary Langerhans' cell histiocytosis is seen predominantly in young adults, the median age in one series being 33 years.[188] When first discovered, 20% to 25% of patients are asymptomatic,[185] and the disease is identified on a screening chest radiograph. When the disease is present, the average duration of symptoms before presentation is about 6 months. Less than one third of patients have only nonspecific constitutional symptoms, such as fatigue, weight loss, and fever.[185] Respiratory symptoms are present in the remaining two thirds and usually consist of dry cough and dyspnea. Hemoptysis is uncommon, occurring in only 6 of 100 patients in one study.[185]

Radiologic Manifestations

Radiologic abnormalities are characteristically bilateral, symmetric, and diffuse throughout the upper and mid lung zones with sparing of the costophrenic angles (Table 9–7).[184, 185] Early on, the radiographic appearance consists of a nodular pattern, with individual lesions 1 to 10 mm in diameter; these may regress or resolve completely.[189, 190] Although cavitated nodules are seen only occasionally on radiograph during this stage,[191] they can be identified on HRCT scan in approximately 10% of cases.[192, 193]

In more advanced disease, the pattern may become reticulonodular (Fig. 9–27). Although this stage usually is considered to be irreversible, one patient has been de-

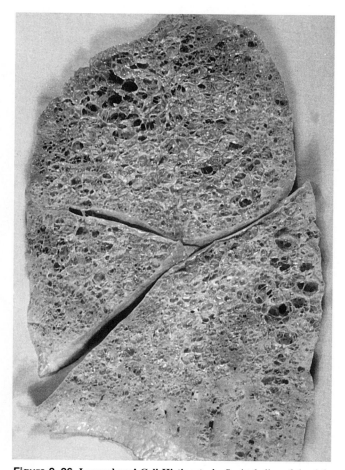

Figure 9–26. Langerhans' Cell Histiocytosis. Sagittal slice of the right lung in its midportion shows innumerable cystic spaces, most measuring about 0.5 to 1 cm in diameter. They are present in central and peripheral regions and are more evident in the upper lobe and superior portions of the lower and middle lobes. Note relative sparing of the tip of the right middle lobe and the lung bases.

Table 9–7. LANGERHANS' CELL HISTIOCYTOSIS: CHARACTERISTIC CLINICAL AND RADIOLOGIC MANIFESTATIONS

Median age 33 years
Slowly progressive dyspnea
Usually smokers
Bilaterally symmetric distribution
Upper and middle lung zones
Relative sparing of lung base
Nodular or reticulonodular pattern
HRCT shows nodules and thin-walled cysts
Cysts often have bizarre shapes

HRCT, high-resolution computed tomography.

scribed in whom the radiographic abnormalities resolved completely within 3 years after smoking cessation.[194] The end stage of disease is characterized by a coarse reticular pattern that, in the upper lung zones particularly, often assumes a cystic appearance characteristic of honeycombing. Usually the cysts are about 1 cm in diameter but may measure 3 cm.

Several investigators have reviewed the CT findings in pulmonary Langerhans' cell histiocytosis.[192, 193, 196] The most common abnormalities on HRCT scan are cysts (present in approximately 80% of patients) and nodules (present in 60% to 80%). Less common findings, each seen in approximately 10% of cases, include cavitated nodules, reticulation, and areas of ground-glass attenuation. As might be expected, the incidence of these abnormalities depends on the stage of the disease. In patients who have recent symptoms, the predominant abnormality consists of small nodules, which may vary from a few in number to a myriad (Fig. 9–28).[192, 193] Most nodules measure 1 to 5 mm in diameter, although larger nodules are seen in approximately 30% of cases. The nodules tend to have a centrilobular distribution corresponding to the peribronchiolar distribution of the cellular infiltrate seen histologically.[193] Their margins may be smooth or irregular. Follow-up CT scans show that cavitation of small nodules may occur within a few weeks of the initial CT scan and that larger nodules may be replaced by cysts;[192, 193] occasionally, small nodules disappear.

With progression of disease, cysts become a more prom-

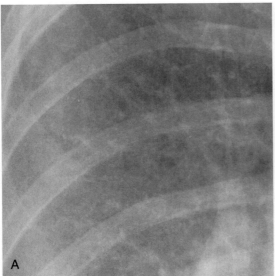

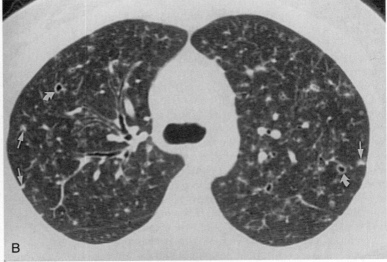

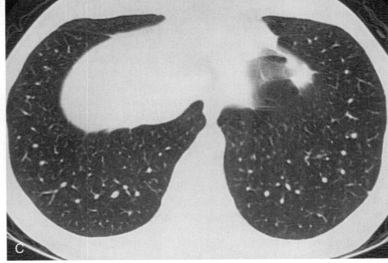

Figure 9–27. Langerhans' Cell Histiocytosis. View of the right upper lobe *(A)* from a posteroanterior chest radiograph shows poorly defined reticulonodular pattern. HRCT scan at the level of the tracheal carina *(B)* shows small nodules *(straight arrows)*, small cysts *(curved arrows)*, and a few irregular linear opacities. HRCT scan through the lower lung zones *(C)* shows only minimal abnormalities. The patient was a 39-year-old woman. (Case courtesy of Dr. Jim Barrie, University of Alberta Medical Centre, Edmonton, Alberta, Canada.)

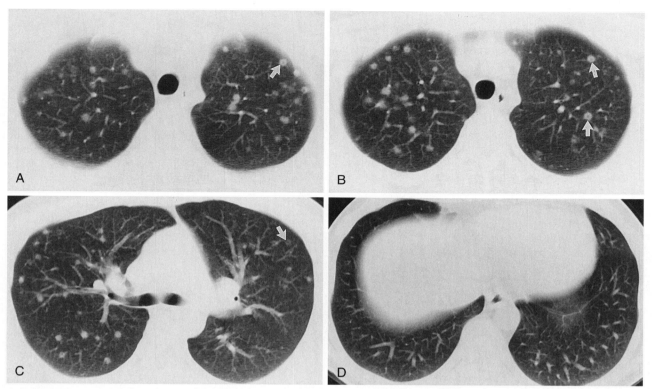

Figure 9–28. Pulmonary Langerhans' Cell Histiocytosis: Cavitating Nodules. A 30-year-man presented with a pathologic fracture of the right first rib. The chest radiograph showed poorly defined small nodular opacities. Conventional 10-mm collimation CT scan shows multiple bilateral nodules measuring 3 to 7 mm in diameter. Central lucencies can be seen in several of the nodules near the lung apices *(A and B)*, suggesting central cavitation. Similar findings are present at the level of the right upper lobe bronchus *(C)*. No nodules were identified in the lung bases *(D)*. Diagnosis of Langerhans' cell histiocytosis was proved by biopsy of the right first rib.

inent feature. They range from a few millimeters to several centimeters in diameter and may be round, oval, or bizarre in shape.[192, 195] The reticular and reticulonodular opacities that are identified frequently on chest radiograph are relatively uncommon on CT scan,[192, 193] with many of the opacities probably representing cysts (Fig. 9–29).[192] In many cases, the pulmonary parenchyma between the cysts is remarkably normal on CT scan.[192] With progression of disease, there is evidence of fibrosis and, eventually, extensive honeycombing.[47] Regardless of the stage of the disease, the abnormalities are most severe in the upper and mid lung zone; the lung bases are relatively spared.[47, 198]

The pattern and distribution of abnormalities on HRCT scan are usually characteristic enough to allow a confident diagnosis.[47, 48, 197] In one study of 140 consecutive patients who had chronic infiltrative lung disease, the superiority of HRCT over chest radiography in the assessment of pattern and distribution of abnormalities was the greatest for pulmonary Langerhans' cell histiocytosis.[47] In another investigation of 61 patients who had end-stage lung disease from a variety of causes, a correct first-choice diagnosis of pulmonary Langerhans' cell histiocytosis was made by two independent blinded observers in eight of eight cases.[48] The presence of nodules and cysts throughout the mid and upper lung zones with relative sparing of the lung bases is virtually diagnostic. In patients who have nodules alone, the differential diagnosis is more difficult because the pattern may resemble the findings seen in sarcoidosis, tuberculosis, and metastatic cancer. In patients who have only

cystic changes, the findings can be distinguished easily from idiopathic pulmonary fibrosis because the latter typically shows most severe involvement in the subpleural lung regions and the lower lung zones.[211] In a woman, cystic changes similar to those in pulmonary Langerhans' cell histiocytosis may be seen in lymphangioleiomyomatosis and tuberous sclerosis;[199, 200] however, the cysts in these conditions are present diffusely throughout the lungs, without sparing of the lung bases, and nodules are seen rarely.[199, 200]

In our experience, the progressive loss of lung volume that is so characteristic of idiopathic pulmonary fibrosis is seldom seen in pulmonary Langerhans' cell histiocytosis, perhaps because the development of cysts counteracts the retraction exerted by the fibrous tissue. The tendency for the lungs to maintain normal volume has been observed by others; in one study of 50 patients who had pulmonary Langerhans' cell histiocytosis, none was considered to have a decrease in lung volume, and some were thought to show evidence of overinflation.[184] In another review of 100 patients, 60 were considered to have lung volumes within the normal range, 31 to be overinflated, and only 9 to have a lung volume below normal.[185]

Hilar and mediastinal node enlargement and pleural effusion are rare in adults,[201–204] although the former is relatively common in children.[202, 205] Spontaneous pneumothorax is a relatively common complication; in two series comprising 150 patients, it developed in 18 (12%) patients.[184, 185] Spontaneous pneumothorax may be the first

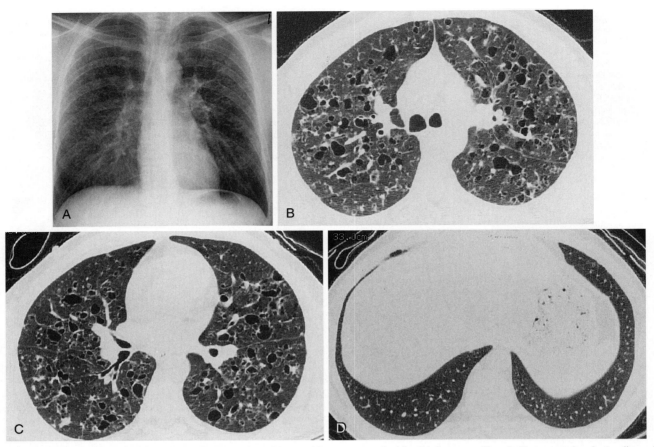

Figure 9–29. Pulmonary Langerhans' Cell Histiocytosis. A 30-year-old man presented with mild shortness of breath. Posteroanterior chest radiograph *(A)* shows a coarse reticular pattern as well as several cysts. Although the abnormalities are relatively diffuse in upper and middle lung zones, there is sparing of the costophrenic sulci. HRCT scan at the level of the main bronchi *(B)* shows numerous bilateral cystic lesions of various sizes. Note relatively normal intervening lung parenchyma. The apparent reticular opacities on radiograph are shown on CT scan to be due to cysts, there being little evidence of additional fibrosis. The visualized bronchi are normal in diameter, and these do not communicate with the cysts. HRCT scan at the level of the right middle lobe bronchus *(C)* shows numerous bilateral cysts. A few irregularly marginated small nodules are visible. HRCT scan through the lung bases *(D)* shows only a few localized cysts.

manifestation of the disease[184] and occasionally occurs in the absence of radiographic abnormalities in the lungs.[202] Concomitant involvement of bones and lungs can occur[206, 207] but is uncommon in adults, being evident in only 5 of 100 patients in one series.[185]

References

1. Yamamoto M, Sharma OP, Hosada Y: The 1991 descriptive definition of sarcoidosis. Sarcoidosis 9(Suppl):33, 1993.
2. Nagai S: Pulmonary sarcoidosis: Pathogenesis and population differences. Intern Med 34:833, 1995.
3. Kirtland SH, Winterbauer RH: Pulmonary sarcoidosis. Semin Respir Med 14:344, 1993.
4. Scadding JG: Sarcoidosis. London, Eyre & Spottiswoode, 1967.
5. Brown JK: Pulmonary sarcoidosis: Clinical evaluation and management. Semin Respir Med 12:215, 1991.
6. Mayock RL, Bertrand P, Morrison CE, et al: Manifestations of sarcoidosis: Analysis of 145 patients, with a review of nine series selected from the literature. Am J Med 35:67, 1963.
7. Rudberg-Roos I: The course and prognosis of sarcoidosis as observed in 296 cases. Acta Tuberc Scand 52(Suppl):1, 1962.
8. Scadding JG: Prognosis of intrathoracic sarcoidosis in England: A review of 136 cases after five years' observation. BMJ 2:1165, 1961.
9. Rybicki BA, Maliarik MJ, Popovich J Jr, et al: Epidemiology, demographics and genetics of sarcoidosis. Semin Respir Infect 13:166, 1998.
10. Rossman MD, Daniele RP, Dauber JH: Nodular endobronchial sarcoidosis: A study comparing blood and lung lymphocytes. Chest 79:427, 1981.
11. Hadfield JW, Page RL, Flower CDR, et al: Localized airways narrowing in sarcoidosis. Thorax 37:443, 1982.
12. De Remee RA: The roentgenographic staging of sarcoidosis: Historic and contemporary perspectives. Chest 83:128, 1983.
13. James DG, Neville E, Siltzbach LE, et al: A worldwide review of sarcoidosis. Ann N Y Acad Sci 278:321, 1976.
14. Chiles C, Putman CE: Pulmonary sarcoidosis. Semin Respir Med 13:345, 1992.
15. Berkmen YM: Radiologic aspects of intrathoracic sarcoidosis. Semin Roentgenol 20:356, 1985.
16. Rockoff SD, Rohatgi PK: Unusual manifestations of thoracic sarcoidosis. Am J Roentgenol 144:513, 1985.
17. Kirks DR, McCormick VD, Greenspan RH: Pulmonary sarcoidosis: Roentgenologic analysis of 150 patients. Am J Roentgenol 117:777, 1973.
18. Bein ME, Putman CE, McLoud TC, et al: A reevaluation of intrathoracic lymphadenopathy in sarcoidosis. Am J Roentgenol 131:409, 1978.
19. Schabel SI, Foote GA, McKee KA: Posterior lymphadenopathy in sarcoidosis. Radiology 129:591, 1978.
20. Rabinowitz JG, Ulreich S, Soriano C: The usual unusual manifestations of sarcoidosis and the "hilar-haze"—a new diagnostic aid. Am J Roentgenol 120:821, 1974.
21. Spann RW, Rosenow EC III, DeRemee RA, et al: Unilateral hilar or paratracheal adenopathy in sarcoidosis: A study of 38 cases. Thorax 26:296, 1971.

22. Scadding JG: The late stages of pulmonary sarcoidosis. Postgrad Med J 46:530, 1970.
23. Weinstein DS: Pulmonary sarcoidosis: Calcified micronodular pattern simulating pulmonary alveolar microlithiasis. J Thorac Radiol 14:218, 1999.
24. Gross BH, Schneider HJ, Proto AV: Eggshell calcification of lymph nodes: An update. Am J Roentgenol 135:1265, 1980.
25. Israel HL, Lenchner G, Steiner RM: Late development of mediastinal calcification in sarcoidosis. Am Rev Respir Dis 124:302, 1981.
26. Wurm K, Reindell H: On the differential roentgenological diagnosis of sarcoidosis (Boeck's disease) and lymphogranulomatosis. Radiologe 2:134, 1962.
27. Wurm K: The stages of pulmonary sarcoidosis. Geriatr Med Monthly 5:386, 1960.
28. Müller NL, Kullnig P, Miller RR: The CT findings of pulmonary sarcoidosis: Analysis of 25 patients. Am J Roentgenol 152:1179, 1989.
29. Sider L, Horton Jr ES: Hilar and mediastinal adenopathy in sarcoidosis as detected by computed tomography. J Thorac Imaging 5:77, 1990.
30. Kuhlman JE, Fishman EK, Hamper UM, et al: The computed tomographic spectrum of thoracic sarcoidosis. Radiographics 9:449, 1989.
31. Saksouk FA, Haddad MC: Detection of mesenteric involvement in sarcoidosis using computed tomography. Br J Radiol 60:1135, 1987.
32. Warshauer DM, Dumbleton SA, Molina PL, et al: Abdominal CT findings in sarcoidosis: Radiologic and clinical correlation. Radiology 192:93, 1994.
33. Murdoch J, Müller NL: Pulmonary sarcoidosis: Changes on follow-up CT examination. Am J Roentgenol 159:473, 1992.
34. Gawne-Cain ML, Hansell DM: The pattern and distribution of calcified mediastinal lymph nodes in sarcoidosis and tuberculosis: A CT study. Clin Radiol 51:263, 1996.
35. Epler GR, McLoud TC, Gaensler EA, et al: Normal chest roentgenograms in chronic diffuse infiltrative lung disease. N Engl J Med 298:934, 1978.
36. Schlossberg O, Sfedu E: Disseminated sarcoidosis. Sarcoidosis 4:149, 1987.
37. Rosen Y, Amorosa JK, Moon S, et al: Occurrence of lung granulomas in patients with stage I sarcoidosis. Am J Roentgenol 129:1083, 1977.
38. Brauner MW, Grenier P, Mompoint D, et al: Pulmonary sarcoidosis: Evaluation with high-resolution CT. Radiology 172:467, 1989.
39. Hillerdal G, Nöu E, Osterman K, et al: Sarcoidosis: Epidemiology and prognosis. Am Rev Respir Dis 130:29, 1984.
40. Symmons DPM, Woods KL: Recurrent sarcoidosis. Thorax 35:879, 1980.
41. Baughman RP: Sarcoidosis: Usual and unusual manifestations (clinical conference). Chest 94:165, 1988.
42. Ellis K, Renthal G: Pulmonary sarcoidosis: Roentgenographic observations on course of disease. Am J Roentgenol 88:1070, 1962.
43. Stone DJ, Schwartz A: A long-term study of sarcoid and its modification by steroid therapy: Lung function and other factors in prognosis. Am J Med 41:528, 1966.
44. Israel HL, Sperber M, Steiner RM: Course of chronic hilar sarcoidosis in relation to markers of granulomatous activity. Invest Radiol 18:1, 1983.
45. Kirks DR, McCormick VD, Greenspan RH: Pulmonary sarcoidosis: Roentgenologic analysis of 150 patients. Am J Roentgenol 117:777, 1979.
46. Mathieson JR, Mayo JR, Staples CA, et al: Chronic diffuse infiltrative lung disease: Comparison of diagnostic accuracy of CT and chest radiography. Radiology 171:111, 1989.
47. Grenier P, Valeyre D, Cluzel P, et al: Chronic diffuse interstitial lung disease: Diagnostic value of chest radiography and high-resolution CT. Radiology 179:123, 1991.
48. Primack SL, Hartman TE, Hansell DM, et al: End-stage lung disease: CT findings in 61 patients. Radiology 189:681, 1993.
49. Padley SPG, Padhani AR, Nicholson A, et al: Pulmonary sarcoidosis mimicking cryptogenic fibrosing alveolitis on CT. Clin Radiol 51:807, 1996.
50. Mesbahi SJ, Davies P: Unilateral pulmonary changes in the chest x-ray in sarcoidosis. Clin Radiol 32:283, 1981.
51. Müller NL, Mawson JB, Mathieson JR, et al: Sarcoidosis: Correlation of extent of disease at CT with clinical, functional, and radiographic findings. Radiology 171:613, 1989.
52. McLoud TC, Epler GR, Gaensler EA, et al: A radiographic classification for sarcoidosis: Physiologic correlation. Invest Radiol 17:129, 1982.
53. Traill ZC, Maskell GF, Gleeson FV: High-resolution CT findings of pulmonary sarcoidosis. Am J Roentgenol 168:1557, 1997.
54. Grenier P, Chevret S, Beigelman C, et al: Chronic diffuse infiltrative lung disease: Determination of the diagnostic value of clinical data, chest radiography, and CT with Bayesian analysis. Radiology 191:383, 1994.
55. Remy-Jardin M, Giraud F, Remy J, et al: Pulmonary sarcoidosis: Role of CT in the evaluation of disease activity and functional impairment and in prognosis assessment. Radiology 191:675, 1994.
56. Gruden JF, Webb WR: Identification and evaluation of centrilobular opacities on high-resolution CT. Semin Ultrasound CT MRI 16:435, 1995.
57. Nishimura K, Itoh H, Kitaichi M, et al: Pulmonary sarcoidosis: Correlation of CT and histopathologic findings. Radiology 189:105, 1993.
58. Rubinstein I, Solomon A, Baum GL, et al: Pulmonary sarcoidosis presenting with unusual roentgenographic manifestations. Eur J Respir Dis 67:335, 1985.
59. Chao DC, Hassenpflug M, Sharma OP: Multiple lung masses, pneumothorax, and psychiatric symptoms in a 29-year-old African-American woman. Chest 108:871, 1995.
60. Pinsker KL: Solitary pulmonary nodule in sarcoidosis. JAMA 240:1379, 1978.
61. Rose RM, Lee RG, Costello P: Solitary nodular sarcoidosis. Clin Radiol 36:589, 1985.
62. Lynch DA, Webb WR, Gamsu G, et al: Computed tomography in pulmonary sarcoidosis. J Comput Assist Tomogr 13:405, 1989.
63. Glazer HS, Levitt RG, Shackelford GD: Peripheral pulmonary infiltrates in sarcoidosis. Chest 86:741, 1984.
64. Teirstein AS, Siltzbach LE: Sarcoidosis of the upper lung fields simulating pulmonary tuberculosis. Chest 64:303, 1973.
65. Johkoh T, Ikezoe J, Takeuchi N, et al: CT findings in "pseudoalveolar" sarcoidosis. J Comput Assist Tomogr 16:904, 1992.
66. Leung AN, Brauner MW, Caillat-Vigneron N, et al: Sarcoidosis activity: Correlation of HRCT findings with those of ^{67}Ga scanning, bronchoalveolar lavage, and serum angiotensin-converting enzyme assay. J Comput Assist Tomogr 22:229, 1998.
67. Marlow TJ, Krapiva PI, Schabel SI, et al: The "Fairy Ring": A new radiographic finding in sarcoidosis. Chest 115:275, 1999.
68. Tazi A, Desfemmes-Baleyte T, Soler P, et al: Pulmonary sarcoidosis with a diffuse ground glass pattern on the chest radiograph. Thorax 49:793, 1994.
69. Leung AN, Miller RR, Müller NL: Parenchymal opacification in chronic infiltrative lung diseases: CT-pathologic correlation. Radiology 188:209, 1993.
70. Nishimura K, Itoh H, Kitaichi M, et al: CT and pathological correlation of pulmonary sarcoidosis. Semin Ultrasound CT MRI 16:361, 1995.
71. Thomas PD, Hunninghake GW: Current concepts of the pathogenesis of sarcoidosis. Am Rev Respir Dis 135:747, 1987.
72. Brauner MW, Lenoir S, Grenier P, et al: Pulmonary sarcoidosis: CT assessment of lesion reversibility. Radiology 182:349, 1992.
73. Miller A: The vanishing lung syndrome associated with pulmonary sarcoidosis. Br J Dis Chest 75:209, 1981.
74. Ichikawa Y, Fujimoto K, Shiraishi T, et al: Primary cavitary sarcoidosis: High-resolution CT findings. Am J Roentgenol 163:745, 1994.
75. Canessa PA, Torraca A, Lavecchia MA, et al: Primary acute pulmonary cavitation in asymptomatic sarcoidosis. Sarcoidosis 6:158, 1989.
76. Biem J, Hoffstein V: Aggressive cavitary pulmonary sarcoidosis. Am Rev Respir Dis 143:428, 1991.
77. Gorske KJ, Fleming RJ: Mycetoma formation in cavitary pulmonary sarcoidosis. Radiology 95:279, 1970.
78. Freundlich IM, Libshitz HI, Glassman LM, et al: Sarcoidosis: Typical and atypical thoracic manifestations and complications. Clin Radiol 21:376, 1970.
79. Hansell DM, Milne DG, Wilsher ML, et al: Pulmonary sarcoidosis: Morphologic associations of airflow obstruction at thin-section CT. Radiology 209:697, 1998.
80. Judson MA, Strange C: Bullous sarcoidosis: A report of three cases. Chest 114:1474, 1998.
81. Dorman RL Jr, Whitman GJ, Chew FS: Thoracic sarcoidosis. Am J Roentgenol 164:1368, 1995.

82. Henry DA, Kiser PE, Scheer CE, et al: Multiple imaging evaluation of sarcoidosis. Radiographics 6:75, 1986.

83. Gleeson FV, Traill ZC, Hansell DM: Evidence on expiratory CT scans of small-airway obstruction in sarcoidosis. Am J Roentgenol 166:1052, 1996.

84. Wilen SB, Rabinowitz JG, Ulreich S, et al: Pleural involvement in sarcoidosis. Am J Med 57:200, 1974.

85. Knox AJ, Wardman AG, Page RL: Tuberculous pleural effusion occurring during corticosteroid treatment of sarcoidosis. Thorax 41:651, 1986.

86. Lum GH, Poropatich RK: Unilateral pleural thickening. Chest 110:1348, 1996.

87. Loughney E, Higgins BG: Pleural sarcoidosis: A rare presentation. Thorax 52:200, 1997.

88. Whitcomb ME, Hawley PC, Domby WR, et al: The role of fiberoptic bronchoscopy in the diagnosis of sarcoidosis: Clinical conference in pulmonary disease from Ohio State University, Columbus. Chest 74:205, 1978.

89. Gomm SA: An unusual presentation of sarcoidosis: Spontaneous haemopneumothorax. Postgrad Med J 60:621, 1984.

90. Ross RJ, Empey DW: Bilateral spontaneous pneumothorax in sarcoidosis. Postgrad Med J 59:106, 1983.

91. Rizzato G, Montemurro L: The locomotor system. *In* James DG (ed): Sarcoidosis and Other Granulomatous Disorders. New York, Marcel Dekker, 1994.

92. Yaghmai I: Radiographic, angiographic and radionuclide manifestations of osseous sarcoidosis. Radiographics 3:375, 1983.

93. Rizzato G, Montemurro L, Fraioli P: Bone mineral content in sarcoidosis. Semin Respir Med 13:411, 1992.

94. Chiles C, Adams GW, Ravin CE: Radiographic manifestations of cardiac sarcoid. Am J Roentgenol 145:711, 1985.

95. Riedy K, Fisher MR, Belic N, et al: MR imaging of myocardial sarcoidosis. Am J Roentgenol 151:915, 1988.

96. Mazzone P, Arroliga A: Acute dyspnea and hypoxia in a 37-year-old woman with sarcoidosis. Chest 113:830, 1998.

97. Folz SJ, Johnson CD, Swensen SJ: Abdominal manifestations of sarcoidosis in CT studies. J Comput Assist Tomogr 19:573, 1995.

98. Siltzbach LE, James DG, Neville E, et al: Course and prognosis of sarcoidosis around the world. Am J Med 57:847, 1974.

99. Ebright JR, Soin JS, Manoli RS: The gallium scan: Problems and misuse in examination of patients with suspected infection. Arch Intern Med 142:246, 1982.

100. Myslivecek M, Husak V, Kolek V, et al: Absolute quantitation of gallium-67 citrate accumulation in the lungs and its importance for the evaluation of disease activity in pulmonary sarcoidosis. Eur J Nucl Med 19:1016, 1992.

101. Okada M, Takahashi H, Nukiwa T, et al: Correlative analysis of longitudinal changes in bronchoalveolar lavage, 67 gallium scanning, serum angiotensin-converting enzyme activity, chest x-ray, and pulmonary function tests in pulmonary sarcoidosis. Jpn J Med 26:360, 1987.

102. Line BR, Hunninghake GW, Keogh BA, et al: Gallium-67 scanning to stage the alveolitis of sarcoidosis: Correlation with clinical studies, pulmonary function studies and bronchoalveolar lavage. Am Rev Respir Dis 123:440, 1981.

103. Klech H, Kohn H, Kummer F, et al: Assessment of activity in sarcoidosis: Sensitivity and specificity of 67 gallium scintigraphy, serum ACE levels, chest roentgenography, and blood lymphocyte populations. Chest 82:732, 1982.

104. Sulavik SB, Spencer RP, Palestro CJ, et al: Specificity and sensitivity of distinctive chest radiographic and/or GA images in the noninvasive diagnosis of sarcoidosis. Chest 103:403, 1993.

105. Liebow AA, Carrington CB: The interstitial pneumonias. *In* Simon M, Potchen EJ, LeMay M (eds): Frontiers of Pulmonary Radiology. New York, Grune & Stratton, 1969, p 102.

106. Katzenstein AA, Myers JL: State of the art: Idiopathic pulmonary fibrosis. Am J Respir Crit Care Med 157:1301, 1998.

107. Scadding JG, Hinson KFW: Diffuse fibrosing alveolitis (diffuse interstitial fibrosis of the lungs). Thorax 28:680, 1973.

108. Bjoraker JA, Ryu JH, Edwin MK, et al: Prognostic significance of histopathologic subsets in idiopathic pulmonary fibrosis. Am J Respir Crit Care Med 157:199, 1998.

109. Tierney LM Jr: Idiopathic pulmonary fibrosis. Semin Respir Med 12:229, 1991.

110. Westcott JL, Cole SR: Traction bronchiectasis in end-stage pulmonary fibrosis. Radiology 161:665, 1986.

111. Carrington CB, Gaensler EA, Coutu RE, et al: Natural history and treated course of usual and desquamative interstitial pneumonia. N Engl J Med 298:801, 1978.

112. McLoud TC, Carrington CB, Gaensler EA: Diffuse infiltrative lung disease: A new scheme for description. Radiology 149:353, 1983.

113. Müller NL, Guerry-Force ML, Staples CA, et al: Differential dignosis of bronchiolitis obliterans with organizing pneumonia and usual interstitial pneumonia: Clinical, functional, and radiologic findings. Radiology 162:151, 1987.

114. Grenier P, Chevret S, Beigelman C, et al: Chronic diffuse infiltrative lung disease: Determination of the diagnostic value of clinical data, chest radiography and CT and Bayesian analysis. Radiology 191:383, 1994.

115. Staples CA, Müller NL, Vedal S, et al: Usual interstitial pneumonia: Correlation of CT with clinical, functional and radiological findings. Radiology 162:377, 1987.

116. McAdams HP, Rosado de Christenson ML, Wehunt WD, et al: The alphabet soup revisited: The chronic interstitial pneumonias in the 1990's. Radiographics 16:1009, 1996.

117. Picado C, Gomez de Almeida R, Xaubet A, et al: Spontaneous pneumothorax in cryptogenic fibrosing alveolitis. Respiration 48:77, 1985.

118. Feigin DS: New perspectives on interstitial lung disease. Radiol Clin North Am 21:683, 1983.

119. Mathieson JR, Mayo JR, Staples, CA, et al: Chronic diffuse infiltrative lung disease: Comparison of diagnostic accuracy of CT and chest radiography. Radiology 171:111, 1989.

120. Padley SPG, Hansell DM, Flower CDR, et al: Comparative accuracy of high resolution computed tomography and chest radiography in the diagnosis of chronic diffuse infiltrative lung disease. Clin Radiol 44:222, 1991.

121. Orens JB, Kazerooni DA, Martinez FJ, et al: The sensitivity of high-resolution CT in detecting idiopathic pulmonary fibrosis proved by open lung biopsy: A prospective study. Chest 108:109, 1995.

122. Müller NL, Miller RR, Webb WR: Fibrosing alveolitis: CT-pathologic correlation. Radiology 160:585, 1986.

123. Nishimura K, Kitaichi M, Izumi T, et al: Usual interstitial pneumonia: Histologic correlation with high-resolution CT. Radiology 182:342, 1992.

124. Müller NL, Miller RR: State of the art: Computed tomography of chronic diffuse infiltrative lung disease: Part 1. Am Rev Respir Dis 142:1206, 1990.

125. Müller NL, Colby TV: Idiopathic interstitial pneumonias: High-resolution CT and histologic findings. Radiographics 17:1016, 1997.

126. Akira M, Sakatani M, Ueda E: Idiopathic pulmonary fibrosis: Progression of honeycombing at thin-section CT. Radiology 189:687, 1993.

127. Wells AU, Rubens MB, du Bois RM, et al: Serial CT in fibrosing alveolitis: Prognostic significance of the initial pattern. Am J Roentgenol 161:1159, 1993.

128. Terriff BA, Kwan SY, Chan-Yeung M, et al: Fibrosing alveolitis: Chest radiography and CT as predictors of clinical and functional impairment at follow-up in 26 patients. Radiology 184:445, 1992.

129. Hartman TE, Primack SL, Kang EY, et al: Disease progression in usual interstitial pneumonia compared with desquamative interstitial pneumonia: Assessment with serial CT. Chest 110:378, 1996.

130. Gay SE, Kazerooni EA, Towes GB, et al: Idiopathic pulmonary fibrosis: Predicting response to therapy and survival. Am J Respir Crit Care Med 157:1063, 1998.

131. Lee JS, Gong G, Song K-S, et al: Usual interstitial pneumonia: Relationship between disease activity and the progression of honeycombing at thin-section computed tomography. J Thorac Imaging 13:199, 1998.

132. Aquino SL, Webb WR, Zaloudek CJ, et al: Lung cysts associated with honeycombing: Change in size on expiratory CT scans. Am J Roentgenol 162:583, 1994.

133. Worthy SA, Brown MJ, Müller NL: Cystic air spaces in the lung: Change in size on expiratory high-resolution CT in 23 patients. Clin Radiol 53:515, 1998.

134. Gevenois PA, Abehsera M, Knoop C, et al: Disseminated pulmonary ossification in end-stage pulmonary fibrosis: CT demonstration. Am J Roentgenol 162:1303, 1994.

135. Müller NL, Staples CA, Miller RR, et al: Disease activity in idiopathic pulmonary fibrosis: CT and pathologic correlation. Radiology 165:731, 1987.

136. Niimi H, Kang EY, Kwong JS, et al: CT of chronic infiltrative lung disease: Prevalence of mediastinal lymphadenopathy. J Comput Assist Tomogr 20:305, 1996.

137. Bergin C, Castellino RA: Mediastinal lymph node enlargement on CT scans in patients with usual interstitial pneumonitis. Am J Roentgenol 154:251, 1990.

138. Franquet T, Gimenez A, Alegret X, et al: Mediastinal lymphadenopathy in cryptogenic fibrosing alveolitis: The effect of steroid therapy on the prevalence of nodal enlargement. Clin Radiol 53:435, 1998.

139. Tung KT, Wells AU, Rubens MB, et al: Accuracy of the typical computed tomographic appearances of fibrosing alveolitis. Thorax 48:334, 1993.

140. Nishimura K, Izumi T, Kitaichi M, et al: The diagnostic accuracy of high-resolution computed tomography in diffuse infiltrative lung diseases. Chest 104:1149, 1993.

141. Swensen SJ, Aughenbaugh GL, Myers JL: Diffuse lung disease: Diagnostic accuracy of CT in patients undergoing surgical biopsy of the lung. Radiology 205:229, 1997.

142. Johnston ID, Prescott RJ, Chalmers JC, et al: British Thoracic Society study of cryptogenic fibrosing alveolitis: Current presentation and initial management. Fibrosing alveolitis subcommittee of the research committee of the British Thoracic Society. Thorax 52:38, 1997.

143. Kanematsu T, Kitaichi M, Nishimura K, et al: Clubbing of the fingers and smooth-muscle proliferation in fibrotic changes in the lung of patients with idiopathic pulmonary fibrosis. Chest 105:339, 1994.

144. Bjoraker JA, Ryu HJ, Edwin MK, et al: Prognostic significance of histopathologic subsets in idiopathic pulmonary fibrosis. Am J Respir Crit Care Med 157:199, 1998.

145. Stack BHR, Choo-Kang YFJ, Heard BE: The prognosis of cryptogenic fibrosing alveolitis. Thorax 27:535, 1972.

146. Louw SJ, Bateman ED, Benatar SR: Cryptogenic fibrosing alveolitis: Clinical spectrum and treatment. S Afr Med J 65:195, 1984.

147. Hubbard R, Johnston I, Britton J: Survival in patients with cryptogenic fibrosing alveolitis: A population-based cohort study. Chest 113:396, 1998.

148. Mapel DW, Hunt WC, Utton R, et al: Idiopathic pulmonary fibrosis: Survival in population based and hospital based cohorts. Thorax 53:469, 1998.

149. Kondoh Y, Taniguchi H, Kawabata Y, et al: Acute exacerbation in idiopathic pulmonary fibrosis: Analysis of clinical and pathologic findings in three cases. Chest 103:1808, 1993.

150. Johkoh T, Ikezoe J, Kohno N, et al: High-resolution CT and pulmonary function tests in collagen vascular disease: Comparison with idiopathic pulmonary fibrosis. Eur J Radiol 18:113, 1994.

151. Aberle DR, Gamsu G, Ray CS, et al: Asbestos-related pleural and parenchymal fibrosis: Detection with high-resolution CT. Radiology 166:729, 1988.

152. King TE Jr, Costabel U, Cordier J-F, et al: Idiopathic pulmonary fibrosis: Diagnosis and treatment. International Consensus Statement. Am J Respir Crit Care Med 161:646, 2000.

153. Lynch DA, Newell JD, Logan PM, et al: Can CT distinguish idiopathic pulmonary fibrosis from hypersensitivity pneumonitis? Am J Roentgenol 165:807, 1995.

154. Lynch DA, Rose C, Way DE, et al: Hypersensitivity pneumonitis: Sensitivity of high-resolution CT in a population-based study. Am J Roentgenol 159:469, 1992.

155. Liebow AA, Steer A, Billingsley J: Desquamative interstitial pneumonia. Am J Med 39:369, 1965.

156. Bone RC, Wolfe J, Sobonya RE, et al: Desquamative interstitial pneumonia following long-term nitrofurantoin therapy. Am J Med 60:697, 1976.

157. Goldstein JD, Godleski JJ, Herman PG: Desquamative interstitial pneumonitis associated with monomyelocytic leukemia. Chest 81:321, 1982.

158. Abraham JL, Hertzberg MA: Inorganic particulates associated with desquamative interstitial pneumonia. Chest 80:67S, 1981.

159. Herbert A, Sterling G, Abraham J, et al: Desquamative interstitial pneumonia in an aluminum welder. Hum Pathol 13:694, 1982.

160. Lougheed MD, Roos JO, Waddell WR, et al: Desquamative interstitial pneumonitis and diffuse alveolar damage in textile workers. Chest 108:1196, 1995.

161. Yousem SA, Colby TV, Gaensler EA: Respiratory bronchiolitis-associated interstitial lung disease and its relationship to desquamative interstitial pneumonia. Mayo Clin Proc 64:1373, 1989.

162. Gaensler EA, Goff AM, Prowse CM: Desquamative interstitial pneumonia. N Engl J Med 274:113, 1966.

163. Feigin DS, Friedman PJ: Chest radiography in desquamative interstitial pneumonitis: A review of 37 patients. Am J Roentgenol 134:91, 1980.

164. Cruz E, Rodriguez J, Lisboa C, et al: Desquamative alveolar disease (desquamative interstitial pneumonia): Case report. Thorax 24:186, 1969.

165. Hartman TE, Primack SL, Swensen SJ, et al: Desquamative interstitial pneumonia: Thin-section CT findings in 22 patients. Radiology 187:787, 1993.

166. Akira M, Yamamoto S, Hara H, et al: Serial computed tomographic evaluation in desquamative interstitial pneumonia. Thorax 52:333, 1997.

167. Tubbs RR, Benjamin SP, Reich NE, et al: Desquamative interstitial pneumonitis. Chest 72:159, 1977.

168. Katzenstein ALA, Fiorelli RF: Nonspecific interstitial pneumonia/fibrosis: Histologic features and clinical significance. Am J Surg Pathol 18:136, 1994.

169. Travis WD, Matsui K, Moss JE, et al: Idiopathic nonspecific interstitial pneumonia: Prognostic significance of cellular and fibrosing patterns: Survival comparison with usual interstitial pneumonia and desquamative interstitial pneumonia. Am J Surg Pathol 24:19, 2000.

170. Park JS, Lee KS, Kim JS, et al: Nonspecific interstitial pneumonia with fibrosis: Radiographic and CT findings in seven patients. Radiology 195:645, 1995.

171. Hartman TE, Swensen SJ, Hansell DM, et al: Non-specific interstitial pneumonitis: Variable appearance at high resolution chest CT. Radiology 217:701, 2000.

172. Kim TS, Lee KS, Chung MP, et al: Nonspecific interstitial pneumonia with fibrosis: High-resolution CT and pathologic findings. Am J Roentgenol 171:1645, 1998.

173. Katoh T, Andoh T, Mikawa K, et al: Computed tomographic findings in nonspecific interstitial pneumonia/fibrosis. Respirology 3:69, 1998.

174. Johkoh T, Müller NL, Cartier Y, et al: Idiopathic interstitial pneumonias: Diagnostic accuracy of thin-section CT in 129 patients. Radiology 211:555, 1999.

175. Chan-Yeung M, Müller NL: Cryptogenic fibrosing alveolitis. Lancet 350:651, 1997.

176. Park CS, Jeon JW, Park SW, et al: Nonspecific interstitial pneumonia/fibrosis: Clinical manifestations, histologic and radiologic features. Korean J Intern Med 11:122, 1996.

177. Cottin V, Donsbeck A, Revel D, et al: Nonspecific interstitial pneumonia. Am J Respir Crit Care Med 158:1286, 1998.

178. Hamman L, Rich AR: Fulminating diffuse interstitial fibrosis of the lungs. Trans Am Clin Climatol Assoc 51:154, 1935.

179. Olson J, Colby TV, Elliot CG: Hamman-Rich syndrome revisited. Mayo Clin Proc 65:1538, 1990.

180. Katzenstein A-LA, Myers JL, Mazur MT: Acute interstitial pneumonia: A clinicopathologic, ultrastructural, and cell kinetic study. Am J Surg Pathol 10:256, 1986.

181. Porte A, Stoeckel ME, Mantz JM, et al: Acute interstitial pulmonary fibrosis: Comparative light and electron microscopic study of 19 cases: Pathogenic and therapeutic implications. Intensive Care Med 4:181, 1978.

182. Primack SL, Hartman TE, Ikezoe J, et al: Acute interstitial pneumonia: Radiographic and CT findings in nine patients. Radiology 188:817, 1993.

183. Chu T, Jaffe R: The normal Langerhans' cell and the LCH cell. Br J Cancer 23:4, 1994.

184. Lacronique J, Roth C, Battesti J-P, et al: Chest radiological features of pulmonary histiocytosis X: A report based on 50 adult cases. Thorax 37:104, 1982.

185. Friedman PJ, Liebow AA, Sokoloff J: Eosinophilic granuloma of lung: Clinical aspects of primary pulmonary histiocytosis in the adult. Medicine 60:385, 1981.

186. Colby TV, Lombard C: Histiocytosis X in the lung. Hum Pathol 14:847, 1983.

187. Hance AJ, Basset F, Saumon G, et al: Smoking and interstitial lung disease: The effect of cigarette smoking on the incidence of pulmonary histiocytosis X and sarcoidosis. Ann N Y Acad Sci 465:643, 1986.

188. Travis WD, Borok Z, Roum JH, et al: Pulmonary Langerhans' cell granulomatosis (histiocytosis X): A clinicopathologic study of 48 cases. Am J Surg Pathol 17:971, 1993.

189. Williams AW, Dunnington WG, Berte SJ: Pulmonary eosinophilic granuloma: A clinical and pathologic discussion. Ann Intern Med 54:30, 1961.

190. Bickers JN, Buechner HA, Ekman PJ: Pulmonary eosinophilic granuloma: Its natural history and prognosis. Am Rev Respir Dis 85:211, 1962.

191. Clark RL, Margulies SI, Mulholland JH: Histiocytosis X: A fatal case with unusual pulmonary manifestations. Radiology 95:631, 1970.

192. Moore ADA, Godwin JD, Müller NL, et al: Pulmonary histiocytosis X: Comparison of radiographic and CT findings. Radiology 172:249, 1989.

193. Brauner MW, Grenier P, Mouelhi MM, et al: Pulmonary histiocytosis X: Evaluation with high-resolution CT. Radiology 172:255, 1989.

194. Von Essen S, West W, Sitorius M, et al: Complete resolution of roentgenographic changes in a patient with pulmonary histiocytosis X. Chest 98:765, 1990.

195. Kulwiec EL, Lynch DA, Aguayo SM, et al: Imaging of pulmonary histiocytosis X. Radiographics 12:515, 1992.

196. Grenier P, Valeyre D, Cluzel P, et al: Chronic diffuse interstitial lung disease: Diagnostic value of chest radiography and high resolution CT. Radiology 179:123, 1991.

197. Bonelli FS, Hartman TE, Swensen SJ, et al: Accuracy of high-resolution CT in diagnosing lung diseases. Am J Roentgenol 170:1507, 1998.

198. Müller NL, Miller RR: Computed tomography of chronic diffuse infiltrative lung disease: Part 2. Am Rev Respir Dis 142:1440, 1990.

199. Müller NL, Chiles C, Kullnig P: Pulmonary lymphangiomyomatosis: Correlation of CT with radiographic and functional findings. Radiology 175:335, 1990.

200. Lenoir S, Grenier P, Brauner MW, et al: Pulmonary lymphangiomyomatosis and tuberous sclerosis: Comparison of radiographic and thin-section CT findings. Radiology 175:329, 1990.

201. Takahashi M, Martel W, Oberman HA: The variable roentgenographic appearance of idiopathic histiocytosis. Clin Radiol 17:48, 1966.

202. Carlson RA, Hattery RR, O'Connell EJ, et al: Pulmonary involvement by histiocytosis X in the pediatric age group. Mayo Clin Proc 51:542, 1976.

203. Tittel PW, Winkler CF: Chronic recurrent pleural effusion in adult histiocytosis X. Br J Radiol 54:68, 1981.

204. Guardia J, Pedreira J-D, Esteban R, et al: Early pleural effusion in histiocytosis X. Arch Intern Med 139:934, 1979.

205. Matlin AH, Young LW, Klemperer MR: Pleural effusion in two children with histiocytosis X. Chest 61:33, 1972.

206. Konno K, Hayashi I, Oka S: Eosinophilic granuloma (histiocytosis X) involving anterior chest wall and lung. Am Rev Respir Dis 100:391, 1969.

207. Meier B, Rhyner K, Medici TC, et al: Eosinophilic granuloma of the skeleton with involvement of the lung: A report of three cases. Eur J Respir Dis 64:551, 1983.

208. Hunninghake GW, Costable U, Ando M, et al: American Thoracic Society, Statement on Sarcoidosis. Am J Respir Crit Care Med 160:736, 1999.

209. Mañá J, Gómez-Vaquero C, Montero A, et al: Löfgren's syndrome revisited: A study of 186 patients. Am J Med 107:240, 1999.

210. Daniil ZD, Gilchrist FC, Nicholson AG, et al: A histologic pattern of nonspecific interstitial pneumonitis is associated with a better prognosis than usual interstitial pneumonia in patients with cryptogenic fibrosing alveolitis. Am J Respir Crit Care Med 160:899, 1999.

211. Primack SL, Hartman TE, Hansell DM, et al: End-stage lung disease: CT findings in 61 patients. Radiology 189:681, 1993.

212. Arakawa H, Niimi H, Kurihara Y, et al: Expiratory high-resolution CT: Diagnostic value in diffuse lung diseases. Am J Roentgenol 175:1537, 2000.

213. Bartz RR, Stern EJ: Airways obstruction in patients with sarcoidosis: Expiratory CT scan findings. J Thorac Imag 15:285, 2000.

214. Johkoh T, Müller NL, Taniguchi H, et al: Acute interstitial pneumonia: Thin-section CT findings in 36 patients. Radiology 211:859, 1999.

215. Ichikado K, Johkoh T, Ikezoe J, et al: Acute interstitial pneumonia: High-resolution CT findings correlated with pathology. Am J Roentgenol 168:333, 1997.

CHAPTER 10

The Pulmonary Manifestations of Human Immunodeficiency Virus Infection

GENERAL EPIDEMIOLOGIC FEATURES

Since it was first described in 1981, the acquired immunodeficiency syndrome (AIDS) has become a pandemic associated with significant morbidity and mortality.[15] An estimated 42 million people have been infected with human immunodeficiency virus (HIV); more than 12 million have died.[8, 9] Two thirds of the more than 30 million people who have AIDS or HIV infection live in sub-Saharan Africa,[8] and more than 95% of new infections are occurring in developing countries.[9] In urban centers in the sub-Saharan region of Africa, western Europe, and North America, AIDS has become the leading cause of death for men and women between 15 and 49 years of age[15] and is the fourth leading cause of death worldwide.[9]

The two most important risk factors for HIV infection are sexual contact with an infected person and intravenous drug use. Approximately 45% of cases of AIDS in the United States occur in male homosexuals, 30% occur in intravenous drug users, 20% occur in individuals who had heterosexual contact with an infected person, and 5% occur in male homosexual intravenous drug users.[16]

From the beginning of the AIDS epidemic, pulmonary disease has been a major cause of morbidity and mortality, particularly in developed countries. A review of the medical records of more than 18,000 HIV-infected patients who received care in 10 American cities confirmed an association between the degree of immunosuppression, as reflected in the blood CD4$^+$ lymphocyte count, and the risk of developing particular respiratory disorders.[19] Common respiratory tract illnesses, such as bronchitis, sinusitis, and pharyngitis, were seen in association with all CD4$^+$ T-lymphocyte counts, although at a greater frequency than that in a seronegative population.[18] With lower counts, pulmonary infections occurred with increasing frequency. Approximately 80% of cases of bacterial pneumonia and pulmonary tuberculosis were associated with a CD4$^+$ count less than 400 cells/μl. With counts less than 300 cells/μl, bacterial pneumonia was often recurrent, and infection by nontuberculous mycobacteria was seen; counts less than 200 cells/μl often were associated with *Pneumocystis carinii* pneumonia, disseminated tuberculosis, or Kaposi's sarcoma (KS). Patients who had the most severe degree of immunosuppression (counts <100 cells/μl) tended to develop disseminated infection caused by *Mycobacterium avium-intracellulare* complex (MAC), cytomegalovirus (CMV), and various fungi. Similar observations have been made in the Pulmonary Complications of HIV Infection Study, in which a cohort of 1,353 HIV-infected patients was followed prospectively for 5 years.[20]

PULMONARY INFECTION

Many organisms have been found to cause pulmonary disease in patients who are HIV positive. Although some, such as *Mycobacterium tuberculosis*, *P. carinii*, and CMV, are seen in other immunodeficient patients, they tend to be particularly prevalent in the AIDS population; HIV-infected patients often have higher organism loads. Many unusual organisms, such as *Rhodococcus equii* and cryptosporidia, are seen almost exclusively in the setting of HIV infection. Simultaneous infection by more than one organism is relatively common, particularly in patients who have advanced disease;[21] there is evidence that the incidence of such multiple infections has increased since the beginning of the AIDS epidemic.[21] Despite this evidence, the incidence of the major opportunistic infections historically associated with AIDS (e.g., *P. carinii* pneumonia, CMV retinitis, and disseminated MAC infection) decreased from 21.9 per 100 person-years in 1994 to 3.7 per 100 person-years in 1997;[17] this improvement is largely attributable to the effectiveness of intensive antiretroviral therapy. The clinical manifestations of pulmonary infection caused by all these organisms may differ from those in other HIV-negative patients, even those who have other forms of immunodeficiency.

Nontuberculous Bacteria

Bacterial pneumonia is more frequent in HIV-positive individuals than in seronegative controls, the risk being highest among those whose CD4+ lymphocyte counts are less than 200 cells/μl.[22] The clinical and radiologic features of bacterial pneumonia are similar to those in the normal host (*see* Chapter 5);[24–26] however, pneumonia in HIV-positive patients more frequently is multilobar and more frequently is associated with bacteremia.[1]

Streptococcus pneumoniae is the leading cause of bacterial respiratory disease associated with bacteremia among HIV-infected adults.[27] Another relatively common cause of bacterial pneumonia is *Haemophilus influenzae*;[24, 28] *Staphylococcus aureus* has been reported uncommonly.[23] Approximately 50% of HIV-positive patients who have bacterial pneumonia have lobar or segmental consolidation, 30% have diffuse consolidation, and 20% have nodules.[2, 3] Bacterial infections are the most common cause of lobar and segmental consolidation in HIV-positive patients.[26] A similar appearance may be caused by other organisms, however, particularly *P. carinii* and *M. tuberculosis* and, occasionally, by noninfectious diseases, particularly KS and lymphoma.[26]

R. equi (*Corynebacterium equi*) is a common pulmonary pathogen in foals and is being recognized increasingly in humans. Infection is most frequent in immunocompromised individuals, particularly those who have AIDS;[29, 30] the identification of the organism should prompt consideration of concomitant HIV infection.[24] Radiologic manifestations usually consist of a round opacity or area of consolidation limited to one lobe, most commonly an upper lobe.[31] Several opacities may coalesce and undergo cavitation associated with a fluid level.[32, 33] Pleural effusion is present in approximately 20% of cases. In most patients, the abnormality persists for more than 1 month despite antibiotic therapy.

Bartonella (Rochalimaea) henselae and *Bartonella quintana* are the causative agents of bacillary angiomatosis, a reactive vasoproliferative lesion that occurs almost exclusively in patients who have AIDS.[35, 36] The mode of transmission of the disease is not known; however, because *B. henselae* is the most common cause of cat-scratch disease,[34, 37] it is likely that it involves animal or insect vectors. Symptoms include fever, chills, night sweats, weight loss,

anemia, and (occasionally) hemoptysis or chest pain.[36, 38] Lymphadenopathy in the axilla, neck, or groin is common.[36] In a review of the radiologic findings in nine patients, eight were found to have lung nodules measuring 1 mm to 1.5 cm in diameter.[36] The nodules had smooth margins and either well-defined or ill-defined borders; they had a propensity to be located adjacent to vascular structures.[36] One patient presented with a 6-cm peripheral mass that invaded the adjacent chest wall and showed marked enhancement after intravenous administration of contrast material (Fig. 10–1).[39] Most patients have hilar or mediastinal lymph node enlargement;[36] evidence of intra-abdominal lymph node involvement also is common. The enlarged nodes show marked enhancement after intravenous administration of contrast material.[36] Pleural effusions may be present and often are large. Less common findings include enhancing soft tissue masses in the skin and low attenuation lesions in the liver or spleen.[36]

Mycobacteria

Mycobacterium tuberculosis

Because the development of tuberculosis after infection by *M. tuberculosis* depends largely on a CD4 lymphocyte–mediated increase in the ability of macrophages to phagocytose and kill the organisms,[41] it is not surprising that HIV infection is associated with an increased prevalence of the disease. In 1995, the overall annual incidence of tuberculosis in the United States was 8.7 per 100,000 persons.[43] By contrast, in a study of 1,130 HIV-positive patients followed prospectively for a median of 53 months, 31 developed tuberculosis (0.7 cases per 100 person-years, a relative risk almost 100 times that of the general population).[43] Although most cases appear to be the result of reactivation of latent disease,[42] new infection has been important in some populations.[10, 11, 44]

The clinical features of tuberculosis in patients who have AIDS vary with the degree of immunosuppression.[40] When immune function is relatively preserved, the manifestations tend to be the same as those in patients who are not HIV positive.[40] In patients in whom CD4+ counts are depressed, the likelihood of atypical features is increased. Extrapulmonary tuberculosis is significantly more common in patients who are infected with HIV than in seronegative patients; it is seen in more than 50% at some point in the course of the disease, and it is the sole manifestation of the disease in about one quarter.[60] Gastrointestinal symptoms, disseminated disease (more than one noncontiguous extrapulmonary site or a positive culture from blood, bone marrow, or liver biopsy), and miliary disease are significantly more common in HIV-infected than in seronegative patients.[40, 62] An unusual systemic inflammatory reaction has been described in some patients who have been treated with combination antiretroviral therapy during the course of therapy for tuberculosis.[12]

Radiologic Manifestations

The patterns of abnormality seen in patients who have AIDS differ from those seen in other patients,[45, 46] the former having a greater likelihood of lymph node enlarge-

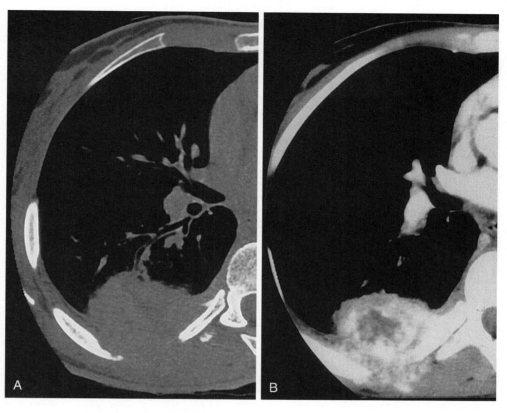

Figure 10–1. Bacillary Angiomatosis. A 26-year-old woman who had AIDS presented with chest pain, low-grade fever, and weight loss. Chest radiograph showed a mass in the right lung. CT scan *(A)* shows a peripheral right lower lobe mass, which is invading the chest wall. A scan after intravenous administration of contrast material *(B)* shows marked heterogeneous enhancement of the mass. Histologic assessment showed features of bacillary angiomatosis. (From Coche et al: Am J Roentgenol 165:56, 1995. Courtesy of Dr. Philippe Grenier, Hôpital Pitie-Salpétrière, Paris, France.)

ment, lower lobe disease, and extensive parenchymal involvement and a lower likelihood of cavitation (Table 10–1, Fig. 10–2).[4, 48, 49] In one investigation of 67 HIV-seropositive and 158 HIV-seronegative patients who had smear-positive or culture-positive pulmonary tuberculosis, parenchymal opacities were seen in 56 of the 67 (83%) HIV-positive patients, cavitation was seen in 40 (60%), and pleural effusion was seen in 6 (9%);[49] lymph node enlargement was evident in 46% of patients in whom the hila were not obscured by confluent parenchymal opacities (13 of 29). Of the 158 HIV-negative patients, parenchymal opacities were seen in 156 (99%), cavitation was seen in 136 (87%), and pleural effusion was seen in 19 (12%); lymphadenopathy was evident in 16% of patients in whom the hila were not obscured by confluent parenchymal disease (11 of 70). The chest radiograph was normal in 5 of

67 (7%) HIV-positive patients and in only 1 (0.6%) of 158 HIV-negative patients.

In a second investigation of 67 HIV-positive and 31 HIV-negative patients who had cultures positive for *M. tuberculosis*, findings seen more commonly in the former patients included mediastinal lymph node enlargement (60% versus 23%) and an atypical distribution of parenchymal opacities (55% versus 10%);[46] less common findings included parenchymal opacities characteristic of reactivation tuberculosis (30% versus 77%) and cavitation (18% versus 52%). There was no significant difference in the prevalence of pleural effusion (30% versus 23%) or normal radiographs (3% versus 10%).

There is considerable variation in the reported frequency of the various radiographic manifestations of tuberculosis in HIV-positive patients. Hilar or mediastinal lymph node enlargement has been reported in 20% to 60% of patients;[49–51] cavitary disease, in 0% to 40%;[49–53] atypical distribution (middle or lower lobe predominance) or atypical pattern (diffuse reticulation or miliary nodules), in 40% to 60%;[46, 49, 50] and pleural effusion, in 10% to 40%.[46, 49, 50] Normal radiographs have been documented in 3% to 15% of cases.[46, 54, 55]

The prevalence of radiologic abnormalities is influenced by the country of origin of the patient and by the degree of immunosuppression. Cavitation is seen less commonly in patients from the United States than in patients from North and Central Africa.[49, 51, 56] In patients who have a relatively normal immune status (>200 CD4+ cells/μl), the appearance is generally similar to that seen in postprimary tuberculosis in the normal host (Fig. 10–3); markedly immunosuppressed patients tend to have a pattern similar to

Table 10–1. PULMONARY TUBERCULOSIS IN AIDS: CHARACTERISTIC RADIOLOGIC MANIFESTATIONS

Patients with >200 CD4+ cells/μl
    Pattern resembles reactivation tuberculosis
    Cavitation present in most cases
    Lymphadenopathy relatively uncommon
    Enlarged nodes have low attenuation on CT scan
Patients with <200 CD4+ cells/μl
    Pattern resembles primary tuberculosis
    Cavitation relatively uncommon
    Lymphadenopathy present in most patients
    Enlarged nodes have low attenuation on CT scan
    About 20% of patients have a normal radiograph

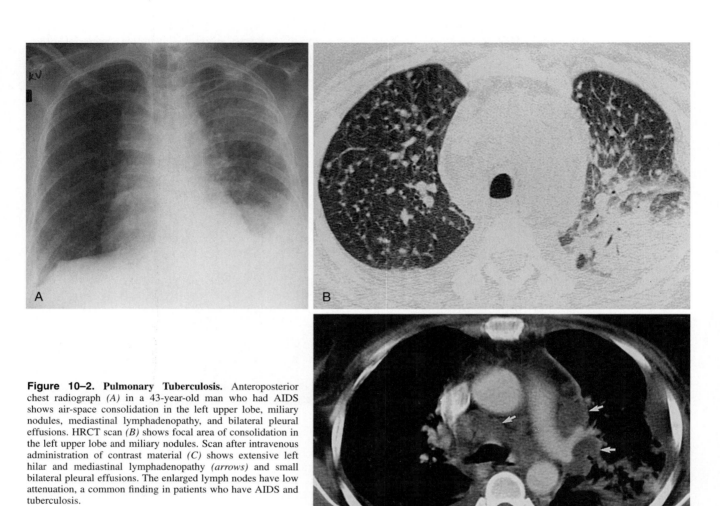

Figure 10–2. Pulmonary Tuberculosis. Anteroposterior chest radiograph *(A)* in a 43-year-old man who had AIDS shows air-space consolidation in the left upper lobe, miliary nodules, mediastinal lymphadenopathy, and bilateral pleural effusions. HRCT scan *(B)* shows focal area of consolidation in the left upper lobe and miliary nodules. Scan after intravenous administration of contrast material *(C)* shows extensive left hilar and mediastinal lymphadenopathy *(arrows)* and small bilateral pleural effusions. The enlarged lymph nodes have low attenuation, a common finding in patients who have AIDS and tuberculosis.

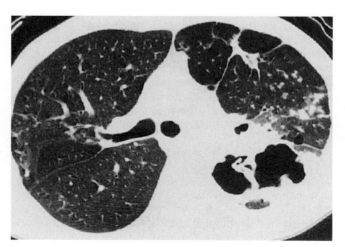

Figure 10–3. Tuberculosis. HRCT scan in a 39-year-old patient who had AIDS shows a large cavity in the superior segment of the left lower lobe, localized areas of scarring in the left upper lobe, and focal centrilobular nodules in the left upper and right upper lobes. The findings are characteristic of reactivation tuberculosis with endobronchial spread.

primary tuberculosis in the normal host or miliary disease.[4, 48, 54] In one investigation of 97 HIV-positive patients, hilar or mediastinal lymph node enlargement was evident on chest radiograph in 20 of 58 (34%) patients who had CD4[+] cell counts less than 200 cells/μl compared with 4 of 29 (14%) patients who had counts greater than 200 cells/μl.[48] Patients who have lower cell counts are more likely to have normal chest radiographs; in one investigation, 10 (21%) of 48 patients who had fewer than 200 CD4[+] cells/μl had normal chest radiographs, compared with only 1 of 20 (5%) patients with more than 200 CD4[+] cells/μl.[54]

The computed tomography (CT) findings have been described in several reports.[45, 46, 59] The most common abnormality consists of enlarged hilar and mediastinal lymph nodes, typically associated with low attenuation (*see* Fig. 10–2).[47, 57, 58] In one review of 25 patients, extensive node enlargement was present in 23 (92%) and focal hilar lymphadenopathy in 2 patients.[58] In 20 of the 25 (80%) patients, the enlarged nodes had low attenuation; in 5 of these, the periphery showed marked enhancement after intravenous administration of contrast material. In another investigation of 29 HIV-positive and 47 HIV-negative patients, the most common abnormalities in the former patients were lymph node enlargement (in 22 [76%]), nodules less than 1 cm in diameter (in 20 [69%]), dense consolidation (in 11 [38%]), and pleural effusion (in 7 [24%]);[59] lymphadenopathy was seen more commonly in HIV-positive than HIV-negative patients (76% versus 55%). Findings seen less commonly in HIV-positive patients included cavitation (24% versus 49%), 1- to 3-cm diameter nodules (14% versus 47%), and bronchial wall thickening (14% versus 45%). A linear correlation between the CD4[+] cell count and the number of lobes involved ($r = 0.84$) and between the CD4[+] cell count and the number of nodules ($r = 0.97$) was seen in the HIV-positive patients. Patients who had more than 200 CD4[+] cells/μl were more likely to have cavitation than patients who had lower cell counts (50% versus 13%) and less likely to have lymphadenopathy (33% versus 70%). Two patients, both with CD4[+] cells counts of less than 20/μl, had normal CT scans.

The presence of low attenuation or rim enhancing hilar or mediastinal lymph nodes in patients with AIDS is most suggestive of tuberculosis or MAC infection.[66] In one investigation, the authors reviewed the CT findings in 102 patients who had AIDS.[66] Hilar or mediastinal lymph node enlargement was present in 12 of 16 (75%) patients with mycobacterial infection, 13 of 26 (50%) patients with KS, 4 of 5 (80%) patients with lymphoma, and 3 of 5 (60%) patients with fungal infection. Low attenuation lymph nodes with or without rim enhancement were seen only in patients with tuberculosis or MAC infection.[66]

Nodule size and distribution on high-resolution computed tomography (HRCT) are helpful in the differential diagnosis of pulmonary complications in patients with AIDS.[13] In one investigation, 36 of 43 (86%) patients with opportunistic infection had a predominance of nodules smaller than 1 cm in diameter, whereas 14 of 17 (82%) patients with KS or lymphoma had a predominance of nodules larger than 1 cm.[13] The nodules had a centrilobular distribution in 28 of 43 (65%) patients with opportunistic infection compared with only 1 of 17 (6%) patients with KS or lymphoma. Nodules were seen rarely in *P. carinii*

pneumonia. Nodule size and distribution were not helpful in distinguishing mycobacterial from other bacterial infections, however.[13]

In HIV-positive patients who have pulmonary tuberculosis and normal radiographs, CT scan usually shows subtle parenchymal abnormalities.[4, 45] In one series of 40 HIV-positive patients with pulmonary tuberculosis, 6 (15%) had normal radiographs; CT scan was abnormal in all 6 patients.[45] Abnormalities seen on CT scan included miliary nodules in two patients, centrilobular nodules resulting from endobronchial spread in one, tuberculomas in two, and lymphadenopathy in one patient.[45]

Chest radiographs in AIDS patients with pulmonary tuberculosis often show transient worsening after antiretroviral therapy. This worsening presumably is related to improvement in immune function and inflammatory response.[14] The worsening of the radiographic abnormalities usually occurs 1 to 5 weeks after initiation of antiretroviral therapy and improves 2 weeks to 3 months later.[14]

Mycobacterium avium-intracellulare Complex

Disseminated infection by MAC organisms is the most common systemic bacterial infection in patients who have AIDS, occurring in 50%.[40, 64] Most patients have an advanced degree of immunosuppression, with CD4[+] lymphocyte counts less than 50 cells/μl.[40] Persistent fever and fatigue are the most common symptoms; night sweats, anorexia, chronic abdominal pain, and chronic diarrhea are present occasionally.[40, 65] Organisms may be cultured from respiratory tract secretions before the onset of bacteremia and in patients who have disseminated infection.[70, 71] Radiographically evident pulmonary disease is uncommon, however;[61, 65] in a study of 48 patients in whom the organism was isolated from respiratory specimens, only 2 patients had focal lung disease attributed to the organism.[72]

The radiographic and CT findings resemble those of tuberculosis and include focal areas of air-space consolidation, nodules, and mediastinal lymph node enlargement (Fig. 10–4).[61, 67] One group studied 53 patients who had AIDS and culture-proven mycobacterial pulmonary disease (29 with *M. tuberculosis*, 20 with MAC, and 4 with other nontuberculous organisms);[67] only patients who were free of concurrent infection and whose symptoms improved after appropriate mycobacterial therapy alone were included in the analysis. The most common abnormalities were small nodules (usually centrilobular, in 15 patients), areas of ground-glass attenuation (in 11 patients), and enlarged mediastinal lymph nodes (in 10 patients). Compared with patients who had tuberculosis, patients who had nontuberculous infection were more likely to have extensive disease or bilateral involvement and less likely to have lymphadenopathy (43% versus 76%). MAC also has been reported as a cause of endobronchial obstruction.[68, 69]

Fungi

P. carinii is the most important fungus to cause pulmonary disease in patients who are HIV-positive; however, other organisms account for a significant number of AIDS-defining illnesses.[73, 74]

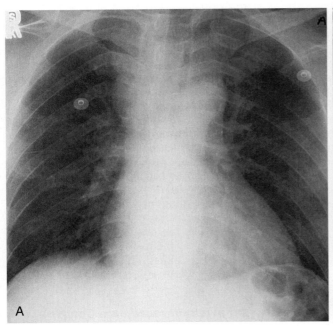

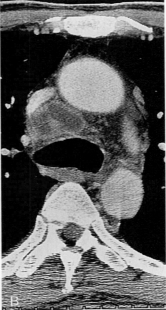

Figure 10–4. *Mycobacterium avium-intracellulare.* Anteroposterior chest radiograph *(A)* in a 47-year-old patient who had AIDS shows widening of the right superior mediastinum. Contrast-enhanced CT scan *(B)* shows an enlarged right paratracheal lymph node. The enlarged node has central low attenuation and rim enhancement. The patient had culture-proven disseminated *M. avium-intracellulare* complex. (From Kang EY, et al: Am J Roentgenol 166:15, 1996.)

Pneumocystis carinii

From the early 1980s to the early 1990s, *P. carinii* pneumonia occurred in 75% of patients who had AIDS[75] and constituted the most common AIDS-defining illness and the most common cause of life-threatening disease.[76, 77] Coinciding with the increased use of primary and secondary prophylaxis against the complication and of effective antiretroviral therapy in the late 1980s, the incidence of *P. carinii* pneumonia began to decline.[75, 78] Among 1,182 HIV-seropositive patients followed prospectively for a 52-month period as part of the Pulmonary Complications of HIV Infection Study, only 145 (12%) developed *P. carinii* pneumonia.[79] Despite the decrease in its incidence, *P. carinii* pneumonia is still an important infection; it is the AIDS-defining illness in 25% of all patients infected with HIV.[80] It has been the first opportunistic infection in about 15% of HIV-infected individuals who have received prophylaxis and in 45% of those who have not.[75] In two series from the United States, 25% of patients admitted to the hospital with the infection died.[81, 82]

The clinical features of *P. carinii* pneumonia are nonspecific. Patients commonly complain of fever, nonproductive cough, and progressive dyspnea on exertion.[77] Sputum production has been noted in less than 25% of patients.[114]

Table 10–2. *PNEUMOCYSTIS CARINII* PNEUMONIA: CHARACTERISTIC RADIOLOGIC MANIFESTATIONS

Ground-glass or granular pattern on radiograph
Perihilar predominance or diffuse distribution
Pneumothorax in 5%–10% of patients
Ground-glass pattern on HRCT
Symmetric, bilateral distribution
Cystic changes in about 30% of patients

HRCT, high-resolution computed tomography.

Radiologic Manifestations

The most common radiographic presentation of *P. carinii* pneumonia consists of bilateral and symmetric ground-glass, finely granular, or reticular opacities (Table 10–2, Fig. 10–5).[86, 88] The abnormalities can be diffuse but often have a perihilar, lower lung zone predominance or, less commonly, upper lung zone predominance.[86, 88] If left untreated, the opacities usually progress to predominantly perihilar or diffuse air-space consolidation (Fig. 10–6).[84]

The development of air-filled cysts or pneumatoceles

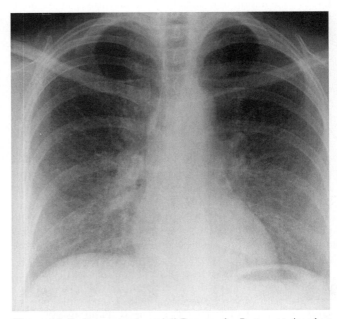

Figure 10–5. *Pneumocystis carinii* **Pneumonia.** Posteroanterior chest radiograph in a 41-year-old woman who had AIDS and proven *P. carinii* pneumonia shows bilateral symmetric ground-glass opacities involving mainly the middle and lower lung zones.

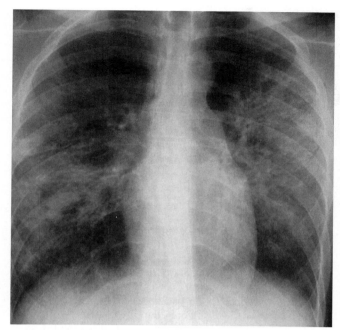

Figure 10–6. *Pneumocystis carinii* **Pneumonia**. Posteroanterior chest radiograph in a 31-year-old patient who had AIDS and *P. carinii* pneumonia shows bilateral areas of air-space consolidation involving mainly the midlung zones.

(Fig. 10–7) has been reported in about 5% to 35% of patients.[86, 89, 91] The cysts can be seen anywhere in the lungs, although they are more common in the upper lobes. They range from 1 to 10 cm in diameter and generally have walls 1 mm or less in thickness.[89–91] The cysts are usually spherical. In one study of 34 patients, the cysts

varied from 1 to 5 cm in diameter and were seen most commonly in the upper lung zones;[91] they were multiple in 32 of the 34 patients. Follow-up of the patients who survived the acute episode of pneumonia showed that most cysts resolved completely over a period of 5 days to 1 year (average, 5 months); a few showed no significant change in the size of the cysts on follow-up.

Pneumothorax occurs in about 5% to 10% of patients.[86, 88, 96] Factors associated with the complication include the presence of cysts on the chest radiograph,[83, 94] a history of cigarette smoking,[95] and the use of aerosolized pentamidine.[83, 96] In one investigation, pneumothorax developed in 12 (35%) of the 34 patients who had radiographically evident cysts compared with only 2 (7%) patients who did not.[91] The pneumothorax may be unilateral or bilateral[97, 98] and may be recurrent.[93] Pneumomediastinum occurs occasionally, either by itself or in association with pneumothorax.[86, 92]

Additional radiographic abnormalities seen in a small percentage of patients include focal parenchymal consolidation,[85, 86] single or multiple nodules,[99, 100] miliary nodules,[87, 101] cavitation,[99, 102] hilar or mediastinal lymph node enlargement,[86, 87] lymph node and visceral calcification,[103, 104] and pleural effusion.[85, 88] Radiographs have been reported to be normal in about 5% to 10% of patients.[5–7]

The characteristic HRCT findings of *P. carinii* pneumonia consist of symmetric bilateral areas of ground-glass attenuation.[105, 106] Similar to findings on radiographs, the abnormalities can be diffuse; however, they often involve mainly the perihilar regions or have a patchy distribution with intervening areas of normal parenchyma that frequently are sharply marginated by the interlobular septa (Fig. 10–8).[105, 106] Other common findings include cyst formation (Fig. 10–9), small nodules, irregular linear opacities (Fig. 10–10), and interlobular septal thickening.

In one series of 24 patients, areas of ground-glass attenuation were present on HRCT scan in 22 (92%); consolidation, in 9 (38%); cyst formation, in 8 (33%); small nodules,

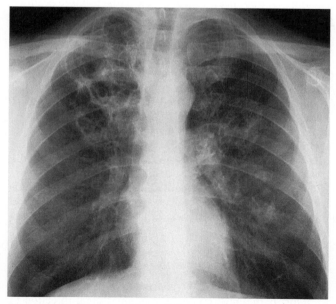

Figure 10–7. *Pneumocystis carinii* **Pneumonia: Pneumatoceles**. Posteroanterior chest radiograph in a 53-year-old patient who had AIDS shows numerous cystic lesions involving mainly the right upper lobe. These pneumatoceles had not been present on a chest radiograph performed 3 months previously.

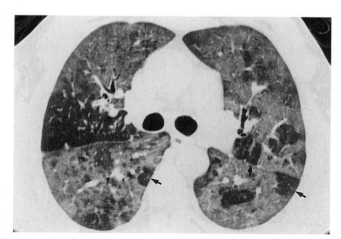

Figure 10–8. *Pneumocystis carinii* **Pneumonia**. HRCT scan in a 46-year-old man who had AIDS shows bilateral areas of ground-glass attenuation with a mosaic pattern. There is sharp demarcation between normal and abnormal lung parenchyma, with the areas of spared lung parenchyma having a size and configuration that corresponds to that of secondary pulmonary lobules *(arrows)*.

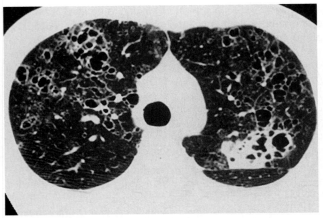

Figure 10–9. *Pneumocystis carinii* **Pneumonia with Cystic Changes.** HRCT scan through the upper lobes in a 30-year-old patient who had AIDS shows numerous irregularly shaped cysts in a random distribution. Focal areas of ground-glass attenuation and consolidation are evident.

in 6 (25%); irregular linear opacities, in 4 (17%); interlobular septal thickening, in 4 (17%); lymph node enlargement, in 6 (25%); pleural effusion, in 4 (17%); and pneumothorax, in 4 (17%).[66] In a second series of 39 patients, areas of ground-glass attenuation were present in 86% of patients, cystic changes were present in 38%, a reticular interstitial pattern was present in 18%, and small nodules were present in 18%.[106] The prevalence of these findings is related to the stage of disease;[47, 87] the initial abnormalities usually consist of areas of ground-glass attenuation that progress to consolidation, whereas irregular linear opacities (reticulation) and interlobular septal thickening are seen most commonly in patients who have subacute or resolving disease.[47, 87]

Most patients who have AIDS and *P. carinii* pneumonia have characteristic radiographic findings, obviating the need for CT.[6] CT can be helpful in the assessment of patients who have symptoms of pulmonary disease and normal or nonspecific radiographic findings, however.[107–109] As might be expected, HRCT may show parenchymal abnor-

malities in patients who have normal radiographs.[107–109] In one investigation of 13 such patients who had a high clinical index of suspicion for *P. carinii* pneumonia, all 4 patients who had patchy areas of ground-glass attenuation on HRCT had *P. carinii* identified in bronchoalveolar lavage fluid specimens;[108] the bronchoalveolar lavage fluid in the 9 patients who had normal HRCT scans was negative. In a second prospective investigation of 51 patients who had a high clinical pretest probability of *P. carinii* pneumonia and normal, equivocal, or nonspecific chest radiograph findings, HRCT scan showed parenchymal abnormalities in all 6 patients who had *P. carinii* pneumonia proved by bronchoalveolar lavage (sensitivity, 100%) and was falsely positive in 5 of 45 patients with negative bronchoalveolar lavage (specificity 89%).[109]

HRCT is superior to chest radiography in differentiating *P. carinii* pneumonia from other pulmonary infections and from malignancy in patients who have AIDS.[107] In one review of the radiographs and HRCT scans from 139 HIV-positive patients (including 106 who had proven thoracic complications and 33 who had no evidence of active intrathoracic disease), 96% were identified correctly by two observers as having intrathoracic abnormalities on CT scan compared with 90% on radiograph.[107] Among the patients who had no pulmonary complications, 73% were identified correctly as such at radiography and 86% at CT. A confident first-choice diagnosis was made in 47% of CT interpretations (correct in 87%) compared with 34% on radiograph (correct in 67%). A correct diagnosis of *P. carinii* pneumonia was made in 87% of 19 cases. The diagnosis of *P. carinii* pneumonia in these cases was based on the presence of areas of ground-glass attenuation. The value of this finding was assessed in a study that included 102 patients who had AIDS and proven thoracic complications and 20 HIV-positive patients without active intrathoracic disease.[66] A correct first-choice diagnosis of *P. carinii* pneumonia was made based on the HRCT findings in 29 (83%) of 35 patients; the diagnosis was made with a high degree of confidence in 25 patients. Although ground-glass attenuation in patients who have AIDS can be the result of several other abnormalities, such as CMV pneumonia or lymphocytic interstitial pneumonitis, in most cases, it is a manifestation of *P. carinii* pneumonia.

Scintigraphy plays a limited role in the diagnosis of *P. carinii* pneumonia.[47, 63] Although gallium 67 citrate scintigraphy has a relatively high sensitivity (80% to 95%), its specificity is low (50% to 75%).[111–113] The procedure requires 48 to 72 hours after intravenous injection for the blood pool to clear the chest and allow optimal imaging.[113] Other parenchymal abnormalities that can increase pulmonary gallium uptake in patients who have AIDS include tuberculosis, MAC infection, CMV pneumonia, and lymphoma.[110, 111, 113]

Cryptococcus neoformans

Cryptococcosis, usually caused by *Cryptococcus neoformans*, is the most common systemic fungal infection in HIV-infected patients.[73] It is seen in about 10% of patients who have AIDS,[115] usually when the CD4[+] count is less than 200 cells/μl.[116] Although central nervous system disease dominates the clinical picture, the lungs commonly are affected. In one study of 31 HIV-infected patients

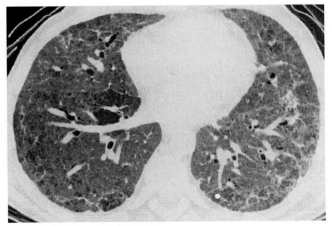

Figure 10–10. *Pneumocystis carinii* **Pneumonia.** HRCT scan in a 42-year-old patient who had AIDS and proven *P. carinii* pneumonia shows extensive bilateral areas of ground-glass attenuation. Focal areas of normal lung parenchyma, areas of decreased attenuation, and irregular linear opacities involving mainly the subpleural lung regions are evident.

who developed cryptococcal infection, 12 had cryptococcal pneumonia;[117] 11 of these patients had evidence of extrapulmonary disease.

Most cases of pneumonia are clinically silent and discovered serendipitously during the course of investigation of central nervous system or systemic complaints.[74] Pulmonary signs and symptoms are nonspecific. Fever, cough, dyspnea, sputum production, and pleuritic chest pain all have been described.[118] Hemoptysis is uncommon.[118]

The most common radiologic manifestations consist of a reticular or reticulonodular interstitial pattern (seen in about 50% to 60% of patients) or discrete nodules (seen in 30%).[119–121] The latter tend to occur early in the course of AIDS and in patients who have less severe immunosuppression.[47, 121] Less common manifestations include ground-glass opacities, air-space consolidation, miliary nodules, lymph node enlargement, and pleural effusions.[47, 119, 121]

Histoplasma capsulatum

In the United States, histoplasmosis occurs in approximately 2% of patients who have AIDS, a prevalence that increases to 5% in endemic areas.[47] About 75% of these patients have disseminated disease and are markedly immunosuppressed, typically having CD4+ counts of less than 100 cells/μl.[122]

More than half of affected individuals have radiographic evidence of pulmonary involvement at the time of diagnosis.[123–125] In one review of 27 patients, the chest radiograph was abnormal in 23 (85%);[122] findings included diffuse nodular opacities 3 mm or less in diameter seen in 9 (39%) patients, nodules greater than 3 mm in diameter seen in 1 patient, small linear or irregular opacities seen in 7 (30%) patients, and focal or patchy areas of consolidation seen in 7 (30%) patients. Small pleural effusions were present in five patients, and hilar or paratracheal lymph node enlargement was present in one patient. The radiographic and HRCT findings of miliary histoplasmosis are similar to those of miliary tuberculosis.[122, 126]

Coccidioides immitis

Coccidioidomycosis is common among HIV-infected patients who live in areas endemic for the infection. In one study from Arizona, the cumulative incidence of active disease among 170 patients followed prospectively was 25% by 41 months.[127] Risk factors included a CD4+ lymphocyte count of less than 250 cells/μl and a diagnosis of AIDS at entry into the study; evidence of prior infection did not appear to predict the development of disease.

Presenting symptoms are nonspecific and include fever, weight loss, cough, and fatigue.[77] The identification of an abnormal chest radiograph usually triggers investigation that leads to the diagnosis. The usual manifestations consist of focal or diffuse areas of air-space consolidation;[128] less common findings include nodules, cavitation, hilar lymph node enlargement, and pleural effusion.

Blastomyces dermatitidis

Blastomycosis has been recognized uncommonly as an opportunistic infection in HIV-infected patients; fewer than 60 patients were described by 1997.[129] The chest radiograph may show focal consolidation, diffuse interstitial or miliary changes and (rarely) bilateral nodules, cavitary disease, or pleural effusion.[129, 130]

Aspergillus Species

Invasive pulmonary aspergillosis is uncommon in patients who have AIDS, occurring in only about 0.1% to 0.5%.[116] Most cases have been described after 1990, however, making this organism an *emerging pathogen* in this clinical context.[131, 132] Most patients who develop pulmonary aspergillosis have neutropenia and a history of broad-spectrum antibiotic and glucocorticoid use.[132, 134, 187] In the absence of these factors, patients who develop invasive lung disease usually have advanced HIV infection, generally with a CD4+ lymphocyte count less than 50 cells/μl.[187] Symptoms consist of fever, cough, chest pain, and dyspnea;[133] they tend to be insidious in onset and progression.[132] Occasionally, there is complicating pneumothorax;[116] fatal hemoptysis is common.[133]

As has been described in non-AIDS patients, pulmonary aspergillosis in patients who have AIDS is manifested in several ways that can be categorized broadly as saprophytic, allergic, or invasive. Invasive aspergillosis is probably the most common and may present as upper lobe cavitary disease, which may resemble chronic necrotizing aspergillosis (Fig. 10–11)[133, 135] or which may be characterized by one or two large cavities without surrounding infiltration).[116, 135] Such cavitary disease has been reported in approximately one third of cases.[132, 133, 187] Other common findings include focal areas of consolidation and single or multiple nodules.[135, 187] CT may demonstrate nodules and cavitary lesions not apparent on the radiograph.[135]

Viruses

The clinical significance of the identification of a viral organism in the lung often is uncertain in HIV-infected patients. Nevertheless, a variety of viruses can cause pulmonary disease,[136] the most commonly implicated being CMV.

Cytomegalovirus

CMV frequently can be detected on culture of bronchoalveolar lavage fluid obtained from patients infected with HIV.[136–138] The presence of the organism seldom is associated with significant morbidity and mortality, and it is likely that it is not pathogenic in most cases. The organism does cause pulmonary damage, however, and is associated with disseminated disease in some patients. In one review of 54 autopsies performed on patients who had AIDS, 39 (72%) had histologic evidence of CMV infection, of whom 31 (80%) had pneumonitis;[139] CMV was the only organism identified in 2 of these patients, both of whom had severe lung disease. In a second study of 75 autopsies, histologic evidence for CMV pneumonia was identified in 81%;[140] CMV was thought to have caused significant disease in 21 patients, and 5 were considered to have died as a direct result of the pneumonia. Fever, dyspnea, and dry cough are common findings in patients who have pneumonitis.

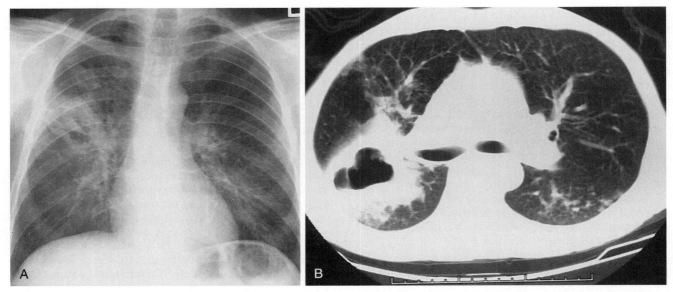

Figure 10–11. Angioinvasive Aspergillosis. Posteroanterior chest radiograph *(A)* in a 42-year-old patient who had AIDS shows a poorly defined irregular, thick-walled cavity in the right upper lobe and patchy areas of consolidation. Conventional CT scan *(B)* shows a well-defined irregular, thick-walled cavity in the posterior segment of the right upper lobe and patchy surrounding consolidation. The diagnosis was pathologically proven angioinvasive aspergillosis.

The most common radiologic findings consist of bilateral ground-glass opacities or areas of consolidation.[141, 142] Less common manifestations include reticular opacities, discrete nodules or masses, and, rarely, miliary nodules.[142, 143] Similar findings have been described on CT scan (Fig. 10–12).[141]

PULMONARY NEOPLASIA

About 25% of patients who have AIDS develop a malignant neoplasm at some point in the course of the disease.[143] Three cancers—KS, non-Hodgkin's lymphoma, and cervical carcinoma—are indicator conditions for the diagnosis of AIDS.[143] Several other neoplasms, including pulmonary carcinoma, may be increased in frequency in patients who have HIV infection.

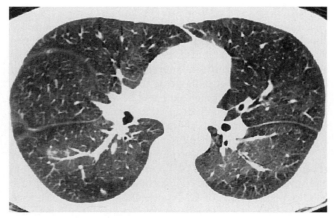

Figure 10–12. Cytomegalovirus Pneumonia. HRCT scan in a 38-year-old woman who had AIDS shows bilateral areas of ground-glass attenuation with relative sparing of the subpleural lung regions. Repeated bronchoalveolar lavage showed large numbers of cytomegalovirus organisms and no other organisms.

Kaposi's Sarcoma

KS occurs in approximately 15% to 20% of HIV-infected male homosexuals and in 1% to 3% of other HIV-infected patients.[143] Since the beginning of the AIDS epidemic, the incidence of the tumor as an AIDS-defining illness has declined progressively;[144] whether more intense antiretroviral therapy would alter the incidence of this tumor further remains to be determined. The neoplasm is more common in patients whose immune function is impaired. A strong association with herpesvirus 8 has been found in many studies.[146] Most patients who have pulmonary KS have respiratory symptoms.[143] Dyspnea and cough have been reported most commonly;[152] occasionally, blood streaking of sputum, fever, and chest pain are present.[145]

Pathologically, pulmonary lesions typically are most prominent in the bronchovascular or pleural interstitium. This distribution may result in an appearance similar to lymphangitic carcinomatosis except that involved regions are red or purplish rather than white and usually are larger. Expansion of tumor outside the bronchovascular interstitium may result in nodules or, occasionally, in ill-defined areas of parenchymal consolidation.

Radiologic Manifestations

The characteristic radiographic findings consist of bilateral, symmetric, poorly defined nodular or linear opacities (Table 10–3, Fig. 10–13). Although sometimes diffuse, these opacities often have a predominantly perihilar distribution.[149–151] The nodules measure 0.5 to 3 cm in diameter and tend to coalesce.[147, 150] Bronchovascular bundles may show thickening, which often progresses to perihilar consolidation.[151] Other radiographic findings include thickening of the interlobular septa (Kerley B lines), pleural effusions (in 30% to 70% of patients[147–149]), and hilar or mediastinal lymph node enlargement (in 5% to 15%).[151, 152] In 5% to 15% of patients who have pulmonary parenchy-

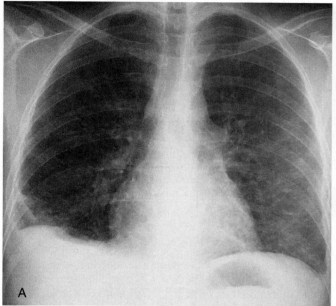

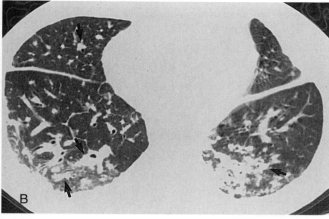

Figure 10–13. Kaposi's Sarcoma. Anteroposterior chest radiograph *(A)* shows bilateral, symmetric, poorly defined nodular and linear opacities and small bilateral pleural effusions. HRCT scan *(B)* shows nodular thickening of the bronchoarterial bundles *(arrows)*, interlobular septal thickening, and small bilateral pleural effusions. (From Kang EY, et al: Am J Roentgenol 166:15, 1996.)

mal involvement at autopsy or endoscopy, the radiograph is normal.[147, 149, 151]

The characteristic HRCT findings consist of irregularly shaped, spiculated or poorly defined nodules in a predominantly perihilar and peribronchoarterial distribution (Fig. 10–14).[66, 154, 155] Other common findings include bronchial wall thickening (Fig. 10–15), interlobular septal thickening, focal areas of ground-glass attenuation or air-space consolidation, and pleural effusion. The areas of ground-glass attenuation may be the result of hemorrhage,[6, 156] but the finding should raise the possibility of concomitant *P. carinii* pneumonia. In one review of the findings in 26 patients who had KS, nodules were seen on CT scan in 22 (85%) patients; peribronchoarterial thickening, in 21 (81%); hilar or mediastinal lymph node enlargement, in 13 (50%); interlobular septal thickening, in 10 (38%); consolidation, in 9 (35%); ground-glass attenuation, in 6 (23%); and pleural effusion, in 9 (35%).[66] Hilar or mediastinal lymph node enlargement is evident on CT scan in 30% to 50% of patients.[66, 149, 154] Affected nodes usually measure less than 2 cm in diameter.[149] Less common findings include a focal parenchymal mass; cavitation; involvement of the sternum, ribs, or thoracic spine; and pericardial effusion.[66, 153]

The characteristic appearance of KS on CT scan allows a confident radiologic diagnosis in most cases. In one investigation of 102 patients who underwent the procedure, a correct first-choice diagnosis of KS was made in 26

(83%) of 32 patients who had the disease.[66] Although CT permits accurate assessment of the presence, pattern, and distribution of parenchymal abnormalities in KS, however, it is relatively insensitive in the detection of endobronchial lesions.[47] Tumors large enough to cause atelectasis or stridor may be identified as intraluminal soft tissue lesions,[47, 149] but smaller lesions seldom are seen.

Non-Hodgkin's Lymphoma

Non-Hodgkin's lymphoma develops in about 5% to 10% of HIV-infected patients, an incidence that is more than 60-fold higher than that described in the general population.[157] Pulmonary involvement has been recognized clinically in approximately 1% to 15% of affected patients.[158] Most patients have an advanced degree of immunosuppression; the mean CD4$^+$ count in one series of 38 patients was only 67 cells/μl.[158] Tumors generally are high grade, widely

Table 10–3. KAPOSI'S SARCOMA: CHARACTERISTIC RADIOLOGIC MANIFESTATIONS

Bilateral, symmetric nodular opacities
Nodules have irregular, spiculated margins
Perihilar and peribronchoarterial distribution
Interlobular septal thickening
Lymphadenopathy evident on CT scan in 30%–50% of cases
Enlarged nodes usually 1–2 cm in diameter
Pleural effusion in about 30% of cases

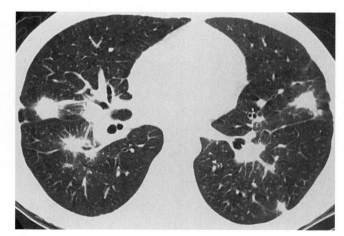

Figure 10–14. Kaposi's Sarcoma. HRCT scan in a 34-year-old man who had AIDS shows bilateral nodules with spiculated margins and peribronchial thickening. (Courtesy of Dr. Andrew Mason, Department of Radiology, St. Paul's Hospital, Vancouver, BC.)

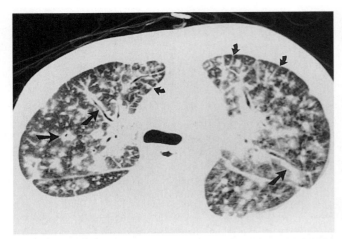

Figure 10–15. Kaposi's Sarcoma. HRCT scan in a 28-year-old man who had AIDS shows extensive bilateral thickening of the bronchoarterial bundles *(straight arrows)*, irregularly marginated nodules, and thickening of the interlobular septa *(curved arrows)*. (From Worthy S, Kang KY, Müller NL: Semin Ultrasound CT MRI 16:353, 1995.)

Table 10–4. NON-HODGKIN'S LYMPHOMA: CHARACTERISTIC RADIOLOGIC MANIFESTATIONS

Single or multiple nodules
Nodules usually have smooth margins
Masslike areas of consolidation
Pleural effusions in about 50% of patients
Lymphadenopathy evident on CT scan in 30% of cases

disseminated, and extranodal at presentation;[159] about 20% present in the central nervous system.[160]

The most common radiologic findings in the thorax consist of single or multiple pulmonary nodules and pleural effusions (Table 10–4, Fig. 10–16).[163, 164] The nodules usually are well circumscribed and range from 0.5 to 5 cm in diameter.[47, 163] On CT scan, they may have smooth or spiculated margins and often contain air bronchograms. Other common manifestations include reticular or reticulonodular opacities and bilateral areas of consolidation.[47, 163] The nodules and the masslike areas of consolidation may cavitate.[163, 164] Pleural effusions have been reported in 25% to 75% of patients[158, 163, 164] and usually are seen in association with parenchymal abnormalities; occasionally, they are the only finding.[161, 165] The prevalence of lymph node enlargement has ranged from 0[162, 164] to 55%[158] in various studies; a reasonable overall estimate is 30%.[161, 163] Abnor-

malities described in a few patients include tracheal irregularity or polypoid endobronchial tumors,[163, 166] extrathoracic masses spreading into the mediastinum,[164] and rib destruction.[47]

Pulmonary Carcinoma

Initial reports in which pulmonary carcinoma was found to occur at a young age and to behave in an aggressive fashion in a number of patients who were HIV seropositive raised the possibility of a pathogenic association between the two conditions.[167–169] The results of extensive epidemiologic surveys subsequently confirmed the link between HIV infection and an increased risk for the development of pulmonary carcinoma.[170–172] The clinical and radiologic manifestations of pulmonary carcinoma in patients who have AIDS are similar to those in HIV-negative individuals.[173–175]

MISCELLANEOUS PULMONARY ABNORMALITIES

Nonspecific Interstitial Pneumonitis

Nonspecific interstitial pneumonitis is a relatively common disorder in HIV-positive patients that is characterized histologically by a mild-to-moderate infiltrate of lymphocytes and plasma cells in the peribronchiolar, perivascular, and interlobular septal interstitial tissue;[176] in contrast to

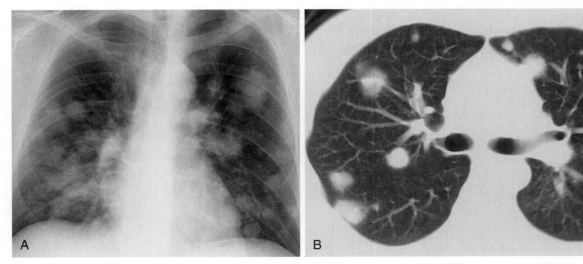

Figure 10–16. Non-Hodgkin's Lymphoma. Posteroanterior chest radiograph *(A)* in a 41-year-old man who had AIDS shows numerous bilateral nodules of varying sizes. CT scan *(B)* shows that the nodules have smooth or slightly irregular margins and are distributed randomly throughout both lungs. There was no evidence of lymphadenopathy on radiograph or CT scan.

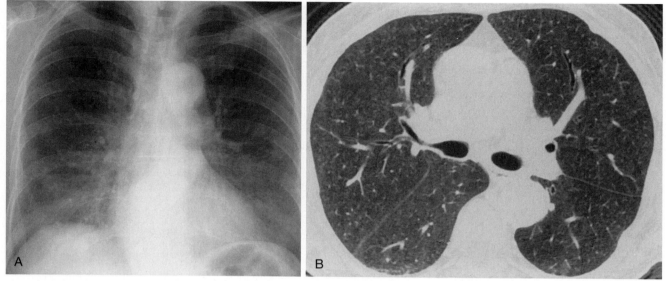

Figure 10–17. Lymphocytic Interstitial Pneumonia. Posteroanterior chest radiograph *(A)* in a 74-year-old man who had AIDS shows bilateral hazy increase in opacity of both lungs. HRCT scan *(B)* shows diffuse ground-glass attenuation and poorly defined small nodules. The diagnosis of lymphocytic interstitial pneumonia was confirmed at open-lung biopsy.

lymphocytic interstitial pneumonitis (*see* farther on), involvement of the alveolar interstitium is relatively mild or absent altogether. Associated clinical findings are diverse but in general terms are indistinguishable from those seen with opportunistic infection.[177, 178] Most patients have fever, cough, and dyspnea that usually is mild; mild-to-moderate deficits in gas exchange are common.[177]

The radiologic findings usually consist of a fine reticular or reticulonodular pattern or ground-glass opacities in the perihilar regions or diffusely distributed throughout both lungs.[179, 180] The appearance resembles that of *P. carinii* pneumonia. In one series of 36 patients in whom the diagnosis was made by transbronchial or open-lung biopsy, 16 (44%) had normal chest radiographs.[179]

Lymphocytic Interstitial Pneumonitis

Lymphocytic interstitial pneumonitis is characterized histologically by more or less diffuse infiltration of the pulmonary parenchymal interstitium by cytologically mature mononuclear cells (predominantly lymphocytes) (*see* page 258).[176, 181] Although rare in HIV-infected adults,[145] lymphocytic interstitial pneumonitis is relatively common in children,[182, 183] in whom it is an AIDS-defining disease.[184]

Radiographic findings consist of fine or coarse reticular or reticulonodular opacities,[184] multiple nodules measuring 2 to 5 mm in diameter,[25] or poorly defined hazy (ground-glass) opacities (Fig. 10–17). Occasionally, areas of consolidation are superimposed on a background reticulonodular pattern.[185] HRCT scans show areas of ground-glass attenuation[163] or ill-defined 2- to 4-mm nodules, frequently in a peribronchial distribution.[186] Cysts similar to those seen in *P. carinii* pneumonia have been noted in some patients.[163] The abnormalities may resemble those of other lymphoproliferative disorders; in one series of five adult patients who had lymphocytic interstitial pneumonitis, the HRCT findings (ill-defined 2- to 4-mm nodules) were similar to those seen in three patients who had an *atypical lympho-*

proliferative disorder and to the one patient who had mucosa-associated lymphoma.[186]

References

1. Haramati LB, Jenny-Avital ER: Approach to the diagnosis of pulmonary disease in patients infected with the human immunodeficiency virus. J Thorac Imaging 13:247, 1998.
2. Amorosa JK, Nahass RG, Nosher JL, et al: Radiologic distinction of pyogenic pulmonary infection from *Pneumocystis carinii* pneumonia in AIDS patients. Radiology 175:721, 1990.
3. Polsky B, Gold JW, Whimbey E, et al: Bacterial pneumonia in patients with the acquired immunodeficiency syndrome. Ann Intern Med 104:38, 1986.
4. Leung AN: Pulmonary tuberculosis: The essentials. Radiology 210:307, 1999.
5. Kennedy CA, Goetz Bidwell M: Atypical roentgenographic manifestations of *Pneumocystis carinii* pneumonia. Arch Intern Med 152:1390, 1992.
6. Mason AC, Müller NL: The role of computed tomography in the diagnosis and management of human immunodeficiency virus (HIV)-related pulmonary diseases. Semin Ultrasound CT MRI 19:154, 1998.
7. Boiselle PM, Tocino I, Hooley RJ, et al: The accuracy of chest radiograph interpretation in the diagnosis of PCP, bacterial pneumonia and TB in HIV positive patients. J Thorac Imaging 12:47, 1997.
8. Horowitz HW, Telzak EE, Sepkowitz KA, et al: Human immunodeficiency virus infection, Part I. Dis Mon 44:545, 1998.
9. Fauci AS: The AIDS epidemic. N Engl J Med 341:1046, 1999.
10. van Rie A, Warren R, Richardson M, et al: Exogenous reinfection as cause of recurrent tuberculosis after curative treatment. N Engl J Med 341:1174, 1999.
11. Barnes PF, Yang Z, Pogoda JM, et al: Foci of tuberculosis transmission in central Los Angeles. Am J Respir Crit Care Med 159:1081, 1999.
12. Furrer H, Malinverni R: Systemic inflammatory reaction after starting highly active antiretroviral therapy in AIDS patients treated for extrapulmonary tuberculosis. Am J Med 106:371, 1999.
13. Edinburgh KJ, Jasmer RM, Huang L, et al: Multiple pulmonary nodules in AIDS: Usefulness of CT in distinguishing among potential causes. Radiology 214:427, 2000.
14. Fishman JE, Saraf-Lavi E, Narita M, et al: Pulmonary tuberculosis in AIDS patients: Transient chest radiographic worsening after initiation of antiretroviral therapy. Am J Roentgenol 174:43, 2000.

15. Quinn TC: Global burden of the HIV pandemic. Lancet 348:99, 1996.

16. Anonymous: Update: Trends in AIDS incidence—United States, 1996. MMWR Morb Mortal Wkly Rep 46:861, 1997.

17. Bollinger RC, Tripathy SP, Quinn TC: The human immunodeficiency virus epidemic in India: Current magnitude and future projections. Medicine 74:97, 1995.

18. Rosen MJ: Overview of pulmonary complications. Clin Chest Med 4:621, 1996.

19. Hanson DL, Chu SY, Farizo KM, et al: Distribution of CD4+ T lymphocytes at diagnosis of acquired immunodeficiency syndrome-defining and other human immunodeficiency virus-related illnesses. Arch Intern Med 155:1537, 1995.

20. Wallace JM, Hansen NI, Lavange L, et al: Respiratory disease trends in the pulmonary complications of HIV infection study cohort. Am J Respir Crit Care Med 155:72, 1997.

21. Sehonanda A, Choi YJ, Blum S: Changing patterns of autopsy findings among persons with acquired immunodeficiency syndrome in an inner-city population: A 12-year retrospective study. Arch Pathol Lab Med 120:459, 1996.

22. Hirschtick RE, Glassroth J, Jordan MC, et al: Bacterial pneumonia in persons infected with the human immunodeficiency virus. N Engl J Med 333:845, 1995.

23. Daley CL: Bacterial pneumonia in HIV-infected patients. Semin Respir Infect 8:104, 1993.

24. Noskin GA, Glassroth J: Bacterial pneumonia associated with HIV-1 infection. Clin Chest Med 17:713, 1996.

25. Richards PJ, Armstrong P, Parkin JM, et al: Chest imaging in AIDS. Clin Radiol 53:554, 1998.

26. Amin Z, Miller RF, Shaw PJ: Lobar or segmental consolidation on chest radiographs of patients with HIV infection. Clin Radiol 52:541, 1997.

27. Janoff EN, Breiman RF, Daley CL, et al: Pneumococcal disease during HIV infection: Epidemiologic, clinical and immunologic perspectives. Ann Intern Med 117:314, 1992.

28. Falco V, Fernandez de Sevilla T, Alegre J, et al: Bacterial pneumonia in HIV-infected patients: A prospective study of 68 episodes. Eur Respir J 7:235, 1994.

29. Scott MA, Graham BS, Verrall R, et al: *Rhodococcus equi*: An increasingly recognized opportunistic pathogen: Report of 12 cases and review of 65 cases in the literature. Am J Clin Pathol 103:649, 1995.

30. Verville TD, Huycke MM, Greenfield RA, et al: *Rhodococcus equi* infections of humans: 12 cases and a review of the literature. Medicine 73:119, 1994.

31. Scannell KA, Portoni EJ, Finkle HI, et al: Pulmonary malacoplakia and *Rhodococcus equi* infection in a patient with AIDS. Chest 97:1000, 1990.

32. MacGregor JH, Samuelson WM, Sane DC, et al: Opportunistic lung infection caused by *Rhodococcus (Corynebacterium) equi*. Radiology 160:83, 1986.

33. Van Etta LL, Filce GA, Ferguson RM, et al: *Corynebacterium equi*: A review of 12 cases of human infection. Rev Infect Dis 5:1012, 1983.

34. Slater LN, Welch DF, Hensel D, et al: A newly recognized fastidious gram-negative pathogen as a cause of fever and bacteremia. N Engl J Med 323:1587, 1990.

35. Adal KA, Cockerell CJ, Petri WA: Cat scratch disease, bacillary angiomatosis, and other infections due to *Rochalimaea*. N Engl J Med 330:1509, 1994.

36. Moore EH, Russell LA, Klein JS, et al: Bacillary angiomatosis in patients with AIDS: Multiorgan imaging findings. Radiology 197:67, 1995.

37. Koehler JE, LeBoit PE, Egbert BM, et al: Cutaneous vascular lesions and disseminated cat-scratch disease in patients with the acquired immunodeficiency syndrome (AIDS) and AIDS-related complex. Ann Intern Med 109:449, 1988.

38. Foltzer MA, Guiney WB, Wager GC, et al: Bronchopulmonary bacillary angiomatosis. Chest 104:973, 1993.

39. Coche E, Beigelman C, Lucidarme O, et al: Thoracic bacillary angiomatosis in a patient with AIDS. Am J Roentgenol 165:56, 1995.

40. Chin DP, Hopewell PC: Mycobacterial complications of HIV infection. Clin Chest Med 17:697, 1996.

41. Barnes PF, Bloch AB, Davidson PT, et al: Tuberculosis in patients with human immunodeficiency virus infection. N Engl J Med 324:1644, 1991.

42. Selwyn PA, Hartel D, Lewis VA, et al: A prospective study of the risk of tuberculosis among intravenous drug users with human immunodeficiency virus infection. N Engl J Med 320:545, 1989.

43. Markowitz N, Hansen NI, Hopewell PC, et al: Incidence of tuberculosis in the United States among HIV-infected persons. Ann Intern Med 126:123, 1997.

44. Small PM, Hopewell PC, Singh SP, et al: The epidemiology of tuberculosis in San Francisco: A population-based study using conventional and molecular methods. N Engl J Med 330:1703, 1994.

45. Leung AN, Brauner MW, Gamsu G, et al: Pulmonary tuberculosis: Comparison of CT findings in HIV-seropositive and HIV-seronegative patients. Radiology 198:687, 1996.

46. Haramati LB, Jenny-Avital ER, Alterman DD: Effect of HIV status on chest radiographic and CT findings in patients with tuberculosis. Clin Radiol 52:31, 1997.

47. McGuinness G: Changing trends in the pulmonary manifestations of AIDS. Radiol Clin North Am 35:1029, 1997.

48. Jones BE, Young SMM, Antoniskis D, et al: Relationship of the manifestations of tuberculosis to CD4 cell counts in patients with human immunodeficiency virus infection. Am Rev Respir Dis 148:1292, 1993.

49. Long R, Maycher B, Scalcini M, et al: The chest roentgenogram in pulmonary tuberculosis patients seropositive for human immunodeficiency virus type 1. Chest 99:123, 1991.

50. Harries AD: Tuberculosis in human immunodeficiency virus infection in developing countries. Lancet 335:387, 1990.

51. Saks AM, Posner R: Tuberculosis in HIV positive patients in South Africa: A comparative radiological study with HIV negative patients. Clin Radiol 46:387, 1992.

52. Louie E, Rice LB, Holzman RS: Tuberculosis in non-Haitian patients with acquired immunodeficiency syndrome. Chest 90:542, 1986.

53. Rieder HL, Cauthen GM, Bloch AB, et al: Tuberculosis and acquired immunodeficiency syndrome—Florida. Arch Intern Med 149:1268, 1989.

54. Greenberg SD, Frager D, Suster B, et al: Active pulmonary tuberculosis in patients with AIDS: Spectrum of radiographic findings (including a normal appearance). Radiology 193:115, 1994.

55. Keiper MD, Beumont E, Elshami A, et al: CD4 T lymphocyte count and the radiographic presentation of pulmonary tuberculosis: A study of the relationship between these factors in patients with human immunodeficiency virus infection. Chest 107:74, 1995.

56. Colebunders RL, Ryder RW, Nzilambi N, et al: HIV infection in patients with tuberculosis in Kinshasa, Zaire. Am Rev Respir Dis 139:1082, 1989.

57. Perich J, Ayuso MC, Vilana R, et al: Disseminated lymphatic tuberculosis in acquired immunodeficiency syndrome: Computed tomography findings. Can Assoc Radiol J 41:353, 1990.

58. Pastores SM, Naidich DP, Aranda CP, et al: Intrathoracic adenopathy associated with pulmonary tuberculosis in patients with human immunodeficiency virus infection. Chest 103:1433, 1993.

59. Laissy JP, Cadi M, Boudiaf ZE, et al: Pulmonary tuberculosis: Computed tomography and high-resolution computed tomography patterns in patients who are either HIV-negative or HIV-seropositive. J Thorac Imaging 13:58, 1998.

60. Chaisson RE, Schecter GF, Theuer CP, et al: Tuberculosis in patients with the acquired immunodeficiency syndrome. Am Rev Respir Dis 136:570, 1987.

61. Hocqueloux L, Lesprit P, Herrmann J-L, et al: Pulmonary *Mycobacterium avium* complex disease without dissemination in HIV-infected patients. Chest 113:542, 1998.

62. Shafer RW, Goldberg R, Sierra M, et al: Frequency of *Mycobacterium tuberculosis* bacteremia in patients with tuberculosis in an area endemic for AIDS. Am Rev Respir Dis 140:1611, 1989.

63. Gourevitch MN, Hartel D, Schoenbaum EE, et al: Lack of association of induration size with HIV infection among drug users reacting to tuberculin. Am J Respir Crit Care Med 154:1029, 1996.

64. Dore GJ, Hoy JF, Mallal SA, et al: Trends in incidence of AIDS illnesses in Australia from 1983 to 1994. The Australian AIDS cohort. J Acquir Immune Defic Syndr Hum Retrovirol 16:39, 1997.

65. Horsburgh CR: *Mycobacterium avium* complex infection in the acquired immunodeficiency syndrome. N Engl J Med 324:1332, 1991.

66. Hartman TE, Primack SL, Müller NL, et al: Diagnosis of thoracic complications in AIDS: Accuracy of CT. Am J Roentgenol 162:547, 1994.

67. Laissy JP, Cadi M, Cinqualbre A, et al: *Mycobacterium tuberculosis* versus nontuberculous mycobacterial infection of the lung in AIDS patients: CT and HRCT patterns. J Comput Assist Tomogr 21:312, 1997.

68. Mehle ME, Adamo JP, Mehta AC, et al: Endobronchial *Mycobacterium avium-intracellulare* infection in a patient with AIDS. Chest 96:119, 1989.

69. Packer SJ, Cesario T, Williams JH: *Mycobacterium avium* complex infection presenting as endobronchial lesions in immunosuppressed patients. Ann Intern Med 109:389, 1988.

70. Nassos PS, Yajko DM, Sanders CA, et al: Prevalence of *Mycobacterium avium* complex in respiratory specimens from AIDS and non-AIDS patients in a San Francisco Hospital. Am Rev Respir Dis 143:66, 1991.

71. Chin DP, Hopewell PC, Yajko DM, et al: *Mycobacterium avium* complex in the respiratory or gastrointestinal tract and the risk of *M. avium* complex bacteremia in patients with human immunodeficiency virus infection. J Infect Dis 169:289, 1994.

72. Rigsby MO, Curtis AM: Pulmonary disease from nontuberculous mycobacteria in patients with human immunodeficiency virus. Chest 106:913, 1994.

73. American Thoracic Society: Fungal infection in HIV-infected persons. Am J Respir Crit Care Med 152:816, 1995.

74. Stansell JD: Pulmonary fungal infections in HIV-infected persons. Semin Respir Infect 8:116, 1993.

75. Hoover DR, Saah AJ, Bacellar H, et al: Clinical manifestations of AIDS in the era of *Pneumocystis* prophylaxis. N Engl J Med 329:1922, 1993.

76. Buckley RM, Braffman MN, Stern JJ: Opportunistic infections in the acquired immunodeficiency syndrome. Semin Oncol 17:335, 1990.

77. Murray JF, Mills J: Pulmonary infectious complications of human immunodeficiency virus infection. Am Rev Respir Dis 141:1582, 1990.

78. Delmas MC, Schwoebel V, Heisterkamp SH, et al: Recent trends in *Pneumocystis carinii* pneumonia as AIDS-defining disease in nine European countries. Coordinators for AIDS Surveillance. J Acquir Immune Defic Syndr Hum Retrovirol 9:74, 1995.

79. Stansell JD, Osmond DH, Charlebois E, et al: Predictors of *Pneumocystis carinii* pneumonia in HIV-infected persons. Am J Respir Crit Care Med 155:60, 1997.

80. Levine SJ: *Pneumocystis carinii*. Clin Chest Med 17:665, 1996.

81. Curtis JR, Ullman M, Collier AC, et al: Variations in medical care for HIV-related *Pneumocystis carinii* pneumonia: A comparison of process and outcome at two hospitals. Chest 112:398, 1997.

82. Curtis JR, Greenberg DL, Hudson LD, et al: Changing use of intensive care for HIV-infected patients with *Pneumocystis carinii* pneumonia. Am J Respir Crit Care Med 150:1305, 1994.

83. Watts JC, Chandler FW: Evolving concepts of infection by *Pneumocystis carinii*. *In* Rosen PP, Fechner RE (eds): Pathology Annual. Part 1. Vol 26. Norwalk, CT, Appleton & Lange, 1991, p 93.

84. Gamsu G, Hecht ST, Birnberg FA, et al: *Pneumocystis carinii* pneumonia in homosexual men. Am J Roentgenol 139:647, 1982.

85. Suster B, Akerman M, Orenstein M, et al: Pulmonary manifestations of AIDS: Review of 106 episodes. Radiology 161:87, 1986.

86. DeLorenzo LJ, Huang CT, Maguire GP, et al: Roentgenographic patterns of *Pneumocystis carinii* pneumonia in 104 patients with AIDS. Chest 91:323, 1987.

87. Naidich DP, McGuinness G: Pulmonary manifestations of AIDS: CT and radiographic correlations. Radiol Clin North Am 29:999, 1991.

88. Goodman PC: *Pneumocystis carinii* pneumonia. J Thorac Imaging 6:16, 1991.

89. Sandhu JS, Goodman PC: Pulmonary cysts associated with *Pneumocystis carinii* pneumonia in patients with AIDS. Radiology 173:33, 1989.

90. Gurney JW, Bates FT: Pulmonary cystic disease: Comparison of *Pneumocystis carinii* pneumatoceles and bullous emphysema due to intravenous drug abuse. Radiology 173:27, 1989.

91. Chow C, Templeton PA, White CS: Lung cysts associated with *Pneumocystis carinii* pneumonia: Radiographic characteristics, natural history, and complications. Am J Roentgenol 161:527, 1993.

92. Takahashi T, Hoshino Y, Nakamura T, et al: Mediastinal emphysema with *Pneumocystis carinii* pneumonia in AIDS. Am J Roentgenol 169:1465, 1997.

93. Beers MF, Sohn M, Swartz M: Recurrent pneumothorax in AIDS patients with *Pneumocystis* pneumonia: A clinicopathologic report of three cases and review of the literature. Chest 98:266, 1990.

94. McClellan MD, Miller SB, Parsons PE, et al: Pneumothorax with *Pneumocystis carinii* pneumonia in AIDS: Incidence and clinical characteristics. Chest 100:1224, 1991.

95. Metersky ML, Colt HG, Olson LK, et al: AIDS-related spontaneous pneumothorax: Risk factors and treatment. Chest 108:946, 1995.

96. Sepkowitz KA, Telzak EE, Gold JW, et al: Pneumothorax in AIDS. Ann Intern Med 114:455, 1991.

97. Coker RJ, Moss F, Peters B, et al: Pneumothorax in patients with AIDS. Respir Med 87:43, 1993.

98. Alkhuja S, Badhey K, Miller A: Simultaneous bilateral pneumothorax in an HIV-infected patient. Chest 112:1417, 1997.

99. Klein JS, Warnock M, Webb WR, et al: Cavitating and noncavitating granulomas in AIDS patients with *Pneumocystis* pneumonitis. Am J Roentgenol 152:753, 1989.

100. Eagar GM, Friedland JA, Sagel SS: Tumefactive *Pneumocystis carinii* infection in AIDS: Report of three cases. Am J Roentgenol 160:1197, 1993.

101. Wasser LS, Brown E, Talavera W: Miliary PCP in AIDS. Chest 96:693, 1989.

102. Chechani V, Zaman MK, Finch PJP: Chronic cavitary *Pneumocystis carinii* pneumonia in a patient with AIDS. Chest 95:1347, 1989.

103. Radin DR, Baker EL, Klatt EC, et al: Visceral and nodal calcification in patients with AIDS-related *Pneumocystis carinii* infection. Am J Roentgenol 154:27, 1990.

104. Groskin SA, Massi AF, Randall PA: Calcified hilar and mediastinal lymph nodes in an AIDS patient with *Pneumocystis carinii* infection. Radiology 175:345, 1990.

105. Bergin CJ, Wirth RL, Berry GJ, et al: *Pneumocystis carinii* pneumonia: CT and HRCT observations. J Comput Assist Tomogr 14:756, 1990.

106. Kuhlman JE, Kavuru M, Fishman EK, et al: *Pneumocystis carinii* pneumonia: Spectrum of parenchymal CT findings. Radiology 175:711, 1990.

107. Kang EY, Staples CA, McGuinness G, et al: Detection and differential diagnosis of pulmonary infections and tumors in patients with AIDS: Value of chest radiography versus CT. Am J Roentgenol 166:15, 1996.

108. Richards PJ, Riddell L, Reznek RH, et al: High resolution computed tomography in HIV patients with suspected *Pneumocystis carinii* pneumonia and a normal chest radiograph. Clin Radiol 51:689, 1996.

109. Gruden JF, Huang L, Turner J, et al: High-resolution CT in the evaluation of clinically suspected *Pneumocystis carinii* pneumonia in AIDS patients with normal, equivocal, or nonspecific radiographic findings. Am J Roentgenol 169:967, 1997.

110. Woolfenden JM, Carrasquillo JA, Larson SM: Acquired immunodeficiency syndrome: Ga-67 citrate imaging. Radiology 162:383, 1987.

111. Kramer EL, Sanger JJ, Garay SM, et al: Gallium-67 chest scan patterns in HIV seropositive patients: Diagnostic implications. Radiology 170:671, 1989.

112. Goldenberg DM, Sharkey RM, Udem S, et al: Immunoscintigraphy of *Pneumocystis carinii* pneumonia in AIDS patients. J Nucl Med 35:1028, 1994.

113. Kramer EL, Divgi CR: Pulmonary applications of nuclear medicine. Clin Chest Med 12:55, 1991.

114. Kovacs JA, Hiemenz JW, Macher AM, et al: *Pneumocystis carinii* pneumonia: A comparison between patients with the acquired immunodeficiency syndrome and patients with other immunodeficiencies. Ann Intern Med 100:663, 1984.

115. Zuger A, Louie E, Holzman RS, et al: Cryptococcal disease in patients with the acquired immunodeficiency syndrome: Diagnostic features and outcome of treatment. Ann Intern Med 104:234, 1986.

116. Davies SF, Sarosi GA: Fungal pulmonary complications. Clin Chest Med 17:725, 1996.

117. Cameron ML, Bartlett JA, Gallis HA, et al: Manifestations of pulmonary cryptococcosis in patients with acquired immunodeficiency syndrome. Rev Infect Dis 13:64, 1991.

118. Chechani V, Kamholz SL: Pulmonary manifestations of disseminated cryptococcosis in patients with AIDS. Chest 98:1060, 1990.

119. Miller WT Jr, Edelman JM, Miller WT: Cryptococcal pulmonary infection in patients with AIDS: Radiographic appearance. Radiology 175:725, 1990.

120. Sider L, Westcott MA: Pulmonary manifestations of cryptococcosis in patients with AIDS: CT features. J Thorac Imaging 9:78, 1994.

121. Friedman EP, Miller RF, Severn A, et al: Cryptococcal pneumonia in patients with the acquired immunodeficiency syndrome. Clin Radiol 50:756, 1995.

122. Conces DJ Jr, Stockberger SM, Tarver RD, et al: Disseminated histoplasmosis in AIDS: Findings on chest radiographs. Am J Roentgenol 160:15, 1993.

123. Salzman SH, Smith RL, Aranda CP: Histoplasmosis in patients at risk for the acquired immunodeficiency syndrome in a nonendemic setting. Chest 93:916, 1988.

124. Sarosi GA, Johnson PC: Progressive disseminated histoplasmosis in the acquired immunodeficiency syndrome: A model for disseminated disease. Semin Respir Infect 5:146, 1990.

125. Johnson PC, Khadori N, Najjar A, et al: Progressive disseminated histoplasmosis in patients with acquired immunodeficiency syndrome. Am J Med 85:152, 1988.

126. McGuinness G, Naidich DP, Jagirdar J, et al: High resolution CT findings in miliary lung disease. J Comput Assist Tomogr 16:384, 1992.

127. Ampel NM, Dols CL, Galgiani JN: Coccidioidomycosis during human immunodeficiency virus infection: Results of a prospective study in a coccidioidal endemic area. Am J Med 94:235, 1993.

128. Fish DG, Ampel NM, Galgiani JN, et al: Coccidioidomycosis during human immunodeficiency virus infection: A review of 77 patients. Medicine 69:384, 1990.

129. Pappas PG: Blastomycosis in the immunocompromised patient. Semin Respir Infect 12:243, 1997.

130. Pappas PG, Pottage JC, Powderly WG, et al: Blastomycosis in patients with the acquired immunodeficiency syndrome. Ann Intern Med 116:847, 1992.

131. Nash G, Irvine R, Kerschmann RL, et al: Pulmonary aspergillosis in acquired immune deficiency syndrome: Autopsy study of emerging pulmonary complication of human immunodeficiency virus infection. Hum Pathol 28:1268, 1997.

132. Denning DW, Follansbee SE, Scolaro M, et al: Pulmonary aspergillosis in the acquired immunodeficiency syndrome. N Engl J Med 324:654, 1991.

133. Miller WT Jr, Sais GJ, Frank I, et al: Pulmonary aspergillosis in patients with AIDS: Clinical and radiographic correlations. Chest 105:37, 1994.

134. Minamoto GY, Barlam TF, Vander Els NJ: Invasive aspergillosis in patients with AIDS. Clin Infect Dis 14:66, 1992.

135. Staples CA, Kang EY, Wright JL, et al: Invasive pulmonary aspergillosis in AIDS: Radiographic, CT, and pathologic findings. Radiology 196:409, 1995.

136. Wallace JM: Viruses and other miscellaneous organisms. Clin Chest Med 17:745, 1996.

137. De La Hoz RE, Hayashi S, Cook D, et al: Investigation of the role of the cytomegalovirus as a respiratory pathogen in HIV-infected patients. Can Respir J 3:235, 1996.

138. Baughman RP: Cytomegalovirus: The monster in the closet? Am J Respir Crit Care Med 156:1, 1997.

139. Wallace JM, Hannah J: Cytomegalovirus pneumonitis in patients with AIDS: Findings in an autopsy series. Chest 92:198, 1987.

140. McKenzie R, Travis WD, Dolan SA, et al: The causes of death in patients with human immunodeficiency virus infection: A clinical and pathologic study with emphasis on the role of pulmonary diseases. Medicine 70:326, 1991.

141. Waxman AB, Goldie SJ, Brett-Smith H, et al: Cytomegalovirus as a primary pulmonary pathogen in AIDS. Chest 111:128, 1997.

142. McGuinness G, Scholes JV, Garay SM, et al: Cytomegalovirus pneumonitis: Spectrum of parenchymal CT findings with pathologic correlation in 21 AIDS patients. Radiology 192:451, 1994.

143. White DA: Pulmonary complications of HIV-associated malignancies. Clin Chest Med 17:755, 1996.

144. Lifson AR, Darrow WW, Hessol NA, et al: Kaposi's sarcoma in a cohort of homosexual and bisexual men: Epidemiology and analysis for cofactors. Am J Epidemiol 131:221, 1990.

145. White DA, Matthay RA: Noninfectious pulmonary complications of infection with the human immunodeficiency virus. Am Rev Respir Dis 140:1763, 1989.

146. Cesarman E, Knowles DM: Kaposi's sarcoma-associated herpesvirus: A lymphotropic human herpesvirus associated with Kaposi's sarcoma, primary effusion lymphoma and multicentric Castleman's disease. Semin Diagn Pathol 14:54, 1997.

147. Davis SD, Henschke CI, Chamides BK, et al: Intrathoracic Kaposi sarcoma in AIDS patients: Radiographic-pathologic correlation. Radiology 163:495, 1987.

148. Sivit CJ, Schwartz AM, Rockoff SD: Kaposi's sarcoma of the lung in AIDS: Radiologic-pathologic analysis. Am J Roentgenol 148:25, 1987.

149. Naidich DP, Tarras M, Garay SM, et al: Kaposi's sarcoma: CT-radiographic correlation. Chest 96:723, 1989.

150. Goodman PC: Kaposi's sarcoma. J Thorac Imaging 6:43, 1991.

151. Gruden JF, Huang L, Webb WR, et al: AIDS-related Kaposi sarcoma of the lung: Radiographic findings and staging system with bronchoscopic correlation. Radiology 195:545, 1995.

152. Huang L, Schnapp LN, Gruden JF, et al: Presentation of AIDS-related pulmonary Kaposi's sarcoma diagnosed by bronchoscopy. Am J Respir Crit Care Med 153:1385, 1996.

153. Wolff SD, Kuhlman JE, Fishman EK: Thoracic Kaposi sarcoma in AIDS: CT findings. J Comput Assist Tomogr 17:60, 1993.

154. Khalil AM, Carette MF, Cadranel JL, et al: Intrathoracic Kaposi's sarcoma: CT findings. Chest 108:1622, 1995.

155. Traill ZC, Miller RF, Shaw PJ: CT appearances of intrathoracic Kaposi's sarcoma in patients with AIDS. Br J Radiol 69:1104, 1996.

156. Primack SL, Hartman TE, Lee KS, et al: Pulmonary nodules and the CT halo sign. Radiology 190:513, 1994.

157. Lynch JW Jr: AIDS-related non-Hodgkin's lymphoma: Useful techniques for diagnosis. Chest 110:585, 1996.

158. Eisner MD, Kaplan LD, Herndier B, et al: The pulmonary manifestations of AIDS-related non-Hodgkin's lymphoma. Chest 110:729, 1996.

159. Raphael BG, Knowles DM: Acquired immunodeficiency syndrome-associated non-Hodgkin's lymphoma. Semin Oncol 17:361, 1990.

160. Knowles DM: Molecular pathology of acquired immunodeficiency syndrome-related non-Hodgkin's lymphoma. Semin Diagn Pathol 14:67, 1997.

161. Sider L, Weiss AJ, Smith MD, et al: Varied appearance of AIDS-related lymphoma in the chest. Radiology 171:629, 1989.

162. Polish LB, Cohn DL, Ryder JW, et al: Pulmonary non-Hodgkin's lymphoma in AIDS. Chest 96:1321, 1989.

163. Carignan S, Staples CA, Müller NL: Intrathoracic lymphoproliferative disorders in the immunocompromised patient: CT findings. Radiology 197:53, 1995.

164. Blunt DM, Padley SPG: Radiographic manifestations of AIDS related lymphoma in the thorax. Clin Radiol 50:607, 1995.

165. Morassut S, Vaccher E, Balestreri L, et al: HIV-associated human herpes virus 8-–positive primary lymphomatous effusions: Radiologic findings in six patients. Radiology 205:459, 1997.

166. Mason AC, White CS: CT appearance of endobronchial non-Hodgkin lymphoma. J Comput Assist Tomogr 18:559, 1994.

167. Alshafie MT, Donaldson B, Oluwole SF: Human immunodeficiency virus and lung cancer. Br J Surg 84:1068, 1997.

168. Mady BJ: Poorly differentiated non-small cell carcinoma of the lung in acquired immunodeficiency syndrome. Respiration 62:232, 1995.

169. Karp J, Profeta G, Marantz PR, et al: Lung cancer in patients with immunodeficiency syndrome. Chest 103:410, 1993.

170. Parker MS, Leveno DM, Campbell TJ, et al: AIDS-related bronchogenic carcinoma: Fact or fiction? Chest 113:154, 1998.

171. Gabutti G, Vercelli M, De Rosa MG, et al: AIDS related neoplasms in Genoa, Italy. Eur J Epidemiol 11:609, 1995.

172. Barchielli A, Buiatti E, Galanti C, et al: Linkage between AIDS surveillance system and population-based cancer registry data in Italy: A pilot study in Florence, 1985–1990. Tumori 81:169, 1995.

173. White CS, Haramati LB, Elder KH, et al: Carcinoma of the lung in HIV-positive patients: Findings on chest radiographs and CT scans. Am J Roentgenol 164:593, 1995.

174. Fishman JE, Schwartz DS, Sais GJ, et al: Bronchogenic carcinoma in HIV-positive patients: Findings on chest radiographs and CT scans. Am J Roentgenol 164:57, 1995.

175. Gruden JF, Webb WR, Yao DC, et al: Bronchogenic carcinoma in 13 patients infected with the human immunodeficiency virus (HIV): Clinical and radiographic findings. J Thorac Imaging 10:99, 1995.

176. Travis WD, Fox CH, Devaney KO, et al: Lymphoid pneumonitis in 50 adult patients infected with the human immunodeficiency virus: Lymphocytic interstitial pneumonitis versus nonspecific pneumonitis. Hum Pathol 23:529, 1992.

177. Suffredini AF, Ognibene FP, Lack EE, et al: Nonspecific interstitial pneumonitis: A common cause of pulmonary disease in the acquired immunodeficiency syndrome. Ann Intern Med 107:7, 1987.

178. Sattler F, Nichols L, Hirano L, et al: Nonspecific interstitial pneumonitis mimicking *Pneumocystis carinii* pneumonia. Am J Respir Crit Care Med 156:912, 1997.

179. Simmons JT, Suffredini AF, Lack EE, et al: Nonspecific interstitial pneumonitis in patients with AIDS: Radiologic features. Am J Roentgenol 149:265, 1987.

180. Griffiths MH, Miller RF, Semple SJG: Interstitial pneumonitis in patients infected with the human immunodeficiency virus. Thorax 50:1141, 1995.

181. Schneider RF: Lymphocytic interstitial pneumonitis and nonspecific interstitial pneumonitis. Clin Chest Med 17:763, 1996.

182. Sharland M, Gibb DM, Holland F: Respiratory morbidity from lymphocytic interstitial pneumonitis (LIP) in vertically acquired HIV infection. Arch Dis Child 76:334, 1997.

183. Marks MJ, Haney PJ, McDermott MP, et al: Thoracic disease in children with AIDS. Radiographics 16:1349, 1996.

184. Centers for Disease Control and Prevention: Revision of case definitions of acquired immunodeficiency syndrome for national reporting—United States. MMWR Morb Mortal Wkly Rep 34:373, 1985.

185. Kramer MR, Saldana MJ, Ramos M, et al: High titers of Epstein-Barr virus antibodies in adult patients with lymphocytic interstitial pneumonitis associated with AIDS. Respir Med 86:49, 1992.

186. McGuinness G, Soles JV, Jagirdar JS, et al: Unusual lymphoproliferative disorders in nine adults with HIV or AIDS: CT and pathologic findings. Radiology 197:59, 1995.

187. Mylonakis E, Barlam TF, Flanigan T, et al: Pulmonary aspergillosis and invasive disease in AIDS. Chest 114:251, 1998.

CHAPTER 11

Transplantation

LUNG AND HEART-LUNG TRANSPLANTATION
  Complications
    Reperfusion Edema
    Acute Rejection
    Obliterative Bronchiolitis
    Post-Transplantation Lymphoproliferative Disorder
    Infection
    Recurrence of Primary Disease
    Pleural Complications
    Bronchial Complications
BONE MARROW TRANSPLANTATION
  Complications
    Pulmonary Edema
    Diffuse Alveolar Hemorrhage
    Idiopathic Pneumonia Syndrome
    Obliterative Bronchiolitis
    Infection

LUNG AND HEART-LUNG TRANSPLANTATION

Since the mid-1980s, lung and heart-lung transplantations have passed from the status of experimental procedures to standard therapy for a wide variety of otherwise fatal pulmonary conditions (Table 11–1). By 1998,

Table 11–1. LUNG DISEASES TREATED BY TRANSPLANTATION

Interstitial lung disease
  Idiopathic pulmonary fibrosis
  Drug-induced lung disease
  Sarcoidosis
  Langerhans' cell histiocytosis
  Pneumoconiosis
  Lymphangioleiomyomatosis
  Lung disease as part of a systemic illness (selected cases)
Obstructive lung disease
  Nonsuppurative
    Emphysema
    Obliterative bronchiolitis
  Suppurative
    Cystic fibrosis
    Bronchiectasis
Vascular disease
  Primary pulmonary hypertension
  Secondary pulmonary hypertension, including chronic
    thromboembolic pulmonary hypertension
Miscellaneous lung disease
  Alveolar microlithiasis

approximately 8,000 lung transplants had been performed worldwide.[98]

Current options for lung transplantation include single-lung transplantation, double-lung transplantation (usually by bilateral sequential single-lung transplantation), heart-lung transplantation,[2] and lobar transplantation from living related donors.[4, 105] Single-lung transplantation is suitable for most patients requiring lung transplantation and is preferred whenever possible because it increases the pool of donor organs and decreases the waiting time that otherwise would be required for procuring two healthy lungs for double-lung transplantation.[2] Double-lung transplantation is necessary in patients who have septic lung disease, such as cystic fibrosis, because of the possibility of infection in the transplanted lung or elsewhere if the residual lung were left in place.[2, 3] Heart-lung transplantation is indicated in patients who have Eisenmenger's complex without correctable cardiac defects, pulmonary disease associated with unrelated heart disease, and chronic thromboembolic pulmonary hypertension when thromboendarterectomy is not feasible.[3]

Complications

Reperfusion Edema

Noncardiogenic pulmonary edema commonly occurs in the transplanted lung shortly after its reimplantation (reperfusion injury, *pulmonary reimplantation response*) (Table 11–2).[1, 9] The edema is the result of increased pulmonary vascular permeability, the severity of which is related closely to the time interval between excision of the lung from the donor and its implantation in the recipient (ischemia time).[8] Pathologic features include air-space and interstitial edema;[11] in severe cases, the appearance is that of diffuse alveolar damage.[2]

Abnormalities typically are evident first on the chest

Table 11–2. REPERFUSION EDEMA

Noncardiogenic pulmonary edema
Develops immediately after transplantation
Peaks in severity 2–4 days after transplant
Radiologic features mimic hydrostatic pulmonary edema
Common radiologic findings
  Perihilar haze
  Thickening of peribronchial and perivascular interstitium
  Thickening of interlobular septa

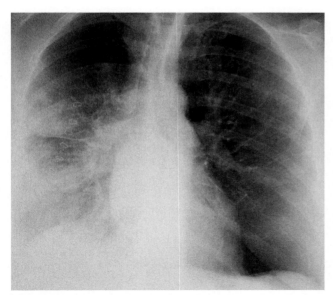

Figure 11–1. Pulmonary Transplantation: Reperfusion Injury. An anteroposterior chest radiograph shows ground-glass opacification and poorly defined areas of consolidation in the transplanted right lung. A small right pleural effusion also is present. The native left lung shows findings consistent with panacinar emphysema. The patient was a 50-year-old woman with the clinical diagnosis of reperfusion edema 3 days after single-lung transplantation for emphysema.

radiograph 24 to 48 hours after transplantation, reach a peak by day 3 or 4, and usually resolve between days 5 and 14.[106] Radiologic findings are nonspecific and are similar to those seen in patients who have left ventricular failure, fluid overload, and acute rejection. Findings range from a subtle perihilar haze to patchy or confluent air-space consolidation involving mainly the middle and lower lung zones (Fig. 11–1).[13, 14] Interstitial abnormalities, including peribronchial and perivascular thickening and a reticular pattern, are seen in most patients.

The spectrum of radiographic findings and the time course of reperfusion injury have been assessed in several studies. In one review of 105 consecutive patients who underwent lung transplantation, radiographic abnormalities were identified on the first postoperative chest radiograph in 141 of 148 (95%) transplanted lungs; by day 3, findings were noted in 144 (97%).[13] In most cases, the abnormalities consisted predominantly of a perihilar haze or mild interstitial thickening. They were usually maximal in the first 3 days and decreased gradually thereafter; most patients had normal radiographs or only mild residual interstitial abnormalities by day 10. In another investigation of 45 patients (20 who had undergone single-lung transplantation and 25 who had undergone double-lung transplantation), reperfusion edema was evident on chest radiograph on day 1 in 39 (87%) and by day 3 in 44 (98%).[16] The edema was asymmetric in 9 (36%) of the 25 patients who had undergone double-lung transplantation. There was poor correlation between the severity of radiographic findings and the alveolar-arterial oxygen gradient. A poor correlation between the extent of radiographic abnormalities in the transplanted lung and deficits in gas has been shown by another group of investigators.[17]

Acute Rejection

Acute rejection is an almost invariable complication of lung transplantation and an important cause of morbidity;[18, 19] in one investigation of 69 patients who had single-lung, double-lung, or heart-lung transplants and who survived at least 5 days, all had at least one episode of rejection.[20] Although the reaction may be seen 3 days after transplantation, it usually is manifested first after 1 to 2 weeks (Table 11–3).[18] Frequency of acute rejection diminishes with time from transplantation;[21] 60% of all cases occur during the first 3 postoperative months,[18] and acute rejection after 4 years is uncommon.[21]

Acute rejection is predominantly a cell-mediated immune response that results from the activation and proliferation of effector T cells directed against the HLA complex of donor cells.[19, 22] The principal histologic finding is a mononuclear inflammatory cell infiltrate that, in the lower grades, is located predominantly in the interstitial tissue surrounding venules, arterioles, and small veins and arteries.[23] In more severe disease, the infiltrate extends throughout the vessel wall to involve the endothelium (*endotheliitis*) and into the adjacent alveolar interstitium. Air spaces usually are unaffected except in severe disease. Clinical manifestations are nonspecific, consisting of cough, dyspnea, fever, and tachypnea.

Radiographic abnormalities in patients who have acute lung rejection include a fine reticular interstitial pattern, interlobular septal thickening, ground-glass opacities, patchy or confluent air-space consolidation, and new or increasing pleural effusions (Fig. 11–2).[15, 25, 26] These findings tend to involve mainly the mid and lower lung zones.[99] Several groups of investigators have shown that these abnormalities are present in approximately 50% of patients who have biopsy-proven acute rejection after heart-lung or lung transplantation.[12, 13, 99] In one study of 100 chest radiographs performed within 24 hours before transbronchial biopsy, acute rejection was associated with the presence of reticular interstitial or air-space disease in 21 of 42 instances of rejection (sensitivity 50%).[99] Similar radiographic abnormalities were present in 18 of 58 instances unassociated with rejection (specificity 69%).

Radiographic parenchymal abnormalities are more likely when rejection occurs early in the postoperative course than when it occurs later. In one study, 45 episodes of acute rejection were evaluated in 20 patients, 23 occurring within the first month after transplantation and 22 after the first month.[24] The diagnosis of rejection was based on transbronchial biopsy in 33 episodes and on clinical findings in 12; all patients had symptoms. Radiographic abnor-

Table 11–3. ACUTE REJECTION

Cell-mediated immune response
Interstitial mononuclear cell infiltrate
First manifested 1–2 wk after transplantation
Most commonly seen in first 3 mo after transplantation
Radiologic features mimic hydrostatic pulmonary edema
Common radiologic findings
    Perihilar haze
    Thickening of peribronchial and perivascular interstitium
    Thickening of interlobular septa
    New or increasing pleural effusions

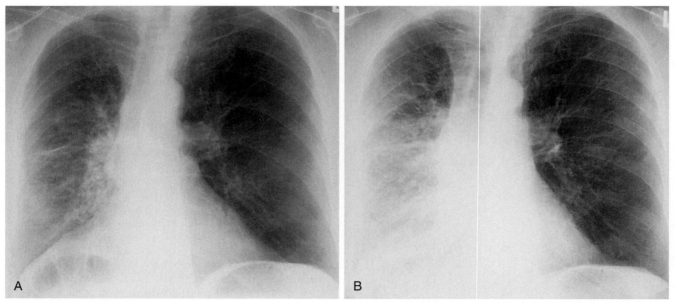

Figure 11–2. Pulmonary Transplantation: Acute Rejection. A 62-year-old woman underwent right lung transplantation for emphysema. Posteroanterior chest radiograph performed 6 days later *(A)* shows mild interstitial thickening involving mainly the right perihilar region and right lower lobe. Radiograph 2 days later *(B)* shows an increase in the parenchymal abnormalities associated with the development of septal lines, ground-glass opacities throughout the right middle and lower lung zones, and focal areas of consolidation. The diagnosis of acute rejection was confirmed by transbronchial biopsy.

malities were detected in 22 of 45 (49%) episodes; radiographs were abnormal in 17 of 23 (74%) episodes occurring during the first month but in only 5 of 22 episodes (23%) occurring later than the first month after transplantation. The parenchymal abnormalities consisted mainly of poorly defined perihilar nodular opacities (airspace nodules), which sometimes coalesced and progressed to frank consolidation involving mainly the perihilar regions and lower lung zones.

Pleural effusions are common in acute rejection and are occasionally the only radiographic manifestation. In one study, the radiographic findings in 22 episodes of acute rejection included a combination of parenchymal abnormalities and pleural effusion in 15 (68%) cases, pulmonary changes alone in 4 (18%) cases, and pleural effusion alone in 3 (14%) cases.[24]

High-resolution computed tomography (HRCT) findings of acute lung rejection were reviewed in a study of 32 patients who had undergone single-lung, double-lung, or heart-lung transplantation.[27] A total of 190 transbronchial biopsy specimens and concurrent HRCT scans were obtained. Of the biopsy specimens, 40 (21%) showed evidence of acute rejection, 111 (58%) were normal, and 39 (21%) were inconclusive. The most common abnormality seen in patients who had acute rejection was localized or widespread areas of ground-glass attenuation. This finding was identified in 26 of 40 cases (65%) diagnosed as acute rejection compared with 5 of 11 (45%) with biopsy findings suggestive but not diagnostic of rejection, 7 of 28 (25%) with nonspecific biopsy findings, and 10 of 111 (9%) with normal biopsy results. Ground-glass attenuation was more likely to be present in patients who had higher grades of rejection on transbronchial biopsy specimens. Septal lines were identified in 11 (27%) cases of acute rejection, 1 of 11 (9%) cases with suggestive findings of rejection, 4 of

28 (14%) cases with nonspecific biopsy findings, and 7 of 111 (6%) cases with normal biopsy results (Fig. 11–3). Less common abnormalities seen in acute rejection included recent or increased size of pleural effusions, basal consolidation, and peribronchial cuffing, each seen in 10 patients (25%). Although these three findings also were seen in association with reperfusion injury, in this situation they usually were limited to the lower lung zones. The HRCT findings do not distinguish acute rejection from reperfusion injury or fluid overload.

Obliterative Bronchiolitis

Progressive air-flow obstruction as a result of bronchiolar fibrosis (obliterative bronchiolitis) has been reported in 70% of patients after lung transplantation (Table 11–4).[28, 29] Of affected individuals, 55% die from the complication, making it the major cause of late graft failure.[30, 31] The complication has occurred after heart-lung, double-lung, and single-lung transplantation.[32]

Although the precise pathogenesis of obliterative bronchiolitis is uncertain, most evidence points to an immunologically mediated airway injury. Most authorities use the terms *post-transplantation obliterative bronchiolitis* or *obliterative bronchiolitis syndrome* (the latter to refer to patients who have pulmonary dysfunction in the absence of histologic evidence of obliterative bronchiolitis and other apparent reasons for air-flow obstruction[33]) interchangeably with chronic rejection.[6, 30] Histologically, obliterative bronchiolitis is manifested by an eccentric or, more often, concentric increase in the connective tissue between the muscle and epithelium of membranous and proximal respiratory bronchioles.[34]

Although obliterative bronchiolitis has developed as early as 2 months and as late as 4 years after transplanta-

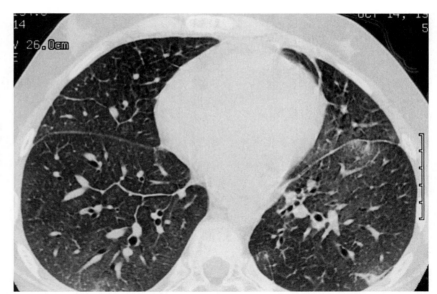

Figure 11–3. Pulmonary Transplantation: Acute Rejection. HRCT scan performed 10 days after double-lung transplantation shows interlobular septal thickening and patchy bilateral areas of ground-glass attenuation. The diagnosis of acute rejection was confirmed by transbronchial biopsy.

tion, the mean time between transplantation and its recognition is 6 to 12 months.[10, 18] The clinical course is variable; in some patients, the disease has an insidious onset and indolent progress, whereas in others, the onset and course are rapid.[41] Some patients are asymptomatic, and the disease is detected by the discovery of abnormalities of surveillance lung function and lung histology.[10] Symptoms include malaise, dry cough, and shortness of breath on exertion.[10] As lung function deteriorates, dyspnea worsens.[1]

Radiologic findings include decreased peripheral vascular markings, decreased or increased lung volumes, and, less commonly, bronchial dilation.[35, 36] The last-named is considered to be present when the internal diameter of the bronchus is greater than that of the adjacent pulmonary artery and is seen most commonly on HRCT scan (Fig. 11–4);[37] in one study of seven patients who had obliterative bronchiolitis syndrome, two had bronchial dilation evident on radiograph, and six had bronchial dilation evident on HRCT scan.[37] The dilation involved mainly the segmental and subsegmental branches of the lower lobes. Lower lobe bronchial dilation was not seen in any of nine otherwise healthy heart-lung transplant recipients who were used as controls.

In another investigation of 15 patients who had biopsy-proven obliterative bronchiolitis after lung transplantation

Table 11–4. OBLITERATIVE BRONCHIOLITIS

Immunologically mediated airway injury
Concentric narrowing of bronchioles
Usually develops ≥6 mo after transplantation
Radiographic findings
   Hyperinflation
   Attenuation of peripheral vascular markings
HRCT findings
   Bronchial dilation
   Mosaic attenuation and perfusion
   Air-trapping
Most reliable radiologic finding
   Air-trapping on expiratory HRCT

HRCT, high-resolution computed tomography.

and 18 control subjects, 13 patients (87%) had one or more abnormalities seen on HRCT scan.[38] These abnormalities included bronchial dilation in 12 (80%) patients, bronchial wall thickening in 4 (27%) patients, and mosaic perfusion in 6 (40%) patients. Findings present in the control subjects included bronchial dilation in 4 (22%) and mosaic perfusion in 4 (22%); bronchial wall thickening was not seen. Five of the patients who had obliterative bronchiolitis and 16 of the control subjects also underwent expiratory HRCT scans; air-trapping was seen in 4 (80%) of the patients and only 1 (6%) of the controls. The combination of bronchial dilation on the inspiratory HRCT scans and air-trapping on expiratory scans was not seen in any of the control subjects.[38] In another investigation of 21 lung transplant recipients (including 11 who had biopsy-proven obliterative bronchiolitis and 10 who had no histologic or functional evidence of airway disease), bronchial dilation was present on inspiratory HRCT scan in 4 of the 11 (36%) patients who had obliterative bronchiolitis and 2 of the 10 (20%) who did not;[38] a mosaic attenuation was present in 7 (64%) of the obliterative bronchiolitis patients compared with 1 of 10 (10%) of the others. On expiratory HRCT scan, air-trapping was present in 10 of 11 patients who had obliterative bronchiolitis compared with only 2 of 10 who did not. The results of these two investigations suggest that air-trapping on expiratory HRCT scan is the most sensitive and accurate radiologic indicator of obliterative bronchiolitis (*see* Fig. 11–4).[38, 39]

The value of repeated HRCT scans in the long-term follow-up of patients who have lung transplants was assessed in a study of 13 consecutive patients.[40] Obliterative bronchiolitis syndrome developed in eight patients, on average within 12 months of transplantation. The first chronic changes identifiable on HRCT scan were a decrease in lung volume, a decrease in the peripheral vascular markings, and interlobular septal thickening, findings that appeared 7 to 11 months postoperatively. The mean interval for the appearance of bronchial dilation was 12 months. Areas of decreased attenuation and mosaic perfusion were identified on average 16 and 21 months after transplantation. Expir-

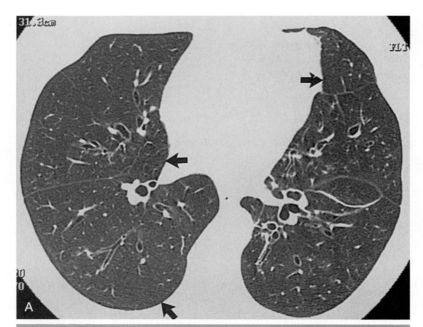

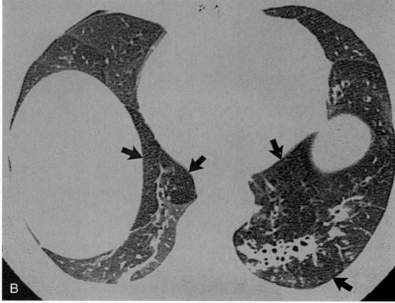

Figure 11–4. Pulmonary Transplantation: Obliterative Bronchiolitis. Inspiratory HRCT scan *(A)* shows marked bronchial dilation and areas of reduced attenuation and vascularity *(arrows)*. Expiratory HRCT scan *(B)* at the level of the domes of the diaphragm shows airtrapping *(arrows)*. The patient was a 60-year-old woman who had biopsy-proven obliterative bronchiolitis 2 years after lung transplantation.

atory HRCT was not performed. A second group of investigators assessed the value of air trapping on expiratory HRCT as a predictor of post-transplantation obliterative bronchiolitis syndrome in a longitudinal study of 38 heart-lung transplant recipients.[109] Air trapping involving more than 32% of the lung parenchyma had a sensitivity of 83% and a specificity of 89% in distinguishing patients with and those without obliterative bronchiolitis syndrome.[109]

Post-Transplantation Lymphoproliferative Disorder

Several histologic patterns of lymphocyte proliferation can occur after bone marrow or solid-organ transplantation (Table 11–5), ranging from apparently benign (hyperplas-

tic) proliferation to frank malignant lymphoma. The abnormalities are known collectively as *post-transplantation lymphoproliferative disorder* (PTLD).[42] Most lesions are the result of a proliferation of Epstein-Barr virus–infected B cells.[43, 44]

The reported prevalence of PTLD in lung transplant recipients varies from about 5% to 20%;[5, 50] most cases present in the first year after transplantation.[5] Most patients who have benign-appearing lesions histologically have clinically unsuspected disease.[50] Lymphoma-like proliferations often present in the allograft as focal or multifocal nodules or masses.[45] Localized disease in organs other than the lung as well as disseminated disease also has been described.[5]

The most common radiologic findings consist of single or multiple pulmonary nodules (Fig. 11–5) and hilar or

Table 11–5. POST-TRANSPLANTATION LYMPHOPROLIFERATIVE DISORDER

Related to EBV infection and immunosuppression
Ranges from benign polyclonal lymphocytic proliferation to malignant lymphoma
Usually develops between 1 mo and 1 yr post transplantation
Most common radiologic manifestations
    Multiple lung nodules
    Hilar and mediastinal lymphadenopathy

EBV, Epstein-Barr virus.

mediastinal lymph node enlargement (Fig. 11–6).[46, 47] In one investigation of 28 patients, nodules were identified on radiograph or computed tomography (CT) scan in 16 (57%).[46] They were relatively well circumscribed, measured 0.3 to 5 cm in diameter, and usually were multiple and distributed randomly throughout the lungs. Patchy, predominantly peribronchial air-space consolidation associated with air bronchograms was seen in three patients, two of whom also had lung nodules. Mediastinal and hilar lymph node enlargement was seen in 17 (61%) of 28 patients; thymic involvement, in 2; pericardial thickening or effusion, in 2; and pleural effusion, in 4. In another investigation of four patients, all had nodules on HRCT scan, two had hilar and mediastinal lymph node enlargement, and one had pleural effusion.[47] In three of the four patients, a halo of ground-glass attenuation was seen surrounding the lung nodules; pathologic correlation in one of these patients showed that the halo was related to infiltration of the adjacent lung by a less dense infiltrate of lymphoid cells.[48] In a third study of 17 patients, 15 (88%) had multiple nodules on CT scan, 6 (35%) had interlobular septal thickening, 5 (29%) had areas of ground-glass attenuation, 4 (23%) had areas of air-space consolidation, and 5 had hilar or mediastinal lymph node enlargement.[49] The nodules most commonly had a predominantly subpleural or peribronchovascular distribution.

Infection

Pulmonary infection is the most common cause of morbidity and mortality in lung transplant recipients.[5, 51] Possibly because the lung is in direct and constant contact with the environment, the infection rate is substantially higher in lung transplant recipients than in other organ recipients.[52] The spectrum of responsible organisms includes a variety of bacteria, fungi, and *Mycoplasma* species.[53, 54] The radiologic manifestations are similar to those seen in other immunocompromised patients and are discussed in Chapter 5. The radiologic findings of respiratory viral infection in lung transplant recipients were evaluated in an investigation of 20 transplant recipients who had 21 proven episodes of respiratory viral infection.[107] The organisms included parainfluenza, influenza, respiratory syncytial, and adenovirus. Chest radiographs were abnormal in 11 (52%) episodes; in the remaining patients, the infection involved predominantly or exclusively the upper respiratory tract. The parenchymal abnormalities included homogeneous or heterogeneous opacities or focal mass–like consolidation. In all cases, the abnormalities were initially confined to the graft (or grafts). Four patients, three of whom had adenoviral infection, showed rapid progression to diffuse homogeneous parenchymal opacification and died as a consequence of the respiratory infection.[107]

The CT manifestations of bacterial, viral, and fungal pneumonia after lung transplantation are similar.[108] One group of investigators reviewed the CT findings of 39 patients who had undergone lung transplantation and who had 45 documented pneumonias.[108] The most common organisms were cytomegalovirus, *Pseudomonas,* and *Aspergillus.* The most common CT findings consisted of consolidation seen in 37 (82%) pneumonias, ground-glass opacities in 34 (76%), septal thickening in 33 (73%), pleural effusion in 33 (73%), and multiple nodules in 25 (56%) cases.[108] CT was not helpful in distinguishing between viral, bacterial, and fungal pneumonias. Of 25 pneumonias in patients with a single transplanted lung, parenchymal abnormalities involved both lungs in 12 (48%), only the

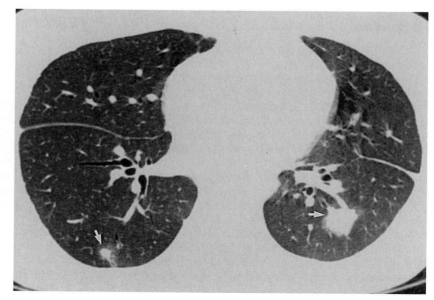

Figure 11–5. Post-Transplantation Lymphoproliferative Disorder. HRCT scan shows bilateral lung nodules *(arrows)* surrounded by a poorly defined halo of ground-glass attenuation. Thickening of the left interlobar fissure as a result of a small pleural effusion also is evident. The diagnosis of post-transplantation lymphoproliferative disorder was confirmed by open-lung biopsy. The patient was a 52-year-old woman who had undergone double-lung transplantation 3 months previously.

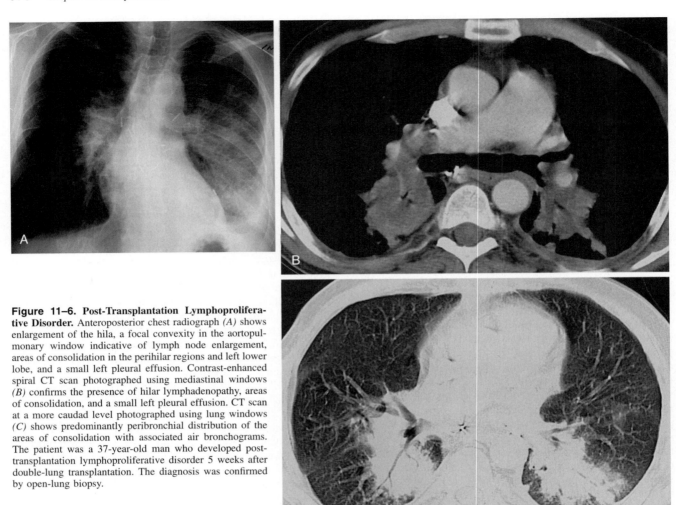

Figure 11–6. Post-Transplantation Lymphoproliferative Disorder. Anteroposterior chest radiograph *(A)* shows enlargement of the hila, a focal convexity in the aortopulmonary window indicative of lymph node enlargement, areas of consolidation in the perihilar regions and left lower lobe, and a small left pleural effusion. Contrast-enhanced spiral CT scan photographed using mediastinal windows *(B)* confirms the presence of hilar lymphadenopathy, areas of consolidation, and a small left pleural effusion. CT scan at a more caudad level photographed using lung windows *(C)* shows predominantly peribronchial distribution of the areas of consolidation with associated air bronchograms. The patient was a 37-year-old man who developed post-transplantation lymphoproliferative disorder 5 weeks after double-lung transplantation. The diagnosis was confirmed by open-lung biopsy.

transplanted lung in 11 (44%), and only the native lung in two (8%).[108]

Recurrence of Primary Disease

Recurrence of the primary disease in the lung allograft has been described for sarcoidosis,[55, 56] lymphangioleiomyomatosis,[58, 59] Langerhans' cell histiocytosis,[60, 63] diffuse panbronchiolitis,[61] alveolar proteinosis,[62] desquamative interstitial pneumonitis,[64, 65] and giant cell pneumonitis in the absence of exposure to cobalt in the post-transplant period.[66] Further reports of disease recurrence are to be expected,[5] given the brief history of lung transplantation relative to the lengthy history of pretransplant morbidity.

Chest radiograph and HRCT scan may be normal, may show nonspecific abnormalities, or may show findings suggestive of the specific recurrent disease. In two patients who developed recurrent sarcoidosis in the lung allograft, one had normal radiologic findings and the other had diffuse miliary nodules on chest radiograph and HRCT scan.[57] In another patient who had recurrent alveolar proteinosis, the presence of parenchymal disease 3 years after double-lung transplantation first was suggested by the presence of poorly defined small, rounded air-space opacities on chest radiograph.[62]

Pleural Complications

Pleural effusion is virtually inevitable immediately after lung transplantation.[7, 68] Effusions generally are small to moderate in size but may be massive.[7] Their pathogenesis likely reflects a combination of the trauma of the surgery, increased pulmonary capillary permeability, and disruption of lymphatic flow in the lung allograft;[7] abnormal postoperative positive fluid balance may be a factor in some patients.

Persistent or recurrent pneumothorax is seen in some patients.[69] In one study of 138 patients who had single-lung and double-lung transplants, it developed in 14 (10%);[69] in 6 patients, it occurred after transbronchial biopsy. Other iatrogenic causes of pneumothorax include transthoracic needle aspiration, thoracentesis, and placement of a central venous catheter.[70] When pneumothorax complicates heart-lung transplantation, it frequently is bilateral because of persistent communications between the exposed left and right pleural cavities.[70] Similar communication may follow sequential double-lung transplant procedures using the clamshell incision approach, as a result of disruption of the anterior pleural reflections.[7]

Bronchial Complications

The two main complications related to the bronchial anastomosis are dehiscence and stenosis. Dehiscence usually occurs in the first few months after transplantation and sometimes is related to infection at the anastomotic site. With current surgical and management techniques, it is rare.[71]

Chest radiographs are of limited value in the diagnosis of bronchial dehiscence or stenosis; however, both conditions usually can be recognized on CT scan.[26, 67] In one study of 23 patients who had single or bilateral lung transplants, CT scans were obtained for suspected or known dehiscence.[72] (CT technique consisted of 10-mm collimation scans performed through the chest and additional 2- to 4-mm-thick sections at the level of the anastomosis.) Twenty-one bronchial dehiscences were identified bronchoscopically in 17 patients; a bronchial defect was identified on CT scan in all 21 (sensitivity 100%) and in one of 18 bronchoscopically proven intact anastomoses (specificity 94%). The size of the bronchial defects on CT scan ranged from 0.1 to 1.5 cm, with most measuring 0.5 cm or less. Although evidence of extraluminal air was identified on CT scan in all bronchoscopically proven dehiscences, it also was present in 5 (28%) of 18 intact anastomoses. In four of these five anastomoses, the CT scans were performed 7 to 12 days after transplantation, and the extraluminal gas represented residual gas from the time of surgery; in the other patient, air was believed to have been introduced iatrogenically at bronchoscopy in an attempt to identify a subsegmental bronchus.[72] Pneumothorax was present in 9 (43%) of 21 bronchial dehiscences and in 6 (33%) of intact anastomoses.

Normal postoperative changes may be misinterpreted as dehiscence on conventional CT images in patients who have undergone telescoping bronchial anastomoses.[74] One of these normal changes is separation of the invaginated bronchial cuff and the recipient bronchus, which can result in an endoluminal flap. The gap between the flap and the wall of the recipient bronchus can simulate a bronchial wall defect, and air dissecting between the two can simulate extraluminal air (Fig. 11–7). These flaps or linear air collections are seen only along the anterior margin of the normal anastomosis because the posterior margin of the anastomosis is sutured end-to-end; any defect or flap along the posterior wall should suggest dehiscence. Another feature of the normal telescoping anastomosis that can be misinterpreted as dehiscence on transverse images is a small anastomotic diverticulum or pseudodiverticulum. This feature is seen as a smoothly marginated, spherical air collection at the inferior and medial aspect of the anastomosis (Fig. 11–8). Distinction of this and other normal features of telescoping anastomosis from true dehiscence can be made most readily on oblique coronal multiplanar reconstructions.[74]

CT allows assessment of the presence and extent of bronchial stenosis (Fig. 11–9).[12, 14] Optimal assessment of bronchial caliber requires that the bronchus be in the same

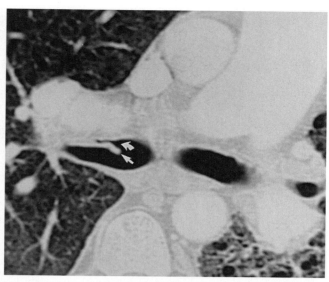

Figure 11–7. Endoluminal Flap at Bronchial Anastomosis. CT scan shows a flap *(straight arrow)* projecting into the lumen of the right bronchus. The flap represents invaginated donor bronchus projecting into the recipient bronchus. A linear air collection *(curved arrow)* is present between the invaginated donor bronchus and the recipient bronchus. This air collection does not extend beyond the external margin of the anastomosis and should not be confused with bronchial dehiscence. The patient was a 40-year-old man who had undergone single right lung transplantation for pulmonary fibrosis. (Courtesy of Drs. Laura Heyneman and Page McAdams, Duke University, Durham, NC.)

horizontal level as the CT image[14] or that spiral CT be performed and multiplanar reconstructions obtained.[73] In one investigation of 27 patients in whom spiral CT was performed using 3-mm collimation from a level approxi-

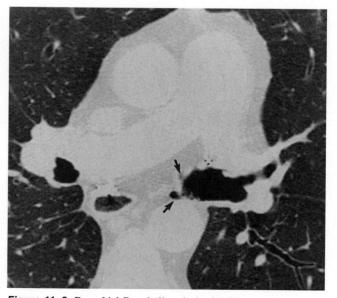

Figure 11–8. Bronchial Pseudodiverticula. HRCT scan shows irregularity of the left bronchial lumen and localized air collections *(arrows)* adjacent to the left bronchus. These abnormalities were shown at bronchoscopy to represent pseudodiverticula. The pseudodiverticula remained unchanged on subsequent CT scans performed over a 3-year period. The patient was a 41-year-old woman who had undergone double-lung transplantation for bronchiectasis.

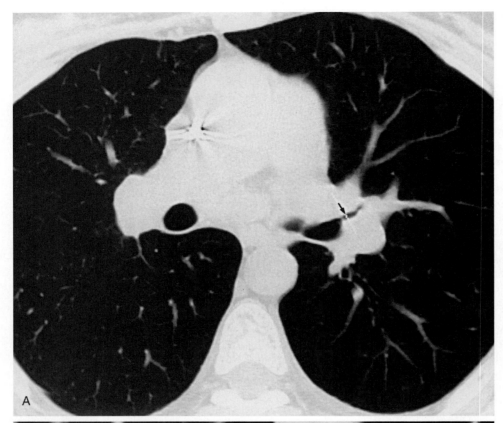

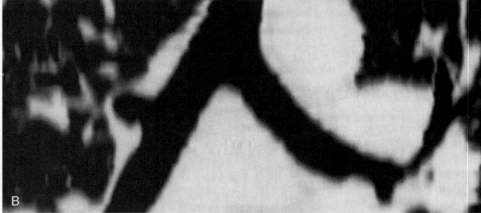

Figure 11–9. Bronchial Stenosis. CT scan *(A)* shows severe stenosis of the left upper lobe bronchus *(arrow)*. Coronal reconstruction *(B)* confirms the presence of stenosis in the left upper lobe bronchus and shows mild focal stenosis of the distal left main bronchus. The patient was a 31-year-old woman who developed left bronchial stenosis 4 months after double-lung transplantation for cystic fibrosis. (Case courtesy of Dr. Ann Leung, Stanford University School of Medicine, Stanford, CA.)

mately 2 cm above the tracheal carina, interpretation of the conventional transverse CT images for the 54 bronchial anastomoses revealed 1 mild stenosis, 1 severe stenosis, 10 anastomoses with a shelf (a common finding of no clinical significance), and 42 normal anastomoses.[73] Multiplanar reconstructions showed mild stenosis in two patients who had normal findings on the conventional transverse images. All four patients who had evidence of stenosis on multiplanar reconstructions had the findings confirmed at bronchoscopy; however, this procedure showed mild stenosis in three patients who had normal findings on CT scan.[73]

Examination of the lumen of the bronchi by CT bronchography (virtual bronchoscopy) has been shown to be superior to review of conventional transverse images.[100] Neither this procedure nor the other CT techniques is 100% accurate, however, and bronchoscopy is required for definitive diagnosis of the various bronchial anastomotic complications.[100]

BONE MARROW TRANSPLANTATION

Bone marrow transplantation is currently a standard therapy for aplastic anemia, acute and chronic leukemia, and some forms of lymphoma. It also has been used in patients who have hemoglobinopathies, immunodeficiency disorders, myelodysplastic syndrome, multiple myeloma, and some solid tumors.[75] The procedure is uncommon but not rare; more than 15,000 autologous and allogeneic transplants occur yearly worldwide.

Pulmonary disease accounts for a substantial part of the

Table 11–6. COMPLICATIONS OF BONE MARROW TRANSPLANTATION

Early Post-Transplantation Period (First 100 days)
 Pre-engraftment period (days 0–30)
  Fungal infection
  Alveolar hemorrhage
  Pulmonary edema
  Drug reactions
 Postengraftment period (days 31–100)
  Drug reactions
  Cytomegalovirus pneumonia
  Pneumocystis carinii pneumonia
  Idiopathic pneumonia
Late Post-Transplantation Period (After 100 days)
 Obliterative bronchiolitis
 Bronchiolitis obliterans organizing pneumonia
 Chronic graft-versus-host disease

morbidity and mortality of the procedure: Greater than 30% of transplantation-related deaths are related to respiratory disorders, and pulmonary complications occur in 40% to 60% of recipients.[75, 76] These complications are classified as early or late according to whether they occur during or after the first 100 days following transplantation (Table 11–6).[75, 76]

Complications

Pulmonary Edema

Pulmonary edema develops commonly after allogeneic and autologous bone marrow transplantation. In one retrospective review of 55 patients, radiographic evidence of the complication was found in 29 (53%);[77] it was accompanied by hepatic dysfunction in 28, renal dysfunction in 22, and central nervous system abnormalities in 17, suggesting that the edema may be a manifestation of a systemic process.

The onset of edema is rapid and usually occurs in the second or third week after transplantation;[75] it develops earlier in patients who have allogeneic grafts than in those who have autologous ones.[75] Clinical manifestations are nonspecific and include dyspnea, weight gain, and crackles on physical examination.[75] Radiographic findings are similar to those of pulmonary edema associated with fluid overload and include enlarged pulmonary vessels, interstitial thickening with peribronchial cuffing and septal lines, and, commonly, small pleural effusions.[78, 79]

Diffuse Alveolar Hemorrhage

Pulmonary hemorrhage is an important complication of bone marrow transplantation. In one review of 141 consecutive patients who had autologous transplants, it occurred in 29 (21%);[80] 23 (79%) died, compared with death in only 14 of 112 patients (13%) who did not have diffuse alveolar hemorrhage. The complication has been described occasionally in patients after allogeneic marrow transplants.[81]

Diffuse alveolar hemorrhage is characterized clinically by progressive dyspnea, cough, and hypoxemia;[80] hemoptysis is rare.[75] Symptoms develop about 12 days after transplantation (range, 7 to 40 days).[80] The characteristic radio-

graphic and HRCT findings consist of bilateral or, less commonly, unilateral ground-glass opacities and patchy or confluent air-space consolidation (Fig. 11–10).[79, 82] These abnormalities tend to involve mainly the perihilar region and lower lung zones.[82]

Idiopathic Pneumonia Syndrome

Idiopathic pneumonia syndrome (interstitial pneumonitis, idiopathic pneumonia) has been defined as diffuse lung injury occurring after bone marrow transplantation for which an infectious cause is not identified.[75] Interstitial pneumonitis of all etiologies accounts for about 40% of transplantation-related deaths; of these, half are noninfectious and meet the definition of idiopathic pneumonia syndrome.[83, 84] The complication develops in about 10% of patients who have bone marrow transplantation.[83] The median time of onset after transplantation has been reported to be 2 to 7 weeks.[85] Most episodes of pneumonia occurring in the first 28 days after transplantation are idiopathic; after this period, the rate of idiopathic pneumonia syndrome is about 20%.[83]

The clinical manifestations are varied: Radiographic changes may be associated with a complete lack of symptoms or with acute and severe respiratory distress.[83] Characteristically, patients complain of dyspnea and nonproductive cough. The radiologic findings are nonspecific, consisting of bilateral interstitial thickening occasionally associated with ground-glass opacities and poorly defined small nodular opacities.[79, 83]

Obliterative Bronchiolitis

Obstructive airway disease caused by obliterative bronchiolitis is an uncommon complication of bone marrow

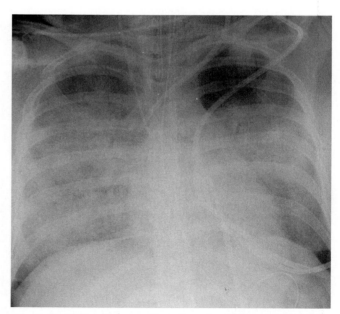

Figure 11–10. Bone Marrow Transplantation: Diffuse Alveolar Hemorrhage. Anteroposterior chest radiograph shows extensive bilateral consolidation with air bronchograms. The patient was a 27-year-old woman who developed diffuse alveolar hemorrhage 2 weeks after bone marrow transplantation.

transplantation;[88] it was found in only 4 of 113 patients (3.5%) in one series[87] and in 9 of 179 (5%) patients in another.[89] The clinical manifestations consist of cough, which is progressively productive, as well as wheezing and exertional dyspnea.[89]

The chest radiograph may be normal or may show evidence of hyperinflation. The characteristic HRCT findings consist of dilation of the segmental and subsegmental bronchi and localized areas of decreased attenuation and perfusion.[79, 86] HRCT scans performed at end-expiration show air-trapping (Fig. 11–11).[79] Recurrent pneumothorax and pneumomediastinum have been described in several patients.[90]

Infection

Specific infections in patients who have bone marrow transplantation tend to occur at particular times, corresponding to specific defects in host defense.[90, 91] Pulmonary infections may be classified as occurring in the pre-engraftment period (days 0 to 30), postengraftment period (days 31 to 100), and late post-transplantation (>100 days).[101]

Because of the widespread use of empiric broad-spectrum antibiotics, bacterial pneumonia is rare in the pre-engraftment period. The most common causes of pulmonary infection during this time are opportunistic fungi, the most frequent pathogen being *Aspergillus*.[101, 102] In the postengraftment period, with recovery of neutrophils but persistent deficits in cellular and humoral immunity, the most common pathogens are viruses, particularly cytomegalovirus. Cytomegalovirus pneumonia occurs in 10% to 40% of allogeneic bone marrow transplant recipients but is rare after autologous transplants.[103] Other important causes of respiratory illnesses during this period include respiratory syncytial virus, influenza virus, and parainfluenza virus.[104] The incidence of *Pneumocystis carinii* pneumonia in bone marrow transplant recipients has decreased considerably since the institution of routine prophylaxis with trimethoprim-sulfamethoxazole.[102] Most pulmonary infections in the late post-transplantation period occur in the

setting of chronic graft-versus-host disease, which predisposes allogeneic transplant recipients to bacterial and opportunistic fungal infection.[102, 103]

The radiologic manifestations of pneumonia in bone marrow transplantation recipients are the same as those in other hosts.[92, 93] CT can provide additional information that either changes patient management or establishes more clearly the pattern and extent of pulmonary disease (Fig. 11–12).[94, 95] In one investigation in which conventional radiographs and HRCT scans were performed prospectively in 33 symptomatic episodes seen in 33 patients, 14 chest radiographs were interpreted as normal and 22 as showing nonspecific changes;[93] however, none of the radiographic findings was considered helpful in providing sufficient information for further management. In 2 of 14 (14%) episodes in patients who had normal chest radiographs and in 9 of 22 (41%) episodes in patients who had nonspecific radiographic findings, abnormalities seen on CT scan resulted in a change in clinical management that included performing bronchoscopy, increasing or changing antibiotic coverage, starting white blood cell transfusions, biopsy, or a combination of these. In another investigation of 18 patients in whom CT scans were reviewed retrospectively after 21 episodes of intrathoracic complications, CT scan showed diagnostically relevant findings that were not apparent at radiography in 12 of 21 cases (57%), including a ground-glass pattern in early pneumonia.[94]

The usefulness of HRCT in the early detection of pneumonia was assessed prospectively in a study of 87 neutropenic patients who had 146 episodes of fever that persisted for more than 2 days despite empiric antibiotic therapy.[95] Chest radiographs and HRCT scans were normal in 56 (38%) of 146 episodes, both were abnormal in 20 (14%) episodes, and chest radiographs were normal and HRCT scans were abnormal in 70 (46%) episodes. Microorganisms were detected in 11 of 20 (55%) patients who had abnormal radiographs and CT scans and in 30 of 70 (43%) patients in whom the HRCT scans showed parenchymal abnormalities and the radiographs were normal. In 22 (31%) of these 70 episodes, abnormalities later became apparent on the radiograph. The median interval (delay)

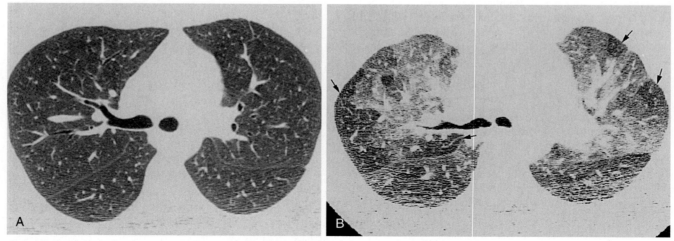

Figure 11–11. Bone Marrow Transplantation: Obliterative Bronchiolitis. HRCT scan at end-inspiration *(A)* is normal, whereas one performed at end-expiration *(B)* shows localized areas of air-trapping *(arrows)*. The patient was a 32-year-old woman who presented with dyspnea 18 months after bone marrow transplantation.

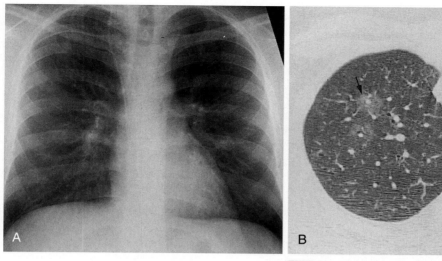

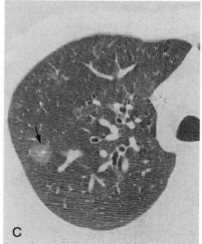

Figure 11–12. Bone Marrow Transplantation: Angioinvasive Aspergillosis. Anteroposterior chest radiograph *(A)* in a 19-year-old man 3 weeks after bone marrow transplantation shows questionable parenchymal opacities. HRCT scan images of the right upper lobe *(B* and *C)* show small nodules with surrounding halos of ground-glass attenuation *(arrows)*. These findings are most suggestive of angioinvasive aspergillosis. The diagnosis was confirmed by open-lung biopsy.

until an opacity became apparent on the chest radiograph in these patients was 5 days (range, 1 to 22 days).

The findings in these studies suggest that HRCT should be performed in bone marrow transplant recipients who have persistent fever and no evidence of pneumonia on chest radiograph. Similar to chest radiograph, however, HRCT findings in the various infectious complications after bone marrow transplantation are relatively nonspecific.[79] The main exception is the presence of a halo of ground-glass attenuation surrounding a pulmonary nodule, a finding that is most suggestive of invasive aspergillosis (*see* Fig. 11–12).[79, 96] Uncommonly, such hemorrhagic nodules are caused by other organisms, such as *Candida*, cytomegalovirus, and herpes simplex.[97]

References

1. Judson MA: Clinical aspects of lung transplantation. Clin Chest Med 14:335, 1993.
2. Davis RD, Pasque M: Pulmonary transplantation. Ann Surg 221:14, 1995.
3. Jenkinson SG, Levine SM: Lung transplantation. Dis Mon 40:1, 1994.
4. Kotloff RM, Zuckerman JB: Lung transplantation for cystic fibrosis. Chest 109:787, 1996.
5. Trulock EP: Lung transplantation. Am J Respir Crit Care Med 155:789, 1997.
6. Report of the ATS Workshop on Lung Transplantation: Lung transplantation. Am Rev Respir Dis 147:772, 1993.
7. Judson MA, Sahn SA: The pleural space and organ transplantation. Am J Respir Crit Care Med 153:1153, 1996.
8. Kaplan JD, Trulock EP, Cooper JD, et al: Pulmonary vascular permeability after lung transplantation. Am Rev Respir Dis 145:954, 1992.
9. Anderson DC, Glazer HS, Semenkovich JW, et al: Lung transplant edema: Chest radiography after lung transplantation—the first 10 days. Radiology 195:275, 1995.
10. Ettinger NA, Trulock EP: Pulmonary considerations of organ transplantation. Am Rev Respir Dis 144:433, 1991.
11. Zenati M, Yousem SA, Dowling RD, et al: Primary graft failure following pulmonary transplantation. Transplantation 50:165, 1990.
12. Herman SJ, Rappaport DC, Weisbrod GL, et al: Single-lung transplantation: Imaging features. Radiology 170:89, 1989.
13. Anderson DC, Glazer HS, Semenkovich JW, et al: Lung transplant edema: Chest radiography after lung transplantation: The first 10 days. Radiology 195:275, 1995.
14. Herman SJ: Radiologic assessment after lung transplantation. Radiol Clin North Am 32:663, 1994.
15. Garg K, Zamora MR, Tuder R, et al: Lung transplantation: Indications, donor and recipient selection, and imaging of complications. Radiographics 16:355, 1996.
16. Kundu S, Herman SJ, Winton TL: Reperfusion edema after lung transplantation: Radiographic manifestations. Radiology 206:75, 1998.

17. Ablett MJ, Grainger AJ, Keir MJ, et al: The correlation of the radiologic extent of lung transplantation edema with pulmonary oxygenation. Am J Roentgenol 171:587, 1998.

18. Trulock EP: Management of lung transplant rejection. Chest 103:1566, 1993.

19. Keenan RJ, Zeevi A: Immunologic consequences of transplantation. Chest Surg Clin N Am 5:107, 1995.

20. Griffith BP, Hardesty RL, Armitage JM, et al: Acute rejection of lung allografts with various immunosuppressive protocols. Ann Thorac Surg 54:846, 1992.

21. Kesten S, Chamberlain D, Maurer J: Yield of surveillance transbronchial biopsies performed beyond two years after lung transplantation. J Heart Lung Transplant 15:384, 1996.

22. Sayegh MH, Turka LA: The role of T-cell activation pathway in transplant rejection. N Engl J Med 338:1813, 1998.

23. Marboe CC: Pathology of lung transplantation. Pathology 4:73, 1996.

24. Millet B, Higenbottam TW, Flower CDR, et al: The radiographic appearances of infection and acute rejection of the lung after heart-lung transplantation. Am Rev Respir Dis 140:62, 1989.

25. Bergin CJ, Castellino RA, Blank N, et al: Acute lung rejection after heart-lung transplantation: Correlation of findings on chest radiographs with lung biopsy results. Am J Roentgenol 155:23, 1990.

26. Erasmus JJ, McAdams HP, Tapson VF, et al: Radiologic issues in lung transplantation for end-stage pulmonary disease. Am J Roentgenol 169:69, 1997.

27. Loubeyre P, Revel D, Delignette A, et al: High-resolution computed tomographic findings associated with histologically diagnosed acute lung rejection in heart-lung transplant recipients. Chest 107:132, 1995.

28. Dauber JH: Posttransplant bronchiolitis obliterans syndrome: Where have we been and where are we going? Chest 109:857, 1996.

29. Reichenspurner H, Girgis RE, Robbins RC, et al: Stanford experience with obliterative bronchiolitis after lung and heart-lung transplantation. Ann Thorac Surg 62:1467, 1996.

30. Sundaresan S, Trulock EP, Mohanakumar T, et al: Prevalence and outcome of bronchiolitis obliterans syndrome after lung transplantation. Washington University Lung Transplant Group. Ann Thorac Surg 60:1341, 1995.

31. Sarris GE, Smith JA, Shumway NE, et al: Long-term results of combined heart-lung transplantation: The Stanford experience. J Heart Lung Transplant 13:940, 1994.

32. Reichenspurner H, Girgis RE, Robbins RC, et al: Obliterative bronchiolitis after lung and heart-lung transplantation. Ann Thorac Surg 60:1845, 1995.

33. Cooper JD, Billingham M, Egan T, et al: A working formulation for the standardization of nomenclature and for clinical staging of chronic dysfunction in lung allografts. International Society for Heart and Lung Transplantation. J Heart Lung Transplant 12:713, 1993.

34. Tazelaar HD, Yousem SA: The pathology of combined heart-lung transplantation: An autopsy study. Hum Pathol 19:1403, 1988.

35. Skeens JL, Fuhrman CR, Yousem SA: Bronchiolitis obliterans in heart-lung transplantation patients: Radiologic findings in 11 patients. Am J Roentgenol 153:253, 1989.

36. Morrish WF, Herman SJ, Weisbrod GL, et al: Bronchiolitis obliterans after lung transplantation: Findings at chest radiography and high-resolution CT. Radiology 179:487, 1991.

37. Lentz D, Bergin CJ, Berry GJ, et al: Diagnosis of bronchiolitis obliterans in heart-lung transplantation patients: Importance of bronchial dilatation on CT. Am J Roentgenol 159:463, 1992.

38. Worthy SA, Park CS, Kim JS, et al: Bronchiolitis obliterans after lung transplantation: High-resolution CT findings in 15 patients. Am J Roentgenol 169:673, 1997.

39. Leung AN, Fisher K, Valentine V, et al: Bronchiolitis obliterans after lung transplantation: Detection using expiratory HRCT. Chest 113:365, 1998.

40. Ikonen T, Kivisaari L, Taskinen E, et al: High-resolution CT in long-term follow-up after lung transplantation. Chest 111:370, 1997.

41. Nathan SD, Ross DJ, Belman MJ, et al: Bronchiolitis obliterans in single-lung transplant recipients. Chest 107:967, 1995.

42. Chadburn A, Cesarman E, Knowles DM: Molecular pathology of posttransplantation lymphoproliferative disorders. Semin Diagn Pathol 14:15, 1997.

43. Mentzer SJ, Longtine J, Fingeroth J, et al: Immunoblastic lymphoma of donor origin in the allograft after lung transplantation. Transplantation 61:1720, 1996.

44. Schenkein DP, Schwartz RS: Neoplasms and transplantation: Trading swords for plowshares. N Engl J Med 336:949, 1997.

45. Aris RM, Maia DM, Neuringer IP, et al: Post-transplantation lymphoproliferative disorder in the Epstein-Barr virus-naive lung transplant recipient. Am J Respir Crit Care Med 154:1712, 1996.

46. Dodd GD III, Ledesma-Medina J, Baron RL, et al: Posttransplant lymphoproliferative disorder: Intrathoracic manifestations. Radiology 184:65, 1992.

47. Carignan S, Staples CA, Müller NL: Intrathoracic lymphoproliferative disorders in the immunocompromised patient: CT findings. Radiology 197:53, 1995.

48. Brown MJ, Miller RR, Müller NL: Acute lung disease in the immunocompromised host: CT and pathologic examination findings. Radiology 190:247, 1994.

49. Collins J, Müller NL, Leung AN, et al: Epstein-Barr-virus-associated lymphoproliferative disease of the lung: CT and histologic findings. Radiology 208:749, 1998.

50. Montone KT, Litzky LA, Wurster A, et al: Analysis of Epstein-Barr virus-associated posttransplantation lymphoproliferative disorder after lung transplantation. Surgery 119:544, 1996.

51. Paradis IL, Williams P: Infection after lung transplantation. Semin Respir Infect 8:207, 1993.

52. Kramer MR, Marshall SE, Starnes VA, et al: Infectious complications in heart-lung transplantation. Arch Intern Med 153:2010, 1993.

53. Lyon GM, Alspaugh JA, Meredith FT, et al: *Mycoplasma hominis* pneumonia complicating bilateral lung transplantation: Case report and review of the literature. Chest 112:1428, 1997.

54. Gass R, Fisher J, Badesch D, et al: Donor-to-host transmission of *Mycoplasma hominis* in lung allograft recipients. Clin Infect Dis 22:567, 1996.

55. Martel S, Carre PC, Carrera G, et al: Tumour necrosis factor-alpha gene expression by alveolar macrophages in human lung allograft recipient with recurrence of sarcoidosis. Toulouse Lung Transplantation Group. Eur Respir J 9:1087, 1996.

56. Muller C, Briegel J, Haller M, et al: Sarcoidosis recurrence following lung transplantation. Transplantation 61:1117, 1996.

57. Kazerooni EA, Jackson C, Cascade PN: Sarcoidosis: Recurrence of primary disease in transplanted lungs. Radiology 192:461, 1994.

58. Nine JS, Yousem SA, Paradis IL, et al: Lymphangioleiomyomatosis: Recurrence after lung transplantation. J Heart Lung Transplant 13:714, 1994.

59. O'Brien JD, Lium JH, Parosa JF, et al: Lymphangiomyomatosis recurrence in the allograft after single-lung transplantation. Am J Respir Crit Care Med 151:2033, 1995.

60. Etienne B, Bertocchi M, Gamondes J-P, et al: Relapsing pulmonary Langerhans cell histiocytosis after lung transplantation. Am J Respir Crit Care Med 157:288, 1998.

61. Baz MA, Kussin PS, Van Trigt P, et al: Recurrence of diffuse panbronchiolitis after lung transplantation. Am J Respir Crit Care Med 151:895, 1995.

62. Parker LA, Novotny DB: Recurrent alveolar proteinosis following double lung transplantation. Chest 111:1457, 1997.

63. Habib SB, Congleton J, Carr D, et al: Recurrence of recipient Langerhans' cell histiocytosis following bilateral lung transplantation. Thorax 53:323, 1998.

64. King MB, Jessrun J, Hertz MI: Recurrence of desquamative interstitial pneumonia after lung transplantation. Am J Respir Crit Care Med 156:2003, 1997.

65. Verleden GM, Sels F, Van Raemdonck D, et al: Possible recurrence of desquamative interstitial pneumonitis in a single lung transplant recipient. Eur Respir J 11:971, 1998.

66. Frost AE, Keller CA, Brown RW, et al: Giant cell interstitial pneumonitis: Disease recurrence in the transplanted lung. Am Rev Respir Dis 148:1401, 1993.

67. Collins J, Kuhlman JE, Love RB: Acute, life-threatening complications of lung transplantation. Radiographics 18:21, 1998.

68. Judson MA, Handy JR, Sahn SA: Pleural effusions following lung transplantation: Time course, characteristics, and clinical implications. Chest 109:1190, 1996.

69. Herridge MS, de Hoyos AL, Chaparro C, et al: Pleural complications in lung transplant recipients. J Thorac Cardiovasc Surg 110:22, 1995.

70. Paranjpe DV, Wittich GR, Hamid LW, et al: Frequency and manage-

ment of pneumothoraces in heart-lung transplant recipients. Radiology 190:255, 1994.

71. Date H, Trulock EP, Arcidi JM, et al: Improved airway healing after lung transplantation: An analysis of 348 bronchial anastomoses. J Thorac Cardiovasc Surg 110:1424, 1995.

72. Semenkovich JW, Glazer HS, Anderson DC, et al: Bronchial dehiscence in lung transplantation: CT evaluation. Radiology 194:205, 1995.

73. Quint L, Whyte R, Kazerooni E, et al: Stenosis of the central airways: Evaluation by using helical CT with multiplanar reconstructions. Radiology 194:871, 1995.

74. McAdams HP, Murray JG, Erasmus JJ, et al: Telescoping bronchial anastomoses for unilateral or bilateral sequential lung transplantation: CT appearance. Radiology 203:202, 1997.

75. Soubani AO, Miller KB, Hassoun PM: Pulmonary complications of bone marrow transplantation. Chest 109:1066, 1996.

76. Breuer R, Lossos IS, Berkman N, et al: Pulmonary complications of bone marrow transplantation. Respir Med 87:571, 1993.

77. Cahill RA, Spitzer TR, Mazumder A: Marrow engraftment and clinical manifestations of capillary leak syndrome. Bone Marrow Transplant 18:177, 1996.

78. Dickout WJ, Chan CK, Hyland RH, et al: Prevention of acute pulmonary edema after bone marrow transplantation. Chest 92:303, 1987.

79. Worthy SA, Flint JD, Müller NL: Pulmonary complications after bone marrow transplantation: High-resolution CT and pathologic findings. Radiographics 17:1359, 1997.

80. Robins RA, Linder J, Stahl MG, et al: Diffuse alveolar hemorrhage in autologous bone marrow transplant recipients. Am J Med 87:511, 1989.

81. Schmidt-Wolf I, Schwerdtfeger R, Schwella N, et al: Diffuse pulmonary alveolar hemorrhage after allogenic bone marrow transplantation. Ann Hematol 67:139, 1993.

82. Witte RJ, Gurney JW, Robbins RA, et al: Diffuse pulmonary alveolar hemorrhage after bone marrow transplantation: Radiographic findings in 39 patients. Am J Roentgenol 157:461, 1991.

83. Clark JG, Hansen JA, Hertz MI, et al: Idiopathic pneumonia syndrome after bone marrow transplantation. Am Rev Respir Dis 147:1601, 1993.

84. Wingard JR, Mellits ED, Sostrin MB, et al: Interstitial pneumonitis after allogeneic bone marrow transplantation. Medicine 67:175, 1988.

85. Crawford SW, Longton G, Storb R: Acute graft-versus-host disease and the risks for idiopathic pneumonia after marrow transplantation for severe aplastic anemia. Bone Marrow Transplant 12:225, 1993.

86. Padley SPG, Adler BD, Hansell DM, et al: Bronchiolitis obliterans: High resolution CT findings and correlation with pulmonary function tests. Clin Radiol 47:236, 1993.

87. Ralph DD, Springmeyer SC, Sullivan KM, et al: Rapidly progressive air-flow obstruction in marrow transplant recipients: Possible association between obliterative bronchiolitis and chronic graft-versus-host disease. Am Rev Respir Dis 129:641, 1984.

88. Clark JG, Crawford SW, Madtes DK, et al: Obstructive lung disease after allogeneic marrow transplantation. Ann Intern Med 111:368, 1989.

89. Philit F, Wiesendanger T, Archimbaud E, et al: Post-transplant obstructive lung disease ("bronchiolitis obliterans"): A clinical comparative study of bone marrow and lung transplant patients. Eur Respir J 8:551, 1995.

90. Krowka MJ, Rosenow EC, Hoagland HC: Pulmonary complications of bone marrow transplantation. Chest 87:237, 1985.

91. Crawford SW: Bone marrow transplantation and related infections. Semin Respir Infect 8:183, 1993.

92. Wise RH Jr, Shin MS, Gockerman JP, et al: Pneumonia in bone marrow transplant patients. Am J Roentgenol 143:707, 1984.

93. Barloon TJ, Galvin JR, Mori M, et al: High-resolution ultrafast chest CT in the clinical management of febrile bone marrow transplant patients with normal or nonspecific chest roentgenograms. Chest 99:928, 1991.

94. Graham NJ, Müller NL, Miller RR, et al: Intrathoracic complications following allogeneic bone marrow transplantation: CT findings. Radiology 181:153, 1991.

95. Heussel CP, Kauczor HU, Heussel G, et al: Early detection of pneumonia in febrile neutropenic patients: Use of thin-section CT. Am J Roentgenol 169:1247, 1997.

96. Kuhlman JE, Fishman EK, Burch PA, et al: Invasive pulmonary aspergillosis in acute leukemia: The contribution of CT to early diagnosis and aggressive management. Chest 92:95, 1987.

97. Primack SL, Hartman TE, Lee KS, et al: Pulmonary nodules and the CT halo sign. Radiology 190:513, 1994.

98. Hosenpud JD, Bennett LE, Keck BM, et al: The registry for the International Society for Heart and Lung Transplantation: Fifteenth Official Report—1998. J Heart Lung Transplant 17:656, 1998.

99. Kundu S, Herman SJ, Larhs A, et al: Correlation of chest radiographic findings with biopsy-proven acute lung rejection. J Thorac Imaging 14:178, 1999.

100. McAdams HP, Palmer SM, Erasmus JJ, et al: Bronchial anastomotic complications in lung transplant recipients: Virtual bronchoscopy for noninvasive assessment. Radiology 209:689, 1998.

101. Choi YH, Leung AN: Radiologic findings: Pulmonary infections after bone marrow transplantation. J Thorac Imaging 14:201, 1999.

102. Soubani AO, Miller KB, Hassoun PM: Pulmonary complications of bone marrow transplantation. Chest 109:1066, 1996.

103. Sable CA, Donowitz GR: Infections in bone marrow transplant recipients. Clin Infect Dis 18:273, 1994.

104. Whimbey E, Champlin RE, Couch RB, et al: Community respiratory virus infections among hospitalized bone marrow transplant recipients. Clin Infect Dis 22:778, 1996.

105. Arcasoy SM, Kotloff RM: Lung transplantation. N Engl J Med 340:1081, 1999.

106. Ward S, Müller NL: Pulmonary complications following lung transplantation. Clin Radiol 55:332, 2000.

107. Matar LD, McAdams HP, Palmer SM, et al: Respiratory viral infections in lung transplant recipients: Radiologic findings with clinical correlation. Radiology 213:735, 1999.

108. Collins J, Müller NL, Kazerooni EA, et al: CT findings of pneumonia after lung transplantation. Am J Roentgenol 175:811, 2000.

109. Bankier AA, Muylem AV, Knoop C, et al: Bronchiolitis obliterans syndrome in heart-lung transplant recipients: Diagnosis with expiratory CT. Radiology 218:533, 2001.

CHAPTER 12

Embolic Lung Disease

PULMONARY THROMBOEMBOLISM

Emboli of fragments of thrombus to the pulmonary vasculature are common and range from minute fibrin-platelet aggregates unassociated with clinical, radiologic, or functional consequences to massive clots that completely occlude the pulmonary trunk or a main pulmonary artery and cause sudden death. Because pulmonary thromboembolism (PTE) by definition implies the formation of thrombus elsewhere than the lungs, the two processes frequently are discussed together under the term *venous thromboembolic disease*. The term *deep venous thrombosis* (DVT) usually implies thrombosis of the deep veins of the leg and it is used here in that sense; although clinically significant thrombosis is most common at this site, many of the factors involved in the pathogenesis of thrombosis and the consequences thereof are similar at other sites.

Epidemiology

It is difficult to be certain of the precise incidence of DVT and PTE and of the importance of the two with respect to morbidity and mortality. Based on extrapolation of limited data concerning the fatality rate of untreated PTE and on autopsy studies that indicate that in-hospital PTE often is not diagnosed before death, Dalen and Alpert[2] concluded that there were approximately 630,000 cases of PTE annually in the United States; of these, it was estimated that 163,000 (about 25%) had a diagnosis and the initiation of therapy. The accuracy of these figures should be questioned, however. It is likely that silent PTE does not have the 30% mortality of untreated PTE to which Dalen and Alpert referred. In one study of 87 patients who had venographically proven DVT and no chest symptoms and who were randomized to receive treatment with anticoagulation or placebo, lung scintigraphy was performed at 10 and 60 days to assess the development of *silent* PTE;[3] no patient died in either group, and there was no significant difference in the rate of silent PTE (13% in the anticoagulated group and 8% in the coagulated group).

In another study, which included data from 16 short-stay community hospitals in Massachusetts, investigators found an average annual incidence of PTE of 23 per 100,000 population and an in-hospital case-fatality rate of 12%.[4] Extrapolation of these data led to the conclusion that there are 170,000 new cases of clinically recognized DVT or PTE in patients treated in short-stay hospitals each year, an estimate for treated PTE substantially less than that proposed by Dalen and Alpert.[2]

Because of the effects of gravity and immobility, the legs are the most vulnerable site for an alteration in venous blood flow, and the frequency of PTE directly parallels thrombosis in this site; more than 90% of cases of PTE originate in the lower extremity.[1] Less common sources of thromboemboli include the pelvic veins, the inferior vena cava, and the right atrium. The right ventricle[5, 6] (rarely in association with a right ventricular myxoma),[7, 8] right-sided heart valves, superior vena cava,[9, 10] and veins of the neck and arms[11] are relatively infrequent sources. The incidence of thrombosis in the arms has been estimated to be less than 2% of all cases of DVT;[12] however, complicating PTE is not uncommon, being reported in 3 of 25 patients in one series[13] and in 4 of 19 patients with catheter-related thrombosis in another.[14]

Clinical Manifestations

Most pulmonary thromboemboli produce no symptoms or cause such minimal distress that they may be recognized only in retrospect, regardless of whether the occlusion has occurred in the smaller vessels, the segmental arteries, or the lobar arteries. The most common symptoms are dyspnea, tachypnea, and pleuritic chest pain. The severity of clinical manifestations varies considerably: At one extreme, an ostensibly healthy individual may die suddenly,[155] and at the other, a large embolus obstructing a major vessel may give rise to only minor disturbance in circulatory dynamics and minimal clinical findings.[156] Attention to symptoms is still important in the diagnosis of PTE. In one study of 104 patients who had PTE, the association of the sudden onset of dyspnea, chest pain, and syncope (singly or in combination) with an electrocardiographic sign of right ventricular overload or a radiographic sign of PTE (oligemia, amputation of a hilar artery, or pulmonary consolidation compatible with infarction) was observed in 87 (84%) patients.[225] The same association was present in only 8 (5%) of 146 patients in whom the diagnosis of PTE had been excluded. The sensitivity and specificity of this algorithm for PTE were 84% and 95%, respectively.

Radiographic Manifestations

Most episodes of PTE produce no symptoms or detectable changes on chest radiograph. Even if the diagnosis is suspected clinically and confirmed angiographically, no abnormalities are seen on radiographs in approximately 10% to 15% of cases. In one review of chest radiographs of 383 patients who had angiographically proven PTE and 680 patients who had negative angiograms, the chest radiograph was interpreted as normal in 12% of patients with pulmonary emboli;[19] the negative predictive value of a normal radiograph was 74%. The radiographic manifestations of PTE can be classified into manifestations without and with pulmonary infarction or hemorrhage. Although many abnormalities have been described (Table 12–1), the chest radiograph is of limited value in diagnosis.

Thromboembolism Without Infarction

Changes related to thromboembolism without infarction include oligemia, change in vessel size, loss of lung volume, and alteration in size and configuration of the heart.

Oligemia

Oligemia may be focal (Westermark's sign), in which case it usually is seen in the periphery of the lung and is

Table 12–1. CHEST RADIOGRAPH IN ACUTE PULMONARY THROMBOEMBOLISM

Limited value in diagnosis
Performed mainly to exclude other diseases that may mimic pulmonary
   thromboembolism clinically
Findings with low sensitivity and relatively high specificity
   Peripheral oligemia (Westermark's sign)
   Enlargement of central pulmonary artery (Fleischner's sign)
   Pleural-based opacity (Hampton's hump)
   Elevated hemidiaphragm
Nonspecific findings
   Air-space consolidation
   Linear atelectasis
   Pleural effusion
Radiograph normal in 10%–15% of cases with proven diagnosis

caused by occlusion of a fairly large lobar or segmental pulmonary artery (Fig. 12–1), or general, as a result of widespread small vessel occlusion.[17, 21] Although oligemia is a reliable sign of massive PTE, it is not sensitive in the detection of smaller emboli. In one review of the radiographic findings in 123 patients who had acute PTE, oligemia was present in only 7 (5%).[20] In another study of 1,063 patients suspected of having acute PTE who underwent pulmonary angiography, oligemia had a sensitivity of 14% and a specificity of 92% in the diagnosis.[19]

Widespread acute PTE may result in extensive areas of oligemia and focal areas of increased vascularity secondary to blood flow redistribution. Occasionally the blood flow redistribution may result in focal pulmonary edema (Fig. 12–2).

Changes in the Pulmonary Arteries

Enlargement of a major pulmonary artery (Fleischner's sign) is a helpful sign in the diagnosis of PTE, particularly when serial radiographs reveal progressive increase in size of the affected vessel (*see* Fig. 12–1).[22] In a study of 25 patients who had massive PTE (defined arteriographically as involvement of at least half the major pulmonary arterial branches), enlarged hilar pulmonary arteries were seen in 14.[17] Of equal diagnostic importance is the abrupt tapering of the occluded vessel distally; the vessel may terminate suddenly, creating the so-called knuckle sign (*see* Fig. 12–1).[16, 25] In the study cited previously of 73 patients who had perfusion scan–confirmed PTE, approximately 25% showed this sign.[24] In addition to abrupt termination, occluded vessels may be delineated more sharply than normal, a sign probably relating to diminished pulsation.

Similar to oligemia, enlargement of a hilar pulmonary artery usually is seen only in patients who have massive PTE, and this sign has a relatively low sensitivity in diagnosis. In one investigation of 123 patients who had angiographically proven acute embolism, a prominent central pulmonary artery was seen in only 20 (16%); the mean pulmonary artery pressure in these patients was 30 ± 14 mm Hg, compared with a mean pressure of 16 ± 5 mm Hg in patients who had normal chest radiographs.[20] In another review of chest radiographic findings in 1,063 patients suspected of having acute PTE who underwent pulmonary angiography, a prominent central pulmonary

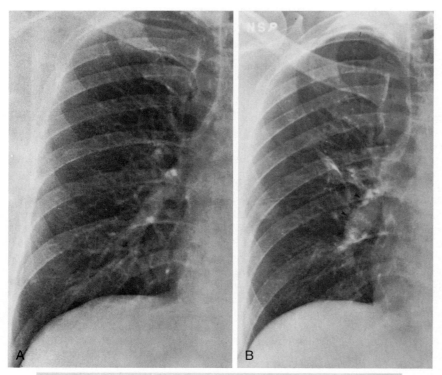

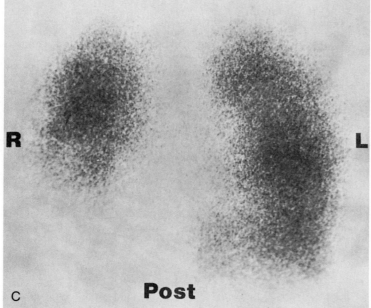

Figure 12–1. Pulmonary Thromboembolism Without Infarction. On admission of a 52-year-old man to the hospital, posteroanterior radiograph *(A)* revealed no significant abnormalities. Several days after abdominal surgery, he experienced abrupt onset of right chest pain and dyspnea. A radiograph at this time *(B)* showed an obvious increase in diameter and a change in configuration of the right interlobar artery *(arrowheads)*; also the distal end of this artery appeared *knuckled* and the vessels peripheral to it diminutive. The right lower zone showed increased radiolucency indicating diminished perfusion (Westermark's sign). Lung scan *(C)* revealed absence of perfusion of the lower half of the right lung.

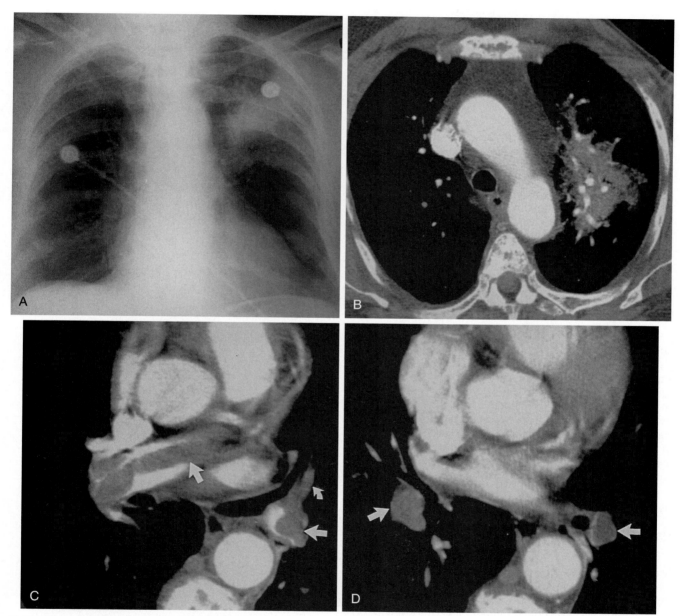

Figure 12–2. Acute Pulmonary Thromboembolism. A 72-year-old woman who had breast carcinoma and extensive metastatic disease presented with acute shortness of breath. Anteroposterior chest radiograph *(A)* shows focal consolidation in the left upper lobe and oligemia throughout the remaining left and right lungs. Contrast-enhanced spiral CT scan *(B)* shows increased size and number of vessels within the area of consolidation. CT scan at the level of the bronchus intermedius *(C)* shows large filling defects *(straight arrows)* in the right pulmonary artery and left lower lobe pulmonary artery and complete occlusion of the lingular artery *(curved arrow)*. CT scan at a more caudad level *(D)* shows almost complete occlusion of the lower lobe pulmonary arteries *(arrows)*. Thromboembolism also was present in the right upper lobe pulmonary artery. Incidental note is made of vertebral body metastases from breast carcinoma. The left upper lobe consolidation represented acute pulmonary edema resulting from blood flow redistribution from obstruction of almost the entire remaining pulmonary arterial system. (Case courtesy of Dr. Cathy Staples, Kelowna General Hospital, Kelowna, BC, Canada.)

artery was found to have a diagnostic specificity of 80% but a sensitivity of only 20%.[19]

Volume Loss

Loss of volume of a lower lobe may be manifested radiographically by elevation of the hemidiaphragm, downward displacement of the major fissure, or both. Elevation of the hemidiaphragm was observed in 25% of 123 patients who had angiographically proven PTE in one study.[20] In another review of the radiographic findings in 1,063 patients, elevation of the diaphragm had a diagnostic sensitivity and specificity of 20% and 85%, respectively.[19] Loss of volume is a more frequent finding when infarction is present (*see* farther on); in one study of eight patients who had massive PTE and who showed loss of volume, seven had infarction.[17]

Another relatively common finding is the presence of line shadows representing linear atelectasis, as described in 22% of cases in one study.[26] These shadows are roughly horizontal, usually occur in the lower lung zones, are 1 to 3 mm thick and several centimeters long, and abut the pleural surface. In a study of 10 patients who had linear atelectasis present on their last antemortem radiograph, 6 had recent thromboemboli at autopsy.[27]

Cardiac Changes

Radiographic findings suggestive of acute pulmonary arterial hypertension are not a common accompaniment of PTE, being observed in only 10% of 126 patients in one study[28] and 12% of 123 patients in another.[20] They occur most often with widespread peripheral emboli and sometimes—when a large enough area of the arterial system is occluded—with massive central embolization. The signs are those of cardiac enlargement as a result of dilation of the right ventricle, increase in size of the main pulmonary artery, and, usually, increase in size and rapidity of tapering of the hilar pulmonary vessels.[22, 25]

Thromboembolism with Infarction or Hemorrhage

Parenchymal Consolidation and Volume Loss

The radiographic changes in PTE with infarction or hemorrhage consist of segmental areas of consolidation associated with volume loss. Their relative frequency is influenced by the time interval between the onset of symptoms and the performance of radiography. In a study of 50 patients who had angiographically documented acute PTE, loss of lung volume as evidenced by elevation of a hemidiaphragm was observed in 50% within 24 hours of onset of symptoms and in only 15% when symptoms had been present longer.[29] By contrast, pulmonary opacities were found in 37% of patients within 24 hours and 57% thereafter.

In the early stages of pulmonary infarction, parenchymal opacities are ill defined. They are most common in the base of the right lower lobe, often nestled in the costophrenic sulcus. Most cases involve one or perhaps two segments, affecting a relatively small volume of lung parenchyma; however, infarction occasionally involves the

whole or a major portion of a lobe.[30, 32] The interval between the embolic episode and the development of an opacity ranges from 10 to 12 hours[33, 34] to several days after vascular occlusion;[33] in one series, the opacity developed within 24 hours in half of the patients.[26]

The configuration of a pulmonary infarct usually has an appearance known as *Hampton's hump*.[15, 19] This configuration consists of homogeneous wedge-shaped consolidation in the lung periphery, with its base contiguous to a visceral pleural surface and its rounded, convex apex directed toward the hilum (Fig. 12–3).[33, 35] The size of the consolidated area varies from patient to patient and, in the case of multiple infarcts, from one area to another. The consolidated areas are usually 3 to 5 cm in diameter but may be 10 cm.[33] An air bronchogram rarely is seen;[36] this absence, combined with the presence of peripheral homogeneous consolidation, should strongly suggest infarction rather than acute air-space pneumonia. An air bronchogram does not rule out infarction, however. Cavitation is rare[37] and usually indicates the presence of septic emboli.[18, 231]

The time course of resolution of infarction varies widely and is a reliable indicator of the nature of the consolidative

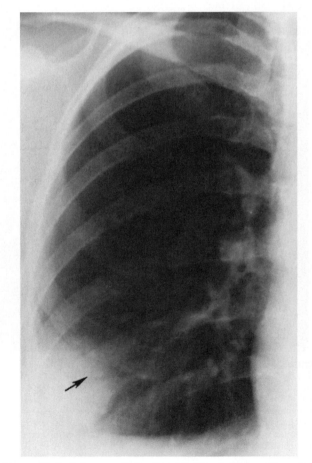

Figure 12–3. Pulmonary Infarction: Hampton's Hump. View of the right lung from posteroanterior chest radiograph reveals a homogeneous opacity in the right costophrenic angle possessing a convex contour *(arrow)* toward the hilum. This constitutes the typical features of Hampton's hump and is highly suggestive of a pulmonary infarct. The patient was a young man who had a history of acute chest pain associated with thrombophlebitis of the right leg.

process. If embolism results only in parenchymal hemorrhage and edema, clearing may occur within 4 to 7 days, often without residua;[38] when it leads to tissue necrosis, radiographic resolution, when it occurs, averages 20 days[23] and may take 5 weeks.[39] The pattern of resolution can be a valuable sign in differentiating a pulmonary infarct from acute pneumonia.[40] In the latter, the shadow appears to break up, rendering an originally homogeneous opacity inhomogeneous as scattered areas of radiolucency appear within it; with infarction, the shadow diminishes gradually while maintaining its homogeneity and (roughly) its original shape. This pattern of resolution of pulmonary infarcts has been likened to a melting ice cube (the *melting sign*).[40] This sign is applicable only in the resolving stages of either lesion, however, and is of no value at a time when the institution of appropriate therapy is vital.

The short-term and long-term appearance of healed infarcts varies considerably. In a follow-up study of 32 patients who had 58 angiographically proven pulmonary infarcts, complete radiographic resolution occurred in 29 (50%) of the 58 infarcts; of the remainder, residual findings included linear scars (14), pleurodiaphragmatic adhesions (9), and localized pleural thickening (6).[41] In all cases, the residual features were diminutive when compared with the original abnormality.

Pleural Disease

Pleural effusion is seen in 35% to 55% of patients who have acute PTE.[19, 20] It is identified most commonly in patients who have infarction or hemorrhage but may be present in patients who do not have parenchymal consolidation.[19] The amount of pleural fluid is usually small, but it may be abundant. It is more often unilateral.[33] Pneumothorax is a rare complication of PTE with infarction.[31]

Validity of Radiographic Findings

Two groups of investigators have assessed the accuracy of the various radiographic findings in the diagnosis of acute PTE.[19, 42] In one study, chest radiographs were reviewed from 152 patients, all of whom were suspected at one time of having acute PTE, but only 108 proved to have embolism on the basis of a positive pulmonary angiogram.[42] The radiographs were randomized and presented for interpretation to nine readers (seven of whom were radiologists specializing in pulmonary disease). The question, "Does this patient have pulmonary embolism?" required a *yes*, *no*, or *don't know* answer. The average true-positive ratio (sensitivity) was 0.33 (range, 0.08 to 0.52), and the average true-negative ratio (specificity) was 0.59 (range, 0.31 to 0.80). A predictive index, reflecting the overall accuracy of diagnosis, was 0.40 (range, 0.17 to 0.57) for the entire group.[42]

In a second study, chest radiographs of 1,063 patients who had suspected acute PTE were interpreted independently by two chest radiologists.[19] The study included 383 patients who had angiographically proven PTE and 680 patients who had a normal pulmonary angiogram.[19] The most common parenchymal abnormalities in patients who had PTE were atelectasis and focal areas of increased opacity. The prevalence of these findings was not significantly different from that in patients who did not have embolism, however. Atelectasis (manifested by elevation of the hemidiaphragm) had a sensitivity of 20% and a specificity of 85%, and pleural-based areas of increased opacity (Hampton's hump) had a sensitivity of 22% and a specificity of 82%. Similarly, oligemia (Westermark's sign), prominent central pulmonary artery (Fleischner's sign), vascular redistribution, and pleural effusion were poor predictors of PTE. Chest radiograph was interpreted as normal in 12% of patients who had PTE and in 18% of patients in whom it was absent.

As these studies show, chest radiography is of limited value in the diagnosis of PTE. Its major importance lies in excluding other disease processes that can mimic it, such as pneumonia and pneumothorax, and in providing correlation with ventilation-perfusion ($\dot{V}/\dot{Q}$) lung scans.[19, 35, 42]

Special Diagnostic Techniques

Despite the hundreds of studies that have been performed since the 1970s, the optimal approach to the diagnosis of PTE remains controversial. As discussed previously, chest radiography is associated with poor sensitivity and specificity. Clinical symptoms and signs and the results of laboratory investigation are of limited diagnostic value. Although it is well recognized that pulmonary angiography is the definitive method of establishing the diagnosis and of showing the extent of embolism, the procedure is expensive and time-consuming and may lead to significant morbidity. For more than two decades, $\dot{V}/\dot{Q}$ scintigraphy was the technique of choice as the initial screening procedure. More recently, contrast-enhanced computed tomography (CT) using spiral or electron-beam technique has become the method of choice in several centers. Other imaging techniques that may play a role include magnetic resonance (MR) imaging (for the diagnosis of PTE and DVT) as well as a variety of other techniques used for the diagnosis of DVT, such as venography, ultrasonography, and CT.

Scintigraphy

$\dot{V}/\dot{Q}$ lung scan has been shown to be a safe, noninvasive technique to evaluate regional pulmonary perfusion and ventilation and has been used widely in the evaluation of patients suspected of having PTE.

Technique

The radiopharmaceuticals of choice for perfusion lung scanning are technetium-99m–labeled human albumin microsphere (Tc-99m HAM) particles or macroaggregated albumin (Tc-99m MAA) particles.[43, 44] Technetium-99m MAA particles vary in size from 10 to 150 μm, with greater than 90% of particles measuring between 10 and 90 μm. Tc-99m HAM particles are more uniform in size (35 to 60 μm). The biologic half-life of Tc-99m MAA within the lung is 2 to 6 hours.

The intravenous administration of Tc-99m HAM or Tc-99m MAA should be performed over 5 to 10 respiratory cycles with the patient in the supine position, which limits the effect of gravity on regional pulmonary arterial blood flow. After injection, particles pass through the right atrium and ventricle and lodge within precapillary arterioles in the lungs. The distribution of particles within the lungs is proportional to regional pulmonary blood flow at the time of injection. The usual dose has an activity between 74 and 148 MBq (2 to 4 mCi) and contains 200,000 to 500,000 particles. It has been estimated that the particles cause transient blocks of approximately 0.1% of precapillary pulmonary arterioles,[45] providing a static image of regional flow. For diagnostic purposes, at least six views of the lungs should be obtained, including anterior, posterior, right and left lateral, and right and left posterior oblique views. Additional right and left anterior oblique views may be helpful in selected cases and are used routinely by many physicians.[43, 44]

Perfusion scintigraphy is a sensitive but nonspecific technique for identifying pulmonary disease: Virtually all parenchymal lung diseases and airway diseases, such as chronic obstructive pulmonary disease (COPD) and asthma, can cause decreased pulmonary arterial blood flow within the affected lung zone. Because thromboemboli characteristically cause abnormal perfusion with preserved ventilation (mismatched defects) (Fig. 12–4), whereas parenchymal lung disease most often causes ventilation and perfusion abnormalities in the same lung region (matched defects), combined $\dot{V}/\dot{Q}$ scintigraphy is performed routinely in most centers to improve diagnostic specificity. Most experience with ventilation imaging has been with xenon 133.[35] Alternative ventilation imaging agents, such as xenon 127, krypton 81m, technetium-99m aerosols, technegas, or pertechnegas, have not been evaluated as exten-

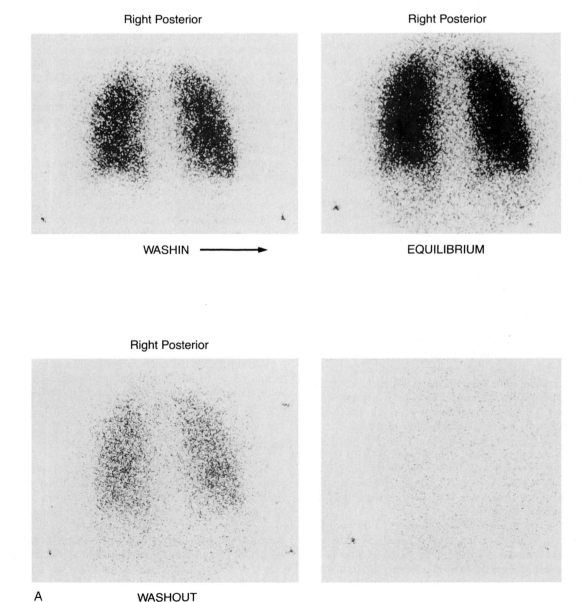

Figure 12–4. Value of Ventilation-Perfusion Lung Scans in the Diagnosis of Thromboembolism. Xenon 133 posterior inhalation lung scan *(A)* shows normal ventilation parameters during the washin, equilibrium, and washout phases.

Anterior

Posterior

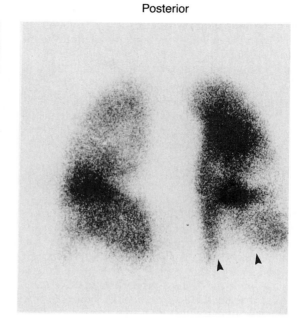

Right Posterior Oblique

Left Posterior Oblique

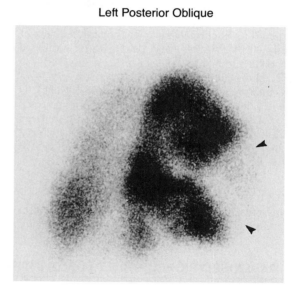

B

Figure 12–4. *Continued* Corresponding technetium-99m MAA perfusion lung scans *(B)* in anterior, posterior, and right and left posterior oblique projections identify multiple segmental filling defects throughout both lungs *(arrowheads)*. These findings, in concert with the ventilation study, are virtually diagnostic (high probability) of pulmonary thromboembolism. The patient was a 65-year-old man who presented with acute dyspnea.

sively;[35, 46] however, the available data suggest that there is no major diagnostic difference among them.

With xenon 133, ventilation imaging generally is performed before perfusion imaging.[35] An initial posterior washin or first breath image is acquired for 100,000 counts or 10 to 15 seconds after the inhalation of 550 to 770 MBq of xenon 133. Equilibrium images then are obtained while the patient rebreathes the gas within a closed system for at least 4 minutes. The washin or breath-hold images show regional lung ventilation. Regions of the lungs that appear

as defects on the washin images may normalize on the equilibrium image because of collateral ventilation. Finally, serial washout images are acquired while the patient breathes ambient air, allowing for regional air-trapping to be detected as focal areas of retained activity. Serial washout images should be performed initially in the posterior projection rather than in the left and right posterior oblique positions to maximize the number of lung segments that can be visualized. To optimize diagnostic performance, images should be taken with patients in the erect position;

however, if necessary, they can be made in patients who are supine or on ventilatory assistance.

Diagnostic Criteria

As indicated, the diagnosis of PTE by scintigraphy is based on the presence of V̇/Q̇ mismatch, that is, the presence of ventilation in the absence of perfusion distal to obstructing emboli. The findings are classified in terms of probability of embolism, the most commonly used reporting terms being *normal*, *near-normal*, *low*, *intermediate*, and *high*.

Several diagnostic criteria have been suggested for the interpretation of V̇/Q̇ lung scans.[47, 48] Many of these criteria were assessed in the Prospective Investigation of Pulmonary Embolism Diagnosis (PIOPED) study, a large prospective multicenter study.[51] In an investigation comparing various diagnostic algorithms, the original PIOPED criteria had the highest likelihood ratio for predicting the presence of emboli on pulmonary angiography.[49] Use of these criteria was associated with the highest proportion of V̇/Q̇ scans being interpreted as intermediate probability, however. Several amendments of the original PIOPED criteria have been made (Table 12–2).[43, 48] By using the revised criteria, it is possible to decrease the number of intermediate-probability interpretations and classify them correctly as low probability. Several criteria have been identified that have a positive predictive value (PPV) of less than 10% for PTE.[226] These include nonsegmental perfusion abnormalities (PPV = 8%), matched V̇/Q̇ abnormalities in two or three zones of a single lung (PPV = 3%), and one to three perfusion defects involving less than 25% of a segment (PPV = 1%). These abnormalities constitute criteria for very low–probability interpretation and increase the utility of V̇/Q̇ scintigraphy in the assessment of patients with suspected acute PTE.[226] Use of the revised PIOPED criteria has been shown in clinical studies to provide a more accurate assessment of angiographically proven PTE than use of the original criteria.[43, 50]

Diagnostic Accuracy

In a random sample of 931 patients who underwent scintigraphy in the PIOPED study, 13% had high-probability scans, 39% had intermediate-probability scans, 34% had low-probability scans, and 14% had normal or near-normal scans.[51] There was good agreement for classifying V̇/Q̇ scans as high probability (95%) or as normal (94%); however, there was a 25% to 75% disagreement in interpreting intermediate-probability and low-probability scans.[51] Of the 931 patients, 755 underwent pulmonary angiography. Of patients who had high-probability scans and definitive diagnosis at angiography, 88% had emboli compared with 33% of patients who had intermediate-probability scans, 16% who had low-probability scans, and 9% who had near-normal or normal scans. The sensitivity, specificity, and PPV of V̇/Q̇ scanning for detecting acute PTE in this study are presented in Table 12–3. The diagnostic value was not significantly different between men and women and among patients of different ages.[52, 53] The diagnostic utility was similar among patients who had pre-existing cardiac or pulmonary disease compared with patients who had no such disease. In a subset of patients who had COPD, the sensitivity of a high-probability scan was significantly lower than that in patients who had no pre-existing cardiopulmonary disease;[54] however, the PPV of a high-probability scan was 100%, and the negative predictive value of a low-probability or very low–probability scan was 94%.

Although clinical assessment of patients who have suspected PTE does not lead to a definitive diagnosis in most instances, the results from the PIOPED study emphasize the importance of incorporating the pretest clinical likelihood of PTE in the overall diagnostic evaluation (Table 12–4). In patients who have low-probability or very low–probability V̇/Q̇ scans and no history of immobilization, recent surgery, trauma to the lower extremities, or central venous instrumentation, the prevalence of PTE was only 4.5%.[55] In patients who had low-probability or very low–probability scan interpretations and one risk factor, the prevalence of PTE was 12%, whereas in patients who had two or more risk factors, the prevalence was 21%. In the PIOPED study, however, most patients had intermediate-probability or low-probability V̇/Q̇ scans and an intermediate clinical likelihood of PTE; for these patients, the combination of clinical assessment and V̇/Q̇ scans does not provide adequate information to direct patient management

Table 12–2. REVISED PIOPED CRITERIA FOR INTERPRETATION OF VENTILATION-PERFUSION IMAGES

Probability of Pulmonary Embolism	Diagnostic Criteria
High probability (≥80%)	Two or more large mismatched segmental perfusion defects or the arithmetic equivalent in moderate or large and moderate defects, i.e., one large plus two or more moderate defects or four or more moderate mismatches
Intermediate probability (20%–79%)	One moderate plus one large mismatched segmental perfusion defect or the arithmetic equivalent in moderate defects
	One matched ventilation-perfusion defect with a normal chest radiograph. Difficult to categorize as low or high or not described as low or high.
Low probability (≤19%)	Nonsegmental perfusion defects (e.g., cardiomegaly, enlarged aorta, enlarged hila, elevated diaphragm). Any perfusion defect with a substantially larger abnormality at chest radiography
	Perfusion defects matched by ventilation abnormality provided that there are (1) normal chest radiographs and (2) some areas of normal perfusion in the lungs
	Any number of small perfusion defects with a normal chest radiograph
Normal	No perfusion defects or perfusion defects that outline exactly the shape of the lungs seen on the chest radiograph (hilar and aortic impressions may be seen, and the chest radiograph and/or ventilation scan may be abnormal)

Modified from Gottschalk A, Sostman HD, Juni JE, et al: Nucl Med 34:1119, 1993; and Sostman HD, Coleman RE, DeLong DM, et al: Radiology 193:103, 1994.

Table 12–3. SENSITIVITY, SPECIFICITY, AND POSITIVE PREDICTIVE VALUE OF VENTILATION-PERFUSION LUNG SCANNING FOR DETECTING ACUTE PULMONARY EMBOLISM USING ORIGINAL PIOPED INTERPRETATION CRITERIA

V̇/Q̇ Scan Interpretation	Sensitivity (%)	Specificity (%)	PPV (%)
High	40	98	87
High, intermediate	82	64	49
High, intermediate, low	98	12	32

V̇/Q̇, ventilation-perfusion; PPV, positive predictive value. Results based on the study by Worsley DF, Palevsky HI, Alavi A: Arch Intern Med 154:2737, 1994.

accurately, and further investigation with peripheral venous studies, spiral CT, or pulmonary angiography is warranted.

The value of V̇/Q̇ scans in patients who have COPD is controversial. In one combined V̇/Q̇-angiographic study of 83 patients who had COPD and suspected PTE, the overall sensitivity and specificity of V̇/Q̇ imaging were 0.83 and 0.92, respectively.[56] False-negative interpretations occurred in 3 of the 16 patients who showed ventilation abnormalities in more than 50% of their lungs, whereas in the 67 patients who had ventilation abnormalities affecting 50% or less of the lungs, the sensitivity (0.95) and specificity (0.94) for detecting PTE were high. The researchers concluded that V̇/Q̇ imaging is a reliable method for detecting PTE in patients who have regions of V̇/Q̇ match as long as ventilation abnormalities are limited in extent.

In a later study aimed at assessing the accuracy of chest radiographs in predicting the extent of airway disease in patients with suspected PTE, investigators found that V̇/Q̇ scans were indeterminate in all 21 patients who had radiographic evidence of widespread COPD, in 35% of patients who had focal obstructive disease, and in only 18% of patients whose chest radiographs revealed no evidence of COPD.[57] The investigators concluded that ventilation imaging probably is not warranted in patients who have radiographic evidence of widespread COPD. When an attempt is made to distinguish V̇/Q̇ matching that is compatible with PTE from that caused by COPD, a computation of the actual V̇/Q̇ ratio may be useful: In one study in which a V̇/Q̇ ratio of 1.25 or higher was used to define an area of mismatch, the percentage of patients classified correctly as having either PTE or COPD increased from 56% to 88%, based simply on a consideration of the matched or mismatched character of perfusion.[58]

Table 12–4. EFFECT OF SELECTED RISK FACTORS ON THE PREVALENCE OF PULMONARY EMBOLISM

V̇/Q̇ Scan Interpretation	0 Risk Factor*	1 Risk Factor*	≥2 Risk Factors*
High	63/77 (82%)	41/49 (84%)	56/58 (97%)
Intermediate	52/207 (25%)	40/107 (37%)	77/173 (45%)
Low/very low	14/315 (4%)	19/155 (12%)	37/179 (21%)

*Risk factors include immobilization, trauma to the lower extremities, surgery, or central venous instrumentation within 3 months of enrollment.
Results based on the study by Worsley DF, Palevsky HI, Alavi A: Arch Intern Med 154:2737, 1994.

In another study of 108 patients who had COPD and who were suspected of having PTE (21 of whom had the diagnosis confirmed by angiography), it was impossible to distinguish between patients who had and who did not have emboli by clinical assessment alone.[54] Among the 108 patients, high-probability, intermediate-probability, low-probability, and normal-probability scan results were present in 5%, 60%, 30%, and 5%, respectively. The frequency of PTE in these categories was 100%, 22%, 2%, and 0, respectively. Although high-probability and low-probability V̇/Q̇ scan results have good predictive values, most patients who have COPD have intermediate-probability scans and require further investigation, which may include spiral CT and angiography.

In summary, approximately 15% of patients who have PTE have high-probability V̇/Q̇ scan results, 40% have intermediate-probability scans, 30% have low-probability scans, and 15% have normal or near-normal scan results.[51] Approximately 90% of patients who have high-probability scan results have PTE, compared with 30% of patients who have intermediate-probability scans, 15% who have low-probability scan results, and 9% who have normal or near-normal scans.[51, 59]

The diagnostic accuracy can be improved by combining the results of V̇/Q̇ scanning with the clinical impression. In the PIOPED study, a clinical probability of PTE was estimated before lung scanning.[51] Three probabilities were considered: low (0 to 19%), intermediate (20% to 79%), and high (80% to 100%). A low-probability scan result paired with a low clinical index of suspicion had a negative predictive value of 96%. Conversely, a concordant high-probability V̇/Q̇ scan result and a high clinical index of suspicion had a PPV of 96%. Only 25% of patients fit into these clinicoscintigraphic categories, however, with 75% of patients having an uncertain diagnosis.[51] Under optimal circumstances of excellent clinical assessment and expert interpretation of lung scans, further investigation often is required to evaluate the presence or absence of emboli.

Computed Tomography

The introduction of spiral CT and ultrafast electron-beam CT technology has made it possible to image the entire chest in a short time, often during a single breath-hold. Pulmonary arteries can be imaged during peak enhancement with intravenous contrast material and direct visualization of emboli. Several groups of investigators have shown a high sensitivity and specificity of these advanced CT techniques (CT angiography) in the detection of emboli in the main, lobar, and segmental pulmonary arteries.[60, 61, 63]

Technique

Optimal assessment of pulmonary vessels on spiral and electron-beam CT requires careful attention to technique. For adequate assessment of the pulmonary arteries, images should be obtained from the level of the aortic arch to 1 cm above the level of the lowest hemidiaphragm.[65] Depending on the severity of the patient's dyspnea, scans may be obtained during a breath-hold at end-inspiration or during shallow breathing. The collimation (section thickness) in various studies has ranged from 3 to 6 mm.[60-62] A section thickness greater than 3 mm leads to suboptimal visualization of segmental and subsegmental arteries as a result of partial volume averaging;[65, 66] because of this, we routinely use 3-mm collimation scans and reconstruct the images at 1.5-mm intervals. The technique is evolving rapidly, however, and preliminary results suggest that visualization of subsegmental emboli may be improved with the use of 2-mm collimation scans.[65] The speed of image acquisition and the spatial resolution in the z axis have been increased considerably with the development of multidetector spiral CT scanners.[232, 233] These scanners allow imaging of the entire thorax during a single breath-hold using 1.25-mm or 2.5-mm collimation scans.

Optimal contrast enhancement of the pulmonary arteries requires selection of the most appropriate contrast agent and optimal concentration, timing, and speed of contrast injection. Injection of highly concentrated contrast material (35% to 40% iodine concentration) may result in streak artifacts originating at the level of the superior vena cava, which may radiate to the adjacent right pulmonary artery and preclude detection of intraluminal filling defects. Injection of low concentrations (12% to 15% iodine) requires rapid intravenous injection (7 ml per second).[60] We recommend using 30% iodinated contrast material (300 mg iodine/ml) injected at a rate of 3 to 4 ml per second for a total dose of 120 to 150 ml. A 12- to 15-second delay between the start of contrast material injection and the start of the scan is recommended.[63, 66] This delay allows adequate contrast enhancement in most cases; however, in patients who have decreased cardiac output, the time delay may have to be increased to 15 seconds or more.[65]

An alternate technique, which we favor, consists of using a test injection to determine the circulation time. The main pulmonary artery is located with preliminary noncontrast images. A total of 20 ml of contrast material is injected at 4 ml per second, and images are obtained at the level of the main pulmonary artery at 3- to 5-second intervals for 20 seconds. A time-density curve is plotted by placing a region of interest (i.e., region in which the computer plots the attenuation values) over the main pulmonary artery to determine the time required for peak contrast enhancement. Current scanners automatically assess the time for enhancement, which can be used to optimize the delay between the start of intravenous contrast material injection and the start of the diagnostic CT scan.

Images are viewed at lung parenchymal (window width 1,500 HU; level −700 HU) and soft tissue (window width 250 to 350 HU; level 35 to 50 HU) window settings.

Vascular Findings

Acute Thromboembolism. The diagnosis of acute PTE on contrast-enhanced CT scan is based on the presence of partial or complete filling defects (Table 12–5).[60, 61] The former is defined as an intravascular central or marginal area of low attenuation surrounded by variable amounts of contrast material (Fig. 12–5); the latter is defined as an intraluminal area of low attenuation that occupies the entire arterial section, that is, by the abrupt absence of contrast material in a visible vessel (Fig. 12–6).[60, 62] The most reliable sign of an acute embolism is a filling defect forming an acute angle with the vessel wall and outlined by contrast material. Although filling defects that form a smooth, obtuse angle with the vessel wall or complete cutoffs of contrast opacification of a vessel may be related to acute emboli, they also may be seen with chronic emboli.

The accuracy of CT angiography in the diagnosis of acute PTE has been assessed in several prospective studies. Initial investigations were limited to evaluation of emboli down to the level of the segmental pulmonary arteries (Fig. 12–7). The results of these studies showed that spiral CT had a sensitivity of 91% to 100% and a specificity of 78% to 96% in the detection of central emboli.[60, 66] Subsequent

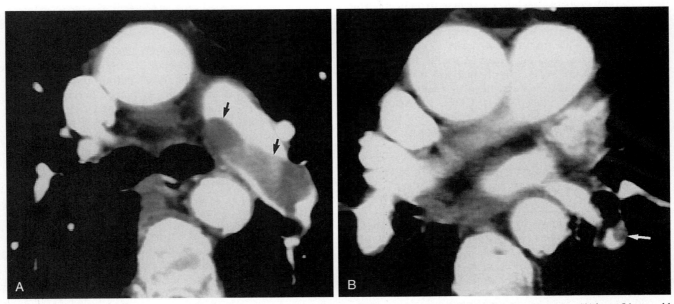

Figure 12–5. Acute Pulmonary Thromboembolism. Contrast-enhanced spiral CT scan at the level of the left pulmonary artery *(A)* in an 84-year-old woman shows large intraluminal filling defect *(arrows)*. Contrast material is present around and distal to the embolus, indicating partial occlusion of the pulmonary artery. CT scan at a more caudad level *(B)* shows embolus *(arrow)* within the left lower lobe pulmonary artery.

Table 12–5. ACUTE PULMONARY THROMBOEMBOLISM: SPIRAL CT

Vascular findings
   Intravascular filling defect
   Acute angles with vessel wall
   Complete cut-off of vascular opacification
   Increased diameter of occluded vessel
Helpful parenchymal findings
   Wedge-shaped nonenhancing pleural-based opacities
   Linear atelectasis
Sensitivity of spiral CT, 80%–90%; specificity, 80%–95%
False-negative interpretations mainly due to subsegmental emboli
False-positive interpretations due to hilar nodes and technical pitfalls

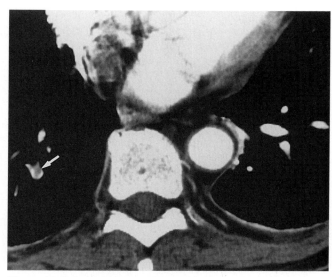

Figure 12–7. Acute Pulmonary Thromboembolism. Contrast-enhanced spiral CT scan in a 65-year-old man shows embolus *(arrow)* in the posterobasal segmental artery of the right lower lobe. The segmental arteries of the left lower lobe are well seen and are normal.

studies showed that spiral CT was of limited value in the diagnosis of subsegmental emboli.[62, 63] The prevalence of emboli limited to the subsegmental vessels is low, however, being seen in only 14 of 251 patients (5.6%) in the PIOPED study.[51] Even on pulmonary angiography, there is relatively poor agreement among experienced observers in the interpretation of subsegmental pulmonary emboli. Data derived from the PIOPED study showed interobserver agreement on pulmonary angiography of 98% for lobar emboli, 90% for segmental emboli, and 66% for subsegmental emboli.[71, 216] It has recently been shown that spiral CT performed using 1- to 3-mm collimation is comparable to angiography in the detection of segmental and subsegmental-sized pulmonary emboli.[234] Although there has been some controversy,[62, 213] most investigators have shown an overall sensitivity of 80% to 90% and a specificity of 80% to 95% for spiral CT in the diagnosis of acute PTE.[63, 69, 214] Similar results have been reported with the use of ultrafast electron-beam CT.[61, 68]

Several groups of investigators have shown that CT angiography is superior to V̇/Q̇ scintigraphy in the diagno-

sis of acute PTE.[64, 66, 69] In one prospective comparison of spiral CT and V̇/Q̇ scintigraphy in 142 patients, the results of both procedures were assessed independently by two experienced observers.[69] The combination of a high-probability V̇/Q̇ scan result plus a spiral CT finding of PTE was considered diagnostic, and no further imaging studies were performed. The combination of normal-probability, very low–probability, or low-probability V̇/Q̇ scan and a negative spiral CT in a patient who had a low clinical suspicion of PTE was considered sufficient to exclude the disease. All other patients underwent pulmonary angiography. Twelve patients had discordant spiral CT and V̇/Q̇ scans; using angiographic results as the gold standard, the spiral CT interpretation was correct in 11 patients and the V̇/Q̇ scan in 1 patient. Overall, CT angiography had a sensitivity of 87% and a specificity of 98% in the diagnosis of acute PTE, compared with a sensitivity of 65% and a specificity of 94% for a high-probability V̇/Q̇ scan. There was better interobserver agreement in the interpretation of the spiral CT scans than the V̇/Q̇ scans. In a second investigation, the authors compared spiral CT angiography with V̇/Q̇ scintigraphy in 179 patients.[227] CT angiography had a sensitivity of 94% and a specificity of 94%, whereas scintigraphy had a sensitivity of 81% and a specificity of 74% in the diagnosis of acute PTE. Interobserver agreement was much better for interpretation of CT angiography (κ statistic = 0.72) than for scintigraphy (κ = 0.22).[227]

It can be concluded from these studies that CT angiography has a high sensitivity and specificity and is superior to V̇/Q̇ scintigraphy in the diagnosis of acute PTE. The procedure allows not only direct visualization of the intraluminal thrombi, but also assessment of the mediastinum and pulmonary parenchyma and evaluation of vascular changes associated with nonembolic disease, such as carcinoma and emphysema. In a prospective randomized trial of 78 patients who had suspected PTE, spiral CT or V̇/Q̇ scans were performed as part of the initial investigation.[64] A

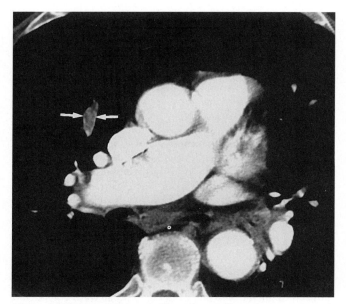

Figure 12–6. Acute Pulmonary Thromboembolism. Contrast-enhanced spiral CT scan in an 83-year-old man shows abrupt absence of contrast material within the medial segmental artery of the right middle lobe *(arrows)* consistent with complete occlusion of the artery by an embolus. Increased diameter of the occluded vessel is apparent.

confident diagnosis of PTE was made in 35 of 39 patients (90%) who underwent spiral CT, compared with 21 of 39 patients (54%) who underwent scintigraphy first. The main reason for this difference was the ability of CT to show lesions other than PTE that were considered to be responsible for the symptoms of 13 of 39 (33%) patients. In another prospective study of 110 patients, spiral CT helped identify correctly 23 of 25 patients who had PTE (sensitivity 92%); in 57 (67%) of the 85 patients who did not have PTE, spiral CT provided additional information that suggested or confirmed the alternate clinical diagnosis.[214] In this series, the most common diagnoses in patients with an abnormal CT scan who did not have PTE were pneumonia, cardiovascular disease, interstitial lung disease, trauma-related chest abnormalities, and pulmonary or pleural malignancy. Potential pitfalls in the diagnosis of PTE on CT include confusion with hilar lymph nodes, poor opacification of the pulmonary arteries, increased image noise in large patients, and obscuration of vessels by surrounding parenchymal opacification.[65, 69, 70]

The clinical validity of a CT-angiography examination interpreted as negative for PTE and the implications for patient outcome were assessed in a study of 132 patients.[215] Findings from clinical follow-up at a minimum of 6 months were assessed, with special focus on the presence of recurrent thromboembolism and mortality in 78 consecutive patients in whom spiral CT scans were interpreted as negative for PTE and anticoagulant therapy was not administered. Nine patients died, one of whom was shown at autopsy performed 7 days after CT scan to have a 1- to 2-mm embolus that may have been missed on spiral CT but that also had been missed at angiography. No evidence of PTE was found in any of the other 77 patients. The negative predictive value for spiral CT in this study was 99%.[215] One group of investigators compared the risk of subsequent pulmonary embolism after a negative spiral CT–angiography examination with that of a negative or low-probability scintigram.[235] Five hundred forty-eight patients who had negative images and were not receiving anticoagulation therapy were prospectively followed for up to 3 months. Subsequent PE was found in two (1%) of 198 patients with negative spiral CT, none of 188 patients with negative ventilation-perfusion scan, and 5 (3%) of 162 patients with low-probability ventilation-perfusion scans.[235] The authors concluded that spiral CT is a reliable test in excluding clinically important PE.

Analysis of a decision model based on the published data has shown that the use of spiral CT is likely to improve cost-effectiveness in the workup of PTE and to be associated with decreased mortality.[72] Investigators assessed various diagnostic algorithms, including various combinations of V̇/Q̇ scintigraphy, ultrasound, D-dimer assay, spiral CT, and conventional angiography; for all realistic values of the pretest probability of PTE and coexisting DVT and of the diagnostic accuracy of spiral CT, all of the best diagnostic strategies included CT angiography.[72]

Although there is little doubt that CT angiography can be helpful in the assessment of patients who have suspected PTE, there is considerable controversy about the specific indications for its use.[73–75] Most authors recommend that the procedure should be performed in patients who have indeterminate V̇/Q̇ scans or low-probability scans and a high clinical index of suspicion for PTE.[60, 63, 69] Various researchers have suggested that spiral CT should replace scintigraphy in the assessment of patients whose symptoms are suggestive of acute PTE and who have no symptoms or signs of DVT (lower extremity ultrasonography being recognized as the primary imaging modality in the assessment of patients who have suspected DVT),[67, 76] in the assessment of all patients whose symptoms are suggestive of acute PTE,[73] or in the assessment of patients who have underlying cardiopulmonary disease and abnormal chest radiograph.[64, 75] Multicenter prospective studies are required to determine the optimal diagnostic strategy in these situations.

Currently, we perform CT angiography in patients who have symptoms that are suggestive of acute PTE who have intermediate-probability V̇/Q̇ scans and in patients who have low-probability or normal scans and a high clinical index of suspicion. We also believe that the procedure is the initial imaging modality of choice and should replace V̇/Q̇ scintigraphy in patients who have severe COPD or who show extensive parenchymal abnormalities on chest radiograph. The diagnostic accuracy of spiral CT scan in the latter group of patients has not been assessed.

Instances of clinically unsuspected PTE occasionally are found incidentally on CT scans performed in the assessment of patients who have a history of trauma, thoracic tumors, aortic disease, or pulmonary abnormalities.[77, 78] In one study, a computer search of reports of 1,879 consecutive contrast-enhanced spiral CT scans identified 18 such patients.[78] (In 11 of the 18 patients, the diagnosis was confirmed by angiography, V̇/Q̇ scintigraphy, or demonstration of DVT; in 6, the diagnosis was considered unequivocal on CT; and in 1, the diagnosis was considered probable on CT, and no further evaluation was performed.) The prevalence was 0.4% (6 of 1,320) among outpatients and 2% (12 of 559) among inpatients. All 18 patients had at least one risk factor for PTE, including carcinoma, atrial fibrillation, hypercoagulable state, or use of birth control pills. In another prospective investigation of 785 patients, the prevalence of PTE was evaluated on routine contrast-enhanced thoracic CT scans.[79] Twelve (1.5%) patients had unsuspected PTE, with an inpatient prevalence of 5% (8 of 160) and an outpatient prevalence of 0.6% (4 of 625). Of the 12 patients who had unsuspected PTE, 10 (83%) had cancer; of the 81 inpatients who had cancer, 7 (9%) had unsuspected PTE.

Chronic Thromboembolism. Although most patients treated for acute PTE improve, some develop chronic disease related to the initial thromboembolic episode, and others have recurrent PTE. In one study of 62 patients, spiral CT scans were performed 1 to 53 months (median, 8 months) after the initial diagnosis of PTE.[80] All patients had been admitted to a cardiology intensive care unit and treated with anticoagulants for massive embolism; 31 had received fibrinolytic therapy initially. On the follow-up spiral CT scan, emboli were considered acute if they partially or completely occluded the arterial lumen and the arterial diameter was not reduced. Emboli were considered chronic if at least two of the following were present: (1) an eccentric location contiguous to the vessel wall (Fig. 12–8), (2) evidence of recanalization within the intraluminal filling defect, (3) arterial stenosis or webs (Fig. 12–9),

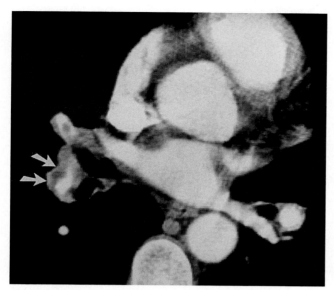

Figure 12–8. Chronic Pulmonary Thromboembolism. Contrast-enhanced spiral CT scan shows an eccentric filling defect along the lateral margin of the right lower lobe pulmonary artery *(arrows)*. A small intraluminal filling defect is present in the middle lobe pulmonary artery. The patient was a 53-year-old man with recurrent pulmonary embolism.

(4) reduction of more than 50% of the arterial diameter, and (5) complete occlusion at the level of the stenosed arteries.[80] In 30 of 62 patients (48%), there was complete resolution of the initial embolus on the follow-up CT scan, and in 24 (39%), there was partial resolution; 8 (13%) patients had features of chronic embolism. The clinical presentations, risk factors at diagnosis, and treatment did not differ among the patients who had or who did not have complete resolution; however, the group of patients that showed residual abnormalities or developed chronic emboli had more extensive embolization at initial diagnosis.

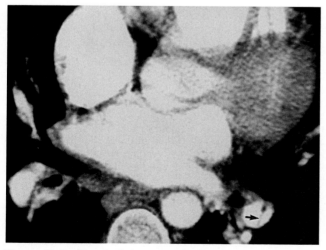

Figure 12–9. Chronic Pulmonary Thromboembolism. Contrast-enhanced spiral CT scan shows a linear filling defect (web) *(arrow)* in the left lower lobe pulmonary artery. The patient was a 39-year-old woman with pulmonary arterial hypertension secondary to chronic pulmonary thromboembolism.

Table 12–6. CHRONIC PULMONARY THROMBOEMBOLISM: SPIRAL CT

Vascular findings
  Intravascular filling defect
  Eccentric location contiguous with vessel wall
  Recanalization of intraluminal filling defect
  Arterial stenosis or webs
  ≥50% reduction of arterial caliber
  Abrupt cut-off of arterial branches
Parenchymal findings
  Localized areas of decreased attenuation and vascularity
  Mosaic pattern of attenuation and perfusion
  Wedge-shaped nonenhancing pleural-based opacities

Similar to acute PTE, contrast-enhanced spiral CT allows confident diagnosis of chronic PTE in most patients (Table 12–6).[81, 82] In one study of 75 patients who had this abnormality, the CT findings were compared with the findings at pulmonary angiography.[82] Chronic PTE was diagnosed on CT scan by visualization of eccentric thrombi within the pulmonary arteries or by indirect signs, such as irregular or nodular arterial walls, abrupt narrowing of the arterial diameter, or abrupt cut-off of distal lobar or segmental artery branches.[82] CT scan showed thrombi in the pulmonary trunk, right and left main arteries, or lobar arteries in 53 patients; thromboendarterectomy performed in 48 of these patients confirmed the CT findings of surgically resectable central chronic embolism. In 22 of the 75 patients, CT scan failed to show central emboli; however, organized thrombi were excised at surgery in 14 of these patients. CT had a 78% sensitivity and a 100% specificity in the diagnosis of surgically resectable chronic PTE.[81]

Parenchymal Findings

Acute Thromboembolism. Parenchymal manifestations of acute PTE on CT are similar to those on chest radiography and include oligemia; loss of lung volume; and wedge-shaped, pleural-based opacities.[84, 85] Localized areas of decreased attenuation secondary to oligemia are uncommon except in patients who have massive emboli (Fig. 12–10). This finding is an unreliable sign of embolization; in a study of 88 patients who had suspected PTE, areas of decreased attenuation were seen in 3 of 26 (11%) patients who had acute PTE but also in 6 of 62 (10%) patients who did not have emboli.[85] In the same study, findings that were seen most commonly in patients who had PTE included wedge-shaped, pleural-based opacities (present in 62% of patients who had emboli compared with 27% of patients who did not) and linear opacities (seen in 46% and 21%). In a second investigation of 92 patients, the only parenchymal abnormality significantly associated with acute PTE was the presence of a peripheral wedge-shaped opacity.[217] This abnormality was seen in 7 of 28 (25%) patients who had PTE compared with 3 of 64 (5%) patients who did not.

As a manifestation of PTE, a wedge-shaped pulmonary opacity abutting the pleural surface is seen more commonly on a CT scan than on a chest radiograph.[83] The opacities may have a configuration of a full triangle or a truncated cone with concave or convex apex (Fig. 12–11). It has been postulated that the latter appearance may be related

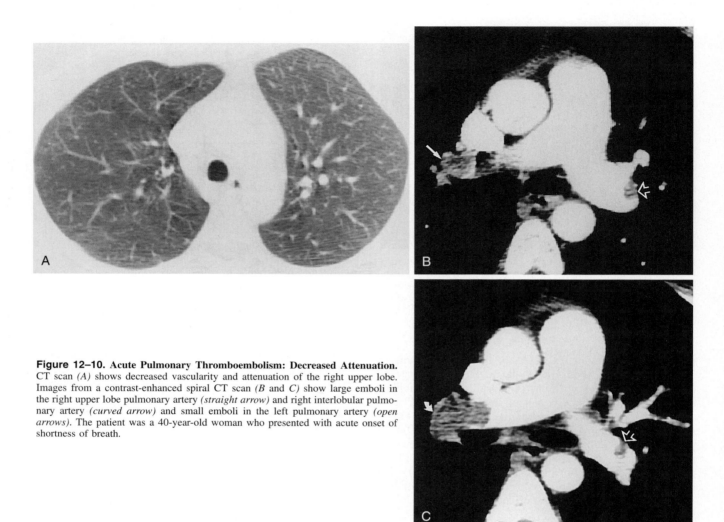

Figure 12–10. Acute Pulmonary Thromboembolism: Decreased Attenuation. CT scan *(A)* shows decreased vascularity and attenuation of the right upper lobe. Images from a contrast-enhanced spiral CT scan *(B and C)* show large emboli in the right upper lobe pulmonary artery *(straight arrow)* and right interlobular pulmonary artery *(curved arrow)* and small emboli in the left pulmonary artery *(open arrows)*. The patient was a 40-year-old woman who presented with acute onset of shortness of breath.

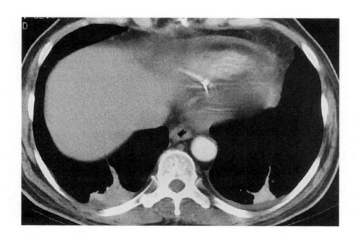

Figure 12–11. Pulmonary Infarcts on CT Scan. Contrast-enhanced spiral CT scan in a 57-year-old patient with acute pulmonary embolism shows pleural-based, wedge-shaped opacities in both lower lobes. The triangular opacity in the right lower lobe did not enhance with intravenous contrast material. A small left pleural effusion is evident.

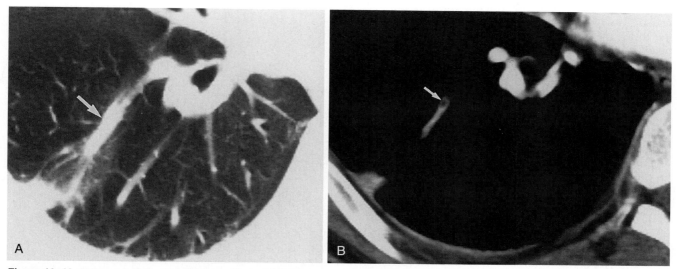

Figure 12–12. Pulmonary Infarct on CT Scan. View of the right lower lobe *(A)* from spiral CT scan in a 65-year-old patient shows a pleural-based opacity. Note the increased diameter of the subsegmental vessel *(arrow)* leading to the subpleural opacity. Soft tissue windows *(B)* show poorly enhancing subsegmental artery with filling defect *(arrow)* consistent with recent thromboembolism.

to sparing of the apex of the cone from infarction as a result of collateral circulation from bronchial arteries.[83] On CT, most infarcts appear to be reabsorbed partially or completely after 1 month, sometimes being manifested only as a scar.[83]

Although characteristic of infarction, a wedge-shaped, pleural-based opacity on CT may be the result of another abnormality, including hemorrhage, pneumonia, neoplasm, or edema.[86] In one study in which high-resolution computed tomography (HRCT) findings were correlated with histologic abnormalities in 83 postmortem lung specimens, a thickened vessel leading to the apex of the pleural-based, wedge-shaped opacity was seen more commonly in patients who had infarction (10 of 12) than in patients who had pneumonia (3 of 20), neoplasm (3 of 18), or hemorrhage (2 of 13) (Fig. 12–12).[86] Rarely, infarcts cavitate.[87]

Chronic Thromboembolism. Although parenchymal findings on CT are of limited value in the diagnosis of acute PTE, they often are characteristic enough to suggest the diagnosis of chronic PTE.[82, 88] The most common abnormality consists of localized areas of decreased attenuation and vascularity that are sharply marginated from adjacent areas with increased or normal attenuation and vessel size, a pattern known as *mosaic perfusion*.[91] Although this pattern also can be seen with airway diseases, particularly obliterative bronchiolitis and asthma, when associated with enlarged central pulmonary arteries or asymmetry in the size of the central or segmental pulmonary arteries, it is suggestive of pulmonary hypertension secondary to chronic PTE (Fig. 12–13).[87, 90, 91]

In a review of the CT findings in 75 patients who had angiographically proven chronic PTE, a mosaic perfusion

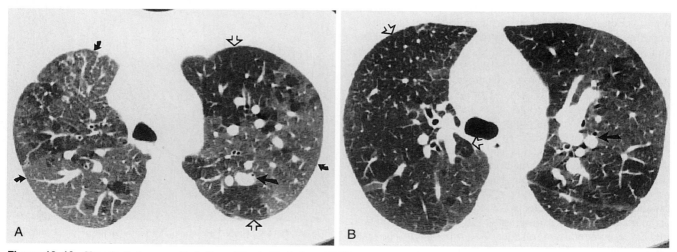

Figure 12–13. Chronic Pulmonary Embolism: Mosaic Perfusion. HRCT scans *(A and B)* show localized areas of decreased attenuation *(open arrows)* and vascularity and areas with increased attenuation and vascularity *(curved arrows)*, a pattern known as *mosaic perfusion*. Markedly increased pulmonary artery-to-bronchus diameter ratios are visible *(straight arrows)*, particularly in the left upper lobe. The patient was a 43-year-old woman with pulmonary arterial hypertension as a result of chronic pulmonary thromboembolism.

pattern was found in 58 (77%).[82] The mean attenuation of the relatively dark areas was − 868 HU, and that of the relatively light areas was − 727 HU. After intravenous administration of contrast material, the areas of decreased attenuation showed less enhancement (mean 30 HU increase after intravenous contrast administration) than the areas of increased attenuation (mean 45 HU). In the same study, 54 of 75 patients (72%) had nodular or wedge-shaped, pleural-based areas of increased attenuation on unenhanced scans that remained unchanged after administration of contrast material; these 54 patients had a total of 76 pleural-based areas of increased attenuation, 10 of which involved the upper lobes; 14, the middle lobe or lingula; and 48, the lower lobes. In another investigation of 33 patients who had chronic PTE, 18 (55%) had areas of mosaic perfusion, and 22 (67%) had linear areas of increased attenuation.[88]

Chronic PTE may be associated with airway abnormalities.[89] In one study, CT findings in 33 patients who had chronic PTE were compared with those in a control group of 19 patients who had acute PTE.[89] Cylindrical bronchiectasis was seen on HRCT in 21 of 33 patients (64%) who had chronic PTE but in only 2 of 19 (11%) who had acute PTE. In the patients who had chronic PTE, the abnormal bronchi were located next to the completely obstructed and retracted pulmonary arteries. Although the pathogenesis of bronchiectasis in these cases is unclear, it has been postulated that it may be similar to that of traction bronchiectasis seen in interstitial pulmonary fibrosis, with the scarring of the severely narrowed pulmonary arteries causing dilation of the adjacent bronchi.[89]

Magnetic Resonance Imaging

Similar to CT, MR imaging allows direct visualization of PTE (Fig. 12–14). MR imaging has the additional advantage of not requiring radiation or the use of iodinated intravenous contrast material; however, it is more expensive and less readily available. Other disadvantages of MR imaging include cardiac and respiratory motion artifacts and complex pulmonary blood flow patterns that may mimic embolism. These problems have been minimized with the development of gradient-recalled echo (GRE) imaging techniques obtained during a single breath-hold. The combination of these techniques with gadolinium enhancement results in good-quality MR angiographic images of the pulmonary arteries (Fig. 12–15).[92, 93, 218]

In one study of 30 consecutive patients who had suspected PTE, MR angiography was performed during the pulmonary arterial phase of an intravenous bolus of gadolinium.[93] The procedure was carried out using a coronal three-dimensional gradient-echo pulse sequence with a slice thickness of 3 to 4 mm and an imaging time of 27 seconds. The images were reviewed by three independent observers, and the results were compared with those of standard pulmonary angiography. All 5 lobar emboli and 16 of 17 segmental emboli identified on conventional pulmonary angiography were identified on MR angiography. Two of the three observers reported one false-positive MR angiogram. Using conventional angiography as the gold standard, the three observers had diagnostic sensitivities of

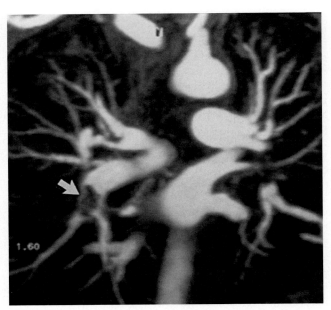

Figure 12–14. MR Imaging of Acute Pulmonary Thromboembolism. Coronal MR image shows filling defect *(arrow)* in the right interlobar pulmonary artery. (Case courtesy of Dr. Jaime Fdez-Cuadrado, Hospital La Paz, Madrid, Spain.)

100%, 87%, and 75% and specificities of 95%, 100%, and 95%.

In a second investigation of 36 consecutive patients, MR angiography was performed during suspended respiration and the pulmonary arterial phase of a gadolinium-based contrast medium injection using a steady-state, GRE sequence.[218] The standard MR images and coronal maximum intensity projection (MIP) images were reviewed on a computer workstation. Using digital subtraction angiogra-

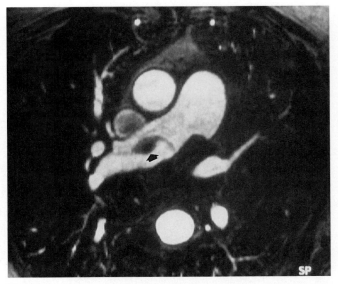

Figure 12–15. Acute Pulmonary Thromboembolism: MR Imaging. MR image shows an embolus *(arrow)* in the right pulmonary artery. The image was obtained using a breath-hold gradient-echo pulse sequence (TR/TE, 7.0/2.2, flip angle 40 degrees) and gadolinium enhancement. (Courtesy of Dr. Pamela Woodard, Mallinckrodt Institute of Radiology, St. Louis, MO.)

phy (DSA) as the gold standard, PTE was identified correctly on MR imaging in 11 of 13 patients (sensitivity 85%) and excluded 22 of 23 patients (specificity 96%). Both cases of false-negative interpretation were in patients who had only small subsegmental emboli.

Preliminary studies suggest that MR imaging may play a role in the assessment of parenchymal abnormalities in acute and chronic PTE.[94, 95] In one investigation, seven patients who had a clinical suspicion of PTE underwent cardiac-gated, spin-echo MR imaging;[94] in three patients who had angiographically confirmed emboli, opacities seen on the plain chest radiograph (presumably representing infarcts) were shown to have increased signal intensity on T1-weighted images. By contrast, in the three patients who had normal pulmonary angiography, opacities on the radiograph did not show high signal intensity on T1-weighted images (in these patients the final diagnosis was *infectious pneumopathy*). One patient had no parenchymal abnormalities on the radiograph or MR imaging.

Pulmonary Angiography

Technique

Pulmonary arteriography is the most definitive technique for diagnosing PTE.[51, 96–98] Best results are obtained if the contrast medium is injected through a catheter whose tip is in the right or left pulmonary artery (Fig. 12–16), a procedure that permits not only a clear view of the ipsilateral arterial tree, but also the measurement of pulmonary artery pressure. The study may reveal partial or complete occlusion of lobar or segmental vessels but seldom is useful when the

obstructed vessels are subsegmental or smaller.[99, 100] The last-named vessels are seen inadequately for several reasons, including dilution of contrast medium during cardiac systole, obscuration of vascular detail because of overlap of opacified vessels, and diversion of blood flow away from embolized vessels. In these situations, it may be necessary to perform segmental arteriography, first in anteroposterior projection, then in other projections if the anteroposterior study is inconclusive.[101] In one review of 57 positive pulmonary arteriograms, additional views—the right posterior oblique projection for the right lung and the left posterior oblique or lateral projection for the left—were found to be necessary in 26 (51%).[102]

In one study, three angiographers reviewed the arteriograms of 60 patients retrospectively, independently, and without benefit of additional data;[103] although the interobserver agreement was 100% for emboli involving the main, lobar, and segmental arteries, it was only 13% for those affecting subsegmental vessels. Among 1,111 patients who underwent catheterization for pulmonary angiography in the PIOPED study, 61% had negative angiograms, 35% had positive angiograms, and 3% had nondiagnostic (poor-quality) angiograms; in 1%, the angiogram was not completed, usually owing to complications. The overall agreement on the interpretation of angiograms as positive, negative, or nondiagnostic among independent readers was 81%. The interobserver agreement was related to the size of the affected vessel—98% for lobar vessels, 90% for segmental vessels, and 66% for subsegmental vessels.[71]

Pulmonary angiography may be performed using conventional film technique or digital subtraction (DSA). The

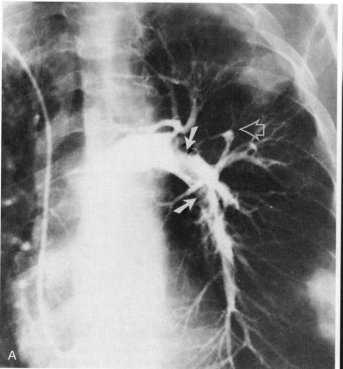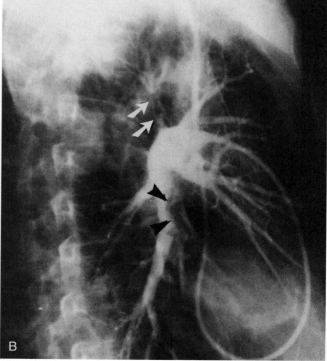

Figure 12–16. Value of Oblique Arteriography in Demonstration of Pulmonary Thromboembolism. Selective left pulmonary arteriograms in left *(A)* and right *(B)* anterior oblique projections show multiple, central *(arrows)* and eccentric *(arrowheads)* intraluminal filling defects. A segmental artery *(open arrow)* in the upper lobe in the left projection *(A)* is amputated. These features are diagnostic of multiple pulmonary thromboemboli.

main advantage of DSA is the elimination of overlapping projection of other structures, allowing better visualization of pulmonary vessels. Use of DSA also allows an approximately 25% reduction in the volume of contrast material that is necessary to obtain optimal images,[104] a feature associated with a reduced risk of right ventricular failure in patients who have severe pulmonary hypertension.[105]

Initial studies in which DSA was used after intravenous injection of contrast material showed it to be inferior to conventional arteriography because dilution of contrast material resulted in poor opacification of small pulmonary arteries.[106, 107] Much better opacification is obtained with the use of selective intra-arterial injection.[108] Developments in digital technique have improved the quality of DSA images markedly, with spatial resolution approaching that of conventional film angiography and image acquisition up to 30 frames per second.[109] These developments provide image quality that is comparable to that of conventional film angiography at a considerably lower cost and with the use of less contrast material. In one study in which intra-arterial DSA and conventional pulmonary angiography were performed in 10 patients, no difference was detected in the degree of visualization of pulmonary artery branches.[110] In another investigation of 397 consecutive patients who had nondiagnostic $\dot{V}/\dot{Q}$ scans, the interobserver agreement in the interpretation of DSA images and conventional angiograms was assessed.[108] All angiograms were read immediately by the attending radiologist, by two radiologists after 6 months, and later by means of consensus of the two radiologists. The percentage agreements on conventional angiography were 80% between immediate and consensus reading, 80% between Observer 1 and consensus reading, 84% between Observer 2 and consensus reading, and 64% between Observer 1 and Observer 2.[108] By comparison, the percentage agreements on DSA images were 88%, 96%, 95%, and 92%. Initial diagnoses were changed after the images were reviewed by consensus in 12% of patients who had DSA images compared with 20% of patients who had conventional angiograms. The authors concluded that interobserver agreement was better with intra-arterial DSA than with conventional pulmonary angiography.

In a more recent investigation, conventional film angiography and DSA were performed in identical posteroanterior and oblique projections in one lung of 80 patients undergoing pulmonary angiography.[111] Diagnoses based on the results of blinded review of each study by three independent observers were compared with the diagnoses made by the physician who performed the procedure and with the consensus diagnoses obtained by group review of both studies. The investigation included 13 patients who had PTE. The sensitivity of DSA (i.e., correct identification of emboli by all three observers) was 92%, and the sensitivity of conventional film angiography was 69%; the specificities of the two modalities were not statistically significantly different. In another investigation of 39 patients, receiver operating characteristic analysis showed similar performance for DSA and conventional film angiography.[112] A limitation of these studies is the weak standard of reference, the final diagnosis being based on review of the angiogram by a group of experts. To overcome this limitation, one

group compared DSA and conventional angiography with the results of histologic examination in a porcine model;[113] no significant difference was found between the two modalities.

Although it has lower spatial resolution, DSA performed using selective intra-arterial injection is comparable or slightly superior to conventional film angiography in the diagnosis of PTE. The main advantages of DSA are lower cost, the need for less contrast material, greater speed, and the ability to magnify electronically and view images in subtracted and nonsubtracted modes.[114]

Complications

Although pulmonary angiography is considered to be the gold standard for the diagnosis of PTE, the procedure is requested in only a small percentage of patients who have clinically suspected emboli. In one review of 316 consecutive cases of suspected PTE in a large university medical center in the United States, only 17% of 141 patients who had indeterminate $\dot{V}/\dot{Q}$ scans underwent angiography.[115] In another survey of 360 acute-care hospitals in the United Kingdom, approximately 47,000 $\dot{V}/\dot{Q}$ lung scans were found to have been obtained compared with only 490 pulmonary angiograms.[116]

The reluctance to request pulmonary angiograms stems to some extent from the concern over the perceived risks of the procedure.[115, 117] This reluctance is still present despite a considerable decrease in the number of complications over the years.[117–119] In one investigation of 1,350 patients who underwent pulmonary angiography at Duke University that was reported in 1980, three deaths (0.2%) were considered to be attributable directly to the procedure;[118] all three were in patients who had pulmonary arterial hypertension (systolic pressures of 75, 100, and 160 mm Hg). The most common serious complications were cardiac perforation and endocardial and myocardial injury, seen in 20 patients (1.5%). In a second study of 1,434 patients from the same institution published in 1987, two deaths attributable directly to the procedure were identified.[119] Additional complications included reversible cardiac arrest in 5 patients and cardiac arrhythmias in 15 patients. Other researchers also reported an increased risk of complications in patients who have pulmonary arterial hypertension. In the study of 1,350 patients undergoing pulmonary angiography, the three deaths attributable directly to the procedure occurred in patients with pulmonary arterial hypertension.[118]

Since 1987, two major technical developments have occurred: (1) the replacement of stiff end-hole catheters by multiple side-hole pigtail[117] or flow-directed catheters[104] and (2) the use of low-osmolar nonionic intravenous contrast medium.[117] In a 1996 review of 1,434 patients who underwent pulmonary angiography with nonionic contrast medium injected through multiple side-hole pigtail catheters (at Duke University), major complications were found in only 4 patients (0.3%);[117] no deaths were attributed to the procedure. The major complications included respiratory arrest requiring ventilatory support (in two patients) and recurrent ventricular arrhythmias (in two patients). Minor complications were seen in 11 patients (0.8%) and included arrhythmias responsive to lidocaine, catheter-induced vasovagal syncope, chest pain, and contrast material–induced urticaria. In another study of 211 patients assessed by selective pulmonary DSA performed with an 8-French Swan-Ganz–type, flow-directed catheter and non-ionic contrast material, no mortality or morbidity as a direct result of pulmonary angiography was observed.[104] In a third investigation of 728 patients who underwent selective angiography with a 7-French pigtail catheter and low-osmolar contrast media, there were no deaths and only one major complication (bleeding in the groin, necessitating surgery).[121]

Angiographic Abnormalities

The angiographic criteria for the diagnosis of PTE include primary and secondary signs.[122] The only primary sign is a filling defect. This defect may be manifested as a persistent intraluminal radiolucency without complete obstruction of blood flow or as a trailing edge of an intraluminal radiolucency when there is complete obstruction of distal blood flow. Secondary signs include abrupt occlusion (*cut-off*) of a pulmonary artery without visualization of an intraluminal filling defect and perfusion defects. The perfusion defects may be manifested as areas of oligemia or avascularity or as abruptly tapering peripheral vessels, with a paucity of branching vessels (*pruning*).[122] The latter reflect nothing more than diminished pulmonary arterial perfusion, a common manifestation of several pulmonary and cardiac diseases from which PTE must be differentiated.[123] These signs may be useful, however, by directing attention to areas in which manifestations of embolism may be subtle; in such cases, segmental arteriography, especially with magnification, may reveal intraluminal defects in smaller vessels. Care must be taken not to misinterpret an opacified artery seen end-on as a blunt obstruction caused by acute thromboembolism.

The angiographic findings of chronic thromboembolic disease were assessed in a study of 250 patients and correlated with findings at pulmonary thromboendarterectomy.[124] Abnormalities consisted of abrupt vascular narrowing, complete vascular obstruction, webs or bands, intimal irregularities, and *pouching* defects. The last-named was defined as the presence of obstructing or partially occlusive chronic thromboemboli that organized in a concave configuration toward the lumen of the artery. Tapering of vessels usually connotes circumferential organization and recanalization—an old thromboembolic episode.[25] Abrupt narrowing of a major pulmonary vessel also is a characteristic finding of chronic PTE, the normal gentle tapering of the vessel being replaced by an abrupt decrease in the diameter of the opacified lumen.[124, 125] Pulmonary artery webs or bands are lines of low opacity that traverse the width of the contrast material within the pulmonary vessel; these often are associated with narrowing of the vessels and poststenotic dilation;[124, 126] they have been shown in follow-up angiographic studies to be present at the precise sites of intra-arterial filling defects previously shown angiographically.[126] Another common finding of chronic PTE is the presence of a scalloped appearance to the pulmonary arterial wall, an abnormality that has been shown to be the

result of irregularly organized thrombus lining the vessel wall.[124]

Methods of Diagnosis of Deep Vein Thrombosis

Conventional Venography

Conventional contrast venography is used to outline the deep veins extending from the calf to the inferior vena cava and has been considered the gold standard imaging modality in the diagnosis of DVT.[127, 128] In one prospective study, 70% of patients who had PTE proved by angiography showed evidence of thrombosis of the deep veins of the legs;[129] it must be assumed that either the remaining 30% had other sources for embolism (e.g., the deep pelvic veins, inferior vena cava, or right atrium) or that all or most of the thrombus in the legs had embolized.[129, 130] Usually, the veins are opacified by injecting contrast medium into a foot vein; the iliac veins can be visualized by femoral vein injection.

Venography has several disadvantages: (1) It can be painful, (2) it induces thrombosis in 3% to 4% of patients when ionic contrast medium is used, (3) inadequate examinations as a result of incomplete venous filling and other technical problems occur in 5% of cases, and (4) there is an approximately 10% interobserver disagreement in the assessment of the presence of thrombus.[132, 133] The incidence of complications is decreased with the use of non-ionic contrast medium.[131, 132] In one study of 463 consecutive patients who underwent venography with a nonionic contrast agent, serious side effects (bronchospasm) were seen in only 2 (0.4%) patients and minor side effects (e.g., local pain and discomfort, nausea and vomiting, and superficial phlebitis) in 83 (18%) patients;[132] postvenographic thrombosis confirmed by repeat venography occurred in 1 of 41 patients (2%) who had a previous normal venogram. Because of the potential complications and limitations of conventional venography, it has been replaced largely by other imaging techniques, particularly ultrasound, in the initial investigation of patients who have suspected DVT.

Ultrasonography

Studies of the use of ultrasound in the diagnosis of DVT in the 1980s were based on the observation that the normal vein lumen is obliterated after compression by the ultrasound probe while a vein containing thrombus remains distended, the thrombus often being seen as an echogenic area within the normal nonechoic vein lumen.[128] Such studies showed a sensitivity of approximately 90% and a specificity of 97% to 100% in the diagnosis of popliteal and femoral vein thrombosis.[134, 135] Assessment of DVT by ultrasound improved greatly with the advent of color flow technology in the late 1980s.[128] In the normal vein, color-coded flow fills the lumen completely. Thrombosis results in the absence of flow or the presence of isoechoic or echogenic thrombus within the lumen with absence or persistent underfilling of color-coded flow.[128] Color Doppler ultrasound has a sensitivity of greater than 95% and a specificity of greater than 98% in the diagnosis of popliteal and femoral vein thrombosis.[136, 137]

Color Doppler ultrasound allows a similar sensitivity and specificity in the diagnosis of calf vein thrombosis as that of above-knee lesions.[139, 140] The clinical value of assessment of calf vein thrombosis is controversial, however.[128, 219] Most investigators believe that thrombosis localized to this site is not associated with a risk of PTE.[138] One group of investigators evaluated retrospectively the findings in 283 patients in whom the initial ultrasound of thigh veins showed no evidence of DVT.[220] Follow-up was available for at least 6 months in 256 patients who survived 6 months or longer after their initial ultrasound examination, and information on the cause of death was available in the remaining patients. Adverse outcomes occurred in only 3 of the 283 patients (1.1%). Two had indeterminate ultrasound scans of the calf, did not receive anticoagulation therapy, and developed nonlethal PTE. The third patient had a negative calf ultrasound and subsequently developed a thrombus in the popliteal vein. All three patients recently had undergone surgery. The authors concluded that ultrasound of the calf is not helpful in identifying patients at increased risk of clinically important PTE or propagation of DVT into the thigh. In a follow-up study of 1,022 patients who had negative thigh ultrasound examinations, another group of investigators showed that about 10% developed DVT of thigh veins within 8 to 33 months of follow-up;[221] all these patients had persistent symptoms related to the lower extremity.

Because of its ready accessibility, low cost, and high diagnostic accuracy, ultrasonography has become the imaging modality of choice in the diagnosis of DVT in most centers. In patients who have symptoms of acute PTE and DVT, lower extremity ultrasound has been recommended as the initial imaging modality of choice.[73, 74, 228] A positive examination in this clinical setting allows confident diagnosis of PTE with no need for further investigation.[73, 74] In patients who do not have symptoms or signs of DVT, lower extremity Doppler ultrasound plays a limited role. Several groups have shown poor sensitivity in the detection of asymptomatic, nonocclusive thrombi in the veins of the leg and calf, including those in postoperative patients.[128, 135, 141]

Computed Tomography

Contrast-enhanced spiral CT assessment of the deep venous system of the legs can be performed using direct CT venography or indirect CT venography. Direct CT venography is performed by placing a 22-gauge intravenous cannula in the dorsal vein of each foot and a tourniquet around each ankle. Diluted intravenous contrast material is injected simultaneously into both legs. After a 35-second delay, spiral CT is performed from the ankle to the inferior vena cava using a collimation of 10 mm and a table increment of 20 mm (pitch of 2). The images are reconstructed at 5-mm intervals.[142] The diagnosis of DVT is based on visualization of a filling defect in an opacified vein or a nonopacified venous segment interposed between a proximally and distally opacified vein.[142]

Preliminary reports suggest that the procedure is sensitive and specific in the diagnosis of DVT.[142–144] In one study, 52 consecutive patients who had clinically suspected DVT were assessed with spiral CT and with conventional venography;[142] in cases in which the latter was nondiagnostic, color-coded duplex ultrasound was performed to establish a definitive diagnosis. CT had a sensitivity of 100%, a specificity of 96%, a PPV of 91%, and a negative predictive value of 100% in the diagnosis of DVT. CT was superior to conventional venography in showing extension of thrombus into the pelvic veins and inferior vena cava.

Adequate visualization of lower extremity veins can be obtained after intravenous injection of contrast material into an arm vein, a technique known as *indirect CT venography.*[144, 229, 230] The main advantage of indirect CT venography is that it can be performed after the CT angiogram of the pulmonary vasculature without the need of another venopuncture or additional intravenous contrast material. The only significant disadvantage compared with direct CT venography is that its peak enhancement is lower.[230] Because of the broad shape of the venous time-density curve, however, near-peak enhancement can be achieved in most patients at 3 minutes after the start of intravenous contrast injection (i.e., 2 minutes after CT pulmonary angiography).[230]

One group of investigators performed spiral CT angiography and indirect CT venography in 71 consecutive patients with suspected acute PTE.[229] Indirect venography was performed 3.5 minutes after the beginning of contrast injection. CT scans were obtained at 5-cm intervals from the upper calves to the diaphragm. DVT was shown by CT venography in 19 patients, 12 of whom also had PTE. CT venography correlated exactly with Doppler ultrasound assessment of the femoropopliteal venous system, where most pulmonary emboli originate, and showed pelvic extension of DVT in six patients.[229] The high sensitivity (90% to 100%) of indirect CT venography in the detection of DVT was confirmed in two other studies, but both also showed occasional false-positive diagnosis resulting in a positive predictive value of approximately 70%.[236, 237] These results suggest that the combination of CT angiography and indirect CT venography may allow a comprehensive evaluation of overall thrombus burden in a single examination.[229] CT venography is particularly useful in patients suspected clinically of having PTE and who have a negative spiral CT scan of the chest. To assess the value of performing indirect CT venography after spiral CT angiography in patients suspected of having pulmonary embolism (PE), one group of investigators prospectively evaluated 541 consecutive patients from seven institutions.[238] Deep vein thrombosis was found at CT venography in 45 (8%) and PE at CT angiography in 91 (17%) patients. DVT occurred in 16 patients who had no PE, which increased the diagnosis of thromboembolic disease by 18%.[238]

Magnetic Resonance Imaging

Several groups have shown that MR imaging is comparable or superior to conventional venography or ultrasound in the diagnosis of DVT.[145–148] In one prospective study of 16 patients, GRE MR imaging was compared with conventional venography;[145] using this MR technique, thrombosed vessels showed decreased to absent signal intensity, whereas patent vessels were characterized by high signal intensity. In 16 of 17 extremities, MR imaging allowed accurate detection and localization of the thrombi that had been identified by venography.[145] In another prospective study, GRE MR imaging was compared with venography in 61 patients who had clinically suspected DVT.[147] The diagnosis on MR imaging was based on the presence of an intravascular filling defect with low signal intensity surrounded by high signal intensity resulting from flowing blood or on the presence of occlusion of an enlarged vein with a clot that had decreased or absent signal intensity. Using venography as the gold standard, MR imaging had a sensitivity and specificity of 87% and 97% for the calf veins, 100% and 100% for the thigh veins, and 100% and 95% for the pelvic veins. In another series of 79 patients, GRE MR imaging had a sensitivity of 97% and specificity of 95% compared with conventional venography.[148] Because of its high diagnostic accuracy, MR imaging is recommended in patients who have suspected DVT and a nondiagnostic ultrasound; in patients who have suspected pelvic vein thrombosis; and in the differential diagnosis of DVT from nonvascular disease, such as ruptured Baker's cyst.

Scintigraphy

Several radionuclide techniques have been assessed for the detection of DVT, including radioactive iodine-125–labeled fibrinogen,[149] radioactive indium–labeled autologous platelets,[150, 151] technetium-99m MAA,[152, 153] and technetium-99m–modified recombinant tissue plasminogen activator.[154] The techniques have many limitations, including difficulty in interpretation, and have been used rarely in clinical practice.

Summary

On the basis of the data reported in the literature and our own experience, we believe that the following recommendations are reasonable for the evaluation of patients suspected of having acute PTE:

1. All patients should have a chest radiograph, its role being mainly to exclude abnormalities, such as acute pneumonia or pneumothorax, that may mimic PTE clinically.

2. Patients who have symptoms or signs of DVT should undergo Doppler ultrasound of the legs; if the result of this examination is positive, the patient can be considered to have PTE, and no further investigation is required.

3. Patients who have no symptoms or signs of DVT and symptomatic patients who have a negative Doppler ultrasound examination and who do not have extensive underlying parenchymal lung disease or COPD should undergo V̇/Q̇ scintigraphy. A high-probability or a normal V̇/Q̇ scan can be considered definitive. A low-probability finding together with a low clinical index of suspicion can be considered adequate to exclude PTE. All other patients should undergo further evaluation with contrast-enhanced spiral CT.

4. Patients who have extensive pulmonary parenchymal disease or COPD and patients who have nondiagnostic V̇/Q̇ scans should undergo contrast-enhanced spiral CT.

5. Patients whose CT scans are suboptimal and patients whose CT scans are negative but for whom there is a high clinical index of suspicion of PTE should undergo pulmonary angiography.

SEPTIC EMBOLISM

Septic embolism occurs when fragments of thrombus contain organisms, usually bacteria and occasionally fungi or parasites. The pulmonary manifestations of such emboli may be the only indication of serious underlying infection; because the radiologic changes often are distinctive, their recognition early in the disease should permit diagnosis and prompt institution of therapy.[157]

Septic embolism occurs most frequently in young adults; in one study of 17 patients, most were younger than 40 years old.[158] The organism most often grown on blood cultures was *Staphylococcus aureus*, streptococci being the next most common; in four patients, blood cultures were negative. A predisposing factor nearly always is present, usually drug addiction, alcoholism, generalized infection in patients who have immunologic deficiencies (particularly lymphoma), congenital heart disease, and skin infection.[159]

Most emboli originate in the heart (in association with endocarditis of the tricuspid valve or a ventricular septal defect)[160, 161] or the peripheral veins (septic thrombophlebitis). Because tricuspid endocarditis may not be associated with signs or symptoms implicating the valve,[162] the identification of pulmonary emboli may be the first clue to this diagnosis. Occasionally, emboli originate in the pharynx, infection extending to the parapharyngeal space and internal jugular venous system, resulting in a clinical presentation referred to as *Lemierre's syndrome* or *postanginal sepsis*.[163, 164] The oral anaerobes, particularly *Bacteroides* and *Fusobacterium* species, are the most common pathogens associated with this form of disease. Symptoms of septic thromboembolism of any etiology include fever, cough (with or without expectoration of purulent material), and hemoptysis.

Radiographically, pulmonary disease usually is manifested by multiple, ill-defined, round or wedge-shaped peripheral opacities (Table 12–7, Fig. 12–17). They may be uniform in size or vary widely, reflecting recurrent showers of emboli. The opacities usually are bilateral, although they may be asymmetric and occasionally are unilateral.[165] The opacities may be migratory in nature, appearing first in one area, then in another as older lesions resolve and new ones appear.[158] Cavitation is frequent and may occur rapidly; the

Table 12–7. SEPTIC EMBOLISM: RADIOLOGIC MANIFESTATIONS

Chest radiograph
    Multiple ill-defined round opacities
    Wedge-shaped pleural-based opacities
    Thin-walled cavities
CT scan
    Multiple discrete nodules
    Often located at end of vessels (*feeding vessel* sign)
    Various stages of cavitation
    Wedge-shaped pleural-based opacities
    Rimlike peripheral enhancement

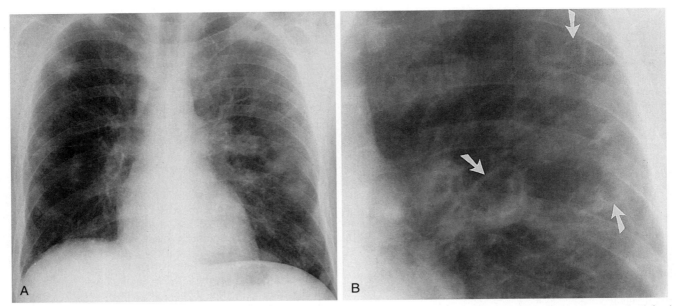

Figure 12–17. Septic Embolism. View of posteroanterior chest radiograph *(A)* in a 28-year-old man presenting with fever shows poorly defined bilateral nodular opacities. Blood cultures grew *Staphylococcus aureus.* Over the following days, the nodules cavitated. View of the left lung *(B)* from chest radiograph performed 1 week later shows multiple thin-walled cavities *(arrows).*

cavities are usually thin-walled, and many have no fluid level. Acute septic embolism may be associated with hilar and mediastinal lymph node enlargement that may be massive;[166] empyema is an infrequent complication.

Radiographs sometimes show multiple, small, poorly defined opacities that simulate diffuse bronchopneumonia, and alertness is necessary to make the diagnosis, particularly if the underlying disease is bacterial endocarditis. In questionable cases, the diagnosis can be confirmed by CT (Fig. 12–18).[165, 167] In one study, the radiographic and CT findings were compared in 15 patients who had documented septic pulmonary emboli.[165] On radiograph, diffuse bilateral nodules in various stages of cavitation were identified in seven (47%) patients, usually in association with focal areas of consolidation in the lower lobes; the remaining patients had only unilateral or bilateral areas of consolidation that were not identified as being subpleural or as suggestive of infarcts. On CT scan, discrete nodules in various stages of cavitation were identified in 10 (67%) patients, in each of whom at least some of the nodules were located at the end of a pulmonary vessel (feeding vessel sign). In 11 (73%) patients, the areas of consolidation were found to be subpleural and wedge-shaped on CT scan. Central areas of heterogeneous lucency or frank cavitation were identified in 91% of the areas of consolidation on CT scan compared with only 7% on radiograph (Fig. 12–19). After administration of intravenous contrast material, a rimlike pattern of peripheral enhancement could be identified along the borders of all the wedgelike areas of consolidation. Of patients, 67% had pleural effusions and 27% had hilar or mediastinal lymphadenopathy identified on CT.

In another study of 18 patients who had documented septic PTE, multiple peripheral nodules ranging in size from 0.5 to 3.5 cm in diameter and wedged-shaped peripheral areas of consolidation abutting the pleura were identi-

fied on CT in 83% and 50% of patients, respectively;[167] 80% of patients who had peripheral nodules had a feeding vessel sign. In 30% of cases, the diagnosis of septic embolism was suggested first by review of the CT findings.

PULMONARY COMPLICATIONS OF SICKLE CELL DISEASE

Pulmonary complications can occur in all of the more common sickle hemoglobinopathies, including homozygous hemoglobin SS and the compound heterozygous states of hemoglobin S/C and hemoglobin S/β-thalassemia.[168] Approximately 85% of affected individuals survive into the second decade of life.[168] The sickle cell gene is carried by 8% of African Americans so that the disease is relatively common in the United States.[169]

The most common pulmonary complication, termed *acute chest syndrome,* is characterized by fever, pleuritic chest pain, dyspnea, leukocytosis, and new lung opacities on radiographs. The abnormality occurs in 50% of patients who have sickle cell disease and often is recurrent.[168, 169] It is second only to pain as a cause for hospitalization and is responsible for 25% of all deaths in sickle cell disease.[168] The radiographic findings consist of bilateral patchy areas of consolidation, which have been attributed to edema and infarction. Rib infarcts are seen rarely.[171] In addition to consolidation, HRCT shows areas of vascular attenuation attributed to hypoperfusion.[170] Patients who have repeated pulmonary infections and episodes of acute chest syndrome may develop focal or, rarely, diffuse interstitial fibrosis.[172, 173]

HRCT findings of chronic sickle cell lung disease were assessed in a prospective study of 29 patients.[173] Patients were solicited from collaborating sickle cell centers and selected for the study based on a history of at least one previous episode of acute chest syndrome or pneumonia.

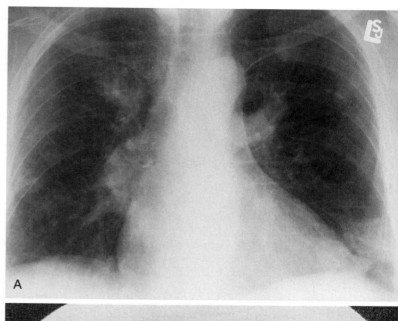

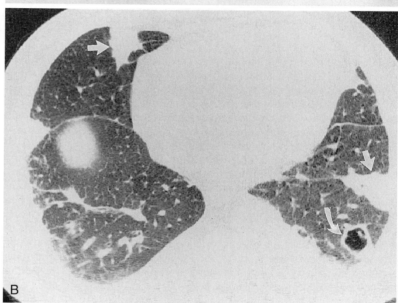

Figure 12–18. Septic Embolism. Posteroanterior chest radiograph *(A)* in a 64-year-old man shows poorly defined bilateral opacities and small bilateral pleural effusions. CT scan at the level of the dome of the right hemidiaphragm *(B)* shows bilateral pleural-based, wedge-shaped opacities *(straight arrows)* and a cavitating nodule *(curved arrow)* in the left lower lobe. Bilateral pleural effusions are evident. Blood cultures grew *Streptococcus viridans*.

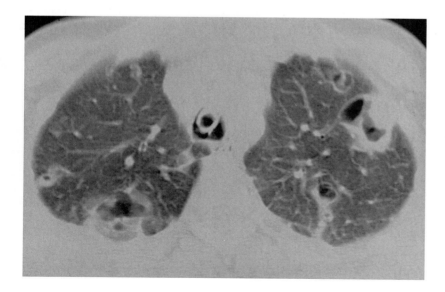

Figure 12–19. Septic Embolism. CT scan shows cavitating nodules in both upper lobes. Also visible is an endotracheal tube in place. Blood cultures grew enterococci. The patient was a 20-year-old drug addict.

They ranged from 5 to 54 years of age (mean, 22 years) and included 27 patients with homozygous sickle cell disease and 2 with hemoglobin SC disease. Twelve of the 29 (41%) patients had multifocal interstitial changes consisting of interlobular septal thickening, parenchymal bands of attenuation, and pleural tags with associated architectural distortion; none had honeycombing or diffuse interstitial fibrosis.

FAT EMBOLISM

Although intact fragments of adipose tissue (usually with admixed hematopoietic cells) often are found in the pulmonary arteries after severe trauma, the term *fat embolism* traditionally refers to the presence of free fat within the vasculature.[176, 177] The precise incidence of fat embolism is difficult to ascertain, partly because diagnostic criteria are variable and partly because most cases do not result in clinical manifestations. The incidence of clinically significant disease in patients who have simple tibial or femoral fractures generally is believed to be about 1% to 3%.[174, 178] In individuals who have more severe trauma, the incidence of embolism is probably 10% to 20%.[174, 175]

The pathogenetic mechanisms involved in the production of the pulmonary fat embolism syndrome are probably twofold. The first is mechanical obstruction of pulmonary vessels by fat globules themselves and, possibly, by platelet or red blood cell aggregates.[180] A second, biochemically mediated, process likely ensues after the initial obstructive effect has subsided. Fat appears to be transported to the lungs as neutral triglycerides,[181] and it is likely that these are converted by endothelial lipases into free fatty acids, which then exert a direct toxic effect on the alveolar wall.[182]

Pathologically, the lungs of patients who have died with fat emboli frequently are heavy and show patchy areas of hemorrhage and edema.[179] Although symptoms may appear almost immediately after the event causing embolization,[190, 191] in most cases there is a delay of 12 to 24 hours (Table 12–8); sometimes, delay is 3 days.[192] The most common pulmonary symptom is dyspnea; cough, hemoptysis, and pleural pain occur occasionally.

Symptoms associated with systemic fat embolism are seen in 85% of patients who have pulmonary disease.[174] They are chiefly related to the central nervous system and include confusion, restlessness, stupor, delirium, seizures, and coma. Skin involvement also is frequent (20% to 50% of cases[174]), typically manifested as a petechial rash appearing 2 to 3 days after embolization.[192] The petechiae are particularly prominent along the anterior axillary folds[193] and in the conjunctiva and retina, a distribution that has been attributed to fat floating on the bloodstream and affecting vessels that are uppermost.[194]

Radiologic Manifestations

As indicated, pulmonary fat embolism is unrecognized in many cases, partly because symptoms are mild or absent, but also because chest radiograph often is normal. A normal radiograph was found in 87% of patients in one series in whom the diagnosis was based on the presence of lipiduria.[183] When present, the radiographic findings are those of adult respiratory distress syndrome of any cause, consisting of widespread air-space consolidation. The distribution is predominantly peripheral rather than central[184, 185] and usually involves the basal regions to a greater degree than does pulmonary edema of cardiac origin. Further differentiation from cardiogenic edema is provided by the absence of cardiac enlargement and signs of pulmonary venous hypertension; however, in one study of 30 patients, diffuse linear opacities resembling interstitial edema were just as common as air-space opacities.[186] Pleural effusions typically are absent.

The time lapse between trauma and radiographic signs is usually 1 to 2 days.[184, 187] This delay differentiates fat embolism from traumatic lung contusion, in which the radiographic opacity invariably appears immediately after injury. In addition, although the latter opacity usually clears rapidly (in about 24 hours), the resolution of fat embolism usually takes 7 to 10 days and occasionally 4 weeks.[188] Further differentiation lies in the extent of lung involvement; contusion seldom affects both lungs diffusely and symmetrically. When both lungs are involved, the radiographic findings usually are more severe in the lung deep to the site of maximal trauma.

In one patient, the initial radiographic findings consisted of poorly defined small nodular opacities.[222] These were shown on HRCT scan to be located predominantly in the centrilobular and subpleural regions. These nodules presumably reflected the presence of alveolar edema or hemorrhage.[222] The nodules, present early in the course of the disease, subsequently were obscured by confluent areas of consolidation. In another case, multiple small nodular opacities developed after fat embolism and adult respiratory distress syndrome that were shown to be calcified on CT scans;[189] most calcifications were interpreted on CT scan as being located in branches of the pulmonary arteries. A technetium-99m diphosphonate bone scan showed diffuse uptake over the lungs. The patient had no symptoms except for mild dyspnea on exertion.

AMNIOTIC FLUID EMBOLISM

Amniotic fluid embolism is a highly lethal complication of pregnancy in which amniotic fluid enters the bloodstream through tears in the uterine veins and results in rapid cardiopulmonary collapse.[175, 195] It has been estimated that about 10% of peripartum maternal deaths in the United States are caused by amniotic fluid embolism.[196]

The clinical manifestations typically are abrupt in onset and rapid in progression.[198] Although symptoms begin during spontaneous labor in most patients, in about 30% they occur after delivery (10% spontaneous and 20% post–

Table 12–8. FAT EMBOLISM

Typically develops 1–2 days after severe trauma
Pulmonary symptoms: dyspnea and cough
Systemic manifestations: confusion, restlessness, petechiae
Radiologic manifestations
    Findings are those of ARDS
    Widespread consolidation
    Basal and peripheral predominance
    Chest radiograph is often normal

ARDS, adult respiratory distress syndrome.

cesarean section).[197] In one series, disease was heralded by dyspnea and cyanosis in 20 patients, sudden profound shock disproportionate to blood loss in 12, and signs of central nervous system irritability (convulsions, hyperreflexia, and other signs) in 8.[198]

The principal radiographic finding is air-space edema indistinguishable from acute pulmonary edema of other cause.[199, 200] Whether cardiac enlargement accompanies the edema depends on the severity of pulmonary arterial hypertension and consequent cor pulmonale with or without left ventricular failure. The consolidation may persist or resolve within a few days.[200] Because the predominant radiographic manifestation is widespread air-space consolidation, the chief differential diagnoses are massive pulmonary hemorrhage and aspiration of liquid gastric contents.

EMBOLISM OF TALC, STARCH, AND CELLULOSE

Emboli of talc, starch, and cellulose are seen almost invariably in individuals who have engaged in intravenous drug abuse over a long period.[201, 202] In most instances, the complication occurs with medications intended solely for oral use; pills are crushed in a spoon or bottle top, water is added, and the mixture is drawn into a syringe and injected. Implicated medications have in common the addition of an insoluble filler to bind the medicinal particles together and to act as a lubricant to prevent the tablets from sticking to punches and dies during manufacture.[204] The most widely used filler is talc. When injected intravenously, the fillers become trapped within pulmonary arterioles and capillaries and cause vascular occlusion. In time, the foreign particles migrate through the vessel wall and come to lie in the adjacent perivascular and parenchymal interstitial tissue, where they engender a foreign body giant cell reaction and fibrosis.

Most addicts who inject oral medications are asymptomatic, granulomas being found incidentally at autopsy in those who die from other causes.[204, 205] Typically, symptoms develop only in very heavy users (not infrequently with a history of injection of thousands of pills) and consist of slowly progressive dyspnea and (occasionally) persistent cough.[201]

The earliest radiologic manifestation is widespread small nodules; the diameter of individual nodules ranges from barely visible to about 1 mm (Fig. 12–20). The pattern does not have a reticular component, the opacities being distinct and *pinpoint* in character, simulating alveolar microlithiasis. Although some authors have described a midzonal predominance of these micronodules,[203, 207] the distribution we have observed has been diffuse and uniform throughout the lungs. In some patients, the widespread nodularity is associated with loss of volume, sometimes severe.

In the later stages of the disease, the opacities in the upper lobes may coalesce to form an almost homogeneous opacity that resembles closely the progressive massive fibrosis of silicosis or coal workers' pneumoconiosis except for the frequent presence of an air bronchogram.[202, 206] Pulmonary arterial hypertension and cor pulmonale may develop.[207, 208] In the late stages of the disease, increasing disability and deteriorating function are associated with radiographic evidence of emphysema and bullae;[202] the

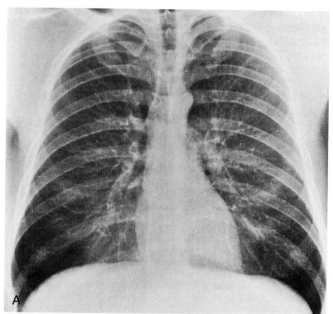

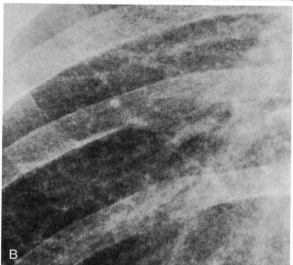

Figure 12–20. Pulmonary Talcosis in Intravenous Drug Abuse. This asymptomatic 22-year-old man had been shooting heroin and methadone for 4 years at the time these radiographs were obtained. There is widespread involvement of both lungs by tiny micronodular opacities *(A)*, seen to better advantage on a magnified image (2:1) of the right lower zone *(B)*. There is no anatomic predominance. The pattern is similar to the discrete opacities of alveolar microlithiasis.

chest radiograph may be diagnostic at this stage, revealing a combination of small nodular opacities, coalescent upper lobe lesions resembling progressive massive fibrosis, and lower lobe emphysema or bullae. Pneumothorax, sometimes recurrent, has been described,[201] and mediastinal lymph node enlargement occurs occasionally.[201, 203] Gallium 67 scans may be positive.[209, 210]

HRCT findings consist of diffuse ground-glass attenuation (Fig. 12–21), a diffuse micronodular pattern, and perihilar upper lobe conglomerate areas of fibrosis.[211, 223, 224] Localized areas of high attenuation consistent with talc deposition can be seen within the conglomerate masses (Fig. 12–22).[211, 223, 224]

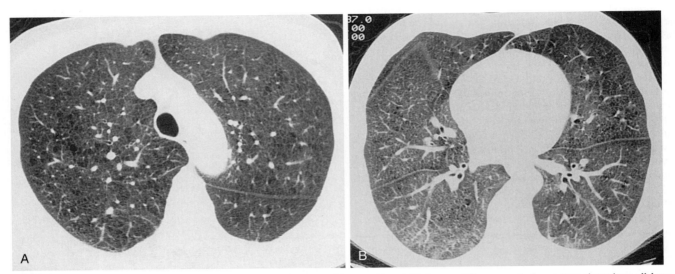

Figure 12–21. Talcosis: Ground-Glass Attenuation on CT Scan. HRCT scans *(A* and *B)* show a diffuse ground-glass pattern throughout all lung zones. No discrete nodules were seen at any level. The diagnosis of talcosis was proved by open-lung biopsy. The patient was a 49-year-old man with a 25-year history of intravenous drug abuse who presented with increasing shortness of breath. Over the years, he had used intravenous heroin, methylphenidate (Ritalin), and pentazocine (Talwin) on a daily basis. He also had a 70-pack-year smoking history.

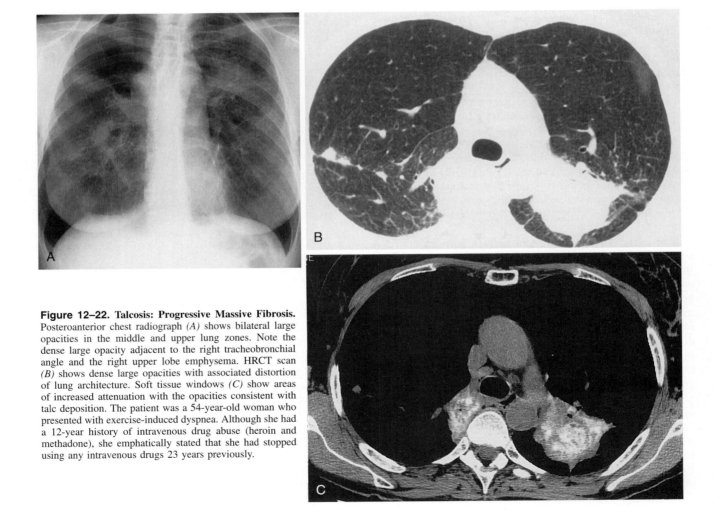

Figure 12–22. Talcosis: Progressive Massive Fibrosis. Posteroanterior chest radiograph *(A)* shows bilateral large opacities in the middle and upper lung zones. Note the dense large opacity adjacent to the right tracheobronchial angle and the right upper lobe emphysema. HRCT scan *(B)* shows dense large opacities with associated distortion of lung architecture. Soft tissue windows *(C)* show areas of increased attenuation with the opacities consistent with talc deposition. The patient was a 54-year-old woman who presented with exercise-induced dyspnea. Although she had a 12-year history of intravenous drug abuse (heroin and methadone), she emphatically stated that she had stopped using any intravenous drugs 23 years previously.

Radiographic and CT findings of intravenous abuse of methylphenidate (crushed Ritalin tablets) differ from those of other types of intravenous drug abuse.[212] The main abnormality consists of emphysema, characteristically bilateral, symmetric, and involving mainly the lower lung zones. There is no associated bulla formation. In one investigation, the authors assessed the CT appearance of talcosis secondary to intravenous abuse of oral medications in 12 patients.[224] Seven patients had abused methylphenidate, and five patients had abused substances other than methylphenidate. The predominant abnormalities seen on CT scan consisted of a fine nodular and lower lobe panacinar emphysema in three patients and ground-glass attenuation in two. Emphysema was the only abnormality seen in the remaining five patients. There was no significant difference in the prevalence of nodules and ground-glass attenuation between the Ritalin and non-Ritalin groups. Lower lobe panacinar emphysema was more common in Ritalin abusers (six of seven patients [86%]) than in non-Ritalin drug abusers (one of five patients [20%]).

References

1. Moser KM: Venous thromboembolism. Am Rev Respir Dis 141:235, 1990.
2. Dalen JE, Alpert JS: Natural history of pulmonary embolism. *In* Sasahara AA, Sonnenblick EH, Lesch M (eds): Pulmonary Emboli: A Progress in Cardiovascular Diseases reprint (Vol XVII, Nos. 3–5). New York, Grune & Stratton, 1975, p 77.
3. Nielsen HK, Husted SE, Krusell LR, et al: Silent pulmonary embolism in patients with deep venous thrombosis: Incidence and fate in a randomized controlled trial of anticoagulation versus no anticoagulation. J Intern Med 235:457, 1994.
4. Anderson FA Jr, Wheeler HB, Goldenberg RJ, et al: A population-based perspective of the hospital incidence and case-fatality rates of deep vein thrombosis and pulmonary embolism. Arch Intern Med 151:933, 1991.
5. Waller BF, Dean PJ, Mann O, et al: Right ventricular outflow obstruction from thrombus with small peripheral pulmonary emboli. Chest 79:224, 1981.
6. Crowell RH, Adams GS, Koilpillai CJ, et al: In vivo right heart thrombus—precursor of life-threatening pulmonary embolism. Chest 94:1236, 1988.
7. Gonzalez A, Altieri PI, Marquez E, et al: Massive pulmonary embolism associated with a right ventricular myxoma. Am J Med 69:795, 1980.
8. Bortolotti U, Mazzucco A, Valfre C, et al: Right ventricular myxoma: Review of the literature and report of 2 patients. Ann Thorac Surg 33:277, 1982.
9. Goldstein MF, Nestico P, Olshan AR, et al: Superior vena cava thrombosis and pulmonary embolus: Association with right atrial mural thrombus. Arch Intern Med 142:1726, 1982.
10. Adelstein DJ, Hines JD, Carter SG, et al: Thromboembolic events in patients with malignant superior vena cava syndrome and the role of anticoagulation. Cancer 62:2258, 1988.
11. Sundqvist S-B, Hedner U, Kullenberg HKE, et al: Deep venous thrombosis of the arm: A study of coagulation and fibrinolysis. BMJ 283:265, 1981.
12. Coon WW, Willis PW III: Thrombosis of axillary and subclavian veins. Arch Surg 94:657, 1967.
13. Adams JT, McEvoy RK, de Weese JA: Primary deep venous thrombosis of upper extremity. Arch Surg 91:29, 1965.
14. Monreal M, Lafoz E, Ruiz J, et al: Upper-extremity deep venous thrombosis and pulmonary embolism. Chest 99:280, 1991.
15. Hampton AO, Castleman B: Correlation of postmortem chest teleroentgenograms with autopsy findings: With special reference to pulmonary embolism and infarction. Am J Roentgenol 43:305, 1940.
16. Llamas R, Swenson EW: Diagnostic clues in pulmonary thromboembolism evaluated by angiographic and ventilation-blood flow studies. Thorax 20:327, 1965.
17. Kerr IH, Simon G, Sutton GC: The value of the plain radiograph in acute massive pulmonary embolism. Br J Radiol 44:751, 1971.
18. Redline S, Tomashefski JF Jr, Altose MD: Cavitating lung infarction after bland pulmonary thromboembolism in patients with the adult respiratory distress syndrome. Thorax 40:915, 1985.
19. Worsley DF, Alavi A, Aronchick JM, et al: Chest radiographic findings in patients with acute pulmonary embolism: Observations from the PIOPED study. Radiology 189:133, 1993.
20. Stein PD, Athanasoulis C, Greenspan RH, et al: Relation of plain chest radiographic findings to pulmonary arterial pressure and arterial blood oxygen levels in patients with acute pulmonary embolism. Am J Cardiol 69:394, 1992.
21. Westermark N: On the roentgen diagnosis of lung embolism. Acta Radiol 19:357, 1938.
22. Fleischner FG: Pulmonary embolism. Clin Radiol 13:169, 1962.
23. Figley MM, Gerdes AJ, Ricketts HJ: Radiographic aspects of pulmonary embolism. Semin Roentgenol 2:389, 1967.
24. Palla A, Donnamaria V, Petruzzelli S, et al: Enlargement of the right descending pulmonary artery in pulmonary embolism. Am J Roentgenol 141:513, 1983.
25. Williams JR, Wilcox WC: Pulmonary embolism: Roentgenographic and angiographic considerations. Am J Roentgenol 89:333, 1963.
26. Stein GN, Chen JT, Goldstein F, et al: The importance of chest roentgenography in the diagnosis of pulmonary embolism. Am J Roentgenol 81:255, 1959.
27. Westcott JL, Cole S: Plate atelectasis. Radiology 155:1, 1985.
28. Laur A: Roentgen diagnosis of pulmonary embolism and its differentiation from myocardial infarction. Am J Roentgenol 90:632, 1963.
29. Szucs MM Jr, Brooks HL, Grossman W, et al: Diagnostic sensitivity of laboratory findings in acute pulmonary embolism. Ann Intern Med 74:161, 1971.
30. Talbot S, Worthington BS, Roebuck EJ: Radiographic signs of pulmonary embolism and pulmonary infarction. Thorax 28:198, 1973.
31. Torrance DJ Jr: Roentgenographic signs of pulmonary artery occlusion. Am J Med Sci 237:651, 1959.
32. Jacoby CG, Mindell HJ: Lobar consolidation in pulmonary embolism. Radiology 118:287, 1976.
33. Fleischner FG: Roentgenology of the pulmonary infarct. Semin Roentgenol 2:61, 1967.
34. Beilin DS, Fink JP, Leslie LW: Correlation of postmortem pathological observations with chest roentgenograms. Radiology 57:361, 1951.
35. Alderson PO, Martin EC: Pulmonary embolism: Diagnosis with multiple imaging modalities. Radiology 164:297, 1987.
36. Bachynski JE: Absence of the air bronchogram sign: A reliable finding in pulmonary embolism with infarction or hemorrhage. Radiology 100:547, 1971.
37. Coke LR, Dundee JC: Cavitation in bland infarcts of the lung. Can Med Assoc J 72:907, 1955.
38. Castleman B: Pathologic observations on pulmonary infarction in man. *In* Sasahara AA, Stein M (eds): Pulmonary Embolic Disease. New York, Grune & Stratton, 1965, pp 86–92.
39. Fleischner FG: Observations on the radiologic changes in pulmonary embolism. *In* Sasahara AA, Stein M (eds): Pulmonary Embolic Disease. New York, Grune & Stratton, 1965, pp 206–213.
40. Woesner ME, Sanders I, White GW: The melting sign in resolving transient pulmonary infarction. Am J Roentgenol 111:782, 1971.
41. McGoldrick PJ, Rudd TG, Figley MM, et al: What becomes of pulmonary infarcts? Am J Roentgenol 133:1039, 1979.
42. Greenspan RH, Ravin CE, Polansky SM, et al: Accuracy of the chest radiography in diagnosis of pulmonary embolism. Invest Radiol 17:539, 1982.
43. Sostman HD, Coleman RE, DeLong DM, et al: Evaluation of revised criteria for ventilation-perfusion scintigraphy in patients with suspected pulmonary embolism. Radiology 193:103, 1994.
44. Miniati M, Pistolesi M, Marini C, et al: Value of perfusion lung scan in the diagnosis of pulmonary embolism: Results of the Prospective Investigative Study of Acute Pulmonary Embolism Diagnosis (PISA-PED). Am J Respir Crit Care Med 154:1187, 1996.
45. Heck LL, Duley JW: Statistical considerations in lung scanning with Tc-99m albumin particles. Radiology 113:675, 1975.
46. James JM, Herman KJ, Lloyd JJ, et al: Evaluation of ^{99}Tcm Technegas ventilation scintigraphy in the diagnosis of pulmonary embolism. Br J Radiol 64:711, 1991.

47. Sostman HD, Rapoport S, Gottschalk A, et al: Imaging of pulmonary embolism. Invest Radiol 21:443, 1986.
48. Gottschalk A, Sostman HD, Juni JE, et al: Ventilation-perfusion scintigraphy in the PIOPED study: II. Evaluation of criteria and interpretations. J Nucl Med 34:1119, 1993.
49. Webber MM, Gomes AS, Roe D, et al: Comparison of Biello, McNeil, and PIOPED criteria for the diagnosis of pulmonary emboli on lung scans. Am J Roentgenol 154:975, 1990.
50. Freitas FE, Sarosi MG, Nagle CC, et al: The use of modified PIOPED criteria in clinical practice. J Nucl Med 36:1573, 1995.
51. PIOPED Investigators: Value of the ventilation/perfusion scan in acute pulmonary embolism: Result of the Prospective Investigation of Pulmonary Embolism Diagnosis (PIOPED). JAMA 263:2753, 1990.
52. Quinn DA, Thompson BT, Terrin ML, et al: A prospective investigation of pulmonary embolism in women and men. JAMA 268:1689, 1992.
53. Worsley DF, Alavi A, Palevsky HI: Comparison of the diagnostic performance of ventilation/perfusion lung scanning in different patient populations. Radiology 199:481, 1996.
54. Lesser BA, Leeper KV Jr, Stein PD, et al: The diagnosis of acute pulmonary embolism in patients with chronic obstructive pulmonary disease. Chest 102:17, 1992.
55. Worsley DF, Palevsky HI, Alavi A: Clinical characteristic of patients with pulmonary embolism and low or very low probability lung scan interpretations. Arch Intern Med 154:2737, 1994.
56. Alderson PO, Biello DR, Sachariah KG, et al: Scintigraphic detection of pulmonary embolism in patients with obstructive pulmonary disease. Radiology 138:661, 1981.
57. Smith R, Ellis K, Alderson PO: Role of chest radiography in predicting the extent of airway disease in patients with suspected pulmonary embolism. Radiology 159:391, 1986.
58. Meignan M, Simonneau G, Oliveira L, et al: Computation of ventilation-perfusion ratio with Kr-81m in pulmonary embolism. J Nucl Med 25:149, 1984.
59. Ralph DD: Pulmonary embolism: The implications of prospective investigation of pulmonary embolism diagnosis. Radiol Clin North Am 32:679, 1994.
60. Remy-Jardin M, Remy J, Wattinne L, et al: Central pulmonary thromboembolism: Diagnosis with spiral volumetric CT with the single-breath-hold technique: Comparison with pulmonary angiography. Radiology 185:381, 1992.
61. Teigen CL, Maus TP, Sheedy PF II, et al: Pulmonary embolism: Diagnosis with electron-beam CT. Radiology 188:839, 1993.
62. Goodman LR, Curtin JJ, Mewissen MW, et al: Detection of pulmonary embolism in patients with unresolved clinical and scintigraphic diagnosis: Helical CT versus angiography. Am J Roentgenol 164:1369, 1995.
63. van Rossum AB, Pattynama PMT, Ton ERTA, et al: Pulmonary embolism: Validation of spiral CT angiography in 149 patients. Radiology 201:467, 1996.
64. Cross JJL, Kemp PM, Walsh CG, et al: A randomized trial of spiral CT and ventilation perfusion scintigraphy for the diagnosis of pulmonary embolism. Clin Radiol 53:177, 1998.
65. Remy-Jardin M, Remy J, Artaud D, et al: Spiral CT of pulmonary embolism: Technical considerations and interpretive pitfalls. J Thorac Imaging 12:103, 1997.
66. Remy-Jardin M, Remy J, Deschildre F, et al: Diagnosis of pulmonary embolism with spiral CT: Comparison with pulmonary angiography and scintigraphy. Radiology 200:699, 1996.
67. Garg K, Welsh CH, Feyerabend AJ, et al: Pulmonary embolism: Diagnosis with spiral CT and ventilation-perfusion scanning—correlation with pulmonary angiographic results or clinical outcome. Radiology 208:201, 1998.
68. Teigen CL, Maus TP, Sheedy PF II, et al: Pulmonary embolism: Diagnosis with contrast-enhanced electron-beam CT and comparison with pulmonary angiography. Radiology 194:313, 1995.
69. Mayo JR, Remy-Jardin M, Müller NL, et al: Prospective comparison of spiral CT and ventilation-perfusion scintigraphy in the diagnosis of pulmonary embolism. Radiology 205:447, 1997.
70. Gefter WB, Hatabu H, Holland GA, et al: Pulmonary thromboembolism: Recent developments in diagnosis with CT and MR imaging. Radiology 197:561, 1995.
71. Stein PD, Athanasoulis C, Alavi A, et al: Complications and validity of pulmonary angiography in acute pulmonary embolism. Circulation 85:462, 1992.

72. van Erkel AR, van Rossum AB, Bloem JL, et al: Spiral CT angiography for suspected pulmonary embolism: A cost-effectiveness analysis. Radiology 201:29, 1996.
73. Goodman LR, Lipchik RJ, Kuzo RS: Acute pulmonary embolism: The role of computed tomographic imaging. J Thorac Imaging 12:83, 1997.
74. Sostman HD: Opinion response to acute pulmonary embolism: The role of computed tomographic imaging. J Thorac Imaging 12:89, 1997.
75. Gefter WB, Palevsky HI: Opinion response to acute pulmonary embolism: The role of computed tomographic imaging. J Thorac Imaging 12:97, 1997.
76. van Rossum AB, Pattynama PMT, Mallens WMC, et al: Can helical CT replace scintigraphy in the diagnostic process in suspected pulmonary embolism? A retrolective-prolective cohort study focusing on total diagnostic yield. Eur Radiol 8:90, 1998.
77. Romano WM, Cascade PN, Korobkin MT, et al: Implications of unsuspected pulmonary embolism detected by computed tomography. Can Assoc Radiol J 46:363, 1995.
78. Winston CB, Wechsler RJ, Salazar AM, et al: Incidental pulmonary emboli detected at helical CT: Effect on patient care. Radiology 201:23, 1996.
79. Gosselin MV, Rubin GD, Leung AN, et al: Unsuspected pulmonary embolism: Prospective detection on routine helical CT scans. Radiology 208:209, 1998.
80. Remy-Jardin M, Louvegny S, Remy J, et al: Acute central thromboembolic disease: Posttherapeutic follow-up with spiral CT angiography. Radiology 203:173, 1997.
81. Tardivon AA, Musset D, Maitre S, et al: Role of CT in chronic pulmonary embolism: Comparison with pulmonary angiography. J Comput Assist Tomogr 17:345, 1993.
82. Schwickert HC, Schweden F, Schild HH, et al: Pulmonary arteries and lung parenchyma in chronic pulmonary embolism: Preoperative and postoperative CT findings. Radiology 191:351, 1994.
83. Sinner WN: Computed tomographic patterns of pulmonary thromboembolism and infarction. J Comput Assist Tomogr 2:395, 1978.
84. Greaves SM, Hart EM, Brown K, et al: Pulmonary thromboembolism: Spectrum of findings on CT. Am J Roentgenol 165:1359, 1995.
85. Coche E, Müller NL, Kim KI, et al: Acute pulmonary embolism: Ancillary findings on spiral CT. Radiology 207:753, 1998.
86. Ren H, Kuhlman JE, Hruban RH, et al: CT of inflation-fixed lungs: Wedge-shaped density and vascular sign in the diagnosis of infarction. J Comput Assist Tomogr 14:82, 1990.
87. King MA, Ysrael M, Bergin CJ: Chronic thromboembolic pulmonary hypertension: CT findings. Am J Roentgenol 170:955, 1998.
88. King MA, Bergin CJ, Yeung DWC, et al: Chronic pulmonary thromboembolism: Detection of regional hypoperfusion with CT. Radiology 191:359, 1994.
89. Remy-Jardin M, Remy J, Louvegny S, et al: Airway changes in chronic pulmonary embolism: CT findings in 33 patients. Radiology 203:355, 1997.
90. Bergin CJ, Rios G, King MA, et al: Accuracy of high-resolution CT in identifying chronic pulmonary thromboembolic disease. Am J Roentgenol 166:1371, 1996.
91. Austin JHM, Müller NL, Friedman PJ, et al: Glossary of terms for CT of the lungs: Recommendations of the Nomenclature Committee of the Fleischner Society. Radiology 200:327, 1996.
92. Loubeyre P, Revel D, Douek P, et al: Dynamic contrast-enhanced MR angiography of pulmonary embolism: Comparison with pulmonary angiography. Am J Roentgenol 162:1035, 1994.
93. Meaney JFM, Weg JG, Chenevert TL, et al: Diagnosis of pulmonary embolism with magnetic resonance angiography. N Engl J Med 336:1422, 1997.
94. Kessler R, Fraisse P, Krause D, et al: Magnetic resonance imaging in the diagnosis of pulmonary infarction. Chest 99:298, 1991.
95. Bergin CJ, Hauschildt J, Rios G, et al: Accuracy of MR angiography compared with radionuclide scanning in identifying the cause of pulmonary arterial hypertension. Am J Roentgenol 168:1549, 1997.
96. Kelley MA, Carson JL, Palevsky HI, et al: Diagnosing pulmonary embolism: New facts and strategies. Ann Intern Med 114:300, 1991.
97. Stein PD, Hull RD, Saltzman HA, et al: Strategy for diagnosis of patients with suspected acute pulmonary embolism. Chest 103:1553, 1993.
98. Oudkerk M, van Beek EJR, van Putten WLJ, et al: Cost-effectiveness analysis of various strategies in the diagnostic management of pulmonary embolism. Arch Intern Med 153:947, 1993.

99. Weidner W, Swanson L, Wilson G: Roentgen techniques in the diagnosis of pulmonary thromboembolism. Am J Roentgenol 100:397, 1967.

100. Ormond RS, Gale HH, Drake EH, et al: Pulmonary angiography and pulmonary embolism. Radiology 86:658, 1966.

101. Bookstein JJ: Segmental arteriography in pulmonary embolism. Radiology 93:1007, 1969.

102. Gomes AS, Grollman JH, Mink J: Pulmonary angiography for pulmonary emboli: Rational selection of oblique views. Am J Roentgenol 129:1019, 1977.

103. Quinn MF, Lundell CJ, Klotz TA, et al: Reliability of selective pulmonary arteriography in the diagnosis of pulmonary embolism. Am J Roentgenol 149:469, 1987.

104. van Rooij WJ, den Heeten GJ, Sluzewski M: Pulmonary embolism: Diagnosis in 211 patients with use of selective pulmonary digital subtraction angiography with a flow-directed catheter. Radiology 195:793, 1995.

105. Nicod P, Peterson K, Levine M, al: Pulmonary angiography in severe chronic pulmonary hypertension. Ann Intern Med 107:565, 1987.

106. Pond GD, Ovitt TW, Capp MP: Comparison of conventional pulmonary angiography with intravenous digital subtraction angiography for pulmonary embolic disease. Radiology 147:345, 1983.

107. Musset D, Rosso J, Petitpretz P, et al: Acute pulmonary embolism: Diagnostic value of digital subtraction angiography. Radiology 166:455, 1988.

108. van Beek EJR, Bakker AJ, Reekers JA: Pulmonary embolism: Interobserver agreement in the interpretation of conventional angiographic and DSA images in patients with nondiagnostic lung scan results. Radiology 198:721, 1996.

109. Matsumoto AH, Tegtmeyer CJ: Contemporary diagnostic approaches to acute pulmonary emboli. Radiol Clin North Am 33:167, 1995.

110. van Rooij WJ, den Heeten GJ: Intra-arterial digital subtraction angiography of the pulmonary arteries using a flow-directed balloon catheter in the diagnosis of pulmonary embolism. Rofo Fortschr Geb Rontgenstr Neuen Bildgeb Verfahr 156:333, 1992.

111. Johnson MS, Stine SB, Shah H, et al: Possible pulmonary embolus: Evaluation with digital subtraction versus cut-film angiography—prospective study in 80 patients. Radiology 207:131, 1998.

112. Hagspiel KD, Polak JF, Grassi CJ, et al: Pulmonary embolism: Comparison of cut-film and digital pulmonary angiography. Radiology 207:139, 1998.

113. Schlueter FJ, Zuckerman DA, Horesh L, et al: Digital subtraction versus film-screen angiography for detecting acute pulmonary emboli: Evaluation in a porcine model. J Vasc Intern Radiol 8:1015, 1997.

114. Darcy MD: Pulmonary digital subtraction angiography: Ready for prime time. Radiology 207:11, 1998.

115. Schluger N, Henschke C, King T, et al: Diagnosis of pulmonary embolism at a large teaching hospital. J Thorac Imaging 9:180, 1994.

116. Cooper TJ, Hayward MWJ, Hartog M: Survey on the use of pulmonary scintigraphy and angiography for suspected pulmonary thromboembolism in the UK. Clin Radiol 43:243, 1991.

117. Hudson ER, Smith TP, McDermott VG, et al: Pulmonary angiography performed with Iopamidol: Complications in 1,434 patients. Radiology 198:61, 1996.

118. Mills SR, Jackson DC, Older RA, et al: The incidence, etiologies, and avoidance of complications of pulmonary angiography in a large series. Radiology 136:295, 1980.

119. Perlmutt LM, Braun SD, Newman GE, et al: Pulmonary arteriography in the high-risk patient. Radiology 162:187, 1987.

120. Dalen JE, Brooks HL, Johnson LW, et al: Pulmonary angiography in acute pulmonary embolism: Indications, techniques, and results in 367 patients. Am Heart J 81:175, 1971.

121. Nilsson T, Carlsson A, Måre K: Pulmonary angiography: A safe procedure with modern contrast media and technique. Eur Radiol 8:86, 1998.

122. Sagel SS, Greenspan RH: Nonuniform pulmonary arterial perfusion: Pulmonary embolism? Radiology 99:541, 1971.

123. Goldhaber SZ, Hennekens CH, Evans DA, et al: Factors associated wth correct antemortem diagnosis of major pulmonary embolism. Am J Med 73:822, 1982.

124. Auger WR, Fedullo PF, Moser KM, et al: Chronic major-vessel thromboembolic pulmonary artery obstruction: Appearance at angiography. Radiology 182:393, 1992.

125. Moser KM, Bloor CM: Pulmonary vascular lesions occurring in patients with chronic major vessel thromboembolic pulmonary hypertension. Chest 103:685, 1993.

126. Peterson KL, Fred HL, Alexander JK: Pulmonary arterial webs: A new angiographic sign of previous thromboembolism. N Engl J Med 277:33, 1967.

127. Weinmann EE, Salzman EW: Deep-vein thrombosis. N Engl J Med 331:1630, 1994.

128. Baxter GM: The role of ultrasound in deep venous thrombosis. Clin Radiol 52:1, 1997.

129. Hull RD, Hirsh J, Carter CJ, et al: Pulmonary angiography, ventilation lung scanning, and venography for clinically suspected pulmonary embolism with abnormal perfusion lung scan. Ann Intern Med 98:891, 1983.

130. Bell WR: Pulmonary embolism: Progress and problems. Am J Med 72:181, 1982.

131. Bettmann MA, Robbins A, Braun SD, et al: Contrast venography of the leg: Diagnostic efficacy, tolerance, and complication rates with ionic and nonionic contrast media. Radiology 165:113, 1987.

132. Lensing AWA, Prandoni P, Büller HR, et al: Lower extremity venography with Iohexol: Results and complications. Radiology 177:503, 1990.

133. McLachlan MSF, Thomas JG, Taylor DW, et al: Observer variation in the interpretation of lower limb venograms. Am J Roentgenol 132:227, 1979.

134. Aitken AGF, Godden DJ: Real time ultrasound diagnosis of deep vein thrombosis: A comparison with venography. Clin Radiol 38:309, 1987.

135. Cronan JJ, Dorfman GS, Scola FH, et al: Deep venous thrombosis: US assessment using vein compression. Radiology 162:191, 1987.

136. Rose SC, Zwiebel WJ, Nelson BD, et al: Symptomatic lower extremity deep venous thrombosis: Accuracy, limitations, and role of color duplex flow imaging in diagnosis. Radiology 175:639, 1990.

137. Lewis BD, Meredith JE, Welch TJ, et al: Diagnosis of acute deep venous thrombosis of the lower extremities: Prospective evaluation of color Doppler flow imaging versus venography. Radiology 192:651, 1994.

138. Moser KM, LeMoine JR: Is embolic risk conditioned by location of deep venous thrombosis? Ann Intern Med 94:439, 1981.

139. Baxter GM, Duffy P, Partridge E: Colour flow imaging of calf vein thrombosis. Clin Radiol 46:198, 1992.

140. Atri M, Herba MJ, Reinhold C, et al: Accuracy of sonography in the evaluation of calf deep vein thrombosis in both postoperative surveillance and symptomatic patients. Am J Roentgenol 166:1361, 1996.

141. Ginsberg JS, Caco CC, Brill-Edwards PA, et al: Venous thrombosis in patients who have undergone major hip or knee surgery: Detection with compression US and impedance plethysmography. Radiology 181:651, 1991.

142. Baldt MM, Zontsich T, Stümpflen A, et al: Deep venous thrombosis of the lower extremity: Efficacy of spiral CT venography compared with conventional venography in diagnosis. Radiology 200:423, 1996.

143. Stehling MK, Rosen MP, Weintraub J, et al: Spiral CT venography of the lower extremity. Am J Roentgenol 163:451, 1994.

144. Lomas DJ, Britton PD: CT demonstration of acute and chronic iliofemoral thrombosis. J Comput Assist Tomogr 15:861, 1991.

145. Spritzer CE, Sussman SK, Blinder RA, et al: Deep venous thrombosis evaluation with limited-flip-angle, gradient-refocused MR imaging: Preliminary experience. Radiology 166:371, 1988.

146. Erdman WA, Jayson HT, Redman HC, et al: Deep venous thrombosis of extremities: Role of MR imaging in the diagnosis. Radiology 174:425, 1990.

147. Evans AJ, Sostman HD, Knelson MH, et al: Detection of deep venous thrombosis: Prospective comparison of MR imaging with contrast venography. Am J Roentgenol 161:131, 1993.

148. Spritzer CE, Norconk JJ Jr, Sostman HD, et al: Detection of deep venous thrombosis by magnetic resonance imaging. Chest 104:54, 1993.

149. Browse NL: Prophylaxis of pulmonary embolism. BMJ 2:780, 1970.

150. Davis HH, Heaton WA, Siegel BA, et al: Scintigraphic detection of atherosclerotic lesions and venous thrombi in man by indium-111 labelled autologous platelets. Lancet 1:1185, 1978.

151. Sostman HD, Neumann RD, Loke J, et al: Detection of pulmonary embolism in man with 111 In-labeled autologous platelets. Am J Roentgenol 138:945, 1982.

152. Gomes AS, Webber MM, Buffkin D: Contrast venography vs. radio-nuclide venography: A study of discrepancies and their possible significance. Radiology 142:719, 1982.

153. Ryo UY, Qazi M, Srikantaswamy S, et al: Radionuclide venography: Correlation with contrast venography. J Nucl Med 18:11, 1977.

154. Butler SP, Boyd SJ, Parker SZ: Technetium-99m-modified recombinant tissue plasminogen activator to detect deep venous thrombosis. J Nucl Med 37:744, 1996.

155. Breckenridge RT, Ratnoff OD: Pulmonary embolism and unexpected death in supposedly normal persons. N Engl J Med 270:298, 1964.

156. Cooley RN: Pulmonary thromboembolism—the case for the pulmonary angiogram. Am J Roentgenol 92:693, 1964.

157. Fred HL, Harle TS: Septic pulmonary embolism. Dis Chest 55:483, 1969.

158. Jaffe RB, Koschmann EB: Septic pulmonary emboli. Radiology 96:527, 1970.

159. Roberts WC, Buchbinder NA: Right-sided valvular infective endocarditis: A clinicopathologic study of twelve necropsy patients. Am J Med 53:7, 1972.

160. Iwama T, Shigemaatsu S, Asami K, et al: Tricuspid valve endocarditis with large vegetations in a non-drug addict without underlying cardiac disease. Intern Med 35:203, 1996.

161. Clifford CP, Eykyn SJ, Oakley CM: Staphylococcal tricuspid valve endocarditis in patients with structurally normal hearts and no evidence of narcotic abuse. QJM 87:755, 1994.

162. Bain RC, Edwards JE, Scheifley CH, et al: Right-sided bacterial endocarditis and endarteritis: A clinical and pathologic study. Am J Med 24:98, 1958.

163. Weesner CL, Cisek JE: Lemierre syndrome: The forgotten disease. Ann Emerg Med 22:256, 1993.

164. Ahkee S, Srinath L, Huang A, et al: Lemierre's syndrome: Postanginal sepsis due to anaerobic oropharyngeal infection. Ann Otol Rhinol Laryngol 103:208, 1994.

165. Huang RM, Naidich DP, Lubat E, et al: Septic pulmonary emboli: CT-radiographic correlation. Am J Roentgenol 153:41, 1989.

166. Gumbs RV, McCauley DI: Hilar and mediastinal adenopthy in septic pulmonary embolic disease. Radiology 142:313, 1982.

167. Kuhlman JE, Fishman EK, Teigen C: Pulmonary septic emboli: Diagnosis with CT. Radiology 174:211, 1990.

168. Dreyer ZE: Chest infections and syndromes in sickle cell disease of childhood. Semin Respir Infect 11:163, 1996.

169. Verdegem TD, Yee SJ: Lung disease in sickle cell anemia: A tropical disease with a twist. Semin Respir Med 12:107, 1991.

170. Bhalla M, Abboud MR, McLoud TC, et al: Acute chest syndrome in sickle cell disease: CT evidence of microvascular occlusion. Radiology 187:45, 1993.

171. Cockshott WP: Rib infarcts in sickling disease. Eur J Radiol 14:63, 1992.

172. Haupt H, Moore GW, Bauer TW, et al: The lung in sickle cell disease. Chest 81:332, 1982.

173. Aquino SL, Gamsu G, Fahy JV, et al: Chronic pulmonary disorders in sickle cell disease: Findings at thin-section CT. Radiology 193:807, 1994.

174. Dudney TM, Elliott CG: Pulmonary embolism from amniotic fluid, fat and air. Prog Cardiovasc Dis 36:447, 1994.

175. King MB, Harmon KR: Unusual forms of pulmonary embolism. Clin Chest Med 15:561, 1994.

176. Richards RR: Fat embolism syndrome. Can J Surg 40:334, 1997.

177. Johnson MJ, Lucas GL: Fat embolism syndrome. Orthopedics 19:41, 1996.

178. Benatar SR, Ferguson AD, Goldschmidt RB: Fat embolism—some clinical observations and a review of controversial aspects. QJM 41:85, 1972.

179. Sevitt S: Fat Embolism. London, Butterworths, 1962.

180. Thompson PL, Williams KE, Walters MN-I: Fat embolism in the microcirculation: An in-vivo study. J Pathol 97:23, 1969.

181. Hallgren B, Kerstall J, Rudenstam C-M, et al: A method for the isolation and chemical analysis of pulmonary fat embolism. Acta Chir Scand 132:613, 1966.

182. Peltier LF: Fat embolism: III. The toxic properties of neutral fat and free fatty acids. Surgery 40:665, 1956.

183. Glas WW, Grekin TD, Musselman MM: Fat embolism. Am J Surg 85:363, 1953.

184. Berrigan TJ Jr, Carsky EW, Heitzman ER: Fat embolism: Roentgenographic pathologic correlation in 3 cases. Am J Roentgenol 96:967, 1966.

185. Heitzman ER: The Lung: Radiologic-Pathologic Correlations. St. Louis, CV Mosby, 1973.

186. Curtis A McB, Knowles GD, Putnam CE, et al: The three syndromes of fat embolism: Pulmonary manifestations. Yale J Biol Med 52:149, 1979.

187. Maruyama Y, Little JP: Roentgen manifestations of traumatic pulmonary fat embolism. Radiology 79:945, 1962.

188. Williams JR, Bonte FJ: Pulmonary damage in nonpenetrating chest injuries. Radiol Clin North Am 1:439, 1963.

189. Hamrick-Turner J, Abbitt PL, Harrison RB, et al: Diffuse lung calcifications following fat emboli and adult respiratory distress syndromes: CT findings. J Thorac Imaging 9:47, 1994.

190. Thomas ML, Tighe JR: Death from fat embolism as a complication of intraosseous phlebography. Lancet 2:1415, 1973.

191. Peter RE, Schopfer A, Le Coultre B, et al: Fat embolism and death during prophylactic osteosynthesis of a metastatic femur using an unreamed femoral nail. J Orthop Trauma 11:233, 1997.

192. Burgher LW, Dines DE, Linscheid RL: Fat embolism and the adult respiratory distress syndrome. Mayo Clin Proc 49:107, 1974.

193. Hoare EM: Platelet response in fat embolism and its relationship to petechiae. BMJ 2:689, 1971.

194. Tachakra SS: Distribution of skin petechiae in fat embolism rash. Lancet 1:284, 1976.

195. Masson RG: Amniotic fluid embolism. Clin Chest Med 13:657, 1992.

196. Philip RS: Amniotic fluid embolism. N Y State J Med 67:2085, 1967.

197. Clark SL, Hankins GD, Dudley DA, et al: Amniotic fluid embolism: Analysis of the national registry. Am J Obstet Gynecol 172:1158, 1995.

198. Peterson EP, Taylor HB: Amniotic fluid embolism: An analysis of 40 cases. Obstet Gynecol 35:787, 1970.

199. Lumley J, Owen R, Morgan M: Amniotic fluid embolism: A report of three cases. Anaesthesia 34:33, 1979.

200. Fidler JL, Patz EF Jr, Ravin CE: Cardiopulmonary complications of pregnancy: Radiographic findings. Am J Roentgenol 161:937, 1993.

201. Paré JA, Fraser RG, Hogg JC, et al: Pulmonary "mainline" granulomatosis: Talcosis of intravenous methadone abuse. Medicine 58:229, 1979.

202. Paré JP, Cote G, Fraser RS: Long-term follow-up of drug abusers with intravenous talcosis. Am Rev Respir Dis 139:233, 1989.

203. Douglas RG, Kafilmout KJ, Patt NL: Foreign particle embolism in drug addicts: Respiratory pathophysiology. Ann Intern Med 75:865, 1971.

204. Hopkins GB: Pulmonary angiothrombotic granulomatosis in drug offenders. JAMA 221:909, 1972.

205. Siegel H, Bloustein P: Continuing studies in the diagnosis and pathology of death from intravenous narcotism. J Forensic Sci 15:179, 1970.

206. Feigin DS: Talc: Understanding its manifestations in the chest. Am J Roentgenol 146:295, 1986.

207. Genereux GP, Emson HE: Talc granulomatosis and angiothrombotic pulmonary hypertension in drug addicts. J Can Assoc Radiol 25:87, 1974.

208. Robertson CH Jr, Reynolds RC, Wilson JE: Pulmonary hypertension and foreign-body granulomas in intravenous drug abusers: Documentation by cardiac catheterization and lung biopsy. Am J Med 61:657, 1976.

209. Farber HW, Fairman RP, Glauser FL: Talc granulomatosis: Laboratory findings similar to sarcoidosis. Am Rev Respir Dis 125:258, 1982.

210. Brown DG, Aguirre A, Weaver A: Gallium-67 scanning in talc-induced pulmonary granulomatosis. Chest 77:561, 1980.

211. Padley SPG, Adler BD, Staples CA, et al: Pulmonary talcosis: CT findings in three cases. Radiology 186:125, 1993.

212. Stern EJ, Frank MS, Schmutz JF, et al: Panlobular pulmonary emphysema caused by IV injection of methylphenidate (Ritalin): Findings on chest radiographs and CT scans. Am J Roentgenol 162:555, 1994.

213. Drucker EA, Rivitz SM, Shepard J-AO, et al: Acute pulmonary embolism: Assessment of helical CT for diagnosis. Radiology 209:235, 1998.

214. Kim K-I, Müller NL, Mayo JR: Clinically suspected pulmonary embolism: Utility of spiral CT. Radiology 210:693, 1999.

215. Garg K, Sieler H, Welsh CH, et al: Clinical validity of helical CT

being interpreted as negative for pulmonary embolism: Implications for patient treatment. Am J Roentgenol 172:1627, 1999.

216. Stein PD, Henry JW, Gottschalk A: Reassessment of pulmonary angiography for the diagnosis of pulmonary embolism: Relation of interpreter agreement to the order of the involved pulmonary arterial branch. Radiology 210:689, 1999.

217. Shah AA, Davis SD, Gamsu G, et al: Parenchymal and pleural findings in patients with and patients without acute pulmonary embolism detected at spiral CT. Radiology 211:147, 1999.

218. Gupta A, Frazer CK, Ferguson JM, et al: Acute pulmonary embolism: Diagnosis with MR angiography. Radiology 210:353, 1999.

219. Fraser JD, Anderson DR: Deep venous thrombosis: Recent advances and optimal investigation with US. Radiology 211:9, 1999.

220. Gottlieb RH, Widjaja J, Mehra S, et al: Clinically important pulmonary emboli: Does calf vein US alter outcomes? Radiology 211:25, 1999.

221. Vaccaro JP, Cronan JJ, Dorfman GS: Outcome analysis of patients with normal compression US examinations. Radiology 179:443, 1990.

222. Heyneman LE, Müller NL: Pulmonary nodules in early fat embolism syndrome: A case report. J Thorac Imaging 15:71, 2000.

223. Demeter S, Raymond GS, Puttagunta L, et al: Intravenous pulmonary talcosis with complicating massive fibrosis. Can Assoc Radiol J 50:413, 1999.

224. Ward S, Heyneman LE, Reittner P, et al: Talcosis secondary to IV abuse of oral medications: CT findings. Am J Roentgenol 174:789, 2000.

225. Miniati M, Prediletto R, Formichi B, et al: Accuracy of clinical assessment in the diagnosis of pulmonary embolism. Am J Respir Crit Care Med 159:864, 1999.

226. Stein PD, Gottschalk A: Review of criteria appropriate for a very low probability of pulmonary embolism on ventilation-perfusion lung scans: A position paper. Radiographics 20:99, 2000.

227. Blachere H, Latrabe V, Montaudon M, et al: Pulmonary embolism revealed on helical CT angiography: Comparison with ventilation-perfusion radionuclide lung scanning. Am J Roentgenol 174:1041, 2000.

228. Sheiman RG, McArdle CR: Clinically suspected pulmonary embolism: Use of bilateral lower extremity US as the initial examination—a prospective study. Radiology 212:75, 1999.

229. Loud PA, Katz DS, Klippenstein DL, et al: Combined CT venography and pulmonary angiography in suspected thromboembolic disease: Diagnostic accuracy for deep venous evaluation. Am J Roentgenol 174:61, 2000.

230. Yankelevitz DF, Gamsu G, Shah A, et al: Optimization of combined CT pulmonary angiography with lower extremity CT venography. Am J Roentgenol 174:67, 2000.

231. Libby LS, King TE, LaForce FM, et al: Pulmonary cavitation following pulmonary infarction. Medicine 64:342, 1985.

232. Rydberg J, Buckwalter KA, Caldemeyer KS, et al: Multisection CT: Scanning techniques and clinical applications. RadioGraphics 20:1787, 2000.

233. Qanadli SD, Hajjam ME, Mesurolle B, et al: Pulmonary embolism detection: Prospective evaluation of dual-section helical CT versus selective pulmonary arteriography in 157 patients. Radiology 217:447, 2000.

234. Baile EM, King GG, Müller NL, et al: Spiral computed tomography is comparable to angiography for the diagnosis of pulmonary embolism. Am J Respir Crit Care Med 161:1010, 2000.

235. Goodman LR, Lipchik RJ, Kuzo RS, et al: Subsequent pulmonary embolism: Risk after a negative helical CT pulmonary angiogram—prospective comparison with scintigraphy. Radiology 215:535, 2000.

236. Garg K, Kemp JL, Wojcik D, et al: Thromboembolic disease: Comparison of combined CT pulmonary angiography and venography with bilateral leg sonography in 70 patients. Am J Roentgenol 175:997, 2000.

237. Duwe KM, Shiau M, Budorick NE, et al: Evaluation of the lower extremity veins in patients with suspected pulmonary embolism: A retrospective comparison of helical CT venography and sonography. Am J Roentgenol 175:1525, 2000.

238. Cham MD, Yankelevitz DF, Shaham D, et al: Deep vein thrombosis: Detection by using indirect CT venography. Radiology 216:744, 2000.

CHAPTER 13

Pulmonary Hypertension

GENERAL FEATURES OF PULMONARY HYPERTENSION

Pulmonary arterial hypertension is an increase in pressure above normally accepted values in the main pulmonary artery at rest or during exercise as measured with a catheter. The generally accepted normal upper limits for these pressures are 30 mm Hg systolic and 18 mm Hg mean.[1] Pulmonary venous hypertension is present when the pressure in the pulmonary veins measured indirectly by a catheter wedged in a pulmonary artery exceeds 12 mm Hg. Slight increases in pulmonary arterial pressure generally cause no clinical, radiographic, or electrocardiographic abnormalities, even with mean pressures of 24 mm Hg.[2] As the pressure rises, however, the increased impedance to right ventricular ejection produces clinical and electrocardiographic signs and, eventually, radiologic changes indicative of hypertrophy of the right ventricle. With a further increase in pressure, catheterization studies may show elevation not only of pulmonary arterial and right ventricular systolic pressures, but also of right ven-

tricular diastolic pressure, indicating the presence of right ventricular failure.

The pressure drop across any vascular bed is related directly to blood flow and viscosity; an increase in either of these causes an increase in pressure for any given vascular geometry. The pressure across the vascular bed also is related indirectly to the radius of its vessels; the total cross-sectional area of the pulmonary vasculature can decrease because of loss or intraluminal occlusion of vessels, vascular smooth muscle contraction and shortening, or vascular wall thickening and remodeling. Pulmonary arterial pressure can be increased as a result of an increase in the downstream or venous pressure.

It is useful conceptually to divide the causes of pulmonary hypertension into three groups, each of which possesses different clinical, physiologic, and radiologic characteristics (Table 13–1): (1) causes in which the major mechanisms of production are precapillary in location, (2) causes in which the significant physiologic disturbance arises from disease in the postcapillary vessels, and (3) causes in which the hypertension reflects a disturbance in vessels on both sides of the capillary bed—combined precapillary and postcapillary hypertension. In each of these groups, the capillaries may be involved to some extent and may contribute considerably to the increase in vascular resistance. A major contribution to increased pulmonary vascular resistance in emphysema is the destruction of the capillary bed; chronic pericapillary edema can be associated with fibrosis, limiting distensibility of the capillary bed in postcapillary venous hypertension.

The radiologic manifestations differ somewhat depending on the cause of the hypertension; however, some findings are common to all causes. These findings are described here; additional features specific to individual causes are discussed in the appropriate sections.

Radiologic Manifestations

Radiography. The characteristic radiologic features of pulmonary arterial hypertension consist of enlargement of the central arteries and rapid tapering of the vessels as they extend to the periphery of the lungs (Table 13–2, Fig. 13–1). This discordance in caliber between central and peripheral vessels is a distinctive feature of pulmonary arterial hypertension regardless of etiology.[5, 6] The heart may be normal in size or enlarged. An unusual manifestation of severe chronic hypertension (most often in association with Eisenmenger's syndrome) is the presence of vas-

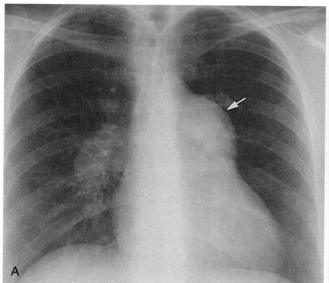

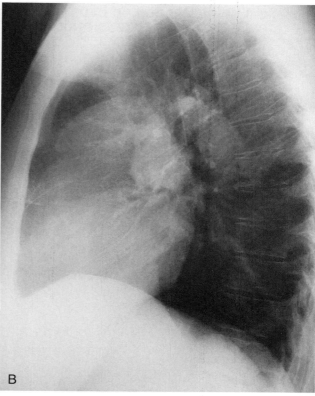

Figure 13–1. Pulmonary Arterial Hypertension. Posteroanterior *(A)* and lateral *(B)* chest radiographs show enlargement of the central pulmonary arteries with rapid tapering of the vessels. On the posteroanterior view, marked enlargement of the main pulmonary artery results in a focal convexity *(arrow)* immediately below the level of the aortic arch. On the lateral view, right ventricular enlargement and dilation of the pulmonary outflow tract result in filling of the lower retrosternal air space. The patient was a 36-year-old woman who had primary pulmonary arterial hypertension.

cular calcification. This calcification usually is located in the main pulmonary artery and its hilar branches; occasionally, it affects the lobar vessels.[7]

Enlargement of the hilar arteries can be assessed by measuring the diameter of the interlobar arteries. The upper limit of the transverse diameter of the right interlobar artery from its lateral aspect to the air column of the intermediate bronchus is 16 mm in men and 15 mm in women.[8] Because the transverse diameter of the left interlobar artery often is impossible to measure on a conventional posteroanterior radiograph, a useful alternative is to measure the vessel on a lateral radiograph from the circular lucency created by the left upper lobe bronchus viewed end-on to the posterior margin of the vessel as it loops over the bronchus; the accepted upper limit of normal for this measurement is 18 mm.

Although the presence of pulmonary arterial hypertension can be recognized radiographically, the sensitivity and degree of accuracy with which its severity can be estimated are controversial.[4, 9, 11] Measurements of the interlobar pulmonary arteries are affected by the variable magnification related to patient size, distance between the x-ray tube and the film, and distance between the pulmonary artery and the film. Accurate measurement may be difficult or impossible in the presence of extensive parenchymal lung disease. Assessment of vascular pruning is subjective, and the degree of pruning does not correlate well with the level of pulmonary hypertension.[13] Rapid tapering usually is a late manifestation, being seen less commonly than enlargement of the central pulmonary arteries in patients who have pulmonary hypertension.[10, 12]

Computed Tomography. Because the main pulmonary artery is intrapericardial, it cannot be measured on conventional radiography; however, it can identified readily on computed tomography (CT) and magnetic resonance (MR) imaging. In a study of 32 patients who had cardiopulmonary disease and 26 age-matched and sex-matched control subjects believed but not proved to have normal pulmonary arterial pressure, the upper limit diameter of the main pulmonary artery in normal subjects was 28.6 mm; in a patient group in which diameters correlated with data from cardiac catheterization, a diameter of the main pulmonary artery greater than 29 mm predicted the presence of pulmonary arterial hypertension.[14]

In another investigation, the findings on CT were compared with those at right heart catheterization in 55 patients being assessed for lung and heart-lung transplantation.[15] The study included 45 patients who had chronic lung disease, including emphysema, idiopathic pulmonary fibrosis, sarcoidosis, systemic sclerosis, cystic fibrosis, and lymphangioleiomyomatosis, and 10 patients who had pulmonary vascular disease (primary pulmonary hypertension, Eisenmenger's syndrome, and chronic thromboembolism). In this study, the cut-off diameter of the main pulmonary artery at or below which there was a 95% certainty of normal mean pressure was 28 mm. Because the diameter in patients who had normal mean arterial pressure ranged from 22 to 36 mm, however, the researchers concluded that the cut-off of 28 mm had questionable clinical utility. Multiple regression analysis revealed that the combination of main and left pulmonary artery cross-sectional area normalized for body surface area showed the best correla-

Table 13–1. MECHANISMS AND CAUSES OF PULMONARY HYPERTENSION

PRECAPILLARY HYPERTENSION
Primary vascular disease
    Increased flow (unrestricted left-to-right shunts)
    Decreased flow (tetralogy of Fallot)
    Primary pulmonary hypertension
    Multiple pulmonary artery stenoses or coarctation[2]
    Compression of the main pulmonary artery or its branches
    Pulmonary thrombotic and embolic disease
        Thromboembolism
        In situ thrombosis
        Metastatic neoplasm
        Parasites
        Miscellaneous (e.g., fat, talc, amniotic fluid)
    Human immunodeficiency virus infection
    Pulmonary capillary hemangiomatosis
    Immunologic abnormalities (e.g., systemic lupus erythematosus,
        progressive systemic sclerosis)
    High altitude
Pleuropulmonary disease
    Emphysema
    Bronchiectasis, bronchiolitis, and cystic fibrosis
    Postpulmonary resection
    Pleural disease (fibrothorax)
    Chest wall deformities
        Thoracoplasty
        Kyphoscoliosis
Alveolar hypoventilation
    Neuromuscular disease
    Obesity
    Obstructive sleep apnea
    Idiopathic (Ondine's curse)
POSTCAPILLARY HYPERTENSION
Cardiac disease
    Left ventricular failure
    Mitral valve disease
    Myxoma (or thrombus) of the left atrium
    Cor triatriatum
Pulmonary venous disease
    Congenital stenosis of the pulmonary veins
    Fibrosing mediastinitis
    Idiopathic veno-occlusive disease
    Anomalous pulmonary venous return
    Neoplasms
    Thrombosis

tion with mean pulmonary artery pressure ($r = 0.81$). The multiple regression equations helped predict mean arterial pressure within 5 mm Hg in 50% of patients who had chronic lung disease but in only 8% of patients who had pulmonary vascular disease. Right interlobar artery diameter did not correlate well with pulmonary arterial pressure; it was postulated that this might have been the result of difficulty in measuring accurately the diameter of the artery because of associated parenchymal lung disease or lymphadenopathy.

In another study of 36 patients who had pulmonary arterial hypertension, main pulmonary artery diameter measurements on CT were correlated with right heart hemodynamic data.[16] Of patients, 20 had hypertension secondary to interstitial lung disease; 4, to chronic obstructive pulmonary disease (COPD); 7, to chronic thromboembolism; and 3, to portal hypertension. Two patients had primary pulmonary hypertension. Nine patients who had normal pulmonary artery pressure were used as controls. A main pulmonary artery diameter on CT equal to or greater than 29 mm had a sensitivity of 87%, a specificity of 89%, and

a positive predictive value of 97% for pulmonary arterial hypertension. There was no linear correlation between the degree of hypertension and main pulmonary artery diameter.

Based on the results of these various studies, we believe that a main pulmonary artery diameter greater than 29 mm is suggestive but not diagnostic of hypertension or increased pulmonary blood flow as a result of a left-to-right shunt. It has been suggested that a segmental artery-to-bronchus diameter ratio greater than 1 in three or more lobes is helpful in predicting the presence of pulmonary arterial hypertension.[16]

A simple and practical method to determine whether the diameter of the main pulmonary artery is increased on CT is to compare its diameter with that of the ascending thoracic aorta at the same level.[17] One group of investigators determined whether the main pulmonary artery-to-thoracic aorta diameter ratio was predictive of pulmonary arterial hypertension in 50 patients.[17] The patients had a wide range of pulmonary and cardiovascular diseases and had undergone pulmonary artery pressure measurements at right heart catheterization. A main pulmonary artery diameter greater than that of the ascending aorta was present in 20 of 37 patients who had pulmonary arterial hypertension (sensitivity 70%) and only 1 of 13 patients who had normal arterial pressure (specificity 92%).[17] There was good correlation between the main pulmonary artery-to-thoracic aorta diameter ratio and the mean pulmonary artery pressure ($r = 0.74$).

Patients who have severe pulmonary arterial hypertension have been shown to have small to moderate degrees of pericardial effusion or thickening.[18, 19] In one investigation of 45 patients who underwent catheterization and CT of the chest, 8 of 15 (53%) who had severe hypertension (mean pressure >35 mm Hg) had abnormal pericardial thickness (>2 mm) because of thickening or effusion.[19] This finding was not seen in any of the patients who had mild or moderate hypertension.

Echocardiography. The most accurate noninvasive method of assessing the presence of pulmonary arterial hypertension is echocardiography. Many variables derived from continuous wave or pulsed Doppler echocardiography can be employed to determine right ventricular peak systolic pressure, which is used as an estimate of pulmonary artery pressure. These variables include calculation of the transtricuspid or transpulmonary valve pressure gradient based on the velocity of the tricuspid or pulmonary regurgitant jets, the evaluation of right ventricular outflow tract

Table 13–2. PULMONARY ARTERIAL HYPERTENSION

Systolic PA pressure >30 mm Hg
    Mean PA pressure >18 mm Hg
Radiologic manifestations
    Enlarged central pulmonary arteries
    Right interlobar artery diameter
        >16 mm in men
        >15 mm in women
    Rapid tapering of vessels
    Diameter of main PA >29 mm (as measured on CT or
        MR imaging)

PA, posteroanterior.

velocity profiles, and the measurement of right ventricular isovolumic relaxation time.[20–22] The use of the tricuspid regurgitant jet probably is the most accurate.

In one study of 100 patients who had pulmonary hypertension secondary to COPD, standard echocardiographic assessment was found to be useful for estimation of pulmonary artery pressure in 30.[20] The number of patients in whom the technique can be employed successfully is increased by injecting a small bolus of agitated saline into a peripheral vein during the test. The saline bolus contains microbubbles, which act as an echocardiographic contrast agent to enhance the detection of small tricuspid regurgitant jets.[23] Using data derived from measurements of pulmonary valve regurgitation, one group reported a correlation of pulmonary artery diastolic pressure and Doppler-derived end-diastolic pressure gradient of 0.91.[24] Using a different approach, another group of investigators found that a combination of right ventricular dimensions, reflecting the presence of chronic pulmonary hypertension, correlated significantly ($r = 0.97$) with mean pulmonary artery pressure in a group of patients who had COPD.[25, 26]

An advantage of the echocardiographic assessment of pulmonary hemodynamics is that the dynamic response of the pulmonary circulation and right side of the heart can be assessed by performing the measurements during increased cardiac work in response to exercise or to an inotropic agent (stress echocardiography).[27] Although the echocardiographic technique may underestimate true peak pulmonary artery pressure in patients who have severe hypertension, it is accurate enough to categorize patients as having mild, moderate, or severe disease.[28] Transesophageal echocardiography is more sensitive than transthoracic echocardiography in detecting the site of intracardiac shunts in patients who present with pulmonary hypertension of unknown cause[29] and often provides additional hemodynamic data in patients who have severe pulmonary hypertension and are being considered for lung transplantation.[30]

Magnetic Resonance Imaging. MR imaging can be used to define the direction and velocity of blood flow within the cardiac chambers and great vessels in addition to providing images of cardiovascular structure (Fig. 13–2).[31] Reviews of MR imaging in pulmonary hypertension and right ventricular dysfunction and in congenital heart disease have been published.[32, 33] The procedure has been shown to predict accurately right heart hemodynamics in patients who have primary pulmonary hypertension.[34] Velocity-encoded cine gradient-echo MR imaging can provide two-dimensional velocity maps of the cross-sectional area of a vessel. Peak systolic pulmonary artery blood velocity estimated by this method correlates well with that measured using Doppler echocardiography;[35] it also shows substantial differences in velocity across the vascular lumen in patients who have pulmonary hypertension. Using MR imaging estimates of pulmonary blood flow ejection velocity, pulmonary arterial pressure has been estimated noninvasively ($r = 0.82$) in a small group of 12 patients who had different pulmonary vascular abnormalities.[36]

One group of investigators compared the cardiac output and indices of pulmonary arterial blood flow estimated by velocity-encoded MR imaging with cardiac output and pulmonary vascular resistance measured at right heart catheterization in 19 patients.[37] There was good correlation ($r = 0.87$) between estimates of cardiac output obtained by velocity-encoded MR imaging and by right heart catheterization. There was good correlation between various MR estimates of pulmonary arterial blood flow and pulmonary vascular resistance measured at catheterization ($r = 0.65$ to 0.89).[37] In another group of 12 subjects who had primary pulmonary hypertension, the mean pulmonary artery-to-aortic caliber ratio was found to correlate significantly with the degree of hypertension ($r = 0.7$).[38] MR imaging has been employed to make measurements of end-systolic and end-diastolic right ventricular volume and to calculate ejection volume and fraction;[39, 40] MR imaging may be useful as a noninvasive supplemental method for evaluating patent ductus arteriosus and pulmonary arterial dissection.[41]

Ventilation-Perfusion Scintigraphy. The role of ventilation-perfusion scintigraphy in patients who have pulmonary hypertension is mainly in distinguishing primary pulmonary hypertension from hypertension associated with chronic thromboembolism, a normal or low-probability scan virtually excluding the latter process. In one study of 75 patients, 24 of 25 (96%) who had chronic thromboembolic disease had high-probability scans, and 1 patient had an intermediate-probability scan;[42] by contrast, of 35 patients who had primary pulmonary hypertension, 33 (94%) had low-probability scans, 1 had an intermediate-probability scan, and 1 had a high-probability scan. Ten of 15 (67%) patients who had nonthromboembolic secondary pulmonary arterial hypertension had low-probability scans, 3 (20%) had intermediate-probability scans, and 2 (13%) had high-probability scans. In patients who have intermediate-probability or high-probability scans, the diagnosis of chronic thromboembolic disease usually can be confirmed using contrast-enhanced spiral CT (Fig. 13–3).[43–45] Preliminary results suggest a role for MR imaging in the assessment of these patients (*see* Fig. 13–3).[46] In a few patients, angiography may be required for definitive diagnosis.

Although fatalities have been reported after lung scanning in patients who have primary pulmonary hypertension,[47, 48] none of the 163 patients who had perfusion scans in the National Institutes of Health (NIH) study reported adverse effects.[11] Similarly, although it has been said that patients who have severe pulmonary hypertension are subject to sudden death during or after cardiac catheterization,[50] only 1 of the 50 patients who had pulmonary angiography in the NIH study had an adverse effect (transient hypotension). Complications are reduced by performing selective left and right main pulmonary artery injections.[51] In one study in which this procedure was performed in 67 consecutive patients who had pulmonary hypertension, either primary or secondary to chronic thromboembolism, no major disturbances in cardiac rhythm, no episodes of significant systemic hypotension, and no fatalities were reported; this approach has become the standard.

PRECAPILLARY PULMONARY HYPERTENSION

Primary Vascular Disease

Increased Flow

Included in this category are the congenital heart defects with left-to-right shunt (atrial septal defect, ventricular septal defect, patent ductus arteriosus, aorticopulmonary window, transposition of the great vessels, and partial anomalous pulmonary venous drainage) and conditions associated

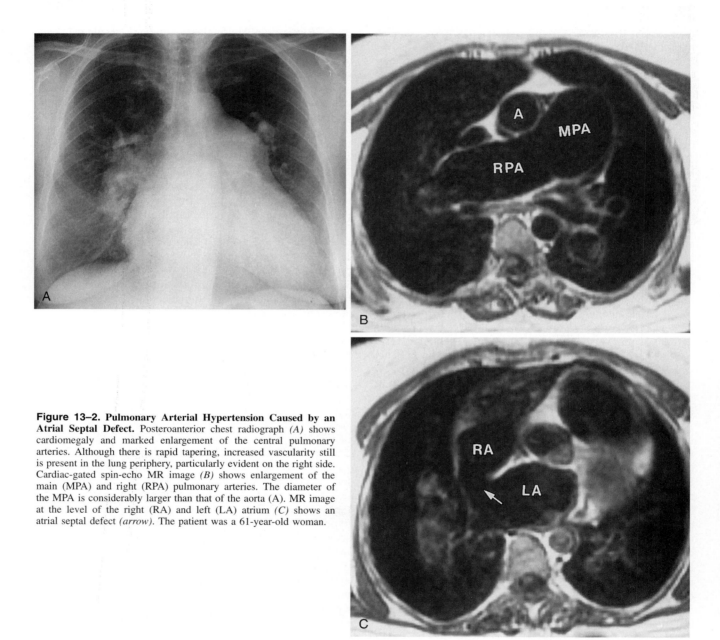

Figure 13–2. Pulmonary Arterial Hypertension Caused by an Atrial Septal Defect. Posteroanterior chest radiograph *(A)* shows cardiomegaly and marked enlargement of the central pulmonary arteries. Although there is rapid tapering, increased vascularity still is present in the lung periphery, particularly evident on the right side. Cardiac-gated spin-echo MR image *(B)* shows enlargement of the main (MPA) and right (RPA) pulmonary arteries. The diameter of the MPA is considerably larger than that of the aorta (A). MR image at the level of the right (RA) and left (LA) atrium *(C)* shows an atrial septal defect *(arrow)*. The patient was a 61-year-old woman.

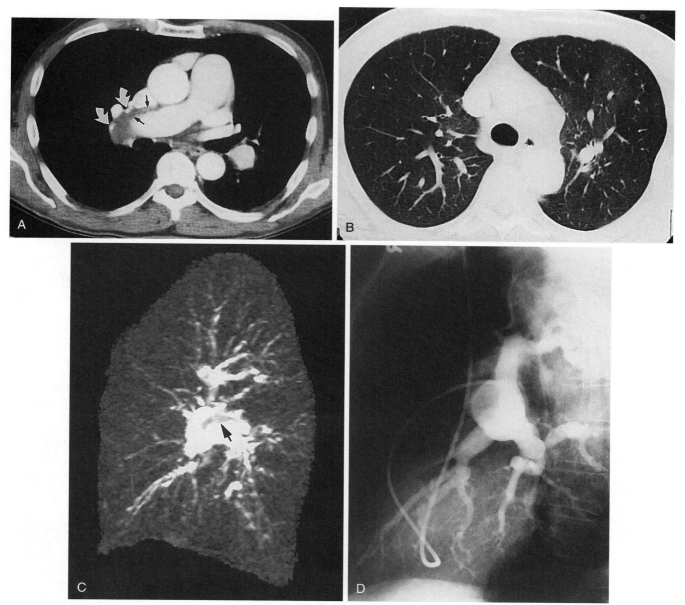

Figure 13–3. Thromboembolic Pulmonary Arterial Hypertension. Contrast-enhanced spiral CT scan *(A)* in a 65-year-old man with pulmonary arterial hypertension shows a thrombus within the right pulmonary artery *(straight arrows)*. The thrombus is contiguous with the arterial wall, a finding that is characteristic of an organized embolus. Focal calcification of the intima also is evident *(curved arrows)*. Lung windows *(B)* show localized areas with decreased attenuation and vascularity and areas with increased attenuation and vascularity (a pattern known as *mosaic perfusion*). This pattern is seen in most patients who have pulmonary arterial hypertension secondary to chronic thromboembolism. Sagittal gradient-recalled-echo (GRE) MR image *(C)* shows thrombus lining the upper aspect of the right pulmonary artery *(arrow)*. Abnormal segmental vessels are evident in the right upper and lower lobes. Sagittal view of a selective right pulmonary angiogram *(D)* shows corresponding abnormal segmental vessels. (Courtesy of Dr. Colleen Bergin, University of California, San Diego Medical Center.)

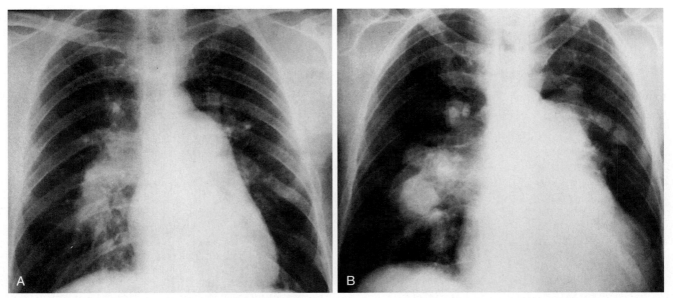

Figure 13–4. Eisenmenger's Syndrome Caused by Atrial Septal Defect. This man presented for the first time at age 32 with a history of increasing shortness of breath on exertion. Radiograph *(A)* showed marked enlargement of the hilar pulmonary arteries, which tapered rapidly as they proceeded distally. The peripheral vasculature was diminished, and the size and configuration of the heart were consistent with cor pulmonale. Cardiac catheterization revealed a secundum-type atrial septal defect. Pressures in the main pulmonary artery were 113/42 mm Hg, and pressures in the ascending aorta were 99/56 mm Hg. Eleven years later *(B)*, the main pulmonary arteries and the heart had undergone remarkable enlargement; the peripheral oligemia was much more evident. The patient showed severe cyanosis and polycythemia. Despite supportive therapy, the patient died shortly after this examination. At autopsy, the lumen of the main pulmonary artery was considerably larger than that of the ascending aorta. Mural thrombi were present in the major pulmonary arteries.

with an increase in total blood volume or cardiac output, or both, such as thyrotoxicosis and chronic renal failure. A relative increase in pulmonary blood flow caused by extensive lung resection can result in hypertension, presumably by similar mechanisms.[52]

Pulmonary arterial flow may be increased greatly for extended periods before increased resistance results in hypertension. It is assumed that the elevated resistance is caused initially by an increase in vasomotor tone and subsequently is related to irreversible morphologic changes in the vasculature. Ultimately, left-to-right shunting can lead to the development of severe irreversible pulmonary arterial hypertension with dilation of the central pulmonary arteries and reversal of the left-to-right shunt at the atrial, ventricular, or aorticopulmonary level (Eisenmenger's syndrome).[53]

Many patients who have left-to-right shunts are asymptomatic. If the shunt is large, some physical underdevelopment and a tendency to respiratory infections may occur. The patient may complain of fatigue, palpitations, and dyspnea on exertion and may exhibit signs of cardiac failure.

Radiologic Manifestations

The main radiographic sign associated with increased flow is an increase in caliber of the pulmonary arteries throughout the lungs. Because the hemodynamic change is one of increased flow, the degree of enlargement of the main and hilar pulmonary arteries usually is proportional to the degree of distention of the intrapulmonary vessels. When peripheral resistance is normal, the arteries taper gradually and proportionately distally. Vascular markings

that normally are invisible in the peripheral 2 cm of the lungs may become visible. Clinical observations[54] as well as the results of some experimental animal studies[55] suggest that the pulmonary veins increase in size to the same extent as the pulmonary arteries. Rarely, large left-to-right shunts are not associated radiographically with enlargement of the pulmonary vascular bed or cardiomegaly. In one study of 596 patients who had atrial septal defects proved by cardiac catheterization or surgery, 14 (2.3%) had a normal heart size and a normal pulmonary vascular pattern;[56] all 14 had secundum atrial septal defects of large size, the smallest shunt amounting to 50%.

It may be difficult radiographically to recognize the presence of pulmonary arterial hypertension in patients who have a left-to-right shunt. Although increased rapidity of tapering, a disparity between proximal and peripheral pulmonary vessel size, or both (Fig. 13–4) are valuable signs when present,[57, 58] peripheral oligemia is a late manifestation usually indicating reversal of the left-to-right shunt secondary to increased vascular resistance.[59] The difficulty is compounded by the fact that other signs of pulmonary arterial hypertension, such as enlargement of the main and hilar pulmonary arteries, are unreliable because these structures may be enlarged greatly when resistance is normal.

The diagnosis of a left-to-right shunt can be made readily using echocardiography or MR imaging (*see* Fig. 13–2).[33, 60] Both modalities can show the presence of shunt and the underlying anatomic features of simple and complex cardiovascular anomalies. Cardiac catheterization, with or without angiocardiography, is often required, however, particularly in the presence of suspected pulmonary arterial hypertension.

Primary Pulmonary Hypertension

Primary pulmonary hypertension is rare,[49] having an incidence of only about 1 per 1 million population. The mean age at presentation is 36 ± 15 years, and there is a female-to-male predominance of 1.7:1.[49] The main symptom is dyspnea on exertion, which often is insidious in onset.[64] Most patients experience progressive dyspnea, cor pulmonale, and death within a few years.[61]

Radiologic Manifestations

The radiographic findings consist of enlargement of the central pulmonary arteries, rapid tapering of vessels, and peripheral oligemia (*see* Fig. 13–1).[49] Overinflation does not occur, permitting ready differentiation from the diffuse pulmonary oligemia associated with emphysema. In one study of 187 patients whose chest radiographs were graded subjectively, prominence of the main pulmonary artery was found in 90%, enlarged hilar vessels in 80%, right ventricular hypertrophy in 74%, and decreased peripheral vascularity in 51%;[49] the appearance was thought to be normal in 6%.

Echocardiography typically shows right ventricular and right atrial enlargement, with a normal or small left ventricle.[62] Echocardiography allows assessment of the systolic pulmonary arterial pressure[63] and exclusion of left-to-right shunts and valvular heart disease. In one study of 187 patients, the procedure showed right ventricular enlargement in 75% and paradoxical septal wall motion in 59%.[11]

Ventilation-perfusion scans may be normal or may show patchy nonsegmental perfusion defects. In the previously mentioned study of 187 patients, perfusion scan results were abnormal in 58%;[11] most of the abnormalities consisted of diffuse, patchy defects that were estimated to have a low probability of representing pulmonary thromboembolism. In another study based on a retrospective assessment of 35 patients who had primary pulmonary hypertension, 33 (94%) had low-probability ventilation-perfusion scan results;[42] one each had intermediate-probability and high-probability scans. Contrast-enhanced spiral CT or pulmonary angiography is required to rule out chronic thromboembolism in such patients.

Pulmonary Hypertension Associated with Hepatic Disease

In 1979, 9 patients were described who had combined portal and pulmonary hypertension, and an additional 14 patients who had this combination of abnormalities were gleaned from the medical literature.[65] Of these 23 patients, 15 had had a surgical portocaval shunt established because of esophageal varices. Since this initial publication, there have been numerous reports of an association of liver disease and pulmonary hypertension, particularly, but not invariably,[66, 67] when accompanied by portal hypertension.[68, 69] The complication can occur a variable time after portosystemic shunting in patients who have noncirrhotic portal hypertension secondary to portal fibrosis[70] or multifocal nodular hyperplasia.[71] As might be expected, the overall prevalence of pulmonary hypertension in patients who have cirrhosis is low; in one large autopsy study, it was 0.73%, and in a clinical series of 2,459 patients who had biopsy-proven cirrhosis, it was 0.61%.[72]

The pathogenesis of the pulmonary hypertension likely is related to several mechanisms. It has been hypothesized that vasoactive or vasotoxic substances produced in the gut and normally metabolized by the liver can reach the pulmonary circulation;[73] however, the nature of such substances is unclear. It is possible that a component of the pulmonary hypertension is secondary to hemodynamic alterations.[74]

The symptoms and signs of pulmonary hypertension in patients who have liver disease are similar to those in patients who have pulmonary hypertension from other causes, although the symptoms and signs may be masked by the inactivity caused by the underlying liver disease. The radiologic manifestations range from normal to the characteristic findings of pulmonary arterial hypertension (Fig. 13–5).[12]

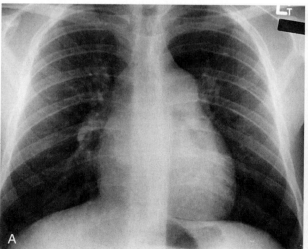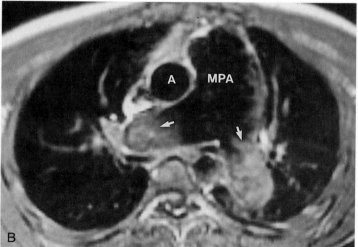

Figure 13–5. Pulmonary Arterial Hypertension Related to Cirrhosis. Posteroanterior chest radiograph *(A)* of a 17-year-old man shows cardiomegaly and enlargement of the central pulmonary arteries. Spin-echo MR image *(B)* shows enlargement of the main pulmonary artery (MPA), which has a greater diameter than that of the aorta (A). Increased signal is evident within the right and left pulmonary arteries *(arrows)*, reflecting the presence of slow blood flow because of hypertension.

Pulmonary Hypertension Associated with Pulmonary Artery Thrombosis and Thromboembolism

Hypertension inevitably develops if a sufficient portion of the pulmonary arterial system is occluded by thrombus. Such a situation can occur by at least three mechanisms: (1) multiple, recurrent embolic episodes involving small thrombi and occurring over a number of months or years; (2) one or a few embolic episodes involving a large thrombus that occludes a significant proportion of the proximal pulmonary vasculature directly or that does so by propagation of clot *in situ*[75, 76]—such thrombi may or may not be associated with evidence of thromboembolism in small vessels; and (3) *in situ* thrombosis of small or large pulmonary arteries unassociated with emboli. Although the first of these mechanisms has been thought to be the most common cause of pulmonary hypertension of thrombotic origin,[77] many clinical and pathologic observations suggest that it may be infrequent[3, 76] and that most cases are the result of the other two mechanisms.

Radiologic Manifestations

The characteristic radiographic findings of thromboembolic pulmonary arterial hypertension include right ventricular enlargement, prominence of the central pulmonary arteries, rapid tapering of vessels, and areas of decreased vascularity (mosaic oligemia) (Table 13–3, *see* Fig. 13–3).[10, 78] In one review of 22 patients, cardiomegaly was identified in 19 (86%), right descending pulmonary artery enlargement was identified in 12 (54%), and localized areas of diminished vascularity were identified in 15 (68%).[10] The areas of decreased vascularity on plain radiographs were confirmed by angiography to be associated with chronic emboli. When either thrombosis or embolism occurs in the major hilar pulmonary arteries, the combination of bulging hilar pulmonary arteries, severe peripheral oligemia, and cor pulmonale constitutes a virtually pathognomonic triad.[79] Large emboli within the main pulmonary arteries occasionally are associated with small hilar vessels, however.[10]

Ventilation-perfusion scintigraphy is a safe, highly sensitive test to evaluate patients suspected of having thromboembolic pulmonary arterial hypertension (Fig. 13–6).[42, 80] The extent of abnormalities on a perfusion lung scan can underestimate significantly the severity of angiographic and hemodynamic compromise, however.[81] In one investigation of 75 patients, including 25 who had chronic thromboembolic hypertension, 35 who had primary hypertension, and 15 who had secondary nonthromboembolic hypertension, a high-probability ventilation-perfusion scan had a sensitivity of 96% and a specificity of 94% for detecting thromboembolic hypertension.[42] A combination of high-probability and intermediate-probability scans had a sensitivity of 100% and a specificity of 86%.

In another study, the usefulness of conventional chest radiography and perfusion scintigraphy using technetium 99m–labeled albumin macroaggregates was assessed in 19 patients who had biopsy-proven plexogenic pulmonary hypertension, thromboembolic pulmonary hypertension, or veno-occlusive disease.[82] Chest radiographs were normal in patients who had plexogenic and thromboembolic hypertension; perfusion lung scans were abnormal in seven of the eight patients who had thromboembolic disease and in none of the nine patients who had plexogenic hypertension. In the two patients who had veno-occlusive disease, the chest radiographs showed evidence of pulmonary venous hypertension. The investigators suggested that a combination of chest radiography and perfusion scintigraphy could be useful in distinguishing these three conditions.

The diagnosis of chronic thromboembolism can be suggested on the basis of alterations in pulmonary vascularity and attenuation on high-resolution computed tomography (HRCT).[83–85] Such alterations consist of patchy areas of decreased vascularity and attenuation associated with blood flow redistribution to uninvolved areas, a pattern known as *mosaic attenuation* or *mosaic perfusion* (Fig. 13–7). In one investigation of 67 patients (17 having chronic thromboembolic hypertension; 6, primary pulmonary hypertension; 5, secondary nonthromboembolic hypertension; and 39, a variety of airway, interstitial, or air-space parenchymal abnormalities), HRCT had a sensitivity and specificity of approximately 97% in separating pulmonary hypertension caused by chronic thromboembolic disease from other pulmonary abnormalities, including other causes of pulmonary hypertension.[85] The two features that allowed the accurate differentiation were disparity in the size of segmental arteries and a mosaic pattern of attenuation. The average ratios of segmental vessel size were 2.2 for patients who had chronic thromboembolic hypertension and 1.1 for the remaining patients.

Another group of investigators showed a lower diagnostic accuracy of HRCT in distinguishing the various causes of pulmonary arterial hypertension.[86] In this study, which included 64 patients who had pulmonary arterial hypertension (15 having chronic thromboembolism; 4, primary pulmonary hypertension; 21, underlying lung disease; 17, cardiac disease; and the remaining miscellaneous causes), a mosaic pattern of lung attenuation was present in 12 of 15 (80%) patients who had thromboembolic disease, 2 of 4 (50%) who had primary pulmonary hypertension, 2 of 2 (100%) who had veno-occlusive disease, 1 of 21 (5%) who had underlying lung disease, and 2 of 17 (12%) who had underlying cardiac disease. The difficulty in distinguishing mosaic attenuation secondary to chronic thromboembolism from mosaic attenuation secondary to parenchymal lung disease or airway disease has been confirmed by another group.[87]

Table 13–3. CHRONIC THROMBOEMBOLIC PULMONARY ARTERIAL HYPERTENSION

Chest radiograph
    Enlarged central pulmonary arteries
    Rapid tapering of vessels
    Areas with decreased vascularity
CT scan
    Enlarged central pulmonary arteries
    Mosaic attenuation and perfusion
Contrast-enhanced spiral CT or angiography
    Eccentric location of pulmonary emboli
    Recanalization within intraluminal filling defects
    Arterial stenosis or web
    Abrupt narrowing of arterial diameter

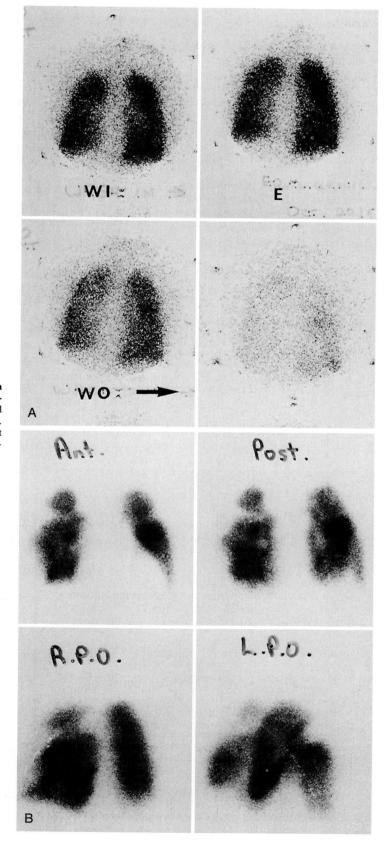

Figure 13–6. Pulmonary Hypertension: Perfusion Pattern on Scintigraphy in Chronic Thromboembolism Without Infarction. Ventilation *(A)* and perfusion *(B)* lung scintigrams reveal features that are considered *high probability* for thromboembolism. WI, E, and WO represent the washin, equilibrium, and washout phases of the perfusion scintigraphic study. The patient was a 64-year-old man.

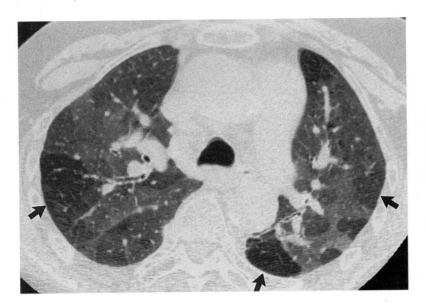

Figure 13–7. Mosaic Perfusion in Thromboembolic Pulmonary Arterial Hypertension. HRCT scan in a 73-year-old woman shows localized areas that have decreased attenuation and vascularity *(arrows)* and areas with increased lung attenuation and increase in size and number of pulmonary vessels (mosaic perfusion). The large size of the pulmonary arteries compared with that of the adjacent bronchi is a finding consistent with pulmonary hypertension.

Contrast-enhanced spiral CT currently is the imaging modality of choice for the evaluation of patients who have pulmonary arterial hypertension and suspected chronic thromboembolism based on a combination of radiographic and scintigraphic findings or HRCT. By this technique, chronic emboli are considered to be present when at least two of the following are identified: (1) an eccentric location contiguous to the vessel wall (Fig. 13–8), (2) evidence of recanalization within the intraluminal filling defect, (3) arterial stenosis or web, (4) abrupt narrowing of the artery with reduction of more than 50% of its diameter (Fig.

13–9), and (5) complete occlusion at the level of the stenosed artery.[88] The most common finding is an eccentric location of the thrombus resulting in a crescentic, often irregularly marginated, filling defect adjacent to the vessel wall.[89, 90] Calcification has been reported in 10% of thrombi.[90, 91]

In one study in which contrast-enhanced CT was compared with pulmonary angiography in 21 consecutive patients who had chronic pulmonary thromboembolism, the former technique was found to be superior in showing the presence and extent of proximal thrombi (confirmed by surgery).[45] It also showed more peripheral thrombi than were apparent on angiography. Angiography was superior to CT in showing vascular distortion and stenosis. In another study of 63 patients who underwent thromboendarterectomy, contrast-enhanced CT had a sensitivity of 77% and a specificity of 100% in the diagnosis of chronic thromboembolism and ensuring operability.[44] In a third study, contrast-enhanced spiral CT was compared with MR imaging and pulmonary angiography in 55 patients who had chronic thromboembolic pulmonary hypertension *(see* Fig. 13–3).[46] MR imaging was performed using gadolinium-enhanced spin-echo and gradient-recalled-echo (GRE) techniques; surgical correlation for the presence of central vessel disease was available in 40 of the 55 patients. Of a total of 56 abnormal central arterial portions, abnormalities were identified on spiral CT in approximately 80%, compared with 70% on angiography and 35% on MR imaging. Central abnormalities were seen more clearly on the GRE MR images than on spin-echo technique. Spiral CT has been used to identify enlarged bronchial arteries in some patients who have chronic thromboembolic hypertension; in one study, the visualization of prominent bronchial arteries was a predictor of a favorable outcome after thromboendarterectomy.[92]

Pulmonary angiography is recommended when there is a discrepancy between the CT and clinical findings and in the assessment of selected patients undergoing thromboendarterectomy.[46] Pulmonary angiography is safe when performed with nonionic contrast medium and selective bolus injection directly into pulmonary arterial branches.[93] In one

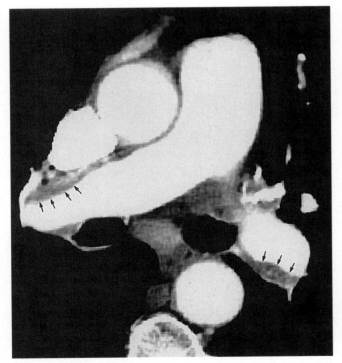

Figure 13–8. Chronic Thromboembolism. Contrast-enhanced spiral CT scan in a 56-year-old woman shows filling defects adjacent to the wall of the right and left interlobar pulmonary arteries *(arrows)*. This eccentric location is characteristic of chronic thromboembolism.

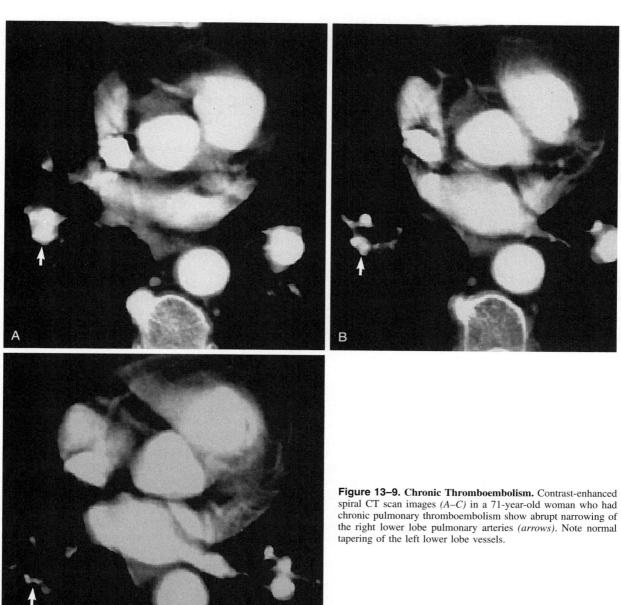

Figure 13–9. Chronic Thromboembolism. Contrast-enhanced spiral CT scan images *(A–C)* in a 71-year-old woman who had chronic pulmonary thromboembolism show abrupt narrowing of the right lower lobe pulmonary arteries *(arrows)*. Note normal tapering of the left lower lobe vessels.

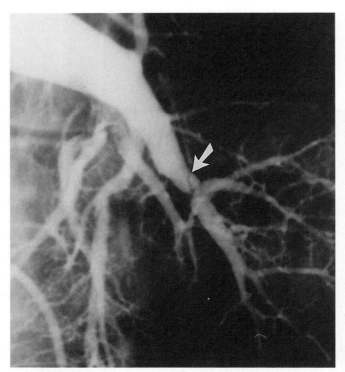

Figure 13–10. Thromboembolic Pulmonary Arterial Hypertension. View from a left pulmonary angiogram shows areas with decreased perfusion, irregularity of the segmental vessels, and a focal linear filling defect (arterial web) *(arrow)*, findings that are characteristic of pulmonary arterial hypertension secondary to chronic thromboembolism.

study of 250 patients in whom pulmonary angiograms were performed for assessment of chronic major vessel thromboembolic pulmonary artery obstruction, the findings most suggestive of the disease were *pouch defects*, webs or bands, intimal irregularities, abrupt vascular narrowing, and complete vascular obstruction (Fig. 13–10).[94] A pouch defect is a partially or completely occlusive chronic thrombus that organizes in a concave configuration toward the lumen. Pulmonary arterial webs or bands are seen as lines of decreased opacity that traverse the width of the pulmonary artery, usually at the lobar or segmental level;[95] they often are associated with vessel narrowing or poststenotic dilation.

Pulsed Doppler echocardiography permits assessment of right ventricular size and systolic function in patients who have recent or chronic pulmonary emboli. Thromboemboli within the heart or pulmonary artery (or both) also may be detected; if a tricuspid regurgitant jet develops as a result of embolization, ultrasonographic assessment of pulmonary artery pressure can be performed.[96] In a study of 60 patients who had pulmonary hypertension, 35 of whom had central pulmonary emboli, transesophageal echocardiography was 97% sensitive and 88% specific in detecting this cause.[97]

Pulmonary Hypertension Associated with Systemic Immunologic Disorders

Pulmonary arterial hypertension, unaccompanied by parenchymal lung disease and manifested pathologically by plexogenic arteriopathy, occurs occasionally in immunologically mediated connective tissue disorders, particularly progressive systemic sclerosis, mixed connective tissue disease, and systemic lupus erythematosus. Raynaud's phenomenon often is present, suggesting that the pulmonary disease represents part of a generalized vasculopathy. Pulmonary hypertension occurs in some individuals with immunologically mediated interstitial lung disease, such as rheumatoid disease and progressive systemic sclerosis; in these cases, radiographic and pathologic features are identical to the features associated with chronic interstitial lung disease of other etiologies. Rarely, hypertension is a complication of pulmonary vasculitis, most often Takayasu's arteritis or Behçet's disease; in these cases, the pathogenesis of the hypertension probably is related to *in situ* arterial thrombosis.

Primary Pleuropulmonary Disease

A wide variety of primary diseases of the lungs, pleura, chest wall, and respiratory control center may cause a rise in pulmonary arterial pressure without significant change in pulmonary venous pressure (*see* Table 13–1). This increase seldom reaches the level attained in cases of primary vascular disease, however. The hypertension may be transient, reflecting episodes of pulmonary infection and its associated hypoxia. Usually, clinical symptoms are attributable to the underlying disease, and the presence of pulmonary hypertension is not detectable clinically until cor pulmonale and cardiac failure develop.

Radiologic Manifestations

The radiographic manifestations of pulmonary hypertension in emphysema are identical to those of primary vascular disease; however, the invariable presence of overinflation permits ready differentiation (Fig. 13–11). In one study of 61 men who had COPD and 42 normal control subjects, a strong positive correlation was found between the diameters of the right and left interlobar arteries and the presence and severity of pulmonary arterial hypertension.[9]

In patients who have diffuse interstitial or air-space disease, the radiologic changes are dominated almost invariably by the underlying pulmonary disease; in many cases, the peripheral vascular markings are obscured. In one study of the radiologic findings in 29 patients who had diffuse interstitial disease (progressive systemic sclerosis in 20, sarcoidosis in 6, and miscellaneous causes in 3) and in whom cardiac catheterization had revealed pulmonary arterial hypertension and normal pulmonary wedge pressures, pulmonary artery pressure was related significantly to the size of the central pulmonary arteries, and pulmonary hemodynamic abnormalities were roughly proportional to the radiologic severity of parenchymal disease.[98]

In another retrospective review of 41 patients who had progressive systemic sclerosis, the degree of pulmonary arterial hypertension was found to be out of proportion to the severity of interstitial pulmonary fibrosis, suggesting the possibility of a concomitant primary vasculopathy.[99] In this series, pulmonary arterial hypertension was evident radiographically or clinically in 15 patients (37%). Hilar pulmonary artery enlargement seldom is as marked as in primary vascular disease; however, evidence of progressive enlargement on serial radiographs should suggest the diagnosis of pulmonary hypertension.

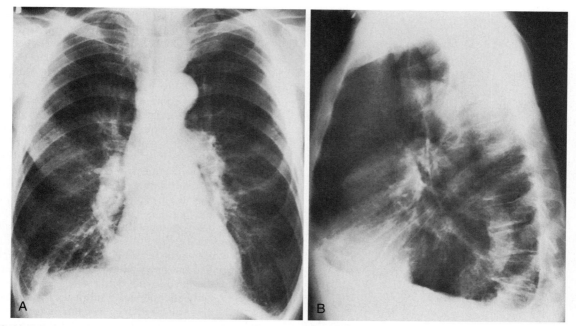

Figure 13–11. Pulmonary Arterial Hypertension Secondary to Emphysema. Posterior *(A)* and lateral *(B)* radiographs show marked overinflation of both lungs, with a low flat position of the diaphragm and an increase in the depth of the retrosternal air space. The lungs are diffusely oligemic, the peripheral vessels being narrow and attenuated. A discrepancy in the size of the central and peripheral pulmonary vessels is caused not only by a decrease in caliber peripherally, but also by an increase in size centrally; the latter constitutes convincing evidence of pulmonary arterial hypertension. At autopsy, the parenchymal changes were predominantly those of panacinar emphysema.

POSTCAPILLARY PULMONARY HYPERTENSION

Postcapillary pulmonary hypertension results from any condition that increases pulmonary venous pressure above a critical level. The most common of these are diseases of the left side of the heart, usually those that cause left ventricular failure, such as systemic hypertension and coronary artery disease. Less common causes include mitral stenosis, congenital cardiac anomalies such as cor triatriatum, capillary hemangiomatosis, fibrosing mediastinitis, atrial myxoma, total anomalous venous drainage, and primary veno-occlusive disease.[100–102]

The symptoms associated with postcapillary hypertension usually are differentiated readily from those of precapillary origin. In left ventricular failure, which is the most common cause, symptoms and signs are predominantly those arising from acute or subacute pulmonary edema, including dyspnea, orthopnea, and paroxysmal nocturnal dyspnea. Expectoration of pink frothy sputum may be present; occasionally (particularly in mitral stenosis), bright red blood is coughed up. Some patients who have chronic congestive heart failure[110] or pulmonary veno-occlusive disease[111] do not present with these typical symptoms, and their radiographic findings and hemodynamic measurements may be equivocal; in such circumstances, an erroneous diagnosis of primary pulmonary arterial or interstitial disease may be made.

Radiologic Manifestations

Normally, pulmonary perfusion and pulmonary vascular caliber increase from apex to base; this occurs because pulmonary venous pressure is higher in the lower than in the upper lobes in erect humans owing to a difference in hydrostatic pressure (averaging approximately 12 to 15 mm

Hg in adults). Pulmonary venous hypertension produces a distinctive alteration in the pulmonary vascular pattern characterized by narrowing of vessels in the lower lobe and distention of vessels in the upper lobe (Fig. 13–12). With continued increase in venous pressure, the reduction in venous caliber progresses upward from the lung bases and eventually involves the upper lobes, constricting the engorged upper lobe veins and producing a pattern of diffuse alteration in the pulmonary vasculature. The inevitable result is generalized elevation of pulmonary arterial vascular resistance and pulmonary arterial hypertension (Fig. 13–13).[103] Blood flow redistribution with an increase in the number and size of upper lobe vessels is most striking in the setting of chronic venous hypertension rather than secondary to an acute hemodynamic change.[5] Other radiologic findings in pulmonary venous hypertension include septal lines (Kerley A and B lines, as a result of interlobular septal edema) and loss of definition of pulmonary vascular markings (as a result of perivascular edema) and small pleural effusions.

It is common to hear the term *upper lobe venous engorgement* used to describe redistribution of blood flow from lower to upper zones. Because the distention of the upper zone vessels is caused by blood flow redistribution to the upper lobes, however, it affects the arteries and the veins. It is preferable conceptually to use the phrase *upper zone vascular distention* to indicate redistribution of blood flow. Because distention of upper zone vessels occurs in five situations other than pulmonary venous hypertension (supine position, predominantly lower zonal parenchymal disease, left-to-right shunts, hypervolemia, and pulmonary arterial hypertension), it is advisable as a first approximation to refer to the abnormality as *recruitment of upper zone vessels*; after other aspects of the radiographic appear-

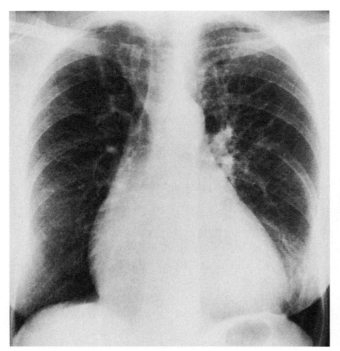

Figure 13–12. Redistribution of Blood Flow to Upper Lung Zones Caused by Pulmonary Venous Hypertension. Posteroanterior radiograph shows unusually prominent vascular markings in the upper zones and sparse markings in the lower zones. The patient, a 42-year-old woman, had recurrent episodes of left ventricular decompensation as a result of a congestive cardiomyopathy.

ance have been evaluated, it may be possible to ascribe the recruitment to a specific cause.

It is customary for radiologists to assess the caliber of upper zone vessels by comparing them with those in the lower zone. Although a disparity must exist for redistribution of flow to be appreciated, we believe that it is difficult to be convinced of an increase in upper zonal vessel caliber by such a comparison. It has been our experience that subjective assessment of the caliber of vessels in the upper zones, based on experience of what constitutes the normal, is more dependable. Such an assessment is facilitated by comparison with previous radiographs, but with few exceptions (chiefly patients who have left-to-right shunts or whose radiographs have been obtained in the recumbent position), subjective assessment possesses considerable reliability even without comparison.

In a review of chest radiographs of 111 patients who had critical mitral stenosis (valve openings of $\leq 1.5 \times 1.0$ cm), dilated upper zone vessels were found in all but 6 patients.[104] The pulmonary artery and left atrial pressures and the degree of valve narrowing were the same in these patients as in the group as a whole. It is apparent that critical mitral stenosis can be present without dilation of the upper lobe vessels, although such an occurrence must be rare.

The alteration in pulmonary vascular pattern that is seen in mitral stenosis may be observed in mild left ventricular failure; in a study of the chest radiographs of 50 consecutive patients admitted to a coronary care unit, redistribution of blood flow to upper zones was found to be the most

common abnormality (76% of patients).[105] Radiographic signs of left ventricular failure may be apparent without clinical evidence of decompensation. In another study of 94 patients who had chest radiographs obtained on admission to a coronary care unit, 31 (33%) were found to have radiographic evidence of pulmonary venous hypertension (manifested most commonly by distention of upper zone vessels) without associated clinical signs;[106] in 23 of these, however, clinically evident failure developed subsequently. In another study of 30 patients who had recent myocardial infarction, the severity of radiographic abnormality generally correlated well with pulmonary capillary wedge pressure.[107] Redistribution of blood flow was the earliest manifestation of elevated wedge pressure, followed sequentially by loss of the normal sharp margins of the pulmonary vessels, the development of perihilar haze, and finally overt air-space edema.

Although it might be anticipated that radiographic evidence of redistribution of blood flow to upper lung zones in patients who have severe mitral stenosis might disappear relatively rapidly after adequate surgical correction by commissurotomy or valve replacement, this is not the case. In a study of 25 patients who had pure mitral stenosis, five radiographic signs were used in an analysis of preoperative and postoperative radiographs:[108] (1) septal (Kerley B) lines, (2) abnormal pulmonary vascular pattern (redistribution of blood flow), (3) left atrial enlargement, (4) the ratio

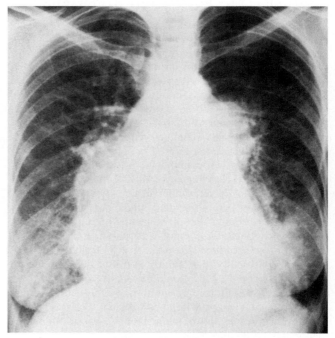

Figure 13–13. Combined Venous and Arterial Hypertension in Mitral Stenosis. Posteroanterior radiograph of a 40-year-old woman with a 20-year history of rheumatic heart disease shows severe pulmonary arterial hypertension as evidenced by a moderate increase in the size of the hilar pulmonary arteries and by the rapid tapering of these vessels as they proceed distally. A slight discrepancy in the size of the upper lobe and lower lobe pulmonary vessels and evidence of interstitial edema indicate associated pulmonary venous hypertension. When these signs are considered in the light of the character of the cardiac enlargement, the diagnosis of chronic mitral valvular disease with pulmonary venous and arterial hypertension may be made with confidence.

of the diameter of the main pulmonary artery to the diameter of the left hemithorax, and (5) the diameter of the right interlobar artery. The most useful changes for predicting postoperative hemodynamic and clinical improvement were left atrial size, the ratio of the width of the main pulmonary artery from the midline divided by the diameter of the left hemithorax at the diaphragm, and the diameter of the right interlobar artery distal to the right middle lobe artery. The use of these signs resulted in prediction of significant hemodynamic and clinical improvement in 100% and 86% of cases.

A change from the abnormal vascular pattern observed preoperatively—that is, a disappearance of signs of redistribution of blood flow—was found to be less reliable, presumably because considerable time is required for relatively fixed anatomic changes in vessels to regress.[109] This observation is important in that the radiographic demonstration of persisting upper zonal vascular distention several months after corrective surgery does not indicate elevated left atrial and pulmonary venous pressure. Persistence of septal (Kerley B) lines also is a poor indicator of hemodynamic or clinical improvement because their thickening may be caused by fibrosis secondary to chronic edema rather than the accumulation of fluid alone.

PULMONARY VENO-OCCLUSIVE DISEASE

Pulmonary veno-occlusive disease is a rare abnormality characterized pathologically by evidence of repeated pulmonary venous thrombosis and clinically by evidence of pulmonary arterial hypertension, pulmonary edema, or both. The condition can occur at any age but is most common during childhood and adolescence. In adolescents, the sex incidence is approximately equal; however, in older individuals, there appears to be a slight male predominance.[112]

The etiology and pathogenesis are unknown and may be related to more than one source or mechanism. A variety of ingested substances have been implicated. The most important of these are medications, including bleomycin and mitomycin.[114, 115] Herbal *bush* teas containing *Senecio*, *Crotalaria*, and *Heliotropium* species may cause hepatic veno-occlusive disease; in some of these cases, pulmonary venous involvement has been described.[116, 117] Pulmonary veno-occlusive disease has been reported after bone marrow transplantation[118] and after radiation therapy to the thorax.[119] The abnormality has been reported with the use of oral contraceptives,[120] an association that has been reported with hepatic veno-occlusive disease.[121]

Pathologically the most prominent feature is stenosis or obliteration of the lumen of small pulmonary veins and venules by intimal fibrous tissue.[112, 113] Larger pulmonary veins usually are spared. Clinically the patients present with slowly progressive dyspnea and orthopnea punctuated by attacks of acute pulmonary edema; hemoptysis may occur.

Radiologic Manifestations

Radiographically, signs of pulmonary arterial hypertension typically are present and are identical to signs associated with primary or thromboembolic disease. Signs of

postcapillary hypertension, chiefly pulmonary edema (Fig. 13–14), are evident.[122, 123] In a review of the radiographic findings in 26 patients, evidence of pulmonary edema was present in 20 (77%). The left atrium is not enlarged, and there is no evidence of redistribution of blood flow to upper lung zones, both important findings in distinguishing pulmonary veno-occlusive disease from mitral stenosis. Similar to radiograph, HRCT scan shows smooth thickening of the interlobular septa and interlobar fissures and areas of ground-glass attenuation consistent with interstitial pulmonary edema (*see* Fig. 13–14).[124, 125] Small pleural effusions are present in most patients.[125] Ventilation-perfusion scans can show segmental areas of ventilation-perfusion mismatch.[126]

PULMONARY ARTERY ANEURYSMS

Aneurysms of the main and lobar branches of the pulmonary artery are rare.[127] Only eight examples were found in a review of 109,571 autopsies, an incidence of 1 in 13,696.[128] The cause and pathogenetic mechanisms are diverse (Table 13–4). Most are secondary to trauma, infection, or Behçet's disease. Trauma to the chest wall or directly to a vessel (e.g., via an intravascular catheter or surgical procedure) can result in pulmonary arterial damage and, occasionally, residual aneurysm formation;[129, 130] however, the walls of many of these lesions probably are formed by blood clot, and they are described better as pseudoaneurysms. Such lesions most commonly are caused by pulmonary artery perforation by a Swan-Ganz catheter.[131]

Infection is an important pathogenetic mechanism. A variety of microorganisms can be responsible. In developed countries, syphilis[128] and tuberculosis (Rasmussen's aneurysm)[132] were relatively common causes until the middle of the twentieth century;[150] with control of these diseases, pyogenic organisms such as *Staphylococcus aureus* and *Streptococcus* have become increasingly important.[133–135] Rarely, fungi such as *Aspergillus* and *Candida* are the cause.[136, 137] Immunologically mediated vasculitis is associated rarely with pulmonary artery aneurysm formation, most often in Behçet's disease (*see* Chapter 8).[138, 139]

Table 13–4. ETIOLOGY AND PATHOGENESIS OF PULMONARY ARTERY ANEURYSMS

Type	Causes	Selected References
Congenital	Deficiency of vessel wall	134
	Postvalvular or arterial stenosis	152
Degenerative/metabolic	Marfan's syndrome	153
	Cystic medial necrosis (dissecting aneurysm)	154
Traumatic		129
Infectious (mycotic)	Syphilis	128
	Tuberculosis	132
	Pyogenic bacteria	134
	Others (e.g., fungi)	136
Immunologic	Behçet's disease	138
Secondary to pulmonary disease	Hypertension (including dissecting aneurysms)	155
	Bronchiectasis	
Idiopathic	Hughes-Stovin syndrome	156

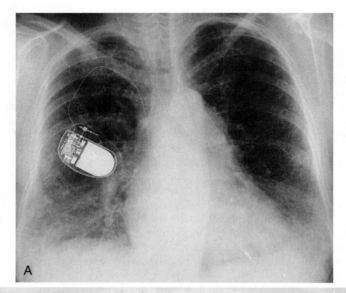

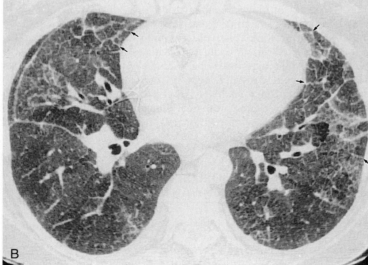

Figure 13–14. Primary Veno-Occlusive Disease. Posteroanterior chest radiograph *(A)* in a 51-year-old woman shows enlargement of the central pulmonary arteries and extensive interstitial pulmonary edema. A permanent pacemaker with a right ventricular lead in place is evident. HRCT scan *(B)* essentially confirms the radiographic findings, showing interlobular septal thickening *(arrows)* and areas of ground-glass attenuation consistent with interstitial pulmonary edema.

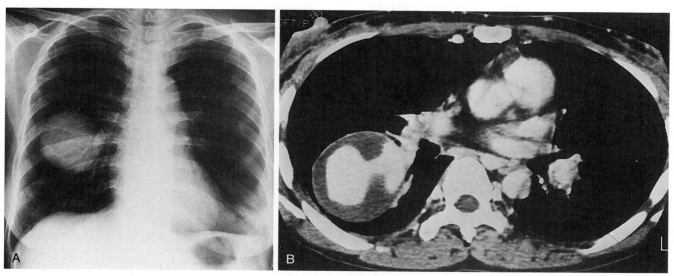

Figure 13–15. Pulmonary Artery Aneurysm: Behçet's Disease. Posteroanterior chest radiograph *(A)* in a 36-year-old woman who had Behçet's disease shows a round, well-defined mass in the right lower lobe and a localized area of consolidation in the left lower lobe. Contrast-enhanced CT scan *(B)* shows a large aneurysm of the right pulmonary artery with enhancement of the patent lumen and a circumferential thrombus. (Courtesy of Dr. Jung-Gi Im, Seoul National University Hospital, Seoul, South Korea. From Radiology 194:199, 1995.)

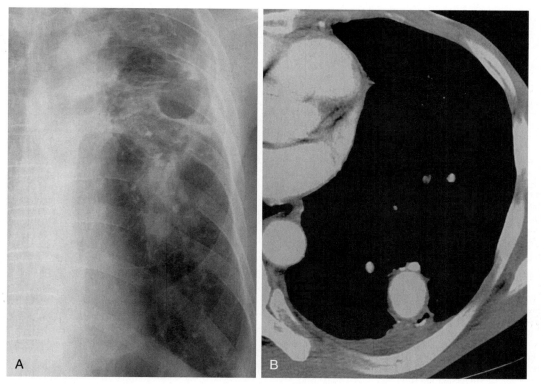

Figure 13–16. Pulmonary Artery Aneurysm in Tuberculosis (Rasmussen's Aneurysm). View of the left lung from posteroanterior chest radiograph *(A)* shows extensive scarring of the left upper lobe with associated superior retraction of the hilum, bullae, and lower lobe emphysema. The patient had been treated previously for tuberculosis. Contrast-enhanced CT scan *(B)* shows peripheral nodular opacity that is isointense with the cardiac chambers and the normal peripheral pulmonary arteries. The findings are diagnostic of pulmonary artery aneurysm. (Case courtesy of Dr. Kyung Soo Lee, Department of Diagnostic Imaging, Samsung Medical Center, Seoul, South Korea.)

In many patients, pulmonary signs and symptoms are absent or are overshadowed by underlying cardiac or pulmonary disease; in some, cough, dyspnea, and hemoptysis are present.[140] Rarely the aneurysm projects into the bronchial lumen as an endobronchial mass.[151] A more common manifestation of such extension is rupture with massive hemorrhage;[139, 140] it has been estimated that 3% to 6% of patients who have massive hemoptysis have an underlying pulmonary artery aneurysm.[150] Hemoptysis is an indicator of aneurysm *instability* and the need for prompt intervention.[150]

Radiologic Manifestations

Radiographic findings include pulmonary nodules ranging from 2 to 8 cm in diameter or dense focal parenchymal consolidation (Fig. 13–15).[141, 143] The nodules may have well-defined or poorly defined margins as a result of associated hemorrhage. Areas of consolidation may persist or may evolve into a nodule or mass.[142] The diagnosis may be confirmed using contrast-enhanced CT,[144, 145] MR imaging,[145, 146] or angiography.[142, 143] Contrast-enhanced spiral CT is the modality of choice and shows the aneurysms as enhancing round opacities that are isointense to the central pulmonary arteries (Fig. 13–16).[131] CT may show a halo of ground-glass attenuation surrounding the aneurysm resulting from pulmonary hemorrhage.[147] In addition to being helpful in diagnosis, angiography is integral to treatment with embolotherapy using wire coils or detachable balloons.[148–150]

References

1. Fowler NO, Westcott RN, Scott RC: Normal pressure in the right heart and pulmonary artery. Am Heart J 46:264, 1953.
2. Sasamoto H, Hosono K, Katayama K, et al: Electrocardiographic findings in patients with chronic cor pulmonale. Respir Circ 9:55, 1961.
3. Palevsky HI, Schloo BL, Pietra GG, et al: Primary pulmonary hypertension: Vascular structure, morphometry, and responsiveness to vasodilator agents. Circulation 80:1207, 1989.
4. Chen JTT, Capp MP, Johnsrude IS, et al: Roentgen appearance of pulmonary vascularity in the diagnosis of heart disease. Am J Roentgenol 112:559, 1971.
5. Ravin CE: Pulmonary vascularity: Radiographic considerations. J Thorac Imaging 3:1, 1988.
6. Randall PA, Heitzman ER, Bull MJ, et al: Pulmonary hypertension: A contemporary review. Radiographics 9:905, 1989.
7. Mallamo JT, Baum RS, Simon AL: Diffuse pulmonary artery calcifications in a case of Eisenmenger's syndrome. Radiology 99:549, 1971.
8. Chang CH: The normal roentgenographic measurement of the right descending pulmonary artery in 1,085 cases. Am J Roentgenol 87:929, 1962.
9. Matthay RA, Schwarz MI, Ellis JH Jr, et al: Pulmonary artery hypertension in chronic obstructive pulmonary disease: Determination by chest radiography. Invest Radiol 16:95, 1981.
10. Woodruff WW III, Hoeck BE, Chitwood WR Jr, et al: Radiographic findings in pulmonary hypertension from unresolved embolism. Am J Roentgenol 144:681, 1985.
11. Rich S, Dantzker DR, Ayres SM, et al: Primary pulmonary hypertension: A national prospective study. Ann Intern Med 107:216, 1987.
12. Chan T, Palevsky HI, Miller WT: Pulmonary hypertension complicating portal hypertension: Findings on chest radiographs. Am J Roentgenol 151:909, 1988.
13. Ormond RS, Drake EH, Hildner FJ: Pulmonary hypertension: An angiographic study. Radiology 88:680, 1967.
14. Kuriyama K, Gamsu G, Stern RG, et al: CT-determined pulmonary artery diameters in predicting pulmonary hypertension. Invest Radiol 19:16, 1984.
15. Haimovici JBA, Trotman-Dickenson B, Halpern EF, et al: Relationship between pulmonary artery diameter at computed tomography and pulmonary artery pressures at right-sided heart catheterization. Acad Radiol 4:327, 1997.
16. Tan RT, Kuzo R, Goodman LR, et al: Utility of CT scan evaluation for predicting pulmonary hypertension in patients with parenchymal lung disease. Chest 113:1250, 1998.
17. Ng CS, Wells AU, Padley SPG: A CT sign of chronic pulmonary arterial hypertension: The ratio of main pulmonary artery to aortic diameter. J Thorac Imaging 14:270, 1999.
18. Park B, Dittrich HC, Polikar R, et al: Echocardiographic evidence of pericardial effusion in severe chronic pulmonary hypertension. Am J Cardiol 63:143, 1989.
19. Baque-Juston MC, Wells AU, Hansell DM: Pericardial thickening or effusion in patients with pulmonary artery hypertension: A CT study. Am J Roentgenol 172:361, 1999.
20. Tramarin R, Torbicki A, Marchandise B, et al: Doppler echocardiographic evaluation of pulmonary artery pressure in chronic obstructive pulmonary disease: A European multicentre study. Working Group on Noninvasive Evaluation of Pulmonary Artery Pressure. Eur Heart J 12:103, 1991.
21. Burghuber OC, Brunner CH, Schenk P, et al: Pulsed Doppler echocardiography to assess pulmonary artery hypertension in chronic obstructive pulmonary disease. Monaldi Arch Chest Dis 48:121, 1993.
22. Brecker SJ, Xiao HB, Stojnic BB, et al: Assessment of the peak tricuspid regurgitant velocity from the dynamics of retrograde flow. Int J Cardiol 34:267, 1992.
23. Torres F, Tye T, Gibbons R, et al: Echocardiographic contrast increases the yield for right ventricular pressure measurement by Doppler echocardiography. J Am Soc Echocardiogr 2:419, 1989.
24. Lei MH, Chen JJ, Ko YL, et al: Reappraisal of quantitative evaluations of pulmonary regurgitation and estimation of pulmonary artery pressure by continuous wave Doppler echocardiography. Cardiology 86:249, 1995.
25. Chotivittayatarakorn P, Pathmanand C, Thisyakorn C, et al: Doppler echocardiographic predictions of pulmonary artery pressure in children with congenital heart disease. J Med Assoc Thai 75:79, 1992.
26. Trivedi HS, Joshi MN, Gamade AR: Echocardiography and pulmonary artery pressure: Correlation in chronic obstructive pulmonary disease. J Postgrad Med 38:24, 1992.
27. Bach DS: Stress echocardiography for evaluation of hemodynamics: Valvular heart disease, prosthetic valve function, and pulmonary hypertension. Prog Cardiovasc Dis 39:543, 1997.
28. Brecker SJ, Gibbs JS, Fox KM, et al: Comparison of Doppler derived haemodynamic variables and simultaneous high fidelity pressure measurements in severe pulmonary hypertension. Br Heart J 71:384, 1994.
29. Chen WJ, Chen JJ, Lin SC, et al: Detection of cardiovascular shunts by transesophageal echocardiography in patients with pulmonary hypertension of unexplained cause. Chest 107:8, 1995.
30. Gorcsan J, Edwards TD, Ziady GM, et al: Transesophageal echocardiography to evaluate patients with severe pulmonary hypertension for lung transplantation. Ann Thorac Surg 59:717, 1995.
31. Frank H, Globits S, Glogar D, et al: Detection and quantification of pulmonary artery hypertension with MR imaging: Results in 23 patients. Am J Roentgenol 161:27, 1993.
32. Boxt LM: MR imaging of pulmonary hypertension and right ventricular dysfunction. Magn Reson Imaging Clin N Am 4:307, 1996.
33. Rebergen SA, Niezen RA, Helbing WA, et al: Cine gradient-echo MR imaging and MR velocity mapping in the evaluation of congenital heart disease. Radiographics 16:467, 1996.
34. Tardivon AA, Mousseaux E, Brenot F, et al: Quantification of hemodynamics in primary pulmonary hypertension with magnetic resonance imaging. Am J Respir Crit Care Med 150:1075, 1994.
35. Kondo C, Caputo GR, Masui T, et al: Pulmonary hypertension: Pulmonary flow quantification and flow profile analysis with velocity-encoded cine MR imaging. Radiology 183:751, 1992.
36. Wacker CM, Schad LR, Gehling U, et al: The pulmonary artery acceleration time determined with the MR-RACE-technique: Comparison to pulmonary artery mean pressure in 12 patients. Magn Reson Imaging 12:25, 1994.
37. Mousseaux E, Tasu JP, Jolivet O, et al: Pulmonary arterial resistance:

Noninvasive measurement with indexes of pulmonary flow estimated at velocity-encoded MR imaging—preliminary experience. Radiology 212:896, 1999.

38. Murray TI, Boxt LM, Katz J, et al: Estimation of pulmonary artery pressure in patients with primary pulmonary hypertension by quantitative analysis of magnetic resonance images. J Thorac Imaging 9:198, 1994.

39. Boxt LM, Katz J, Kolb T, et al: Direct quantitation of right and left ventricular volumes with nuclear magnetic resonance imaging in patients with primary pulmonary hypertension. J Am Coll Cardiol 19:1508, 1992.

40. Boxt LM, Katz J: Magnetic resonance imaging for quantitation of right ventricular volume in patients with pulmonary hypertension. J Thorac Imaging 8:92, 1993.

41. Stern EJ, Graham C, Gamsu G, et al: Pulmonary artery dissection: MR findings. J Comput Assist Tomogr 16:481, 1992.

42. Worsley DF, Palevsky HI, Alavi A: Ventilation-perfusion lung scanning in the evaluation of pulmonary hypertension. J Nucl Med 35:793, 1994.

43. Falaschi F, Palla A, Formichi B, et al: CT evaluation of chronic thromboembolic pulmonary hypertension. J Comput Assist Tomogr 16:897, 1992.

44. Schwickert HC, Schweden F, Schild HH, et al: Pulmonary arteries and lung parenchyma in chronic pulmonary embolism: Preoperative postoperative CT findings. Radiology 191:351, 1994.

45. Tardivon AA, Musset D, Maitre S, et al: Role of CT in chronic pulmonary embolism: Comparison with pulmonary angiography. J Comput Assist Tomogr 17:345, 1993.

46. Bergin CJ, Sirlin CB, Hauschildt JP, et al: Chronic thromboembolism: Diagnosis with helical CT and MR imaging with angiographic and surgical correlation. Radiology 204:695, 1997.

47. Williams JO: Death following injection of lung scanning agent in a case of pulmonary hypertension. Br J Radiol 47:61, 1974.

48. Child JS, Wolfe JD, Tashkin D, et al: Fatal lung scan in a case of pulmonary hypertension due to obliterative pulmonary vascular disease. Chest 67:308, 1975.

49. Rich S, Dantzker DR, Ayres SM, et al: Primary pulmonary hypertension: A national prospective study. Ann Intern Med 107:216, 1987.

50. Caldini P, Gensini GG, Hoffman MS: Primary pulmonary hypertension with death during right heart catheterization: A case report and a survey of reported fatalities. Am J Cardiol 4:519, 1959.

51. Nicod P, Peterson K, Levine M, et al: Pulmonary angiography in severe chronic pulmonary hypertension. Ann Intern Med 107:565, 1987.

52. Cachecho R, Isik FF, Hirsch EF: Pathologic consequences of bilateral pulmonary lower lobectomies: Case report. J Trauma 32:268, 1992.

53. Hopkins WE: Severe pulmonary hypertension in congenital heart disease: A review of Eisenmenger syndrome. Curr Opin Cardiol 10:517, 1995.

54. Ormond RS, Poznanski AK, Templeton AW: Pulmonary veins in congenital heart disease in the adult. Radiology 76:885, 1961.

55. Milne ENC: Some new concepts of pulmonary blood flow and volume. Radiol Clin North Am 16:515, 1978.

56. Baltaxe HA, Amplatz K: The normal chest roentgenogram in the presence of large atrial septal defects. Am J Roentgenol 107:322, 1969.

57. Rees RSO, Jefferson KE: The Eisenmenger syndrome. Clin Radiol 18:366, 1967.

58. Rees S: The chest radiograph in pulmonary hypertension with central shunt. Br J Radiol 41:172, 1968.

59. Doyle AE, Goodwin JF, Harrison CV, et al: Pulmonary vascular patterns in pulmonary hypertension. Br Heart J 19:353, 1957.

60. Wexler L, Higgins CB, Herfkens RJ: Magnetic resonance imaging in adult congenital heart disease. J Thorac Imaging 9:219, 1994.

61. Hughes JD, Rubin LJ: Primary pulmonary hypertension: An analysis of 28 cases and a review of the literature. Medicine 65:56, 1986.

62. Goodman J, Harrison DC, Popp RL: Echocardiographic features of primary pulmonary hypertension. Am J Cardiol 33:438, 1974.

63. Martin-Duran R, Larman M, Trugeda A, et al: Comparison of Doppler-determined elevation pulmonary arterial pressure with pressure measured at cardiac catheterization. Am J Cardiol 57:859, 1986.

64. Selby CL: Living with primary pulmonary hypertension. In Rubin LJ, Rich S (eds): Primary Pulmonary Hypertension. Vol 99. In Lefant C (executive ed): Lung Biology in Health and Disease. New York, Marcel Dekker, 1997, pp 319–325.

65. Lebrec D, Capron JP, Dhumeaux D, et al: Pulmonary hypertension complicating portal hypertension. Am Rev Respir Dis 120:849, 1979.

66. Yoshida EM, Erb SR, Ostrow DN, et al: Pulmonary hypertension associated with primary biliary cirrhosis in the absence of portal hypertension: A case report. Gut 35:280, 1994.

67. Woolf D, Voigt MD, Jaskiewicz K, et al: Pulmonary hypertension associated with non-cirrhotic portal hypertension in systemic lupus erythematosus. Postgrad Med J 70:41, 1994.

68. Schraufnagel DE, Kay JM: Structural and pathologic changes in the lung vasculature in chronic liver disease. Clin Chest Med 17:1, 1996.

69. Mandell MS, Groves BM: Pulmonary hypertension in chronic liver disease. Clin Chest Med 17:17, 1996.

70. Rossi SO, Gilbert-Barness E, Saari T, et al: Pulmonary hypertension with coexisting portal hypertension. Pediatr Pathol 12:433, 1992.

71. Portmann B, Stewart S, Higenbottam TW, et al: Nodular transformation of the liver associated with portal and pulmonary arterial hypertension. Gastroenterology 104:616, 1993.

72. McDonnell PJ, Toye PA, Hutchins GM: Primary pulmonary hypertension and cirrhosis: Are they related? Am Rev Respir Dis 127:437, 1983.

73. Kibria G, Smith P, Heath D, et al: Observations on the rare association between portal and pulmonary hypertension. Thorax 35:945, 1980.

74. Van der Linden P, Le Moine O, et al: Pulmonary hypertension after transjugular intrahepatic portosystemic shunt: Effects on right ventricular function. Hepatology 23:982, 1996.

75. Moser KM, Auger WR, Fedullo PF, et al: Chronic thromboembolic pulmonary hypertenson: Clinical picture and surgical treatment. Eur Respir J 5:334, 1992.

76. Rich S, Levitsky S, Brundage BH: Pulmonary hypertension from chronic pulmonary thromboembolism. Ann Intern Med 108:425, 1988.

77. Benotti JR, Dalen JE: The natural history of pulmonary embolism. Clin Chest Med 5:403, 1985.

78. Chitwood WR Jr, Sabiston DC Jr, Wechsler AS: Surgical treatment of chronic unresolved pulmonary embolism. Clin Chest Med 5:507, 1984.

79. Bernstein RJ, Ford RL, Clausen JL, et al: Membrane diffusion and capillary blood volume in chronic thromboembolic pulmonary hypertension. Chest 110:1430, 1996.

80. Powe JE, Palevsky HI, McCarthy KE, et al: Pulmonary arterial hypertension: Value of perfusion scintigraphy. Radiology 164:727, 1987.

81. Ryan KI, Fedullo PF, Davis GB, et al: Perfusion scan findings understate the severity of angiographic and hemodynamic compromise in chronic thromboembolic pulmonary hypertension. Chest 93:1180, 1988.

82. Rich S, Pietra GG: Primary pulmonary hypertension: Radiograph and scintigraphic patterns of histologic subtypes. Ann Intern Med 105:499, 1986.

83. Martin KW, Sagel SS, Siegel BA: Mosaic oligemia simulating pulmonary infiltrates on CT. Am J Roentgenol 147:670, 1986.

84. King MA, Bergin CJ, Yeung DWC, et al: Chronic pulmonary thromboembolism: Detection of regional hypoperfusion with CT. Radiology 191:359, 1994.

85. Bergin CJ, Rios G, King MA, et al: Accuracy of high-resolution CT in identifying chronic pulmonary thromboembolic disease. Am J Roentgenol 166:1371, 1996.

86. Sherrick AD, Swensen SJ, Hartman TE: Mosaic pattern of lung attenuation on CT scans: Frequency among patients with pulmonary artery hypertension of different causes. Am J Roentgenol 169:79, 1997.

87. Worthy SA, Müller NL, Hartman TE, et al: Mosaic attenuation pattern on thin-section CT scans of the lung: Differentiation among infiltrative lung, airway, and vascular diseases as a cause. Radiology 205:465, 1997.

88. Remy-Jardin M, Louvegny S, Remy J, et al: Acute central thromboembolic disease: Post-therapeutic follow-up with spiral CT angiography. Radiology 203:173, 1997.

89. Teigen CL, Maus TP, Sheedy PE, et al: Pulmonary embolism: Diagnosis with electron-beam CT. Radiology 188:839, 1993.

90. Roberts HC, Kauczor HU, Schweden F, et al: Spiral CT of pulmonary hypertension and chronic thromboembolism. J Thorac Imaging 12:118, 1997.

91. Schwickert H, Schweden F, Schild H, et al: Demonstration of chronic recurrent pulmonary emboli with spiral CT. Fortschr Roentgenstr 158:308, 1993.

92. Kauczor H-U, Schwickert HC, Mayer E, et al: Spiral CT of bronchial arteries in chronic thromboembolism. J Comput Assist Tomogr 18:855, 1994.

93. Pitton MB, Duber C, Mayer E, et al: Hemodynamic effects of nonionic contrast bolus injection and oxygen inhalation during pulmonary angiography in patients with chronic major-vessel thromboembolic pulmonary hypertension. Circulation 94:2485, 1996.

94. Auger WR, Fedullo PF, Moser KM, et al: Chronic major-vessel thromboembolic pulmonary artery obstruction: Appearance at angiography. Radiology 182:393, 1992.

95. Peterson KL, Fred HL, Alexander JK: Pulmonary arterial webs: A new angiographic sign of previous thromboembolism. N Engl J Med 277:33, 1967.

96. Come PC: Echocardiographic evaluation of pulmonary embolism and its response to therapeutic interventions. Chest 101(4 Suppl):151S, 1992.

97. Wittlich N, Erbel R, Eichler A, et al: Detection of central pulmonary artery thromboemboli by transesophageal echocardiography in patients with severe pulmonary embolism. J Am Soc Echocardiogr 5:515, 1992.

98. Austin JHM, Young BG Jr, Thomas HM, et al: Radiologic assessment of pulmonary arterial pressure and blood volume in chronic, diffuse, interstitial pulmonary diseases. Invest Radiol 14:9, 1979.

99. Steckel RJ, Bein ME, Kelly PM: Pulmonary arterial hypertension in progressive systemic sclerosis. Am J Roentgenol 124:461, 1975.

100. Bindelglass IL, Trubowitz S: Pulmonary vein obstruction: An uncommon sequel to chronic fibrous mediastinitis. Ann Intern Med 48:876, 1958.

101. Stovin PGI, Mitchinson MJ: Pulmonary hypertension due to obstruction of intrapulmonary veins. Thorax 20:106, 1965.

102. Singshinsuk SS, Hartman AF Jr, Elliott LP: Stenosis of the individual pulmonary veins: A rare cause of pulmonary hypertension. Radiology 87:514, 1966.

103. Milne ENC: Pulmonary blood flow distribution. Invest Radiol 12:479, 1977.

104. Simon G: The value of radiology in critical mitral stenosis—an amendment. Clin Radiol 23:145, 1972.

105. Tattersfield AE, McNicol MW, Shawdon H, et al: Chest x-ray film in acute myocardial infarction. BMJ 3:332, 1969.

106. Chait A, Cohen HE, Meltzer LE, et al: The bedside chest radiograph in the evaluation of incipient heart failure. Radiology 105:563, 1972.

107. McHugh TJ, Forrester JS, Adler L, et al: Pulmonary vascular congestion in acute myocardial infarction: Hemodynamic and radiologic correlations. Ann Intern Med 76:29, 1972.

108. Seningen RP, Chen JTT, Peter RH, et al: Roentgen interpretation of postoperative changes (clinical and hemodynamic) in pure mitral stenosis. Am J Roentgenol 113:693, 1971.

109. Ramirez A, Grimes ET, Abelmann WH: Regression of pulmonary vascular changes following mitral valvuloplasty: An anatomic and physiologic case study. Am J Med 45:975, 1968.

110. Rosenow EC III, Harrison CE Jr: Congestive heart failure masquerading as primary pulmonary disease. Chest 58:28, 1970.

111. Thadani U, Burrow C, Whittaker W, et al: Pulmonary veno-occlusive disease. QJM 44:133, 1975.

112. Wagenvoort CA, Wagenvoort N, Takahashi T: Pulmonary veno-occlusive disease: Involvement of pulmonary arteries and review of the literature. Hum Pathol 16:1033, 1985.

113. Hasleton PS, Ironside JW, Whittaker JS, et al: Pulmonary veno-occlusive disease: A report of four cases. Histopathology 10:933, 1986.

114. Lombard C, Churg A, Winokur S: Pulmonary veno-occlusive disease following therapy for malignant neoplasms. Chest 92:871, 1987.

115. Waldhorn R, Tsou E, Smith F, et al: Pulmonary veno-occlusive disease associated with microangiopathic hemolytic anemia and chemotherapy of gastric adenocarcinoma. Med Pediatr Oncol 12:394, 1984.

116. Stuart KL, Bras G: Veno-occlusive disease of the liver. QJM 26:219, 1957.

117. Mehta MJ, Karmody AM, McKnealy MF: Mediastinal veno-occlusive disease associated with herbal tea ingestion. N Y State J Med 86:604, 1986.

118. Williams LM, Fussell S, Veith RW, et al: Pulmonary veno-occlusive disease in an adult following bone marrow transplantation: Case report and review of the literature. Chest 109:1388, 1996.

119. Kramer MR, Estenne M, Berkman N, et al: Radiation-induced pulmonary veno-occlusive disease. Chest 104:1282, 1993.

120. Townend JN, Roberts DH, Jones EL, et al: Fatal pulmonary veno-occlusive disease after use of oral contraceptives. Am Heart J 124:1643, 1992.

121. Alpert LI: Veno-occlusive disease of the liver associated with oral contraceptives: Case reports and review of literature. Hum Pathol 7:709, 1976.

122. Shackleford GD, Sacks EJ, Mullins JD, et al: Pulmonary veno-occlusive disease: Case report and review of the literature. Am J Roentgenol 128:643, 1977.

123. Rambihar VS, Fallen EL, Cairns JA: Pulmonary veno-occlusive disease: Ante-mortem diagnosis from roentgenographic and hemodynamic findings. Can Med Assoc J 120:1519, 1979.

124. Cassart M, Gevenois PA, Kramer M, et al: Pulmonary venoocclusive disease: CT findings before and after single-lung transplantation. Am J Roentgenol 160:759, 1993.

125. Swensen SJ, Tashjian JH, Myers JL, et al: Pulmonary venoocclusive disease: CT findings in eight patients. Am J Roentgenol 167:937, 1996.

126. Weisser K, Wyler F, Gloor F: Pulmonary veno-occlusive disease. Arch Dis Child 42:322, 1967.

127. Lopez-Candales A, Kleiger RE, Aleman-Gomes J, et al: Pulmonary artery aneurysm: Review and case report. Clin Cardiol 18:738, 1995.

128. Deterling RA Jr, Clagett OT: Aneurysm of the pulmonary artery: Review of the literature and report of a case. Am Heart J 34:471, 1947.

129. Symbas PN, Scott HW Jr: Traumatic aneurysm of the pulmonary artery. J Thorac Cardiovasc Surg 45:645, 1963.

130. Kumar RV, Roughneen PT, de Leval MR: Mycotic pulmonary artery aneurysm following pulmonary artery banding. Eur J Cardiothorac Surg 8:665, 1994.

131. Remy-Jardin M, Remy J: Spiral CT angiography of the pulmonary circulation. Radiology 212:615, 1999.

132. Auerbach O: Pathology and pathogenesis of pulmonary arterial aneurysm in tuberculous cavities. Am Rev Tuberc 39:99, 1939.

133. Kauffman SL, Lynfield J, Hennigar GR: Mycotic aneurysms of the intrapulmonary arteries. Circulation 35:90, 1967.

134. Jaffe RB, Condon VR: Mycotic aneurysms of the pulmonary artery and aorta. Radiology 116:291, 1975.

135. Navarro C, Dickinson PCT, Kondlapoodi P, et al: Mycotic aneurysms of the pulmonary arteries in intravenous drug addicts. Am J Med 76:1124, 1984.

136. Choyke PL, Edmonds PR, Markowitz RI, et al: Mycotic pulmonary artery aneurysm: Complication of aspergillus endocarditis. Am J Roentgenol 138:1172, 1982.

137. Rousch K, Scala-Barnett DM, Donabedian H, et al: Rupture of a pulmonary artery associated with candidal endocarditis. Am J Med 84:142, 1988.

138. Slavin RE, de Groot WJ: Pathology of the lung in Behçet's disease. Am J Surg Pathol 5:779, 1981.

139. De Montpreville VT, Macchiarini P, Dartevelle PG, et al: Large bilateral pulmonary artery aneurysms in Behçet's disease: Rupture of the contralateral lesion after aneurysmorrhaphy. Respiration 63:49, 1996.

140. Ungaro R, Saab S, Almond CH, et al: Solitary peripheral pulmonary artery aneurysms. J Thorac Cardiovasc Surg 71:566, 1976.

141. Chung CW, Doherty JU, Kotler R, et al: Pulmonary artery aneurysm presenting as a lung mass. Chest 108:1164, 1995.

142. Dieden JD, Friloux LA III, Renner JW: Pulmonary artery false aneurysms secondary to Swan-Ganz pulmonary artery catheters. Am J Roentgenol 149:901, 1987.

143. Loevner LA, Andrews JC, Francis IR: Multiple mycotic pulmonary artery aneurysms: A complication of invasive mucormycosis. Am J Roentgenol 158:761, 1992.

144. Ahn JM, Im JG, Ryoo JW, et al: Thoracic manifestations of Behçet syndrome: Radiographic and CT findings in nine patients. Radiology 194:199, 1995.

145. Numan F, Islak C, Berkmen T, et al: Behçet disease: Pulmonary arterial involvement in 15 cases. Radiology 192:465, 1994.

146. Jeang MK, Adyanthaya AV, Schwepe I, et al: Multiple pulmonary artery aneurysms: New use for magnetic resonance imaging. Am J Med 81:1001, 1986.

147. Guttentag AR, Shepard JAO, McLoud TC: Catheter-induced pulmonary artery pseudoaneurysm: The halo sign on CT. Am J Roentgenol 158:637, 1992.

148. Remy J, Smith M, Lamaitre L, et al: Treatment of massive hemoptysis by occlusion of a Rasmussen aneurysm. Am J Roentgenol 135:605, 1980.

149. Davidoff AB, Udoff EJ, Schonfeld SA: Intraaneurysmal embolism of a pulmonary artery aneurysm for control of hemoptysis. Am J Roentgenol 142:1019, 1984.

150. Bartter T, Irwin RS, Nash G: Aneurysms of the pulmonary arteries. Chest 94:1065, 1988.

151. Gibbs PM, Hami A: Pulmonary arterial aneurysm presenting as an endobronchial mass. Thorax 50:1013, 1995.

152. Baum D, Khoury GH, Ongley PA, et al: Congenital stenosis of the pulmonary artery branches. Circulation 29:680, 1964.

153. Tung H, Liebow AA: Marfan's syndrome. Lab Invest 1:382, 1952.

154. Shilkin KB, Low LP, Chen BTM: Dissecting aneurysm of the pulmonary artery. J Pathol 98:25, 1969.

155. Luchtrath H: Dissecting aneurysm of the pulmonary artery. Virchows Arch 391:241, 1981.

156. Teplick JG, Haskin ME, Nedwich A: The Hughes-Stovin syndrome: Case report. Radiology 113:607, 1974.

CHAPTER 14

Pulmonary Edema

CLASSIFICATION OF PULMONARY EDEMA

It is convenient to classify the causes of pulmonary edema into two major categories on the basis of underlying pathogenetic abnormality (Table 14–1). In the first category are conditions in which the edema results from an increase in the pulmonary microvascular pressure (hydrostatic edema, elevated microvascular pressure edema). Left ventricular failure is the most common cause (cardiogenic edema). A decrease in the serum osmotic pressure or in interstitial fluid pressure can contribute to the development of hydrostatic edema, although these abnormalities do not cause edema by themselves. The basic abnormality in hydrostatic edema is an exaggeration of the normal transvascular fluid flux and an overwhelming of the homeostatic mechanisms that normally control the volume of pulmonary extravascular water.

The second category includes conditions in which edema results from an increase in microvascular permeability (normal pressure pulmonary edema, capillary leakage pulmonary edema, permeability pulmonary edema, noncardiogenic pulmonary edema). We prefer to call this form of pulmonary edema *increased permeability edema* or *permeability edema*. Although many specific insults can cause sufficiently widespread endothelial or epithelial damage (or both) to result in generalized pulmonary edema of this type, the resulting clinical, radiologic, and pathologic manifestations are remarkably similar.[1, 2]

It is not always possible to assign individual patients who have pulmonary edema to one of these two categories; a combination of permeability and cardiogenic edema is common. Coexistence of the two is particularly serious because many of the mechanisms that impede the accumulation of excess extravascular water are lost when the endothelium loses its selectivity for solutes.

Table 14–1. CLASSIFICATION OF PULMONARY EDEMA

HYDROSTATIC PULMONARY EDEMA
Cardiogenic
   Left ventricular failure
   Mitral valve disease
   Left atrial myxoma or thrombus
   Cor triatriatum
Disease of the Pulmonary Veins
   Primary (idiopathic) veno-occlusive disease
   Fibrosing mediastinitis
Neurogenic (Combined Hydrostatic and Permeability Pulmonary Edema)
   Head trauma
   Increased intracranial pressure
   Postictal
Decreased Capillary Osmotic Pressure
   Renal disease
   Fluid overload
   Cirrhosis
INCREASED PERMEABILITY PULMONARY EDEMA (ARDS)
   Systemic sepsis
   Pulmonary infection
   Trauma
   Inhalation of noxious fumes and gases
   Aspiration of noxious fluids
   Ingestion or injection of drugs or poisons

ARDS, adult respiratory distress syndrome.

PULMONARY EDEMA ASSOCIATED WITH ELEVATED MICROVASCULAR PRESSURE (HYDROSTATIC PULMONARY EDEMA)

Cardiogenic Pulmonary Edema

The most common cause of interstitial and air-space pulmonary edema is a rise in pulmonary venous pressure secondary to disease of the left side of the heart. Increased pressure within the left atrium and pulmonary veins can develop as a result of back pressure from the left ventricle (secondary to long-standing systemic hypertension, aortic valvular disease, cardiomyopathy, or coronary artery disease with or without myocardial infarction) or can be caused by obstruction to the left atrial outflow (as a result of mitral valve stenosis, left atrial myxoma, or cor triatriatum). Rarely, pulmonary venous hypertension is the result of stenosis of the pulmonary veins themselves, such as occurs in congenital or acquired veno-occlusive disease or fibrosing mediastinitis.

The clinical manifestations of cardiogenic pulmonary edema depend on whether the onset of edema is acute or insidious. When severe, the acute form is dramatic, with dyspnea developing over minutes to hours. The patient characteristically sits bolt upright in obvious respiratory distress and uses the accessory muscles of respiration. In patients in whom edema develops less precipitously, the onset of symptoms may be insidious, and there may be few physical findings. Dyspnea may occur only during exertion; a history of orthopnea and paroxysmal nocturnal dyspnea is a helpful diagnostic feature in such patients, although these symptoms, accompanied by cough, also are common in patients who have asthma or chronic obstructive pulmonary disease.

Radiologic Manifestations

Hydrostatic pulmonary edema results in two principal radiologic patterns, depending on whether edema fluid remains relatively localized in the interstitial space or whether it also occupies the air spaces of the lung (Table 14–2).

Predominantly Interstitial Edema

Transudation of fluid into the interstitial spaces of the lung inevitably constitutes the first stage of pulmonary edema because the capillaries are situated in this compartment. Although this transudation of fluid constitutes the

Table 14–2. HYDROSTATIC PULMONARY EDEMA: CHARACTERISTIC RADIOLOGIC MANIFESTATIONS

Increased caliber of upper lobe vessels
Loss of definition of subsegmental and segmental vessels
Septal (Kerley) lines
Thickening of interlobar fissures
Perihilar or diffuse consolidation
Air bronchograms uncommon
Small pleural effusions commonly evident on radiograph
Widening of vascular pedicle
Cardiomegaly common

first stage of fluid accumulation in the lungs, it is not the first radiographic sign of cardiac decompensation or pulmonary venous hypertension. Pulmonary venous hypertension usually is evidenced by redistribution of blood flow from lower to upper lung zones so that an increase in caliber of upper zone vessels typically precedes evidence of overt edema (Fig. 14–1).[4, 5] Upper lobe vessel *recruitment* occurs in many other situations (e.g., pulmonary arterial hypertension), however, and is seen more commonly in patients who have chronic venous hypertension than in those who have acute left ventricular failure.[5, 6] Redistribution of blood flow can be assessed reliably only on radiographs performed at maximal inspiration in the erect position.[4, 5] Usually, this assessment is done subjectively by comparing the number and size of upper lung zone vessels to lower zone vessels at an equal distance from the hila.[4, 5] The earliest stage at which redistribution can be recognized is when the number and caliber of upper zone vessels are similar to those in the lower zone.[4, 7] As the redistribution becomes more pronounced, the upper zone vessels become larger.

A more objective assessment of arterial enlargement is based on the measurement of the diameter of bronchi and adjacent pulmonary arteries seen end-on. Normally the diameter of the pulmonary arteries in the upper lung zones is the same or less than the external diameter of the companion bronchi.[4, 8] When there is blood flow redistribution, the artery becomes larger than the accompanying bronchus (Fig. 14–2). In one investigation in which the pulmonary artery-to-bronchus diameter ratios were measured on upright chest radiographs, the mean ratio in 30 normal subjects was 0.85 (standard deviation [SD] 0.15), compared with 1.62 (SD 0.31) in 30 patients who had fluid overload and 1.50 (SD 0.25) in 30 patients who had left ventricular failure.[8] The mean ratio in normal subjects in the supine position was 1.01 (SD 0.13) compared with 1.49 (SD 0.31) for patients who had left ventricular failure.

When pulmonary venous hypertension is moderate in degree, fluid accumulates in the perivascular and interlobular septal interstitial tissue.[9, 10] As a result of this localization, edema fluid produces the typical radiographic pattern of loss of the normal sharp definition of subsegmental and segmental pulmonary vessels, thickening of the interlobular septa, and interlobar fissures (Fig. 14–3). Several groups of investigators have shown that this pattern tends to develop when pulmonary venous pressure (wedge pressure) reaches about 17 to 20 mm Hg.[4, 11, 12] Although the presence of septal lines can be valuable in confirming the diagnosis when other signs are equivocal, in our experience the frequency with which they can be identified is low compared with loss of definition of pulmonary vascular markings; their absence should not be construed as evidence against the diagnosis.

When edema fluid accumulates in the parenchymal interstitial tissue (the alveolar wall phase[3]) before the development of air-space edema, radiographic findings usually are absent or manifested only as a faintly discernible *haze*, which tends to be predominantly lower zonal or perihilar in distribution. In one investigation, a sequence of redistribution of blood flow, loss of the sharp marginal contour of pulmonary vessels, and perihilar haze and air-space consolidation was observed in 30 patients who had recent

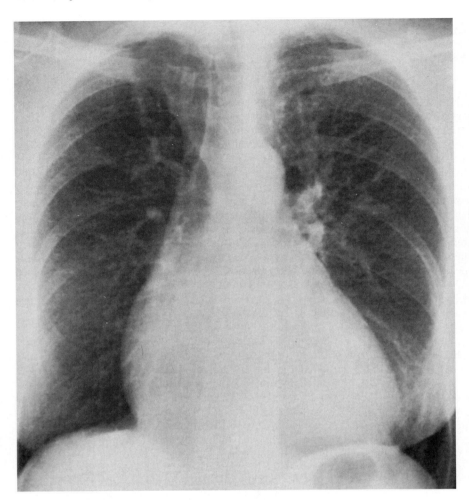

Figure 14–1. Redistribution of Blood Flow to Upper Lung Zones Caused by Pulmonary Venous Hypertension. Posteroanterior radiograph shows unusually prominent vascular markings in the upper zones and sparse markings in the lower zones. The patient was a 42-year-old woman who had recurrent episodes of left ventricular decompensation as a result of cardiomyopathy.

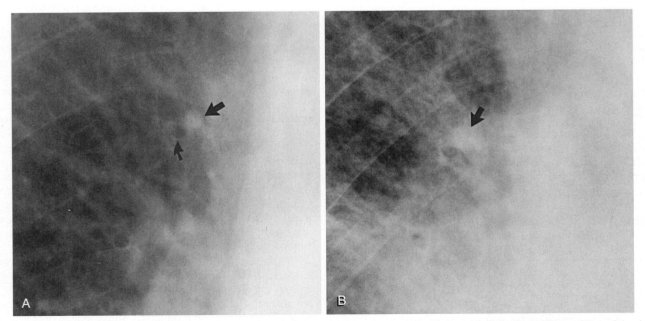

Figure 14–2. Increased Upper Lung Zone Pulmonary Artery-to-Bronchus Diameter Ratio in Hydrostatic Pulmonary Edema. View of the right upper lung zone from anteroposterior chest radiograph *(A)* in a healthy 87-year-old man shows a normal pulmonary artery-to-bronchus diameter ratio. The external diameter of the pulmonary artery *(straight arrow)* is similar to that of the external diameter of its accompanying bronchus *(curved arrow)*. Three years later, the patient developed acute pulmonary edema after myocardial infarction. Erect anteroposterior chest radiograph *(B)* shows increased diameter of the pulmonary artery *(arrow)*. Perihilar haze also is evident.

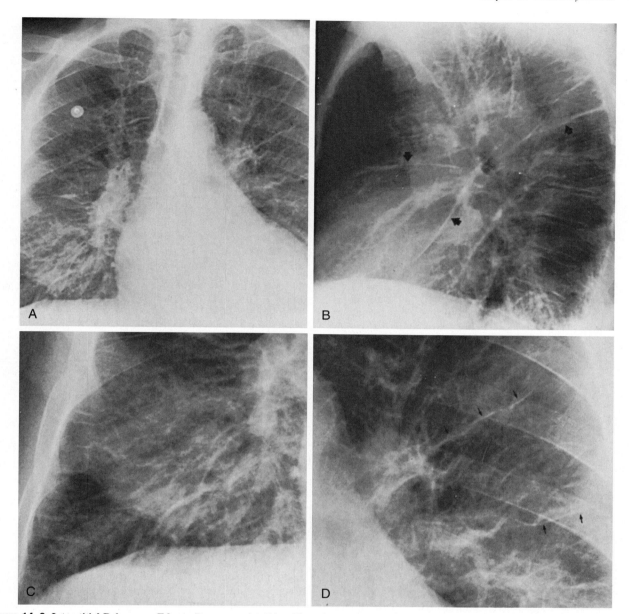

Figure 14–3. Interstitial Pulmonary Edema. Posteroanterior *(A)* and lateral *(B)* radiographs show multiple linear opacities throughout both lungs that are seen to better advantage in magnified view of the right lower *(C)* and left upper *(D)* lungs. These lines consist of a combination of long septal lines (Kerley A), predominantly in the midlung zones *(arrows in D)*, and shorter peripheral septal lines (Kerley B). In lateral projection *(B)*, the interlobar fissures are prominent *(arrows)* and represent pleural edema. The edema had cleared completely 24 hours later.

myocardial infarction;[12] generally the severity of radiographic abnormalities correlated well with pulmonary wedge pressure. Despite these observations, there is often a phase lag between elevation of pulmonary wedge pressure and radiographic signs of pulmonary edema, possibly because of the time required for transudation of fluid into the extravascular space.[13] The heart usually is enlarged but may not be when the cause of the edema is recent myocardial infarction, coronary artery insufficiency,[14] restrictive cardiomyopathy, left atrial myxoma, cor triatriatum, tachyarrhythmias, acute systemic hypertension such as that occasioned by an adrenal pheochromocytoma, or, occasionally, mitral stenosis or aortic stenosis.

Evidence for interstitial pulmonary edema is provided by an increase in the thickness of the walls of bronchi seen end-on in the perihilar zones. In the absence of chronic airway disease, such as bronchitis or asthma, these structures measure less than 1 mm in thickness. When fluid accumulates in the interstitial tissue surrounding them, their shadow thickens and loses its sharp definition (Fig. 14–4). Similar thickening can occur in large central airways, such as the intermediate bronchus. This sign has been employed to advantage in some patients in whom other signs of interstitial edema have not been convincing;[15] however, it is important to exclude airway disease, such as chronic bronchitis or asthma. Another sign of interstitial edema is thickening of the interlobar fissures (*see* Fig. 14–3).[5, 16] Because the pleura is in continuity with the interlobular septa, when fluid accumulates in the latter sites (creating Kerley B lines), it often collects in the pleural interstitium

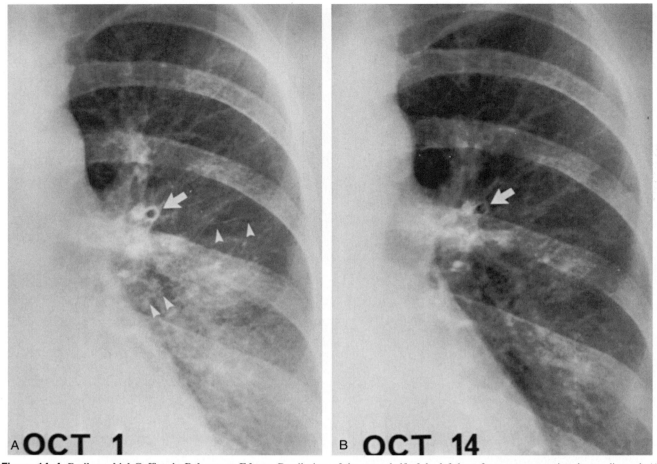

Figure 14–4. Peribronchial Cuffing in Pulmonary Edema. Detail view of the upper half of the left lung from posteroanterior chest radiograph *(A)* shows distended upper lobe vessels, perihilar haze, septal A lines *(arrowheads)*, and thickened bronchial wall viewed end-on *(arrow)*. A few days later, after diuretic therapy *(B)*, signs of pulmonary edema had resolved. The decreased thickness of the bronchial wall is apparent *(arrow)*. The patient was a middle-aged woman with renal failure.

as well. In such circumstances, the excess fluid causes not only a thickening of the interlobar fissures, but also a widening of the pleural layer over the convexity of the lungs, particularly in the costophrenic recesses, an abnormality that sometimes is confused with pleural effusion. Small pleural effusions may be present in addition.

When there is adequate treatment of the edema, radiologic signs may disappear within hours. A delay in resolution is seen in some patients, however.[12] In both of the studies cited previously, investigators observed a time lag between the fall of pressure and radiologic improvement, in some cases 12 to 22 hours after left ventricular filling pressure had returned to normal as the result of treatment.[17, 18] Persistence of septal lines after adequate therapy (such as mitral commissurotomy for mitral stenosis) usually indicates irreversible fibrosis. The radiographic features that help to distinguish hydrostatic from permeability edema are the normal heart size and infrequent interstitial edema or pleural effusion in edema associated with increased microvascular permeability.[19]

Although the diagnosis of hydrostatic pulmonary edema usually is based on clinical information and chest radiography, it is important to recognize the appearance of hydrostatic edema on computed tomography (CT) because it can mimic other diseases and sometimes occurs as an unsuspected finding in patients who are having CT for a different reason.[20, 21] As on radiographs, there is disproportionate enlargement of nondependent pulmonary arteries and veins and smooth thickening of the interlobular septa, interlobar fissures, and peribronchovascular connective tissue (Fig. 14–5).[20, 21] Areas of ground-glass attenuation can result from interstitial or air-space edema; consolidation reflects the presence of air-space edema. Pleural and pericardial effusions are detected more easily than on standard radiographs.[22] Other findings that can be seen on CT in association with hydrostatic pulmonary edema include enlarged mediastinal lymph nodes and inhomogeneous attenuation of mediastinal fat.[23]

Air-Space Edema

Although interstitial edema invariably precedes air-space edema pathologically, in some patients chest radiograph shows evidence of both simultaneously.[19, 24] The characteristic radiographic abnormality is the presence of patchy or confluent bilateral areas of consolidation that tend to be symmetric and to involve mainly the perihilar regions and the lower lung zones. Air bronchograms are seen in 10% to 30% of patients.[19, 24] In most cases, the shadows are confluent, creating irregular, rather poorly

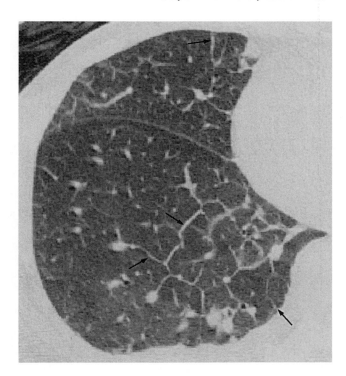

Figure 14–5. Interstitial Pulmonary Edema. View of the right lung from HRCT scan shows increased diameter of the pulmonary vessels, smooth thickening of the interlobular septa *(arrows)*, and localized areas of ground-glass attenuation in the dependent lung regions. A small pleural effusion also is present. The patient was a 49-year-old woman who developed interstitial pulmonary edema as a result of fluid overload.

defined, patchy opacities of unit density scattered randomly throughout the lungs; in the medial third of the lungs particularly, coalescence of areas of consolidation is common. The distribution varies from patient to patient but may be surprisingly similar during different episodes in the same individual. Patchy air-space consolidation sometimes extends to the subpleural zone or *cortex* of the lung (Fig. 14–6); however, the cortex may be spared completely, creating the *bat's wing* or *butterfly* pattern of edema.

Like hydrostatic interstitial pulmonary edema, air-space edema usually clears fairly rapidly in response to adequate treatment, and resolution appears complete radiographically in not more than 3 days in most cases.

Bat's Wing or *Butterfly* Pattern of Edema

The terms *bat's wing* and *butterfly* describe an anatomic distribution of air-space edema in which the hilum and *medulla* of the lungs are consolidated fairly uniformly, and the peripheral 2 to 3 cm of lung parenchyma—the *cortex*—is relatively uninvolved (Fig. 14–7). Definition of the margin of consolidated parenchyma often is indistinct but may be remarkably sharp. Localization of the edema to the central lung regions may be apparent in posteroanterior and lateral radiographic projections[35] and can be seen in the interstitium as well as the air spaces, particularly on CT. The uninvolved cortex usually extends along the interlobar lung fissures as well as around the convexity of the thorax, creating a waistlike indentation visible in posteroanterior projection in the region of the minor fissure. Similarly the upper and lower paramediastinal zones may be relatively free of involvement. Resolution of the edema generally begins in the periphery and spreads medially.[36] The pattern is uncommon; in one series of 110 cases of moderate to severe edema of varying etiology, it was identified in only 5%.[26] This pattern of edema occurs most commonly in acute severe cardiac failure as seen with massive myocardial infarction and in renal failure.[10]

Asymmetric Distribution of Pulmonary Edema

Although edema caused by cardiac disease usually is bilateral and fairly symmetric, it may be predominantly unilateral.[10, 25] The mechanisms underlying the development of this pattern were described in a study of 15 patients,[27] and the literature has been reviewed.[10, 28] The causes have been divided into ipsilateral and contralateral groups (Table 14–3).[28] The former refers to conditions in which the pathogenetic mechanism leading to the asymmetry is on the same side as the edema. In patients who have cardiac decompensation, unilateral edema probably is seen most often when the affected lung is dependent for a prolonged period (Fig. 14–8). In one review of 357 chest radiographs

Table 14–3. UNILATERAL PULMONARY EDEMA: COMMON CAUSES

Ipsilateral
    Prolonged lateral decubitus position
    Unilateral aspiration
    Pulmonary contusion
    Rapid thoracentesis
    Bronchial obstruction
    Obstruction of pulmonary vein
Contralateral
    COPD
    Swyer-James syndrome
    Acute pulmonary thromboembolism
    Unilateral or asymmetric lung destruction and fibrosis
    Pleural disease
Right upper lobe
    Mitral regurgitation

COPD, chronic obstructive pulmonary disease.

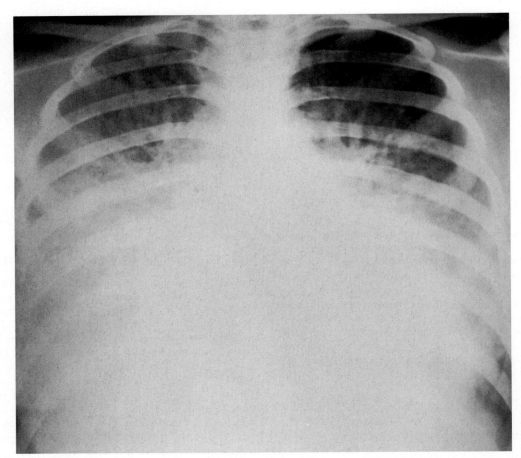

Figure 14–6. Acute Pulmonary Edema Secondary to Left Ventricular Failure. Posteroanterior radiograph shows extensive consolidation of both lungs extending to the visceral pleural surfaces. The heart is moderately enlarged. Six hours before this radiograph, the patient had abrupt onset of severe dyspnea, pleuritic pain, and cough productive of copious frothy sputum. The clinical and radiographic pictures are typical of acute pulmonary edema secondary to left ventricular failure.

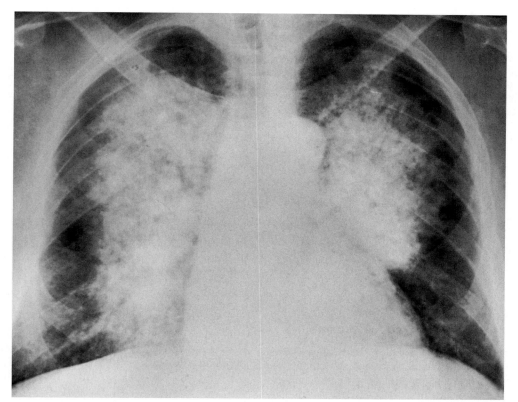

Figure 14–7. *Bat's Wing* **Pattern of Pulmonary Edema.** Posteroanterior radiograph shows consolidation of the perihilar and *medullary* portions of both lungs, creating a *bat's wing* or *butterfly* appearance; the *cortex* of both lungs is relatively unaffected. The margins of the edematous lung are defined sharply. The consolidation is fairly homogeneous and is associated with well-defined air bronchograms on both sides. This 59-year-old man had suffered a massive myocardial infarct 48 hours previously.

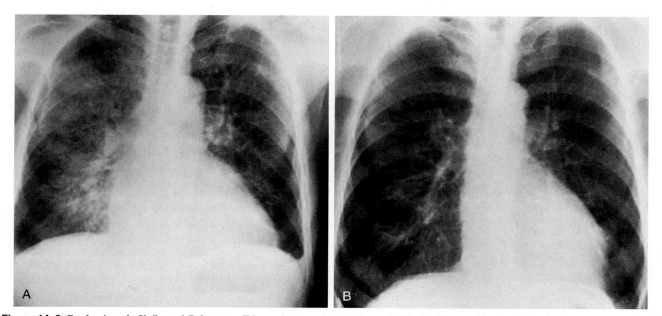

Figure 14–8. Predominantly Unilateral Pulmonary Edema. Posteroanterior radiograph *(A)* of a 70-year-old man admitted with an acute myocardial infarct shows patchy air-space consolidation occupying the medial two thirds of the right lung characteristic of acute pulmonary edema. The left lung is unaffected, although there is a small left pleural effusion. The heart is moderately enlarged. A visit to the patient's bedside revealed the fact that he lay on his right side most of the time because other positions seemed to intensify his shortness of breath. A radiograph after resolution of the edema *(B)* shows a marked increase in volume of both lungs characteristic of diffuse pulmonary emphysema. The unilaterality of the edema was related to the influence of gravity. It cannot be explained on the basis of emphysema because this disease is bilateral and symmetric.

from 25 patients who had pulmonary edema, were receiving assisted ventilation, and often were positioned on their side to promote drainage of tracheobronchial secretions, 68% showed gravity-dependent asymmetric edema;[34] only 18% showed edema predominantly in the *up* lung.

Edema localized to the right upper lobe sometimes is seen in patients in whom mitral regurgitation is the cause of the edema;[32, 33] in one study of 131 patients who had severe regurgitation, 12 (9%) showed this pattern.[33] We have seen this pattern most commonly in acute mitral regurgitation after myocardial infarction (Fig. 14–9). The mechanism underlying this distribution has been shown to be a predominant orientation of the regurgitant jet toward the right superior pulmonary vein.[29]

Contralateral edema refers to the accumulation of excess water in a *normal* lung opposite to the abnormality (*see* Table 14–3). The most common cause is asymmetric parenchymal involvement in chronic obstructive pulmonary disease.[10]

Pulmonary Edema Associated with Renal Disease, Hypervolemia, or Hypoproteinemia

Acute and chronic renal disease—with or without uremia—can be associated with acute pulmonary edema.[8, 37] It is likely that the major contributing cause to the development of pulmonary edema in these cases is left ventricular failure, although it is probable that decreased protein osmotic pressure, hypervolemia, and increased capillary permeability also have a role. In some patients who have uremia, normal pulmonary capillary pressures have been recorded in the presence of pulmonary edema.[38]

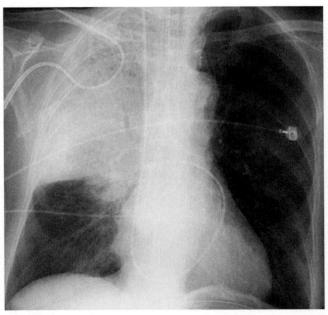

Figure 14–9. Right Upper Lobe Pulmonary Edema Resulting from Acute Mitral Regurgitation. Anteroposterior chest radiograph in a 66-year-old woman shows diffuse right upper lobe consolidation. Although the appearance is most suggestive of a pneumonia, it was proved to be due to air-space pulmonary edema secondary to acute mitral regurgitation after myocardial infarction. This is an extreme example of localized right upper lobe edema resulting from mitral regurgitation.

The administration of large volumes of intravenous fluids has been shown to cause pulmonary edema in patients who do not have underlying heart disease,[39, 41] particularly during the postoperative period and in the elderly. In many of these patients, the edema develops in the absence of known pulmonary injury and usually has been attributed to volume overload of the left ventricle, resulting in temporary high-output left ventricular failure. It has been shown, however, that in some patients, fluid infusion results in pulmonary edema without functional impairment of the left ventricle and without an increase in left ventricular filling pressures or pulmonary arterial wedge pressure;[40] in these cases, the edema has been attributed at least in part to a decrease in colloid osmotic pressure.

Pulmonary Edema Secondary to Abnormalities of the Pulmonary Veins

Obstructive disease of the pulmonary veins is a relatively rare cause of pulmonary venous hypertension and edema that has many causes, including (1) congenital heart disease of high-flow and low-flow types; (2) congenital stenosis or atresia of the pulmonary veins at their junction with the left atrium; (3) idiopathic veno-occlusive disease involving the small-sized and medium-sized veins; (4) fibrosing mediastinitis; (5) anomalous pulmonary venous drainage, above or below the diaphragm, in which venous compression, stenosis, or increased resistance of the hepatic sinusoids leads to a rise in pulmonary venous pressure;[42] (6) invasion or compression of pulmonary veins (e.g., by a malignant neoplasm such as left atrial leiomyosarcoma,[43] by enlarged lymph nodes,[44] or by a bronchogenic cyst [Fig. 14–10]); and (7) pulmonary vein thrombosis (as in cases of postlobectomy edema).[31]

Radiographic manifestations usually are indistinguishable from manifestations of pulmonary venous hypertension from cardiac causes except that the heart is usually of normal size, and in cases in which only one or two veins are affected, the edema may be localized to a specific portion of lung (e.g., a single lobe or lung). The edema is predominantly interstitial in location, although it may be associated periodically with air-space disease. The chronic elevation of venous pressure may result in pulmonary arterial hypertension indistinguishable from that associated with chronic mitral stenosis.

Neurogenic and Postictal Pulmonary Edema

Acute pulmonary edema in association with raised intracranial pressure, head trauma, and seizures is a well-described but infrequent phenomenon. Although its mechanism is poorly understood, clinical and experimental studies indicate that increased microvascular pressure and increased permeability are involved.[45–47] This combination of increased pressure and increased permeability led to the following hypothesis:[50] An acute increase in intracranial pressure causes a generalized sympathetic discharge that results in a massive increase in pulmonary vascular pressures, barotrauma to the endothelium, and consequent increased permeability; by the time microvascular pressures have been measured, they may have returned to control levels, leaving barotrauma-induced changes in permeability

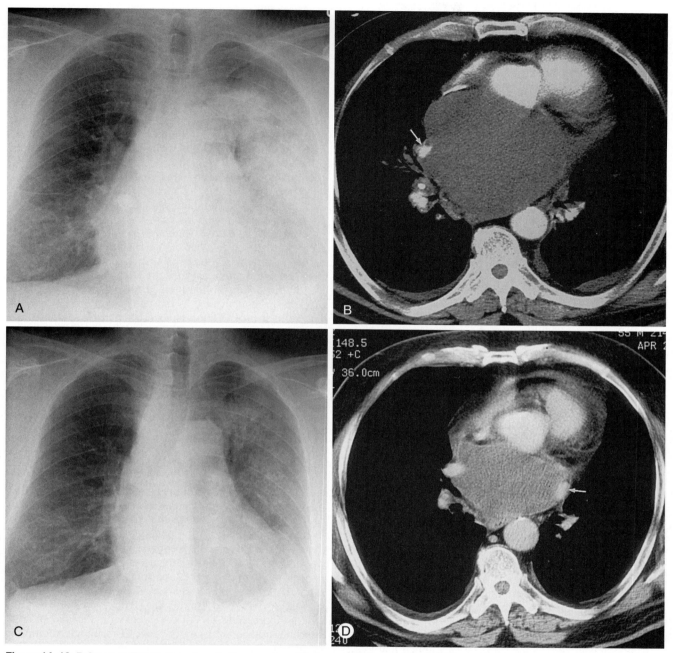

Figure 14–10. Pulmonary Edema Secondary to Compression of Pulmonary Vein by Mediastinal Bronchial Cyst. Posteroanterior chest radiograph *(A)* in a 55-year-old man shows extensive consolidation in the left upper lobe and a small left pleural effusion. CT scan *(B)* shows a large cystic mass with homogeneous water density in the subcarinal region consistent with a mediastinal bronchial cyst. The right superior pulmonary vein is seen *(arrow)*, but the left superior pulmonary vein is not visualized, being compressed by the mass. Small bilateral pleural effusions are evident. Chest radiograph performed 3 days later *(C)* shows marked improvement in the left upper lobe consolidation. In the interval, the patient developed increased opacity in the right paratracheal region with associated displacement of the trachea as a result of accumulation of fluid from spontaneous rupture of the bronchial cyst. Contrast-enhanced CT scan *(D)* shows marked decrease in size of the subcarinal cyst. The left superior pulmonary vein now shows contrast enhancement *(arrow)*. The consolidation in the left upper lobe presumably represented pulmonary edema caused by compression of the left superior pulmonary vein; it resolved within 3 days after spontaneous rupture of the cyst. (Case courtesy of Dr. Carole Dennie, Department of Radiological Sciences, Ottawa Civic Hospital, Ottawa, Canada.)

as the major culprit. This hypothesis has been supported by individual case reports in which patients who had neurogenic pulmonary edema have been observed to develop episodic systemic and pulmonary vascular hypertensive crises during which pulmonary arterial wedge pressure increased to 50 mm Hg.[51] Neurogenic edema after trauma and in postoperative patients may be difficult or impossible to differentiate from edema caused by fluid overload.[10] The diagnosis is made by exclusion of other causes.

The radiographic manifestations consist of homogeneous or, less commonly, inhomogeneous bilateral airspace consolidation.[10, 49] The edema usually is generalized;[48] however, an atypical pattern (e.g., predominantly upper zonal or unilateral) is seen in some patients.[30] The atypical distribution could be related to positional factors and gravity effects. Characteristically the edema disappears within several days after surgical relief of increased intracranial pressure. Most patients are comatose and experience frequent periods of apnea when pulmonary edema develops. They are likely to aspirate gastric secretions and to suffer prolonged hypoxemia. It is possible that aspiration is the cause of the edema in some cases.

PULMONARY EDEMA ASSOCIATED WITH NORMAL MICROVASCULAR PRESSURE (PERMEABILITY PULMONARY EDEMA)

After a variety of direct or indirect pulmonary insults, some patients develop progressive respiratory distress characterized by tachypnea, dyspnea, cough, and physical findings of air-space consolidation. Chest radiograph reveals diffuse air-space disease, blood gas analysis shows severe arterial desaturation that is resistant to high concentrations of inhaled oxygen, the lungs become stiff and difficult to ventilate, pulmonary vascular pressures and resistance increase, and it becomes necessary to institute prolonged ventilatory support. Pathologic changes are similar despite the varying inciting events, consisting of necrosis of type I epithelial cells, interstitial and alveolar edema, hyaline membrane formation, and in the later stages interstitial and air-space fibrosis. This group of clinicopathologic abnormalities generally is called *adult respiratory distress syndrome* (ARDS).[2] A second relatively common designation is *permeability edema*; although *increased permeability edema* is more appropriate, the abbreviated nomenclature serves to distinguish this form of edema from that resulting primarily from increased microvascular pressure. Because of their familiarity and brevity, the terms *permeability edema* and *ARDS* are used throughout this text.

Although estimates in the early 1970s implied that there were 150,000 new cases of ARDS each year in the United States (75 per 100,000 population),[52] more recent evidence suggests that the incidence of the disorder, as presently defined, is about 1.5 per 100,000 people per year.[53] Major risk factors include sepsis, aspiration of liquid gastric contents, severe trauma (including long bone and pelvic fractures and pulmonary contusion), multiple blood transfusions, near-drowning, pancreatitis, prolonged hypotension, overwhelming pneumonia, and disseminated intravascular coagulation (often associated with sepsis).[54, 55] Less common risk factors are drug overdose, major burns,[56] and coronary artery bypass surgery.[55]

Pathologic Characteristics

As indicated, the pathologic changes in the lungs of patients who have ARDS are virtually the same regardless of cause and usually are described by the term *diffuse alveolar damage*. Although a continuum of histologic abnormalities exists, for purposes of discussion the changes can be described conveniently in three phases: exudative, proliferative, and fibrotic.[58–60]

Exudative Phase. In the early exudative phase, which in most cases occurs within hours after the initial pulmonary insult, there is interstitial edema (affecting perivascular and interlobular interstitium as well as the alveolar wall), capillary congestion, and air-space filling by a proteinaceous exudate and a variable number of red blood cells. Later (2 to 7 days), intra-alveolar fluid appears compact and eosinophilic and may contain macrophages; similar material in alveolar ducts and distal respiratory bronchioles tends to become flattened against the airway wall, producing hyaline membranes.

Proliferative Phase. Although it is not possible to put a precise time on the end of the exudative phase, changes of the proliferative phase usually are seen 7 to 28 days after the initial pulmonary insult. This process is characterized by fibroblast proliferation, predominantly within alveolar air spaces, but also in the parenchymal interstitium.[61] The cellular proliferation is accompanied by synthesis and deposition of proteoglycan molecules in the interstitium.[62] In time, collagen is laid down within this provisional matrix.

Fibrotic Phase. In some patients, sufficient collagen is deposited to result in a significant degree of interstitial fibrosis. In patients who have less severe disease, healing is unassociated with functionally or histologically significant residual fibrosis.

Clinical Manifestations

The clinical manifestations of ARDS can develop insidiously, hours or days after the initiating event (e.g., sepsis or fat emboli), or acutely, coincident with the causative event (e.g., aspiration of liquid gastric contents). Typical symptoms are dyspnea, tachypnea, dry cough, retrosternal discomfort, and agitation; cyanosis may be present. The expectoration of copious, blood-tinged fluid signifies severe disease. Arterial blood analysis shows hypoxemia and a normal or decreased arterial P_{CO_2}. The hypoxemia is difficult or impossible to correct even with the use of high concentrations of inspired oxygen. Clinical deterioration is usual, requiring endotracheal intubation to maintain adequate oxygenation (oxygen saturation >90%).

Comparing studies of prognosis, treatment, and outcome in ARDS has been hampered by a lack of consistent diagnostic criteria. This deficiency stimulated individuals at an American-European consensus conference to develop criteria to define groups of patients on the basis of disease severity.[80] According to these criteria, patients can be separated into two groups, one that has less severe disease (termed *acute lung injury*) and one that has the more severe features of full-blown ARDS. As shown in Table 14–4, the criteria are based on clinical, radiographic, and physiologic findings.

Table 14–4. DIAGNOSTIC CRITERIA FOR ADULT RESPIRATORY DISTRESS SYNDROME

Injury	Criteria
Acute lung injury	Acute onset Pao_2/Fio_2 ≤300 mm Hg Bilateral pulmonary infiltrates on frontal chest radiograph Pulmonary artery wedge pressure ≤18 mm Hg (when measured) or no clinical evidence of left atrial hypertension
Adult respiratory distress syndrome	Acute onset Pao_2/Fio_2 ≤200 mm Hg Bilateral pulmonary infiltrates on frontal chest radiograph Pulmonary artery wedge pressure ≤18 mm Hg (when measured) or no clinical evidence of left atrial hypertension

Radiologic Manifestations

Radiography

Remarkably good correlation has been reported between the radiographic patterns observed during life and the pathologic changes observed at autopsy.[58, 63, 65]

Exudative Phase. All observers report a characteristic delay of 12 hours from the clinical onset of respiratory failure to the appearance of abnormalities on the chest radiograph. The earliest radiographic findings consist of patchy, ill-defined opacities throughout both lungs. In one study, evidence of interstitial edema was remarkably infrequent (5 of 75 patients);[63] however, in two other series, it was more common (Fig. 14–11).[58, 64] The appearance is similar to air-space edema of cardiac origin except that the heart size usually is normal; the edema tends to show a more peripheral distribution (Table 14–5).

The patchy zones of consolidation rapidly coalesce to a point of massive air-space consolidation (Fig. 14–12). Characteristically, involvement is diffuse, affecting all lung zones from apex to base and to the extreme periphery of each lung; in our experience, this widespread distribution can be of considerable value in distinguishing ARDS from cardiogenic pulmonary edema, whose distribution is seldom as extensive. Similarly, in contrast to cardiogenic edema, an air bronchogram frequently is visible. Pleural effusion is characteristically inapparent on supine radiographs; its presence suggests complicating acute pneumonia or pulmonary infarction.

It is important to be aware of the potential effects of

Table 14–5. PERMEABILITY PULMONARY EDEMA: CHARACTERISTIC RADIOLOGIC MANIFESTATIONS

Normal size of upper lobe vessels
Diffuse or predominantly peripheral consolidation
Air bronchograms common
Effusions seldom evident on conventional radiographs (small effusions commonly seen on decubitus view or CT scan)
Septal lines uncommon (when present suggest concomitant hydrostatic edema)
Normal vascular pedicle
Cardiomegaly uncommon

mechanical ventilation and positive end-expiratory pressure ventilation (PEEP) on the radiographic appearance.[66] The institution of PEEP can result in dramatic variations in the appearance of parenchymal opacities in technically identical radiographs exposed over a 10- to 15-minute period; patients who show radiographic evidence of diffuse pulmonary edema in the absence of mechanical ventilation can show an almost complete disappearance of radiographic abnormality within minutes of the institution of PEEP. Knowledge of ventilator settings is essential to the correct interpretation of the severity of pulmonary abnormalities in patients who have ARDS. Continuous positive-pressure ventilation also can lead to diffuse interstitial emphysema that may be visible against the background of extensive parenchymal consolidation. It is important to recognize this development because of the frequency of subsequent pneumomediastinum, pneumothorax, or both.

Proliferative and Fibrotic Phases. After approximately 1 week, the lungs remain diffusely abnormal, but the pattern tends to become reticular or *bubbly*,[58, 64] corresponding to the onset of interstitial and air-space fibrosis. In most patients who survive, radiograph shows improvement within the first 10 to 14 days. Failure to improve may indicate the development of a superimposed process (e.g., pneumonia) and carries a poor prognosis.[67] Of 46 patients who were followed in one study, 8 who had a relatively long survival and continuous assisted ventilation developed a coarse reticular pattern.[58]

Computed Tomography

The findings on CT and high-resolution computed tomography (HRCT) depend on the stage of ARDS. Early in the exudative phase, CT commonly shows diffuse, but not uniform, ground-glass opacification or consolidation, which often does not conform to a gravity-dependent distribution (Fig. 14–13). The interspersed areas of relative sparing are not appreciated easily on chest radiographs.[6] Later in the exudative phase, the consolidation becomes more homogeneous and gravity dependent. During the organizing phase, there is often a decrease in overall lung density and the appearance of interstitial reticulation.[22] Examination at this time often shows evidence of complications of ARDS and its treatment, such as interstitial emphysema, pneumomediastinum, pneumothorax, and subpleural bullae or cysts (Fig. 14–14).[6, 69] In one investigation of 74 patients at various stages of the disease, pulmonary opacities were bilateral in 92% and gravity dependent in 86%;[68] only 25% showed a homogeneous increase in attenuation, and most showed patchy consolidation or mixed air-space and ground-glass opacification. Air bronchograms were almost invariable (89%), and small pleural effusions were common; 22% had unilateral pleural effusions and 28% had bilateral pleural effusions.

Another group of investigators compared the pattern and distribution of findings on CT in 22 patients who had pulmonary causes of ARDS (e.g., pneumonia) and 11 who had extrapulmonary causes (e.g., sepsis).[70] In the first group, ground-glass opacities and air-space consolidation were equally prevalent, whereas the predominant finding in the second group was ground-glass attenuation. The ground-glass opacities were distributed evenly, whereas the

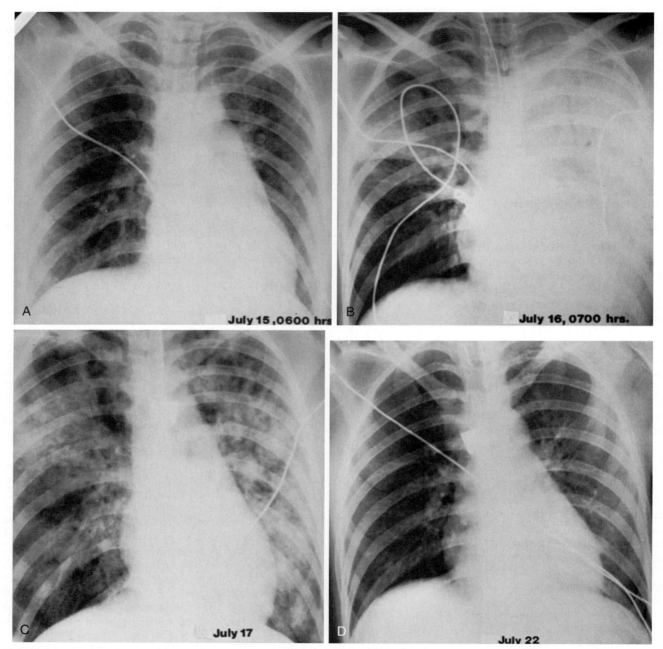

Figure 14–11. Adult Respiratory Distress Syndrome Associated with Gram-Negative Septicemia. Several hours before presenting for a radiograph, a 31-year-old woman had noted the onset of respiratory distress, which had increased in severity in this interval. This radiograph *(A)* reveals diffuse interstitial edema but no evidence of air-space edema or of major pulmonary consolidation. A radiograph taken 24 hours later *(B)* shows that the right upper lobe and the whole of the left lung were extensively consolidated by acute air-space edema. A radiograph taken 48 hours later *(C)* shows the lungs were uniformly involved, although in more patchy distribution. With the institution of vigorous supportive therapy and positive end-expiratory pressure ventilation, the patient's condition improved slowly to a point where 5 days later *(D)* the lungs were almost clear. Gram-negative septicemia followed laparotomy.

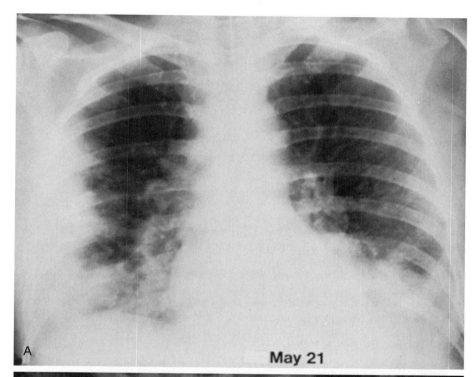

Figure 14–12. Adult Respiratory Distress Syndrome. This 18-year-old woman was admitted to the intensive care unit in severe shock after a motor vehicle accident. Radiograph the day after admission *(A)* showed homogeneous consolidation of the left lower lobe and the axillary portion of the right lung. Two days later *(B)*, both lungs were massively consolidated; note the prominent air bronchogram. The diagnosis was confirmed at autopsy.

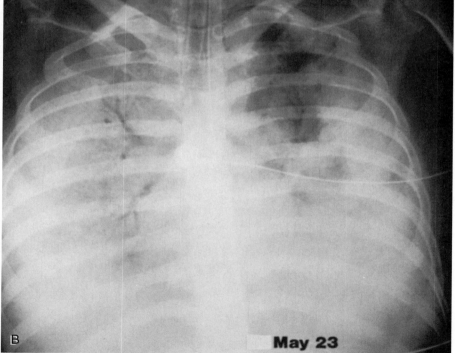

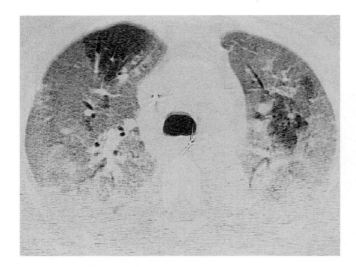

Figure 14–13. Adult Respiratory Distress Syndrome. HRCT scan shows extensive bilateral areas of ground-glass attenuation, air bronchograms, areas of consolidation in the dependent lung regions, and focal areas of relatively normal lung. The patient was a 45-year-old woman who developed adult respiratory distress syndrome secondary to cytotoxic drug reaction. The diagnosis was proved at autopsy.

consolidation involved mainly the dorsal portions of the lower lung zones. Ten of 11 (91%) patients who had ARDS of extrapulmonary origin had a bilateral symmetric distribution of findings compared with 16 of 22 (73%) patients with ARDS of pulmonary origin. Grossly asymmetric disease with a greater than 50% difference in involvement between right and left lung always was associated with asymmetric consolidation and was seen only in ARDS of pulmonary origin. In both groups of patients,

small pleural effusions and air bronchograms were seen commonly, whereas interlobular septal thickening and pneumatoceles were infrequent.[70]

Because air has an attenuation of $-1,000$ HU and water has a value of 0 HU, CT densitometry and area measurement can be used to calculate lung water, lung weight, and lung density. When these calculations were used in patients who had ARDS and compared with an assessment of the severity of edema based on the subjective

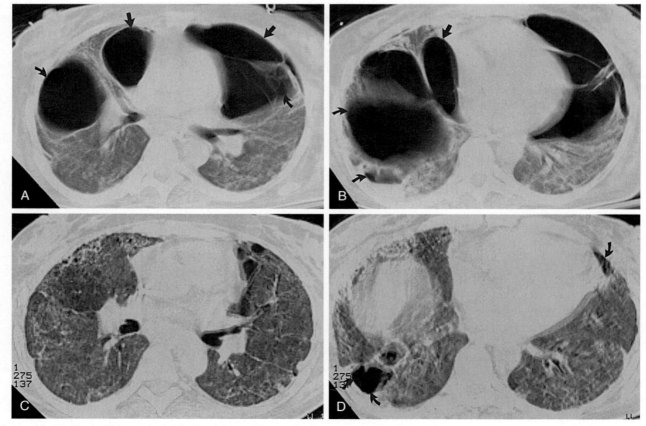

Figure 14–14. Cystic Changes in Adult Respiratory Distress Syndrome. A 30-year-old woman developed sepsis and adult respiratory distress syndrome after cesarean section. HRCT scans 1 week later *(A and B)* show bilateral loculated pneumothoraces *(straight arrows)* and cystic changes *(curved arrows)* in both lungs. HRCT scans 1 month later *(C and D)* show bilateral areas of ground-glass attenuation, irregular linear opacities, and residual cystic changes *(curved arrows)*. (Case courtesy of Dr. Maura Brown, Surrey Memorial Hospital, Surrey, British Columbia.)

examination of a portable chest radiograph, however, a highly significant correlation was found, indicating the robustness of the plain radiograph.[71] CT can be used to calculate the vertical gradient in lung inflation in patients who have ARDS. In one study of 17 patients, a significant decrease in the calculated milliliters of gas per gram of tissue was found at all levels;[72] however, as in normal individuals, a vertical gradient persisted.

Similar to radiography, the CT features of ARDS are altered when the patient's lungs are inflated by the application of PEEP. Because the involvement of the lung often is patchy, PEEP tends to inflate the uninvolved, normally compliant regions but does not alter the volume of the densely consolidated regions. Less consolidated (ground-glass) or atelectatic areas of lung may show an increase in aeration if the applied PEEP exceeds a critical opening pressure.[66, 73] This patchy inflation of the lung is the reason that application of high levels of PEEP or high tidal volumes frequently result in barotrauma in these patients.

The major conditions to be considered in radiologic differential diagnosis are severe cardiogenic pulmonary edema and widespread bacterial pneumonia. The latter may be impossible to differentiate from ARDS except on clinical grounds. Although involvement of the lungs seldom is as widespread and uniform in cardiogenic edema as in ARDS, differentiation between the two in the most severe cases can be made only by measuring the pulmonary arterial wedge pressure with a Swan-Ganz catheter, bearing in mind that left ventricular failure and consequent elevation of the wedge pressure also can occur as a complication of ARDS itself.

Follow-up CT in survivors of ARDS frequently shows residual reticular opacities (*see* Fig. 14–14).[74, 75] One group of investigators compared the HRCT findings during the acute illness and at follow-up 4 to 9 months later in 27 patients.[75] A coarse reticular pattern was the most prevalent (23 patients [85%]) and extensive abnormality at follow-up. The reticular pattern had a striking anterior predominance and was associated with distortion of parenchymal architecture and traction bronchiectasis, findings indicative of fibrosis. Multivariate analysis showed correlation between the extent of reticular pattern at follow-up and the duration of mechanical ventilation. Less common findings on follow-up CT included ground-glass opacities, areas of decreased attenuation resulting from small airway disease or emphysema, and pleural thickening.[75]

Radiographic Differentiation of Cardiogenic and Permeability Edema

The diagnosis of pulmonary edema usually can be made readily on chest radiograph. There is considerable controversy, however, regarding the ability to distinguish high-pressure (cardiogenic) from low-pressure (permeability) pulmonary edema on the basis of radiographic abnormalities.[5, 77, 78] Investigators have found a high degree of variability in diagnostic accuracy and in the features that are considered to constitute the most helpful signs in making the distinction. Some of this variability is related to different patient populations, difference in data analysis, use of posteroanterior as compared with anteroposterior chest radiographs, and assessment of upright versus supine chest radiographs.[24, 76] In general, the distinction is made more reliably in patients who have mild to moderate edema, on radiographs performed in posteroanterior projection, in erect or seated positions and by analysis of changes seen in sequential radiographs.[5, 76, 78]

Based on the results of the various studies in the literature, we believe that the most helpful radiographic findings in differential diagnosis are the number and caliber of pulmonary vessels (distribution of pulmonary blood flow); the distribution of pulmonary edema; the vascular pedicle width; and the presence or not of cardiomegaly, septal lines, air bronchograms, and pleural effusion.

Pulmonary Vascular Caliber. Pulmonary vascular caliber may be categorized as normal, balanced (equal size of upper and lower lung zone vessels), or inverted (upper zone vessels larger than lower zone vessels).[19] In one study in which most radiographs were performed in the posteroanterior projection with the patient upright or seated, approximately 50% of 61 patients who had cardiogenic pulmonary edema had an inverted blood flow pattern compared with none of 30 patients who had fluid overload and 10% of 28 patients who had permeability pulmonary edema.[19] A balanced blood flow pattern was not found to be helpful in distinguishing the various forms of edema. Distribution of blood flow has not been found to be helpful in distinguishing the various forms of pulmonary edema in supine patients.[76, 78]

Distribution of Pulmonary Edema. In one study, the distribution of edema was even (homogeneous from chest wall to heart) in 90% of patients who had cardiac failure, 30% of patients who had renal failure, and 35% of patients who had high permeability edema.[19] A perihilar distribution was seen in 10% of patients who had cardiac failure, 70% who had renal failure, and none who had permeability edema; a peripheral predominance was seen in 45% of patients who had permeability edema. In a second investigation, a peripheral predominance was seen in 12 of 25 (48%) patients who had increased permeability edema compared with 2 of 15 (13%) patients who had hydrostatic pulmonary edema.[78]

Width of the Vascular Pedicle. A large portion of the superior mediastinal opacity on posteroanterior chest radiograph is caused by the great systemic vessels and has been called the *vascular pedicle*.[19] The width of this *structure* is measured from the point at which the superior vena cava crosses the right main bronchus to the point at which the left subclavian artery arises from the aortic arch. In one study in which most radiographs were performed on posteroanterior projection in erect or seated patients, the width of the vascular pedicle was increased (>53 mm on erect posteroanterior radiographs) in 60% who had cardiac failure, 85% who had fluid overload, and 20% who had increased permeability pulmonary edema.[19] In two other studies in which the radiographs were performed with patients supine, differences in the width of the vascular pedicle were not considered helpful in diagnosis.[76, 78]

Septal Lines. The presence of septal lines is one of the most useful findings in differential diagnosis. In one investigation, septal lines were observed in approximately 30% of patients who had cardiac or renal-overhydration edema but in none of the patients who had ARDS.[19] In a second series, the lines were identified in 21 of 49 (43%) patients who had cardiac failure and in only 3 of 33 (9%) with permeability edema.[76] Although not all workers have found similar results,[78] we consider septal lines to be highly suggestive of hydrostatic pulmonary edema or a combination of hydrostatic and increased permeability edema.

Air Bronchogram. In one investigation, air bronchogram was identified in 70% of patients who had capillary permeability edema and in only 20% of patients who had cardiac and renal-overhydration edema.[19] In a second study, it was seen in 23 of 33 (70%) patients who had permeability edema and in 13 of 49 (26%) patients who had hydrostatic pulmonary edema.[76]

Pleural Effusion. As might be expected, pleural effusion is generally more common in association with cardiogenic edema. In one review, pleural effusion was identified in approximately 40% of patients who had this condition, as compared with only 10% of patients who had permeability edema.[19] When specifically looked for on decubitus or upright radiographs or on CT scan, however, small effusions are common in permeability edema; in one investigation, they were identified on radiograph in 14 of 49 (29%) patients who had hydrostatic pulmonary edema and 9 of 33 (27%) patients who had permeability edema.[78]

Heart Size. In one study, after application of a 12.5% correction factor necessitated by the supine position of patients, the anteroposterior projection, and the shortened 40-inch distance, cardiac enlargement was identified in 72% of patients who had cardiogenic edema but in only 32% of patients who had capillary permeability edema.[19] In another investigation, 9 of 15 (60%) patients with hydrostatic edema had cardiomegaly compared with 11 of 25 (44%) patients with permeability edema.[78]

Summary. As the results of these studies show, no single radiographic criterion allows reliable distinction between hydrostatic and permeability edema. A *combination* of findings permits correct identification of hydrostatic pulmonary edema in 80% to 90% of patients,[19, 77, 78] however, and correct identification of permeability edema in 60% to 90%.[19, 77, 78] In cases in which the diagnosis is equivocal, measurement of the pulmonary arterial wedge pressure with a Swan-Ganz catheter may be required, bearing in mind that elevation of the wedge pressure secondary to left ventricular dysfunction can occur as a complication of ARDS itself.

Natural History and Prognosis

ARDS is a serious disease, having a mortality rate of greater than 50% despite the availability of modern diagnostic techniques and therapies.[81, 82] In one study of 57 patients, 37 (65%) died;[57] in 90% of these, death occurred within 14 days of the onset of symptoms. Patients who die of pulmonary insufficiency usually show a progressive decrease in lung compliance and worsening gas exchange; in the terminal stages, barotrauma and hypercapnia may develop despite an enormous minute ventilation.

Specific Forms of Permeability Edema

High-Altitude Pulmonary Edema

Many individuals develop a symptom complex known as *high-altitude pulmonary edema* or *mountain* or *altitude sickness*, while becoming acclimatized to high altitudes.[67, 92]

Clinical features of the condition include headache, giddiness, dizziness, tiredness, weakness, body aches, anorexia, nausea, vomiting, abdominal pain, insomnia, restlessness, cough, dyspnea on exertion, and fever.[68] All symptoms and signs characteristically disappear on descent to sea level.

The illness may become manifest on acute[84] and prolonged[85] exposure at 3,500 to 4,000 m (11,500 to 13,000 feet); rare cases have been documented to develop at 2,750 m (9,000 feet).[86, 87] Usually the move from sea level to high altitude is abrupt; all but 3 of 101 patients in one report had arrived at an altitude of 3,500 m by airplane.[83] Affected individuals characteristically are young and otherwise healthy. Edema usually develops within 2 to 3 days and almost always within the first month after arrival at high altitude.

The pathogenesis of high-altitude pulmonary edema is uncertain and controversial.[88] The results of many studies have shown that increased capillary permeability is a contributing factor.[89] One hypothesis suggests that hypoxia secondary to the low FIO_2 causes intense, but inhomogeneous, vasoconstriction of a large proportion of the pulmonary arteries, forcing blood flow at high pressures through the remaining patent vessels.[89, 90] In regions where arterial constriction is deficient, there is high flow and transmission of the increased pulmonary arterial pressure directly to the capillary bed. The high capillary pressure and the shear stress caused by the high flow in the unconstricted areas result in pulmonary microvascular endothelial damage and permeability edema.

The radiographic appearances are those of acute pulmonary edema of any etiology. In a retrospective study of radiographic findings in 60 patients who had high-altitude pulmonary edema severe enough to warrant admission to the hospital, 55 (92%) had air-space consolidation (homogeneous in 40 and patchy in distribution in 15).[91] In about 45%, the consolidation was bilaterally symmetric; in 45%, it affected mainly the right lung; and in 10%, it was seen mainly in the left lung. The consolidation tended to be most severe in the lower lobes and most commonly involved central and peripheral lung regions; in some patients, it was predominantly central or, less commonly, peripheral in distribution. Nearly all patients had some peribronchial and perivascular cuffing and perihilar haze, and nine (15%) patients had Kerley B lines. No patients had pleural effusion at presentation; however, four developed small effusions within 24 to 48 hours. The cardiothoracic ratio was normal or minimally increased. On CT, high-altitude pulmonary edema has a patchy and predominantly peripheral distribution.[92] Although the central pulmonary vessels may be prominent as a result of acute pulmonary hypertension, cardiac enlargement has not been noted. The edema usually resolves within 1 to 2 days[30, 93] but may be present for 10 days.[79]

Postpneumonectomy Pulmonary Edema

Acute pulmonary edema is a well-recognized complication of lung resection, especially pneumonectomy.[94, 95] In one study of 197 patients who underwent pneumonectomy, acute pulmonary edema was diagnosed in 2.5%;[96] in another investigation of 402 patients who had a lobectomy or pneumonectomy, it was recognized in 1% of the former and in about 5% of the latter. Although fluid overload formerly was believed to be the major contributing factor, it is clear now that the edema is related to increased pulmonary capillary permeability.[97] Postpneumonectomy edema has a poor prognosis with a mortality rate exceeding 80%.[96]

Postpneumonectomy pulmonary edema occurs early in the postoperative period.[10] The patients typically present with marked dyspnea in the first 2 to 3 days after surgery. The radiographic findings in mild edema resemble those of interstitial pulmonary edema with ill-defined vascular markings and presence of septal lines. In patients who have severe edema, the radiologic manifestations are identical to those of ARDS.[10]

Pulmonary Edema After Lung Re-Expansion

Numerous case reports have been documented of unilateral pulmonary edema developing after rapid removal of air or liquid from the pleural space in the presence of pneumothorax or hydrothorax.[100, 101] Based on a summary of 12 cases, three features were considered common to almost all cases:[99] (1) The pneumothorax or hydrothorax is moderate or large in size (amounting to at least 50% of the affected hemithorax); (2) the pulmonary edema is localized strictly to the ipsilateral lung; and (3) the pneumothorax or hydrothorax has been present for a considerable period, usually several days, before rapid re-expansion. In the 12 cases, the duration of pneumothorax, as judged from the onset of dyspnea, averaged 18 days, with a minimum of 3 days. Although these features are applicable to most patients, they are not seen in all. Cases have been documented in which edema has developed in association with pneumothoraces that have been present for only one or a few hours[98] and in which the edema has developed contralateral to the re-expanded lung.[102, 103] The edema usually develops immediately or within 1 hour or re-expansion, and all cases occur within a 24-hour period.[104]

The pathogenesis of this form of edema is unclear. Increased capillary permeability appears to be at least one factor, as indicated by the elevated protein content of the edema fluid.[105, 106] The radiographic manifestations usually consist of unilateral air-space consolidation, which typically develops within 2 to 4 hours after re-expansion of the lung.[100] The consolidation usually affects the entire re-expanded lung, although occasionally it involves only one lobe.[100] Rarely, both lungs are affected.[101] CT scan shows a patchy distribution of the areas of consolidation. The consolidation resolves after 5 to 7 days.

Pulmonary Edema Secondary to Parenteral Contrast Media

Pulmonary edema has been described after the parenteral administration of the oil-based medium used for lymphangiography and the water-based media employed in urography, arteriography, and contrast-enhanced CT. It has been shown that the injection of an oil-based contrast medium in rabbits results in hemorrhagic pulmonary edema several days after embolization.[107] The fatty acids used in ethiodized oil are esterified; although a major proportion of the content of this material is oleic acid, esterification

makes it less toxic than the free fatty acid. The oil microemboli may be acted on by esterases in the lung, causing a breakdown of the esterified compounds to free fatty acids and resultant pulmonary capillary damage.

Pulmonary edema can accompany the anaphylactic shock that occasionally occurs after intravenous administration of water-based contrast media.[108, 110] The onset of the edema is characteristically acute, occurring minutes to hours after the injection, and is associated with evidence of systemic hypotension and complement activation.[109] The complication has been reported after the administration of high-osmolality contrast material[111] as well as ionic low-osmolality[112] and nonionic low-osmolality contrast material.[113] The prognosis is generally good.[114]

References

1. Ashbaugh DG, Bigelow DB, Petty TL, et al: Acute respiratory distress in adults. Lancet 2:319, 1967.
2. Petty TL, Ashbaugh DG: The adult respiratory distress syndrome: Clinical features, factors influencing prognosis and principles of management. Chest 60:233, 1971.
3. Staub NC, Nagano H, Pearce ML: Pulmonary edema in dogs, especially the sequence of fluid accumulation in lungs. J Appl Physiol 22:227, 1967.
4. Ravin CE: Pulmonary vascularity: Radiographic considerations. J Thorac Imaging 3:1, 1988.
5. Morgan PW, Goodman LR: Pulmonary edema and adult respiratory distress syndrome. Radiol Clin North Am 29:943, 1991.
6. Ketai LH, Godwin JD: A new view of pulmonary edema and acute respiratory distress syndrome. J Thorac Imaging 13:147, 1998.
7. Turner AF, Lau FYK, Jacobson G: A method for the estimation of pulmonary venous and arterial pressures from the routine chest roentgenogram. Am J Roentgenol 116:97, 1972.
8. Woodring JH: Pulmonary artery-bronchus ratios in patients with normal lungs, pulmonary vascular plethora, and congestive heart failure. Radiology 179:115, 1991.
9. Stender HS, Schermuly W: Das interstitielle Lungenödem im Röntgenbild. [Roentgen findings in interstitial pulmonary edema.] Fortschr Roentgensstr 95:461, 1961.
10. Gluecker T, Capasso P, Schnyder P, et al: Clinical and radiologic features of pulmonary edema. Radiographics 19:1507, 1999.
11. Simon M: The pulmonary vessels: Their hemodynamic evaluation using routine radiographs. Radiol Clin North Am 1:363, 1963.
12. McHugh TJ, Forrester JS, Adler L, et al: Pulmonary vascular congestion in acute myocardial infarction: Hemodynamic and radiologic correlations. Ann Intern Med 76:29, 1972.
13. Slutsky RA, Higgins CB: Intravascular and extravascular pulmonary fluid volumes: II. Response to rapid increases in left atrial pressure and the theoretical implications for pulmonary radiographic and radionuclide imaging. Invest Radiol 18:33, 1983.
14. Dodek A, Kassebaum DG, Bristow JD: Pulmonary edema in coronary-artery disease without cardiomegaly: Paradox of the stiff heart. N Engl J Med 286:1347, 1972.
15. Heitzman ER: The Lung: Radiologic-Pathologic Correlations. St. Louis, CV Mosby, 1973, pp 127, 137.
16. Heitzman ER, Ziter FM: Acute interstitial pulmonary edema. Am J Roentgenol 98:291, 1966.
17. Heikkilä J, Hugenholtz PG, Tabakin BS: Prediction of left heart filling pressure and its sequential change in acute myocardial infarction from the terminal force of the P wave. Br Heart J 35:142, 1973.
18. Bennett ED, Rees S: The significance of radiological changes in the lungs in acute myocardial infarction. Br J Radiol 47:879, 1974.
19. Milne EN, Pistolesi M, Miniati M, et al: The radiologic distinction of cardiogenic and noncardiogenic edema. Am J Roentgenol 144:879, 1985.
20. Primack SL, Müller NL, Mayo JR, et al: Pulmonary parenchymal abnormalities of vascular origin: High-resolution CT findings. Radiographics 14:739, 1994.
21. Storto ML, Kee ST, Golden JA, et al: Hydrostatic pulmonary edema: High-resolution CT findings. Am J Roentgenol 165:817, 1995.

22. Goodman LR: Congestive heart failure and adult respiratory distress syndrome: New insights using computed tomography. Intensive Care Radiol 34:33, 1996.

23. Slanetz PJ, Truong M, Shepard JAO, et al: Mediastinal lymphadenopathy and hazy mediastinal fat: New CT findings of congestive heart failure. Am J Roentgenol 171:1307, 1998.

24. Milne ENC: Letter to the editor: Hydrostatic versus increased permeability pulmonary edema. Radiology 170:891, 1989.

25. Richman SM, Godar TJ: Unilateral pulmonary edema. N Engl J Med 264:1148, 1961.

26. Nessa CG, Rigler LG: The roentgenological manifestations of pulmonary edema. Radiology 37:35, 1941.

27. Azimi F, Wolson AH, Dalinka MK, et al: Unilateral pulmonary edema: Differential diagnosis. Australas Radiol 19:20, 1975.

28. Calenoff L, Kruglik GD, Woodruff A: Unilateral pulmonary edema. Radiology 126:19, 1978.

29. Roach JM, Stajduhar KC, Torrington KG: Right upper lobe pulmonary edema caused by acute mitral regurgitation: Diagnosis by transesophageal echocardiography. Chest 103:1286, 1993.

30. Felman AH: Neurogenic pulmonary edema: Observations in 6 patients. Am J Roentgenol 112:393, 1971.

31. Gyves-Ray KM, Spizarny DL, Gross BH: Case report: Unilateral pulmonary edema due to postlobectomy pulmonary vein thrombosis. Am J Roentgenol 148:1078, 1987.

32. Alarcon JJ, Guembe P, de Miguel E, et al: Localized right upper lobe edema. Chest 107:274, 1995.

33. Schnyder PA, Sarraj AM, Duvoisin BE, et al: Pulmonary edema associated with mitral regurgitation: Prevalence of predominant involvement of the right upper lobe. Am J Roentgenol 161:33, 1993.

34. Leeming BWA: Gravitational edema of the lungs observed during assisted respiration. Chest 64:719, 1973.

35. Hughes RT: The pathology of butterfly densities in uraemia. Thorax 22:97, 1967.

36. Herrnheiser G, Hinson KFW: An anatomical explanation of the formation of butterfly shadows. Thorax 9:198, 1954.

37. Macpherson RI, Banerjee AK: Acute glomerulonephritis: A chest film diagnosis? J Can Assoc Radiol 25:58, 1974.

38. Gibson DG: Hemodynamic factors in the development of acute pulmonary oedema in renal disease. Lancet 2:1217, 1966.

39. Cooperman LH, Price HL: Pulmonary edema in the operative and postoperative period. Ann Surg 172:883, 1970.

40. daLuz PL, Weil MH, et al: Pulmonary edema related to changes in colloid osmotic and pulmonary artery wedge pressure in patients after acute myocardial infarction. Circulation 51:350, 1975.

41. Stein L, Beraud J, Cavonilles J, et al: Pulmonary edema during fluid infusion in the absence of heart failure. JAMA 229:65, 1974.

42. Hacking PM, Simpson W: Partially obstructed total anomalous pulmonary venous return. Clin Radiol 18:450, 1967.

43. Sande MA, Alonso DR, Smith JP, et al: Left atrial tumor presenting with hemoptysis and pulmonary infiltrates. Am Rev Respir Dis 102:258, 1970.

44. Montreal General Hospital Case Records: Dyspnea and lymphadenopathy in a patient with two PH-1 chromosomes. N Engl J Med 289:524, 1973.

45. Benowitz NL, Simon RP, Copeland JR: Status epilepticus: Divergence of sympathetic activity and cardiovascular response. Ann Neurol 19:197, 1986.

46. Johnston SC, Darragh TM, Simon RP: Postictal pulmonary edema requires pulmonary vascular pressure increases. Epilepsia 37:428, 1996.

47. Melon E, Bonnet F, Lepresle E, et al: Altered capillary permeability in neurogenic pulmonary oedema. Intensive Care Med 11:323, 1985.

48. Ducker TD: Increased intracranial pressure and pulmonary edema: I. Clinical study of 11 patients. J Neurosurg 28:112, 1968.

49. Ell SR: Neurogenic pulmonary edema: A review of the literature and a perspective. Invest Radiol 26:499, 1991.

50. Theodore J, Robin E: Speculations on neurogenic pulmonary edema. Am Rev Respir Dis 113:404, 1976.

51. Wray NP, Nicotra MB: Pathogenesis of neurogenic pulmonary edema. Am Rev Respir Dis 118:783, 1978.

52. Respiratory Diseases: Task Force Report on Problems, Research Approaches, Needs. DHEW publication No. NIH73-432. Bethesda, MD, National Heart and Lung Institute, 1972, pp 167–180.

53. Villar J, Slutsky AS: The incidence of adult respiratory distress syndrome. Am Rev Respir Dis 140:814, 1989.

54. Petty TL: Indicators of risk, course, and prognosis in adult respiratory distress syndrome (ARDS). Am Rev Respir Dis 132:471, 1985.

55. Connelly KG, Repine JE: Markers for predicting the development of acute respiratory distress syndrome. Annu Rev Med 48:429, 1997.

56. Wittram C, Kenny JB: The admission chest radiograph after acute inhalation injury and burns. Br J Radiol 67:751, 1994.

57. Fowler AA, Hamman RF, Good JT, et al: Adult respiratory distress syndrome: Risk with common predisposition. Ann Intern Med 98:593, 1983.

58. Ostendorf P, Birzle H, Vogel W, et al: Pulmonary radiographic abnormalities in shock: Roentgen-clinical pathological correlation. Radiology 115:257, 1975.

59. Hasleton PS: Adult respiratory distress syndrome—a review. Histopathology 7:307, 1983.

60. Blennerhasset JB: Shock lung and diffuse alveolar damage: Pathological and pathogenetic considerations. Pathology 17:239, 1985.

61. Fukuda Y, Ishizaki M, Masuda Y, et al: The role of intraalveolar fibrosis in the process of pulmonary structural remodeling in patients with diffuse alveolar damage. Am J Pathol 126:171, 1987.

62. Bensadoun ES, Burke AK, Hogg JC, et al: Proteoglycan deposition in pulmonary fibrosis. Am J Respir Crit Care Med 154:1819, 1996.

63. Joffe N: The adult respiratory distress syndrome. Am J Roentgenol 122:719, 1974.

64. Dyck DR, Zylak CJ: Acute respiratory distress in adults. Radiology 106:497, 1973.

65. Greene R: Adult respiratory distress syndrome: Acute alveolar damage. Radiology 163:57, 1987.

66. Zimmerman JE, Goodman LR, Shahvari MBG: Effect of mechanical ventilation and positive end-expiratory pressure (PEEP) on chest radiographs. Am J Roentgenol 133:811, 1979.

67. Wheeler AP, Carroll FE, Bernard GR: Radiographic issues in adult respiratory distress syndrome. New Horiz 1:471, 1993.

68. Tagliabue M, Casella TC, Zincone GE, et al: CT and chest radiography in the evaluation of adult respiratory distress syndrome. Acta Radiol 35:230, 1994.

69. Gattinoni L, Bombino M, Pelosi P, et al: Lung structure and function in different stages of severe adult respiratory distress syndrome. JAMA 271:1772, 1994.

70. Goodman LR, Fumagalli R, Tagliabue P, et al: Adult respiratory distress syndrome due to pulmonary and extrapulmonary causes: CT, clinical, and functional correlations. Radiology 213:545, 1999.

71. Bombino M, Gattinoni L, Pesenti A, et al: The value of portable chest roentgenography in adult respiratory syndrome. Chest 100:762, 1991.

72. Pelosi P, D'Andrea L, Vitale G, et al: Vertical gradient of regional lung inflation in adult respiratory distress syndrome. Am J Respir Crit Care Med 149:8, 1994.

73. Gattinoni L, D'Andrea L, Pelosi P, et al: Regional effects and mechanism of positive end-expiratory pressure in early adult respiratory distress syndrome. JAMA 269:2122, 1993.

74. Finfer S, Rocker G: Alveolar overdistension is an important mechanism of persistent lung damage following severe protracted ARDS. Anaesth Intensive Care 24:569, 1996.

75. Desai SR, Wells AU, Rubens MB, et al: Acute respiratory distress syndrome: CT abnormalities at long-term follow-up. Radiology 210:29, 1999.

76. Smith RC, Mann H, Greenspan RH, et al: Radiographic differentiation between different etiologies of pulmonary edema. Invest Radiol 22:859, 1987.

77. Miniati M, Pistolesi M, Paoletti P, et al: Objective radiographic criteria to differentiate cardiac, renal, and injury lung edema. Invest Radiol 23:433, 1988.

78. Aberle DR, Wiener-Kronish JP, Webb WR, et al: Hydrostatic versus increased permeability pulmonary edema: Diagnosis based on radiographic criteria in critically ill patients. Radiology 168:73, 1988.

79. Im JG, Yu YJ, Ahn JM, et al: Hydrostatic versus oleic acid-induced pulmonary edema: High-resolution computed tomography findings in the pig lung. Acta Radiol 1:364, 1994.

80. Bernard GR, Artigas A, Brigham KL, et al: The American-European Consensus Conference on ARDS: Definitions, mechanisms, relevant outcomes, and clinical trial coordination. Am J Respir Crit Care Med 149:818, 1994.

81. Bernard GR, Brigham KL: The adult respiratory distress syndrome. Annu Rev Med 36:195, 1985.

82. Lee J, Turner JS, Morgan CJ, et al: Adult respiratory

syndrome: Has there been a change in outcome predictive measures? Thorax 49:596, 1994.

83. Menon ND: High-altitude pulmonary edema: A clinical study. N Engl J Med 273:66, 1965.

84. Kamat SR, Banerjil BC: Study of cardiopulmonary function on exposure to high altitude: I. Acute acclimatization to an altitude of 3500 to 4000 meters in relation to altitude sickness and cardiopulmonary function. Am Rev Respir Dis 106:404, 1972.

85. Kamat SR, Rao TL, Sama BS, et al: Study of cardiopulmonary function on exposure to high altitude: II. Effects of prolonged stay at 3500 to 4000 meters and reversal on return to sea level. Am Rev Respir Dis 106:414, 1972.

86. Kleiner JP, Nelson WP: High altitude pulmonary edema: A rare disease? JAMA 234:491, 1975.

87. Anonymous: Pulmonary oedema of mountains. BMJ 3:65, 1972.

88. Richalet JP: High altitude pulmonary oedema: Still a place for controversy? Thorax 50:923, 1995.

89. Hultgren HN: High-altitude pulmonary edema: Current concepts. Annu Rev Med 47:267, 1996.

90. Hultgren HN: High altitude pulmonary edema: Hemodynamic aspects. Int J Sports Med 18:20, 1997.

91. Vock P, Brutsche MH, Nanzer A, et al: Variable radiomorphologic data of high altitude pulmonary edema: Features from 60 patients. Chest 100:1306, 1991.

92. Bärtsch P: High altitude pulmonary edema. Respiration 64:435, 1997.

93. Colice GL, Matthay MA, Bass E, et al: Neurogenic pulmonary edema: Clinical commentary. Am Rev Respir Dis 130:941, 1984.

94. Shapira OM, Shahian DM: Postpneumonectomy pulmonary edema. Ann Thorac Surg 56:190, 1993.

95. Kopec SE, Irwin RS, Umali-Torres CB, et al: The postpneumonectomy state. Chest 114:1158, 1998.

96. van der Werff YD, van der Houwen HK, Heijmans PJ, et al: Postpneumonectomy pulmonary edema: A retrospective analysis of incidence and possible risk factors. Chest 111:1278, 1997.

97. Williams EA, Evans TW, Goldstraw P: Acute lung injury following lung resection: Is one lung anaesthesia to blame? Thorax 51:114, 1996.

98. Humphreys RL, Berne AS: Rapid reexpansion of pneumothorax: A cause of unilateral pulmonary edema. Radiology 96:509, 1970.

99. Waqaruddin M, Bernstein A: Re-expansion pulmonary oedema. Thorax 30:54, 1975.

100. Tarver RD, Broderick LS, Conces DJ: Reexpansion pulmonary edema. J Thorac Imaging 11:198, 1996.

101. Trachiotis GD, Vricella LA, Aaron BL, et al: As originally published in 1988: Reexpansion pulmonary edema. Updated in 1997. Thorac Surg 63:1206, 1997.

102. Steckel RJ: Unilateral pulmonary edema after pneumothorax. N Engl J Med 289:621, 1973.

103. Gascoigne A, Appleton A, Taylor R, et al: Catastrophic circulatory collapse following re-expansion pulmonary oedema. Resuscitation 31:265, 1996.

104. Mahfood S, Hix WR, Aaron BL, et al: Reexpansion pulmonary edema. Ann Thorac Surg 45:340, 1988.

105. Buczko GB, Grossman RF, Goldberg M: Re-expansion pulmonary edema: Evidence for increased capillary permeability. Can Med Assoc J 125:459, 1981.

106. Sprung CL, Loewenherz JW, Baier H, et al: Evidence for increased permeability in reexpansion pulmonary edema. Am J Med 71:497, 1981.

107. Silvestri RC, Huseby JS, Rughani I, et al: Respiratory distress syndrome from lymphangiography contrast medium. Am Rev Respir Dis 122:543, 1980.

108. Solomon DR: Anaphylactoid reaction and non-cardiac pulmonary edema following intravenous contrast injection. Am J Emerg Med 4:146, 1986.

109. Boden WE: Anaphylactoid pulmonary edema ("shock lung") and hypotension after radiologic contrast media injection. Chest 81:759, 1982.

110. Bouachour G, Varache N, Szapiro N, et al: Noncardiogenic pulmonary edema resulting from intravascular administration of contrast material. Am J Roentgenol 157:255, 1991.

111. Borish L, Matloff SM, Findlay SR: Radiographic contrast media-induced noncardiogenic pulmonary edema: Case report and review of the literature. J Allergy Clin Immunol 74:104, 1984.

112. Delacour JL, Floriot C, Wagschal G, et al: Non-cardiac pulmonary edema following intravenous contrast injection. Intensive Care Med 15:49, 1988.

113. Goldsmith SR, Steinberg P: Noncardiogenic pulmonary edema induced by non-ionic low-osmolality radiographic contrast media. J Allergy Clin Immunol 96:698, 1995.

114. Ramesh S, Reisman R: Noncardiogenic pulmonary edema due to radiocontrast media. Ann Allergy Asthma Immunol 75:308, 1995.

CHAPTER 15

Disease of the Airways

UPPER AIRWAY OBSTRUCTION

The upper airway can be considered the conduit for inspired and expired gas that extends from the external nares (during nose breathing) or the lips (during mouth breathing) to the tracheal carina.

Acute Upper Airway Obstruction

Acute upper airway obstruction occurs most commonly in infants and young children because of the small intraluminal caliber and greater compliance of their upper airways. The principal causes are infection, edema, hemorrhage, foreign body aspiration, laryngeal dysfunction, and faulty placement of an endotracheal tube.

Infection

Infection can cause severe narrowing of the upper airways, particularly in infants and young children. Acute pharyngitis and tonsillitis, which may be complicated by retropharyngeal abscess, are caused most commonly by β-hemolytic streptococci.[1] Rarely, tonsillitis or infection of the supraglottic region, especially Epstein-Barr virus–related mononucleosis,[3] causes life-threatening acute upper airway obstruction in adults.[2] Acute bacterial tracheitis is a rare but potentially life-threatening cause of upper airway obstruction that usually affects children[5] but has been reported in adults.[5]

Acute epiglottitis usually is caused by *Haemophilus influenzae* and occasionally by *Staphylococcus aureus* or *Streptococcus pneumoniae*.[7, 8] Although acute epiglottitis most commonly affects infants and young children, it also occurs in adults, in whom it often is unrecognized.[6, 7] In one series of 47 patients who had acute epiglottitis, 10 (21%) were adults; of these, an initial diagnosis of epiglottitis was made in only 4.[6] The presenting symptoms include severe sore throat, difficulty in breathing, stridor, and hoarseness.[6] Radiographic findings include swelling of the epiglottis, aryepiglottic folds, arytenoids, uvula, and prevertebral soft tissues; the hypopharynx and oropharynx tend to be ballooned and the valleculae obliterated. In one investigation of 27 adults who had acute epiglottitis and 15 adults without symptoms, a ratio of the width of the epiglottis to the anteroposterior width of the C4 vertebral body greater than 0.33 had a sensitivity of 96% and a specificity of 100% in the diagnosis.[8] In another investigation in which 31 patients who had epiglottitis were compared with age-matched and sex-matched controls, a ratio of epiglottic width to C3 vertebral body width greater than 0.5 and a ratio of aryepiglottic fold width to C3 body width greater than 0.35 had a 100% sensitivity and specificity for the diagnosis.[9] Although the findings are seen well on computed tomography (CT),[10] this imaging modality seldom is indicated.

An acute retropharyngeal abscess can result in severe upper airway obstruction (Fig. 15–1) and can extend into the mediastinum and cause a mediastinal abscess. Laryngeal stenosis as a result of tuberculous infection usually is subacute rather than acute, but it may be the sole manifestation of disease.[11] Acute necrotizing pseudomembranous tracheobronchitis caused by *Aspergillus* species can be seen in immunosuppressed patients,[12] including those who have acquired immunodeficiency syndrome (AIDS).[13]

Edema

As a cause of acute upper airway obstruction, edema of noninfective origin characteristically affects the larynx. Underlying causes include trauma, inhalation of irritating noxious gases, and angioneurotic edema. The last-named condition is perhaps the most common cause and has a variable etiology, including allergy (anaphylaxis) and heredity;[15] some cases are idiopathic. The edema often is associated with multiple pruritic and usually nonpainful swellings in the subcutaneous tissues of the face, hands, feet, and genitalia; urticaria sometimes is seen. The heredi-

tary form usually begins in childhood and is characterized by recurrent attacks, often in association with abdominal cramps.[16] The form of inheritance is autosomal dominant. The prognosis in the hereditary form of angioneurotic edema is grave: About one third of individuals die from acute upper airway obstruction.[16, 17]

Faulty Placement of an Endotracheal Tube

Complications of endotracheal intubation are uncommon and occur more often in association with emergency resuscitation than with routine respiratory therapy.[17] The chief complication is large airway obstruction resulting from malpositioning of the tube too low in the trachea and major bronchi. In most instances, the endotracheal tube enters the right main bronchus (in 27 of 28 cases in one series),[17] and the orifice of the left main bronchus is occluded by the balloon cuff, resulting in atelectasis of the left lung (Fig. 15–2). If the tube is advanced sufficiently far down the right main bronchus, the right upper lobe bronchus may be occluded, with resultant atelectasis of this lobe as well as the left lung or of the right middle lobe alone.[17] Occasionally the tube enters the left rather than the right main bronchus, leading to obstruction of the latter. The rate at which atelectasis occurs depends on the gas content of the lung at the moment of occlusion. Total collapse requires 18 to 24 hours if the parenchyma contains air but can occur in a matter of minutes if the lung contains 100% oxygen (as is often the case in acute respiratory emergencies). Withdrawal of the tube typically results in rapid re-expansion of the collapsed lung or lobe.

It has been recommended that with the head and neck in a neutral position, the ideal distance between the tip of the endotracheal tube and the tracheal carina is 5 ± 2 cm.[18] Flexion and extension of the neck can cause a 2-cm descent and ascent of the tip of the endotracheal tube; if the position of the neck can be established from the radiograph (through visualization of the mandible), the ideal distance

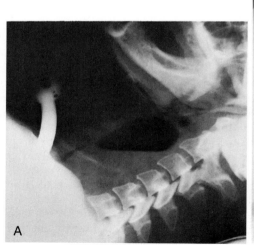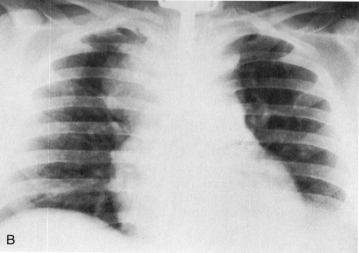

Figure 15–1. Acute Retropharyngeal and Mediastinal Abscess. A 29-year-old woman was admitted to the hospital with an 8-day history of increasing dyspnea, difficulty in swallowing, and loss of voice. An emergency tracheostomy was performed. Lateral radiograph of the soft tissues of the neck with a horizontal x-ray beam *(A)* showed a large accumulation of gas and fluid in the retropharyngeal space associated with complete obliteration of the air space of the hypopharynx and anterior displacement of the cervical trachea. Anteroposterior chest radiograph *(B)* showed a large mediastinal soft tissue density projecting predominantly to the right of the midline. The retropharyngeal and mediastinal abscesses were drained surgically.

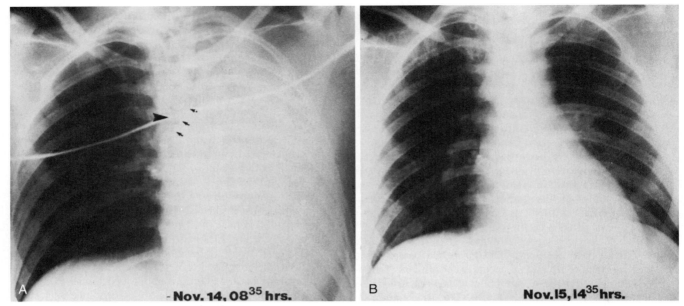

Figure 15–2. Acute Atelectasis of the Left Lung Resulting from Faulty Insertion of a Cuffed Tracheostomy Tube. Anteroposterior radiograph in the supine position *(A)* reveals complete airlessness of the left lung associated with slight displacement of the mediastinum to the left. A tracheostomy tube is in position, its tip *(arrowhead)* situated in the right main bronchus just beyond the carina (the medial wall of the right main bronchus is indicated by *arrows*). This atelectasis occurred over a brief period because a high-oxygen mixture was being administered. After withdrawal of the tracheostomy tube *(B)*, the left lung reinflated spontaneously and rapidly.

between the tip of the endotracheal tube and the carina should be 3 ± 2 cm with the neck flexed and 7 ± 2 cm with the neck extended. If the carina is not visualized, the endotracheal tube can be assumed to be in adequate position if its tip is aligned with the fifth, sixth, or seventh thoracic vertebra.[19]

Chronic Upper Airway Obstruction

General Features

In contrast to acute upper airway obstruction, the cause of which is often apparent, chronic obstructive disease of the pharynx, larynx, and trachea frequently is misdiagnosed as asthma or chronic obstructive pulmonary disease (COPD). Dyspnea is the usual presenting complaint, often first noted on exertion and sometimes exacerbated when the patient assumes a recumbent position.

A variety of conditions affecting the upper airway from the nasopharynx to the tracheal carina can cause chronic upper airway obstruction. The most common conditions are hypertrophy of the tonsils and adenoids, vocal cord paralysis, tracheal stenosis after tracheostomy or prolonged tracheal intubation, and primary and secondary neoplasms. Each of these conditions possesses fairly characteristic radiologic manifestations that permit their differentiation (*see* farther on); however, certain radiologic manifestations are common to all, regardless of their precise nature, and these are described first.

Radiologic Manifestations

Plain radiography plays a limited role in the assessment of patients who have pharyngeal or laryngeal abnormalities. The main exceptions are the use of lateral radiographs of

the soft tissues in the neck in the evaluation of patients suspected of having acute epiglottitis, retropharyngeal abscess, or foreign body obstruction. Imaging of intrinsic abnormalities of the pharynx and larynx usually is performed using CT or magnetic resonance (MR) imaging.[21, 22] CT has been shown to be helpful in assessing extralaryngeal causes of vocal cord paralysis; in one investigation of 20 patients who had left vocal cord palsy, CT showed a tumor in the aortopulmonary window (presumably involving the recurrent laryngeal nerve) in 18 (90%).[23] Chest radiography showed an abnormality at this site in only 5 of the 18 patients. In the same study, 8 of 11 cases of right vocal cord paralysis were the result of malignant tumors involving the recurrent laryngeal nerve in the lower neck or lung apex; in all 8, CT showed a mass in the expected course of the right recurrent laryngeal nerve.

The initial radiologic examination in patients suspected of having a tracheal abnormality usually consists of frontal and lateral chest radiographs.[24, 25] Adequate visualization of the trachea, mediastinum, and lungs requires the use of high (120 to 150) kilovolts (peak). The trachea often is a *blind spot* for the radiologist, a deficiency that can be corrected only by paying particular attention to this region. An example of this diagnostic difficulty is provided by one investigation of 44 patients who had primary tracheal carcinoma;[26] prospectively the tumor was detected on the chest radiograph in only 8 (18%) patients, whereas it could be identified retrospectively in 29 (66%). As might be expected, CT improves detection of tracheal abnormalities significantly; in one study of 35 patients who had focal or diffuse disease of the trachea or main bronchi and 5 normal controls, an abnormality was detected on radiograph in 23 (66%) patients and on conventional CT scan in 33 (94%).[25]

CT allows assessment of the location and extent of

tracheal abnormalities as well as the presence of mediastinal involvement.[25–27] Conventional CT provides excellent resolution in the transverse plane but leads to underestimation of the cephalocaudad extent of tracheal stenosis or tumor involvement.[20, 29] Better assessment of the extent of disease in this plane is obtained using spiral CT with multiplanar and three-dimensional reconstructions (Fig. 15–3).[30–32] In one investigation, spiral CT with multiplanar reconstruction was compared with bronchoscopy in 25 patients who had known or suspected stenosis of the trachea or main bronchi.[31] Spiral CT showed the presence, site, degree, and extent of tracheal and main bronchial stenosis with a sensitivity of 93% (14 true-positive results, 1 false-negative) and a specificity of 100% (3 true-negative results, 0 false-positive); in one patient, focal narrowing as a result of tracheomalacia was detected at bronchoscopy but missed on CT. Spiral CT with multiplanar reconstructions shows focal abnormalities that may not be apparent on conventional transverse sections.[33, 35]

Optimal assessment of tracheal abnormalities on spiral CT requires the use of relatively thin sections (≤3-mm collimation) and reconstructions at 1- to 2-mm intervals.[31, 35, 232] The combination of spiral technique, thin sections, and volume rendering allows depiction of endoluminal-surface views similar to those obtained with bronchography.[36] Volume-rendered, three-dimensional images have been shown to improve recognition of mild tracheal abnormalities not readily apparent on conventional cross-sectional images.[36]

The presence and extent of tracheal abnormalities, including intrinsic stenosis, extrinsic compression, and primary and secondary neoplasms, can be assessed using MR imaging.[24, 37] It has been suggested that dynamic MR imaging may be helpful in the diagnosis of tracheomalacia.[38] Because of its inferior spatial resolution and high cost, however, dynamic MR imaging has a limited role.

Specific Causes

Thyroid Disease

Goiter is a relatively common cause of upper airway obstruction.[39] The radiographic manifestations consist of

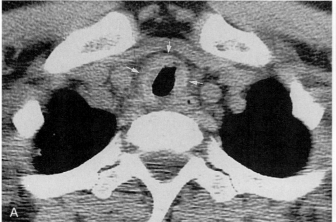
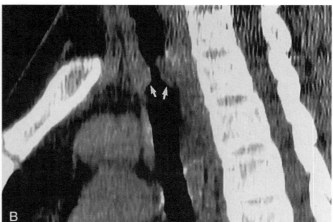
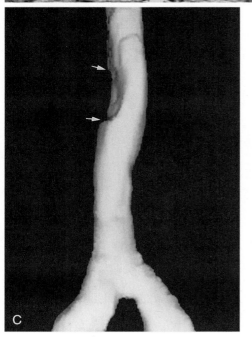

Figure 15–3. Spiral CT with Sagittal and Three-Dimensional Reconstructions in Endotracheal Tuberculosis. A 3-mm collimation spiral CT scan *(A)* shows circumferential thickening of the trachea *(arrows)*. The sagittal reconstruction *(B)* allows better assessment of the focal nature of the thickening as well as narrowing of the lumen *(arrows)*. The focal narrowing is seen well on the coronal three-dimensional reconstruction *(arrows in C)* of the trachea and main bronchi. The patient was a 27-year-old woman. (Courtesy of Dr. Kyung Soo Lee, Department of Radiology, Samsung Medical Center, Seoul, South Korea.)

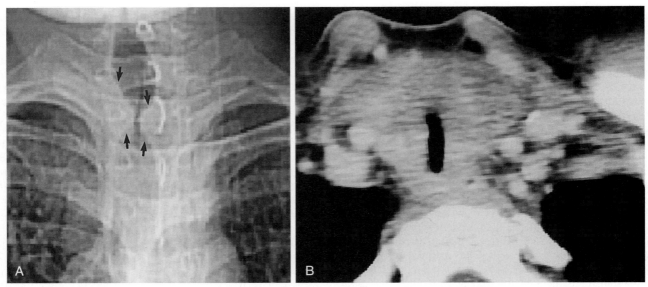

Figure 15–4. Tracheal Narrowing Secondary to Medullary Carcinoma of the Thyroid. View of the thoracic inlet in a 26-year-old man *(A)* shows focal circumferential narrowing of the lower cervical trachea *(arrows)*. Contrast-enhanced CT scan *(B)* shows diffuse enlargement of the thyroid. The gland has poorly defined margins and lower than normal attenuation. Note the associated compression of the trachea.

a paratracheal mass associated with smooth eccentric or circumferential tracheal narrowing. On CT, the thyroid often is enlarged asymmetrically, shows inhomogeneous areas of attenuation, contains foci of calcification, and shows marked enhancement after intravenous administration of contrast material.[40–42] Tracheal narrowing may result from thyroiditis and thyroid carcinoma. Riedel's thyroiditis is a chronic inflammatory condition associated with a marked desmoplastic reaction; it can be associated with tracheal narrowing and fibrosing mediastinitis;[42, 226] on CT, the enlarged thyroid has poorly defined margins. Thyroid carcinomas usually present as a focal mass, which may have homogeneous or inhomogeneous attenuation and often can contain foci of low attenuation as a result of cystic degeneration.[42–44] Occasionally, carcinomas cause diffuse enlargement of the thyroid (Fig. 15–4). The appearance of thyroid carcinomas can mimic that of benign conditions, such as goiter or adenomas, and definitive diagnosis usually requires biopsy. Rarely, marked tracheal narrowing is secondary to an ectopic intratracheal thyroid tissue mass.[45]

Tracheal Stenosis

Assuming a normative range that encompasses three standard deviations about the mean (i.e., pertaining to 99.7% of the normal population), the upper limits of normal for coronal and sagittal tracheal diameters, respectively, in men are 25 mm and 27 mm; in women, they are 21 mm and 23 mm (Table 15–1).[49] The lower limits of normal for both dimensions are 13 mm in men and 10 mm in women. Deviation from these figures indicates the presence of pathologic widening or narrowing of the caliber of the tracheal air column.

The diameters of the extrathoracic trachea increase during Valsalva's maneuver and decrease during Müller's maneuver.[46, 47] By contrast, the diameters of the intrathoracic trachea are not influenced by changes in pleural pressure[46]

but are affected markedly by changes in lung volume.[48] In one investigation of 10 normal individuals, the mean cross-sectional area of the trachea at the level of the aortic arch as measured on CT decreased from 280 mm^2 at total lung capacity (TLC) (range, 221 to 382 mm^2) to 178 mm^2 at residual volume (range, 115 to 236 mm^2), a mean ± standard deviation decrease of 35% ± 18%.[48]

One of the most common causes of chronic upper airway obstruction is tracheal stenosis occurring as a complication of intubation or tracheostomy. In one study of 342 patients who required prolonged endotracheal intubation, 5% manifested stridor after extubation, and 1.8% required reintubation or tracheostomy.[50] Although reversible laryngeal edema and inflammation were the major causes of

Table 15–1. TRACHEA

Normal diameters at TLC	
Men	13–27 mm
Women	10–23 mm
Normal cross-sectional area	
At TLC	221–382 mm^2
At residual volume	115–236 mm^2
Causes of tracheal narrowing	
Goiter, thyroiditis, thyroid neoplasms	
Tracheal stenosis (e.g., postintubation)	
Tracheal neoplasms	
Saber-sheath trachea	
Relapsing polychondritis	
Tracheobronchopathia osteochondroplastica	
Tracheobronchial amyloidosis	
Wegener's granulomatosis	
Tracheomalacia	
Tracheal dilation (tracheomegaly)	
Idiopathic (Mounier-Kuhn syndrome)	
In association with	
Pulmonary fibrosis	
Ankylosing spondylosis	
Cutis laxa	

TLC, total lung capacity.

the stridor, stricture developed as a result of fibrosis in four patients.

Tracheal stenosis after prolonged use of cuffed tracheostomy or endotracheal tubes may occur at the level of the stoma, at the level of the inflatable cuff, or, rarely, where the tip of the tube impinges on the tracheal mucosa. The frequency with which stenosis occurs at these sites seems to vary from series to series; in one group of 25 clinically significant tracheal strictures, 18 occurred at the stoma and 7 at the inflatable cuff;[51] in another group of 55 patients, the incidences of stoma (24 cases) and inflatable cuff (23 cases) stenosis were almost equal (the remaining 8 cases were at various other locations, mostly in the cervical trachea).[52]

Radiographically, postintubation tracheal stenosis extends for several centimeters and typically affects the trachea above the level of the thoracic inlet (Fig. 15–5).[54] The narrowing often is concentric; multiple stenotic areas may be seen.[54] Stenosis after tracheostomy typically begins 1 to 1.5 cm distal to the inferior margin of the tracheostomy stoma and involves 1.5 to 2.5 cm of tracheal wall (including two to four cartilaginous rings).[53] Three radiographic appearances have been described: (1) circumferential narrowing of the tracheal lumen over a distance of about 2 cm; (2) a thin membrane or diaphragm (caused by granulation tissue rather than mature fibrous tissue) that may project almost at right angles from the tracheal wall; and (3) a long, thickened, eccentric opacity of soft tissue density that compromises the tracheal lumen.[53] The last-named condition results most often from impingement of the tip of the tracheostomy tube on the tracheal wall (or from an eccentric cuff) so that mucosal necrosis and subsequent fibrosis are local rather than circumferential.

The degree and extent of tracheal narrowing often are difficult to assess on radiograph and on conventional cross-sectional CT scan (Fig. 15–6).[20] With conventional CT, a focal area of stenosis may be missed, the severity of stenosis overestimated, and the cephalocaudad extent often underestimated.[20] Optimal assessment of focal trachea stenosis requires the use of spiral technique, thin sections (3- to 5-mm collimation), image reconstruction at 1- to 3-mm intervals, and multiplanar reconstructions;[31, 34] this procedure allows accurate assessment of the presence, extent, and severity of stenosis in most cases (Fig. 15–7).[31]

Occasionally, focal stenosis of the cervical trachea is idiopathic. In one series of 15 patients, the stenosis was 2 to 4 cm long and resulted in a tracheal lumen 3 to 5 mm in diameter at the narrowest portion.[55] The radiologic appearance was similar to that of postintubation or posttraumatic tracheal strictures: The narrowing was circumferential in eight patients (53%) and eccentric in seven; the margins of the stenosis were smooth in nine patients (60%) and irregular and lobulated in six.

Sometimes, thinning of the trachea results in tracheomalacia rather than stenosis, usually as a result of excessive removal of cartilage at the time of tracheostomy or its destruction as a result of pressure and infection.[56, 57] The presence of such tracheomalacia can be missed on CT scans performed at end-inspiration,[31] and the diagnosis requires the use of dynamic CT or comparison of images obtained at end-inspiration and at the end of maximal expiration.[48, 467] In one investigation of 10 normal individuals, the cross-sectional area of the intrathoracic trachea decreased by 11% to 61% from TLC to residual volume;[48] in 1 patient who had tracheomalacia, the tracheal cross sectional area decreased from 256 to 54 mm^2, an 80% decrease.[48]

Tracheal Neoplasms

Compared with the larynx and bronchi, the trachea is a rare site of primary cancer. At the Mayo Clinic, only 53 primary cancers of the trachea were diagnosed during 30 years; the relative incidence compared with laryngeal cancer was 1 to 75 and with lung cancer 1 to 180.[58] The most common primary tumor is squamous cell carcinoma, constituting 50% or more of cases in various series and being about four times as common in men as in women.[62–64] Adenoid cystic carcinoma is slightly less common and shows no sex predilection. Other neoplasms, such as lymphoma, leukemia, plasmacytoma, benign and malignant soft tissue neoplasms, and other types of primary and secondary carcinomas, are much less common.

Patients who have tracheal neoplasms often are treated for asthma for a long time before the correct diagnosis is made.[62, 63] Although dyspnea may be noted initially only on exertion, eventually its paroxysmal occurrence at night may suggest the diagnosis of asthma. Hoarseness, cough, and wheezing are common; hemoptysis also may occur.

Radiologically, tracheal tumors are manifested as intraluminal nodules that may have smooth, irregular, or lobu-

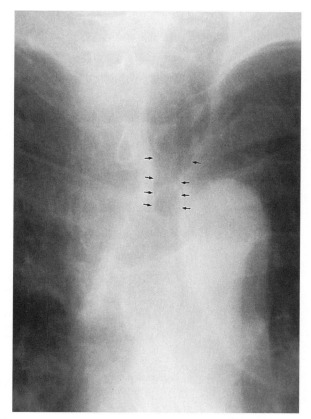

Figure 15–5. Tracheal Stenosis After Intubation. View of the trachea from posteroanterior chest radiograph shows focal circumferential tracheal narrowing *(arrows)*. The patient was a 45-year-old man who developed tracheal stenosis after intubation for 24 hours.

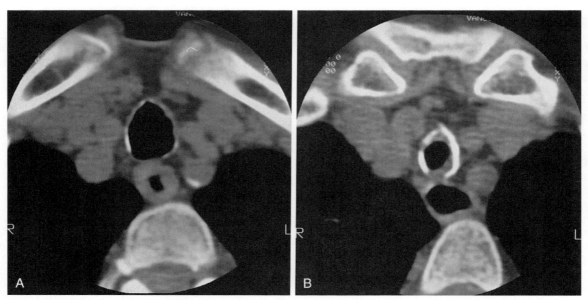

Figure 15–6. Tracheal Stenosis After Intubation. CT scan through the level of the thoracic inlet *(A)* shows a normal diameter of the trachea. CT scan at a more caudad level *(B)* shows circumferential narrowing. The patient presented with stridor 3 months after extubation. (From Kwong JS, Müller NL, Miller RR: Radiographics 12:645, 1992.)

lated margins or as eccentric or circumferential thickening of the tracheal wall associated with narrowing of the lumen.[28, 61] Benign neoplasms, such as schwannomas, neurofibromas, and leiomyomas, most commonly appear as well-circumscribed, round soft tissue masses measuring 2 cm or less in diameter (Fig. 15–8).[28] On CT, such lesions usually are sessile or polypoid and do not extend beyond the tracheal wall.[28] Malignant tumors most commonly appear as focal or circumferential tracheal narrowing or as a relatively flat or polypoid mass; most measure 2 to 4 cm (Fig. 15–9).[28] Associated findings include a paratracheal mass

secondary to extratracheal extension, mediastinal lymph node enlargement, pulmonary nodules related to metastases, and, rarely, tracheoesophageal fistula.[27, 28]

CT is helpful in assessing the extent of tracheal neoplasms but may underestimate the cephalocaudad intramural and extratracheal tumor extent and not allow reliable distinction of a benign from a malignant process.[25, 28] Spiral CT is superior to conventional CT.[30, 33, 34] Tumor extent can be assessed using MR imaging.[24, 28] Endotracheal metastases may manifest as single or multiple polypoid lesions (Fig. 15–10).

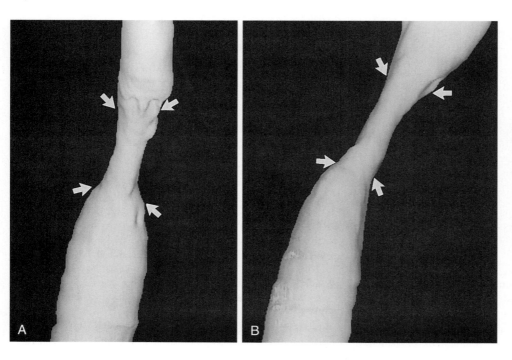

Figure 15–7. Post-tracheotomy Tracheal Stenosis. Three-dimensional reconstructions from spiral CT scan in anteroposterior *(A)* and lateral *(B)* projections show tracheal stenosis *(between arrows).* The reconstructions were performed using surface shading technique. (Courtesy of Dr. Martine Remy-Jardin, Centre Hospitalier Regional et Universitaire de Lille, Lille, France.)

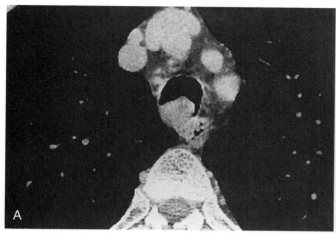

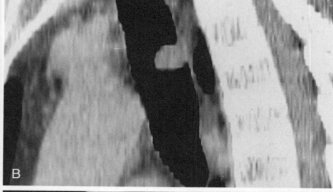

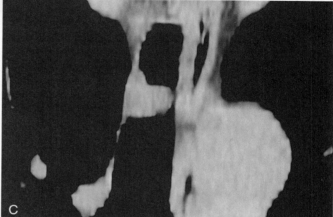

Figure 15–8. Tracheal Neurilemoma. CT scan *(A)* in a 62-year-old man shows a polypoid endotracheal tumor. The origin of the tumor from the posterior and lateral walls of the trachea is shown well on the sagittal *(B)* and coronal *(C)* reconstructions from a spiral CT scan. (Courtesy of Dr. Kyung Soo Lee, Department of Radiology, Samsung Medical Center, Seoul, Korea.)

Saber-Sheath Trachea

In cross-section, the resting trachea is roughly horseshoe shaped, with the open end of the cartilage rings closed by the compliant posterior sheath. Considerable variation exists in the shape of the tracheal cartilage rings, the most common being a C shape; U and V shapes also occur.[66] On posteroanterior and lateral radiographs, the coronal and sagittal diameters of the tracheal air column are approximately equal. Occasionally the coronal diameter of the intrathoracic trachea is reduced markedly, and the sagittal diameter correspondingly is increased, a condition called *saber-sheath trachea* (Fig. 15–11).

In the initial description of 13 patients who had saber-sheath trachea, the only criterion for selection was an internal coronal diameter of the intrathoracic trachea one half or less of the corresponding sagittal diameter;[65] measurements were made 1 cm above the level of the top of the aortic arch. All patients were men 52 to 75 years old. The coronal tracheal diameter was 7 to 13 mm (mean, 10.5 mm), and the *tracheal index* (the ratio of coronal to sagittal diameter) was 0.5 to 0.25 (mean, 0.4). Generally the narrow coronal diameter extended the length of the intrathoracic trachea; at the thoracic outlet, the coronal diameter increased abruptly, and the sagittal diameter narrowed, the air column assuming a normal configuration. This abrupt change in configuration from intrathoracic to extrathoracic trachea was a consistent finding and almost certainly reflected the influence of intrathoracic transmural pressures. Rarely, the presence of mediastinal lipomatosis in associa-tion with a saber-sheath trachea simulates a mediastinal tumor causing tracheal compression on chest radiograph; the correct diagnosis can be made readily on CT.[66] It is unclear whether saber-sheath trachea is a result or a cause of air-flow obstruction; many investigators have suggested that it is a consequence of hyperinflation in patients who have COPD.[67, 68]

Relapsing Polychondritis

Relapsing polychondritis is an uncommon systemic disease that affects cartilage in many sites throughout the body, including the ribs, tracheobronchial tree, ear lobes, nose, and central or peripheral joints. It is recognized as one of the autoimmune connective tissue diseases, and its characteristics are discussed in greater detail in Chapter 8. The typical radiographic finding consists of diffuse narrowing of the trachea and main bronchi;[69, 70] CT shows mild thickening of the anterior and lateral tracheal walls with sparing of the posterior membranes and diffuse thickening of the involved bronchial walls (Fig. 15–12).[72, 232] Similar findings are seen on MR imaging.[71] The stenosis can be fixed[27, 72] or variable,[70, 73] single and localized,[74] multiple,[75] or diffuse.[72, 76] Expiratory CT shows marked narrowing of the trachea.[466, 467] It has been shown that the degree of dynamic collapse seen on multidetector CT with inspiratory and expiratory imaging correlates well with the bronchoscopic findings.[467] *Active* lesions have been reported to take up gallium 67.[77]

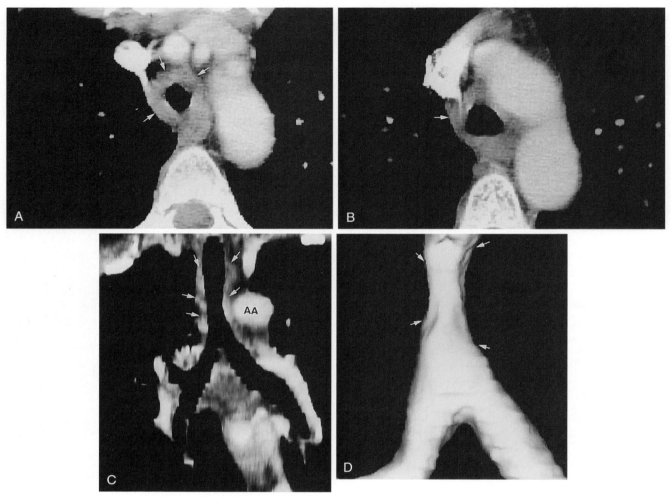

Figure 15–9. Adenoid Cystic Carcinoma: Spiral CT with Coronal and Three-Dimensional Reconstructions. Contrast-enhanced CT scans *(A and B)* in a 53-year-old woman show circumferential thickening of the tracheal wall extending for several centimeters *(arrows)* with associated narrowing of the tracheal lumen. The cephalocaudad extension of tumor can be appreciated better on the coronal reconstruction *(C)*, which shows tracheal wall thickening *(arrows)* extending from above the level of the aortic arch (AA) to just above the level of the tracheal carina. The patient also had subcarinal lymphadenopathy. A three-dimensional reconstruction using surface-shading technique *(D)* shows the cephalocaudad extent of the tracheal narrowing *(arrows)*.

Tracheobronchopathia Osteochondroplastica

Tracheobronchopathia osteochondroplastica is a rare condition characterized by the development of nodules or spicules of cartilage and bone in the submucosa of the trachea and bronchi.[78] It occurs most frequently in men older than 50 years, although it has been reported in younger individuals and women.[79, 80] In most reported cases, the condition was diagnosed as an incidental finding at autopsy or during bronchoscopy.[81] The cause and pathogenesis are unknown. Most patients do not have symptoms; occasionally, there is dyspnea, hoarseness, cough, expectoration, wheezing, and hemoptysis.[82, 89]

The typical radiographic manifestation consists of nodular or undulating thickening of the tracheal and bronchial walls (Fig. 15–13).[83, 84] Foci of calcification often are not apparent on radiograph;[76, 85] in fact, the radiograph may be normal.[86, 87] When apparent, the calcification is seen best on a lateral view.[76] Occasionally the first radiologic abnormalities consist of recurrent pneumonia or atelectasis.[85, 88]

The characteristic CT findings consist of nodular thickening of the trachea, resulting in irregular or undulating narrowing of its lumen (Fig. 15–14). In most cases, foci of calcification also are present within the submucosal nodules;[27, 87] occasionally, minimal calcification is evident.[85] These CT abnormalities typically are seen in the anterior and lateral walls of the trachea and spare the posterior membranous portion; the presence of multiple calcified nodules protruding into the tracheal lumen in this distribution is considered diagnostic of the condition.[71]

Tracheomalacia

Tracheomalacia (tracheobronchomalacia) is a descriptive term that refers to weakness of the tracheal walls and supporting cartilage with resultant easy collapsibility. Tracheomalacia may or may not be accompanied by tracheomegaly. It most often is secondary to pressure necrosis of cartilage resulting from intubation, thyroid lesions,[39, 90] vascular abnormalities,[91] trauma, chronic or recurrent infec-

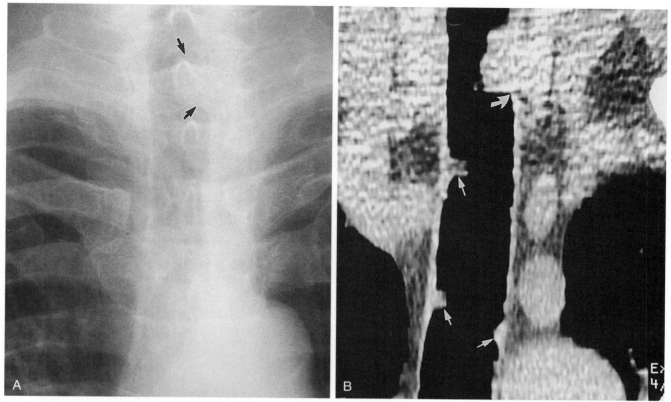

Figure 15–10. Tracheal Metastases from Squamous Cell Carcinoma of the Oropharynx. View of the trachea from posteroanterior radiograph *(A)* shows a focal tracheal lesion *(arrows)*. Coronal reconstruction *(B)* from spiral CT scan shows several endotracheal polypoid lesions *(straight arrows)*. The largest nodule extends beyond the tracheal wall *(curved arrow)*. The patient developed tracheal metastases 2 years after surgical resection of a squamous cell carcinoma of the oropharynx.

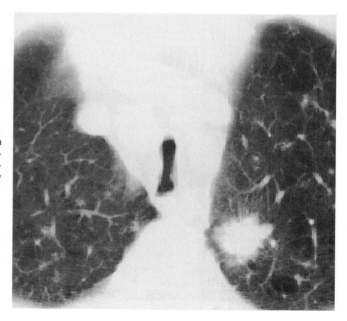

Figure 15–11. Saber-Sheath Trachea. CT scan in a 73-year-old man shows narrowing of the coronal diameter and increase in the anteroposterior (sagittal) diameter of the trachea. Evidence of emphysema and a 2-cm-diameter left upper lobe nodule (subsequently shown to be a pulmonary carcinoma) are visible.

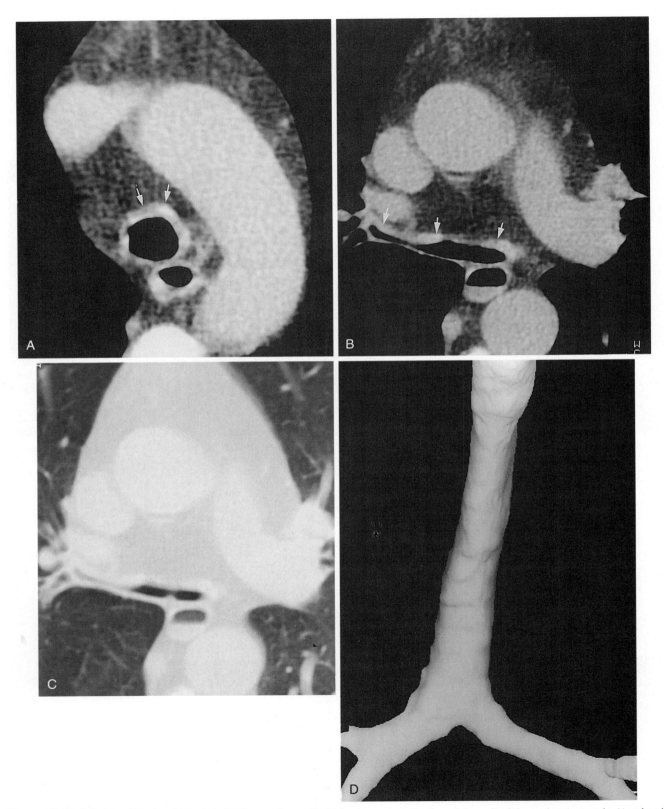

Figure 15–12. Relapsing Polychondritis. Spiral CT scans show mild thickening and calcification of the wall of the trachea *(arrows in A)* and main and right upper lobe bronchi *(arrows in B)*. Lung windows *(C)* show narrowing of the bronchial lumen. Three-dimensional reconstruction using surface shading technique *(D)* shows relatively mild but extensive narrowing of the trachea and main bronchi, particularly the left. (Courtesy of Dr. Martine Remy-Jardin, Centre Hospitalier Regional et Universitaire de Lille, Lille, France.)

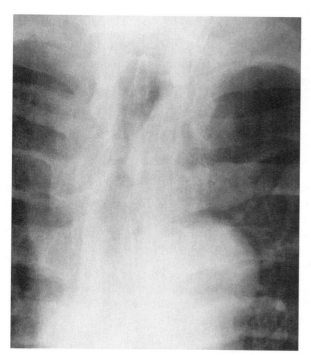

Figure 15–13. Tracheobronchopathia Osteochondroplastica. View of the trachea from posteroanterior chest radiograph in a 69-year-old man shows irregular narrowing of the trachea. The wall has a nodular appearance; no definite calcification is evident.

tion, radiation therapy,[91] or relapsing polychondritis.[92] It also can be seen as a primary condition, most often in children and usually associated with a deficiency of cartilage in the tracheobronchial tree.[92, 93] Symptoms include stridor and shortness of breath. Dilation of the airways may be seen during inspiration, and premature collapse may be seen during expiration.[94]

Tracheobronchomegaly

Tracheobronchomegaly (Mounier-Kuhn syndrome) is characterized by dilation of the tracheobronchial tree that may extend from the larynx to the periphery of the lung.[27, 95, 96] Although surveys of the literature do not suggest a high prevalence,[97] some investigators have found that the condition is an often unrecognized contributor to obstructive lung disease.[94] According to these researchers, tracheobronchomegaly occurs predominantly in men, most of whom are in their twenties or thirties.

The cause and pathogenesis are unclear. An association of tracheobronchomegaly with Ehlers-Danlos syndrome has been reported in adults,[98, 99] and it has been found in children who have congenital cutis laxa,[100] suggesting the presence of an underlying defect in elastic tissue. A case has been reported of an adult marfanoid patient who developed hypercapnic respiratory failure secondary to tracheobronchomegaly.[101] An acquired form of the condition has been reported as a complication of diffuse pulmonary fibrosis[102, 103] and in association with ankylosing spondylitis.[104, 105] Localized disease has been reported in association with relapsing polychondritis.[76]

The increased compliance of the trachea in tracheobronchomegaly results in abnormal flaccidity and easy collapsibility during forced expiration and coughing. The inefficient cough mechanism leads to retention of mucus with resultant recurrent pneumonia, emphysema, bronchiectasis, and pulmonary fibrosis.[111]

Radiographically the diagnosis usually is apparent at a glance. The calibers of the trachea and major bronchi generally are increased, and the air columns have an irregular corrugated appearance caused by the protrusion of mucosal and submucosal tissue between the cartilaginous rings (an appearance that has been termed *tracheal diverticulosis*). This appearance often is visualized best in lateral projection.[95] In the appropriate clinical setting, tracheobron-

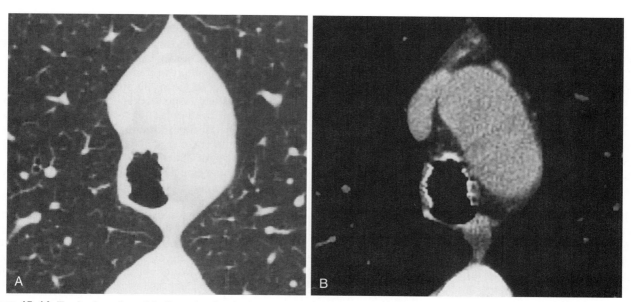

Figure 15–14. Tracheobronchopathia Osteochondroplastica. CT scan *(A)* in a 64-year-old man shows nodular thickening of the tracheal wall. Soft tissue windows *(B)* show extensive calcification of the submucosal nodules. The lack of involvement of the posterior membranous portion of the trachea is a characteristic finding of tracheobronchopathia osteochondroplastica.

chomegaly can be diagnosed on chest radiograph in women when the transverse and sagittal diameters of the trachea exceed 21 and 23 mm and when the transverse diameters of the right and left main bronchi exceed 19.8 and 17.4 mm. In men, tracheobronchomegaly can be considered to be present when the transverse and sagittal diameters of the trachea exceed 25 and 27 mm and when the transverse diameters of the right and left main bronchi exceed 21.1 and 18.4 mm.[106]

CT and MR imaging can be used to identify the tracheal and bronchial dilation.[27, 107] Cinefluoroscopy and dynamic CT show collapse of the dilated trachea and bronchi on expiration;[114, 115] CT may reveal dilation of the intrapulmonary bronchi.[27, 109] In patients who have bronchiectasis, the trachea tends to be larger than that in normal individuals. In one study in which measurements of airway dimensions were made on CT and compared with normal tracheal dimensions derived from radiographs, 7 (17%) of 42 patients who had bronchiectasis were found to fulfill criteria for tracheobronchomegaly, compared with less than 5% of control subjects.[116] In contrast to bronchiectasis, however, the dilated bronchi of patients who have tracheobronchomegaly typically have thin walls.

Obstructive Sleep Apnea

The results of many studies indicate that obstructive sleep apnea (OSA) is a common abnormality in the general population: The prevalence approaches that of asthma.[113] The strongest risk factors for OSA are obesity, older age, and male gender.[114] It is generally accepted that OSA is caused by the normal loss of upper airway muscle tone during sleep superimposed on a degree of upper airway narrowing.[115, 116] The principal symptoms are snoring, apneas witnessed by a bed partner, and excessive daytime sleepiness.[112]

Although imaging techniques have greatly enhanced understanding of the pathogenesis of OSA, there is no ideal method of examining upper airway structure, especially the changes that occur during sleep apnea;[118, 119] as a result, imaging plays a limited role in the assessment of the disorder in individual patients.[120] Despite this limited role, cephalometry, CT, or a combination of these techniques has been used to characterize the abnormalities of soft tissue and bone structures in patients who have proven OSA, and these procedures have been reported to aid in the planning of the most appropriate therapy.[121–123]

A lateral radiograph of the head and neck using a soft tissue technique (also referred to as *lateral cephalometry*) allows assessment of the upper airways, soft tissues, and bone structures (Fig. 15–15). The procedure has shown a variety of abnormalities of craniofacial and upper airway soft tissue anatomy that may predispose to upper airway obstruction during sleep and that relate to the severity of OSA.[117, 124] Some investigators have found that the technique allows separation of snorers who do or do not have OSA with a precision of approximately 80%;[125] however, others have not been able to distinguish reliably between patients who have sleep apnea and nonapneic, habitual snorers.[126] In one investigation of 117 patients referred for evaluation of heavy snoring and possible OSA, a lateral view of the airway obtained after swallowing contrast ma-

terial was used to measure pharyngeal diameters at three sites along the airway;[127] all measurements were performed with the patient standing and supine. Apneic and nonapneic snorers showed a significant reduction in the retropalatal distance on assumption of the supine posture. Stepwise multiple linear regression analysis showed that the retropalatal distance and airway diameter at the tip of the palate and 1 cm distal to it were significant predictors of snoring but not apnea.

The dimensions of the upper airway can be assessed using CT (Fig. 15–16). In one study of 25 men in whom three-dimensional CT reconstructions were performed, measurement of the cross-sectional area of the upper airway at different levels showed the narrowest point to be in the oropharynx (0.52 ± 0.18 cm^2) in most;[128] in some subjects, a second narrowing was seen at the level of the hypopharynx. The investigators measured the volume of the tongue and found that subjects who had larger tongues experienced more severe OSA and had a smaller airway lumen. In another investigation of 36 patients who had OSA and 10 control subjects, measurements of the cross-sectional area of the oropharyngeal lumen were taken at the level of the narrowing;[123] 27 patients who had severe OSA (defined as a high number and prolonged episodes of OSA and $\geq$22% decrease in oxygen saturation) had an oropharyngeal cross-sectional area measuring less than 50 mm^2. By comparison, patients who had moderate OSA had an oropharyngeal cross-sectional area of 60 to 100 mm^2, and the control subjects had a minimal pharyngeal cross-sectional area of 110 mm^2.

In another investigation of the effects of respiration on upper airway caliber using cine CT in 15 normal subjects, 14 snorer/mildly apneic subjects, and 13 patients who had OSA, all subjects were scanned in the supine position during awake nasal breathing.[129] CT images were obtained at four anatomic levels from the nasopharynx to the retroglossal region every 0.4 seconds during a respiratory cycle. The investigators found that the upper airway was significantly smaller in apneic than in normal subjects, especially at the low retropalatal and retroglossal anatomic levels; however, little airway narrowing occurred during inspiration in all three subject groups, suggesting that the action of the upper airway dilator muscles balanced the effects of negative intraluminal pressure. Using dynamic CT imaging, another group found the mean airway cross-sectional area to be largest at end-inspiration and smallest at end-expiration, consistent with relaxation of upper airway dilator muscle activity during expiration.[130] Additional findings on CT include an increase in nonfatty tissues in the pharyngeal wall, thickening of the mucosa of the nasopharynx and oropharynx, enlargement of the lymphoid tissue, and hypertrophy of the tongue, soft tissue palate, or muscles.[120]

Upper airway dimensions can be assessed using MR imaging. T1-weighted spin-echo sequences show deposition of fat adjacent to the pharyngeal airway in patients who have OSA.[131, 132] Ultrafast MR imaging has great potential for providing dynamic three-dimensional images;[133, 134] the procedure can detect sites of airway narrowing and closure and has shown considerable differences among individuals who have OSA.[141, 142] MR imaging is sensitive in detecting changes in upper airway water content. In one study, five patients who had moderate to severe

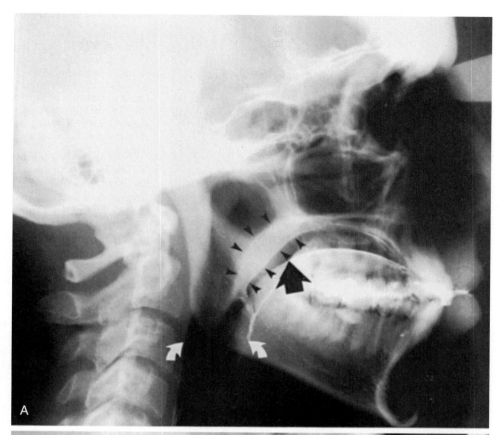

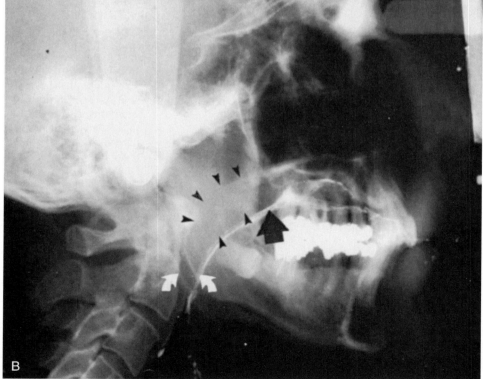

Figure 15–15. Radiography of the Upper Airway in a Normal Subject and a Patient with Obstructive Sleep Apnea. Lateral radiograph of the face and neck *(A)* of a normal subject after ingestion of barium paste to outline the top of the tongue *(large arrows)* reveals a widely patent oropharynx, normal uvula *(arrowheads)*, and hypopharynx *(curved arrows)*. Similar view in a patient who has obstructive sleep apnea *(B)* shows a markedly narrowed oropharynx *(large arrow)* and hypopharynx *(curved arrows)* and a large uvula *(arrowheads)*.

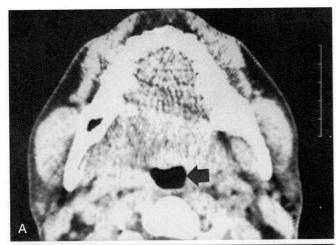

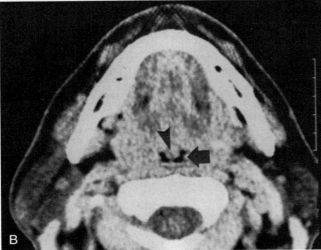

Figure 15–16. CT Scan of the Upper Airway in a Normal Subject and a Patient with Obstructive Sleep Apnea. CT scan at the level of the oropharynx in a normal subject *(A)* shows a widely patent oropharynx *(arrow)*. In a patient who has obstructive sleep apnea, a CT image at approximately the same level *(B)* shows a markedly reduced cross-sectional area of the airway *(arrowhead)* and a prominent uvula *(arrow)*.

OSA were studied with MR imaging before and 4 to 6 weeks after beginning nasal continuous positive airway pressure therapy; the results showed a significant increase in pharyngeal lumen volume (while off continuous positive airway pressure) and reductions in tongue volume and pharyngeal mucosal water content.[137]

ASTHMA

Asthma is "a disease characterized by wide variations over short periods of time in resistance to air flow in intrapulmonary airways."[138] The changes in severity of airway narrowing can occur spontaneously or as a result of therapy. In addition to brevity, this definition has the advantage of being easily applicable to clinical practice. These features are found in other conditions, however, such as cystic fibrosis and congestive heart failure. Because of this problem, other definitions of asthma have been proposed based on the recognition that the airways of asthmatic persons show an increased responsiveness to a variety of stimuli[139] and evidence of a chronic inflammatory reaction.[140] One example of such an extended definition is that proposed by the Global Initiative for Asthma:[141]

Asthma is a chronic inflammatory disorder of the airways in which many cells play a role, in particular mast cells, eosinophils, and T lymphocytes. In susceptible individuals this inflammation causes recurrent episodes of wheezing, breathlessness, chest tightness, and cough, particularly at night and/or in the early morning. These symptoms are usually associated with widespread but variable airflow limitation that is at least partly reversible either spontaneously or with treatment. The inflammation also causes an associated increase in airway responsiveness to a variety of stimuli.

The basic pathophysiologic abnormality that determines the functional and symptomatic status of an asthmatic patient is airway narrowing. This narrowing can occur by four main mechanisms: (1) airway smooth muscle contraction and shortening; (2) edema, inflammatory cell infiltration, and congestion of the airway wall; (3) mucous hypersecretion and plugging of the airway lumen; and (4) airway wall remodeling. For the most part, it is difficult, if not impossible, to determine in a given patient at a given time what proportion of airway obstruction is caused by each of these mechanisms. As a generalization, however, it can be concluded reasonably that when obstruction is rapidly reversible after inhalation of cholinergic antagonists or β-adrenergic agonists, the pathogenesis is smooth muscle shortening, whereas when it responds over days to steroids and other therapeutic interventions, it is caused by edema, inflammatory cell infiltration, and mucous plugging.[142, 143] When given over prolonged periods, anti-inflammatory therapy may be associated with some reversal of airway remodeling.[144]

The diagnosis of asthma is based largely on a history of periodic paroxysms of dyspnea, usually at rest as well as on exertion, interspersed with intervals of complete or nearly complete remission. Some patients have a more chronic form of the disease characterized by more persistent symptoms; however, periodic exacerbation and remission occur in almost all cases. Cough can be a prominent symptom, and nonsmoking patients who have asthma can fulfill the diagnostic criteria for chronic bronchitis.[171] The diagnosis is strengthened by a history of eczema or hay fever or by a family history of allergic phenomena.

Complications of asthma are much more common in children than in adults and consist of pneumonia, atelectasis, mucoid impaction, pneumomediastinum, and (rarely) arterial air embolism. Lower respiratory tract viral infection occurs more frequently and tends to be more severe among asthmatic patients than in the population at large.[172] Atelectasis occurs predominantly in children and is the result of mucoid impaction.[173, 174]

Radiologic Manifestations

The most common radiographic abnormalities of asthma are bronchial wall thickening and hyperinflation; less frequent manifestations include peripheral oligemia, increased central lung markings, and prominence of the hila (Table 15–2).[145, 146] The prevalence of these abnormalities is influenced by several factors, including age at onset and severity of asthma as well as the presence of other disease or

Table 15–2. ASTHMA: RADIOLOGIC MANIFESTATIONS

Chest Radiograph

Bronchial wall thickening
Hyperinflation
Peripheral oligemia

HRCT Scan

Bronchial wall thickening
Narrowing of bronchial lumen
Bronchiectasis
Mosaic perfusion
Air-trapping on expiratory HRCT scan

HRCT, high-resolution computed tomography.

complications of asthma.[145, 146] The influence of age at onset on the presence or absence of radiographic abnormalities was assessed in one investigation of 117 patients older than 15 years of age;[148] radiographic abnormalities were identified in 31% of the patients whose asthma had its onset before the age of 15 years but in none of the patients in whom it occurred after age 30.

The incidence of radiographic abnormalities is affected by disease severity. In a study of 58 patients ranging in age from 10 to 69 years (mean, 33 years) in whom the asthma was categorized as *severe*, evidence of pulmonary overinflation was detected in 42 (73%).[150] In this report, the author drew attention to the rapidity with which signs of overinflation can disappear after appropriate therapy, sometimes in 24 hours.[150]

In the presence of acute, severe asthma or during a prolonged, intractable attack, the most characteristic radiographic signs are pulmonary hyperinflation and expiratory air-trapping (Fig. 15–17). The former is manifested by an increase in the depth of the retrosternal space and in lung height and flattening of the diaphragm. In one investigation of 12 asthmatic patients in whom the presence of hyperinflation was assessed by the subjective evaluation of chest radiographs as well as planimetric measurement, the latter studies revealed a mean increase in TLC of 0.46 liter during acute exacerbation;[155] the only subjective radio-

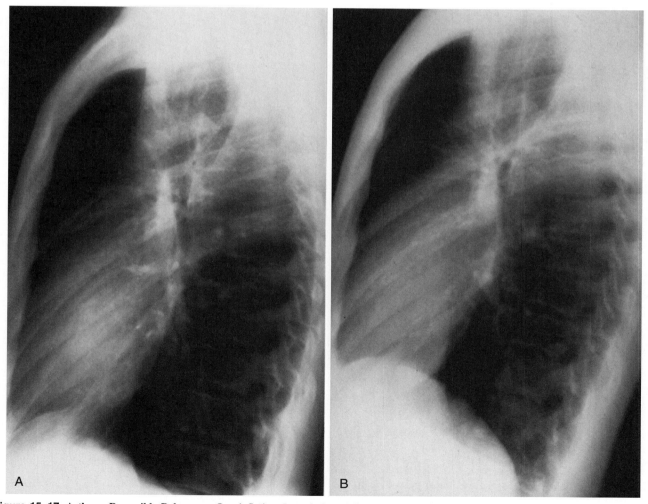

Figure 15–17. Asthma: Reversible Pulmonary Overinflation. Lateral chest radiograph *(A)* of an adult asthmatic patient during an attack of severe bronchospasm shows a low position and flat configuration of the diaphragm, indicating severe pulmonary overinflation. Approximately 1 year later during a remission *(B)*, lung volume had returned to normal. The curvature of the sternum and thoracic spine did not change because these structures do not participate in acute hyperinflation in the adult.

graphic variable that allowed reliable distinction of acute exacerbation from recovery was an increase in lung height.

Cardiac size almost invariably is normal, although the long, narrow cardiac silhouette commonly seen in patients who have emphysema is observed occasionally. Prominence of the main pulmonary artery and its hilar branches with rapid tapering is probably indicative of transient precapillary pulmonary arterial hypertension secondary to hypoxia and occurs in approximately 10% of patients (Fig. 15–18).[151] Abnormal vascular patterns include diffuse narrowing and relative dilation of upper lobe vessels (the latter in the absence of other signs of postcapillary hypertension), and paucity of vessels in the outer 2 to 4 cm of the lungs (Fig. 15–19). This *subpleural oligemia* is especially evident when accompanied by an increased prominence of the hilar and midlung vessels and is reversible with treatment.

The prevalence of bronchial wall thickening in chronic asthma was assessed in one investigation of 57 nonsmoking patients with disease of variable severity.[145] The clinical severity of asthma was assessed using a scoring system that graded the disease from mild (score of 1) to incapacitating (score of 5).[152] Bronchial wall thickening was evident on chest radiograph in 22% of patients who had grade 1 asthma, 26% who had grade 2, 35% who had grade 3, and 46% who had grade 4 or 5. The thickening occurs in segmental and subsegmental bronchi and can be seen as ring shadows when viewed end-on or as *tramline* opacities when viewed *en face*. Smaller bronchi measuring 3 to 5 mm in diameter, normally invisible on conventional chest radiographs, may be identified (Fig. 15–20). These findings probably represent intramural and peribronchial inflammation, fibrosis, or both. Although the thickening usually is permanent, it may decrease or disappear after treatment.

Despite the observations just outlined, chest radiograph has a limited role in the diagnosis of asthma. It often is normal, even during an acute attack; when chest radiograph is abnormal, the findings are nonspecific. There are two main indications for chest radiograph in the assessment of a patient who has a presumptive or confirmed diagnosis of asthma: (1) to exclude other conditions that cause wheezing, particularly emphysema, congestive heart failure, and obstruction of the trachea or major bronchi, and (2) to identify complications such as pneumothorax. Several studies have been conducted to evaluate the efficacy of radio-

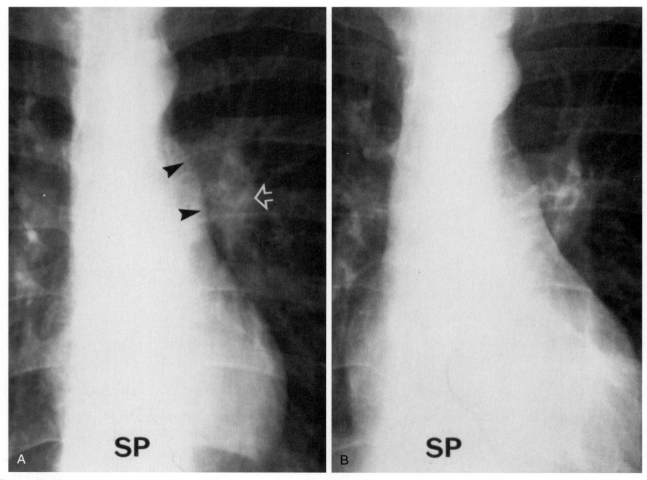

Figure 15–18. Asthma: Reversible Precapillary Pulmonary Hypertension. Detailed view of the heart and left hilum from a posteroanterior radiograph *(A)* shows enlargement of the main pulmonary artery *(arrowheads)* and left interlobar artery *(open arrow)*, consistent with the presence of pulmonary arterial hypertension. At the time of this study, the patient, a young man, was experiencing a severe attack of acute bronchospasm. Approximately 2 years later during a period of remission, a repeat radiograph *(B)* shows a return to normal of the configuration of the main and interlobar arteries. The heart has increased in size during this interval, presumably reflecting the high transpulmonary pressure that existed during the acute attack and the consequent reduction in venous return.

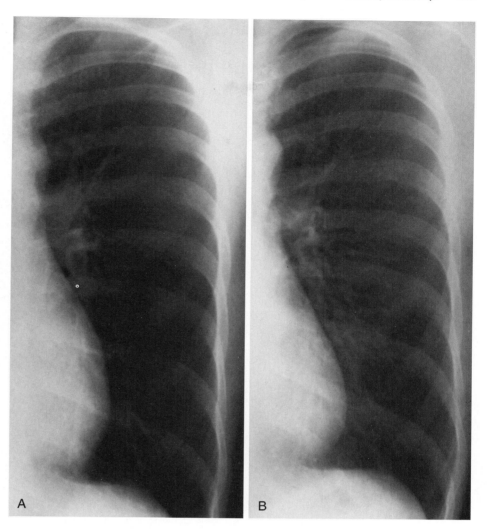

Figure 15–19. Asthma: Peripheral Oligemia. Detailed view of the left lung from posteroanterior chest radiograph *(A)* of a young man during an episode of acute bronchospasm shows moderate hyperinflation. The vasculature in the outer 2 to 3 cm of lung is inconspicuous and barely visible, creating a subpleural shell of oligemic lung. A repeat study 1 year later during remission *(B)* shows less hyperinflation; the pulmonary vessels now taper normally, and most are visible well into the lung periphery.

graphic examination in asthmatic patients, and the conclusions are not unanimous. In one study of 117 adults admitted to the hospital with acute severe asthma, investigators found radiographic abnormalities other than those directly related to asthma that affected management in 10 patients (9%);[153] in 9 of these patients, the presence of consolidation or atelectasis was not detected on clinical examination. In another investigation, 528 chest radiographs from 122 adults were reviewed; each film represented a separate acute asthmatic attack.[154] Only 2.2% of the radiographs showed parenchymal opacities, atelectasis, pneumothorax, or pneumomediastinum (pulmonary overinflation was not included as an abnormal finding).

In another investigation of adult asthmatic patients admitted to the hospital for exacerbations of the disease, chest radiographs showed some abnormality in 50%;[155] detection of the abnormality resulted in a change in management strategy in 5%. In a fourth, retrospective investigation of 1,016 adults admitted to the hospital with acute asthma, radiographic findings were classified into the following groups:[146] (1) normal, 536 patients (53%); (2) features compatible with obstructive lung disease, 323 patients (32%); (3) complications of asthma, including infection, atelectasis, pneumomediastinum, and pneumothorax, 83 pa-

tients (8%); and (4) important incidental findings, including tuberculosis, heart failure, and pulmonary neoplasm, 68 patients (7%). Approximately 15% of patients presenting with symptoms severe enough to require hospital admission had clinically significant radiographic abnormalities. The authors concluded, and we concur, that an admission chest radiograph is indicated in adults presenting with severe asthma.

High-resolution computed tomography (HRCT) allows visualization of airways in asthmatic patients in much greater detail than plain radiography and has made possible the investigation of the site, magnitude, and distribution of airway narrowing (Fig. 15–21). In addition to providing more accurate and detailed images, the digital nature of the data from which the CT image is generated allows a quantitative approach to the analysis of airway dimensions. The most common abnormalities seen on HRCT are bronchial wall thickening, narrowing of the bronchial lumen, bronchiectasis, patchy areas of decreased attenuation and vascularity, and air-trapping.[156–158] The distribution of bronchial abnormalities often is heterogeneous; some airways have normal thickness and diameter, whereas others have thick walls and are narrowed or dilated. As with the findings on chest radiograph, the prevalence of HRCT abnor-

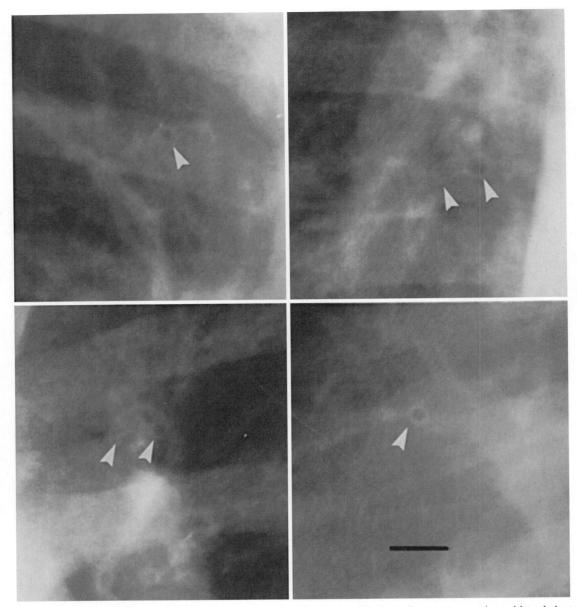

Figure 15–20. Asthma: Bronchial Wall Thickening. Detailed views from four areas of the lungs from posteroanterior and lateral chest radiographs show thick-walled airways measuring 3 to 5 mm in diameter that are not normally visible *(arrowheads)*. The bar represents 1 cm.

malities increases with increased severity of symptoms.[145, 158] Considerable variation exists, however, in the reported frequency and patterns of abnormality. This variation is related to many factors, including differences in technique, data analysis, diagnostic criteria, and patient selection (e.g., smokers or nonsmokers).

Window level, window width, size of the field of view (FOV), and the reconstruction algorithm affect the quality of the CT image and the accuracy of the measurements of airway lumen and wall dimensions (*see* Chapter 2). Many investigators have used phantom airways in an attempt to determine the window levels and widths that would provide the most accurate measurements; on the basis of the results, it is accepted that a window level of −450 HU is ideal.[159, 160] The optimal window width for measurements

of bronchial wall thickness is 1,000 to 1,400 HU. In a study of inflation-fixed lungs, window widths more narrow than 1,000 HU led to substantial magnification of bronchial wall thickness, whereas a window width of 1,500 HU resulted in slight underestimation.[161] Several investigators showed that at the appropriate window level and width, the smallest airways on which reasonably accurate measurements of lumen diameter can be made are 1.5 to 2 mm in diameter.[157, 162, 163] The accuracy of the measurements of airway wall area can be improved by using an analysis algorithm, which improves airway wall edge detection.[233]

Many investigators have described the HRCT findings in asthmatic patients.[156, 158, 164] In one investigation, bronchial wall thickening was present in 44 of 48 (92%) asthmatic patients, compared with 5 of 27 (19%) healthy indi-

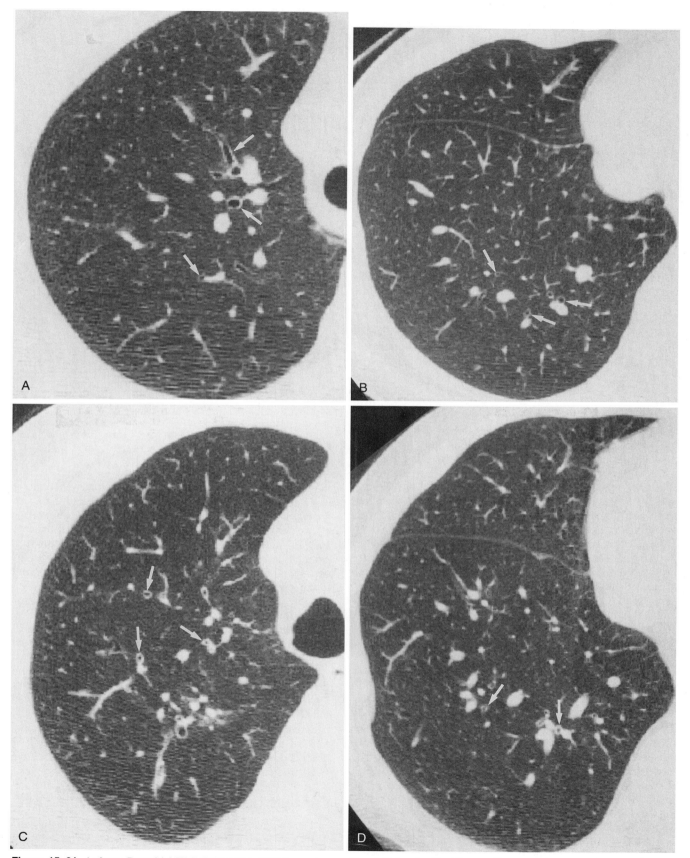

Figure 15–21. Asthma: Bronchial Wall Thickening. HRCT scan images *(A and B)* in a healthy 34-year-old woman show normal upper and lower lobe bronchi *(arrows)*. HRCT scans in a patient who has chronic asthma *(C and D)* show thickening of the bronchial walls *(arrows)*. Decreased diameter of the lumen of several bronchi also is evident, particularly in the right lower lobe.

viduals.[156] In a second investigation, bronchial thickening was seen in 44% of HRCT scans from 39 asthmatic patients, compared with only 4% of scans from 14 normal persons.[158] In a third investigation, bronchial wall thickening was reported in 16 of 17 asthmatic patients who had clinical evidence of allergic bronchopulmonary aspergillosis and in 9 of 11 asthmatic persons who did not.[166] The asthmatic airway wall thickening may not be reversible, at least in the short term; in an investigation of 10 patients who underwent scanning during an acute attack and then 2 weeks later after receiving an intensive course of corticosteroid therapy, no change in wall dimensions was evident.[145]

Airway narrowing in asthmatics can be estimated on HRCT by assessment of the distribution of lumen areas in randomly selected airways. In one investigation, the frequency distribution of airway lumen areas was shifted to the left (a preponderance of smaller lumen sizes) in asthmatic patients compared with age-matched normal individuals.[157] Another method of measuring airway lumen area is to compare it with that of the accompanying blood vessel and calculate a ratio, as is done for the detection of bronchiectasis. In one investigation in which this calculation was performed, the mean inner bronchial-to-arterial diameter ratio in asthmatics who had a normal forced expiratory volume in 1 second (FEV_1) or a moderately reduced FEV_1 (>60% of predicted) was 0.60 ± 0.16 or 0.60 ± 0.18 and was not significantly different from that in normal persons (ratio of 0.65 ± 0.16).[158] In asthmatic patients whose FEV_1 was less than 60% of that predicted, the mean ratio (0.48 ± 0.11) was significantly lower than that in normal persons. In this study, there was no difference in the ratios measured in different lobes or segments. Patients who have moderate or severe asthma have a greater airway wall thickness–to–outer bronchial diameter ratio and a greater percentage of wall area (defined as [wall area/total airway area] × 100) than patients who have mild asthma or normal individuals.[165]

Airways can be dilated excessively in asthmatic patients, as assessed by measurement of the bronchial-to-arterial diameter ratio (Fig. 15–22).[156, 158] The reported prevalence of bronchial dilation in asthmatic patients who do not have clinical evidence of allergic bronchopulmonary aspergillosis is 18% to 77% in these studies and is significantly higher than that in appropriate control subjects. In one of these studies, 36% of all airways examined from 48 asthmatic patients had bronchial dilation (defined as an internal diameter greater than that of the accompanying artery);[156] 77% had at least one dilated bronchus. (Bronchial dilation also was found in 19% of all airways examined in 27 healthy persons, and 59% of the subjects had at least one dilated bronchus.) In another study, bronchial dilation was observed in 31% of CT scans in 39 asthmatic patients, compared with 4% of CT scans in 14 normal persons.[158]

The significance of bronchial dilation in asthmatic patients is uncertain. The fact that about 5% to 20% of airways are bigger than the accompanying artery in healthy individuals[156, 158] illustrates that there is a wide normal variation in this ratio.[167] There is significant heterogeneity between airways in their degree of dilation or narrowing in the same person. This heterogeneity could be between parallel airways, or it could be distributed serially along

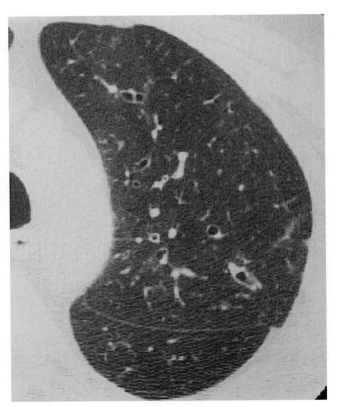

Figure 15–22. Asthma: Bronchial Dilation. HRCT scan in a 57-year-old man with chronic asthma shows left upper lobe bronchiectasis. The patient was a nonsmoker who did not have a history of recurrent infections.

the airway. An alternative explanation for airway dilation is a narrowing of the accompanying artery resulting in an apparent increase in the bronchial diameter. Pulmonary arteries are reactive to changes in alveolar oxygen tension, and an increased bronchial-to-arterial diameter ratio has been observed in HRCT studies performed at altitude compared with those performed at sea level, presumably owing to the reduced ambient oxygen tension at altitude.[168]

Other findings on HRCT include localized areas of low attenuation and vascularity and air-trapping (Fig. 15–23).[147, 158] These areas are the result of abnormalities of ventilation-perfusion distribution that are common even during clinically stable periods and have been described well by scintigraphy.[169, 170] In one investigation, air trapping was shown on expiratory HRCT in approximately 50% of 39 asthmatic patients, compared with 14% of 14 normal individuals;[158] air trapping was seen in 45% of asthmatic patients who had an FEV_1 of greater than 80% predicted, 50% of patients who had an FEV_1 between 60% and 79% predicted, and 67% of patients who had an FEV_1 less than 60% predicted.

CHRONIC OBSTRUCTIVE PULMONARY DISEASE

Chronic respiratory disease related to cigarette smoking had an enormous impact on society in the twentieth century. In the United States, COPD is the fifth most important cause of death.[175]

The definition of COPD is based solely on functional

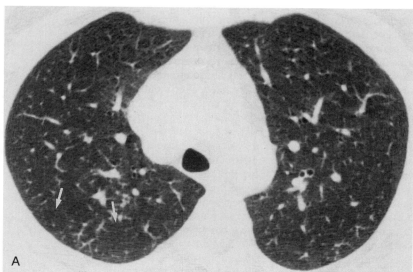
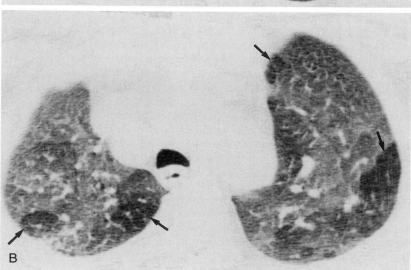

Figure 15–23. Asthma: Air-Trapping. HRCT scan performed at end-inspiration *(A)* shows subtle localized areas of decreased attenuation and vascularity *(arrows)*. HRCT scan performed at the end of maximal expiration *(B)* shows several bilateral areas of air-trapping *(arrows)*. The patient was a 45-year-old lifelong non-smoker who had chronic asthma.

abnormalities. COPD has been defined as "persistent, largely irreversible airway obstruction in which the underlying pathophysiology is not precisely known,"[177] or "a chronic, slowly progressive airway obstructive disorder resulting from some combination of pulmonary emphysema and irreversible reduction in the caliber of small airways in the lung."[180] To retain any usefulness, the term *COPD* should exclude specific, well-defined entities characterized by persistent obstruction, such as asthma, bronchiectasis, bronchiolitis, and cystic fibrosis.

Abundant evidence indicates that several causative factors are involved in the development of COPD. Clinical and epidemiologic studies have focused on the contributions of cigarette smoke (active and passive), air pollution (occupational or urban), infection (especially during childhood), climate, heredity, socioeconomic status, atopy, nonspecific airway hyper-responsiveness, diet, and nutrition.[181] Cigarette smoking is the most important of these factors; many of the other factors simply represent modifiers of the host response to cigarette smoke. Despite these observations, it has been estimated that only 10% to 20% of chronic heavy smokers develop symptomatic COPD;[182, 183]

factors other than cigarette smoking are involved in many cases.

COPD is defined by the presence of significant, largely irreversible air-flow obstruction. This obstruction is frequently, but not invariably, associated with a persistent, productive cough, which defines chronic bronchitis, and lung parenchymal destruction, which defines emphysema.

Chronic Bronchitis. In clinical practice, the diagnosis of chronic bronchitis is based on a history of excessive expectoration of mucus. Because standardization of the quantity of mucus produced is necessary to compare populations, semiquantitative (and somewhat arbitrary) estimates have been incorporated into the clinical definition—for example, one popular definition states that "expectoration must occur on most days during at least 3 consecutive months for not less than 2 consecutive years."[139] All other causes of chronic coughing and expectoration must be eliminated before a diagnosis of chronic bronchitis is made clinically.

Emphysema. Emphysema is abnormal permanent enlargement of air spaces distal to the terminal bronchioles, accompanied by destruction of their walls without obvious fibrosis.[179] Inclusion of the last proviso is controversial because it excludes irregular emphysema and some cases of paraseptal emphysema from the definition and because centrilobular emphysema is associated commonly with microscopic foci of fibrosis. Irregular emphysema and paraseptal emphysema often are associated with localized pulmonary injury, such as pneumonia, or with chronic pulmonary diseases, such as sarcoidosis or silicosis; because the air-space enlargement in such cases is focal, an effect on pulmonary function typically is absent or minimal, and these conditions are not included under the *COPD umbrella*.[178] From a descriptive point of view, we believe it is appropriate to consider them variants of emphysema. For the purposes of definition, air-space enlargement can occur without tissue destruction, such as that which occurs in Down's syndrome; such enlargement is not considered to be emphysema because tissue destruction is not present.

Although, strictly speaking, emphysema can be diagnosed only pathologically, certain alterations in pulmonary function and certain radiologic features allow its detection and an estimation of its severity. The use of CT in particular has allowed a fairly precise quantification of the extent of emphysema, although this modality is insensitive to minor degrees of alveolar destruction.

Depending on the predominant site of parenchymal destruction, several morphologic subtypes of emphysema can be identified. Predominant involvement of the proximal respiratory bronchioles (proximal acinar emphysema) (Fig. 15–24) results in a characteristic distribution near the center of the secondary lobule. It is known most commonly as centrilobular emphysema. This type is found predominantly in cigarette smokers and is the most common form of clinically and functionally significant emphysema.

Predominant involvement of the alveolar ducts and sacs in the peripheral portion of the acinus is referred to as *distal acinar (paraseptal) emphysema* (Fig. 15–25). Grossly, it is usually focal and consists of small emphysematous spaces in a more or less continuous zone of variable length located in the periphery of the lung adjacent to the pleura or interlobular septa.

Involvement of the entire acinus is termed *panacinar*

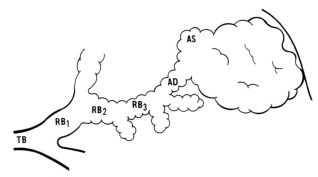

Figure 15–25. Paraseptal Emphysema. In paraseptal (distal acinar) emphysema, the peripheral part of the acinus (alveolar ducts and sacs) predominantly is involved. See Figure 15–24 for abbreviations. (From Thurlbeck WM: Chronic Airflow Obstruction in Lung Disease. Philadelphia, WB Saunders, 1976, p 16.)

(panlobular) emphysema (Fig. 15–26). This variant characteristically is seen in association with α_1-protease inhibitor deficiency; for unknown reasons, it also is seen in patients who have emphysema secondary to intravenous talcosis (*see* page 403). Although panacinar emphysema often is associated with cigarette smoking, such exposure may be absent or minimal. Panacinar emphysema is the form of the disease seen most often in nonsmokers.[184, 185]

Irregular emphysema shows no consistent relationship to any portion of the acinus. It always is associated with fibrosis; according to some definitions, it should not be classified as emphysema.[179] Similar to some cases of paraseptal emphysema, the association of irregular emphysema with fibrosis suggests a relationship with a previous episode of pneumonia.

Radiologic Manifestations

As discussed previously, chronic bronchitis is defined clinically, emphysema pathologically, and COPD functionally. As diagnostic tools that reveal predominantly morphologic abnormalities, the chest radiograph and CT scan can show structural abnormalities attributable to chronic bronchitis or emphysema but can disclose variations caused by

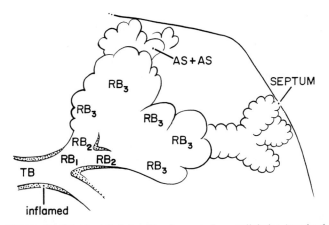

Figure 15–24. Centrilobular Emphysema. In centrilobular (proximal acinar) emphysema, respiratory bronchioles predominantly are involved. (From Thurlbeck WM: Chronic Airflow Obstruction in Lung Disease. Philadelphia, WB Saunders, 1976, p 15.) (TB, terminal bronchiole; RB, respiratory bronchiole; AS, alveolar sac.)

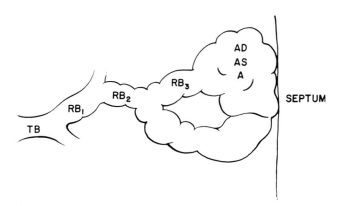

Figure 15–26. Panacinar Emphysema. In panacinar emphysema, the enlargement and destruction of air spaces involve the acinus more or less uniformly. A, alveolus; see Figure 15–24 for other abbreviations. (From Thurlbeck WM: Chronic Airflow Obstruction in Lung Disease. Philadelphia, WB Saunders, 1976, p 15.)

Table 15–3. CHRONIC BRONCHITIS

Clinical diagnosis
History of excessive expectoration of mucus
Not a radiologic diagnosis
Radiologic manifestations
    Bronchial wall thickening
    Prominent lung markings
    Air-trapping on expiratory HRCT scan

HRCT, high-resolution computed tomography.

COPD only by inference. Emphysema, chronic bronchitis, or both can be present in the absence of functional impairment required for the diagnosis of COPD and vice versa. Only chronic bronchitis and emphysema are addressed here.

Chronic Bronchitis

The radiographic manifestations of uncomplicated chronic bronchitis are documented poorly because correlation of radiographic findings with pathologic specimens generally has not been performed and because investigators have not systematically excluded patients who have emphysema. The principal abnormalities are bronchial wall thickening and an increase in lung markings, sometimes referred to as *dirty chest* (Table 15–3).[187–189] The latter term refers to a general accentuation of linear markings throughout the lungs associated with loss of definition of vascular margins.[191] The abnormality was observed in 18% of 119 patients who had chronic bronchitis in one study.[186] The increased markings presumably result from an increase in lung density secondary to accumulation of inflammatory cells and fibrous tissue in the airway walls.[191] Such accumulation may be evident as ring shadows (representing bronchi seen end on, Fig. 15–27) or as tubular shadows (*tram tracks*, when the airways are seen *en face*).[186, 188]

Limited information is available about the HRCT findings in chronic bronchitis. In one investigation of 175 healthy adults, including 98 current smokers, 26 ex-smokers, and 51 nonsmokers, no evidence of bronchial wall thickening was found on radiographs from any of the subjects;[192] however, on HRCT scans, it was considered to be present in 32 (33%) smokers, 4 (16%) ex-smokers, and 9 (18%) nonsmokers.

As with other airway diseases, chronic bronchitis may result in air-trapping. In one investigation of 20 patients who had emphysema, 20 who had chronic bronchitis, and 20 healthy individuals, spirometrically triggered CT images at 90% of vital capacity showed similar mean lung attenuation for patients who had chronic bronchitis and for normal individuals, and decreased attenuation in the patients who had emphysema.[193] At 10% of vital capacity, patients who had chronic bronchitis and those who had emphysema had lower mean lung attenuation than that in the normal individuals. As the authors pointed out, however, the study was based on "relatively extreme selection criteria" and included only patients who had chronic bronchitis and an FEV$_1$ of less than 70% of that predicted; the results may not be applicable to patients who have less severe air-flow obstruction.

Chronic bronchitis is not a radiologic diagnosis. Although changes may be observed on radiograph or an HRCT scan suggesting that bronchitis is present, it is inappropriate for the radiologist to do anything other than indicate that the findings are compatible with that diagnosis.

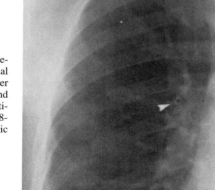

Figure 15–27. Chronic Bronchitis. Posteroanterior chest radiograph shows thickened bronchial walls viewed end-on in the right and left upper lobes *(arrowheads)*. Lung volume, vasculature, and cardiac size are normal. These features are compatible with chronic bronchitis. The patient was a 58-year-old man who had a 15-year history of chronic productive cough.

S.R.

Table 15–4. EMPHYSEMA

Defined pathologically
Enlargement of air spaces secondary to destruction of alveolar walls
Radiologic manifestations
    Bullae
    Areas of radiolucency
    Hyperinflation
Good correlation between inspiratory HRCT and histologic findings
Good correlation between expiratory HRCT and air-flow obstruction

    HRCT, high-resolution computed tomography.

Emphysema

Radiographic abnormalities in emphysema reflect the presence of lung destruction, secondary alterations in the vascular pattern, and increased lung volume (Table 15–4). Direct signs of emphysema, such as bullae and irregular areas of radiolucency related to tissue loss, can be seen on chest radiograph in some patients (Fig. 15–28).[191, 194, 195] Bullae may be single or multiple. Their walls usually are of no more than hairline thickness so that it may be difficult to distinguish them from uninvolved parenchyma. Large bullae can be observed pathologically that are invisible on chest radiograph, even in retrospect;[196] such bullae usually are situated anteriorly or posteriorly, where their presence is masked by a normal lung, or in the subpleural zone, where the absence of visible blood vessels prevents appreciation of vascular distortion.[196]

In most cases, radiographic findings reflect secondary alterations in the vascular pattern and the presence of overinflation (Fig. 15–29).[194, 196, 197] Vascular abnormalities related to emphysema include local avascular areas, distortion of vessels, increased branching angles and loss of normal sinuosity, a decrease in the peripheral vascular markings, and enlargement of the main pulmonary arteries.[196, 198, 199] Diminution in the caliber of the pulmonary vessels, with increased rapidity of tapering distally, has a relatively high specificity for the diagnosis;[190, 196] however, it has a sensitivity of only 15% for the detection of mild to moderate disease and 40% for the detection of severe disease.[198] Although localized avascular areas, narrowing of midlung vessels, and an enlarged pulmonary arterial trunk have been shown to be associated significantly with the extent of emphysema observed pathologically, these parameters are inferior to the presence of overinflation.[200]

The most reliable sign of overinflation is flattening of the diaphragmatic domes (*see* Fig. 15–29).[194, 195, 201] When the configuration of the diaphragm is concave superiorly, the presence of emphysema is virtually certain in adults (*see* Fig. 15–28). The diaphragm is considered flattened when the highest level of the diaphragmatic contour is less than 1.5 cm above a line connecting the costophrenic and vertebrophrenic junctions on the posteroanterior radiograph or a line connecting the sternophrenic and posterior costophrenic angles on the lateral view or when the sternodiaphragmatic angle on the lateral radiograph is 90 degrees or greater.[191, 194, 195] In one investigation, a flattened diaphragm on the posteroanterior chest radiograph was present in 94% of patients who had severe emphysema, 76% of patients who had moderate emphysema, and 21% of patients who had mild emphysema;[201] only 4% of patients without emphysema showed the abnormality.

Other helpful signs of overinflation include an increase in the retrosternal air space, an increase in lung height, and a low position (depression) of the diaphragm. The retrosternal air space is the space between the anterior

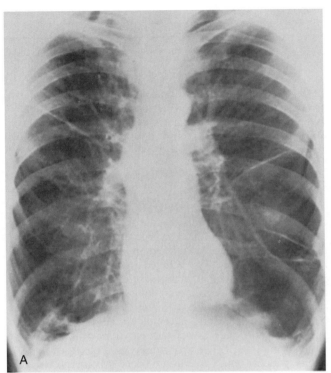

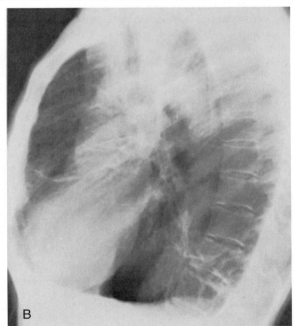

Figure 15–28. Emphysema Associated with Bullae. Posteroanterior *(A)* and lateral *(B)* chest radiographs from a 43-year-old woman show severe overinflation of both lungs. The diaphragm is low, and its superior surface is concave. Note the prominent costophrenic muscle slips. The retrosternal air space is deepened. Numerous bullae are present in both lower lung zones, particularly the left. The peripheral vasculature of the lungs is diminished severely, but there is no evidence of pulmonary arterial hypertension. (It is probable that the upper lung zones are involved less severely than the lower zones, permitting redistribution of blood flow and minimizing the risk of development of hypertension.)

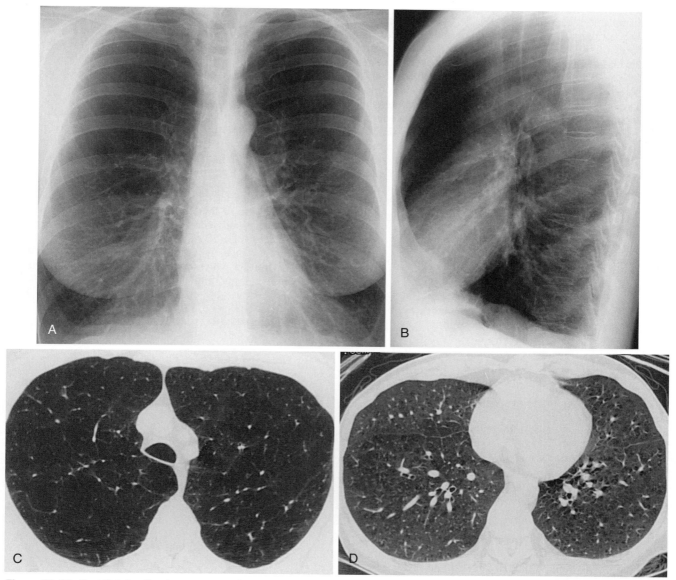

Figure 15–29. Centrilobular Emphysema. Posteroanterior *(A)* and lateral *(B)* chest radiographs show increased lucency and decreased vascularity in the upper lobes, marked overinflation with flattening of the diaphragm, and increased retrosternal air space. HRCT scan through the upper lobes *(C)* shows severe emphysema; a scan at a more caudad level *(D)* shows relatively mild centrilobular emphysema. The patient was a 49-year-old smoker.

margin of the ascending aorta and the sternum. It is considered to be increased when the horizontal distance between the sternum and the most anterior margin of the ascending aorta is greater than 2.5 cm.[194, 195] The lung height is considered to be increased when it measures 30 cm or more from the dome of the right hemidiaphragm to the tubercle of the first rib.[202] The identification of the dome of the right hemidiaphragm at or below the anterior end of the seventh rib is suggestive of hyperinflation;[198, 203] however, this finding has a low sensitivity[213] and is less helpful in diagnosis than is a change in contour.[194, 195]

The greatest diagnostic accuracy on the radiograph is obtained by using a combination of findings. In one investigation, a combination of hyperinflation and vascular changes allowed the correct diagnosis of emphysema in 29 (97%) of 30 autopsy-proven cases in which the patients had been symptomatic as well as 8 (47%) of 17 autopsy-

proven cases involving asymptomatic individuals.[197] In another investigation, the presence of emphysema was assessed in 60 patients (33 who had emphysema and 27 normal controls) using the following criteria: (1) depression or flattening of the diaphragm on posteroanterior radiograph, (2) irregular radiolucency of the lungs, (3) increased retrosternal space on lateral radiograph, and (4) flattening of the diaphragm on lateral radiograph. At least two of the four criteria had to be present for a diagnosis of emphysema. Using these criteria, all 14 symptomatic and 13 of 19 (68%) asymptomatic patients who had emphysema were diagnosed correctly;[194] no false-positive diagnoses were made. Based on these and other data,[196, 205] it can be calculated that the presence of two or more of the four radiographic features listed usually implies a pathologic emphysema score of 30 out of 100 or greater.[206]

Pulmonary arterial hypertension secondary to emphysema usually is recognizable easily by a combination of a deficiency in the peripheral vasculature and an increase in the size of the hilar pulmonary arteries. In cases in which previous chest films are available for comparison, the latter should be readily apparent; when no previous films exist, a diameter of the right interlobar artery exceeding 16 mm should be regarded as convincing evidence of hypertension. Peripheral arterial deficiency often is localized to certain areas of the lungs, vessels elsewhere being of normal or increased caliber. In such cases, the hilar arteries usually are of normal size, suggesting that the relatively uninvolved portions of the lungs are the sites of redistributed blood flow, delaying the development of pulmonary hypertension at least temporarily. In cases of general arterial deficiency, in which redistribution of blood flow to normal regions is impossible, the development of hypertension is manifested by an increase in the size of the hilar arteries and a greater discrepancy in the caliber of central and peripheral vessels.

Computed Tomography

On CT scans, emphysema is characterized by the presence of areas of abnormally low attenuation, usually with-

out visible walls (Fig. 15–30);[206, 208, 209] occasionally, walls 1 mm or less are seen. On HRCT scans, vessels can be seen within the areas of low attenuation.[210] Several groups of investigators have shown that CT, particularly HRCT, findings correlate closely with the presence and severity of emphysema.[208, 214, 216] In one study of 25 patients in which the findings on conventional 1-cm collimation CT scans were compared with findings derived from pathologic assessment, three radiologists independently assessed the CT scans for the extent of areas of low attenuation, pulmonary vascular pruning, and pulmonary vascular distortion.[211] The finding that correlated best with the presence and severity of emphysema was areas of low attenuation ($r = 0.84$ in the upper part of the lung and $r = 0.78$ in the lower part of the lung); use of this criterion allowed the identification of 13 of 15 patients who had centrilobular emphysema and produced only 2 of 10 false-positive results.

In another investigation, preoperative CT scans were obtained from 38 patients who were to undergo lobectomy or pneumonectomy, and the findings on conventional CT and HRCT scans were compared with the pathologic findings in the corresponding transverse slice of lung.[208] The scans were assessed by two independent observers; the

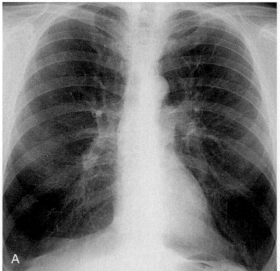

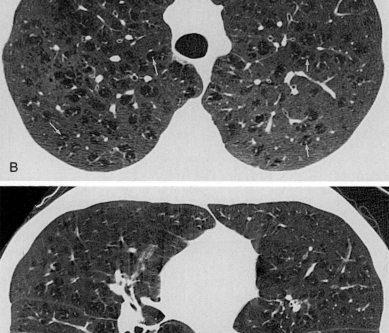

Figure 15–30. Centrilobular Emphysema. Posteroanterior chest radiograph *(A)* shows overinflation and attenuation of the peripheral vascular markings. HRCT scan through the upper lobes *(B)* shows localized areas of low attenuation, characteristic of centrilobular emphysema. Persistent vessels *(arrows)* can be seen in the center of several of the areas of low attenuation; this feature is characteristic of emphysema and helpful in the distinction from cystic lung disease. An HRCT scan obtained at a more caudad level *(C)* shows slightly less severe emphysema. The patient was a 49-year-old man.

diagnosis was based on the presence of areas of low attenuation. Correlation between the CT assessment of emphysema and the pathologic panel score was high for conventional 10-mm collimation CT ($r = 0.81$) and HRCT (1.5-mm collimation) ($r = 0.85$) scans. Lower correlations were found between the scans and the pathologic scores ($r = 0.70$ for conventional CT, $r = 0.72$ for HRCT). Although use of HRCT resulted in only a slight improvement in the correlation with the pathologic extent of emphysema, the emphysema was more conspicuous on HRCT scans than on conventional CT scans. The extent and severity of emphysema were underestimated consistently, however, on conventional CT and HRCT scans. In one of five patients who had no emphysema on pathologic examination, the conventional CT scan was interpreted by one of the observers as showing mild emphysema; in 6 of 33 patients who had emphysema, the emphysema was missed on the CT scans by both observers.

In another investigation of 42 patients who had undergone lobectomy, the accuracy of scans obtained using HRCT (1-mm collimation) and conventional CT (5-mm collimation) was evaluated.[214] The extent of emphysema was assessed on CT scans and in the resected lobes using a panel of standards; the diagnosis of emphysema on CT scans was based on the presence of areas of low attenuation and vascular disruption. The correlations between the CT emphysema scores and the pathologic findings were 0.68 for HRCT and 0.76 for 5-mm collimation CT scans. The severity of emphysema found pathologically was underestimated consistently on 5-mm collimation scans; however, there was no significant difference between the HRCT emphysema scores and the pathology scores. The greater sensitivity of HRCT compared with conventional CT in the detection of emphysema was confirmed in a subsequent study.[193] Additional studies using 1-mm collimation HRCT scans showed no significant difference between the extent of emphysema as assessed on HRCT scans and gross specimens.[216–218] Mild disease can be missed on HRCT scans, however.[206, 208, 219]

Visualization of small, subtle areas of emphysema on CT scans can be improved by the use of narrow window widths ($\leq 1,000$ HU) and low window levels (-600 to -800 HU)[206, 212, 220] or by the use of spiral CT with reconstruction of contiguous sections using the minimum-intensity projection technique.[219, 221] This technique consists of spiral CT performed using 1-mm collimation through a volume of lung ranging from a few millimeters to several centimeters in thickness (sliding thin-slab technique). The images can be reconstructed individually or as a single slab. The minimum intensity projection technique reconstructs the images based on the lowest attenuation values present within the slab and has the effect of suppressing the visualization of pulmonary vessels and optimizing visualization of low-attenuation areas (Fig. 15–31). In one investigation of 29 patients who had no radiographic evidence of emphysema, 10 contiguous 1-mm-thick CT sections were examined before lobectomy.[219] Minimum intensity projection images were generated, including three to eight contiguous sections; slab thicknesses used were 3, 5, and 8 mm. Of the 29 patients, 21 had emphysema on pathologic examination; the emphysema was detected on the minimum intensity projection images in 17 (85%)

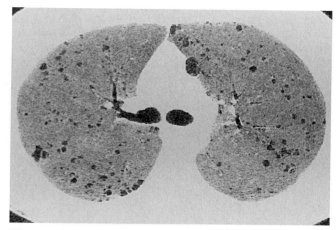

Figure 15–31. Emphysema: Minimum Intensity Projection. Minimum intensity projection reconstruction image from a sliding thin-slab spiral CT study (1-mm collimation, slab thickness 10 mm) shows localized areas of emphysema. The technique suppresses hyperattenuating structures, such as pulmonary vessels, and allows better visualization of areas of decreased attenuation related to emphysema. The patient was a 41-year-old woman.

cases, compared with 13 (62%) on HRCT scans. The specificity of both techniques was 100%. Emphysema was easier to detect on 8-mm-thick slabs than it was on thinner ones because of better suppression of vascular structures.

On HRCT, centrilobular emphysema is characterized by the presence of multiple localized small areas of low attenuation, which often measure less than 1 cm in diameter; when small, they can be seen to be in the central portion of the lobule.[209, 212, 220] The emphysema can be diffuse but typically involves mainly the upper lobes (*see* Fig. 15–29). In most cases, the areas of low attenuation lack visible walls; however, thin walls may be seen, particularly when emphysema is extensive. The walls probably represent interlobular septa. Severe centrilobular emphysema may be indistinguishable from panlobular emphysema on HRCT (compare Figs. 15–29*C* and 15–32*B*).

Panlobular emphysema involves mainly the lower lobes.[222–224] It is characterized on CT scans by areas of low attenuation and a paucity of vessels (Fig. 15–32).[206, 213, 225] Severe panlobular emphysema leads to diffuse, low attenuation and paucity of vascular markings; although these features allow ready identification of advanced disease, mild or moderately severe disease may be difficult to distinguish from normal parenchyma.[208, 213] In one investigation of 10 patients who had panlobular emphysema, the correlation with pathologic findings was 0.90 for conventional CT and 0.96 for HRCT;[213] however, the extent of emphysema was underestimated consistently, although less so on HRCT scans than on conventional CT scans. The diagnosis was missed in three patients on conventional CT scans and in two patients on HRCT scans. In another investigation of 17 patients who had moderate to severe panlobular emphysema associated with α_1-antiprotease inhibitor deficiency, all patients were found to have areas of low attenuation corresponding to parenchymal destruction and reduced vascularity.[225] Bulla formation was seen in 7 of 17 patients. The emphysema could be seen to involve all lung zones on the chest radiographs and HRCT scans, with only a slight lower lung zone predominance.

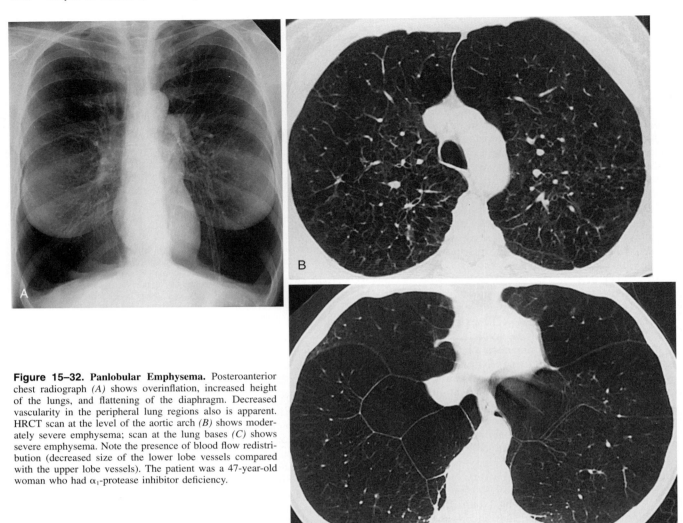

Figure 15–32. Panlobular Emphysema. Posteroanterior chest radiograph *(A)* shows overinflation, increased height of the lungs, and flattening of the diaphragm. Decreased vascularity in the peripheral lung regions also is apparent. HRCT scan at the level of the aortic arch *(B)* shows moderately severe emphysema; scan at the lung bases *(C)* shows severe emphysema. Note the presence of blood flow redistribution (decreased size of the lower lobe vessels compared with the upper lobe vessels). The patient was a 47-year-old woman who had α_1-protease inhibitor deficiency.

Bronchiectasis may be seen on CT scans from patients who have panlobular emphysema. It was identified in 6 of the 17 patients (35%) in the study just cited.[225] In another investigation of 14 patients who had α_1-antitrypsin deficiency, 6 (43%) had evidence of bronchiectasis on CT scans, including 2 who had cystic bronchiectasis.[235] Patients who had bronchiectasis had significantly higher infection rates than patients who did not. Occasionally, bronchiectasis is present before the development of emphysema.[236, 237]

Paraseptal (distal acinar) emphysema is characterized on CT scans by the presence of areas of low attenuation in the subpleural lung regions separated by intact interlobular septa (Fig. 15–33).[206, 207] Because centrilobular emphysema and paraseptal emphysema produce localized areas of low attenuation, they are easier to recognize on CT scans than is panlobular disease.[206, 208, 213]

Objective Quantification of Emphysema

The extent of emphysema can be assessed objectively by CT using a computer program that quantifies the volume of lung that has abnormally low attenuation (Fig. 15–34).[215,] [216, 238] One such program involves the use of a *density mask*, which highlights areas of attenuation below a given threshold. One group of investigators compared density mask estimates with the visual assessment of emphysema in 28 patients who underwent conventional CT before lung resection for tumor.[215] The pathologic score was obtained using a modification of the panel grading system; according to this method, 7 patients had no emphysema, and 21 had emphysema scores ranging from 5 to 100. In each patient, a single representative CT scan was compared with the corresponding pathologic specimen. The investigators assessed the accuracy of density masks, highlighting all voxels with attenuation values less than -920, -910, and -900 HU.

Correlation between the three different density mask scores and the pathologic assessment of emphysema was good (all $r > 0.83$, $P < 0.001$). The best correlations were observed when all voxels with attenuation values between -910 and -1024 HU were highlighted. The correlation between the mean density mask score and the pathologic score for emphysema was 0.89. By comparison, the correlation between the mean of visual scores by two independent

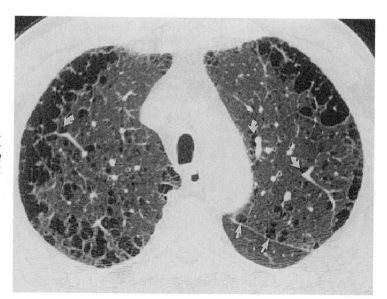

Figure 15–33. Paraseptal Emphysema. HRCT scan shows emphysema, predominantly in subpleural distribution and focally along the interlobar fissure *(straight arrows)* and vessels *(curved arrows)*. The appearance is characteristic of paraseptal (distal acinar) emphysema.

observers and the pathologic score for emphysema was 0.90. There was excellent correlation between the extent of emphysema assessed using the density mask at −910 HU and the subjective assessment of extent of emphysema ($r = 0.95$). When the density mask at −910 HU was used, three cases with mild emphysema were missed, and emphysema was diagnosed in one normal lung; by compar-ison, two independent chest radiologists on two separate occasions missed two cases of similarly mild emphysema. The first observer missed one additional case, and the second observer missed four additional cases with mild emphysema.[215]

Spiral CT allows rapid quantification of the volume of lung involved with emphysema.[239, 240] The use of predeter-

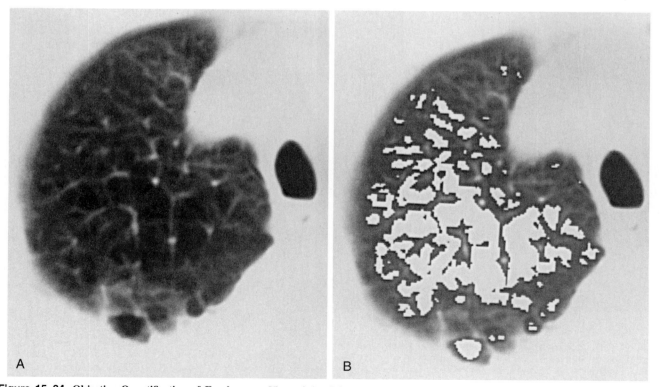

Figure 15–34. Objective Quantification of Emphysema. View of the right upper lobe from a conventional CT scan *(A)* shows the presence of emphysema. Using a computer program *(density mask)*, all voxels below a given threshold are highlighted automatically *(B)*. The highlighted areas correspond to voxels with attenuation values less than −910 HU. The CT program automatically quantifies the volume of lung that contains areas with attenuation below the given threshold as well as the volume of the remaining lung.

mined threshold attenuation values with this technique enables display of the distribution of emphysema in multiple planes and in three dimensions (Fig. 15–35).[239, 240]

The optimal threshold for the assessment of the presence of emphysema depends on the slice thickness and on whether the CT scan is obtained at end-inspiration or at end-expiration. One group of investigators performed HRCT using 1-mm collimation at 1-cm intervals before surgery in 63 patients.[216] They measured the relative areas associated with attenuation values lower than eight thresholds ranging from -900 to -970 HU and compared the results with those obtained from the corresponding pathologic specimens cut in the same plane as that used for the HRCT scans. The optimal threshold value for objective quantification of emphysema on HRCT scans was -950 HU; using this threshold value, there was no significant difference between the extent of emphysema as assessed by HRCT or by morphometry.

Subsequently, the same group confirmed that inspiratory HRCT scans obtained using -950 HU as the threshold correlate best with the macroscopic extent of emphysema.[217] These investigators also showed that HRCT scans obtained at the end of maximal expiration correlate better with measurements of air-flow obstruction than do inspiratory HRCT scans, a finding that may reflect the presence of airway disease in addition to emphysema.[241] The correlation between inspiratory HRCT scans (threshold value, -950 HU) and vital capacity and FEV_1 (per cent of predicted) were -0.24 and -0.50, compared with -0.48 and -0.68 for expiratory HRCT scans (threshold value, -910 HU).

Lung density as measured by CT is affected by many variables, including patient size, location of the areas of emphysema, depth of inspiration, type of CT scanner, collimation, kilovoltage, and the reconstruction algorithm.[215, 242] Despite these limitations, objective assessment of emphysema using a threshold CT attenuation value has been shown to correlate closely with the visual assessment of emphysema[215] and with the pathologic extent of emphysema.[215, 216, 218] CT also allows measurement of overall lung volumes.[243–245] In one investigation of 85 patients, including 60 who had emphysema, there was good correlation between lung volumes determined using conventional CT and the functional residual capacity as determined by plethysmography ($r = 0.79$).[243] As the authors pointed out, the CT lung volumes correlate better with functional residual capacity than with TLC because the CT scans are obtained while the patient is supine, usually after a normal inspiratory effort, whereas plethysmographic lung volumes are determined with the patient in the sitting position and include a maximal inspiration.[243]

Lung volume and thoracic dimensions can be measured using single breath-hold MR imaging.[245] In one investigation in which measurements of lung volume obtained using spiral CT and single breath-hold MR imaging and TLC obtained using plethysmography were compared in 15 patients who had severe emphysema, good correlation was found between the CT-determined lung volume and TLC

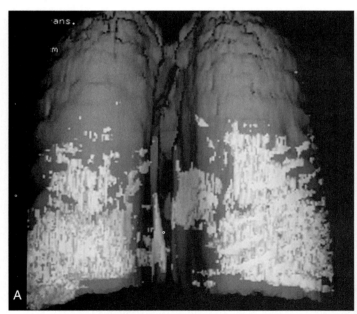

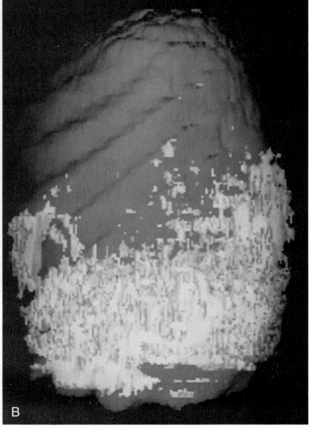

Figure 15–35. Objective Quantification of Panacinar Emphysema. Posterior *(A)* and left lateral *(B)* three-dimensional reconstruction images from a spiral CT study show the areas of emphysema highlighted in white and normal lung tissue as areas of gray. The emphysema involves almost exclusively the lower lung zones. The areas that are highlighted have attenuation values equal to or less than -910 HU. (Courtesy of Dr. Ella Kazerooni, University of Michigan Medical Center, Ann Arbor, MI.)

(r = 0.87) and between the MR imaging–determined lung volume and TLC (r = 0.71).[245] The mean lung volumes (L) were 6.71 ± 1.04 for CT, 7.00 ± 1.13 for MR imaging, and 8.12 ± 1.47 for plethysmographic TLC.

The main advantage of CT over MR imaging and plethysmography is in the assessment of the volume of lung involved with emphysema and regional changes in lung volume after lung volume reduction surgery or bullectomy. Decreases in lung volume and changes in thoracic dimensions after lung volume reduction surgery have been measured using chest radiography,[246] CT,[244, 245, 247] and MR imaging;[245] measurements of changes in lung volume after surgery using these various techniques have been shown to correlate closely with the decrease in lung volumes as determined by plethysmography.

Bullous Disease

A bulla is a sharply demarcated, air-containing space 1 cm or greater in diameter that possesses a smooth wall 1 mm or less in thickness. The space may be unilocular or separated into several compartments by thin septa. The walls are formed by pleura, connective tissue septa, or compressed lung parenchyma. The lesion may arise *de novo*, in which case the surrounding lung tissue is normal; however, it occurs more commonly in association with other disease, usually emphysema or remote infection.

It is useful and traditional to divide patients who have bullous disease into two groups: patients who have COPD and patients judged to have normal pulmonary parenchyma between the bullae and who are free of airway obstruction (primary bullous disease).[248–250] A familial occurrence has been reported in patients who have the latter form.[253] The incidence of bullae is increased in patients who have connective tissue diseases, such as Marfan's syndrome[254] and Ehlers-Danlos syndrome.[255]

Radiologic Manifestations

Bullae are manifested on chest radiograph as thin-walled, sharply demarcated areas of avascularity (Fig. 15–36). The walls are apparent characteristically as hairline

shadows; however, because bullae most often are located at or near the lung surface, only a portion of the wall usually is visible. A location within the substance of the lung renders identification much more difficult, and even peripheral bullae may be missed on radiograph.[256] Bullae are evident much more commonly in the upper lobes than elsewhere, particularly in asymptomatic individuals;[249, 250] however, in patients who have widespread emphysema, there is only a slight predilection for the upper lobes.[464]

As might be expected, CT allows greatly improved visibility of a bulla identified on a radiograph and may reveal one that was not suspected.[207, 256] CT is particularly valuable in defining the anatomy of bullae and in determining the extent of emphysema or parenchymal compression of adjacent lung tissue (Fig. 15–37).[257–259] In one investigation of nine patients (eight smokers and one lifelong nonsmoker) who had bullae that occupied at least one third of a hemithorax, the bullae ranged in diameter from 1 to 20 cm.[258] In all patients, the lesions were predominantly subpleural in distribution; intraparenchymal bullae, present in seven patients, were less than 3 cm in diameter. The predominant abnormality on HRCT was paraseptal emphysema, although eight of the nine patients had evidence of mild to moderately severe centrilobular emphysema.

Bullae may be large enough to compress the adjacent lung parenchyma; although such compression is usually mild,[258] it may result in sufficient atelectasis to cause a masslike opacity. In one investigation of 11 patients who had such opacities, the areas of atelectasis involved mainly the upper lobes;[259] smaller foci of atelectasis were present in the remaining lobes. Re-expansion of the atelectatic lung with resolution of the masslike appearance occurred in seven of the eight patients who underwent resection of bullae. CT allows assessment of the volume of the bullae at TLC and residual volume. In one investigation of 43 patients, bullae were found to contribute little to expired lung volume;[256] residual volume/TLC for the bullae averaged approximately 90%, whereas total lung residual volume/TLC was approximately 60%. Most bullae decrease in size between CT scans performed at end-inspiration and scans performed at the end of maximal expiration; occasionally, bullae remain unchanged in size.[260]

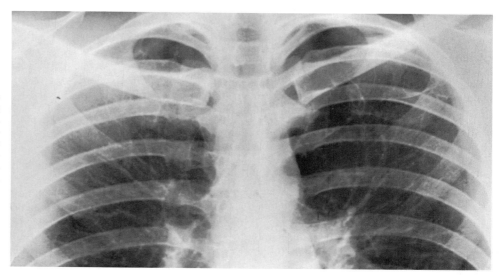

Figure 15–36. Multiple Bullae in Otherwise Normal Lung. View of the upper half of the thorax from posteroanterior radiograph reveals numerous curved hairline shadows in the upper portion of the left lung representing the walls of multiple large bullae. A single bulla is present in the right paramediastinal area.

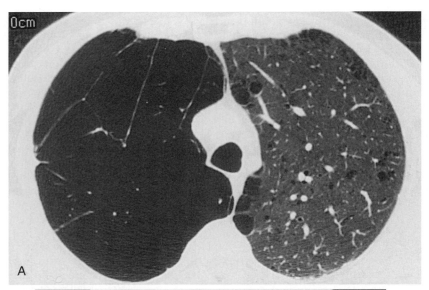

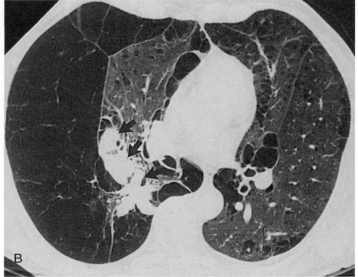

Figure 15–37. Asymmetric Bullous Lung Disease. HRCT scan through the upper lobes *(A)* shows replacement of the parenchyma on the right side by large bullae, associated with a shift of the mediastinum to the left. Mild emphysema is present in the left upper lobe. HRCT scan obtained at a more caudad level *(B)* shows compressive atelectasis *(arrows)* in the right middle and lower lobes and a shift of the mediastinum to the left. The patient was a 68-year-old smoker.

Rarely, bullae disappear as a result of secondary infection[249, 262] or because of inflammatory stenosis of their subtending airways.[238] In many cases, bullae enlarge progressively and may come to occupy most of a hemithorax (Fig. 15–38). In one investigation of 49 patients for whom serial radiographs were available for 1 to more than 10 years, the lesions enlarged consistently;[249] some increased slowly and continuously, whereas others remained constant in size for several years and then for no obvious reason, enlarged. In many patients, bullae were apparent radiographically for many years before the onset of symptoms; this has been our experience also.

Infection usually is manifested radiologically by a fluid level within the bulla,[251, 261] with or without evidence of pneumonitis in the surrounding lung parenchyma. Occasionally, fluid accumulation is caused by hemorrhage,[263] a complication that may be suspected when there is an accompanying drop in the blood hemoglobin level; rarely, hemorrhage may be severe enough to necessitate emergency surgery.[264]

Because bullae commonly do not produce any symptoms, their presence may become evident only when chest radiography is carried out during investigation of acute lower respiratory tract infection. In such circumstances, the radiographic appearance may be misinterpreted as a lung cavity secondary to abscess formation; differentiation is aided by the fact that most patients who have infected bullae are much less ill than patients who have acute lung abscess. Infected bullae usually have much thinner walls (Fig. 15–39), are surrounded by lesser degrees of pneumonitis, and contain much less fluid than cavitated lung abscesses.[265, 266] Complete clearing of fluid from an infected bulla may be protracted, in one series averaging about 6 weeks.[267]

Spontaneous pneumothorax commonly occurs in association with localized areas of emphysema or bullae affecting the lung apices. In one investigation of 116 patients who had surgically treated pneumothorax, 69 had parenchymal abnormalities identified on radiograph;[268] the most common findings consisted of apical bullae (seen in 51 patients),

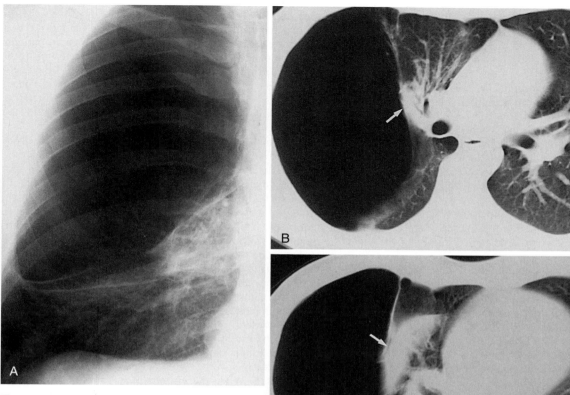

Figure 15–38. Bullous Lung Disease. View of the right lung from posteroanterior radiograph of the right lung *(A)* shows almost complete replacement of the upper lobe by a large bulla. There is associated compression of the adjacent lung. CT scan at the level of the bronchus intermedius *(B)* shows a large bulla and associated compressive atelectasis *(arrow)* in the right upper lobe. CT scan at a more caudad level *(C)* shows areas of atelectasis *(arrows)* in the right middle and lower lobes; the left lung is normal. The patient was a 32-year-old man.

Figure 15–39. Infected Bullae. View of the right lung from a posteroanterior chest radiograph *(A)* shows typical features of emphysema. The supradiaphragmatic portion of the right lower lobe is severely oligemic, and there is displacement of vessels upward, backward, and laterally by one or more large bullae; a faint curvilinear opacity may represent the wall of a bulla *(arrowheads)*. View from a chest radiograph obtained 3 months later *(B)* shows two long fluid levels *(arrowheads)* in adjacent bullae. The walls of the bullae are outlined more clearly *(open arrows)*, presumably as a result of thickening of adjacent tissue by an inflammatory reaction. The fluid levels regressed slowly during 6 weeks.

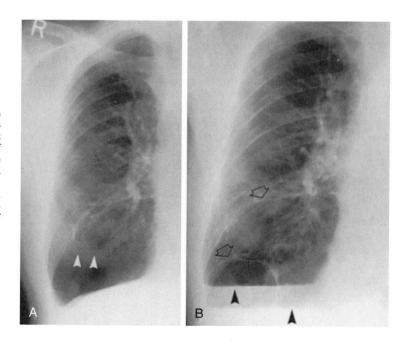

apical scarring (seen in 17 patients), and diffuse emphysema (seen in 9 patients). Bullae and localized areas of emphysema not apparent on the radiograph can be seen on CT scan in greater than 80% of patients who have spontaneous pneumothorax.[269–271] In one investigation of 35 patients who had this abnormality, bullae or smaller localized areas of emphysema were identified on CT scan in 31 (89%) and on radiograph in only 11 (31%);[269] in all of these patients, chest radiograph had been interpreted initially as showing no parenchymal abnormalities. In another investigation of 27 nonsmoking patients who had spontaneous pneumothorax, 21 (81%) had localized bullae or smaller areas of emphysema visible on the CT scan;[271] focal areas of emphysema were identified at surgery in 3 additional patients. In none of these patients were the parenchymal abnormalities visible on chest radiograph. Rarely, pneumothorax is associated with large bullae involving the lower lobes.[253]

When spontaneous pneumothorax develops in association with bullae, it may be identified much more easily when the lung is collapsed than when it is inflated fully; this improved visibility results from the tendency of bullae to remain air-containing while the surrounding lung collapses. Sometimes the distinction of spontaneous pneumothorax from large bullae occupying much of the volume of one lung can be difficult; in such circumstances, CT can be helpful.[272]

Primary bullous disease characteristically is unassociated with symptoms or signs and causes minimal or no abnormality in pulmonary function. Sometimes patients complain of dyspnea on exertion[252] or, rarely, present with severe pulmonary insufficiency and cor pulmonale;[273] in such cases, the lung function impairment may be the result of concomitant COPD.[251] Enlargement occurring as a result of decreased ambient pressure in an airliner can cause air emboli and sudden death.[274]

BRONCHIECTASIS AND OTHER BRONCHIAL ABNORMALITIES

Bronchiectasis

General Features

Bronchiectasis is irreversible dilation of a portion of the bronchial tree. Although it has decreased in importance as a clinically significant affliction—particularly one requiring surgical resection—since the advent of antibiotic therapy,[275, 276] the abnormality has engendered a resurgence of interest as a result of several factors: (1) Advances in medical therapy have led to relatively prolonged survival in patients who have cystic fibrosis, ciliary dyskinetic syndromes, and some immune deficiency syndromes, increasing the pool of patients with these disorders in the population; (2) recurrent bacterial infection, *Pneumocystis carinii* pneumonia, and tuberculosis in human immunodeficiency virus (HIV)–infected subjects can lead to the rapid development of bronchiectasis;[277] (3) the condition has been recognized as an important complication of heart, lung,[278] and bone marrow[279] transplantation; and (4) advances in radiologic imaging have made the recognition of relatively minor degrees of bronchiectasis much easier.[280] The increased ability to detect bronchiectasis by HRCT means that the

spectrum of clinical manifestations associated with the diagnosis has been broadened, and it is now recognized that it may be seen in asymptomatic individuals or in patients who complain only of mild cough unassociated with copious production of purulent sputum. As a result, bronchiectasis detected solely by HRCT is associated with many conditions, such as rheumatoid disease and obliterative bronchiolitis, that were not associated previously with the condition.

The most important cause of clinically significant bronchiectasis in North America and Europe today is cystic fibrosis. In areas of the world where this disease is rare and in developing societies in which the incidence of serious childhood infection is appreciable, postinfective bronchiectasis is still of great significance. Hereditary immunologic and structural abnormalities are much less common, but still important, causes.

The three most important mechanisms that contribute to the pathogenesis of bronchiectasis are infection, airway obstruction, and peribronchial fibrosis. In some cases, all three mechanisms are involved; in others, one is the principal or sole pathogenetic process. Although bronchial infection is present in many patients at some point in the disease, the extent to which it is a cause or an effect of the bronchiectasis is not always clear. Many patients who have bronchiectasis have no symptoms referable to the bronchiectasis itself. When present, the main symptoms are cough and expectoration or purulent sputum; hemoptysis and recurrent fever are less common.

Radiologic Manifestations

Radiography

A variety of radiographic abnormalities characterize bronchiectasis (Table 15–5), including the following:[280, 284, 285]

1. Parallel line opacities (*tram tracks*), representing thickened bronchial walls (Fig. 15–40)
2. Tubular opacities, representing mucus-filled bronchi
3. Ring opacities or cystic spaces and sometimes containing air-fluid levels (Fig. 15–41), usually localized but rarely associated with destruction of an entire lung[286]

Table 15–5. BRONCHIECTASIS

Irreversible bronchial dilation
Chest radiograph manifestations
  Direct signs
    Parallel line opacities (tram tracks)
    Tubular opacities
    Ring opacities or cystic shadows
  Indirect signs
    Atelectasis
    Crowding of pulmonary vascular markings
    Oligemia
HRCT scan findings
  Bronchial lumen diameter greater than adjacent pulmonary artery
  Lack of bronchial tapering
  Visualization of bronchus within 1 cm of costal pleura
  Visualization of bronchus abutting mediastinal pleura
  Bronchial wall thickening

HRCT, high-resolution computed tomography.

Figure 15–40. Bronchiectasis with Tram Tracks. View of the right lower chest from posteroanterior radiograph in a 46-year-old man who had chronic productive cough shows parallel line opacities (tram tracks) *(arrows)* as a result of thickened, dilated bronchi. The diagnosis of bronchiectasis was confirmed on HRCT.

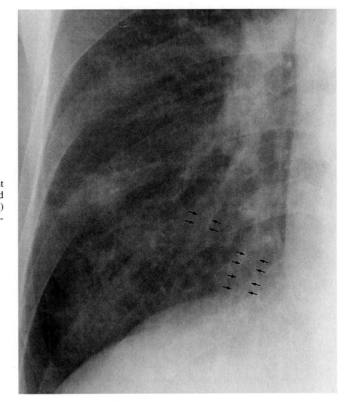

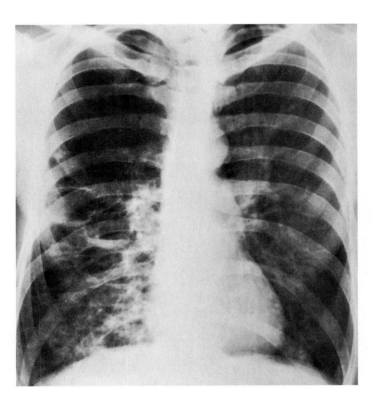

Figure 15–41. Cystic Bronchiectasis. Posteroanterior chest radiograph of a 38-year-old man shows extensive replacement of the right lower lobe by multiple thin-walled cysts, many of which contain air-fluid levels. The left lung is normal; the right upper lobe shows severe oligemia.

4. Increase in size and loss of definition of pulmonary markings in specific segmental areas of the lungs, a change that has been shown to be the result of peribronchial fibrosis and (to a lesser extent) retained secretions[282, 283]

5. Crowding of the pulmonary vascular markings, indicating the almost invariable loss of volume associated with the condition (Fig. 15–42); such atelectasis usually is caused by mucus obstruction of peripheral rather than central bronchi[282, 283]

6. Evidence of oligemia as a result of reduction in pulmonary artery perfusion, a finding usually noted in more severe disease

7. Signs of compensatory overinflation of the remainder of the lung (*see* Fig. 15–42)

Because of the greater prevalence of severe disease in the past, radiographs of patients who had bronchiectasis were usually abnormal and often allowed a confident diagnosis of the condition; in a review of 112 patients published in 1955, only 7% had normal chest radiographs.[283] As the result of a decrease in the number of patients who have severe disease (at least in developed countries) and the availability of HRCT to identify cases of relatively mild bronchiectasis, more recent studies have shown that the radiograph is often normal or shows nonspecific findings.[280, 287] The most illustrative findings in this regard are derived from a prospective study of 84 patients who were suspected of having bronchiectasis on the basis of clinical manifestations.[285] Thirty-seven patients had normal radiographs; on HRCT, 32 had normal findings and 5 (14%) had cylindrical bronchiectasis. Of the 47 patients who had abnormal radiographs, 36 (77%) had bronchiectasis at HRCT, and 11 (23%) had normal findings. The sensitivity of the chest radiograph in this study was 88% (41 of

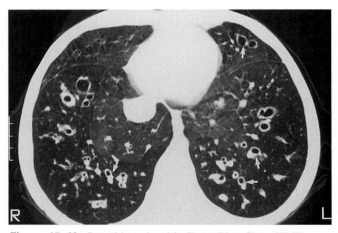

Figure 15–43. Bronchiectasis with Signet-Ring Sign. HRCT scan shows numerous bronchi with an internal diameter greater than that of the adjacent pulmonary artery (signet-ring sign) in the lower lobes and lingula *(arrows)*. The patient was a 15-year-old boy who had cystic fibrosis.

46 cases of bronchiectasis diagnosed by HRCT), and the specificity was 74%. There was a significant correlation between the severity of abnormalities seen on chest radiograph and the severity of bronchiectasis at HRCT ($r = 0.62$).

Computed Tomography

On the basis of the results of the previously mentioned study and other investigations, it generally is accepted that HRCT is the imaging modality of choice to establish the presence of bronchiectasis and to determine its extent. Characteristic findings include the following:[291, 292]

1. An internal bronchial diameter greater than that of the adjacent pulmonary artery (Fig. 15–43)

2. Lack of bronchial tapering, defined as a bronchus that has the same diameter as its parent branch for a distance of more than 2 cm (Fig. 15–44)

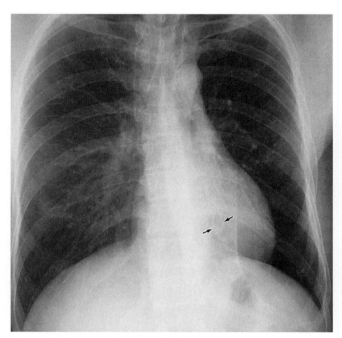

Figure 15–42. Bronchiectasis with Left Lower Lobe Atelectasis. Posteroanterior chest radiograph in a 27-year-old man shows left lower lobe atelectasis. Ectatic thick-walled bronchi *(arrows)* can be seen within the atelectatic lobe. Compensatory overinflation of the left upper lobe is apparent.

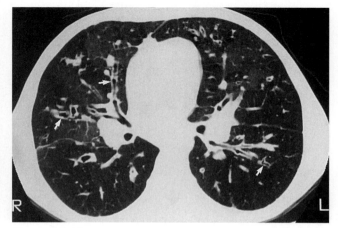

Figure 15–44. Bronchiectasis with Lack of Bronchial Tapering. HRCT scan shows lack of tapering *(arrows)* and thickening of the walls of bronchi in the right middle and left lower lobes. Ectatic bronchi are evident in cross-section (signet-ring sign). The patient was a 15-year-old boy who had cystic fibrosis.

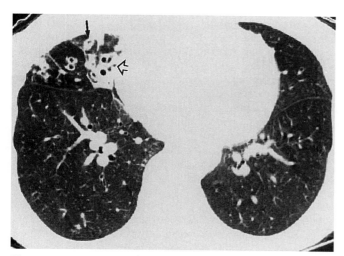

Figure 15–45. Bronchiectasis. HRCT scan in a 50-year-old woman who had bronchiectasis shows bronchi within 1 cm of the costal pleura *(straight arrow)* and abutting the mediastinal pleura *(open arrow)*. The bronchiectasis was presumed to be the result of previous tuberculosis.

3. Visualization of bronchi within 1 cm of the costal pleura (Fig. 15–45)

4. Visualization of bronchi abutting the mediastinal pleura (*see* Fig. 15–45)

5. Bronchial wall thickening (*see* Figs. 15–43 to 15–45)

The HRCT appearance of ectatic bronchi varies depending on the type of bronchiectasis and on the orientation of the airways relative to the plane of the scan. In cylindrical bronchiectasis, bronchi coursing horizontally are visualized as parallel lines (tram tracks) (*see* Fig. 15–44), whereas vertically oriented bronchi appear as circular lucencies larger than the diameter of the adjacent pulmonary artery, resulting in a signet-ring appearance (*see* Fig. 15–43).[292, 293] Varicose bronchiectasis is characterized by the presence of nonuniform bronchial dilation (Fig. 15–46),

whereas cystic bronchiectasis results in a cluster of thin-walled cystic spaces often containing air-fluid levels (Fig. 15–47). HRCT allows ready distinction of cylindrical from cystic bronchiectasis; however, distinction of varicose from cystic bronchiectasis often is difficult,[288] unless the affected bronchus courses in the same horizontal plane as the CT section. The size of the ectatic bronchi decreases on end-expiratory HRCT scans compared with end-inspiratory HRCT scans;[260] occasionally, they collapse completely because of their increased compliance.[281]

Several groups have assessed the accuracy of HRCT in the diagnosis of bronchiectasis.[288–291] In one study of 36 patients who had a characteristic clinical history or radiographic findings, bronchography was performed in 44 lungs and the results used as the gold standard;[288] the sensitivity of HRCT was 96% and the specificity 93%. Analysis of the results showed that HRCT and bronchography were normal in 15 patients and showed a similar presence and extent of bronchiectasis in 25. In two cases, bronchiectasis was seen better on HRCT than on bronchography; in one, bronchography showed cylindrical bronchiectasis when HRCT was normal, and in another, HRCT showed cylindrical bronchiectasis, whereas bronchography, in retrospect, had been misinterpreted as negative.[288]

In a second investigation of 259 segmental bronchi from 70 lobes of 27 lungs, HRCT was positive in 87 of 89 segmental bronchi shown to have bronchiectasis at bronchography (sensitivity, 98%) and negative in 169 of 170 segmental bronchi without bronchiectasis (specificity, 99%).[289] In a third investigation in which the results of preoperative HRCT scans were compared with the pathologic findings in 47 lobes from 22 patients who had undergone surgical resection, abnormalities were detected on HRCT in all lobes;[290] however, bronchiectasis was identified clearly on HRCT in only 41 of the 47 (87%). Three of the remaining six cases had extensive consolidation but no evidence of bronchial dilation on HRCT; in two cases, focal mucoid impaction was misinterpreted as a lung nodule, and in one case, focal cystic bronchiectasis containing a mycetoma was misinterpreted as a cavitating carcinoma.

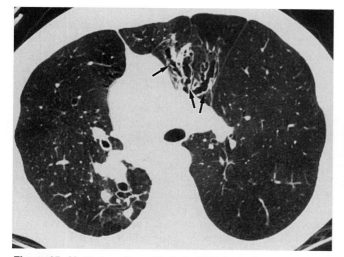

Figure 15–46. Varicose Bronchiectasis. HRCT scan shows ectatic bronchi that have an undulating wall *(arrows)* characteristic of varicose bronchiectasis. Bronchiectasis is evident in the right lung also. The patient was a 46-year-old man who had long-standing central bronchiectasis as a result of allergic bronchopulmonary aspergillosis.

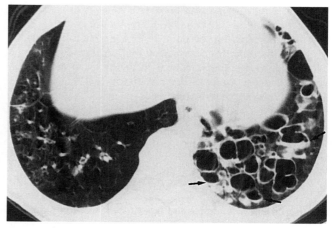

Figure 15–47. Cystic Bronchiectasis. HRCT scan shows thin-walled cystic spaces throughout the left lower lobe and lingula; several have air-fluid levels *(arrows)*. Mild bronchiectasis is present in the right lower lobe. The patient was a 32-year-old man who had bronchiectasis following childhood viral infection.

Although HRCT allows confident diagnosis of the presence and extent of bronchiectasis in most patients, as with most other diseases, it is not 100% sensitive and specific, and several limitations of the technique need to be recognized, as follows:[290, 291]

1. There is a normal variability in the bronchoarterial diameter ratio depending on the population being assessed, the altitude at which the examination is performed, and the window levels and window widths at which scans are photographed. In a study done in Denver (altitude 1,600 m), 16 of 27 (59%) normal individuals had at least one bronchus with an internal diameter greater than that of the adjacent pulmonary artery.[156] In a subsequent investigation, bronchoarterial diameter ratios at altitude were found to be significantly greater than those at sea level, presumably as a result of hypoxic vasoconstriction.[168] In this study, 9 of 17 (57%) normal individuals living at altitude and only 2 of 16 (12%) individuals living at sea level had at least one bronchus that had an internal diameter equal to or greater than that of the adjacent pulmonary artery on HRCT images photographed at a window level of −450 HU. At a window level of −700 HU, only 2 of 17 (12%) normal individuals living at altitude and none of those living at sea level had bronchoarterial ratios equal to or greater than 1. These results show the important influence of the HRCT window level in the assessment of bronchial and arterial diameters and the diagnosis of bronchiectasis.

The analysis in the last-named study was based on careful measurement of the diameters of the bronchi and pulmonary artery using a Vernier caliper. The authors pointed out that subjective visual assessment tends to overestimate the internal diameter of the bronchus relative to that of the pulmonary artery.[168] In a study performed at sea level and based on subjective assessment, bronchoarterial diameter ratios greater than 1 were identified in 21% of 26 normal individuals and in 95% of 59 patients who had bronchiectasis.[291] In this and other[156] studies, no normal individual had a bronchoarterial diameter ratio equal to or greater than 1.5. A bronchoarterial diameter ratio can be considered a reliable sign of bronchiectasis by itself only when it is at least 1.5; when it is greater than 1 and less than 1.5, it must be present in several airways or associated with other findings, such as bronchial wall thickening, lack of bronchial tapering, or both.[156, 291] Care should be taken to assess the smallest cross-sectional airway diameter to avoid making comparisons near bifurcations of bronchi or vessels (because the two may not divide at the same level) and not to overcall bronchiectasis in areas that have decreased vessel size as a result of local vasoconstriction. Because of the difficulty in appreciating the presence of bronchial or vascular bifurcation, the diagnosis of cylindrical bronchiectasis should be made only when bronchial dilation is seen on more than one CT level.

2. Visualization of peripheral bronchi is more specific in the diagnosis of bronchiectasis than increased bronchoarterial diameter ratios but has a slightly lower sensitivity. In one study of 26 normal individuals, none had bronchi visualized within 1 cm of the costal pleura or abutting the mediastinal pleura.[291] Of 49 patients who had bronchiectasis, bronchi were visualized within 1 cm of the costal pleura in 81% and abutting the mediastinal pleura in 53%.

3. Bronchial wall thickening on HRCT is fairly common in bronchiectasis; in one investigation of 47 lobes in which there was surgically proven disease, it was considered to be present in 32 (68%).[290] The abnormality is a nonspecific finding, however, that may be seen in other conditions, particularly asthma,[158] and in asymptomatic smokers.[192] Although measurements of normal bronchial wall thickness have been published, in clinical practice the analysis is based on subjective assessment.[288, 290, 292] Such estimates are influenced by the window level and width at which the HRCT images are photographed.[160, 161] Optimal assessment is obtained using a window level of −700 HU and a width of 1,000 HU; higher window levels are too dark and other window widths, particularly widths less than 1,000 HU, lead to substantial artifactual wall thickening.[161]

4. Bronchi that course obliquely, such as the segmental bronchi of the middle lobe and lingula, are not visualized optimally on routine cross-sectional CT images. Visualization of these bronchi can be optimized by using oblique HRCT scans obtained by angling the CT gantry 20 degrees cranially.[294]

5. Bronchi filled with secretions are visualized as tubular or branching structures when they course horizontally or as nodules when they are oriented perpendicular to the plane of section (Fig. 15–48). These structures usually can be recognized by careful analysis of adjacent HRCT sections. Mucoceles may be confused with a pulmonary tumor, however.[290]

6. In patients who have parenchymal consolidation or atelectasis, ectatic bronchi filled with secretions or blood may not be apparent on HRCT.[290] More commonly, bronchi are air filled and dilated because of a local increase in lung elastic recoil. This reversible bronchial dilation is particularly frequent in the resolving phase of acute pneumonia.[295, 296] With complete resolution of the pneumonia, the dilation disappears gradually, although it may take 3 to 4 months before the normal dimensions of the bronchial tree can be appreciated. An interval of 3 to 6 months should be allowed to elapse after an episode of pneumonia before a definitive diagnosis of bronchiectasis is made on HRCT.

7. Cardiac and respiratory motion may lead to suboptimal bronchial visualization; the resultant image artefacts can obscure the features of bronchiectasis or may result in changes that mimic bronchiectasis.[297] Such motion artefacts can be minimized by using short scan times (≤1 second).

As a result of these considerations, the recommended HRCT technique for the assessment of the potential of bronchiectasis consists of 1- to 2-mm collimation scans at 10-mm intervals through the chest photographed using a window level of −700 HU and a window width of 1,000 HU. It has been suggested that improved visualization may be obtained by using thin-section spiral CT. In one investigation of 50 consecutive patients who had clinical symptoms suggestive of bronchiectasis, HRCT was performed at 10-mm intervals, and spiral CT was carried out using 3-mm collimation volumetric scanning during a 24-second breath-hold.[298] Bronchiectasis was noted in 22 patients on HRCT compared with 26 on spiral CT (including all patients in whom it was identified on HRCT). HRCT showed evidence of bronchiectasis in 77 segments, whereas

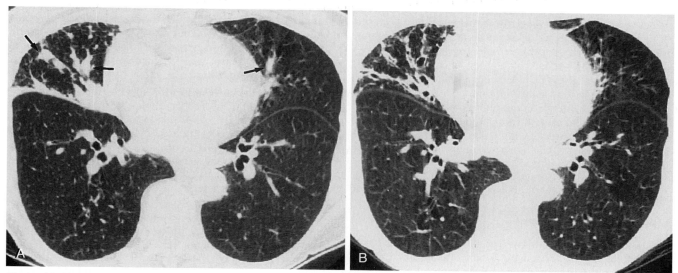

Figure 15–48. Mucus-Filled Bronchi. HRCT scan *(A)* shows tubular and nodular *(arrows)* opacities in the right middle lobe and lingula. HRCT scan performed after expectoration of the mucus *(B)* shows that the opacities represented ectatic bronchi filled with secretions. The patient was an 80-year-old woman who had bronchiectasis as a result of previous tuberculosis.

spiral CT documented it in 90. The radiation dose delivered using spiral CT was 3.5 times greater, however, than that delivered using HRCT. On the basis of these observations, the authors recommended that spiral CT be used in patients in whom there is high clinical suspicion of bronchiectasis and questionable findings on HRCT. Use of thicker sections (e.g., 4- to 5-mm collimation scans) results in a slight decrease in sensitivity compared with HRCT,[285, 299] whereas the use of 10-mm collimation scans decreases the sensitivity to about 60%.[300, 301]

There is a weak but significant correlation between the severity of morphologic abnormalities seen on HRCT and the functional impairment.[227] In one investigation of 261 patients who had symptomatic bronchiectasis, the severity and extent of bronchiectasis correlated with the reduction in FEV$_1$ ($r = -0.36$, $P < 0.001$) and forced vital capacity ($r = -0.36$, $P < 0.001$). Patients who had cystic bronchiectasis were shown to be more likely to grow *Pseudomonas* from sputum samples and to have purulent sputum than were patients who had cylindric or varicose bronchiectasis.[227]

Many other abnormalities are seen with increased frequency in patients who have bronchiectasis, including areas of decreased lung attenuation and perfusion, tracheomegaly, and mediastinal lymph node enlargement. In one investigation of 70 patients who had chronic purulent sputum production and in whom HRCT scans were obtained at full inspiration and at end-expiration, bronchiectasis was identified in approximately 52% of lobes.[302] Areas of decreased attenuation were identified on HRCT performed at end-inspiration in 20% of lobes and on expiratory scans in 34%. These areas were more prevalent in lobes that had bronchiectasis, and their extent correlated with the extent and severity of bronchiectasis; specifically, they were most prevalent in lobes that had extensive or widespread cystic bronchiectasis. Areas of decreased attenuation were seen in lobes without overt bronchiectasis. Multiple regression analysis showed that the extent of areas that had decreased

attenuation was related inversely to the FEV$_1$ ($r = -0.57$) and FEV$_1$/forced vital capacity ($r = -0.49$) and correlated positively with the residual volume ($r = 0.49$). The degree of attenuation was related independently and positively to the extent and severity of bronchiectasis but was unrelated to age, smoking history, clinical evidence of asthma, age at onset of sputum production, or presence of an underlying cause. In another investigation, in which HRCT scans were compared with the pathologic findings in 47 lobes that had been resected for complications of bronchiectasis, areas of decreased attenuation were identified in 21 of the lobes (45%);[304] these areas were seen only in patients who had bronchiolitis in association with bronchiectasis.

Lymph node enlargement is seen relatively commonly on CT in patients who have bronchiectasis, particularly when it is associated with cystic fibrosis. In one investigation, lymph node enlargement was detected in 12 of 42 (29%) patients who had bronchiectasis.[303] In a review of the radiographic findings in 48 adult patients who had cystic fibrosis, lymph node enlargement was found in 25 (52%), hilar enlargement in 22 (46%), and mediastinal enlargement in 21 (44%).[304] The lymphadenopathy was chronic and slowly progressive in all patients, and in no case did it resolve. Hypertrophied bronchial arteries result in tubular or nodular areas of soft tissue attenuation around the central airways and in the mediastinum;[305] their vascular nature can be recognized readily after intravenous administration of contrast material.

Bronchography

Bronchography was the radiologic gold standard for the demonstration of the presence and extent of bronchiectasis. Because of the risks of allergic reaction to the bronchographic medium—ranging from bronchospasm to iodism to anaphylaxis and death—and the temporary impairment of ventilation and gas exchange, the procedure has been replaced by HRCT. It has been suggested, however, that selective bronchography performed through the fiberoptic bronchoscope and using an iso-osmolar, nonionic contrast medium might be helpful in selected patients.[306, 307] (A dimeric contrast medium is required because monomeric nonionic agents at iso-osmolar concentrations do not provide sufficient iodine concentration.) This procedure appears to be well tolerated, although some patients develop headaches, nausea, and flushing.[308] The technique should be reserved for patients who have recurrent hemoptysis and in whom the HRCT scan result is normal or shows questionable abnormalities.[309]

Specific Causes

Dyskinetic Cilia Syndrome

Dyskinetic cilia syndrome (primary ciliary dyskinesia) is a disorder characterized by absent or, more commonly, uncoordinated and ineffective ciliary motion.[312] The syndrome results from ultrastructural abnormalities of the cilia. Individuals who have the full-blown syndrome have chronic sinusitis, otitis, recurrent bronchitis, bronchiectasis, sterility (in males), and corneal abnormalities. Approximately 50% have situs inversus.[312, 317] The combination of situs inversus, paranasal sinusitis, and bronchiectasis is known as Kartagener's syndrome.[310]

The incidence of dyskinetic cilia syndrome in whites is estimated to be between 1 in 12,500[313] to 40,000.[311] The proportion of cases of bronchiectasis that are attributed to dyskinetic cilia syndrome has been reported to be higher in North Africans (36%) than in Europeans (4%).[314] The mode of inheritance best fits with an autosomal recessive pattern.[315] The variety of ultrastructural defects associated with the syndrome suggests considerable genetic heterogeneity.[316]

The radiographic manifestations of dyskinetic cilia syndrome have been described in a study of 30 patients, 15 of each sex.[317] Ages ranged from newborn to 26 years. Radiographic abnormalities were evident in all patients, including bronchial wall thickening, hyperinflation, segmental atelectasis or consolidation, and segmental bronchiectasis. Except for the presence of situs inversus, the radiologic features are not specific and resemble those of bronchiectasis from a variety of other causes. Although the bronchiectasis can be widespread on HRCT, it involves predominantly or exclusively the lower lobes in approximately 50% of patients.[318]

Young's Syndrome

Young's syndrome (obstructive azoospermia) is characterized by infertility related to mechanical obstruction of the genital tract accompanied by sinusitis and bronchiectasis.[319, 320] This combination of abnormalities may suggest a diagnosis of cystic fibrosis or dyskinetic cilia syndrome.[321, 322]

Syndrome of Yellow Nails, Lymphedema, Pleural Effusion, and Bronchiectasis

Of 12 patients reported from the Mayo Clinic who had this syndrome, 8 had recurrent pleural effusion, and 5 had bronchiectasis;[324] in this series, the first manifestation of the syndrome was lymphedema or yellow nails, with pleural effusion appearing somewhat later in all cases. In two other series, bronchiectasis and yellow nails were reported as developing simultaneously in three patients aged 10, 18, and 20 years; lymphedema became manifest later in each patient.[324, 325]

Williams-Campbell Syndrome

Williams-Campbell syndrome is a congenital form of bronchiectasis in which the pathophysiologic mechanism is believed to be a deficiency in the amount of airway cartilage. HRCT findings are characteristic and consist of cystic bronchiectasis limited to the fourth-, fifth-, and sixth-generation bronchi (i.e., distal to the first-generation segmental bronchi).[326–328] Expiratory HRCT shows collapse of the bronchi and distal air-trapping.[326] This combination of findings is virtually diagnostic of the syndrome.[326] Affected individuals usually present in infancy with repeated chest infections and evidence of bronchiectasis; the clinical course may be one of rapid deterioration or prolonged survival.

Broncholithiasis

The term *broncholithiasis* is used to denote the presence of calcified or ossified material within the lumen of the tracheobronchial tree. It usually is caused by erosion and extrusion of calcified necrotic material from a bronchopulmonary lymph node into the bronchial lumen. The underlying cause usually is associated with long-standing foci of necrotizing granulomatous lymphadenitis; any organism leading to such inflammation, including *Mycobacterium tuberculosis*, *Histoplasma capsulatum*, *Coccidioides immitis*, and a variety of others,[329] theoretically can cause the complication. In North America, the most common agent probably is *H. capsulatum*, a feature most likely related to the high incidence of lymphadenitis in endemic areas.[331, 332] The typical clinical manifestation is hemoptysis.

The effects of broncholithiasis are variable and depend on the size and degree of calcification of the stone. Stones that contain relatively little calcium may disintegrate easily and be manifested by recurrent lithoptysis with or without hemoptysis. Stones that are heavily calcified or ossified are less likely to break up and can cause occlusion with distal bronchiectasis and obstructive pneumonitis.

Radiographic manifestations include change of position or disappearance of a calcific focus on serial radiographs or development of airway obstruction, resulting in lobar or segmental atelectasis, mucoid impaction, or expiratory air-trapping.[330–332] Although a specific diagnosis seldom can be made on plain chest radiograph, broncholiths usually can be identified readily on CT scan (Fig. 15–49).[333, 334]

Bronchial Fistulas

Bronchial fistulas can be established with many structures within the thorax and outside it. The principal underlying causes are infection and carcinoma; either may originate in the lung or in the organ with which the fistula is associated. Trauma, other noninfectious inflammatory

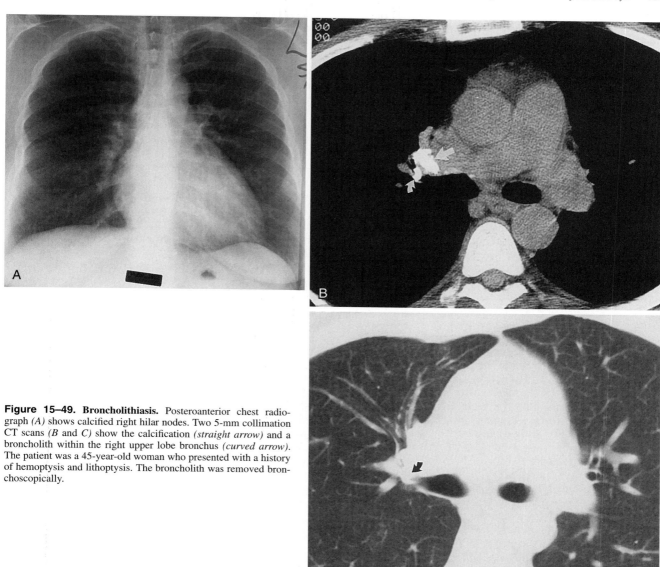

Figure 15–49. Broncholithiasis. Posteroanterior chest radiograph *(A)* shows calcified right hilar nodes. Two 5-mm collimation CT scans *(B* and *C)* show the calcification *(straight arrow)* and a broncholith within the right upper lobe bronchus *(curved arrow).* The patient was a 45-year-old woman who presented with a history of hemoptysis and lithoptysis. The broncholith was removed bronchoscopically.

processes, and foreign bodies (either aspirated or introduced for therapeutic or diagnostic purposes) are occasional causes.

The most common form probably is bronchopleural fistula, usually after lobectomy or pneumonectomy for pulmonary carcinoma.[335] Radiographic manifestations of this complication include an increase in the amount of gas in the pleural or pneumonectomy space, lack of normal shift of the mediastinum, or reappearance of gas in a previously fluid-filled hemithorax.[336–338] Peripheral airway bronchopleural fistulas can present radiographically as persistent pneumothorax, tension pneumothorax, or hydropneumothorax.[336, 337] CT often allows direct visualization and localization of the fistula as well as assessment of the underlying cause.[338, 339] In one investigation of 20 patients who had bronchopleural fistulas involving segmental bronchi or more distal airways, the fistula was identified on CT scan in 10.[339] Five of the 10 patients had acute bacterial

pneumonia with peripheral areas of necrosis or abscess formation that contained fluid and air bubbles that were shown on CT to communicate directly with the pleural space; 4 had ectatic peripheral airways that communicated with the pleural space. In the remaining patient, the communication was between peripheral air spaces within a bronchioloalveolar carcinoma and the pleural space.

HRCT is superior to conventional CT in the demonstration of bronchopleural fistulas.[338, 339] The optimal method consists of volumetric spiral CT imaging using an HRCT technique (1- to 2-mm collimation scans) through the areas of parenchymal abnormality. Three-dimensional reconstruction of the data allows display of the entire course of the fistula.[338, 340]

CYSTIC FIBROSIS

Cystic fibrosis is a hereditary disease of recessive transmission. The fundamental abnormality consists of the pro-

Table 15–6. CYSTIC FIBROSIS

Occurs in 1 per 2,000–3,500 whites
Uncommon in nonwhite population
Autosomal recessive transmission
Abnormal secretions of exocrine glands
Recurrent respiratory infections
Bronchiectasis
Predominantly upper lobe involvement
Hyperinflation
Pancreatic insufficiency
Elevated sweat chlorides >60 mEq/liter

duction of abnormal secretions from a variety of exocrine glands, including the salivary and sweat glands and glands of the pancreas, large bowel, and tracheobronchial tree. The disease is the most common lethal genetically transmitted disease among whites; the estimated incidence in this group is about 1 per 2,000 to 3,500 live births (Table 15–6).[343, 344] The disease is uncommon in nonwhites. Although cystic fibrosis most often is identified during infancy or childhood, many cases first are recognized in adolescents or adults;[345] in 80%, the diagnosis is made before the age of 5 years and in 10% during adolescence.[343, 346]

The major clinical manifestations are obstructive pulmonary disease, which is found in varying degrees of severity in almost all patients, and pancreatic insufficiency (present in 80% to 90%).[341, 342] Involvement of the lungs is manifested clinically principally by recurrent chest infections associated with wheezing, dyspnea, productive cough, and hemoptysis. Malnutrition and protein depletion are consequences of recurrent lung infection, which can accelerate the course of pulmonary disease.[376] Infection is caused predominantly by bacteria, although viruses, mycoplasma, and fungi occasionally are responsible. The most common organisms are *P. aeruginosa* of the mucoid and nonmucoid types, *S. aureus*, and *H. influenzae*; sputum culture shows good correlation with cultures obtained by quantitative culture of distal airway secretions.[377] The isolation of gram-negative bacilli other than *P. aeruginosa* from the tracheobronchial tree has increased;[348] the presence of *Burkholderia cepacia* in particular is associated with the terminal stages of the disease.

Although the diagnosis of cystic fibrosis may be suggested by family history, persistent respiratory disease, or clinical evidence of pancreatic insufficiency, confirmation requires a positive sweat test. Values for sodium and chloride concentrations in sweat increase with advancing age.[378] In children, a chloride concentration of 60 mEq/liter or higher indicates the presence of cystic fibrosis; a value of 50 mEq/liter requires a repeat test. Because healthy normal adults may have values greater than 60 mEq/liter, a diagnosis of cystic fibrosis should not be made at this level in the absence of an appropriate clinical history and unless repeated values of sodium and chloride are at or above this level.[342, 347] Genotyping is an alternative method of diagnosis; however, the large number of uncommon mutations that can lead to cystic fibrosis make it difficult to provide a routine screen that is comprehensive enough to rival the sensitivity of sweat testing.

Radiologic Manifestations

The earliest manifestations of cystic fibrosis on chest radiograph consist of round or poorly defined linear opacities measuring 3 to 5 mm in diameter and located within 2 to 3 cm of the pleura;[350, 351] thickened bronchial walls without bronchial dilation, mild hyperinflation, and hilar lymph node enlargement are seen less commonly.[350] The thickened bronchial walls usually are seen as ring shadows.[350]

Progression of disease is characterized by increases in bronchial diameter, bronchial wall thickness, lung volume, and number and size of peripheral nodular opacities and by the development of mucoid impaction and focal areas of consolidation (Fig. 15–50).[350] Bronchiectasis, bronchial wall thickening, and mucous plugging are particularly frequent and are evident on radiograph in 90% to 100% of adult patients.[350, 364, 465] Bronchiectasis—identified as parallel lines or as ring shadows larger than the accompanying pulmonary artery—usually is widespread on radiograph but tends to affect mainly the upper lobes.[350, 353] When filled with secretions or inspissated mucus, these bronchi are seen as nodular, finger-like, or branching, bandlike opacities.[354, 364] Cystic spaces are seen in about 25% to 30% of adult patients, particularly in the upper lobes, representing cystic bronchiectasis, bullae, or acute or healed abscesses.[349, 355, 356] Hyperinflation is seen in about 80% of adult patients and tends to involve mainly the lower lobes.[350]

Recurrent foci of consolidation occur in most patients, and lobar or segmental atelectasis occurs in about 50%.[350, 355] In one study of 50 patients in whom serial radiographs obtained during a 1- to 5-year or longer period were reviewed, lobar atelectasis was detected in 16 and segmental atelectasis in 12;[350] the former affected the right upper lobe in about 45% of cases, the left upper lobe in 35% of cases, and the right middle lobe in 20% of cases. Other radiographic manifestations include enlarged hila,[350] tracheal dilation,[357] pneumothorax, and pneumomediastinum.[355] Hilar enlargement may be due to lymph node enlargement, seen in 30% to 50% of adult patients,[304, 355] or dilation of the central pulmonary arteries secondary to pulmonary arterial hypertension.[355] Mediastinal lymph node enlargement is seen commonly on radiographs and CT scans.[304, 355] In one study of 48 adults, CT showed hilar lymphadenopathy in 46% and mediastinal lymphadenopathy in 44%; the latter most commonly involved the paratracheal, aortopulmonary window, and subcarinal regions.[304] Patients who had lymphadenopathy had more severe pulmonary involvement than patients who did not.[304]

Chest radiographic abnormalities have been incorporated into many semiquantitative clinical scoring schemes that are believed to be of value in predicting prognosis and directing therapy.[358] The Brasfield system is a 25-point score based on a 0 to 4 grading of air-trapping, linear markings, nodular cystic lesions, large lesions (atelectasis or consolidation), and general severity (an extra point is given for cardiomegaly or evidence of pulmonary hypertension). This system has been used extensively and shows good interobserver reproducibility and correlation with abnormalities of pulmonary function.[359, 360] In one review, 3,038 chest radiographs were obtained from 230 patients aged 3 days to 50 years and scored using the Brasfield system.[382] The scores from all the patients were plotted against age, and a single age-based severity curve was derived in which the mean scores, 95% confidence limits,

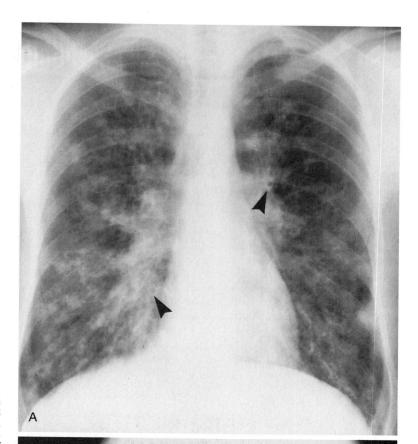

Figure 15–50. **Cystic Fibrosis.** Posteroanterior *(A)* and lateral *(B)* chest radiographs show diffuse bronchial wall thickening *(arrowheads)*; peribronchial thickening; diffuse, small, patchy opacities; and areas of inhomogeneous airspace consolidation. Note thickening of the posterior wall of the bronchus intermedius (IS). The lungs are moderately overinflated. Both hila are enlarged, almost certainly as a result of lymph node enlargement rather than pulmonary arterial hypertension. The patient was a 24-year-old man.

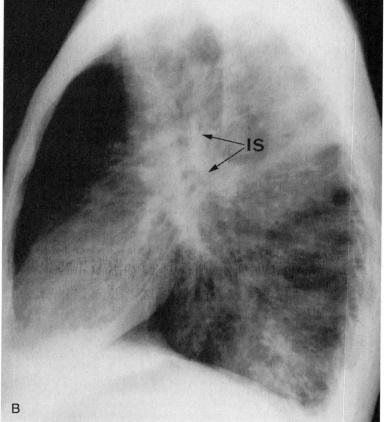

and percentiles could be appreciated. The rate in decline of Brasfield points was slightly less than 1% per year. Additional radiographic scoring systems include the National Institutes of Health chest radiographic score,[361] which has operating characteristics similar to the Brasfield system;[362] the Chrispin and Norman system;[363] and the Northern score,[364] which can be performed on posteroanterior radiograph.

As discussed earlier, HRCT has become the diagnostic method of choice for the detection of bronchiectasis; in patients who have cystic fibrosis, the added anatomic detail afforded by HRCT can be striking. HRCT is particularly useful for identifying early involvement of peripheral airways, manifested by small nodular opacities in the center of secondary lobules anatomically remote from areas affected by bronchiectasis (Fig. 15–51). This tree-in-bud pattern corresponds to branching bronchioles whose walls are thickened by fibrous tissue and inflammatory cells and whose lumens are filled with secretions.[365, 366] The other feature of small airway involvement in cystic fibrosis that can be appreciated using HRCT is a mosaic pattern of attenuation, with areas of decreased attenuation often in a lobular distribution (*see* Fig. 15–51). Correlation of HRCT and pathologic findings in three patients undergoing lung transplantation has shown that this pattern is caused by the presence of obliterative bronchiolitis.[290] The decreased attenuation is secondary to lobular hypoperfusion or gas-trapping. The presence of such gas-trapping is appreciated best on images obtained after expiration to residual volume.

HRCT is more sensitive than radiography in detecting mild disease in cystic fibrosis.[367, 368] In one study of 38 adult patients who had mild disease and were examined with both methods, mild bronchiectasis was detected in 23 of the patients by HRCT but in only 4 by radiography.[367] HRCT has been shown to reveal additional abnormalities not visible on conventional chest radiographs, particularly mucoid impaction.[369] A detailed scoring system for pulmonary abnormalities detected on HRCT has been proposed that involves a 0 to 2 or 0 to 3 score for the presence and extent of bronchiectasis, peribronchial thickening, mucous plugging, atelectasis or consolidation, and cystic or emphysematous changes.[370] It also is based on a 25-point system and can be interchanged with the Brasfield scoring method.

Patients who have cystic fibrosis may experience an

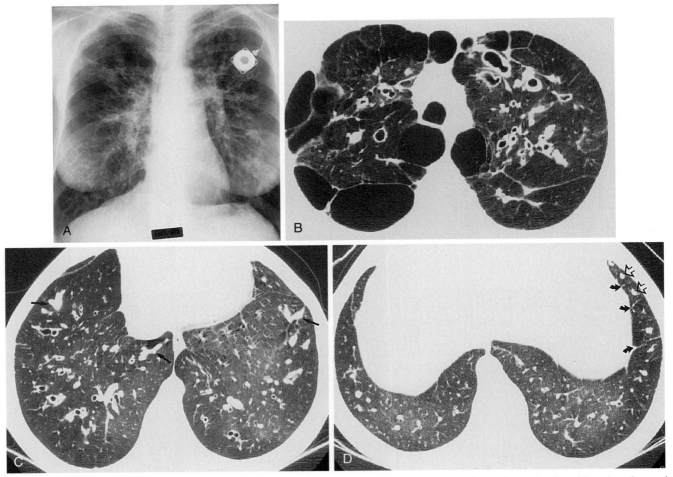

Figure 15–51. Cystic Fibrosis. Posteroanterior chest radiograph *(A)* in a 39-year-old woman shows evidence of extensive bronchiectasis and several large bullae, particularly in the right upper lobe. HRCT scan at the level of the upper lobes *(B)* shows bullae, more severe on the right, and widespread bronchiectasis. HRCT scan at the level of the lower lung zones *(C)* shows less severe bronchiectasis; branching opacities representing mucoid impaction *(straight arrows)*; and areas of decreased attenuation and vascularity, particularly in the dependent lung regions and in the medial segment of the right lower lobe. HRCT scan at a more caudad level *(D)* shows centrilobular nodular opacities *(open arrows)* measuring 3 to 5 mm in diameter and representing dilated, fluid-filled bronchioles. Decreased attenuation and vascularity within the secondary lobules demarcated by interlobular septa *(curved arrows)* also can be identified.

acute worsening of cough and sputum production without any change in the pattern or extent of parenchymal abnormalities on radiograph.[371] Similarly, there is usually no change in the pattern of findings on HRCT during an acute exacerbation, although the extent of abnormalities is increased.[372] In a prospective study of 19 adult patients who underwent HRCT after the onset of an exacerbation and who had follow-up HRCT after 2 weeks of hospitalization with treatment, the only finding limited to the time of the exacerbation was the presence of air-fluid levels in bronchiectatic cavities; however, this abnormality was seen in only 2 of the 19 patients.[372] Findings that improved with therapy included centrilobular nodules, mucous plugging, peribronchial thickening, and air-fluid levels; bronchiectasis and mosaic perfusion were not reversible.

The extent and severity of the airway abnormalities increase with age.[228] In one investigation of 117 patients who had cystic fibrosis, 45% between 0 and 5 years of age had bronchiectasis evident on HRCT compared with 80% 6 to 16 years of age and all patients 17 years and older.[237] The investigators noted an increase in severity and extent of bronchiectasis and mucous plugging with age.

Although the bronchiectasis in cystic fibrosis tends to be most severe in the upper lobes,[229, 234, 353] in most adult patients it is widespread;[234, 318] occasionally, it is limited to the upper or middle lobes[318] or is asymmetric in distribution. This predominant upper lobe distribution is distinct from that seen in patients who have impaired mucociliary clearance, hypogammaglobulinemia, and idiopathic bronchiectasis, which tends to have a lower lobe predominance.[318] By itself, distribution of bronchiectasis is of limited value in the differential diagnosis of the etiology in any individual patient.[229, 318] Based on a bilateral, predominantly upper lobe distribution of bronchiectasis on HRCT, the correct diagnosis of cystic fibrosis was suggested in adult patients only 50% of the time in one series[318] and in 68% of cases in a second study.[229] The differential diagnosis includes severe asthma, especially when complicated by allergic bronchopulmonary aspergillosis and mucous plugging, and other causes of diffuse bronchiectasis, such as the dyskinetic cilia syndromes and hypogammaglobulinemia.[318, 374]

In a study in which MR imaging and conventional radiographs were compared for the detection of thoracic abnormalities, the former proved superior in revealing hilar and mediastinal node enlargement and in distinguishing nodes from prominent hilar vessels.[375] Because of the superior spatial resolution of HRCT, however, MR imaging plays a limited, if any, role in the assessment of these patients.

BRONCHIOLITIS

Classification and Pathologic Characteristics

A variety of pulmonary diseases are characterized predominantly by inflammation of membranous and respiratory bronchioles. Such bronchiolitis can be classified in two ways: (1) according to its proven or presumed cause or the pulmonary or systemic diseases with which it is often associated and (2) according to its histologic features (Table 15–7).

Although an etiologic classification is useful for reminding the physician when to suspect the presence of bronchiolitis, in our opinion the more convenient scheme is based on the histologic characteristics for two important reasons: (1) The histologic patterns of bronchiolitis generally show a better correlation with the clinical and radiologic manifestations of disease than the various etiologies, and (2) the histologic classification shows better correlation with the natural history of disease and the response to therapy. For example, bronchiolitis obliterans organizing pneumonia (BOOP) or follicular bronchiolitis in rheumatoid disease can be expected to respond favorably to corticosteroid therapy, whereas obliterative bronchiolitis usually progresses inexorably to respiratory failure despite treatment.

The classification scheme presented in Table 15–7 is based on a consideration of two pathologic processes: inflammation and fibrosis. The first process is related simply to the traditional separation of inflammation into acute and chronic forms. The acute form typically is associated with processes that cause bronchiolar injury during a short period, such as viral or mycoplasmal infection or the inhalation of toxic gases (Fig. 15–52). The chronic form typically is associated with more prolonged injury and may itself have a variety of pathologic forms. Some of these variants

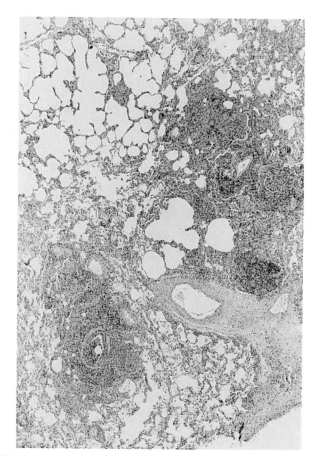

Figure 15–52. Acute Bronchiolitis: *Mycoplasma pneumoniae.* Section from an open-lung biopsy of a 32-year-old man shows several foci of inflammation centered on membranous bronchioles. Neutrophilic and lymphocytic components were evident at higher magnification.

Table 15–7. BRONCHIOLITIS: PATHOLOGIC CLASSIFICATION WITH CORRESPONDING CLINICAL, HISTOLOGIC, AND RADIOLOGIC FEATURES

Forms of Bronchiolitis	Histologic Characteristics	Clinical Features	Radiographic Features	HRCT Features
Acute bronchiolitis	Predominantly acute inflammation associated with a variable degree of inflammation in the adjacent lung parenchyma	Characteristic of infection (particularly viruses and *Mycoplasma pneumoniae*). Also seen as an early reaction after inhalation of toxic fumes or gases	Reticulonodular opacities	Centrilobular nodules and branching lines; patchy or diffuse distribution
Chronic bronchiolitis	Chronic inflammation and fibrosis. Several relatively specific clinicopathologic variants can be seen	This pattern is the major pathologic finding in the membranous bronchioles of cigarette smokers. It also can be seen after chronic irritation of the airways caused by a variety of inhaled substances (e.g., grain dust and some minerals) and in bronchiectasis and hypersensitivity pneumonitis	Reticulonodular opacities	Centrilobular nodules
Respiratory bronchiolitis	Accumulation of macrophages within membranous and respiratory bronchioles accompanied by a variable degree of lymphocyte infiltration and fibrosis in the bronchiolar wall and peribronchiolar interstitium	This is the earliest lesion seen in cigarette smokers. Patients usually are young and asymptomatic. When dyspnea is associated with radiographic abnormalities and restrictive lung function, the abnormality has been termed *respiratory bronchiolitis–associated interstitial pneumonia*	Ground-glass opacities	Ground-glass attenuation and poorly defined centrilobular nodular opacities; upper lobe predominance
Follicular bronchiolitis	Abundant lymphoid tissue, frequently with prominent germinal centers, situated in the walls of bronchioles and, to some extent, bronchi	Most often described in association with rheumatoid arthritis but may be seen in immunodeficiency syndromes and hypersensitivity reactions	Reticulonodular opacities	Centrilobular nodules and branching lines
Diffuse panbronchiolitis	Mural and intraluminal infiltrates of acute and chronic inflammatory cells. The lesions are centered predominantly on respiratory bronchioles and are associated with a striking accumulation of foamy macrophages within the airway wall and adjacent parenchyma	Typically seen in patients from Japan and Southeast Asia	Reticulonodular opacities	Centrilobular nodules and branching lines; bronchiolectasis, bronchiectasis, diffuse distribution
Obliterative bronchiolitis	Fibrous tissue predominantly between the muscularis mucosa and epithelium of membranous bronchioles resulting in more or less concentric airway narrowing	Characteristically seen in bone marrow and lung transplant recipients and in some connective tissue diseases (particularly rheumatoid disease)	Hyperinflation and peripheral areas of vascular attenuation	Low attenuation and mosaic perfusion; air-trapping on expiratory HRCT scan
Bronchiolitis obliterans organizing pneumonia	Focal necrosis of the respiratory bronchiolar and alveolar duct epithelium associated with partial or complete air-space occlusion by fibroblast proliferation. Mild to moderate interstitial pneumonitis and air-space fibrosis in adjacent parenchyma	The lesion is most often of unknown etiology but may occur in association with many causes, including connective tissue diseases, viral and bacterial pneumonia, drugs, aspiration, and airway obstruction	Patchy, usually bilateral air-space consolidation	Multifocal consolidation, often predominantly peribronchial or subpleural; ground-glass opacities

HRCT, high-resolution computed tomography.

are histologically distinctive and have been described by specific terms, such as *respiratory bronchiolitis, follicular bronchiolitis,* and *diffuse panbronchiolitis.* The histologic diagnosis of these conditions depends on the availability of tissue; however, the clinical and radiologic features associated with specific histologic patterns often are sufficiently characteristic to permit a strong presumptive diagnosis.

Although there is some degree of overlap between the acute and chronic forms of bronchiolitis, bronchiolitis can be subdivided histologically into two forms on the basis of the pattern of fibrosis. The first form, which we prefer to call *obliterative bronchiolitis* but which also has been termed *constrictive bronchiolitis,* is characterized by a proliferation of fibrous tissue predominantly between the epithelium and the muscularis mucosa; the proliferation results in a more or less concentric narrowing of the airway lumen, which in its most extreme form results in complete obliteration (Fig. 15–53). Although fibrous tissue can be seen in the submucosal and peribronchial tissue, it is typically a relatively minor factor in causing airway narrowing.[394] The epithelium overlying the abnormal fibrous tissue may be flattened or metaplastic but usually is intact (i.e., without evidence of ulceration). In cases of the second form of bronchiolitis, the epithelium is invariably absent, at least focally. Granulation tissue or plugs of fibroblastic tissue extend from these areas of epithelial damage into the airway lumen, resulting in partial or, occasionally, complete obstruction. Although this histologic pattern may be the only abnormality seen in the lung, in most cases it is associated with a similar epithelial injury and fibroblastic reaction in the adjacent parenchyma. For practical purposes, the bronchiolitis occurs in association with pneumonitis; as a result, BOOP frequently is used to describe this form of disease (Fig. 15–54).[380, 381] (Although we and others believe the term *cryptogenic organizing pneumonia* is a more appropriate label for the abnormality,[382–384] because of the widespread use of the former terms we continue to use it in this text.)

Radiologic Manifestations

The radiographic features of bronchiolitis are highly variable and are related to many factors, including the extent of airway involvement, the chronicity of the disorder, and the presence or absence of underlying parenchymal disease. The abnormalities essentially are limited to two patterns: hyperinflation and peripheral attenuation of vascular markings (Fig. 15–55), associated with obliterative bronchiolitis, and air-space consolidation in BOOP (Fig. 15–56).[381, 385, 386]

The degree of reproducibility in the radiographic detection of hyperinflation, peribronchial wall thickening, perihilar linear opacities, atelectasis, and consolidation was compared in one study of 40 patients who had bronchiolitis. There was considerable interobserver and intraobserver variability in interpretation; the finding of hyperinflation was the most reproducible.[387] The interpretation is influenced strongly by the clinical information provided to the radiologist; if bronchiolitis is mentioned on the requisition, features of bronchiolitis are reported even on radiographs that are normal.[388] In another study, there was no correlation between the clinical severity of the bronchiolitis and the degree of radiologic change.[389]

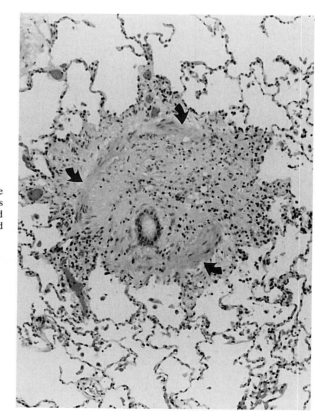

Figure 15–53. Obliterative Bronchiolitis. Section of membranous bronchiole shows marked narrowing of the airway lumen by fibrous tissue that more or less completely surrounds intact epithelium (residual muscularis mucosa is indicated by *arrows*). The patient had long-standing rheumatoid disease and had developed progressive dyspnea associated with obstructive lung function.

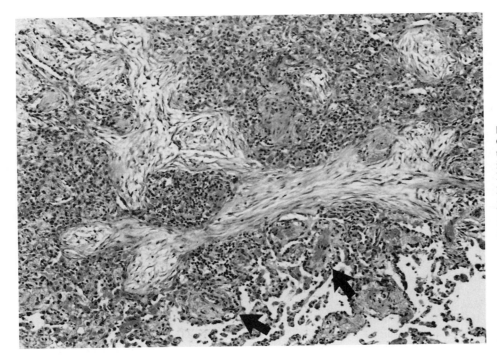

Figure 15–54. Bronchiolitis Obliterans Organizing Pneumonia. Histologic section of lung parenchyma shows chronic inflammation (organizing pneumonia). Branching of connective tissue plugs implies that they are present in the lumens of alveolar ducts and respiratory bronchioles. The interstitial nature of the chronic inflammatory infiltrate is apparent at the junction with normal lung *(arrows).* (×100.)

The anatomic detail that can be revealed using HRCT allows an appreciation of greater radiologic variability; many radiologic and pathologic correlative studies have shown that HRCT can suggest the predominant histologic pattern of bronchiolitis.[390–392] Because of this ability, HRCT is the radiologic method of choice for investigating a patient suspected on clinical or radiographic grounds of having bronchiolitis.

The bronchioles are located near the center of the secondary lobules (Fig. 15–57). Thickening of the bronchiolar wall or filling of bronchioles with granulation tissue, mucus, or pus results in a pattern of small centrilobular nodules and branching lines (tree-in-bud appearance, Fig. 15–58). These abnormalities represent enlarged bronchioles coursing perpendicular and parallel to the CT plane of section. This pattern is characteristic of acute infectious bronchiolitis; in some cases, it is accompanied by scattered areas of ground-glass attenuation or consolidation (Fig. 15–59).[391] A similar CT appearance can be seen in immunocompromised patients who develop acute *Aspergillus* bronchiolitis (Fig. 15–60)[393] or endobronchial spread of tuberculosis.[394] A pattern of centrilobular nodules and branching lines (tree-in-bud) is seen in diffuse panbronchiolitis.[395–397] Small centrilobular nodules reflecting bronchiolar inflammation and wall thickening sometimes can be seen in patients who have diseases that affect the larger airways, such as asthma, COPD, and bronchiectasis.[290, 431] The centrilobular nodules in infectious bronchiolitis and panbronchiolitis usually have well-defined, sharp margins,[391, 396, 398] whereas nodules seen in patients who have respiratory bronchiolitis typically have poorly defined margins (Fig. 15–61).[391, 399]

Narrowing of the bronchiolar lumen, as seen in obliterative (constrictive) bronchiolitis, results in decreased ventilation and reflex vasoconstriction (i.e., areas of decreased attenuation and vascularity). Redistribution of blood flow to uninvolved lung results in a heterogeneous pattern of attenuation (mosaic attenuation) (Fig. 15–62).[400–402] The variation in attenuation of individual lobules is accentuated when images are obtained after the patient exhales to residual volume[402–404] (Fig. 15–63).

Small, focal areas of low attenuation as well as small areas of air-trapping can be seen in healthy subjects.[158, 401, 405] Although these areas can affect one or several lobules at various sites, they most commonly are seen in the superior segments of the lower lobes and near the tip of the lingula. Usually, areas of low attenuation involve less than 25% of the cross-sectional area of one lung at one scan level.[405] Mosaic attenuation and air-trapping can be considered abnormal when they affect a volume of lung equal to or greater than a pulmonary segment and are not limited to the superior segment of the lower lobe or the lingula tip.[158, 401] Mosaic attenuation and air-trapping are seen on HRCT in patients who have obliterative bronchiolitis regardless of etiology,[391, 401, 406] hypersensitivity pneumonitis,[407, 408] asthma,[158, 409] and bronchiectasis.[290, 313] Similar findings occasionally are seen in patients who have pulmonary vascular abnormalities, particularly hypertension secondary to chronic thromboembolism.[410]

Unilateral or bilateral areas of consolidation are characteristic of BOOP (Fig. 15–64). The consolidation often is patchy; although it may have a random distribution, in about 50% of cases it affects mainly the peribronchial or subpleural lung regions.[411, 412] The consolidation reflects the presence of organizing pneumonia. Centrilobular nodular opacities may reflect the presence of intrabronchiolar granulation tissue polyps or peribronchiolar consolidation. Focal areas of consolidation can be seen in association with centrilobular nodular and branching linear opacities in infectious bronchiolitis and bronchopneumonia.[391, 393]

Ground-glass attenuation can be seen in association with respiratory bronchiolitis,[391, 399] respiratory bronchiolitis with

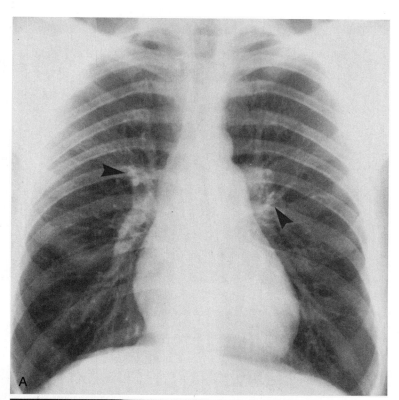

Figure 15–55. Obliterative Bronchiolitis of Unknown Etiology. Posteroanterior *(A)* and lateral *(B)* chest radiographs show pulmonary overinflation. The vasculature in the lower lung zones appears attenuated and in the upper lung zones more prominent than normal, indicating recruitment. When these changes are considered in conjunction with prominence of the main pulmonary artery and probable right ventricular enlargement, the findings are consistent with pulmonary arterial hypertension. Bronchial walls are thickened *(arrowheads).* Histologic examination of the lungs at autopsy showed typical changes of obliterative bronchiolitis and pulmonary artery hypertension. The patient was a young man who presented with progressive dyspnea and right-sided heart failure.

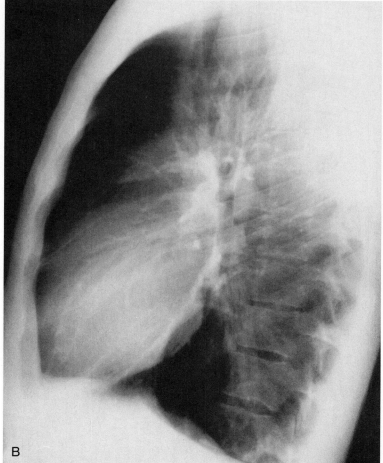

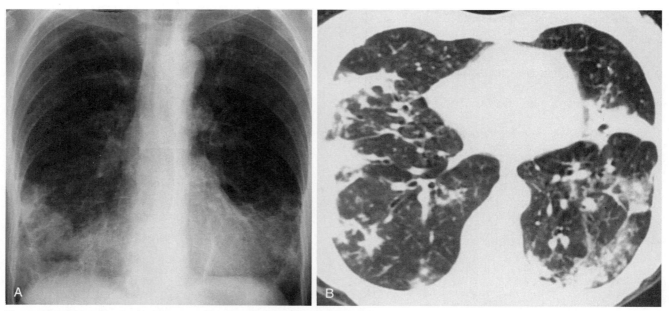

Figure 15–56. Bronchiolitis Obliterans Organizing Pneumonia. Posteroanterior chest radiograph *(A)* in a 64-year-old woman shows bilateral areas of consolidation involving the lower lung zones. CT scan *(B)* shows the predominantly peribronchial and subpleural distribution of the areas of consolidation. The diagnosis of idiopathic bronchiolitis obliterans organizing pneumonia was confirmed by open-lung biopsy.

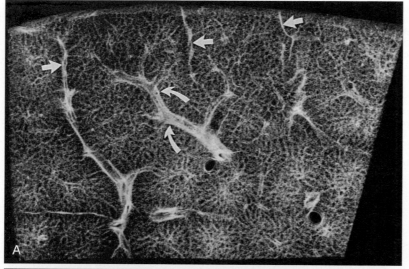

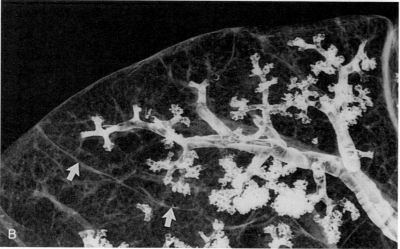

Figure 15–57. Anatomy of the Bronchioles and Secondary Pulmonary Lobules. Radiograph of a 1-mm-thick lung slice *(A)* shows interlobular septa *(straight arrows)* marginating the secondary pulmonary lobules. The lobular and terminal bronchioles *(curved arrows)* and adjacent pulmonary arteries can be seen to course near the center of the pulmonary lobule. Radiograph of specimen with bronchioles filled with barium *(B)* shows the pattern of centrilobular branching lines and nodular opacities that can be expected from bronchiolar and peribronchiolar inflammation. The bronchioles and alveolar ducts are located a few millimeters away from the pleural surface and interlobular septa *(arrows)*. (Courtesy of Dr. Harumi Itoh, Department of Radiology, Fukui Medical University, Fukui, Japan.)

interstitial lung disease,[390, 413] and BOOP.[411, 412] In respiratory bronchiolitis, the abnormality is bilateral, may be diffuse or patchy in distribution, and tends to involve predominantly or exclusively the upper lung zones.[230, 391] Ground-glass attenuation often is seen in association with areas of consolidation in BOOP.[411, 412, 414] Occasionally, particularly in immunocompromised patients who have BOOP, ground-glass attenuation is the only abnormality.[412] Hypersensitivity pneumonitis is characterized on HRCT by the presence of poorly defined centrilobular opacities and extensive bilateral areas of ground-glass attenuation. Localized areas of low attenuation have been observed in 50% to 70% of patients.[407, 408] These areas have been confirmed to represent air-trapping on expiratory CT scan[408] and to correlate with an increase in residual volume and residual volume–to–total lung capacity ratio;[407] they are presumed to be secondary to bronchiolitis.[407]

Specific Clinicopathologic Forms of Bronchiolitis

Acute bronchiolitis characteristically is the result of infection by organisms such as viruses, *Mycoplasma pneumoniae*, and *Chlamydia* species. These diseases are discussed in Chapter 5. A variety of inorganic and organic agents can cause inhalational lung injury; bronchiolitis may

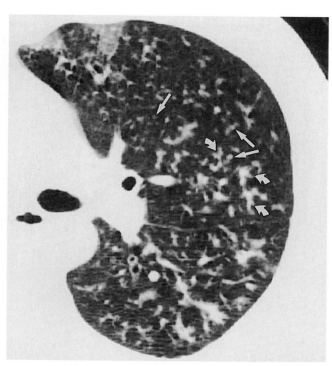

Figure 15–59. Bronchiolitis Related to *Mycoplasma pneumoniae*. View of the left upper lung from HRCT scan shows small centrilobular nodules *(straight arrows)* and branching linear opacities *(curved arrows)* (tree-in-bud pattern). Localized areas of ground-glass attenuation are evident anteriorly. These areas have a lobular distribution characteristic of bronchopneumonia. Open-lung biopsy showed an exquisitely bronchiolocentric process, with inflammation of the bronchiolar wall and the presence of intraluminal exudate. Serologic tests were positive for *M. pneumoniae*. (From Müller NL, Miller RR: Radiology 196:3, 1995.)

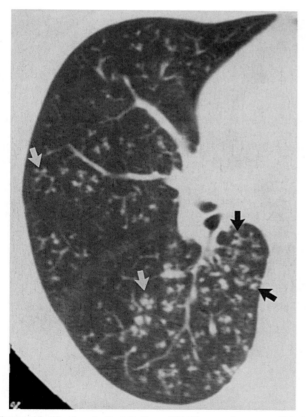

Figure 15–58. Tree-in-Bud Pattern. HRCT scan shows centrilobular branching linear and nodular opacities *(arrows)*, giving an appearance resembling a *tree in bud*. This pattern is seen most commonly in bronchiolitis resulting from infection and in endobronchial spread of tuberculosis. The diagnosis was proved to be endobronchial tuberculosis. (Case courtesy of Dr. Jim Barrie, Department of Radiology, University of Alberta Medical Centre, Edmonton, Alberta.)

be the major manifestation or a minor component of such injury.[415] Acute exposure to smoke,[416] sulfur dioxide, the oxides of nitrogen, and a variety of other gases and fumes can cause bronchiolitis that is associated with severe airflow obstruction. These entities are discussed in Chapter 16. The various forms of bronchiolitis associated with connective tissue disease are discussed in Chapter 8. Obliterative bronchiolitis is an important complication of bone marrow, lung, and heart-lung transplantation (*see* Chapter 11).

Swyer-James Syndrome

Swyer-James syndrome is an uncommon abnormality characterized radiographically by a hyperlucent lobe or lung and functionally by normal or reduced volume during inspiration and air-trapping during expiration.[417] The condition also has been termed *Macleod's syndrome*,[418] *unilateral* or *lobar emphysema*, and *unilateral hyperlucent lung*. As some of these terms suggest, the abnormality has been considered by some to represent a variant of emphysema. However, the hyperlucency of the affected lung or lobe is primarily the result of decreased pulmonary blood volume secondary to bronchiolar obliteration, rather than of destruction of pulmonary parenchyma; as a result, we prefer to include a discussion of the syndrome in a chapter on bronchiolitis.

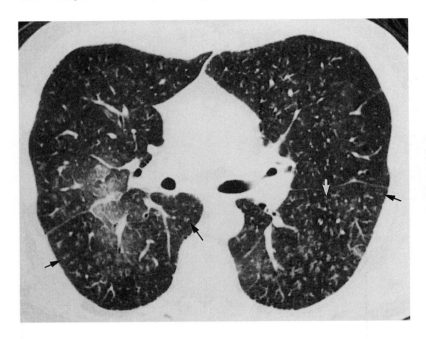

Figure 15–60. Bronchiolitis Related to *Aspergillus* Species. HRCT scan shows bilateral centrilobular nodular and branching opacities *(arrows)*. Focal area of ground-glass attenuation is visible in the right lung. The diagnoses of *Aspergillus* bronchiolitis and early bronchopneumonia were confirmed by open-lung biopsy. The patient was a 52-year-old man who had leukemia.

Use of the terms *unilateral emphysema* and *unilateral hyperlucent lung* has directed attention to a single radiographic feature of a disease that has a variety of modes of expression. The condition may occur in various anatomic distributions, including one segment,[419] one lobe, two lobes in the right lung, and the lower lobe of one lung and the upper lobe of the other. Other disease entities, such as proximal interruption of a pulmonary artery and massive thromboembolism, can cause unilateral hyperlucency and decreased lung volume;[420] however, in contrast to Swyer-James syndrome, these conditions are not associated with air-trapping.

There is substantial evidence that the syndrome is initiated by viral bronchiolitis. In many cases, the disease is recognized (or at least suspected) in childhood when chest radiography is carried out in the investigation of repeated respiratory infections. In others, the condition does not become apparent until adulthood on the basis of a screening chest radiograph of a completely asymptomatic patient. Inquiry into these cases often reveals a history of acute lower respiratory tract infection, generally during childhood.[421, 422] For example, a baseline normal chest radiograph was obtained in a child shortly before the development of an adenoviral pneumonia; after resolution of the pneumonia, the affected lung was hyperlucent, and on subsequent follow-up, it was of reduced volume and exhibited air-trapping and bronchographic evidence of bronchiectasis.[424] In another report, six children who developed the syndrome had definite or highly suggestive evidence of previous adenoviral pneumonia.[425]

The clinical presentation is highly variable. Some patients have no symptoms,[423] and some complain of dyspnea on exertion;[435] others present with a history of repeated lower respiratory tract infections.[417]

Radiologic Manifestations

The radiographic manifestations usually are recognized easily and are virtually pathognomonic. A posteroanterior radiograph of the chest exposed at TLC shows a remarkable difference in the radiolucency of the two lungs (or of the affected and unaffected lobes), caused not by a relative increase in air in the affected lung but by decreased perfu-

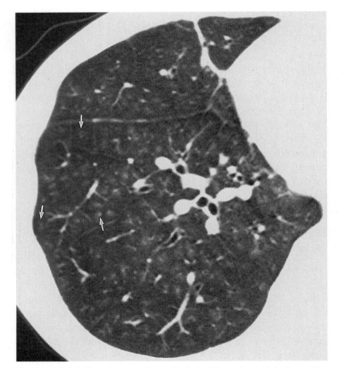

Figure 15–61. Respiratory Bronchiolitis. View of the right lower lung from HRCT scan shows poorly defined centrilobular nodular opacities *(arrows)* and localized areas of ground-glass attenuation. The diagnosis of respiratory bronchiolitis was confirmed by transbronchial biopsy. The patient was a 54-year-old heavy smoker who subsequently stopped the habit; follow-up CT scan performed 5 years later was normal. (Courtesy of Dr. Takeshi Johkoh, Osaka University Medical School, Osaka, Japan.)

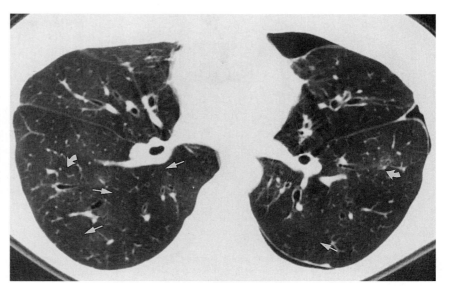

Figure 15–62. Obliterative Bronchiolitis. HRCT scan shows localized areas of decreased attenuation *(straight arrows)* and areas of slightly increased attenuation *(curved arrows)*, a pattern known as *mosaic attenuation*. Note the greater number and size of vessels within the areas that have increased attenuation. The patient was a 29-year-old woman who developed bronchiolitis as a result of chronic graft-versus-host disease. A small left pneumothorax also is noticeable.

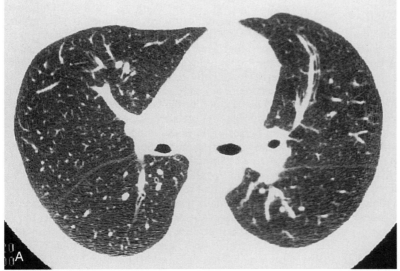

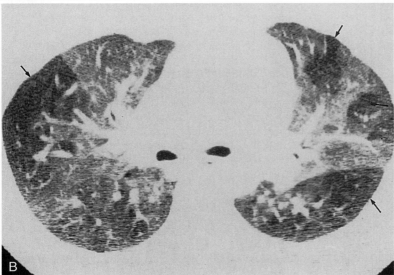

Figure 15–63. Obliterative Bronchiolitis: Value of Expiratory HRCT. A 32-year-old woman presented with progressive shortness of breath and airway obstruction 1 year after bone marrow transplantation. Inspiratory HRCT scan *(A)* shows questionable localized areas of low attenuation. HRCT scan performed at end-expiration *(B)* shows several areas of air-trapping *(arrows)*. These areas can be distinguished readily from the normal increased attenuation seen at end-expiration in the normal lung. (From Worthy SL, Müller NL: Radiol Clin North Am 36:163, 1998.)

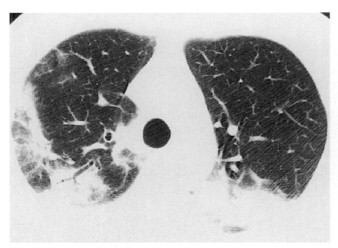

Figure 15–64. Bronchiolitis Obliterans Organizing Pneumonia. HRCT scan at the level of the aortic arch shows bilateral areas of consolidation in a predominantly subpleural and peribronchial distribution. The patient was a 46-year-old man who had idiopathic bronchiolitis obliterans organizing pneumonia diagnosed at video-assisted thoracoscopic biopsy. (From Worthy SL, Müller NL: Radiol Clin North Am 36:163, 1998.)

sion. The peripheral pulmonary markings are diminutive as a result of vascular narrowing and attenuation. The ipsilateral hilum also is diminutive but is present, a valuable feature in the differentiation from proximal interruption of a pulmonary artery (pulmonary artery agenesis). In radiographs exposed at TLC, the volume of the affected lung (or lobe) is comparable to that of the normal contralateral lung or is reduced (Fig. 15–65); it is seldom, if ever, increased. The volume of the affected lung depends to a large extent on the age of the patient at the time of the infectious insult: The younger the patient at the time of the bronchiolitis or pneumonia, the smaller the fully developed lung, presumably because the insult retards further maturation.[427, 428] The volume probably relates also to the presence of focal atelectasis and fibrosis.[426]

One of the characteristic radiologic features of Swyer-James syndrome—a *sine qua non* for diagnosis—is the presence of air-trapping during expiration (*see* Fig 15–65). This air-trapping is a reflection of airway obstruction and is extremely valuable in differentiating the syndrome from other conditions that may give rise to unilateral or lobar hyperlucency. Because the contralateral lung is normal, expiration (particularly if rapid) causes the mediastinum to swing abruptly toward the normal lung; excursion of the hemidiaphragms is markedly asymmetric because it is severely diminished on the affected side. Radiographs exposed at residual volume accentuate the disparity in radiolucency of the two lungs; the density of the normal lung is much greater. This disparity is related to the fact that the normal lung contains less air and, perhaps more importantly, to the fact that its blood flow is virtually the total output of the right ventricle. The hilar vessels on the affected side are diminutive, a finding that can be shown readily on CT or spiral CT angiography.[429–431]

In one study of nine patients who had Swyer-James syndrome, 8- to 10-mm collimation CT scans were compared with bronchography (in seven patients) and angiogra-

phy (in five patients).[430] Eight of the nine affected lungs had decreased attenuation on CT; the other was small but had normal attenuation. Air-trapping was present in all cases; on the expiratory CT scan, there was no appreciable change in the volume of the affected lung, whereas the normal lung decreased in volume. All nine patients had evidence of bronchiectasis and decreased size of the pulmonary vessels. The CT findings were similar to those seen at bronchography and arteriography. In another study of eight patients (of whom seven had 1.5- to 2-mm collimation HRCT scans and one had conventional CT scan), seven had unilateral hyperlucent lung on the radiograph, and one had asymmetric areas of hyperlucency.[431] On CT scans, five patients showed bilateral areas of decreased attenuation, and five had areas of normal attenuation within the hyperlucent lung, indicating that the process was much more heterogeneous than previously suspected. Air-trapping within the hyperlucent lung was confirmed with expiratory CT scan in five patients. Bronchiectasis was seen in only three of the eight patients.

Ventilation-perfusion lung scans may provide useful information in selected cases.[432, 433] In one review of 607 perfusion lung scans performed during a 1-year period, 13 revealed total absence of perfusion of one lung. Only one of these cases was due to the Swyer-James syndrome; the remainder were the result of pulmonary thromboembolism, parenchymal lung disease, pulmonary carcinoma, congenital heart disease, and pneumonectomy. Radionuclide ventilation-perfusion scans may show additional areas of involvement, as in a patient in whom an area of diminished perfusion was detected in the contralateral lung, which did not appear hyperlucent on conventional chest radiograph.[434] Ventilation-perfusion lung scanning is preferable to perfusion scanning alone because the latter does not exclude purely vascular abnormalities, such as thromboembolism.[434]

Although many conditions can have a radiographic appearance similar to that of Swyer-James syndrome, in only one is there a serious potential difficulty in differential diagnosis. A partly obstructing lesion situated within a main bronchus can create a triad of radiographic signs that are indistinguishable—a smaller than normal lung volume, air-trapping on expiration, and diffuse oligemia as a result of hypoxic vasoconstriction (Fig. 15–66). Consequently, in any patient presenting with these signs, the presence of a lesion within the ipsilateral main bronchus must be excluded before a diagnosis of Swyer-James syndrome is accepted; the easiest way to accomplish this is by bronchoscopy, although spiral CT probably is just as effective (*see* Fig. 15–66). Other conditions that give rise to unilateral or lobar radiolucency, such as proximal interruption of a pulmonary artery, hypogenetic lung syndrome, and obstruction of a large pulmonary artery by a thromboembolus, are differentiated readily by the absence of air-trapping during expiration and by other radiographic signs that characterize these conditions.

Bronchiolitis Obliterans Organizing Pneumonia (Cryptogenic Organizing Pneumonia)

The histologic reaction pattern of BOOP can be seen in association with many etiologies, including connective tissue disease, drugs, infection, and aspiration; the following

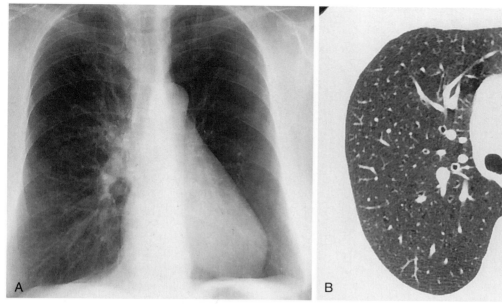

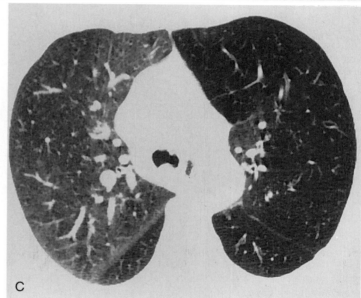

Figure 15–65. Swyer-James Syndrome. Posteroanterior chest radiograph *(A)* shows increased radiolucency and decreased vascularity and size of the left lung. HRCT scan *(B)* at end-inspiration confirms the radiographic findings. The left lung is decreased in volume and is associated with a shift of the mediastinum and of the anterior junction line to the left. HRCT scan performed at end-expiration *(C)* shows air-trapping in the left lung, associated with shift of the mediastinum and of the junction line to the midline. The patient was a 61-year-old woman.

discussion refers mainly to cases in which an etiology is not identified (idiopathic BOOP or cryptogenic organizing pneumonia).

Pathologically, BOOP typically is distributed in a patchy fashion throughout the lung grossly and microscopically within secondary lobules. Plugs of fibroblastic connective tissue can be identified within respiratory bronchioles and alveolar ducts. The parenchyma adjacent to the affected bronchioles shows filling of alveolar air spaces by similar fibroblastic tissue; occasionally a proteinaceous exudate can be identified in the central portion of the fibroblastic tissue, representing a more direct manifestation of prior epithelial or endothelial injury. A variable degree of nonspecific chronic inflammation and interstitial fibrosis also is evident.

Clinically, BOOP usually appears as a subacute illness, with symptoms lasting about 2 to 6 months before diagno-

sis.[381, 446, 447] The most common symptoms are cough (90%), dyspnea (80%), fever (60%), sputum expectoration, malaise, and weight loss (50%). Most patients who have diffuse BOOP show restrictive disease and gas exchange impairment.[391, 446]

Radiologic Manifestations

BOOP can be associated with four distinctive radiographic and CT patterns: (1) multiple, usually bilateral, symmetric, patchy air-space opacities; (2) diffuse, bilateral interstitial opacities, which may be reticular, nodular, or reticulonodular; (3) focal consolidation; and (4) multiple large nodules or masses.[436–438] A mixed pattern of combined air-space and interstitial opacities also has been described.

Patchy air-space consolidation is the most characteristic and the most common of these patterns (Fig. 15–67): Of

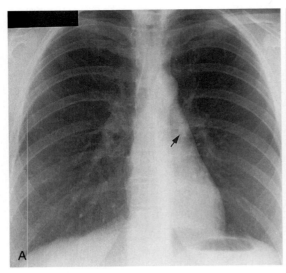

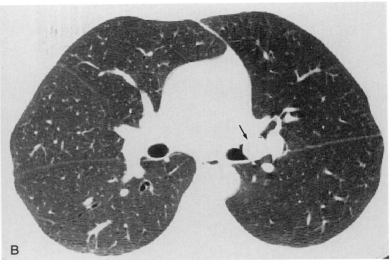

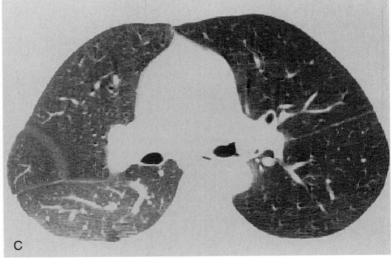

Figure 15–66. Unilateral Radiolucency Caused by a Partly Obstructing Endobronchial Mass. Posteroanterior chest radiograph *(A)* in a 35-year-old woman shows increased radiolucency and decreased vascularity and size of the left lung. An endobronchial tumor *(arrow)* is present in the distal left main bronchus. HRCT scan at end-inspiration *(B)* shows the tumor *(arrow)*, decreased vascularity of the left lung, and a slight decrease in attenuation. Note the decrease in size of the left lung with a shift of the mediastinum and anterior junction line to the left. HRCT scan at end-expiration *(C)* shows air-trapping distal to the endobronchial tumor with a shift of the mediastinum and anterior junction line to the right.

124 patients reported in five studies, 89 (72%) had this manifestation.[381, 439–442] The opacities most often are peripheral and pleural based *(see* Fig. 15–56). They may decrease in size in one area and appear in previously unaffected regions.[443] An unusual case of *levitating* lesions has been described; the bilateral areas of consolidation migrated cephalad during a period of months and gradually disappeared after reaching the lung apices.[444] The size of individual opacities ranges from about 3 cm to almost an entire lobe. Their margins are indistinct, and they may contain air bronchograms. The lung volume may appear preserved or decreased. Concomitant pleural disease is frequent; in one study of 24 patients, it was seen in 5 (21%).[439] In another study of 14 patients, small pleural effusions were detected in 4 (29%).[440] Although the bilateral air-space pattern of BOOP is reasonably characteristic, it is not specific, and the differential diagnosis includes chronic eosinophilic pneumonia, bronchioalveolar carcinoma, lymphoma, pulmonary alveolar proteinosis, and alveolar hemorrhage.[436]

A pattern of reticular or reticulonodular opacities may be seen in association with air-space opacities or, occasionally, as an isolated finding. In two series of 24 and 14

patients, it was reported in 42%[439] and 18%, respectively.[440] A less common radiologic presentation is as a focal area of consolidation. The differential diagnosis includes pulmonary carcinoma, a suspicion that may be enhanced by the presence of fever, weight loss, and hemoptysis; the diagnosis is established most often by resection of the lesion, which tends not to recur.[441] The last and least common manifestation is as multiple large nodules or masses, which may simulate metastatic disease.[438]

On HRCT, most patients show areas of air-space consolidation *(see* Fig. 15–64), small nodules, or both (Fig. 15–68);[411, 412, 445] peripheral reticular areas of increased attenuation and ground-glass opacities are seen less often.[411, 445] In one study of 43 patients (of whom 32 were immunocompetent and 11 were immunocompromised secondary to a variety of conditions), consolidation was more common in immunocompetent (91%) than in immunocompromised (45%) patients;[412] in the immunocompetent group, such consolidation most frequently was subpleural or peribronchial in distribution. Ground-glass attenuation and nodules were more common in immunocompromised patients (73% and 55%, respectively) than in immunocompetent patients (56% and 23%). Occasionally, patients in whom BOOP is

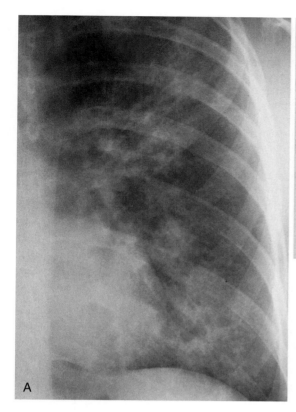

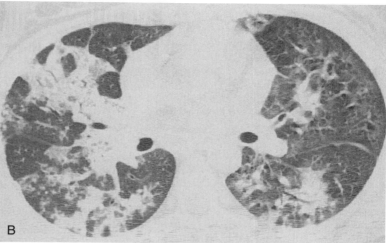

Figure 15–67. Idiopathic Bronchiolitis Obliterans Organizing Pneumonia. View of the left lung from posteroanterior chest radiograph *(A)* in a 20-year-old woman shows patchy areas of consolidation. HRCT scan *(B)* shows a predominantly peribronchial and subpleural distribution of the consolidation. Air bronchograms, focal areas of ground-glass attenuation, and a few centrilobular nodules are evident.

confirmed by biopsy have a CT pattern of small centrilobular nodules and branching shadows that is more characteristic of acute infectious bronchiolitis or diffuse panbronchiolitis (*see* Fig. 15–68).[376]

Respiratory Bronchiolitis

The term *respiratory bronchiolitis* has been used to describe a variety of histologic abnormalities, including accumulation of pigment-laden macrophages in the respira-

tory bronchioles and adjacent alveoli[448] and thickening of the respiratory bronchial walls by inflammatory cells and fibrous tissue.[449] The lesion invariably is associated with cigarette smoking[450] and has been considered to be one of the earliest pathologic reactions to this agent.

In its mildest form, respiratory bronchiolitis is associated with few, if any, symptoms and minimal abnormalities of lung function. In this situation, it typically is discovered as an incidental finding on histologic examination of lungs removed at autopsy or for transplantation. Rarely, a patient

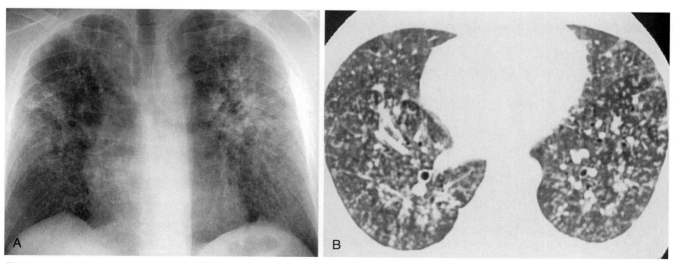

Figure 15–68. Idiopathic Bronchiolitis Obliterans Organizing Pneumonia. Posteroanterior chest radiograph *(A)* in a 47-year-old man shows an extensive bilateral reticulonodular pattern. CT scan *(B)* shows numerous small bilateral nodules in a predominantly centrilobular distribution. The diagnosis of idiopathic bronchiolitis obliterans organizing pneumonia was confirmed by open-lung biopsy.

presents with cough, dyspnea, crackles, and a combined restrictive and obstructive pattern on lung function testing. When associated with typical radiologic and pathologic findings (*see* farther on), this clinicopathologic syndrome has been called *respiratory bronchiolitis–interstitial lung disease*.[230, 451, 452] Patients who have this syndrome may constitute a subset of individuals who have a more severe form of cigarette smoke–induced respiratory bronchiolitis. The lesion also has been considered to represent part of a histologic spectrum of disease that includes desquamative interstitial pneumonitis (*see* Chapter 9).[452]

The radiologic features of respiratory bronchiolitis consist of poorly defined centrilobular nodules or ground-glass opacities (*see* Fig. 15–61).[230, 391, 399] These nodules or opacities may be diffuse but often involve predominantly or exclusively the upper lobes. The findings in respiratory bronchiolitis–interstitial lung disease are similar to those of desquamative interstitial pneumonitis and consist of ground-glass opacities with or without associated fine reticular or reticulonodular interstitial opacities; in contrast to desquamative interstitial pneumonitis, lung volumes usually are normal.[391, 451, 453] On HRCT, the abnormalities consist of diffuse or patchy areas of ground-glass attenuation or poorly defined nodular opacities often superimposed on a background of centrilobular emphysema (Fig 15–69).[230, 391, 413] Occasionally a fine reticular pattern resulting from fibrosis may be seen.

One group of investigators compared the HRCT findings in 16 patients who had pathologically proven respiratory bronchiolitis, eight who had respiratory bronchiolitis–interstitial lung disease and 16 who had desquamative interstitial pneumonitis.[230] The predominant abnormalities in respiratory bronchiolitis were centrilobular nodules seen in 12 (75%) patients and ground-glass attenuation in 6 (38%). No single abnormality predominated in the respiratory bronchiolitis–interstitial lung disease group; findings included ground-glass attenuation (four [50%] patients), centrilobular nodules (three [38%] patients), and mild fibrosis (two [25%] patients). All patients who had desquamative interstitial pneumonia showed ground-glass attenuation, and 10 (63%) of the 16 showed evidence of fibrosis.

Follicular Bronchiolitis

The term *follicular bronchiolitis* refers to a form of bronchiolar disease characterized histologically by the presence of abundant lymphoid tissue, frequently with prominent germinal centers, situated in the walls of bronchioles and, to some extent, bronchi.[454] The most common clinical finding is progressive shortness of breath;[454] cough, fever, and recurrent pneumonia occasionally are present. The lesion is not specific and can be found in association with connective tissue diseases (particularly adult and juvenile rheumatoid disease and Sjögren's syndrome), immunodeficiency diseases, systemic hypersensitivity reactions, and infection by *M. pneumoniae* or viruses.[454, 455]

Chest radiograph characteristically shows a diffuse reticulonodular pattern.[454, 455] HRCT scan may show nodular opacities mainly in a peribronchovascular or subpleural distribution, consistent with the presence of lymphoid aggregates; these opacities usually are small (1 to 3 mm in diameter)[456] but occasionally are 1 to 2 cm in diameter (Fig. 15–70).[231] Other findings include centrilobular branching structures, bronchial wall thickening, and (occasionally) patchy areas of low attenuation.[231, 456] In one investigation of 12 patients, the main abnormalities evident on HRCT scan consisted of bilateral centrilobular nodules seen in all 12 patients, patchy ground-glass opacities in 9 (75%), peribronchial nodules in 5 (42%), and subpleural nodules in 3 (25%).[231]

Diffuse Panbronchiolitis

Diffuse panbronchiolitis is a disease of unknown etiology and pathogenesis associated with chronic inflammation of the paranasal sinuses and respiratory bronchioles, the latter characterized histologically by luminal obliteration and a striking accumulation of foamy macrophages.[457, 458] The disease has been recognized almost exclusively in Japan and South Korea.[459, 460] The chief clinical manifestations are dyspnea on exertion and cough, often with sputum production. Sinusitis is common.[459, 461] Progressive disease is common and sometimes accompanied by respiratory failure.

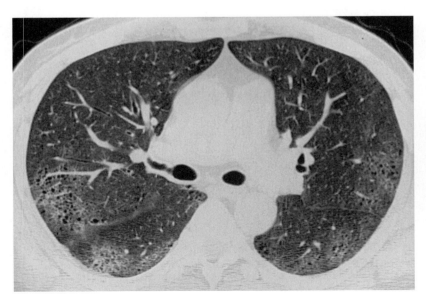

Figure 15–69. Respiratory Bronchiolitis–Interstitial Lung Disease. HRCT scan shows patchy bilateral areas of ground-glass attenuation and mild centrilobular emphysema. The diagnosis of respiratory bronchiolitis–interstitial lung disease was confirmed at surgical biopsy. The patient was a heavy smoker. (Case courtesy of Dr. Kyung Soo Lee, Department of Diagnostic Imaging, Samsung Medical Center, Seoul, South Korea.)

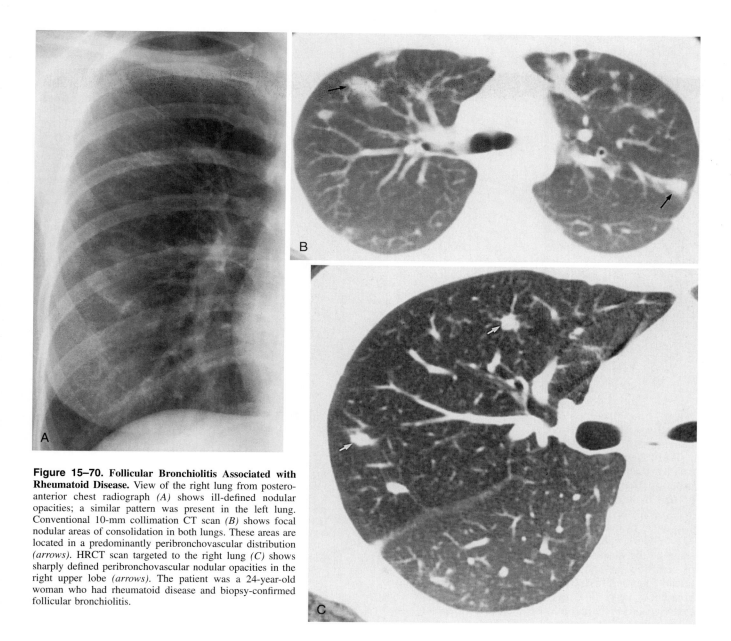

Figure 15–70. Follicular Bronchiolitis Associated with Rheumatoid Disease. View of the right lung from postero-anterior chest radiograph *(A)* shows ill-defined nodular opacities; a similar pattern was present in the left lung. Conventional 10-mm collimation CT scan *(B)* shows focal nodular areas of consolidation in both lungs. These areas are located in a predominantly peribronchovascular distribution *(arrows)*. HRCT scan targeted to the right lung *(C)* shows sharply defined peribronchovascular nodular opacities in the right upper lobe *(arrows)*. The patient was a 24-year-old woman who had rheumatoid disease and biopsy-confirmed follicular bronchiolitis.

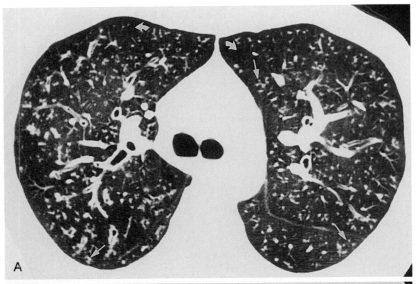

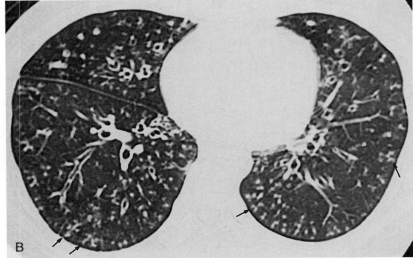

Figure 15–71. Diffuse Panbronchiolitis. HRCT scan in a 32-year-old man with panbronchiolitis *(A)* shows centrilobular nodules *(straight arrows)*, marked bronchial wall thickening, bronchiectasis, and localized areas of decreased attenuation and perfusion *(curved arrows)*. HRCT scan in another patient *(B)* shows centrilobular nodules and branching lines, giving a characteristic tree-in-bud appearance *(arrows)*. Extensive bronchial wall thickening and bronchiectasis are evident. (Courtesy of Dr. Kyung Soo Lee, Samsung Medical Center, Seoul, South Korea.)

Radiographic abnormalities consist of diffuse nodules smaller than 5 mm in diameter and mild to moderate hyperinflation.[459, 462] The findings on HRCT are characteristic and include small centrilobular nodules and branching linear opacities, bronchiolectasis, bronchiectasis, and mosaic areas of decreased parenchymal attenuation (Fig. 15–71).[395–397] The presence of these findings is related to the stage of the disease:[397] The earliest manifestation consists of centrilobular nodular opacities, followed by branching linear opacities that connect to the nodules, followed by bronchiolectasis, and, eventually, bronchiectasis.[397] Large cystic spaces or bullae may be seen in the late stage.

In addition to diagnosis, HRCT has been useful in following the evolution of disease.[463] In one study of 17 patients, centrilobular and branching linear areas of soft tissue attenuation progressed to dilation of proximal airways in 5 untreated patients, whereas these lesions decreased in number and size after erythromycin therapy in 12 patients.[396]

References

1. Evans AS: Clinical syndromes in adults caused by respiratory infections. Med Clin North Am 51:803, 1967.
2. Deeb ZE: Acute supraglottitis in adults: Early indicators of airway obstruction. Am J Otolaryngol 18:112, 1997.
3. Stone CK, Thomas SH: Upper airway obstruction from tonsillar infection in adults. Eur J Emerg Med 1:37, 1994.
4. Seigler RS: Bacterial tracheitis: Recognition and treatment. J S C Med Assoc 89:83, 1993.
5. Valor RR, Polnitsky CA, Tanis DJ, et al: Bacterial tracheitis with upper airway obstruction in a patient with the acquired immunodeficiency syndrome. Am Rev Respir Dis 146:1598, 1992.
6. Schabel SI, Katzberg RW, Burgener FA: Acute inflammation of epiglottis and supraglottic structures in adults. Radiology 122:601, 1977.
7. Ossoff RH, Wolff AP: Acute epiglottitis in adults. JAMA 244:2639, 1980.
8. Nemzek WR, Katzberg RW, Van Slyke MA, et al: A reappraisal of the radiologic findings of acute inflammation of the epiglottis and supraglottic structures in adults. Am J Neuroradiol 16:495, 1995.
9. Rothrock SG, Pignatiello GA, Howard RM: Radiologic diagnosis of epiglottitis: Objective criteria for all ages. Ann Emerg Med 19:978, 1990.
10. Walden CA, Rogers LF: CT evaluation of adult epiglottitis. J Comput Assist Tomogr 13:883, 1989.
11. Ramadan HH, Tarazi AE, Baroudy FM: Laryngeal tuberculosis: Presentation of 16 cases and review of the literature. J Otolaryngol 22:39, 1993.
12. Hines DW, Haber MH, Yaremko L, et al: Pseudomembranous tracheobronchitis caused by *Aspergillus*. Am Rev Respir Dis 143:1408, 1991.

13. Kemper CA, Hostetler JS, Follansbee SE, et al: Ulcerative and plaque-like tracheobronchitis due to infection with *Aspergillus* in patients with AIDS. Clin Infect Dis 17:344, 1993.

14. Scheffer AL: Urticaria and angioedema. Pediatr Clin North Am 22:193, 1975.

15. Michel RG, Hudson WR, Pope TH: Angioneurotic edema: A review of modern concepts. Arch Otolaryngol 101:544, 1975.

16. Frank MM, Gelfand JA, Atkinson JP: Hereditary angioedema: The clinical syndrome and its management. Ann Intern Med 84:580, 1976.

17. Twigg HL, Buckley CE: Complications of endotracheal intubation. Am J Roentgenol 109:452, 1970.

18. Conrardy PA, Goodman LR, Laing F, et al: Alteration of endotracheal tube position: Flexion and extension of the neck. Crit Care Med 4:7, 1976.

19. Goodman LR, Conrardy PA, Laing F, et al: Radiographic evaluation of endotracheal tube position. Am J Roentgenol 127:433, 1976.

20. Gamsu G, Webb WR: Computed tomography of the trachea: Normal and abnormal. Am J Roentgenol 139:321, 1982.

21. Hermans R, Verschakelen JA, Baert AL: Imaging of laryngeal and tracheal stenosis. Acta Otorhinolaryngol Belg 49:323, 1995.

22. Becker M, Moulin G, Kurt A-M, et al: Non-squamous cell neoplasms of the larynx: Radiologic-pathologic correlation. Radiographics 18:1189, 1998.

23. Glazer HS, Aronberg DJ, Lee JKT, et al: Extralaryngeal causes of vocal cord paralysis: CT evaluation. Am J Roentgenol 141:527, 1983.

24. Shepard JAO, McLoud TC: Imaging the airways: Computed tomography and magnetic resonance imaging. Clin Chest Med 12:151, 1991.

25. Kwong JS, Adler BD, Padley SPG, et al: Diagnosis of diseases of the trachea and main bronchi: Chest radiography vs CT. Am J Roentgenol 161:519, 1993.

26. Manninen MP, Paakkala TA, Pukander JS, et al: Diagnosis of tracheal carcinoma at chest radiography. Acta Radiol 33:546, 1992.

27. Kwong JS, Müller NL, Miller RR: Diseases of the trachea and main-stem bronchi: Correlation of CT with pathologic findings. Radiographics 12:645, 1992.

28. McCarthy MJ, Rosado-de-Christenson ML: Tumors of the trachea. J Thorac Imaging 10:180, 1995.

29. Spizarny DL, Shepard JAO, McLoud TC, et al: CT of adenoid cystic carcinoma of the trachea. Am J Roentgenol 146:1129, 1986.

30. Newmark GM, Conces DJ Jr, Kopecky KK: Spiral CT evaluation of the trachea and bronchi. J Comput Assist Tomogr 18:552, 1994.

31. Whyte RI, Quint LE, Kazerooni EA, et al: Helical computed tomography for the evaluation of tracheal stenosis. Ann Thorac Surg 60:27, 1995.

32. Lacrosse M, Trigaux JP, Van Beers BE, et al: 3D spiral CT of the tracheobronchial tree. J Comput Assist Tomogr 19:341, 1995.

33. Quint LE, Whyte RI, Kazerooni EA, et al: Stenosis of the central airways: Evaluation by using helical CT with multiplanar reconstructions. Radiology 194:871, 1995.

34. Tello R, Kruskal J, Dupuy D, et al: In vivo three-dimensional evaluation of the tracheobronchial tree. J Thorac Imaging 10:291, 1995.

35. Lee KS, Yoon JH, Kim TK, et al: Evaluation of tracheobronchial disease with helical CT with multiplanar and three-dimensional reconstruction: Correlation with bronchoscopy. Radiographics 17:555, 1997.

36. Remy-Jardin M, Remy J, Artaud D, et al: Volume rendering of the tracheobronchial tree: Clinical evaluation of bronchographic images. Radiology 208:761, 1998.

37. Fletcher BD, Dearborn DG, Mulopulos GP: MR imaging in infants with airway obstruction: Preliminary observations. Radiology 160:245, 1986.

38. Suto Y, Tanabe Y: Evaluation of tracheal collapsibility in patients with tracheomalacia using dynamic MR imaging during coughing. Am J Roentgenol 171:393, 1998.

39. Newman E, Shaha AR: Substernal goiter. J Surg Oncol 60:207, 1995.

40. Bashist B, Ellis K, Gold RP: Computed tomography of intrathoracic goiters. Am J Roentgenol 140:455, 1983.

41. Glazer GM, Axel L, Moss AA: CT diagnosis of mediastinal thyroid. Am J Roentgenol 138:495, 1982.

42. Yousem DM: Parathyroid and thyroid imaging. Neuroimag Clin N Am 6:435, 1996.

43. Som PM, Sacher M, Lanzieri CF, et al: Two benign CT presentations of thyroid-related papillary adenocarcinoma. J Comput Assist Tomogr 9:162, 1985.

44. Swartz JD, Yussen PS, Popky GL: Imaging of soft tissues of the neck: Non-nodal acquired disease. Crit Rev Diag Imaging 31:471, 1991.

45. Muysoms F, Boedts M, Claeys D: Intratracheal ectopic thyroid tissue mass. Chest 112:1684, 1997.

46. Griscom NT, Wohl MEB: Tracheal size and shape: Effects of change in intraluminal pressure. Radiology 149:27, 1983.

47. Moreno R, Taylor R, Müller N, et al: In vivo human tracheal pressure-area curves using computerized tomographic scans: Correlation with maximal expiratory flow rates. Am Rev Respir Dis 134:585, 1986.

48. Stern EJ, Graham CM, Webb WR, et al: Normal trachea during forced expiration: Dynamic CT measurements. Radiology 187:27, 1993.

49. Breatnach E, Abbott GC, Fraser RG: Dimensions of the normal human trachea. Am J Roentgenol 141:903, 1984.

50. Dixon TC, Sando MJW, Bolton JM, et al: A report of 342 cases of prolonged endotracheal intubation. Med J Aust 2:529, 1968.

51. Pearson FG, Goldberg M, da Silva AJ: Tracheal stenosis complicating tracheostomy with cuffed tubes: Clinical experience and observations from a prospective study. Arch Surg 97:380, 1968.

52. Hemmingsson A, Lindgren PG: Roentgenologic examination of tracheal stenosis. Acta Radiol Diagn 19:753, 1978.

53. James AE Jr, MacMillian AS Jr, Eaton SB, et al: Roentgenology of tracheal stenosis resulting from cuffed tracheostomy tubes. Am J Roentgenol 109:455, 1970.

54. Goodman LR: Post intubation tracheal stenosis. *In* Proto AW (ed): Chest Disease (4th series, test and syllabus). Reston, VA, American College of Radiology, 1989, p 337.

55. Bhalla M, Grillo HC, McLoud TC, et al: Idiopathic laryngotracheal stenosis: Radiologic findings. Am J Roentgenol 161:515, 1993.

56. Harley HRS: Laryngotracheal obstruction complicating tracheostomy or endotracheal intubation with assisted respiration: A critical review. Thorax 26:493, 1971.

57. Silva LU, Wood GJ: Tracheomalacia from excessive cuff pressure of an endotracheal tube. King Faisal Specialist Hosp Med 4:201, 1984.

58. Houston HW, Payne WS, Harrison EG Jr, et al: Primary cancers of the trachea. Arch Surg 99:132, 1969.

59. Hadju SI, Huvos AG, Goodner JT, et al: Carcinoma of the trachea: Clinicopathologic study of 41 cases. Cancer 25:1448, 1970.

60. McCafferty GJ, Parker LS, Suggit SC: Primary malignant disease of the trachea. J Laryngol Otol 78:441, 1964.

61. Dennie CJ, Coblentz CL: The trachea: Pathologic conditions and trauma. Can Assoc Radiol J 44:157, 1993.

62. Spivey CG Jr, Walsh RE, Perez-Guerra F, et al: Central airway obstruction: Report of seven cases. JAMA 226:1186, 1973.

63. Baydur A, Gottlieb LS: Adenoid cystic carcinoma (cylindroma) of the trachea masquerading as asthma. JAMA 234:829, 1975.

64. Mackenzie CF, McAslan TC, Shin B, et al: The shape of the human adult trachea. Anesthesiology 49:48, 1978.

65. Greene R, Lechner GL: "Saber-sheath" trachea: A clinical and functional study of marked coronal narrowing of the intrathoracic trachea. Radiology 115:265, 1975.

66. Hoskins MC, Evans RA, King SJ, et al: "Sabre sheath" trachea with mediastinal lipomatosis mimicking a mediastinal tumour. Clin Radiol 44:417, 1991.

67. Trigaux JP, Hermes G, Dubois P, et al: CT of saber-sheath trachea: Correlation with clinical, chest radiographic and functional findings. Acta Radiol 35:247, 1994.

68. Tsao TC, Shieh WB: Intrathoracic tracheal dimensions and shape changes in chronic obstructive pulmonary disease. J Formos Med Assoc 93:30, 1994.

69. Booth A, Dieppe PA, Goddard PL, et al: The radiological manifestations of relapsing polychondritis. Clin Radiol 40:147, 1989.

70. Goddard P, Cook P, Laszlo G, et al: Relapsing polychondritis: Report of an unusual case and a review of the literature. Br J Radiol 64:1064, 1991.

71. McLoud TC: Diffuse tracheal abnormalities. *In* Siegel BA (ed): Chest Disease (5th series, test and syllabus). Reston, VA, American College of Radiology, 1996, p 259.

72. Müller NL, Miller RR, Ostrow DN, et al: Clinico-radiologic-pathologic conference: Diffuse thickening of the tracheal wall. Can Assoc Radiol J 40:213, 1989.

73. Gibson GJ, Davis P: Respiratory complications of relapsing polychondritis. Thorax 29:726, 1973.

74. McAdam LP, O'Hanlon MA, Bluestone R, et al: Relapsing polychondritis: Prospective study of 23 patients and a review of the literature. Medicine 55:193, 1976.

75. Mohsenifar Z, Tashkin DP, Carson SA, et al: Pulmonary function in patients with relapsing polychondritis. Chest 81:711, 1982.

76. Choplin RH, Wehunt WD, Theros EG: Diffuse lesions of the trachea. Semin Roentgenol 18:38, 1983.

77. Dupont A, Bossuyt A, Sommers G, et al: Relapsing polychondritis: Gallium-67 uptake in recurrent lung lesions. J Nucl Med Allied Sci 27:57, 1983.

78. Van Nierop MA, Wagenaar SS, Van den Bosch JM, et al: Tracheobronchopathia osteochondroplastica: Report of four cases. Eur J Respir Dis 64:129, 1983.

79. Vilkman S, Keistinen T: Tracheobronchopathia osteochondroplastica: Report of a young man with severe disease and retrospective review of 18 cases. Respiration 62:151, 1995.

80. Nienhuis DM, Prakash UB, Edell ES: Tracheobronchopathia osteochondroplastica. Ann Otol Rhinol Laryngol 99:689, 1990.

81. Coetmeur D, Bovyn G, Leroux P, et al: Tracheobronchopathia osteochondroplastica presenting at the time of a difficult intubation. Respir Med 91:496, 1997.

82. Clee MD, Anderson JM, Johnston RN, et al: Clinical aspects of tracheobronchopathia osteochondroplastica. Br J Dis Chest 77:308, 1983.

83. Young RH, Sandstrom RE, Mark GJ: Tracheopathia osteochondroplastica: Clinical, radiologic and pathologic correlations. J Thorac Cardiovasc Surg 79:537, 1980.

84. Onitsuka H, Hirose N, Watanabe K, et al: Computed tomography of tracheopathia osteoplastica. Am J Roentgenol 140:268, 1983.

85. Williams SM, Jones ET: Tracheobronchopathia osteochondroplastica. Radiographics 17:797, 1997.

86. Lundgren R, Stjernberg NL: Tracheobronchopathia osteochondroplastica: A clinical bronchoscopic and spirometric study. Chest 80:706, 1981.

87. Mariotta S, Pallone G, Pedicelli G, et al: Spiral CT and endoscopic findings in a case of tracheobronchopathia osteochondroplastica. J Comput Assist Tomogr 21:418, 1997.

88. Hodges MK, Israel E: Tracheobronchopathia osteochondroplastica presenting as right middle lobe collapse: Diagnosis by bronchoscopy and computerized tomography. Chest 94:842, 1988.

89. Park SS, Shin DH, Lee DH, et al: Tracheopathia osteoplastica simulating asthmatic symptoms: Diagnosis by bronchoscopy and computerized tomography. Respiration 62:43, 1995.

90. Krishnan H, May RE: An unusual cause for respiratory difficulty after thyroidectomy. Br J Clin Pract 47:47, 1993.

91. van Son JA, Julsrud PR, Hagler DJ, et al: Surgical treatment of vascular rings: The Mayo Clinic experience. Mayo Clin Proc 68:1056, 1993.

92. Feist JH, Johnson TH, Wilson RJ: Acquired tracheomalacia, etiology and differential diagnosis. Chest 68:340, 1975.

93. Santoli E, Di Biasi P, Vanelli P, et al: Tracheal obstruction due to congenital tracheomalacia in a child: Case report. Scand J Thorac Cardiovasc Surg 25:227, 1991.

94. Campbell AH, Young IF: Tracheobronchial collapse, a variant of obstructive respiratory disease. Br J Dis Chest 57:174, 1963.

95. Johnston RF, Green RA: Tracheobronchiomegaly: Report of five cases and demonstration of familial occurrence. Am Rev Respir Dis 91:35, 1965.

96. Mounier-Kuhn P: Dilatation de la trachee: Constations radiographiques et bronchoscopiques. (Tracheal dilatation: Roentgenographic and bronchographic findings.) Lyon Med 150:106, 1932.

97. Bateson EM, Woo-Ming M: Tracheobronchomegaly. Clin Radiol 24:354, 1973.

98. Aaby GV, Blake HA: Tracheobronchomegaly. Ann Thorac Surg 2:64, 1966.

99. Ayres J, Rees J, Cochrane GM, et al: Hemoptysis and non-organic upper airways obstruction in a patient with previously undiagnosed Ehlers-Danlos syndrome. Br J Dis Chest 75:309, 1981.

100. Wonderer AA, Elliot FE, Goltz RW, et al: Tracheobronchomegaly and acquired cutis laxa in the child: Physiologic and immunologic studies. Pediatrics 44:709, 1969.

101. Shivaram U, Shivaram I, Cash M: Acquired tracheobronchomegaly resulting in severe respiratory failure. Chest 98:491, 1990.

102. Woodring JH, Barrett PA, Rehm SR, et al: Acquired tracheomegaly in adults as a complication of diffuse pulmonary fibrosis. Am J Roentgenol 152:743, 1989.

103. Vidal C, Pena F, Rodriguez Mosquera M, et al: Tracheobronchomegaly associated with interstitial pulmonary fibrosis. Respiration 58:207, 1991.

104. Padley S, Varma N, Flower CD: Tracheobronchomegaly in association with ankylosing spondylitis. Clin Radiol 43:139, 1991.

105. Fenlon HM, Casserly I, Sant SM, et al: Plain radiographs and thoracic high-resolution CT in patients with ankylosing spondylitis. Am J Roentgenol 168:1067, 1997.

106. Woodring JH, Howard R II, Rehm SR: Congenital tracheobronchomegaly (Mounier-Kuhn syndrome): A report of 10 cases and review of the literature. J Thorac Imaging 6:1, 1991.

107. Dunne MG, Reiner B: CT features of tracheobronchomegaly. J Comput Assist Tomogr 12:388, 1988.

108. Gay S, Dee P: Tracheobronchomegaly: The Mounier-Kuhn syndrome. Br J Radiol 57:640, 1984.

109. Shin MS, Jackson RM, Ho K-J: Tracheobronchomegaly (Mounier-Kuhn syndrome): CT diagnosis. Am J Roentgenol 150:777, 1988.

110. Roditi GH, Weir J: The association of tracheomegaly and bronchiectasis. Clin Radiol 49:608, 1994.

111. Smith DL, Withers N, Holloway B, et al: Tracheobronchomegaly: An unusual presentation of a rare condition. Thorax 49:840, 1994.

112. McNamara SG, Grunstein RR, Sullivan CE: Obstructive sleep apnea. Thorax 48:754, 1993.

113. National Heart, Lung and Blood Institute: Fact Book: Fiscal Year 1993. Bethesda, MD, U.S. Department of Health and Human Services, U.S. Public Health Service, National Institutes of Health, 1994.

114. Wittels EH: Obesity and hormonal factors in sleep and sleep apnea. Med Clin North Am 69:1265, 1985.

115. White DP: Pathophysiology of obstructive sleep apnoea. Thorax 50:797, 1995.

116. Deegan PC, McNicholas WT: Pathophysiology of obstructive sleep apnoea. Eur Respir J 8:1161, 1995.

117. Nelson S, Hans M: Contribution of craniofacial risk factors in increasing apneic activity among obese and nonobese habitual snorers. Chest 111:154, 1997.

118. Douglas NJ: Upper airway imaging. Clin Phys Physiol Meas 11:117, 1990.

119. Fleetham JA: Upper airway imaging in relation to obstructive sleep apnea. Clin Chest Med 13:399, 1992.

120. Stark P, Norbash A: Imaging of the trachea and upper airways in patients with chronic obstructive airway disease. Radiol Clin North Am 36:91, 1998.

121. Tangugsorn V, Skatvedt O, Krogstad O, et al: Obstructive sleep apnoea: A cephalometric study: Part II. Uvulo-glossopharyngeal morphology. Eur J Orthod 17:57, 1995.

122. Tangugsorn V, Skatvedt O, Krogstad O, et al: Obstructive sleep apnoea: A cephalometric study: Part I. Cervico-craniofacial skeletal morphology. Eur J Orthod 17:45, 1995.

123. Avrahami E, Englender M: Relation between CT axial cross-sectional area of the oropharynx and obstructive sleep apnea syndrome in adults. Am J Neuroradiol 16:135, 1995.

124. Lowe AA, Ozbek MM, Miyamoto K, et al: Cephalometric and demographic characteristics of obstructive sleep apnea: An evaluation with partial least squares analysis. Angle Orthod 67:143, 1997.

125. Pracharktam N, Nelson S, Hans MG, et al: Cephalometric assessment in obstructive sleep apnea. Am J Orthod Dentofacial Orthop 109:410, 1996.

126. Frohberg U, Naples RJ, Jones DL: Cephalometric comparison of characteristics in chronically snoring patients with and without sleep apnea syndrome. Oral Surg Oral Med Oral Pathol Oral Radiol Endod 80:28, 1995.

127. Hoffstein V, Weiser W, Haney R: Roentgenographic dimensions of the upper airway in snoring patients with and without obstructive sleep apnea. Chest 100:81, 1991.

128. Lowe AA, Gionhaku N, Takeuchi K, et al: Three dimensional CT reconstructions of tongue and airway in adult subjects with obstructive sleep apnea. Am J Orthod Dentofacial Orthop 90:364, 1986.

129. Schwab RJ, Gefter WB, Hoffman EA, et al: Dynamic upper airway imaging during awake respiration in normal subjects and patients with sleep disordered breathing. Am Rev Respir Dis 148:1385, 1993.

130. Shepard JW Jr, Stanson AW, Sheedy PF, et al: Fast-CT evaluation

of the upper airway during wakefulness in patients with obstructive sleep apnea. Prog Clin Biol Res 345:273, 1990.

131. Shelton KE, Woodson H, Gay S, et al: Pharyngeal fat in obstructive sleep apnea. Am Rev Respir Dis 148:462, 1993.

132. Shelton KE, Woodson H, Gay SB, et al: Adipose tissue deposition in sleep apnea. Sleep 16:S103, 1993.

133. Suto Y, Inoue Y: Sleep apnea syndrome: Examination of pharyngeal obstruction with high-speed MR and polysomnography. Acta Radiol 37:315, 1996.

134. Suto Y, Matsuda E, Inoue Y: MRI of the pharynx in young patients with sleep disordered breathing. Br J Radiol 69:1000, 1996.

135. Suto Y, Matsuo T, Kato T, et al: Evaluation of the pharyngeal airway in patients with sleep apnea: Value of ultrafast MR imaging. Am J Roentgenol 160:311, 1993.

136. Okada T, Fukatsu H, Ishigaki T, et al: Ultra-low-field magnetic resonance imaging in upper airways obstruction in sleep apnea syndrome. Psychiatr Clin Neurosci 50:285, 1996.

137. Ryan FC, Lowe AA, Li D, et al: Magnetic resonance imaging of the upper airway in obstructive sleep apnea before and after chronic nasal continuous positive airway pressure therapy. Am Rev Respir Dis 144:939, 1991.

138. Scadding JG: Definition and the clinical categories of asthma. *In* Clark TJH, Godfrey S (eds): Asthma. 2nd ed. London, Chapman & Hall, 1983, pp 1–11.

139. American Thoracic Society (Statement by Committee on Diagnostic Standards for Nontuberculous Respiratory Diseases): Definitions and classification of chronic bronchitis, asthma, and pulmonary emphysema. Am Rev Respir Dis 85:762, 1962.

140. Matthys H: Definition and assessment of asthma. Lung 168:51, 1990.

141. Global Initiative for Asthma: Global Strategy for Asthma Management and Prevention. NHLBI/WHO Workshop Report. NIH publication No. 95-3659. Bethesda, MD, National Institutes of Health, National Heart, Lung, and Blood Institute, 1995.

142. Hogg JC: The pathophysiology of asthma. Chest 82:85, 1982.

143. Leff A: Pathophysiology of asthmatic bronchoconstriction. Chest 82:135, 1982.

144. Jeffrey PK, Godfrey RW, Adelroth E, et al: Effects of treatment on airway inflammation and thickening of basement membrane reticular collagen in asthma. Am Rev Respir Dis 145:890, 1992.

145. Paganin F, Trussard V, Seneterre E, et al: Chest radiography and high resolution computed tomography of the lungs in asthma. Am Rev Respir Dis 146:1084, 1992.

146. Pickup CM, Nee PA, Randall PE: Radiographic features in 1016 adults admitted to hospital with acute asthma. J Accid Emerg Med 11:234, 1994.

147. Lynch DA: Imaging of asthma and allergic bronchopulmonary mycosis. Radiol Clin North Am 36:129, 1998.

148. Hodson ME, Simon G, Batten JC: Radiology of uncomplicated asthma. Thorax 29:296, 1974.

149. Blackie SP, Al-Majed S, Staples CA, et al: Changes in total lung capacity during acute spontaneous asthma. Am Rev Respir Dis 142:79, 1990.

150. Rebuck AS: Radiological aspects of severe asthma. Australas Radiol 14:264, 1970.

151. Genereux GP: Radiology and pulmonary immunopathologic lung disease. *In* Steiner RE (ed): Recent Advances in Radiology and Medical Imaging. New York, Churchill Livingstone, 1983, pp 213–240.

152. Bousquet J, Chanez P, Lacoste JY, et al: Eosinophilic inflammation in asthma. N Engl J Med 323:1033, 1990.

153. Petheram IS, Kerr IH, Collins JV: Value of chest radiographs in severe acute asthma. Clin Radiol 32:281, 1981.

154. Zieverink SE, Harper AP, Holden RW, et al: Emergency room radiography of asthma: An efficacy study. Radiology 145:27, 1982.

155. Rossi OV, Lahde S, Laitinen J, et al: Contribution of chest and paranasal sinus radiographs to the management of acute asthma. Int Arch Allergy Immunol 105:96, 1994.

156. Lynch DA, Newell JD, Tschomper BA, et al: Uncomplicated asthma in adults: Comparison of CT appearance of the lungs in asthmatic and healthy subjects. Radiology 188:829, 1993.

157. Okazawa M, Müller NL, McNamara AE, et al: Human airway narrowing measured using high resolution computed tomography. Am J Respir Crit Care Med 154:1557, 1996.

158. Park CS, Müller NL, Worthy SA, et al: Airway obstruction in asthmatic and healthy individuals: Inspiratory and expiratory thin-section CT findings. Radiology 203:361, 1997.

159. Webb WR, Gamsu G, Wall SD, et al: CT of a bronchial phantom: Factors affecting appearance and size measurements. Invest Radiol 19:394, 1984.

160. McNamara AE, Müller NL, Okazawa M, et al: Airway narrowing in excised canine lungs measured by high-resolution computed tomography. J Appl Physiol 73:307, 1992.

161. Bankier AA, Fleischmann D, Mallek R, et al: Bronchial wall thickness: Appropriate window settings for thin-section CT and radiologic-anatomic correlation. Radiology 199:831, 1996.

162. Amirav I, Kramer S, Grunstein M, et al: Assessment of methacholine-induced airway constriction with ultrafast high-resolution computed tomography. J Appl Physiol 75:2239, 1993.

163. Herold C, Brown R, Mitzner W, et al: Assessment of pulmonary airway reactivity with high-resolution CT. Radiology 181:369, 1991.

164. Grenier P, Mourey-Gerosa I, Benali K, et al: Abnormalities of the airways and lung parenchyma in asthmatics: CT observations in 50 patients and inter- and intraobserver variability. Eur Radiol 6:199, 1996.

165. Awadh N, Müller NL, Park CS, et al: Airway wall thickness in patients with near fatal asthma and control groups: Assessment with high resolution computed tomographic scanning. Thorax 53:248, 1998.

166. Angus R, Davies M-I, Cowan M, et al: Computed tomographic scanning of the lung in patients with allergic bronchopulmonary aspergillosis and in asthmatic patients with a positive skin test to *Aspergillus fumigatus.* Thorax 49:586, 1994.

167. Kim S, Im J, Kim I, et al: Normal bronchial and pulmonary arterial diameters measured by thin section CT. J Comput Assist Tomogr 19:365, 1995.

168. Kim J, Müller NL, Park CS, et al: Broncho-arterial ratio on thin-section CT: Comparison between high altitude and sea level. J Comput Assist Tomogr 21:306, 1997.

169. Wagner PD, Hedenstierna G, Bylin G: Ventilation-perfusion inequality in chronic asthma. Am Rev Respir Dis 136:605, 1987.

170. Ferrer A, Roca J, Wagner PM, et al: Airway obstruction and ventilation-perfusion relationships in acute severe asthma. Am Rev Respir Dis 147:579, 1993.

171. Simonsson BG: Chronic cough and expectoration in patients with asthma and in patients with alpha$_1$-antitrypsin deficiency. Eur J Respir Dis 118:123, 1982.

172. Bendkowski B: Asian influenza (1957) in allergic patients. BMJ 2:1314, 1958.

173. Eggleston PA, Ward BH, Pierson WE, et al: Radiographic abnormalities in acute asthma in children. Pediatrics 54:442, 1974.

174. Lecks HI, Whitney T, Wood D, et al: Newer concepts in occurrence of segmental atelectasis in acute bronchial asthma and status asthmaticus in children. J Asthma Res 4:65, 1966.

175. Deaths from chronic obstructive pulmonary disease in the United States, 1987. Stat Bull Metrop Insur Co 71:20, 1990.

176. Murray CJL, Lopez AD: Global mortality, disability, and the contribution of risk factors—global burden of disease study. Lancet 349:1436, 1997.

177. Fletcher CM, Pride NB: Definitions of emphysema, chronic bronchitis, asthma, and airflow obstruction: 25 years on from the CIBA symposium (editorial). Thorax 39:81, 1984.

178. Snider GL: What's in a name? Names, definitions, descriptions, and diagnostic criteria of diseases, with emphasis on chronic obstructive pulmonary disease. Respiration 62:297, 1995.

179. Snider GL, Kleinerman JL, Thurlbeck WM, et al: The definition of emphysema—report of a National Heart, Lung, and Blood Institute Division of Lung Diseases Workshop. Am Rev Respir Dis 132:182, 1985.

180. Pride NB, Burrows B: Development of impaired lung function: Natural history and risk factors. *In* Calverley P, Pride N (eds): Chronic Obstructive Pulmonary Disease. London, Chapman & Hall, 1995, pp 69–91.

181. Silverman EK, Speizer FE: Risk factors for the development of chronic obstructive pulmonary disease. Med Clin North Am 80:501, 1996.

182. Fletcher C, Peto R, Tinker C, Speizer FE: The Natural History of Chronic Bronchitis: An Eight Year Follow-up Study of Working Men in London. Oxford, Oxford University Press, 1976.

183. Bascom R: Differential susceptibility to tobacco smoke: Possible mechanisms. Pharmacogenetics 1:102, 1991.

184. Anderson AE Jr, Furlaneto JA, Foraker AG: Bronchopulmonary derangements in nonsmokers. Am Rev Respir Dis 101:518, 1970.

185. Sutinen S, Vaajalahti P, Pääkkö P, et al: Prevalence, severity and types of pulmonary emphysema in a population of deaths in a Finnish city: Correlation with age, sex and smoking. Scand J Respir Dis 59:101, 1978.

186. Bates DV, Gordon CA, Paul GI, et al: Chronic bronchitis: Report on the third and fourth stages of the co-ordinated study of chronic bronchitis in the Department of Veterans Affairs, Canada. Med Serv J Can 22:5, 1966.

187. Simon G: Chronic bronchitis and emphysema: A symposium: III. Pathological findings and radiological changes in chronic bronchitis and emphysema: (b) Radiological changes in chronic bronchitis. Br J Radiol 32:292, 1959.

188. Fraser RG, Fraser RS, Renner JW, et al: The roentgenologic diagnosis of chronic bronchitis: A reassessment with emphasis on parahilar bronchi seen end-on. Radiology 120:1, 1976.

189. Webb WR: Radiology of obstructive pulmonary disease. Am J Roentgenol 169:637, 1997.

190. Simon G: Principles of Chest X-Ray Diagnosis. 3rd ed. London, Butterworth, 1971.

191. Takasugi JE, Godwin JD: Radiology of chronic obstructive pulmonary disease. Radiol Clin North Am 36:29, 1998.

192. Remy-Jardin M, Remy J, Boulenguez C, et al: Morphologic effects of cigarette smoking on airways and pulmonary parenchyma in healthy adult volunteers: CT evaluation and correlation with pulmonary function tests. Radiology 186:107, 1993.

193. Lamers RJ, Thelissen GR, Kessels A, et al: Chronic obstructive pulmonary disease: Evaluation with spirometrically controlled CT lung densitometry. Radiology 193:109, 1994.

194. Sutinen S, Christoforidis AJ, Klugh GA, et al: Roentgenologic criteria for the recognition of non-symptomatic pulmonary emphysema: Correlation between roentgenologic findings and pulmonary pathology. Am Rev Respir Dis 91:69, 1965.

195. Pratt PC: Role of conventional chest radiography in diagnosis and exclusion of emphysema. Am J Med 82:998, 1987.

196. Laws JW, Heard BE: Emphysema and the chest film: A retrospective radiological and pathological study. Br J Radiol 35:750, 1962.

197. Thurlbeck WM, Henderson JA, Fraser RG, et al: Chronic obstructive lung disease: A comparison between clinical, roentgenologic, functional and morphological criteria in chronic bronchitis, emphysema, asthma and bronchiectasis. Medicine 49:81, 1970.

198. Thurlbeck WM, Simon G: Radiographic appearance of the chest in emphysema. Am J Roentgenol 130:429, 1978.

199. Miniati M, Filippi E, Falaschi F, et al: Radiologic evaluation of emphysema in patients with chronic obstructive pulmonary disease. Am J Respir Crit Care Med 151:1359, 1995.

200. Katsura S, Martin CJ: The roentgenologic diagnosis of anatomic emphysema. Am Rev Respir Dis 96:700, 1967.

201. Nicklaus TM, Stowell DW, Christiansen WR, et al: The accuracy of the roentgenologic diagnosis of chronic pulmonary emphysema. Am Rev Respir Dis 93:889, 1966.

202. Reich SB, Weinshelbaum A, Yee J: Correlation of radiographic measurements and pulmonary function tests in chronic obstructive pulmonary disease. Am J Roentgenol 144:695, 1985.

203. Burki NK: Conventional chest films can identify air flow obstruction. Chest 93:675, 1988.

204. Pratt PC: Chest radiographs cannot identify airflow obstruction (letter). Chest 93:1120, 1988.

205. Lohela P, Sutinen S, Pääkkö P, et al: Diagnosis of emphysema on chest radiographs. Fortschr Geb Röntgenstr Nuklearmed Erganzungsband 141:395, 1984.

206. Thurlbeck WM, Müller NL: Emphysema: Definition, imaging, and quantification. Am J Roentgenol 163:1017, 1994.

207. Austin JHM, Müller NL, Friedman PJ, et al: Glossary of terms for CT of the lungs: Recommendations of the Nomenclature Committee of the Fleischner Society. Radiology 200:327, 1996.

208. Miller RR, Müller N, Vedal S, et al: Limitations of computed tomography in the assessment of emphysema. Am Rev Respir Dis 139:980, 1989.

209. Webb WR, Stein MG, Finkbeiner WE, et al: Normal and diseased isolated lungs: High-resolution CT. Radiology 166:81, 1988.

210. Bonelli FS, Hartman TE, Swensen SJ, et al: Accuracy of high-resolution CT in diagnosing lung diseases. Am J Roentgenol 170:1507, 1998.

211. Foster WL Jr, Pratt PC, Roggli VL, et al: Centrilobular emphysema: CT-pathologic correlation. Radiology 159:27, 1986.

212. Hruban RH, Meziane MA, Zerhouni EA, et al: High resolution computed tomography of inflation-fixed lungs: Pathologic-radiologic correlation of centrilobular emphysema. Am Rev Respir Dis 136:935, 1987.

213. Spouge D, Mayo JR, Cardoso W, et al: Panacinar emphysema: CT and pathologic findings. J Comput Assist Tomogr 17:710, 1993.

214. Kuwano K, Matsuba K, Ikeda T, et al: The diagnosis of mild emphysema: Correlation of computed tomography and pathologic scores. Am Rev Respir Dis 141:169, 1990.

215. Müller NL, Miller RR, Abboud RT: "Density mask": An objective method to quantitate emphysema using computed tomography. Chest 94:782, 1988.

216. Gevenois PA, de Maertelaer V, de Vuyst P, et al: Comparison of computed density and macroscopic morphometry in pulmonary emphysema. Am J Respir Crit Care Med 152:653, 1995.

217. Gevenois PA, de Vuyst P, Sy M, et al: Pulmonary emphysema: Quantitative CT during expiration. Radiology 199:825, 1996.

218. Gevenois PA, Koob MC, Jacobovitz D, et al: Whole lung sections for CT-pathologic correlations: Modified Gough-Wentworth technique. Invest Radiol 28:242, 1993.

219. Remy-Jardin M, Remy J, Gosselin B, et al: Sliding thin slab, minimum intensity projection technique in the diagnosis of emphysema: Histopathologic-CT correlation. Radiology 200:665, 1996.

220. Bergin CJ, Müller NL, Miller RR: CT in the qualitative assessment of emphysema. J Thorac Imaging 1:94, 1986.

221. Napel S, Rubin GD, Jeffrey RB: STS-MIP: A new reconstruction technique for CT of the chest. J Comput Assist Tomogr 17:832, 1993.

222. Welch MH, Reinecke ME, Hammarsten JF, et al: Antitrypsin deficiency in pulmonary disease: The significance of intermediate levels. Ann Intern Med 71:533, 1969.

223. Bell RS: The radiographic manifestations of alpha-1 antitrypsin deficiency: An important recognizable pattern of chronic obstructive pulmonary disease (COPD). Radiology 95:19, 1970.

224. Rosen RA, Dalinka MK, Gralino BJ Jr, et al: The roentgenographic findings in alpha-1 antitrypsin deficiency (AAD). Radiology 95:25, 1970.

225. Guest PJ, Hansell DM: High resolution computed tomography (HRCT) in emphysema associated with alpha-1-antitrypsin deficiency. Clin Radiol 45:260, 1992.

226. Cartier Y, Nogueira HA, Müller NL. Fibrosing mediastinitis associated with Riedel's thyroiditis—computed tomographic findings: Case report. Can Assoc Radiol J 49:408, 1998.

227. Lynch DA, Newell J, Hale V, et al: Correlation of CT findings with clinical evaluations in 261 patients with symptomatic bronchiectasis. Am J Roentgenol 173:53, 1999.

228. Helbich TH, Heinz-Peer G, Eichler I, et al: Cystic fibrosis: CT assessment of lung involvement in children and adults. Radiology 213:537, 1999.

229. Cartier Y, Kavanagh P, Johkoh T, et al: Bronchiectasis: Accuracy of high-resolution CT in the differentiation of specific diseases. Am J Roentgenol 173:47, 1999.

230. Heyneman LE, Ward S, Lynch DA, et al: Respiratory bronchiolitis, respiratory bronchiolitis-associated interstitial lung disease, and desquamative interstitial pneumonia: Different entities or part of the spectrum of the same disease process? Am J Roentgenol 173:1617, 1999.

231. Howling SJ, Hansell DM, Wells AU, et al: Follicular bronchiolitis: Thin-section CT and histologic findings. Radiology 212:637, 1999.

232. Webb EM, Elicker BM, Webb WR: Using CT to diagnose nonneoplastic tracheal abnormalities: Appearance of the tracheal wall. Am J Roentgenol 174:1315, 2000.

233. King GG, Müller NL, Whittall KP, et al: An analysis algorithm for measuring airway lumen and wall areas from high-resolution computed tomographic data. Am J Respir Crit Care Med 161:574, 2000.

234. Mason AC, Kakielna BEM: Newly diagnosed cystic fibrosis in adults: Pattern and distribution of bronchiectasis in 12 cases. Clin Radiol 54:507, 1999.

235. King MA, Stone JA, Diaz PT, et al: α_1-Antitrypsin deficiency: Evaluation of bronchiectasis with CT. Radiology 199:137, 1996.

236. Shin MS, Ho KJ: Bronchiectasis in patients with α_1-antitrypsin deficiency: A rare occurrence? Chest 104:1384, 1993.

237. Jones DK, Godden D, Cavanagh P: Alpha-1-antitrypsin deficiency presenting as bronchiectasis. Br J Dis Chest 79:301, 1985.

238. Sakai N, Michima M, Nishimura K, et al: An automated method to assess the distribution of low attenuation areas on chest CT scans in chronic pulmonary emphysema patients. Chest 106:1319, 1994.

239. Kazerooni EA, Whyte RI, Flint A, et al: Imaging of emphysema and lung volume reduction surgery. Radiographics 17:1023, 1997.

240. Mergo PJ, Williams WF, Gonzalez-Rothi R, et al: Three-dimensional volumetric assessment of abnormally low attenuation of the lung from routine helical CT: Inspiratory and expiratory quantification. Am J Roentgenol 170:1355, 1998.

241. Müller NL, Thurlbeck WM: Thin-section CT, emphysema, air trapping and airway obstruction. Radiology 199:621, 1996.

242. Zerhouni EA, Boukadoum M, Siddiky MA, et al: A standard phantom for quantitative CT analysis of pulmonary nodules. Radiology 149:767, 1983.

243. Kinsella M, Müller NL, Abboud RT, et al: Quantitation of emphysema by computed tomography using a "density mask" program and correlation with pulmonary function tests. Chest 97:315, 1990.

244. Bae KT, Slone RM, Gierada DS, et al: Patients with emphysema: Quantitative CT analysis before and after lung volume reduction surgery: Work in progress. Radiology 203:705, 1997.

245. Gierada DS, Hakimian S, Slone RM: MR analysis of lung volume and thoracic dimensions in patients with emphysema before and after lung volume reduction surgery. Am J Roentgenol 170:707, 1998.

246. Takasugi JE, Wood DE, Godwin JD, et al: Lung-volume reduction surgery for diffuse emphysema: Radiologic assessment of changes in thoracic dimensions. J Thorac Imaging 13:36, 1998.

247. Holbert JM, Brown ML, Sciurba FC, et al: Changes in lung volume and volume of emphysema after unilateral lung reduction surgery: Analysis with CT lung densitometry. Radiology 201:793, 1996.

248. Laurenzi GA, Turino GM, Fishman AP: Bullous disease of the lung. Am J Med 32:361, 1962.

249. Boushy SF, Kohen R, Billig DM, et al: Bullous emphysema: Clinical, roentgenologic and physiologic study of 49 patients. Dis Chest 54:327, 1968.

250. Viola AR, Zuffardi EA: Physiologic and clinical aspects of pulmonary bullous disease. Am Rev Respir Dis 94:574, 1966.

251. Stone DJ, Schwartz A, Feltman JA: Bullous emphysema: A long-term study of the natural history and the effects of therapy. Am Rev Respir Dis 82:493, 1960.

252. Richards DW: Pulmonary emphysema: Etiologic factors and clinical forms. Ann Intern Med 53:1105, 1960.

253. Gibson GJ: Familial pneumothoraces and bullae. Thorax 32:88, 1977.

254. Wood JR, Bellamy D, Child AH, et al: Pulmonary disease in patients with Marfan syndrome. Thorax 39:780, 1984.

255. Ayers JG, Pope FM, Reudy JF, et al: Abnormalities of the lungs and thoracic cage in the Ehlers-Danlos syndrome. Thorax 40:300, 1985.

256. Morgan MD, Denison DM, Strickland B, et al: Value of computed tomography for selecting patients with bullous lung disease for surgery. Thorax 41:855, 1986.

257. Gaensler E, Jederlinic P, FitzGerald M: Patient work-up for bullectomy. J Thorac Imaging 1:75, 1986.

258. Stern EJ, Webb WR, Weinacker A, et al: Idiopathic giant bullous emphysema (vanishing lung syndrome): Imaging findings in nine patients. Am J Roentgenol 162:279, 1994.

259. Gierada DS, Glazer HS, Slone RM: Pseudomass due to atelectasis in patients with severe bullous emphysema. Am J Roentgenol 168:85, 1997.

260. Worthy SA, Brown MJ, Müller NL: Cystic air spaces in the lung: Change in size on expiratory high-resolution CT in 23 patients. Clin Radiol 53:515, 1998.

261. Rubin EH, Buchberg AS: Capricious behavior of pulmonary bullae developing fluid. Dis Chest 54:546, 1968.

262. Goodman RB, Lakshminarayan S: Images in clinical medicine: Inflammatory autobullectomy. N Engl J Med 334:1372, 1996.

263. Jay SJ, Johanson WG Jr: Massive intrapulmonary hemorrhage: An uncommon complication of bullous emphysema. Am Rev Respir Dis 110:497, 1974.

264. Berry BE, Ochsner A Jr: Massive hemoptysis associated with localized pulmonary bullae requiring emergency surgery: A case report. J Thorac Cardiovasc Surg 63:94, 1972.

265. Grimes OF, Farber SM: Air cysts of the lung. Surg Gynecol Obstet 113:720, 1961.

266. Bersack SR: Fluid collection in emphysematous bullae. Am J Roentgenol 83:283, 1960.

267. Stark P, Gadziala N, Green R: Fluid accumulation in preexisting pulmonary air spaces. Am J Roentgenol 134:701, 1980.

268. Jordan KG, Kwong JS, Flint J, et al: Surgically treated pneumothorax: Radiologic and pathologic findings. Chest 111:280, 1997.

269. Mitlehner W, Friedrich M, Dissmann W: Value of computed tomography in the detection of bullae and blebs in patients with primary spontaneous pneumothorax. Respiration 59:221, 1992.

270. Lesur O, Delorme N, Fromaget JM, et al: Computed tomography in the etiologic assessment of idiopathic spontaneous pneumothorax. Chest 98:341, 1990.

271. Bense L, Lewander R, Eklund G, et al: Nonsmoking, non-alpha₁-antitrypsin deficiency-induced emphysema in nonsmokers with healed spontaneous pneumothorax, identified by computed tomography of the lungs. Chest 103:433, 1993.

272. Bourgouin P, Cousineau G, Lemire P, et al: Computed tomography used to exclude pneumothorax in bullous lung disease. J Can Assoc Radiol 36:341, 1985.

273. Pierce JA, Growdon JH: Physical properties of the lungs in giant cysts: Report of a case treated surgically. N Engl J Med 267:169, 1962.

274. Neidhart P, Suter PM: Pulmonary bullae and sudden death in a young aeroplane passenger. Intensive Care Med 11:45, 1985.

275. Glauser EM, Cook CD, Harris GBC: Bronchiectasis: A review of 187 cases in children with follow-up pulmonary function studies in 58. Acta Paediatr Scand 165(Suppl):1, 1966.

276. Sanderson JM, Kennedy MCS, Johnson MF, et al: Bronchiectasis: Results of surgical and conservative management (a review of 393 cases). Thorax 29:407, 1974.

277. Bard M, Couderc LJ, Saimot AG, et al: Accelerated obstructive pulmonary disease in HIV infected patients with bronchiectasis. Eur Respir J 11:771, 1998.

278. Loubeyre P, Revel D, Delignette A, et al: Bronchiectasis detected with thin-section CT as a predictor of chronic lung allograft rejection. Radiology 194:213, 1995.

279. Morehead RS: Bronchiectasis in bone marrow transplantation. Thorax 52:390, 1997.

280. Smith IE, Flower CDR: Review article: Imaging in bronchiectasis. Br J Radiol 69:589, 1996.

281. McGuinness G, Naidich DP: Bronchiectasis: CT/clinical correlations. Semin Ultrasound CT MRI 16:395, 1995.

282. Gudbjerg CE: Bronchiectasis: Radiological diagnosis and prognosis after operative treatment. Acta Radiol (Suppl):143, 1957.

283. Gudbjerg CE: Roentgenologic diagnosis of bronchiectasis: An analysis of 112 cases. Acta Radiol 43:209, 1955.

284. Munro NC, Han LY, Currie DC, et al: Radiologic evidence of progression of bronchiectasis. Respir Med 86:397, 1992.

285. van der Bruggen-Bogaarts BAHA, van der Bruggen HMJG, van Waes PFGM, et al: Screening for bronchiectasis: A comparative study between chest radiography and high-resolution CT. Chest 109:608, 1996.

286. Bateson EM, Woo-Ming M: Destroyed lung: A report of cases in West Indians and Australian aborigines. Clin Radiol 27:223, 1976.

287. Currie DC, Cooke JC, Morgan AD, et al: Interpretation of bronchograms and chest radiographs in patients with chronic sputum production. Thorax 42:278, 1987.

288. Grenier P, Maurice F, Musset D, et al: Bronchiectasis: Assessment by thin-section CT. Radiology 161:95, 1986.

289. Young K, Aspestrand F, Kolbenstvedt A: High-resolution CT and bronchography in the assessment of bronchiectasis. Acta Radiol 32:439, 1991.

290. Kang EY, Miller RR, Müller NL: Bronchiectasis: Comparison of preoperative thin-section CT and pathologic findings in resected specimens. Radiology 195:649, 1995.

291. Kim JS, Müller NL, Park CS, et al: Cylindrical bronchiectasis: Diagnostic findings on thin-section CT. Am J Roentgenol 168:751, 1997.

292. McGuinness G, Naidich DP, Leitman BS, et al: Pictorial essay: Bronchiectasis: CT evaluation. Am J Roentgenol 160:253, 1993.

293. Naidich DP, McCauley DI, Khouri NF, et al: Computed tomography of bronchiectasis. J Comput Assist Tomogr 6:437, 1982.

294. Remy-Jardin M, Remy J: Comparison of vertical and oblique CT in evaluation of bronchial tree. J Comput Assist Tomogr 12:956, 1988.

295. Pontius JR, Jacobs LG: The reversal of advanced bronchiectasis. Radiology 68:204, 1957.

296. Nelson SW, Christoforidis A: Reversible bronchiectasis. Radiology 71:375, 1958.

297. Tarver RD, Conces DJ, Godwin JD: Motion artifacts on CT simulate bronchiectasis. Am J Roentgenol 151:1117, 1988.

298. Lucidarme O, Grenier P, Coche E, et al: Bronchiectasis: Comparative assessment with thin-section CT and helical CT. Radiology 200:673, 1996.

299. Joharjy IA, Bashi SA, Abdullah AK: Value of medium-thickness CT in the diagnosis of bronchiectasis. Am J Roentgenol 149:1133, 1987.

300. Müller NL, Bergin CJ, Ostrow DN, et al: Role of computed tomography in the recognition of bronchiectasis. Am J Roentgenol 143:971, 1984.

301. Silverman PM, Godwin DJ: CT-bronchographic correlations in bronchiectasis. J Comput Assist Tomogr 11:52, 1987.

302. Hansell DM, Wells AU, Rubens MB, et al: Bronchiectasis: Functional significance of areas of decreased attenuation at expiratory CT. Radiology 193:369, 1994.

303. Thomas RD, Blaquiere RM: Reactive mediastinal lymphadenopathy in bronchiectasis assessed by CT. Acta Radiol 34:489, 1993.

304. Don CJ, Dales RE, Desmarais RL, et al: The radiographic prevalence of hilar and mediastinal adenopathy in adult cystic fibrosis. Can Assoc Radiol J 48:265, 1997.

305. Song J-W, Im J-G, Shim Y-S, et al: Hypertrophied bronchial artery at thin-section CT in patients with bronchiectasis: Correlation with CT angiographic findings. Radiology 208:187, 1998.

306. Morcos SK, Baudouin SV, Anderson PB, et al: Iotrolan in selective bronchography via the fiberoptic bronchoscope. Br J Radiol 62:383, 1989.

307. Morcos SK, Anderson PB, Kennedy A: Bronchography with iotrolan 300 via the flexible bronchoscope in the evaluation of focal lung opacity. J Bronchol 1:112, 1994.

308. Morcos SK, Anderson PB, Baudouin SV, et al. Suitability of and tolerance to iotrolan 300 in bronchography via the fiberoptic bronchoscope. Thorax 45:628, 1990.

309. Naidich DP, Harkin TJ: Airways and lung: CT versus bronchography through the fiberoptic bronchoscope. Radiology 200:613, 1996.

310. Kartagener M: Zur Pathogenese der bronchiektasien; bronchiektasien bei situs viscerum inversus. Beitr Klin Tuberk 83:489, 1933.

311. Holmes LB, Blennerhassett JB, Austen KF: A reappraisal of Kartagener's syndrome. Am J Med Sci 255:13, 1968.

312. Rossman CM, Forrest JB, Lee RMKW: The dyskinetic cilia syndrome—abnormal ciliary motion in association with abnormal ciliary ultrastructure. Chest 80:860, 1981.

313. Kroon AA, Heij JM, Kuijper WA, et al: Function and morphology of respiratory cilia in situs inversus. Clin Otolaryngol 16:294, 1991.

314. Verra F, Escudier E, Bignon J, et al: Inherited factors in diffuse bronchiectasis in the adult: A prospective study. Eur Respir J 4:937, 1991.

315. Sturgess JM, Thompson MW, Czegledy-Nagy E, et al: Genetic aspects of immotile cilia syndrome. Am J Med Genet 25:149, 1986.

316. Chao J, Turner JA, Sturgess JM, et al: Genetic heterogeneity of dynein-deficiency in cilia from patients with respiratory disease. Am Rev Respir Dis 126:302, 1982.

317. Nadel HR, Stringer DA, Levison H, et al: The immotile cilia syndrome: Radiological manifestations. Radiology 154:651, 1985.

318. Reiff DB, Wells AU, Carr DH, et al: CT findings in bronchiectasis: Limited value in distinguishing between idiopathic and specific types. Am J Roentgenol 165:261, 1995.

319. Handelsman DJ, Conway AJ, Boylan LM, et al: Young's syndrome: Obstructive azoospermia and chronic sinopulmonary infections. N Engl J Med 310:3, 1984.

320. Le Lannou D, Jezequel P, Blayau M, et al: Obstructive azoospermia with agenesis of vas deferens or with bronchiectasia (Young's syndrome): A genetic approach. Hum Reprod 10:338, 1995.

321. Schanker HM, Rajfer J, Saxon A: Recurrent respiratory disease, azoospermia, and nasal polyposis: A syndrome that mimics cystic fibrosis and immotile cilia syndrome. Arch Intern Med 145:2201, 1985.

322. Hughes TM, Skolnick JL, Belker AM: Young's syndrome: An often unrecognized correctable cause of obstructive azoospermia. J Urol 137:1238, 1987.

323. Hiller E, Rosenow EC III, Olsen AM: Pulmonary manifestations of the yellow nail syndrome. Chest 61:452, 1972.

324. Bowers D: Unequal breasts, yellow nails, bronchiectasis and lymphedema. Can Med Assoc J 100:437, 1969.

325. Dilley JJ, Kierland RR, Randall RV, et al: Primary lymphedema associated with yellow nails and pleural effusions. JAMA 204:670, 1968.

326. Kaneko K, Kudo S, Tashiro M, et al: Case report: Computed tomography findings in Williams-Campbell syndrome. J Thorac Imaging 6:11, 1991.

327. Hartman TE, Primack SL, Lee KS, et al: CT of bronchial and bronchiolar diseases. Radiographics 14:991, 1994.

328. McAdams HP, Erasmus J: Chest case of the day: Williams-Campbell syndrome. Am J Roentgenol 165:190, 1995.

329. Weed LA, Andersen HA: Etiology of broncholithiasis. Dis Chest 37:270, 1960.

330. Vix VA: Radiographic manifestations of broncholithiasis. Radiology 128:295, 1978.

331. Gurney JW, Conces DJ Jr: Pulmonary histoplasmosis. Radiology 199:297, 1996.

332. Conces DJ Jr: Histoplasmosis. Semin Roentgenol 1:14, 1996.

333. Adler O, Peleg H: Computed tomography in the diagnosis of broncholithiasis. Eur J Radiol 7:211, 1987.

334. Conces DJ, Tarver RD, Vix VA: Broncholithiasis: CT features in 15 patients. Am J Roentgenol 157:249, 1991.

335. Hollaus PH, Lax F, el-Nashef BB, et al: Natural history of bronchopleural fistula after pneumonectomy: A review of 96 cases. Ann Thorac Surg 63:1391, 1997.

336. Lauckner ME, Beggs I, Armstrong RF: The radiological characteristics of bronchopleural fistula following pneumonectomy. Anaesthesia 38:452, 1983.

337. Powner DJ, Bierman MI: Thoracic and extrathoracic bronchial fistulas. Chest 100:480, 1991.

338. Stern EJ, Sun H, Haramati LB: Peripheral bronchopleural fistulas: CT imaging features. Am J Roentgenol 167:117, 1996.

339. Westcott JL, Volpe JP: Peripheral bronchopleural fistula: CT evaluation in 20 patients with pneumonia, empyema, or postoperative air leak. Radiology 196:175, 1995.

340. Vogel N, Wolcke B, Kauczor HU, et al: Detection of a bronchopleural fistula with spiral CT and 3D reconstruction. Aktuelle Radiol 5:176, 1995.

341. Wood RE, Boat TF, Doershuk CF: Cystic fibrosis. Am Rev Respir Dis 113:833, 1976.

342. Addington WW, Cugell DW, Zelkowitz PS, et al: Cystic fibrosis of the pancreas: A comparison of the pulmonary manifestations in children and young adults. Chest 59:306, 1971.

343. Rosenstein BJ, Langbaum TS, Metz SJ, et al: Cystic fibrosis: Diagnostic considerations. Johns Hopkins Med J 150:113, 1982.

344. Bye MR, Ewig JM, Quittell LM: Cystic fibrosis. Lung 172:251, 1994.

345. Hunt B, Geddes DM: Newly diagnosed cystic fibrosis in middle and later life. Thorax 40:23, 1985.

346. Fitzpatrick SB, Rosenstein BJ, Langbaum TS, et al: Diagnosis of cystic fibrosis during adolescence. J Adolesc Health Care 7:38, 1986.

347. Bowman BH, Mangos JA: Current concepts in genetics: Cystic fibrosis. N Engl J Med 294:937, 1976.

348. Klinger JD, Thomassen MJ: Occurrence and antimicrobial susceptibility of gram-negative nonfermentative bacilli in cystic fibrosis patients. Diagn Microbiol Infect Dis 3:149, 1985.

349. Tomashefski JF Jr, Bruce M, Stern RC, et al: Pulmonary air cysts in cystic fibrosis: Relation of pathologic features to radiologic findings and history of pneumothorax. Hum Pathol 16:253, 1985.

350. Friedman PJ, Harwood IR, Ellenbogen PH: Pulmonary cystic fibrosis in the adult: Early and late radiologic findings with pathologic correlation. Am J Roentgenol 136:1131, 1981.

351. Mitchell-Heggs P, Mearns M, Batten JC: Cystic fibrosis in adolescents and adults. QJM 179:479, 1976.

352. Cleveland RH, Neish AS, Zurakowski D, et al: Cystic fibrosis: A system for assessing and predicting progression. Am J Roentgenol 170:1067, 1998.

353. Wood BP: Cystic fibrosis: 1997. Radiology 204:1, 1997.

354. Waring WW, Brunt CH, Hilman BC: Mucoid impaction of the bronchi in cystic fibrosis. Pediatrics 39:166, 1967.

355. Friedman PJ: Chest radiographic findings in the adult with cystic fibrosis. Semin Roentgenol 22:114, 1987.

356. Grum CM, Lynch JP III: Chest radiographic findings in cystic fibrosis. Semin Respir Infect 7:193, 1992.

357. Griscom NT, Vawter GF, Stigol LC: Radiologic and pathologic abnormalities of the trachea in older patients with cystic fibrosis. Am J Roentgenol 148:691, 1987.

358. Shale DJ: Chest radiology in cystic fibrosis: Is scoring useful? Thorax 49:847, 1994.

359. Lewiston N, Moss R, Hindi R, et al: Interobserver variance in clinical scoring for cystic fibrosis. Chest 91:879, 1987.

360. Rosenberg SM, Howatt WF, Grum CM: Spirometry and chest roentgenographic appearance in adults with cystic fibrosis. Chest 101:961, 1992.

361. Taussig LM, Kattwinkel J, Friedwald WT, et al: A new prognostic score and clinical evaluation system for cystic fibrosis. J Pediatr 82:380, 1973.

362. Sawyer SM, Carlin JB, DeCampo M, et al: Critical evaluation of three chest radiographic scores in cystic fibrosis. Thorax 49:863, 1994.

363. Crispin A, Norman A: The systematic evaluation of the chest radiograph in cystic fibrosis. Pediatr Radiol 2:101, 1974.

364. Conway SP, Pond MN, Bowler I, et al: The chest radiograph in cystic fibrosis: A new scoring system compared with the Chrispin-Norman and Brasfield scores. Thorax 49:860, 1994.

365. Murata K, Itoh H, Todo G: Centrilobular lesions of the lung: Demonstrated by high-resolution CT and pathologic correlation. Radiology 161:641, 1986.

366. Friedman PJ: Radiology of the airways with emphasis on the small airways. J Thorac Imaging 1:7, 1986.

367. Santis G, Hodson ME, Strickland B: High-resolution computed tomography in adult cystic fibrosis patients with mild lung disease. Clin Radiol 44:20, 1991.

368. Lynch DA, Brasch RC, Hardy KA, et al: Pediatric pulmonary disease: Assessment with high-resolution ultrafast CT. Radiology 176:243, 1990.

369. Jacobsen LE, Houston CS, Habbick BF, et al: Cystic fibrosis: A comparison of computed tomography and plain chest radiographs. J Can Assoc Rad 37:17, 1986.

370. Bhalla M, Turcios N, Aponte N, et al: Cystic fibrosis: Scoring system with thin section CT. Radiology 179:783, 1991.

371. Greene KE, Takasugi JE, Godwin JD, et al: Radiographic changes in acute exacerbations of cystic fibrosis in adults: A pilot study. Am J Roentgenol 163:557, 1994.

372. Shah RM, Sexauer W, Ostrum BJ, et al: High-resolution CT in the acute exacerbation of cystic fibrosis: Evaluation of acute findings, reversibility of those findings, and clinical correlation. Am J Roentgenol 169:375, 1997.

373. Amorosa JK, Laraya-Cuasay LR, Sohn L, et al: Radiologic diagnosis of cystic fibrosis in adults and children. Acad Radiol 2:222, 1995.

374. Shah RM, Friedman AC, Ostrum BJ, et al: Pulmonary complications of cystic fibrosis in adults. Crit Rev Diagn Imaging 36:441, 1995.

375. Fiel SB, Friedman AC, Caroline DF, et al: Magnetic resonance imaging in young adults with cystic fibrosis. Chest 91:181, 1987.

376. Shepherd RW, Holt TL, Thomas BJ, et al: Nutritional rehabilitation in cystic fibrosis: Controlled studies of effects on nutritional growth retardation, body protein turnover, and course of pulmonary disease. J Pediatr 109:788, 1986.

377. Gilljam H, Malmborg AS, Strandvik B: Conformity of bacterial growth in sputum and contamination free endobronchial samples in patients with cystic fibrosis. Thorax 41:641, 1986.

378. Jones JD, Steige H, Logan GB: Variations of sweat sodium values in children and adults with cystic fibrosis and other diseases. Mayo Clin Proc 45:768, 1970.

379. Bai T, Eidelman DH, Hogg JC, et al: Proposed nomenclature for quantifying subdivisions of the bronchial wall. J Appl Physiol 77:1011, 1994.

380. Epler GR, Colby TV: The spectrum of bronchiolitis obliterans. Chest 83:161, 1983.

381. Epler GR, Colby TV, McLoud TC, et al: Bronchiolitis obliterans organizing pneumonia. N Engl J Med 312:152, 1985.

382. Davison AG, Heard BE, McAllister WAC, et al: Steroid-responsive relapsing cryptogenic organising pneumonitis. Thorax 37:785, 1982.

383. Davison AG, Heard BE, McAllister WAC, et al: Cryptogenic organizing pneumonia. QJM 52:382, 1983.

384. du Bois RM, Geddes DM: Obliterative bronchiolitis, cryptogenic organizing pneumonia and bronchiolitis obliterans organizing pneumonia: Three names for two different conditions. Eur Respir J 4:774, 1991.

385. McLoud T, Epler G, Colby T, et al: Bronchiolitis obliterans. Radiology 159:1, 1986.

386. Sweatman M, Millar A, Strickland B, et al: Computed tomography in adult obliterative bronchiolitis. Clin Radiol 41:116, 1990.

387. Davies HD, Wang EE, Manson D, et al: Reliability of the chest radiograph in the diagnosis of lower respiratory infections in young children. Pediatr Infect Dis J 15:600, 1996.

388. Babcook CJ, Norman GR, Coblentz CL: Effect of clinical history on the interpretation of chest radiographs in childhood bronchiolitis. Invest Radiol 28:214, 1993.

389. Dawson KP, Long A, Kennedy J, et al: The chest radiograph in acute bronchiolitis. J Paediatr Child Health 26:209, 1990.

390. Lynch DA: Imaging of small airways diseases. Clin Chest Med 14:623, 1993.

391. Müller NL, Miller RR: Diseases of the bronchioles: CT and histopathologic findings. Radiology 196:3, 1995.

392. Worthy SA, Flint JD, Müller NL: Pulmonary complications after bone marrow transplantation: High-resolution CT and pathologic findings. Radiographics 17:1359, 1997.

393. Logan PM, Primack SL, Miller RR, et al: Invasive aspergillosis of the airways: Radiographic, CT and pathologic findings. Radiology 193:383, 1994.

394. Im J-G, Itoh H, Shim Y-S, et al: Pulmonary tuberculosis: CT findings: Early active disease and sequential change with antituberculous therapy. Radiology 186:653, 1993.

395. Nishimura K, Kitaichi M, Izumi T, et al: Diffuse panbronchiolitis: Correlation of high-resolution CT and pathologic findings. Radiology 184:779, 1992.

396. Akira M, Higashihara T, Sakatani M, et al: Diffuse panbronchiolitis: Follow-up CT examination. Radiology 189:559, 1993.

397. Akira M, Kitatani F, Yong-Sik L, et al: Diffuse panbronchiolitis: Evaluation with high-resolution CT. Radiology 168:433, 1988.

398. Gruden JF, Webb WR, Warnock M: Centrilobular opacities in the lung on high-resolution CT: Diagnostic considerations and pathologic correlation. Am J Roentgenol 162:569, 1994.

399. Remy-Jardin M, Remy J, Gosselin B, et al: Lung parenchymal changes secondary to cigarette smoking: Pathologic-CT correlations. Radiology 186:643, 1993.

400. Padley SPG, Adler BD, Hansell DM, et al: Bronchiolitis obliterans: High resolution CT findings and correlation with pulmonary function tests. Clin Radiol 47:236, 1993.

401. Worthy SA, Park CS, Kim JS, et al: Bronchiolitis obliterans after lung transplantation: High-resolution CT findings in 15 patients. Am J Roentgenol 169:673, 1997.

402. Leung AN, Fisher K, Valentine V, et al: Bronchiolitis obliterans after lung transplantation: Detection using expiratory HRCT. Chest 113:365, 1998.

403. Stern EJ, Frank MS: Small airway diseases of the lungs: Findings at expiratory CT. Am J Roentgenol 163:37, 1994.

404. Desai SR, Hansell DM: Small airways disease: Expiratory computed tomography comes of age. Clin Radiol 52:332, 1997.

405. Webb WR, Stern EJ, Nanth N, et al: Dynamic pulmonary CT: Findings in healthy adult men. Radiology 186:117, 1993.

406. Brown MJ, English J, Müller NL: Bronchiolitis obliterans due to neuroendocrine hyperplasia: High-resolution CT-pathologic correlation. Am J Roentgenol 168:1561, 1997.

407. Hansell DM, Wells AU, Padley SP, et al: Hypersensitivity pneumonitis: Correlation of individual CT patterns with functional abnormalities. Radiology 199:123, 1996.

408. Small JH, Flower CDR, Traill ZC, et al: Air-trapping in extrinsic allergic alveolitis on computed tomography. Clin Radiol 51:684, 1996.

409. King GG, Müller NL, Paré PD: Pulmonary perspective: Evaluation of airways in obstructive lung disease using high-resolution CT. Am J Respir Crit Care Med 159:992, 1999.

410. Worthy SA, Müller NL, Hartman TE, et al: Mosaic attenuation pattern on thin-section CT scans of the lung: Differentiation among infiltrative lung, airway, and vascular diseases as a cause. Radiology 205:465, 1997.

411. Müller NL, Staples CA, Miller RR: Bronchiolitis obliterans organizing pneumonia: CT features in 14 patients. Am J Roentgenol 154:983, 1990.

412. Lee KS, Kullnig P, Hartman TE, et al: Cryptogenic organizing pneumonia: CT findings in 43 patients. Am J Roentgenol 162:543, 1994.

413. Holt RM, Schmidt RA, Godwin JD, et al: High resolution CT in respiratory bronchiolitis-associated interstitial lung disease. J Comput Assist Tomogr 17:46, 1993.

414. Nishimura K, Itoh H: High-resolution computed tomographic fea-

tures of bronchiolitis obliterans organizing pneumonia. Chest 102(Suppl):26S, 1992.

415. Wright JL: Inhalational lung injury causing bronchiolitis. Clin Chest Med 14:635, 1993.

416. Kirkpatrick B, Bass JB: Severe obstructive lung disease after smoke inhalation. Chest 76:108, 1979.

417. Swyer PR, James GCW: A case of unilateral pulmonary emphysema. Thorax 8:133, 1953.

418. MacLeod WM: Abnormal transradiancy of one lung. Thorax 9:147, 1954.

419. Ohri SK, Rutty G, Foundation SW: Acquired segmental emphysema: The enlarging spectrum of Swyer-James/Macleod's syndrome. Ann Thorac Surg 56:120, 1993.

420. Warrell DA, Hughes JMB, Rosenzweig DY: Cardiopulmonary performance at rest and during exercise in seven patients with increased transradiancy of one lung (Macleod's syndrome). Thorax 25:587, 1970.

421. Reid LM, Millard FJC: Correlation between radiological diagnosis and structural lung changes in emphysema. Clin Radiol 15:307, 1964.

422. Houk VN, Kent DC, Fosburg RG: Unilateral hyperlucent lung: A study in pathophysiology and etiology. Am J Med Sci 253:406, 1967.

423. Leahy DJ: Increased transradiancy of one lung. Br J Dis Chest 55:72, 1961.

424. Peters ME, Dickie HA, Crummy AB, et al: Swyer-James-Macleod syndrome: A case with a baseline normal chest radiograph. Pediatr Radiol 12:211, 1982.

425. Gold RE, Wilt JC, Adhikari TK, et al: Adenoviral pneumonia and its complications in infancy and childhood. J Can Assoc Radiol 20:218, 1969.

426. Culiner MM: The hyperlucent lung, a problem in differential diagnosis. Dis Chest 49:578, 1966.

427. Reid L, Simon G: Unilateral lung transradiancy. Thorax 17:230, 1962.

428. Margolin HN, Rosenberg LS, Felson B, et al: Idiopathic unilateral hyperlucent lung: A roentgenographic syndrome. Am J Roentgenol 82:63, 1959.

429. Ghossain MA, Achkar A, Buy JN, et al: Swyer-James syndrome documented by spiral CT angiography and high resolution inspiratory and expiratory CT: An accurate single modality exploration. J Comput Assist Tomogr 21:616, 1997.

430. Marti-Bonmati L, Perales FR, Catala F, et al: CT findings in Swyer-James syndrome. Radiology 172:477, 1989.

431. Moore ADA, Godwin JD, Dietrich PA, et al: Swyer-James syndrome: CT findings in eight patients. Am J Roentgenol 158:1211, 1992.

432. McKenzie SA, Allison DJ, Singh MP, et al: Unilateral hyperlucent lung: The case for investigation. Thorax 35:745, 1980.

433. Salmanzadeh A, Pomeranz SJ, Ramsingh PS: Ventilation-perfusion scintigraphic correlation with multimodality imaging in a proven case of Swyer-James (Macleod's) syndrome. Clin Nucl Med 22:115, 1997.

434. Daniel TL, Woodring JH, Vandiviere HM, et al: Swyer-James syndrome: Unilateral hyperlucent lung syndrome: A case report and review. Clin Geriatr 23:393, 1984.

435. Nairn JR, Prime FJ: A physiological study of Macleod's syndrome. Thorax 22:148, 1967.

436. Cordier JF: Cryptogenic organizing pneumonia. Clin Chest Med 14:677, 1993.

437. Yamamoto M, Ina Y, Kitaichi M, et al: Clinical features of BOOP in Japan. Chest 102(Suppl):21S, 1992.

438. Akira M, Yamamoto S, Sakatani M: Bronchiolitis obliterans organizing pneumonia manifesting as multiple large nodules or masses. Am J Roentgenol 170:291, 1998.

439. Chandler P, Shin M, Friedman S, et al: Radiographic manifestations of bronchiolitis obliterans with organizing pneumonia vs usual interstitial pneumonia. Am J Roentgenol 147:899, 1986.

440. Müller N, Guerry-Force ML, Staples C, et al: Differential diagnosis of bronchiolitis obliterans with organizing pneumonia and usual interstitial pneumonia: Clinical, functional, and radiologic findings. Radiology 162:151, 1987.

441. Cordier J, Loire R, Brune J: Idiopathic bronchiolitis obliterans organizing pneumonia. Chest 96:999, 1989.

442. Izumi T, Kitaichi M, Nishimura K, et al: Bronchiolitis obliterans organizing pneumonia: Clinical features and differential diagnosis. Chest 102:715, 1992.

443. Spiteri M, Klenerman P, Sheppard M, et al: Seasonal cryptogenic organizing pneumonia with biochemical cholestasis: A new clinical entity. Lancet 340:281, 1992.

444. Reich J, Scott D: Levitating lung lesions due to bronchiolitis obliterans organizing pneumonia. Chest 103:623, 1993.

445. Bouchardy LM, Kuhlman JE, Ball WC, et al: CT findings in bronchiolitis obliterans organizing pneumonia (BOOP) with radiographic, clinical and histologic correlation. J Comput Assist Tomogr 17:352, 1993.

446. Guerry-Force ML, Müller NL, Wright JL, et al: A comparison of bronchiolitis obliterans with organizing pneumonia, usual interstitial pneumonia, and small airway disease. Am Rev Respir Dis 135:705, 1987.

447. King TE Jr, Mortenson RL: Cryptogenic organizing pneumonia: The North American experience. Chest 102(Suppl 1):8S, 1992.

448. Cosio MG, Hale KA, Niewoehner DE: Morphologic and morphometric effects of prolonged smoking on the small airways. Am Rev Respir Dis 122:265, 1980.

449. Wright JL, Lawson LM, Paré PD, et al: Morphology of peripheral airways in current and ex-smokers. Am Rev Respir Dis 127:474, 1983.

450. Yousem SA, Colby TV, Gaensler EA: Respiratory bronchiolitis-associated interstitial lung disease and its relationship to desquamative interstitial pneumonitis. Mayo Clin Proc 64:1373, 1989.

451. King TE: Respiratory bronchiolitis-associated interstitial lung disease. Clin Chest Med 14:693, 1993.

452. Katzenstein AA, Myers JL: Idiopathic pulmonary fibrosis: Clinical relevance of pathologic classification. Am J Respir Crit Care Med 157:1301, 1998.

453. Myers JL, Veal CF, Shin MS, et al: Respiratory bronchiolitis causing interstitial lung disease: A clinico-pathologic study. Am Rev Respir Dis 135:880, 1987.

454. Yousem SA, Colby TV, Carrington CB: Follicular bronchitis/bronchiolitis. Hum Pathol 16:700, 1985.

455. Fortoul TL, Cano-Valle F, Oliva E, et al: Follicular bronchiolitis in association with connective tissue diseases. Lung 163:305, 1985.

456. Hayakawa H, Sato A, Imokawa S, et al: Bronchiolar disease in rheumatoid arthritis. Am J Respir Crit Care Med 154:1531, 1996.

457. Sugiyama Y: Diffuse panbronchiolitis. Clin Chest Med 14:765, 1993.

458. Iwata M, Colby TV, Kitaichi M: Diffuse panbronchiolitis: Diagnosis and distinction from various pulmonary diseases with centrilobular interstitial foam cell accumulations. Hum Pathol 25:357, 1994.

459. Homma H, Yamanaka A, Tanimoto S, et al: Diffuse panbronchiolitis: A disease of the transitional zone of the lung. Chest 83:63, 1983.

460. Kim YW, Han SK, Shim YS, et al: The first report of diffuse panbronchiolitis in Korea: Five case reports. Intern Med 31:695, 1992.

461. Maeda M, Saiki S, Yamanaka A: Serial section analysis of the lesions in diffuse panbronchiolitis. Acta Pathol Jpn 37:693, 1987.

462. Nakata K, Tanimoto H: Diffuse panbronchiolitis. Jpn J Clin Radiol 26:1133, 1981.

463. Ichikawa Y, Hotta M, Sumita S, et al: Reversible airway lesions in diffuse panbronchiolitis: Detection by high-resolution computed tomography. Chest 107:120, 1995.

464. Reid L: The Pathology of Emphysema. London, Lloyd-Luke (Medical Books) Ltd, 1967.

465. Grum CM, Lynch JP: Chest radiographic findings in cystic fibrosis. Semin Respir Infect 7:193, 1992.

466. Luckey P, Kemper J, Niehues T, et al: Diagnostic role of inspiration and expiration CT in a child with relapsing polychondritis. Am J Roentgenol 176:61, 2001.

467. Gilkeson RC, Ciancibello LM, Hejal RB, et al: Tracheobronchomalacia: Dynamic airway evaluation with multidetector CT. Am J Roentgenol 176:205, 2001.

CHAPTER 16

Pulmonary Disease Caused by Inhalation or Aspiration of Particulates, Solids, or Liquids

INHALATION OF ORGANIC DUST

Hypersensitivity Pneumonitis

The term *hypersensitivity pneumonitis* (extrinsic allergic alveolitis) denotes a group of diseases characterized by an abnormal immunologic reaction in the lung to specific antigens contained in a wide variety of organic dusts. The most common diseases are farmer's lung and bird-fancier's lung (Table 16–1) Regardless of the name of the disease and the specific exposure involved, striking similarities exist among the clinical, pathologic, and radiologic features of all these diseases, suggesting that they share a common pathogenesis.

The histologic appearance consists of a combination of bronchiolitis and alveolitis with granuloma formation.[4, 6, 7] The alveolitis consists of interstitial and intra-alveolar components and is seen in virtually all cases. Within the interstitium, there is an inflammatory infiltrate that consists predominantly of lymphocytes accompanied by variable numbers of histiocytes, plasma cells, polymorphonuclear leukocytes, and eosinophils. The infiltrate usually is patchy in distribution with a tendency to more severe involvement of peribronchiolar regions; uncommonly, it is extensive and confluent.

Loosely formed granulomas composed of epithelioid histiocytes, multinucleated giant cells, or both are seen in 65% to 75% of cases.[4, 8] Bronchiolitis is observed in about 50% of patients.[6] Depending on the severity and frequency of individual bouts of lung damage, a variable degree of interstitial fibrosis eventually supervenes.[9] The interstitial fibrosis at first is mild and patchy in distribution at the microscopic level but eventually progresses into grossly visible scars.[6] Such fibrosis can be localized, in which case it may be most prominent in peribronchial or periseptal areas; sometimes, it is more diffuse, resembling advanced idiopathic pulmonary fibrosis with honeycombing.

As more cases of hypersensitivity pneumonitis are reported, involving an increasing variety of organic antigens, the diagnosis must be suspected primarily on the basis of the clinical history, and meticulous inquiry may be required to uncover an exposure coincident with the development of acute respiratory symptoms. A history of exposure to any organic dust, either animal or vegetable, of small enough size and in sufficient concentration should lead to consideration of the diagnosis. Intermittent exposure of susceptible individuals to a high concentration of antigen is accompanied by recurrent episodes of fever, chills, dry cough, and dyspnea, whereas continuous exposure to a lower concentration characteristically results in gradually progressive dyspnea in the absence of systemic symptoms.[3]

Table 16–1. COMMON VARIETIES OF HYPERSENSITIVITY PNEUMONITIS

Disease	Principal Responsible Antigens	Exposure Source
Bird-fancier's (pigeon-breeder's) lung	Avian proteins contained in serum, excreta, or feathers	Pigeons, budgerigars, canaries, parakeets, chickens, ducks, turkeys, geese
Farmer's lung	Thermophilic bacteria (*Micropolyspora faeni, Thermoactinomyces* species)	Affects men aged 40–50 yr; peak incidence during season when stored hay is used for cattle feeding; acute illness in one third of patients, insidious in remainder; prevalence among farmers in different communities 1%–10%
Humidifier lung	Bacteria: *Thermoactinomyces* species Fungi: *Penicillium* species, *Cladosporium* species Amebae: *Sphaeropsidales* species, *Acanthamoeba castellani, Naegleria gruberi*	Air conditioners, humidifiers, damp floors or walls, hot tubs

Table 16–2. HYPERSENSITIVITY PNEUMONITIS: RADIOLOGIC MANIFESTATIONS

Acute stage: hours to a few days after exposure
   Bilateral air-space consolidation
Subacute stage: days to a few months after exposure
   Ground-glass opacities
   Poorly defined nodular opacities
   Diffuse or middle and lower lung predominance
   Nodules have centrilobular distribution on HRCT
   HRCT often shows lobular areas of air-trapping
Chronic stage: after months or years of exposure
   Findings of fibrosis
   Irregular linear opacities, architectural distortion
   Random, peribronchial, or subpleural predominance
   Usually middle or lower lung predominance
   Common superimposed subacute changes

HRCT, high-resolution computed tomography.

Radiologic Manifestations

The radiologic findings vary with the stage of the disease (Table 16–2). Early in the course of the acute stage, chest radiograph may show no discernible abnormality, even in patients who have florid pathologic changes on lung biopsy.[10, 11] Later on, the characteristic finding consists of bilateral areas of consolidation, which may be diffuse or involve mainly the lower lung zones.[12–14] The air-space consolidation may be extensive, particularly in the lower lung zones, and may obscure the nodular pattern characteristic of the subacute stage (Fig. 16–1).

The radiographic abnormalities in subacute disease usually involve mainly the middle and lower lung zones.[12, 13, 15] The most characteristic pattern consists of poorly defined small nodular opacities;[13] another common abnormality is a poorly defined, hazy increase in lung opacity (ground-glass opacity).[12, 15] The evolution of radiographic change—diffuse involvement of both lungs as evidenced by a persistent nodular pattern, superimposition of consolidation with acute exacerbations, and resolution of the latter pattern within a few days of the initial acute clinical presentation (*see* Fig. 16–1)—should suggest the diagnosis.

Hilar lymph node enlargement is seldom is seen on chest radiographs. In studies of 26 patients who had mushroom

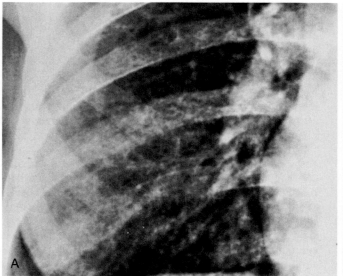
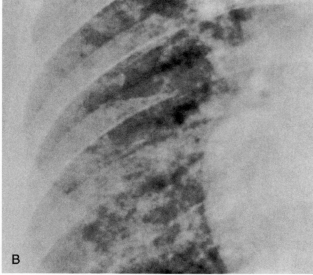

Figure 16–1. Hypersensitivity Pneumonitis (Farmer's Lung). This 25-year-old woman was admitted to the hospital with a 2-week history of moderate dyspnea. Detail view of the lower half of the right lung *(A)* shows poorly defined small nodular opacities consistent with subacute hypersensitivity pneumonitis. Three months after the original episode, the woman was admitted for a second time after the acute onset of dyspnea, cough, and high fever. The chest radiograph at this time *(B)* shows consolidation superimposed on the nodular opacities. This appearance is consistent with an acute exacerbation of hypersensitivity pneumonitis as a result of re-exposure to moldy hay.

worker's lung[16] and 27 who had farmer's lung,[17] no patients had radiographic evidence of hilar or mediastinal lymph node enlargement. In a more recent investigation, node enlargement was evident on radiograph in only 1 of 13 patients.[18] By contrast, mediastinal lymph node enlargement—defined as a short-axis diameter equal to or greater than 10 mm—is seen relatively commonly on computed tomography (CT) scan.[19] Affected nodes seldom measure greater than 15 mm in short-axis diameter and usually involve only one or two nodal stations.[19] In one study of 17 patients, the abnormality was identified in 9 (53%);[19] however, most investigators have found a prevalence of about 5% to 15%.[15, 18, 20] The difference may be related to the underlying cause of hypersensitivity pneumonitis or to the stage of the disease. In one study of patients who had bird-fancier's lung, enlarged nodes were identified on CT scan in 3 of 24 (12%) patients who had chronic disease but in none of 21 patients who had subacute disease.[20]

Although the chest radiograph in subacute disease frequently is abnormal—in greater than 90% of patients in some studies[21–23]—normal findings are not unusual.[23] Normal radiographs have been described in 33% of patients who have bird-fancier's lung[20, 24] or malt worker's lung.[2] By contrast, radiographic abnormalities consistent with hypersensitivity pneumonitis may be present in the absence of clinical symptoms, a situation that pertained in 10 (5%) of 200 pigeon breeders in one series.[1] Although this figure may have been influenced by radiologic over-reading, the association itself is not surprising in view of the evidence on bronchoalveolar lavage of active alveolitis in symptom-free exposed farmers and bird handlers.[25, 26]

Radiographic abnormalities in patients who have subacute hypersensitivity pneumonitis frequently resolve completely within 10 days to 3 months after exposure if the patient is removed from the environment.[5, 13] If exposure is continued or repeated or if the initial exposure is especially severe, the diffuse nodular pattern characteristic of the acute and subacute stages is replaced by changes characteristic of diffuse interstitial fibrosis—a medium to coarse reticular pattern, loss of lung volume, and (sometimes) compensatory overinflation of lung zones that are less affected. Although the fibrosis may be diffuse,[27] frequently there is a definite zonal predominance. Several investigators, including those who have used CT, showed a predominantly middle or lower lung zone involvement (Fig. 16–2).[15, 27, 28] In one study of 16 patients, the fibrosis involved mainly the middle lung zones in 7 (44%), the lower lung zones in 2, and the upper lung zones in 1;[27] no zonal predominance was evident in 7 (44%) patients. In another investigation of 19 patients, the fibrosis involved mainly the lower lung zone in 8 (42%), the middle lung zone in 3 (16%), and the upper lung zone in 3 (16%);[28] no zonal predominance was seen in 5 (26%) patients.

As might be expected, high-resolution computed tomography (HRCT) is superior to chest radiography in the demonstration of parenchymal abnormalities;[14, 15, 20] in particular, HRCT may reveal abnormalities in patients who have clinically or biopsy-proven disease and normal chest radiographs (Fig. 16–3).[20, 22, 29] In one study of 21 patients who had subacute disease and abnormal HRCT scans, 7 (33%) had normal chest radiographs.[20] The sensitivity of HRCT is not 100%,[15] however, as exemplified by a study

of swimming pool employees in which the diagnosis of hypersensitivity pneumonitis was based on two or more work-related signs or symptoms, abnormal findings on transbronchial biopsy specimens, or lymphocytosis in bronchoalveolar lavage fluid[22]—only 1 of 11 subjects (9%) had abnormal findings on chest radiograph, whereas 5 (45%) had abnormal HRCT findings. The HRCT scans in this study were performed at 4-cm slice intervals; because optimal assessment of infiltrative lung disease requires scans at 1-cm intervals, mild localized abnormalities might have been missed.

The improved visualization of parenchymal abnormalities on HRCT in the appropriate clinical context may allow confident diagnosis in patients who have normal or questionable chest radiograph abnormalities. In one study of 208 patients who had various chronic interstitial lung diseases, including 13 who had subacute or chronic disease, a confident correct diagnosis of hypersensitivity pneumonitis was made on a combination of clinical and radiographic findings in 6 patients and on a combination of clinical, radiographic, and HRCT findings in 10 patients.[18]

The HRCT findings of acute hypersensitivity pneumonitis consist of bilateral areas of consolidation superimposed on small centrilobular nodular opacities.[14, 29] The consolidation may be diffuse or involve mainly the lower lung zones. The findings in subacute hypersensitivity pneumonitis consist most often of diffuse bilateral areas of ground-glass attenuation (*see* Fig. 16–3), centrilobular nodular opacities (Fig. 16–4), or both.[14, 15, 20] In one review of 15 patients who had subacute disease, diffuse ground-glass attenuation was present in 11 (73%), and centrilobular nodular opacities were present in 6 (40%).[15] In another review of 21 patients who had subacute bird-breeder's hypersensitivity pneumonitis, the most common finding (seen in 16 patients [76%]) was centrilobular nodules.[20] In this study, 11 patients (52%) had bilateral areas of ground-glass attenuation. Although this finding and the centrilobular opacities usually are diffuse, they often are most marked in the middle and lower lung zones.[15] Another frequent finding in patients who have subacute hypersensitivity pneumonitis is a pattern of mosaic attenuation caused by areas of ground-glass attenuation and focal areas of air-trapping (Fig. 16–5).[30] In one review of 22 patients, this pattern was found in 19 (86%). Such areas frequently have a striking lobular distribution and are associated with evidence of air-trapping on expiratory HRCT scans. Their extent correlates with an increase in residual volume and residual volume-to-total lung capacity ratio.[30]

The chronic stage of hypersensitivity pneumonitis is manifested on HRCT by evidence of fibrosis, frequently associated with features of subacute disease.[14, 20, 27] In one review of HRCT scans in 16 patients, the areas of fibrosis were characterized by the presence of irregular linear opacities and architectural distortion.[27] The irregular lines had a random distribution in the transverse plane in 44% of patients, were predominantly subpleural in 37%, and were peribronchovascular in 19%. Honeycombing was identified in 11 (69%). In 44% of patients, the irregular linear opacities and honeycombing involved mainly the middle lung zones (*see* Fig. 16–2), and in 38%, they were distributed evenly throughout the three lung zones. Upper lobe predominance was present in only 1 of 16 patients (6%).

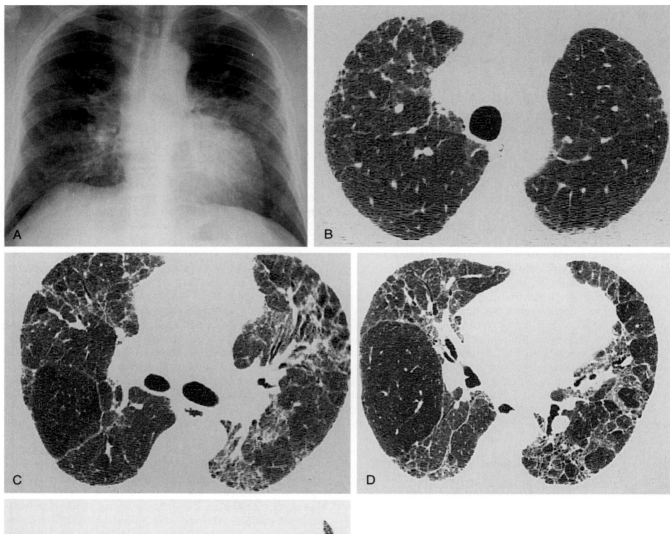

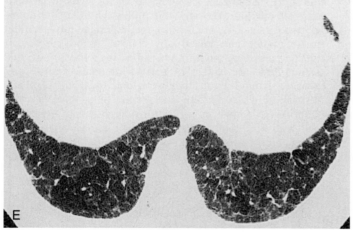

Figure 16–2. Chronic Hypersensitivity Pneumonitis. A postero-anterior chest radiograph *(A)* shows irregular linear opacities involving mainly the middle lung zones. Lung volumes are decreased. HRCT scan (1-mm collimation) at the level of the aortic arch *(B)* shows mild fibrosis. Much more extensive fibrosis is present at the level of the bronchus intermedius *(C)* and the right middle lobe bronchus *(D)*. The fibrosis has a random distribution in the transverse plane and is characterized by the presence of irregular lines of attenuation and distortion of the lung architecture. Mild honeycombing is evident in the posterior basal segments of the lower lobes. HRCT scan through the lung bases *(E)* shows relative sparing. This distribution of disease is characteristic of chronic hypersensitivity pneumonitis. The diagnosis was proved by open-lung biopsy.

Extensive areas of ground-glass attenuation and small centrilobular opacities were present in 15 (94%) and 10 (62%) patients, respectively; these abnormalities were present mainly in the middle and lower lung zones.

In the appropriate clinical context, the HRCT findings in hypersensitivity pneumonitis are characteristic enough to be highly suggestive of the diagnosis.[18] Similar HRCT abnormalities may be seen in other interstitial lung dis-

eases, however. In clinical practice, the main alternative diagnostic considerations are IPF (IPF) and desquamative interstitial pneumonitis (DIP). The accuracy of HRCT in differential diagnosis was assessed in a study of 33 patients who had IPF, 3 who had DIP, and 27 who had hypersensitivity pneumonitis.[28] In all patients, the diagnosis was proved by open-lung biopsy. In 19 patients who had hypersensitivity pneumonitis, the disease was chronic (symptoms

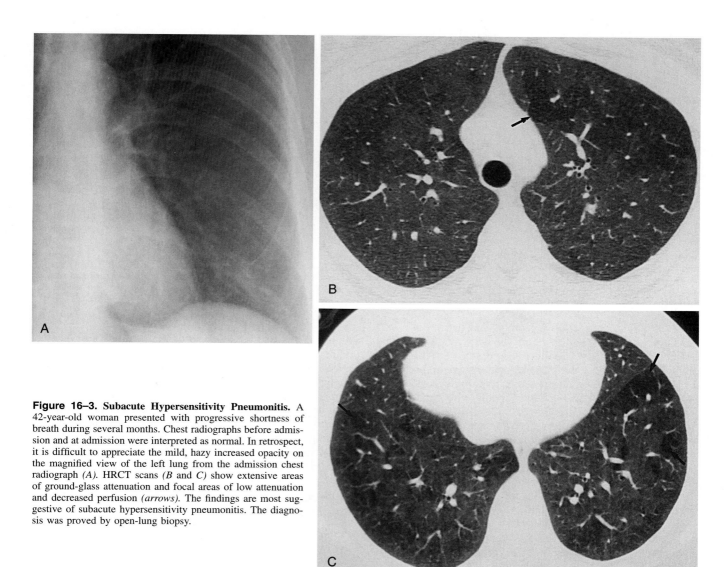

Figure 16–3. Subacute Hypersensitivity Pneumonitis. A 42-year-old woman presented with progressive shortness of breath during several months. Chest radiographs before admission and at admission were interpreted as normal. In retrospect, it is difficult to appreciate the mild, hazy increased opacity on the magnified view of the left lung from the admission chest radiograph *(A)*. HRCT scans *(B* and *C)* show extensive areas of ground-glass attenuation and focal areas of low attenuation and decreased perfusion *(arrows)*. The findings are most suggestive of subacute hypersensitivity pneumonitis. The diagnosis was proved by open-lung biopsy.

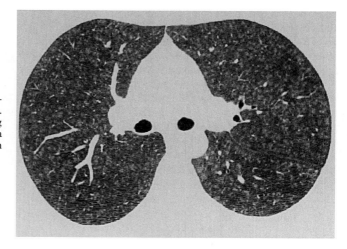

Figure 16–4. Subacute Hypersensitivity Pneumonitis. HRCT scan (1-mm collimation) shows bilateral, poorly defined, small nodular opacities. These opacities are a few millimeters away from the pleura, including interlobar fissures, and a few millimeters away from major vessels, a characteristic distribution of centrilobular nodules. The patient had proven subacute bird-fancier's lung.

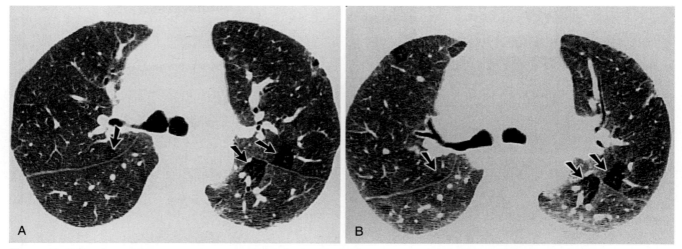

Figure 16–5. Air-Trapping in Hypersensitivity Pneumonitis. HRCT scan (1-mm collimation) obtained at end-inspiration *(A)* shows bilateral areas of ground-glass attenuation. Focal areas of low attenuation and decreased vascularity are evident in right and left lungs *(arrows)*. HRCT scan obtained at end-expiration *(B)* shows expected loss of volume and increased attenuation of both lungs. The focal areas of decreased attenuation have not changed in volume *(arrows)*, a characteristic finding of gas-trapping. The patient had open-lung biopsy–proven subacute disease superimposed on chronic hypersensitivity pneumonitis (bird-breeder's lung).

lasting >1 year); 8 had acute or subacute symptoms. The HRCT findings in subacute hypersensitivity pneumonitis—particularly the presence and distribution of areas of ground-glass attenuation—often were indistinguishable from those of DIP. In 8 of 19 patients who had chronic hypersensitivity pneumonitis (42%), the fibrosis involved mainly the lower lung zones, compared with 27 of 33 patients (81%) who had IPF. In 26% of patients who had chronic hypersensitivity pneumonitis, the fibrosis had no zonal predominance, whereas in 16% it involved mainly the upper zones and in another 16% mainly the middle lung zones. In comparison, the fibrosis showed no zonal predominance in 9% of patients who had IPF and involved mainly the middle lung zones in 6%.

Although there is an overlap of the distribution of fibrosis in patients who have chronic hypersensitivity pneumonitis and IPF, the two conditions often can be distinguished by the relative sparing of the lower half of the lower lung zone, the lack of peripheral predominance of the fibrosis, and the frequent presence of centrilobular nodules in hypersensitivity pneumonitis. These findings permitted a high level of confidence in diagnosis in 39 (62%) patients; in these, the diagnosis was correct in 23 of 26 patients who had IPF and in 12 of 13 patients who had hypersensitivity pneumonitis. The authors concluded that CT allows distinction of hypersensitivity pneumonitis from IPF in most cases; however, subacute hypersensitivity pneumonitis may resemble DIP, and chronic hypersensitivity pneumonitis may resemble IPF.[28]

INHALATION OF INORGANIC DUST (PNEUMOCONIOSIS)

Pneumoconiosis is defined as "the accumulation of dust in the lungs and the tissue reactions to its presence."[31] Such reactions generally take one or both of two clinico-pathologic forms:

1. *Fibrosis*, which can be focal and nodular (as in silicosis) or diffuse (as in asbestosis). This process proba-

bly is related to a toxic effect of the inhaled substance on pulmonary epithelial cells, inflammatory cells, or both;[32] it often results in radiographic abnormalities and, if extensive enough, may lead to significant functional impairment.

2. *Aggregates of particle-laden macrophages*, with minimal or no accompanying fibrosis, a reaction that typically is seen with inert dusts, such as iron, tin, and barium. Although sometimes associated with chronic radiographic abnormalities, this reaction usually results in few, if any, functional or clinical manifestations.

International Classification of Radiographs of the Pneumoconioses

The chest radiograph is an important tool in detecting the effects of dust particle deposition in the lungs and in measuring disease progression.[33] For chest radiograph to be useful in epidemiologic studies, however, it is essential that an acceptable classification of extent of involvement be followed and a standard nomenclature be employed. The most widely used schema is the International Labour Office (ILO) 1980 International Classification of Radiographs of the Pneumoconioses.[34]

The object of this classification is to codify the radiographic changes of the pneumoconioses in a simple, reproducible manner. Although it does not define pathologic entities, this classification possesses the considerable advantage of providing a uniform, semiquantitative method of reporting the type and extent of disease, leading to international comparability of pneumoconiosis statistics. The classification provides a means of systematically recording the radiographic changes in the chest caused by the inhalation of all types of mineral dusts, including coal, silica, carbon, asbestos, and beryllium. It is particularly valuable for epidemiologic studies but also is useful in the evaluation of patients for compensation purposes. Standard reference radiographs have been selected to illustrate the ILO 1980 classification and can be purchased from the ILO office. Because the schema employs radiographic descriptors that are different from those generally used throughout this book, a short glossary of terms follows.

International Labour Office Radiographic Terms

Terms requiring explanation are discussed here. All other terms used in the classification are self-explanatory and identical in context to those used elsewhere in this book.

Small Rounded Opacities. These are well-circumscribed opacities or nodules ranging in diameter from barely visible to 10 mm. The qualifiers *p*, *q*, and *r* subdivide the predominant opacities into three diameter ranges: *p*, up to 1.5 mm; *q*, 1.5 to 3 mm; and *r*, 3 to 10 mm.

Small Irregular Opacities. This term is employed to describe a pattern that, elsewhere in this book, has been designated *linear*, *reticular*, or *reticulonodular*—in other words, a netlike pattern. Although the nature of these opacities is such that the establishment of quantitative dimensions is considerably more difficult than with rounded opacities, the ILO has established three categories: *s*, width up to about 1.5 mm; *t*, width exceeding 1.5 mm and up to about 3 mm; and *u*, width exceeding 3 mm and up to about 10 mm.

To record shape and size, two letters may be used. If the reader considers that all or virtually all opacities are one shape and size, this is noted by recording the symbol twice, separated by a slash (e.g., *q/q*). If another shape or size is seen, this is recorded as the second letter (e.g., *q/t*). The designation *q/t* means that the predominant small opacity is round and of size *q* but that there are, in addition, a significant number of small irregular opacities of size *t*. In this way, any combination of small opacities can be recorded.

Profusion. This term refers to the number of small rounded or small irregular opacities per unit area or zone of lung. There are four basic categories: category *0*, small opacities absent or less profuse than in category *1*; category *1*, small opacities definitely present but few in number (normal lung markings are usually visible); category *2*, numerous small opacities (normal lung markings usually are obscured partly); and category *3*, very numerous small opacities (normal lung markings usually are obscured totally). These categories can be subdivided further by employing a 12-point scale, in which there is a continuum of changes from complete normality to the most advanced category or grade:[35, 36]

0/−	0/0	0/1
1/0	1/1	1/2
2/1	2/2	2/3
3/2	3/3	3/+

Employing this scale, the radiograph is classified first in the usual way into one of the four categories—0, 1, 2, or 3. If the category above or below is considered as a serious alternative during the process, it is recorded (e.g., a radiograph in which profusion is considered to be category 2 but for which category 1 was considered seriously as an alternative would be graded category 2/1). If no alternative is considered (i.e., the profusion was definitely category 2), it would be classified *2/2*.

A subdivision is possible within categories 0 and 3. Category 0/1 is profusion of category 0 with category 1

seriously considered as an alternative. Category 0/0 is a radiograph in which there are no small opacities or one in which a few opacities are thought to be present but are not sufficiently definite or numerous for category 1 to be considered. If the absence of small opacities is particularly obvious, profusion should be recorded as 0/−. Such a category might be seen in a healthy nonsmoking adolescent. A radiograph that shows profusion markedly higher than that classifiable as 3/3 would be recorded as 3/+. The ILO standard films are the final arbitrators of opacity profusion and take precedence over any application of a verbal description of profusion. A film is placed in category 1 if it resembles the ILO standard film of the same category and opacity type. This type of reading always should be done side by side with the ILO standard films.

Large Opacities. This term is used for opacities that are larger than the maximum permitted for small rounded opacities (i.e., >10 mm). Three categories are recognized: category *A*, an opacity having a greatest diameter exceeding 1 cm up to and including 5 cm or several opacities each greater than 1 cm, the sum of whose greatest diameters does not exceed 5 cm; category *B*, comprising one or more opacities larger or more numerous than those in category A whose combined area does not exceed the equivalent of the right upper lung zone; and category *C*, consisting of one or more opacities whose combined area exceeds the equivalent of the right upper lung zone.

Extent. Each lung is divided into three zones—upper, middle, and lower—by horizontal lines drawn at one third and two thirds of the vertical distance between the apex of the lung and the dome of the diaphragm.

Limitations in Radiographic Interpretation

The ILO classification of pneumoconiosis is accepted worldwide as the means for recording the radiographic findings.[274, 275] Several investigators have shown considerable intraobserver and interobserver variability, however, in the interpretation of radiographs for pneumoconiosis.[275–277] In one study of 1,771 radiographs, the percentage of radiographs classified as showing changes consistent with pneumoconiosis (ILO profusion ≥1/0) by three independent readers ranged from 27% to 47%.[278] In another investigation in which a set of 119 radiographs was assessed by six independent experienced readers, five of the readers had good to fair agreement for pleural findings and for profusion as a dichotomous variable (≥1/0 versus ≤0/1) using κ statistics.[275] The percent agreement between these five observers for profusion score ranged from 0.84 to 0.91 with κ values ranging from 0.41 to 0.73. There was poor agreement with the sixth reader, with an agreement for profusion score of only 0.25 and a κ of 0.04. The agreement between the readers was better for normal radiographs than for abnormal radiographs.

Several investigators showed that radiographic changes consistent with dust inhalation can be seen in unexposed populations.[279] A meta-analysis of eight studies published before 1997 yielded a prevalence of profusion scores of 1/0 or greater in unexposed populations of 5.3% (95% confidence interval 2.9% to 7.7%).[279] The prevalence was significantly higher in Europe than in North America (11.3% versus 1.6%), in men than in women, and in individuals 50 years of age or older compared with younger individuals. Given the results of these various investigations, radiographic findings need to be interpreted in the proper clinical context with proper ascertainment of exposure from occupational and environmental sources.

Silica

Silica is a ubiquitous, abundant mineral composed of regularly arranged molecules of silicon dioxide (SiO_2). Exposure to a concentration high enough to result in radiographic and pathologic manifestations of silicosis occurs predominantly in occupational settings. Numerous occupations have been associated with such exposure, including sandblasting, stonecutting, engraving, and polishing. Because of the ubiquity of silica in the earth's crust, mining, tunneling, and quarrying almost inevitably lead to some exposure to the mineral.

The diagnosis of silicosis usually is based on the identification of a diffuse nodular or reticulonodular pattern on chest radiograph of a patient who has an occupational history compatible with exposure to dust containing high concentrations of SiO_2. In contrast to many other inhalation diseases caused by inorganic and organic dusts, the fibrosis and associated disability in silicosis frequently are progressive, even after removal of the patient from the dusty environment.[62] Many patients are asymptomatic when first seen. Some patients complain of shortness of breath, initially on exertion only but becoming increasingly severe as the radiographic abnormalities worsen.

In contrast to classic silicosis, in which most patients are asymptomatic and an exposure of 10 to 20 years is required before the disease becomes evident radiographically,[51] a few patients develop symptomatic disease within 5 to 10 years of exposure (so-called accelerated silicosis). Apart from its relatively early onset and rapid progression, the radiographic, clinical, and pathologic features of this variant are identical to those of more classic disease. Although this form probably is less common today than previously as a result of dust control in the workplace, cases still are observed in conditions of environmental neglect.[41]

Silicoproteinosis is another relatively acute and more rapidly progressive form of disease. This variant was reported initially in quartzite millers[63] and workers in the scouring powder industry;[37, 38] it has been described in tunnel workers, silica flour workers,[63] and sandblasters.[64, 65] When this variant of disease develops, it often leads to death as a result of respiratory failure, commonly with a complicating pneumothorax.[64]

Radiologic Manifestations

The classic radiographic pattern of silicosis consists of multiple nodular opacities ranging from 1 to 10 mm in diameter (Fig. 16–6; Table 16–3). The nodules usually are well circumscribed and of uniform density. Although profusion can be fairly even throughout both lungs, there commonly is considerable upper lobe predominance. The nodules tend to involve mainly the posterior portion of the lungs.[40] Nodules have been identified on pathologic examination that were not seen on premortem chest radio-

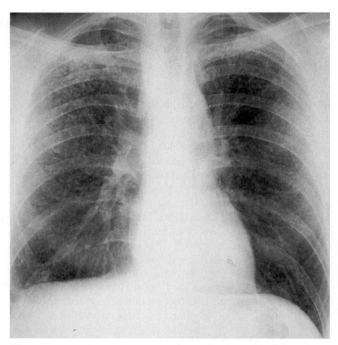

Figure 16–6. Silicosis: Characteristic Radiographic Findings. Posteroanterior chest radiograph shows numerous well-defined small nodules mainly in the upper and middle lung zones. The nodules measure 1.5 to 3 mm in diameter (International Labour Office [ILO] q size nodules), and the profusion is 2/3 (slightly greater than the ILO standard radiograph for profusion 2/2 but considerably less than the standard for profusion 3/3). Early conglomeration is present near the lung apices.

graphs in many cases.[41] Calcification of nodules is evident on radiograph in 10% to 20% of cases.

The radiographic pattern of small round opacities commonly is referred to as *simple* silicosis, in contrast to *complicated* silicosis (progressive massive fibrosis [PMF]). PMF is characterized by large opacities (conglomerate shadows) usually in the upper lobes. By definition, the opacities measure greater than 1 cm in diameter; they may exceed the volume of an upper lobe in aggregate (Fig. 16–7). The shadow margins may be irregular and ill-defined or smooth,[42] creating an interface that parallels the lateral chest wall (*see* Fig. 16–7). The opacities commonly develop in the midzone or periphery of the lung; with time, they tend to migrate toward the hilum, leaving emphysematous lung between the fibrotic tissue and the pleural surface.[43] Although usually bilateral, unilateral opacities may occur and be confused with carcinoma (Fig. 16–8). Cavita-

Table 16–3. SILICOSIS: RADIOLOGIC MANIFESTATIONS

Small nodular opacities
Nodules have well-defined margins
Calcification of nodules in 10–20% of cases
Upper lobe predominance or diffuse
Nodules frequently have posterior (dorsal) predominance
Conglomerate masses (large opacities) usually in upper lobes
Hilar and mediastinal lymph node enlargement common
Calcification of lymph nodes in 5% of cases
Eggshell calcification virtually diagnostic

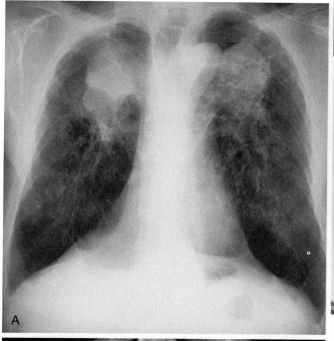

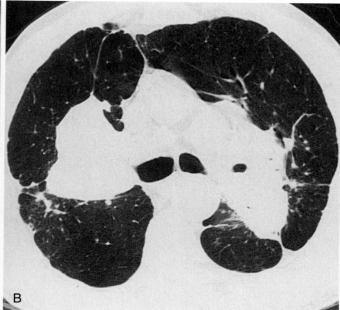

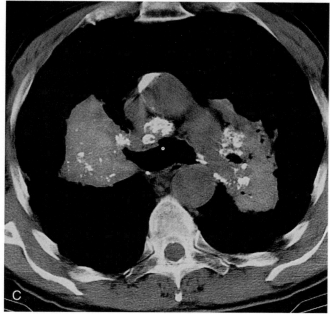

Figure 16–7. Silicosis with Conglomeration. Posteroanterior chest radiograph *(A)* shows large opacities in the upper lung zones associated with marked retraction of the hila superiorly. Several nodular opacities can be seen, mainly in the midlung zones. HRCT scan *(B)* shows conglomerate masses and extensive emphysema. Soft tissue windows *(C)* show calcification within the lung parenchyma and within mediastinal and hilar lymph nodes. The patient was a 70-year-old man with long-standing silicosis related to hard rock mining.

tion develops occasionally. The more extensive the conglomerate fibrosis, the less apparent is nodularity in the remainder of the lungs (*see* Fig. 16–8).[43] There seldom is any radiographic evidence of pleural abnormality.

Hilar lymph node enlargement is common and may occur with or without associated silicosis.[43, 44] Calcification is common—in one series of 1,905 cases, it was identified in 4.7%[47]—and characteristically tends to involve mainly the periphery of the nodes, a finding referred to as *eggshell calcification* (Fig. 16–9). Although occasionally seen in other conditions,[46, 47] this pattern is almost pathognomonic of silicosis; its occurrence in coal and metal miners has been attributed to concomitant exposure to silica.[44] Although most common in the hilar lymph nodes, eggshell

calcification develops rarely in lymph nodes in the mediastinum[45] and the intra-abdominal and retroperitoneal areas.[46]

The enlarged lymph nodes may lead to problems in diagnosis in some patients. In the retroperitoneum, enlarged lymph nodes have been confused with metastatic pancreatic carcinoma.[48] In one patient who had *Mycobacterium avium-intracellulare* infection, bronchial obstruction developed from broncholithiasis as a result of eroding infected silicotic nodes.[49] Mediastinal nodes may encroach on the phrenic nerve, resulting in unilateral diaphragmatic paralysis.[50]

Accelerated silicosis has radiographic features similar to those of the classic form except that they develop during a period of only a few years (Fig. 16–10). Silicoproteinosis is characterized by bilateral parenchymal consolidation

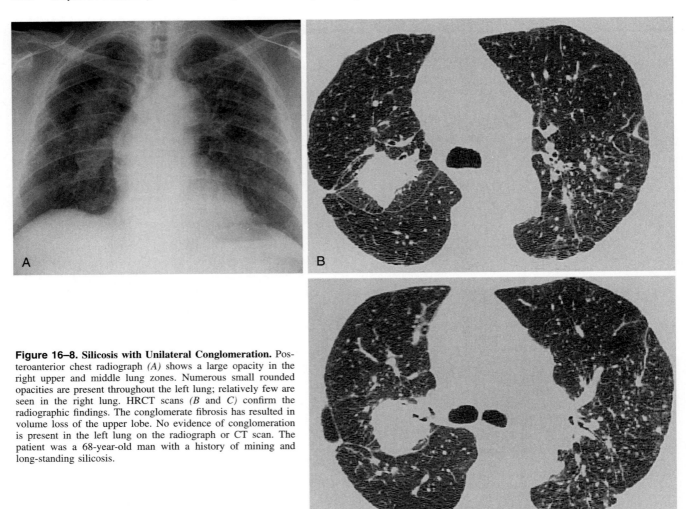

Figure 16–8. Silicosis with Unilateral Conglomeration. Posteroanterior chest radiograph *(A)* shows a large opacity in the right upper and middle lung zones. Numerous small rounded opacities are present throughout the left lung; relatively few are seen in the right lung. HRCT scans *(B* and *C)* confirm the radiographic findings. The conglomerate fibrosis has resulted in volume loss of the upper lobe. No evidence of conglomeration is present in the left lung on the radiograph or CT scan. The patient was a 68-year-old man with a history of mining and long-standing silicosis.

similar to alveolar proteinosis that progresses rapidly during months or 1 or 2 years.[52, 53] Another variant of classic silicosis is Caplan's syndrome, which consists of the presence of large necrobiotic nodules (rheumatoid nodules) superimposed on a background of simple silicosis or coal worker's pneumoconiosis. It is seen more commonly in coal workers' pneumoconiosis than in silicosis. In a controlled study of patients who had silicosis with and without rheumatoid arthritis, the rate of progression of the silicosis was found to be greater in the former, as was the probability that the silicosis was manifested by larger nodules (type r) at the time of presentation.[54] The necrobiotic nodules in Caplan's syndrome can be distinguished from those of silicosis because they tend to occur in crops, measure 0.5 to 5 cm in diameter, and may cavitate.

Radiographic progression of silicosis after removal from exposure has been well established. In one study of 1,902 workers who had no radiographic evidence of PMF a maximum of 4 years before leaving the occupation, 172 subsequently developed this complication on follow-up examination.[55] Despite the development of conglomerate lesions after leaving employment, this cohort of workers showed no overall progression or regression of the grades of simple pneumoconiosis.

The CT findings of silicosis have been described by several investigators.[40, 57, 58] The characteristic abnormalities are similar to those on radiograph: sharply defined small nodules that may be diffuse throughout the lungs but frequently are most numerous in the upper lung zones (Fig. 16–11). In patients who have relatively mild disease, the nodules may be seen only in the posterior aspect of the upper lobes.[40, 287] Nodules adjacent to the visceral pleura may appear as rounded or triangular areas of attenuation, which, when confluent, may simulate pleural plaques (*pseudoplaques*) (Figs. 16–11 and 16–12). Confluent nodules (PMF) usually have irregular margins and may contain areas of calcification (*see* Fig. 16–7); surrounding emphysema usually is present.[56, 57, 61] Hilar or mediastinal lymph node enlargement is apparent in approximately 40% of patients.[18]

Distinction of small nodules from vessels is easier on CT performed using 5- to 10-mm collimation (*see* Fig. 16–11) than on HRCT (*see* Fig. 16–12).[59] HRCT allows better assessment of fine parenchymal detail and of emphysema, however. HRCT may allow detection of nodules in patients who have normal radiographic and thick-section CT findings[57] and is particularly helpful in the assessment of patients who have nodules less than 1.5 mm in diame-

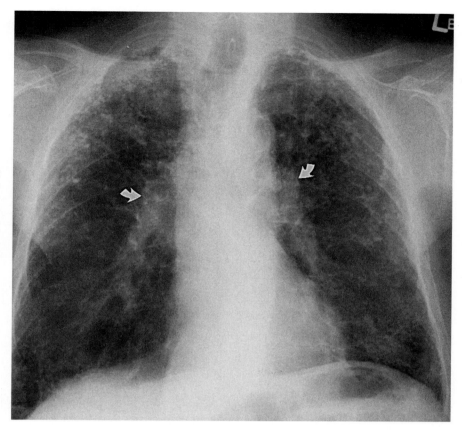

Figure 16–9. Eggshell Calcification of Lymph Nodes in Silicosis. Posteroanterior chest radiograph shows numerous calcified silicotic nodules mainly in the upper and middle lung zones. Several enlarged hilar and mediastinal lymph nodes are present with peripheral (eggshell) calcification *(arrows)*. The patient was a 78-year-old man who had been a miner for more than 20 years.

ter.[58] In one investigation of 49 patients exposed to silica in mines and foundries, 13 (40%) of 32 who had normal radiographs had evidence of silicosis on CT;[57] in three of these (10%), the abnormality was visible only on HRCT. Thick-section CT and HRCT may allow detection of early confluence of nodules not apparent on radiograph.[40, 57] In the assessment of patients who have possible silicosis, it is recommended that 5- to 7-mm collimation CT scans be obtained and be supplemented by HRCT scans obtained at three to five levels through the upper and middle lung zones.[59, 60]

Coal and Carbon

The inhalation and retention in the lung of dust composed predominantly of carbon (often termed *anthracosis*) is seen in many individuals,[66] particularly those who smoke or live in a city or industrial environment. Such innocuous environmental anthracosis is caused by the inhalation of relatively small amounts of dust. Inhalation of large amounts of carbonaceous material, either in the form of coal dust or as substances derived from coal or petroleum products, can be associated with significant pulmonary disease. The most important occupation in terms of the number of individuals affected is coal mining, the resulting disease being appropriately called *coal workers' pneumoconiosis.*

Symptoms of cough, sputum production, and dyspnea are more common in miners who have early coal workers' pneumoconiosis than in miners who have similar smoking and dust exposure histories but no radiographic evidence

of disease.[81] These symptoms are more frequent and severe in workers who have PMF, who also suffer from recurrent attacks of purulent bronchitis. Copious amounts of black sputum may be produced when an ischemic lesion of PMF liquefies and ruptures into a bronchus (*melanoptysis*), in which circumstance a cavity should be visible radiographically.[82–84] With progression of the disease, dyspnea usually worsens; cor pulmonale and right-sided heart failure may ensue.

Radiologic Manifestations

The radiographic pattern of simple pneumoconiosis is typically one of small, round opacities (nodular) (Table 16–4).[69–71] The nodules range from 1 to 5 mm in diameter, tend to be less well defined than those of silicosis, and have a *granular* density in contrast to the homogeneous density of silicotic nodules. Radiographic-pathologic correlative studies suggest that the opacity of individual nod-

**Table 16–4. COAL WORKERS'
PNEUMOCONIOSIS:
RADIOLOGIC MANIFESTATIONS**

Small nodular opacities
Nodules often have poorly defined margins
Calcification of nodules in 10–20% of cases
Upper lobe predominance or diffuse
Nodules often have posterior (dorsal) predominance
Lymph node enlargement in 30% of cases
Most enlarged nodes are calcified

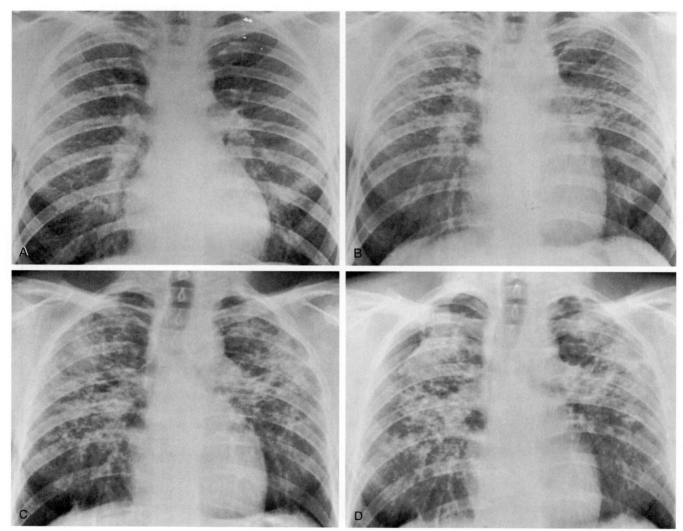

Figure 16–10. Silicosis Showing Rapid Progression. Radiograph of a 27-year-old sandblaster *(A)* shows diffuse, predominantly irregular opacities more prominent in the upper lung zones; hilar lymph nodes are enlarged. Two years later *(B)*, lung volume had reduced, particularly in the upper lung zones (note the upward displacement of both hila). The opacities in the upper lungs were showing early coalescence. Three years later *(C)*, large opacities had developed in the upper lung zones, and 7 years after the patient originally was seen *(D)*, the large opacities had become much larger. Note the sharply defined lateral margin of the large opacity on the right.

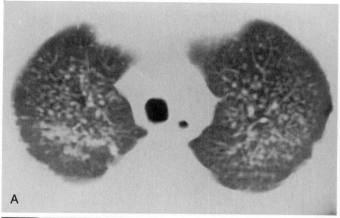

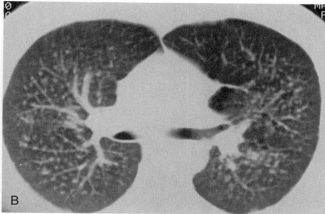

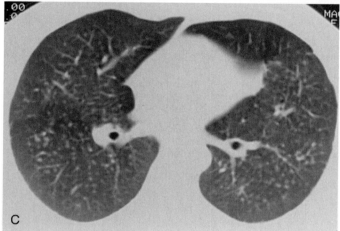

Figure 16–11. Silicosis: Characteristic Findings on Thick-Section CT. 10-mm collimation CT scans show numerous well-defined small nodules, most abundant in the posterior half of the upper lung zones *(A)*. CT scan at this level shows pseudoplaques (i.e., subpleural nodules resulting in an appearance resembling plaques). The nodules have a perivascular distribution, most evident in the scan obtained through the midlung zones *(B)*. CT scan at the level of the inferior pulmonary veins *(C)* shows relatively few nodules. The patient was a 50-year-old miner.

ules cannot be attributed entirely to the coal dust, whose density is only slightly greater than unity.[72] Despite these observations, it generally is agreed that the radiographic manifestations of coal workers' pneumoconiosis cannot be distinguished from those of silicosis with any degree of confidence.

Calcification of pulmonary nodules is identified radiographically in 10% to 20% of older coal miners, particularly anthracite workers.[73, 74] The calcification begins as a central dot, helping to differentiate these nodules from those of silicosis, in which the calcification tends to be diffuse. Eggshell calcification is uncommon; in one study of 1,063 coal miners whose chest radiographs showed evidence of pneumoconiosis, it was evident in only 1.3%, all of whom had worked 20 or more years in the mines.[73]

The appearance of large opacities indicates the development of complicated pneumoconiosis (PMF). These lesions range from 1 cm in diameter to the volume of a whole lobe in aggregate. Although most commonly restricted to the upper half of the lungs, the lesions also may occur in the lower lung zones (Fig. 16–13). They usually are observed on a background of simple pneumoconiosis but have been found to develop in miners whose initial chest radiographs 4 to 5 years earlier were considered to be within normal limits.[75] The complication is said to occur in about 30% of patients who have diffuse bilateral opacities.[67, 76] It typically starts near the periphery of the lung and is manifested as a mass that has a well-defined lateral border that parallels the rib cage and projects 1 to 3 cm from it.[73] The medial margin of the mass often is ill-defined in contrast to its sharp lateral border, a configuration that was observed in 22 of 50 coal miners in one study.[73] The masses of PMF tend to be thicker in one dimension than the other; for example, they tend to produce a broad face on posteroanterior radiograph and a thin shape on lateral radiograph, frequently paralleling the major fissure.[73] As might be expected, this spindle-shaped configuration creates a radiographic opacity that is considerably less dense in one projection than in the other. PMF usually is homogeneous in density, unless cavitation has developed. This complication occurs only occasionally; it may develop after exposure to coal dust has ceased and, in contrast to simple pneumoconiosis, may progress in the absence of further exposure.[67, 70, 77]

As with the conglomerate shadows of silicosis, PMF usually originates in the lung periphery and gradually migrates toward the hilum, leaving a zone of emphysematous lung between it and the chest wall. Particularly when unilateral, a large mass may simulate pulmonary carcinoma closely. Because PMF occasionally is unassociated with radiographic evidence of nodularity,[73] the correct diagnosis in these cases may not be suspected in the absence of an appropriate occupational history. The smooth, sharply defined lateral border and the somewhat flattened configuration characteristic of these lesions are useful clues in differentiation from pulmonary carcinoma, whose borders

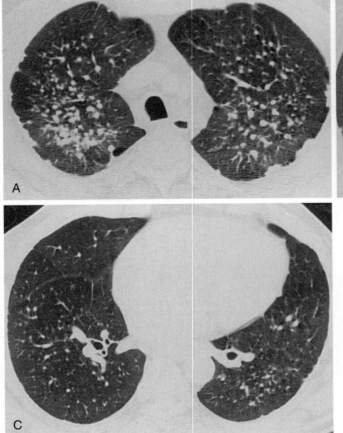

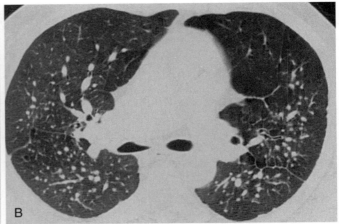

Figure 16–12. Silicosis: Characteristic Findings on HRCT. HRCT scan performed in the same patient as Figure 16–11 shows well-defined nodules mainly involving the upper lung zones *(A)*. The margins of the nodules are defined better on HRCT scan than on the corresponding conventional CT scan, and the pseudoplaques resulting from subpleural nodules are seen better. Because of the thinner section (1.5 mm versus 10 mm), the profusion of nodules appears to be smaller, and the nodules are more difficult to distinguish from vessels. This is particularly evident on the images through the middle *(B)* and lower *(C)* lung zones.

tend to be less well defined and whose configuration typically is spherical. Occasionally, a lesion of PMF contains foci of calcification, an obvious additional aid in radiographic differential diagnosis. Linear calcification may be seen along the border of an area of PMF, invariably along the lateral margin.[73]

Caplan's syndrome consists of the presence of necrobiotic nodules associated with rheumatoid arthritis superimposed on a background of inorganic dust exposure.[68] The nodules are more regular in contour and more peripherally located than the masses of PMF (Fig. 16–14). They range in size from 0.5 to 5 cm in diameter and are seen most often in workers who have subcutaneous rheumatoid nodules and whose chest radiographs are classified as category 0 or 1 simple pneumoconiosis.

The CT findings of coal workers' pneumoconiosis are similar to those of silicosis and consist of small nodules that may be seen diffusely throughout both lungs but are most numerous in the upper lung zone.[58, 78, 79] In patients who have mild disease, the nodules may involve only the upper zone and show a posterior predominance.[78] A random distribution is typical, although HRCT may show a centrilobular predominance in some cases (Fig. 16–15).[60, 78] Subpleural nodules are seen in approximately 80% of patients who have other parenchymal nodules. Confluence of such nodules may result in linear areas of increased attenuation a few millimeters wide (pseudoplaques).[60] Correlation

of HRCT with pathologic specimens has shown that these subpleural micronodules may be associated with localized thickening of the visceral pleura as a result of fibrosis.[80] Calcification of nodules can be identified in approximately 30% of patients. Hilar or mediastinal lymph node enlargement is seen in about 30% of cases; most enlarged nodes are calcified.[78]

Large opacities (PMF) usually have irregular borders associated with distortion of the surrounding lung architecture and emphysema.[60, 78] Less commonly, they have regular borders and are unassociated with emphysema.[78] They occur most commonly in the upper lung zone and, although frequently bilateral, may be unilateral (most commonly on the right).[78]

CT has been shown by several investigators to be superior to radiography in the detection of small nodules.[58, 78, 79] Thick-section CT and HRCT are considered to be complementary in assessment (Fig. 16–16).[60, 78] In one prospective study of 170 coal dust–exposed workers, posteroanterior and lateral chest radiographs, contiguous 10-mm-thick section CT scans, and HRCT scans (2-mm-thick sections) at five selected levels were compared.[78] Findings consistent with coal workers' pneumoconiosis were detected on CT scan in 11 of 48 (23%) workers who had no evidence of pneumoconiosis on chest radiograph (ILO profusion score <1/0); in some patients whose radiographs were interpreted as showing findings consistent with pneu-

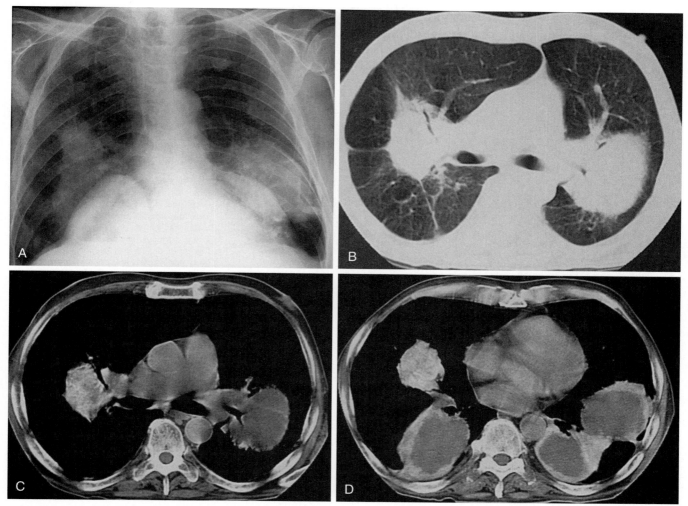

Figure 16–13. Coal Workers' Pneumoconiosis with Conglomerate Masses. Anteroposterior chest radiograph *(A)* shows large opacities in the middle and lower lung zones. A 10-mm collimation CT scan at the level of the right upper lobe bronchus *(B)* shows bilateral perihilar conglomerate masses. Irregular linear opacities and distortion of lung architecture indicative of fibrosis and emphysema are evident. Soft tissue windows *(C and D)* show that three of the conglomerate masses have large central areas of decreased attenuation suggestive of necrosis. The patient was a 65-year-old man with a 30-year history of exposure to coal dust. (Courtesy of Dr. Martine Remy-Jardin, Centre Hospitalier Regional et Universitaire de Lille, Lille, France.)

moconiosis, CT scan showed the abnormalities to consist of bronchiectasis or emphysema, rather than the macules of coal worker's pneumoconiosis.

Asbestos

Asbestos is the general term given to a group of fibrous minerals composed of combinations of silicic acid with magnesium, calcium, sodium, and iron. The word *asbestos* is derived from the Greek, meaning *inextinguishable*,[85] reflecting the resistance of the substance to heat and acid as well as its strength, durability, and flexibility.

Mineralogically, asbestos can be divided into two major groups: the *serpentines*, of which the only member of commercial importance is chrysotile, and the *amphiboles*, which include amosite (brown asbestos), crocidolite (blue asbestos), anthophyllite, tremolite, and actinolite. Chrysotile, tremolite, and crocidolite are responsible for most pleuropulmonary disease, the form and severity of which vary with the different fiber types. Crocidolite and, to a

lesser extent, amosite are considered the most dangerous because of their carcinogenic potential.[85]

The three major sources of exposure to asbestos are (1) the primary occupations of asbestos mining and its processing in a mill; (2) numerous secondary occupations involving its use in a variety of industrial and commercial products; and (3) nonoccupational (environmental or paraoccupational) exposure to contaminated air. In some individuals, such as those living adjacent to asbestos mines, such nonoccupational exposure can be substantial; however, in most, exposure is minimal and is evidenced only by the presence of asbestos fibers in digests of lung tissue.

The secondary uses of asbestos are numerous. The most important are in the construction industry, in which the mineral is incorporated extensively in cement, pipes, tiles, moldings, and paneling; shipbuilding and repair;[90–92] boiler making and repair;[93] railroad-associated occupations;[94] the manufacture of textiles and plastics;[95] the manufacture and repair of gaskets and brake linings (although most insulation and friction materials are now made with nonasbestos

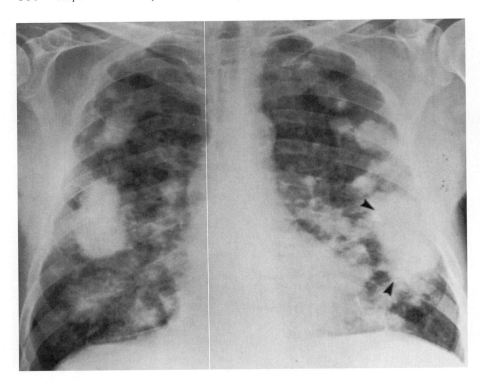

Figure 16–14. Caplan's Syndrome. Posteroanterior radiograph shows a multitude of fairly well-circumscribed nodules ranging in diameter from 1 to 5 cm, scattered randomly throughout both lungs with no notable anatomic predilection. No cavitation is apparent, and there is no evidence of calcification. This patient, a 56-year-old man, had been a coal miner for many years and in recent years had developed arthralgia, which proved to be due to rheumatoid arthritis. As a means of establishing the nature of the pulmonary nodules, a percutaneous needle aspiration was performed on the large mass situated in the lower portion of the left lung *(arrowheads)*: Several milliliters of inky black fluid were aspirated.

fibers[85]); dentistry (affecting dentists and dental technicians);[96] and the jewelry industry.[97] Although the risk of asbestos exposure may be significant during the manufacturing process, it is greater during demolition, such as occurs in construction.[87] Although the fiber generally is assumed to be well bound and harmless once it is incorporated into manufactured products,[98] reports of significant levels of airborne asbestos in buildings with deteriorating insulation leaves this assumption in doubt.[99, 100]

Pathologic Characteristics

Pathologic abnormalities in the chest caused by asbestos inhalation can occur in the pleura, lung parenchyma, airways, and lymph nodes. Pleura disease is the most common and usually takes the form of parietal pleural plaques; localized visceral pleural fibrosis, more or less diffuse pleural fibrosis, and mesothelioma (each of which can be associated with pleural effusion) also occur. Pulmonary manifestations include diffuse interstitial fibrosis (asbestosis), round atelectasis, peribronchiolar fibrosis, and pulmonary carcinoma.

Pleural plaques are the most common form of asbestos-related pleuropulmonary disease and frequently are unassociated with any other pathologic abnormality.[103, 104] These plaques typically consist of well-demarcated, pearly white foci of hard fibrous tissue, 2 to 5 mm thick and several centimeters in diameter.[106] Pleural plaques can have a smooth or nodular surface and be round, elliptical, or irregular in shape.[106] Foci of calcification are common and occasionally are extensive. Characteristically the plaques are located on the parietal pleura overlying the ribs and on the dome of a hemidiaphragm.

Some patients have diffuse pleural thickening.[89] Although this thickening can be restricted to the parietal[89] or visceral[108] pleura, it usually involves both and is accompanied by interpleural adhesions. The fibrosis can extend to adjacent interlobar fissures and interlobular septa[89] and into the mediastinum;[109] however, because the lung parenchyma itself is not affected, asbestosis is by definition not present.

Asbestosis is considered to be present when there is more or less diffuse pulmonary parenchymal interstitial fibrosis. The condition usually is associated with a history of prolonged occupational exposure to asbestos and with a large number of asbestos bodies and fibers in samples of lung tissue analyzed by digestion techniques.[110] Frequently, asbestos bodies are visible in tissue sections, where they may be present in great numbers. The fibrosis is most prominent in the subpleural regions, particularly of the lower lobes, and varies from a slightly coarsened appear-

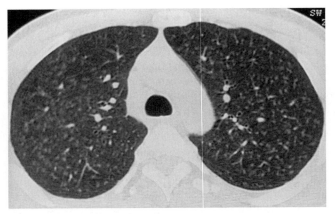

Figure 16–15. Coal Workers' Pneumoconiosis. HRCT scan in a coal worker shows poorly defined small nodular opacities in the upper lobes. The nodules have a predominantly centrilobular distribution. (Case courtesy of Dr. Juan Jimenez, Hospital General de Asturias, Oviedo, Spain.)

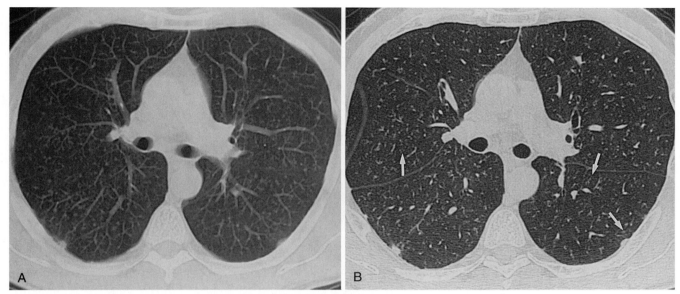

Figure 16–16. Coal Workers' Pneumoconiosis: Thick-Section CT and HRCT Findings. Ten-mm collimation CT scan *(A)* shows small nodules in both lungs. Subpleural nodules mimicking pleural plaques are evident posteriorly. On HRCT scan *(B)*, the nodules are more difficult to distinguish from vessels. The nodular and branching opacities have a centrilobular distribution *(arrows)*. The subpleural pseudoplaques are defined better on the HRCT image. (Courtesy of Dr. Martine Remy-Jardin, Centre Hospitalier Regional et Universitaire de Lille, Lille, France.)

ance of the parenchyma to obvious honeycomb change.[106, 111]

Round atelectasis consists of a focus of atelectatic lung parenchyma partly surrounded by thickened, invaginated pleura.[112, 114] Although the area of collapse usually is only several centimeters in diameter and located in the periphery of the lung, involvement of a whole lobe can be seen.[113]

Clinical Manifestations

Most patients who have pleuropulmonary asbestos-related disease have no symptoms. Benign pleural effusions may or may not be associated with pleural pain.[180] These effusions are recurrent in 15% to 30% of cases,[180, 181] are usually smaller than 500 ml, are often serosanguineous,[180] and persist 2 weeks to 6 months.[180, 181] Although they can occur in the absence of pleural plaques, more often these pleural effusions are present at the time of effusion.[181]

In the absence of underlying chronic obstructive pulmonary disease, breathlessness usually is associated with pulmonary interstitial fibrosis; occasionally, it is caused partly or entirely by diffuse pleural fibrosis.[89, 102, 182] In patients who have asbestosis, shortness of breath seldom develops sooner than 20 to 30 years after initial exposure.[183, 184] It is usually progressive, despite discontinuation of asbestos exposure.

Radiologic Manifestations

Radiologic manifestations of asbestos-related disease are much more common in the pleura than in the parenchyma.[116, 117] In one study of 40 patients, only 5 had parenchymal changes; pleural plaques were the sole manifestation of disease in the other 35 patients.[117] In a second study of 56 patients, 48% showed asbestos pleural disease alone; 41%, combined pleural and parenchymal manifestations;

and 11%, parenchymal changes alone.[115] Radiographic evidence of pleural abnormalities is present in most patients who have asbestosis; in one investigation of 133 such patients, 88 (66%) had pleural changes, including 78 (59%) who had pleural calcification.[118] Overall, it has been estimated that there may be 1.3 million people in the United States who have radiographically detectable asbestos-related pleural thickening.[88]

CT, in particular HRCT, has a higher sensitivity than chest radiography in the detection of pleural and parenchymal abnormalities.[119, 120, 142] In a prospective analysis of 100 asbestos-exposed workers, pleural abnormalities were evident on chest radiograph in 53 and on HRCT scan in 93;[142] parenchymal abnormalities consistent with asbestosis were present on radiograph in 35 and on HRCT scan in 73. Asbestos-related pleural disease can be seen in 95% to 100% of patients who have evidence of asbestosis on HRCT.[119, 121, 142]

Pleural Manifestations

Four types of radiologic abnormality occur in the pleura: (1) focal plaque formation, (2) diffuse thickening, (3) calcification, and (4) effusion. Each type may occur alone or in combination with the others.

Pleural Plaques

Radiographically, pleural plaques usually are more prominent in the lower half of the thorax and tend to follow the ribs when seen *en face*.[107, 122, 123] Pleural plaques may be smooth or nodular in contour and can measure 1 cm in thickness, although they usually are thinner (Fig. 16–17). They are seen most commonly on the domes of the diaphragm, on the posterolateral chest wall between the seventh and tenth ribs, and on the lateral chest wall be-

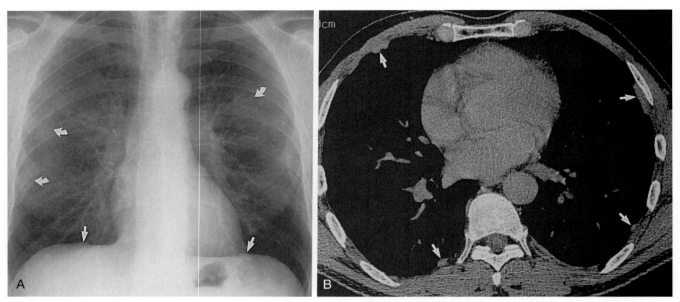

Figure 16–17. Pleural Plaques. Posteroanterior chest radiograph *(A)* shows multiple pleural-based opacities along the chest wall and diaphragm. Several are viewed tangentially *(straight arrows)*, whereas others are ill-defined because they are viewed *en face (curved arrows)*, indicating their origin from the posterolateral or anterolateral chest wall. HRCT scan *(B)* confirms the presence of bilateral plaques *(arrows)*. The patient was a 51-year-old shipyard worker.

tween the sixth and ninth ribs.[116] The earliest manifestation is a thin line of unit density visible under a rib in the axillary region. Although pleural plaques usually are multiple, occasionally only a single plaque is visible.

Because they frequently occur along the posterolateral and anterolateral portion of the thorax, plaques may be difficult to identify on posteroanterior and lateral radiographs, particularly when viewed *en face*. Sometimes, pleural plaques are detected more readily on a tangential 45-degree oblique view.[116, 124, 125] Plaques may be bilateral and symmetric, bilateral and asymmetric, or, less commonly, unilateral.[126–128] For unexplained reasons, unilateral plaques are identified more commonly on the left (Fig. 16–18).[122] In a review of the radiographs of civilian and military employees of the U.S. Navy, of whom 1,914 had plaques, 81% were considered to be bilateral and 19% unilateral;[127] in workers who had unilateral plaques, the left-to-right ratio was 3.5:1. In patients who have bilateral disease, the width and extent of plaques as well as the extent of calcification frequently are greater on the left than on the right, at least on radiographs.[128] In one study of CT scans from 40 patients who had asbestos-related plaques, there was no significant predominance in either hemithorax.[129]

Although plaques usually involve the parietal pleura, they may be seen in the visceral pleura, including the interlobar fissures (Fig. 16–19).[130] Thickening of fissures not related to plaques is common. In a radiographic study of an asbestos-exposed population and a control group, thickening of the interlobar fissures was seen in 54% of asbestos workers compared with 16% in the unexposed control group.[130] Fissural thickening was present in 85% of workers who had parietal pleural plaques and in 36% of workers who did not; it was particularly common in patients who had pulmonary fibrosis (affecting 85%) but also was identified in 45% of workers who did not have evidence of asbestosis.

Although the detection of plaques radiographically is highly specific for a history of asbestos exposure, the sensitivity is relatively poor. Depending on the criteria for diagnosis, the frequency with which plaques are recognized on chest radiograph ranges from 8% to 40% of patients in whom they are demonstrable at autopsy.[104] In one study, the combination of bilateral posterolateral plaques at least 5 mm thick or bilateral calcified diaphragmatic plaques was shown to have a 100% positive predictive value for the diagnosis of autopsy-proven asbestos-related pleural disease;[131] however, these criteria allowed detection of only 12% of plaques. Use of less strict criteria resulted in a considerable number of false-positive diagnoses.

The greatest problem in the radiographic diagnosis of pleural plaques (as well as diffuse pleural thickening) lies in distinguishing them from normal companion shadows of the chest wall—not shadows that are associated with the first three ribs (because this area rarely is involved in asbestos-related pleural disease), but muscle and fat shadows that can be identified in 75% of normal posteroanterior radiographs along the inferior convexity of the thorax. It sometimes is impossible to differentiate pleural plaques from companion shadows on radiograph.

HRCT has a greater sensitivity than conventional CT or chest radiography in the detection of these abnormalities.[119, 132, 142] With this technique, plaques can be identified as circumscribed areas of pleural thickening separated from the underlying rib and extrapleural soft tissues by a thin layer of fat *(see* Figs. 16–17 and 16–18). Normally a 1- to 2-mm-thick stripe of soft tissue attenuation is visible on HRCT scans in the intercostal spaces at the point of contact between the lung and chest wall.[133] This *intercostal stripe* consists of visceral and parietal pleura, endothoracic fascia, and the innermost portion of intercostal muscle. Most of the thickness of the stripe is related to the intercostal muscle because the endothoracic fascia is thin, and the

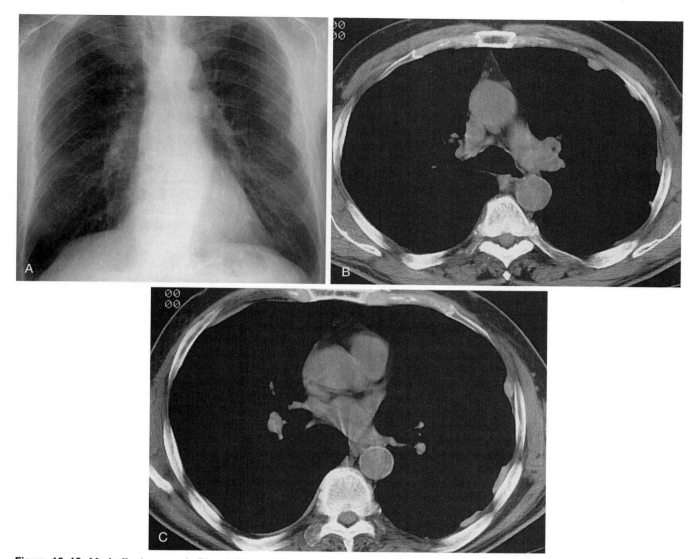

Figure 16–18. Markedly Asymmetric Pleural Plaques. Posteroanterior chest radiograph *(A)* in a 74-year-old shipyard worker shows evidence of pleural plaques only on the left side. HRCT scan at the level of the tracheal carina *(B)* shows only plaques on the left side. HRCT scan through the lower lung zones *(C)* shows prominent plaques on the left and thin plaques on the right.

combined thickness of visceral and parietal pleura and normal fluid is only 0.2 to 0.4 mm.[133] The stripe can be seen because a layer of intercostal fat separates the innermost intercostal muscle from the internal intercostal muscles. Normally, no soft tissue attenuation is seen adjacent to a rib or in the paravertebral regions because the intercostal muscles do not pass internally to the ribs or vertebrae and because the pleura and endothoracic fascia are not thick enough to be seen in these locations. Any distinct stripe of soft tissue attenuation internal to a rib or in the paravertebral region is abnormal.[133]

In one study of 30 patients in whom conventional and oblique radiographs revealed pleural shadows of uncertain origin, CT showed that the opacities were the result of subpleural fat accumulation in 14 (47%);[132] of the remaining 16 patients, 10 had definite pleural plaques, 4 had no evidence of either plaques or fat, and 2 showed shadows that could not be attributed with certainty to either plaques or fat.

Calcification

Although noncalcified pleural plaques are the most common radiographic manifestation of asbestos-related disease, they are more striking when calcified (Fig. 16–20). The frequency of calcification is variable, ranging from 0% to 50% in different series;[101, 115, 117, 134] these differences in prevalence probably are related to differences in the type of inhaled asbestos. As might be expected, the complication is seen more commonly on CT than on radiograph. In a study of 100 asbestos-exposed American workers, calcification was detected on chest radiography in 13, on conventional CT in 16, and on HRCT in 20.[142]

Calcified plaques vary from small linear or circular shadows to shadows that completely encircle the lower portion of the lungs.[135] When calcification is minimal, a radiograph overexposed at maximal inspiration facilitates visibility.[136] Although it may be seen at any location, the most common site is the diaphragm.[137] The complication

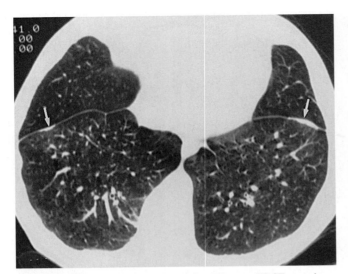

Figure 16–19. Plaques Within Interlobar Fissures. HRCT scan shows pleural plaques in the right and left major fissures *(arrows).* Curvilinear opacities in the right paravertebral region extend to an area of pleural thickening. The patient was a 71-year-old man who previously had worked in a shipyard.

generally does not develop until at least 20 years after the first exposure to asbestos.[116, 137] The exposure can be relatively short, as, for example, in two patients in whom isolated calcified diaphragmatic plaques developed approximately 20 years after occupational exposures of only 8 and 11 months.[138]

Diffuse Pleural Thickening

In contrast to a pleural plaque, diffuse thickening is manifested as a generalized, more or less uniform increase in pleural width. Although the term is not defined precisely in the 1980 ILO classification, the abnormality generally is considered to be present when there is a smooth uninterrupted pleural density extending over at least one fourth of the chest wall with or without obliteration of the costophrenic angles.[139] Diffuse thickening is diagnosed on CT when a continuous area of pleural thickening greater than 3 mm extends for more than 8 cm craniocaudally and 5 cm around the perimeter of the hemithorax.[140]

On HRCT, the margin between an area of diffuse pleural thickening and the adjacent lung frequently is irregular as a result of parenchymal fibrosis, in contrast to the usually sharply circumscribed margins of pleural plaques.[141] The abnormality usually is associated with contralateral pleural abnormalities, either diffuse pleural thickening or plaques.[143] Although calcification may be present, it seldom is extensive.[143, 144] Similar to other causes of fibrothorax, asbestos-related pleural thickening seldom involves the mediastinal pleura (although it frequently affects the parietal pleura abutting the paravertebral gutters, Fig. 16–21).[143, 145] The absence of involvement of the mediastinal pleura can be assessed readily on CT scan and often is helpful in distinguishing benign from malignant pleural thickening; in one study of 19 patients, only 1 of 8 who had fibrothorax had thickening of the mediastinal pleura as compared with 8 of 11 who had mesothelioma.[143]

Pleural Effusion

Asbestos-associated pleural effusion often is not appreciated.[146–148] The most comprehensive report of its prevalence and incidence was a study of 1,135 exposed workers and 717 control subjects in whom benign asbestos effusion was defined by[148] (1) a history of exposure to asbestos; (2) confirmation of the presence of effusion by radiographs,

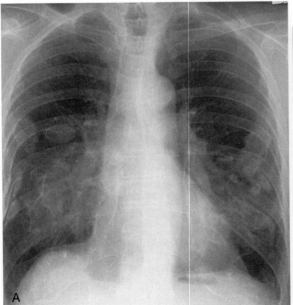

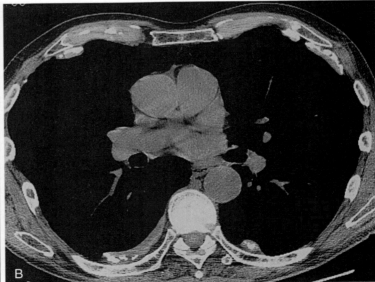

Figure 16–20. Calcified Pleural Plaques. Posteroanterior chest radiograph *(A)* in an 82-year-old man shows numerous bilateral calcified pleural plaques. The patient had worked for many years in a shipyard. HRCT scan *(B)* shows calcified plaques along the posteromedial and anterolateral chest wall.

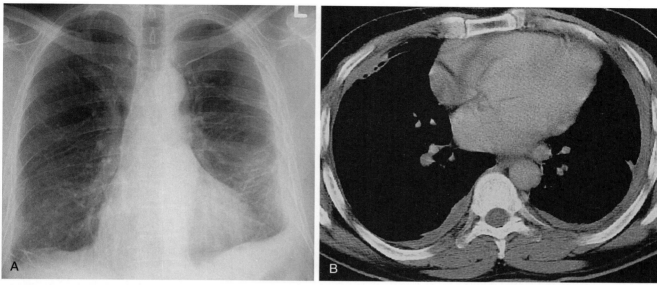

Figure 16–21. Diffuse Asbestos-Related Pleural Thickening. A 47-year-old cement worker presented with progressive shortness of breath. Posteroanterior chest radiograph *(A)* shows diffuse bilateral pleural thickening as well as blunting of the costophrenic sulci. Curvilinear opacities extending to the thickened pleura are present in the left lung. HRCT scan *(B)* confirms the presence of marked pleural thickening. The inner margin of the thickened pleura is irregular because of areas of fibrosis or atelectasis in the adjacent lung. Despite the extensive pleural thickening in the paravertebral portion of the pleura and lateral chest wall, there is no evidence of involvement of the mediastinal pleura.

thoracentesis, or both; (3) absence of other non-neoplastic disease that could have caused the effusion; and (4) absence of malignant tumor within 3 years. According to these criteria, 34 benign effusions (3%) were identified in the exposed workers compared with none in the control subjects. The likelihood of the presence of effusion was dose related. The latency period was shorter than for other asbestos-related disorders, being the most common abnormality during the first 20 years after exposure. Most effusions were small, 28% recurred, and 66% were unassociated with symptoms.

The major differential diagnoses are tuberculosis and mesothelioma. Of 12 patients in one series, mesothelioma was recognized in 1 patient 9 years after the first documented effusion.[146] Of four patients in another series, two eventually developed mesothelioma.[149]

Mesothelioma

The most characteristic radiologic manifestation of mesothelioma consists of diffuse pleural thickening (pleural rind) with associated loss of volume of the ipsilateral hemithorax (Fig. 16–22).[150] Effusion frequently is present and characteristically is not associated with contralateral shift of the mediastinum because of the restrictive action of the tumor. Occasionally the thickening is focal and simulates a pleural plaque.[151, 152] Features that favor mesothelioma include nodular thickening, mediastinal pleural thickening, involvement of the interlobar fissures, and presence of effusion.[143, 152] Pleural plaques are identified on CT scan in about 30% to 70% of patients who have mesothelioma and pleural calcification in 20% to 50%.[143, 151, 152] Calcification is almost invariably within pleural plaques and only rarely within the tumor itself.[153, 154]

In most cases, mesothelioma can be distinguished readily from benign asbestos-related pleural plaques on

radiograph and CT scan. It may be more difficult, however, to distinguish the tumor from diffuse asbestos-related pleural thickening or other causes of benign or malignant pleural disease.[143, 145] In one review of the CT findings in 74 consecutive patients who had diffuse pleural disease, of whom 39 had malignant disease and 35 had benign disease, features that were most suggestive of malignancy included circumferential pleural thickening, nodular thickening, parietal pleural thickening of more than 1 cm, and mediastinal pleural involvement (Fig. 16–23).[143] The sensitivities of these findings in detecting malignant pleural involvement were 41%, 51%, 36%, and 56%; the specificities ranged from 88% to 100%. Of the 39 malignant cases, 28 (sensitivity 72%, specificity 83%) were identified correctly by the presence of one or more of these criteria.

Pulmonary Manifestations

Asbestosis

Asbestosis typically is manifested on chest radiograph by the presence of small, irregular linear opacities (Table 16–5; Fig. 16–24). The development of these abnormalities

Table 16–5. ASBESTOSIS: RADIOLOGIC MANIFESTATIONS

Irregular linear opacities (reticular pattern)
Subpleural predominance
Subpleural dotlike opacities
Curvilinear subpleural lines
Parenchymal bands
Honeycombing may be present
Traction bronchiectasis
Ground-glass opacities
Pleural plaques or diffuse pleural thickening
Lymphadenopathy seldom evident on radiograph

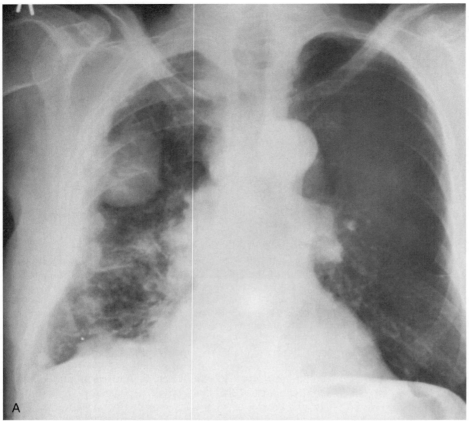

Figure 16–22. Diffuse Mesothelioma. Overpenetrated posteroanterior chest radiograph *(A)* shows a reduction in volume of the right hemithorax. There is marked thickening of the pleura over the whole of the right lung, including its mediastinal surface. The thickening is nodular and is associated with a large pleural-based mass in the upper axillary region. CT scan *(B)* confirms the extensive right pleural thickening *(arrowheads)* and shows enlarged mediastinal lymph nodes (N). The diagnosis of mesothelioma was confirmed at autopsy several months later.

may be divided into three stages:[155] (1) an early stage of fine reticulation occupying predominantly the lower lung zone and associated with a ground-glass appearance that is probably the result of pleural thickening and interstitial fibrosis; (2) a stage in which irregular small opacities become more marked, creating a prominent interstitial reticulation; during this stage, the combination of parenchymal and pleural abnormalities leads to partial obscuration of the heart border—the so-called shaggy heart sign—and of the diaphragm; and (3) a late stage in which reticulation

becomes visible in the middle and upper lung zones, and the cardiac and diaphragmatic contours become more obscured.[43, 155]

Hilar lymph node enlargement seldom is evident on radiograph;[146] however, mediastinal lymph nodes greater than 1 cm in diameter frequently are seen on CT scan.[156] Although asbestosis characteristically exhibits considerable mid and lower zonal predominance, a few patients have been reported in whom slowly progressive pleural and parenchymal fibrosis occurred in the lung apices.[157] Large

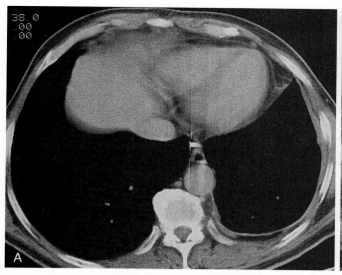
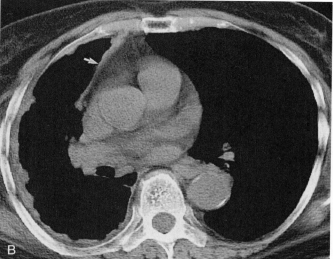

Figure 16–23. Benign Versus Malignant Pleural Thickening. CT scan in a 59-year-old man *(A)* shows extensive thickening of the posteromedial, lateral, and anterior aspects of the left pleura; the mediastinal pleura is uninvolved. The patient had been exposed to asbestos many years before as a carpenter. Pleural biopsy specimens show only fibrosis. CT scan in an 80-year-old woman *(B)* shows extensive right pleural thickening. Involvement of the mediastinal pleura *(arrows)* as well as nodular appearance of the pleural thickening is evident. Biopsy specimen showed mesothelioma.

opacities measuring 1 cm or more in diameter have been described in occasional patients who have asbestosis;[158] however, these patients also have been exposed to quartz, and it is likely that the latter was responsible for the conglomerate shadows.

Although the radiographic findings of asbestosis are not specific, the diagnosis should be suspected when irregular linear opacities are associated with pleural plaques or diffuse pleural thickening. In approximately 20% of patients who have radiographic findings of asbestosis, however, there is no radiographic evidence of asbestos pleural disease.[159] Radiographs fail to show any parenchymal abnormalities in 10% to 20% of patients who have pathologically proven asbestosis.[160, 161]

As with other conditions, CT, particularly HRCT, allows detection of parenchymal abnormalities not evident on chest radiograph.[119, 120, 142] In one prospective study of 100 asbestos-exposed workers, HRCT findings suggestive of asbestosis were present in 43 of 45 (96%) who satisfied clinical criteria of asbestosis, compared with 35 (78%) who had radiographic abnormalities.[142] In another investigation of 60 asbestos workers, characteristic features of asbestosis were found in 100% of patients examined by HRCT, compared with 90% by radiography.[119] In a review of the HRCT findings and pulmonary function tests in 169 asbestos-exposed workers who had normal chest radiographs (ILO profusion score <1/0), CT abnormalities consistent with asbestosis were found in 57;[120] these patients had significantly lower vital capacity and diffusing capacity for carbon monoxide than the workers who had normal CT scans.

The most common HRCT manifestations of asbestosis are intralobular linear opacities, irregular thickening of interlobular septa, subpleural curvilinear opacities, subpleural small rounded or branching opacities, and parenchymal bands *(see* Fig. 16–24).[119, 120, 162] Small, round (dotlike), and branching subpleural opacities are considered to be the earliest manifestation of disease.[162] These opacities typically are visible a few millimeters from the pleural surface

in a centrilobular distribution. HRCT-pathologic correlation showed the opacities to reflect peribronchiolar fibrosis.[162] Subpleural curvilinear opacities are linear areas of increased attenuation of variable length located within 1 cm of the pleura and parallel to the inner chest wall (Fig. 16–25).[163] Most measure 5 to 10 cm in length. They are seen most commonly in early disease, although they may reflect honeycombing; they also may represent atelectasis adjacent to pleural plaques.[144, 162, 164]

Another common HRCT feature seen in asbestos-exposed workers is the presence of parenchymal bands, defined as linear opacities measuring 2 to 5 cm in length coursing through the lung, usually to abut an area of pleural thickening.[142] Pathologic correlation showed these bands to correspond to fibrosis along the bronchovascular sheath or interlobular septa with associated distortion of parenchymal architecture.[164] The bands are more common in asbestosis than in other causes of pulmonary fibrosis; in one study, they were present in 79% of patients who had asbestosis compared with 11% of patients who had IPF.[165] As in other causes of interstitial pulmonary fibrosis, architectural distortion of secondary lobules and irregular thickening of interlobular septa are seen commonly in asbestosis (Fig. 16–26). With progression of fibrosis, irregular linear opacities and honeycombing predominate.[121, 166] At all stages, the abnormalities involve predominantly the subpleural regions of the lower lung zones.[142, 164, 166]

Similar to radiographic abnormalities, HRCT findings are nonspecific, and no single sign can be considered diagnostic of asbestosis.[167] The likelihood of asbestos-related interstitial fibrosis increases, however, with the number of abnormalities identified.[121] The accuracy of HRCT in predicting the presence of asbestosis was assessed in a group of 24 patients and in 6 lungs obtained at autopsy;[121] histologic evidence of asbestosis was present in 25 of the 30 patients or lungs. The most common HRCT findings consisted of intralobular lines or thickened interlobular septa, parenchymal bands, architectural distortion of the

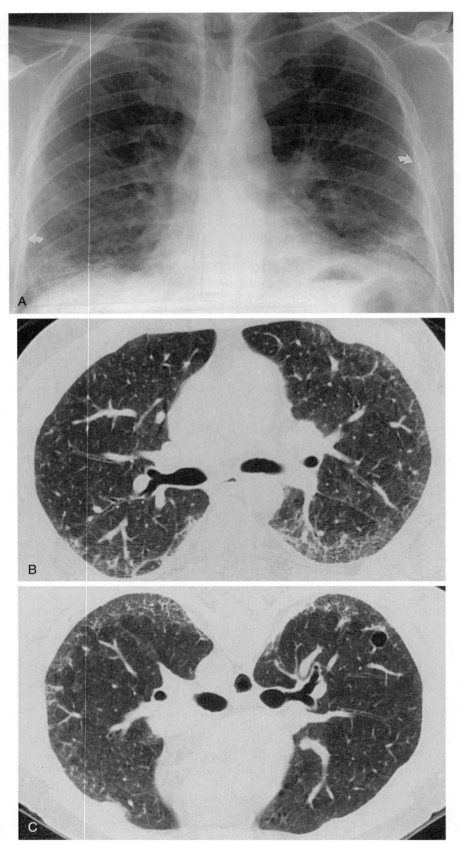

Figure 16–24. Asbestosis. Posteroanterior chest radiograph *(A)* in a 54-year-old shipyard worker shows irregular linear opacities in the lower lung zones. Associated low lung volumes and bilateral pleural plaques *(arrows)* are present. HRCT scans in the supine *(B)* and prone *(C)* positions show irregular linear opacities involving predominantly the subpleural lung regions. The opacities represent intralobular lines and thickening of interlobular septa. Localized areas of ground-glass attenuation in the subpleural lung regions are evident.

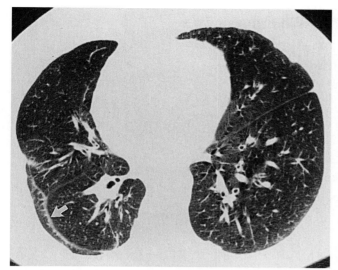

Figure 16–25. Subpleural Curvilinear Opacities in Asbestosis. HRCT scan shows a subpleural curvilinear opacity in the right lung running parallel to the pleura *(arrow)*. Bilateral pleural plaques and evidence of early fibrosis in the posterior aspect of the left lung are present. The parenchymal abnormalities did not change in the prone position. The patient was a 58-year-old shipyard worker.

Table 16–6. ROUND ATELECTASIS: RADIOLOGIC MANIFESTATIONS

Rounded or oval opacity
2–7 cm in diameter
Abuts an area of pleural thickening
Associated with volume loss
Vessels and bronchi curve toward the opacity (comet-tail sign)
Unilateral or bilateral
May progress over months or years

secondary lobules, subpleural lines, and honeycombing. To identify the cases confidently as asbestosis, three of these abnormalities had to be identified on CT; although a positive interpretation based on one or two abnormalities increased the sensitivity, it resulted in a substantial decrease in specificity. The procedure was considered to identify insufficient abnormalities to diagnose asbestosis in 5 of the 25 (20%) cases, whereas 10 radiographs (40%) were nondiagnostic.

Because the abnormalities in patients who have mild asbestosis often are limited to the posterior aspects of the lower lung zones, it is recommended that CT scans in these patients be obtained in supine and prone positions or only in the prone position.[121, 142, 168] Scans with the patient prone are important to distinguish the normal increased opacity in the dependent lung regions from mild fibrosis. It has been shown that taking a small number of prone images at selected levels in the lower lung zones has a high sensitivity in the detection of asbestos-related pulmonary and pleural abnormalities.[168] This procedure, combined with low radiation dose scans, may become a cost-effective method of screening for asbestosis in high-risk populations.[168, 169]

Round Atelectasis

The characteristic radiologic manifestation of round atelectasis is a rounded or oval, pleural-based opacity associated with loss of volume and with curving of adjacent pulmonary vessels and bronchi (the comet-tail sign) (Table 16–6).[170, 171] The opacity typically abuts an area of pleural thickening or a pleural effusion. The comet-tail sign of pulmonary vessels and bronchi as they are swept around and into the focus of atelectasis is easier to identify on CT scan than on radiograph (Fig. 16–27). The abnormality may occur anywhere in the lungs but is most common in the posterior aspect of the lower lobes.[172–175] It may be unilateral or bilateral and may measure 2 to 7 cm in diameter. Significant enhancement may occur with intravenous contrast administration.[176, 177]

As indicated previously, most cases follow asbestos exposure; however, some have been described in association

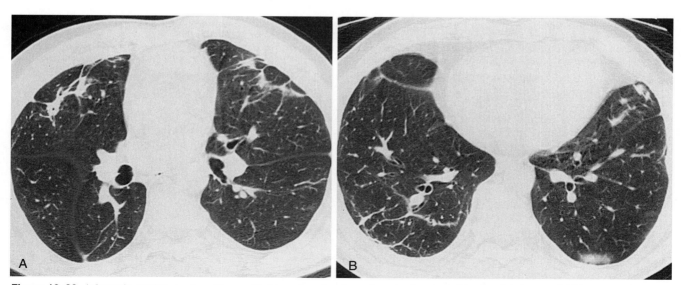

Figure 16–26. Asbestosis. HRCT scan in a 45-year-old shipyard worker shows irregular linear opacities, interlobular septal thickening, and evidence of architectural distortion in the anterior aspect of the midlung zones *(A)*. Irregular thickening of interlobular septa in the right lower lobe *(B)* is evident.

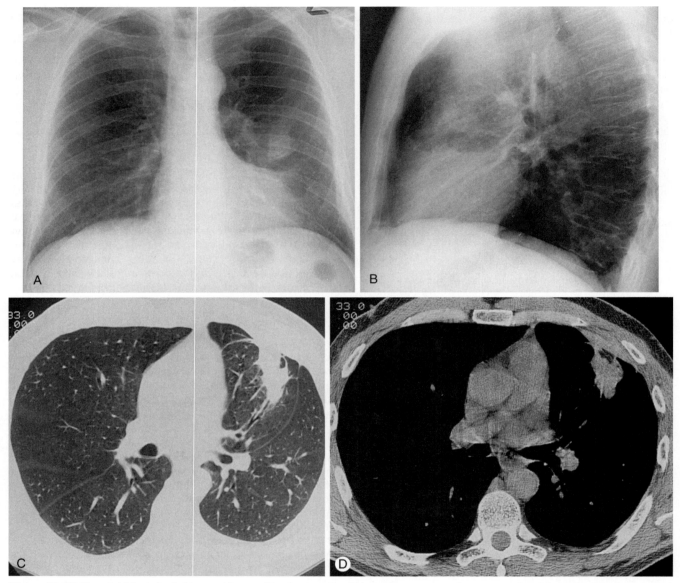

Figure 16–27. Round Atelectasis. A 54-year-old man with a long-standing history of exposure to asbestos was referred for evaluation of a suspected left lung mass. Posteroanterior *(A)* and lateral *(B)* chest radiographs show evidence of left pleural thickening and a 3-cm mass in the left lung. The margins of the mass are defined poorly, indicating that it is pleural based. HRCT scan *(C)* shows an oval soft tissue mass in the lingula associated with loss of volume and anterior displacement of the major fissure. Vessels and bronchi can be seen curving into and sweeping around the area of atelectasis. Soft tissue windows *(D)* show that the area of atelectasis abuts a focal area of pleural thickening. The size of the mass was stable during a 3-year follow-up period.

with other causes of pleural thickening or effusion.[114, 175] The lesion may develop and progress over a few months or several years. In one series of 74 patients, it occurred on a background of benign asbestos pleurisy in 9 and slowly increasing pleural thickening in 13;[114] in the remaining 52 patients, it was a new finding, with earlier radiographs showing only plaques or being normal.

The magnetic resonance (MR) imaging appearance has been described in one patient.[178] Similar to CT, MR imaging showed the abnormality as a peripheral mass abutting an area of pleural thickening with associated vessels curving into the area of atelectasis. Curved low-signal lines within the atelectatic lung were postulated to be caused by indentations of the visceral pleura.[178] Round atelectasis is

not metabolically active on 2-(^{18}F)-fluoro-2-deoxy-D-glucose (FDG) positron emission tomography (PET).[179] FDG-PET imaging can be helpful in differentiating the abnormality from pulmonary carcinoma.[179]

Prognosis and Natural History

The two most important complications of asbestos inhalation are pulmonary fibrosis and pleuropulmonary malignancy. The likelihood of developing clinically evident asbestosis depends (at least in part) on cumulative dust exposure and time from first contact with the mineral. Disabling respiratory disease and cor pulmonale usually develop only in individuals who have a history of heavy dust exposure typically 30 or more years after initial contact.

Of all non-neoplastic pulmonary diseases, those related to asbestos have the highest incidence of associated neoplasia, especially pulmonary carcinoma and pleural mesothelioma.[185, 186] In a cohort study of 11,000 Quebec chrysotile workers, the standardized mortality rates for pulmonary carcinoma and mesothelioma were 1.4 and 25;[187, 188] of the 5,350 individuals who died between 1975 and 1992, approximately 320 died of pulmonary carcinoma, 48 of asbestosis, and 25 of mesothelioma. A latent period of at least 20 years from the time of first exposure to the development of malignancy is characteristic.[189]

ASPIRATION OF SOLID FOREIGN MATERIAL AND LIQUIDS

Aspiration of Solid Foreign Bodies

Aspiration of solid foreign bodies into the tracheobronchial tree occurs most often in infants and small children;[190, 191] 79% of 66 patients investigated in one series were younger than 10 years old.[192] The condition occurs occasionally in older individuals.[193–195] In children, aspiration typically occurs in otherwise healthy individuals. By contrast, adults frequently have an underlying condition associated with impairment of airway protection, such as a neurologic disorder, trauma with loss of consciousness, or drug or alcohol abuse.[194–196] Although the aspirated foreign bodies that have been described are of fascinating variety, including pencils, rubber tubing, pins, needles, thermometers, metallic and plastic toys, and jewelry,[192] the substance most commonly implicated is food, usually vegetable.[192]

The most common symptoms of foreign body aspiration are cough and choking; respiratory failure occurs rarely.[197] In children, choking usually is recognized by parents or guardians.[191, 205] Although many adult patients also give a history of choking at the time of aspiration,[198, 206, 207] it may require much persistence for the physician to elicit this when the episode is not recent. In such individuals, an asymptomatic interval may follow aspiration, especially when bronchi are not obstructed;[193, 208] such a latent period can extend to several months or years, particularly if the aspirated material is bone or inorganic matter.[195] Eventually, disease usually becomes manifest as recurrent pneumonia, chronic cough, or hemoptysis.[195]

Radiologic Manifestations

Although some foreign bodies (such as teeth[198] and coins[194]) are discovered incidentally on routine chest radiograph, in most cases, radiographic findings reflect the effects of partial or complete airway obstruction. Although the aspirated foreign bodies can be seen in all lobes,[194, 195] the most common site is the right lower lobe in children[198] and adults.[194] In one series of 60 adult patients, 17 foreign bodies (28%) were located in the right lower lobe, 11 (18%) in the left lower lobe, 10 (17%) in the left main bronchus, 8 (13%) in the bronchus intermedius, 6 (10%) in the right main bronchus, 2 (3%) in the left upper lobe bronchus, 1 in the trachea, and 1 in the right upper lobe bronchus.[194]

The standard chest radiograph is helpful in locating the site of foreign body impaction in about 70% of patients;[194, 195] in the remainder, it is normal or shows nonspecific air-space opacities. In adults, the most common radiographic findings consist of atelectasis, obstructive pneumonitis (Fig. 16–28), or visualization of a radiopaque foreign body (Fig. 16–29).[194, 195] Other abnormalities include air-trapping on expiratory radiograph, abscess distal to the impacted foreign body, and occasionally lung torsion.[194, 195] In most adults, the lung volume distal to an impacted foreign body is decreased;[194] hyperinflation is rare.[194, 195] Although hyperinflation has been said to occur in most patients in some studies of children,[198] because it can be difficult to obtain radiographs of the chest in infants and young children at the point of maximal inspiration, we suspect that the hyperinflation represented *air-trapping* on radiographs exposed at the position of slight expiration.

CT is not recommended routinely, but can be valuable in selected cases.[201, 280, 289] CT usually shows the foreign body and its precise location within the bronchial tree, even when it is radiolucent (Fig. 16–30).[202, 280]

Bronchiectasis is an occasional complication of long-standing retention of a foreign body.[192, 200, 203] In one series of 500 patients who had this disorder, foreign bodies were considered to be the cause in 8 (four of the foreign bodies were vegetable, and four were mineral).[204]

Aspiration of Gastric or Oropharyngeal Secretions

The term *aspiration pneumonia* is employed by some to denote pulmonary infection caused by aspiration of bacteria-laden oropharyngeal secretions. This form of pneumonia frequently is caused by anaerobic organisms in patients who have poor oral hygiene and commonly is associated with abscess formation. Although occasionally complicated by such anaerobic bacterial infection, aspiration of oropharyngeal or gastric secretions, with or without admixed food particles, also can cause significant pulmonary disease in the absence of infection. Almost invariably, this disease occurs in individuals who have an underlying condition predisposing to aspiration, most commonly one of the following:

- Chronic debilitating disease, such as cancer
- Oropharyngeal or airway instrumentation
- General anesthesia, epileptic seizure, cardiopulmonary resuscitation,[209] electroconvulsive therapy, trauma, alcohol-induced or drug-induced stupor,[210] or cerebrovascular accident[211, 212]
- Disorders affecting swallowing,[213] such as esophageal or pharyngeal carcinoma, hypopharyngeal (Zenker's) diverticulum, and neuromuscular disease involving the esophagus or pharynx[214]

The pathogenesis of pulmonary damage depends on the amount and nature of the aspirated material. The hydrochloric acid of the gastric juice appears to be an important mediator of disease. The results of some experimental studies suggest that pulmonary damage occurs predominantly when the pH of the aspirate is less than 2.5; it has been shown that prior neutralization of acid solutions instilled intratracheally reduces the severity of the pulmo-

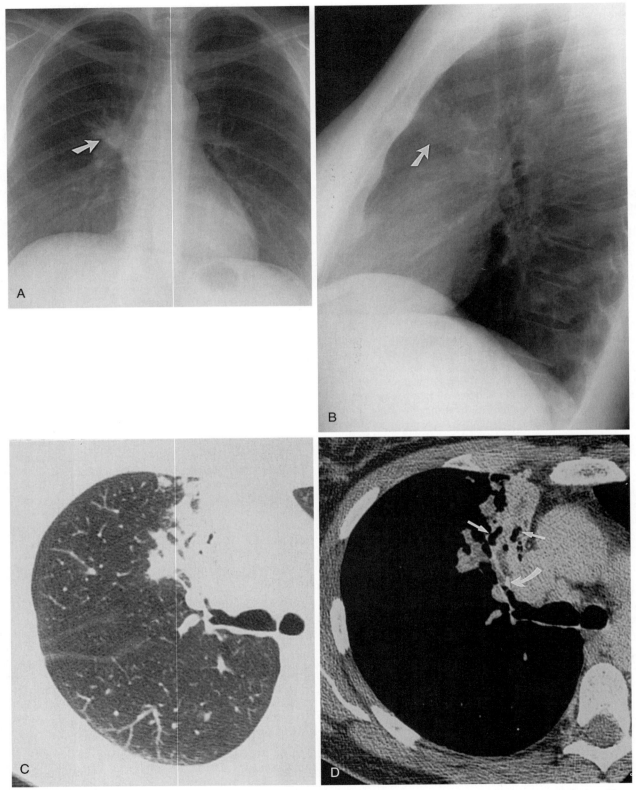

Figure 16–28. Obstructive Pneumonitis Caused by Foreign Body Aspiration. Posteroanterior *(A)* and lateral *(B)* chest radiographs in a 44-year-old woman show localized consolidation and atelectasis involving the anterior segment of the right upper lobe *(arrows)*. HRCT scans *(C* and *D)* show evidence of obstructive pneumonitis and bronchiectasis *(straight arrows)* in the anterior segment of the right upper lobe. The localized area of high attenuation *(curved arrow)* within the bronchial lumen represents an aspirated popcorn kernel.

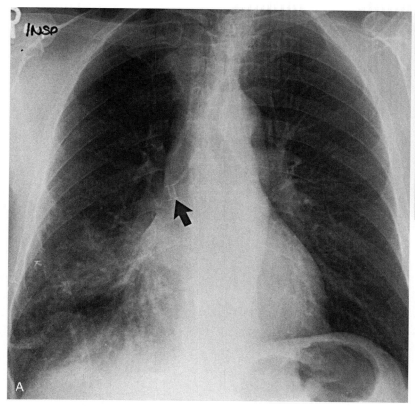

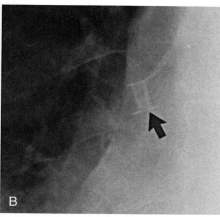

Figure 16–29. Aspiration of Esophageal Speech Device. This 59-year-old man developed areas of atelectasis and consolidation in the right middle and lower lobes after radical laryngectomy. Chest radiograph *(A)* and magnified view of the right lower chest *(B)* show an esophageal speech device *(arrows)* in the bronchus intermedius. The device was removed bronchoscopically.

nary reaction.[215] In humans, it generally is assumed that the risk of pulmonary disease from gastric acid aspiration is related to the pH and the volume of aspirated stomach contents; risk is greatest when the pH is less than 2.5 and the volume is greater than 25 ml. Pulmonary damage also occurs, however, when the pH of aspirated fluid is greater than 2.5.[216-218]

Respiratory distress may be noted before radiographic abnormalities become manifest. In this situation, fiberoptic bronchoscopy may reveal erythema of the tracheal mucosa.[224] In the early stages, diffuse crackles may be heard; once consolidation develops, patchy areas of bronchial breathing may be detected. Hypoxemia may be severe. If the patient survives the stage of acute pulmonary edema, a

Figure 16–30. Foreign Body Aspiration. A 23-year-old drug addict presented with a 3-month history of cough productive of increasing amounts of green sputum. HRCT scan shows tubing within the lumen of the right main bronchus *(arrows).* A small amount of secretions within the bronchial lumen and decreased attenuation, vascularity, and volume of the right lung are evident. The plastic tube was removed bronchoscopically.

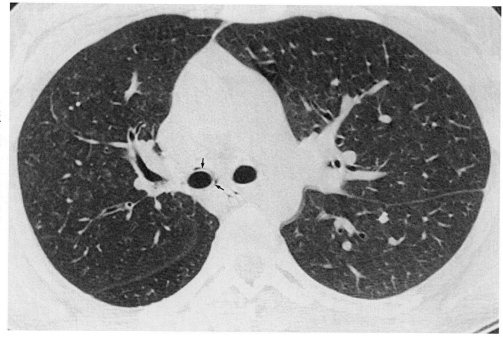

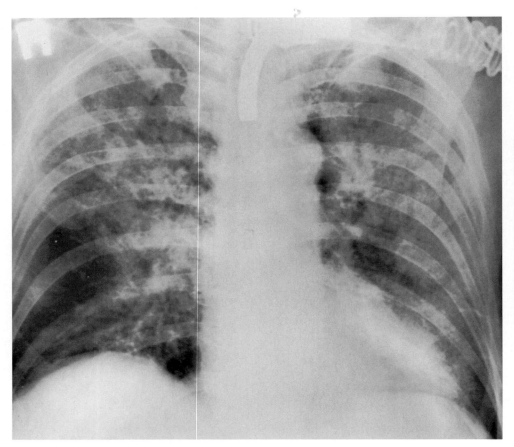

Figure 16–31. Acute Aspiration Pneumonia. While lying in a supine position after anesthesia, a 68-year-old man aspirated considerable quantities of vomitus. Anteroposterior chest radiograph performed within 2 hours shows extensive involvement of both lungs by patchy air-space consolidation typical of acute pulmonary edema. Although a few patchy shadows are present in the lower lung zones, the predominant involvement is in the upper zones, a distribution that can be explained, at least partly, by the position of the patient at the time of aspiration.

dry cough may supervene and eventually become productive of copious purulent sputum; a variety of aerobic and anaerobic pathogens may be cultured from this material.

Radiologic Manifestations

In the patient who has aspirated a large amount of relatively pure gastric secretion at a low pH, chest radiograph typically reveals general involvement of both lungs by patchy air-space consolidation, similar to pulmonary edema of cardiac origin or to the more diffuse permeability edema observed in adult respiratory distress syndrome.[219] Although discrete air-space shadows can be apparent, most opacities are confluent (Fig. 16–31). Distribution typically is bilateral and multicentric but usually favors perihilar or basal regions (Table 16–7).[219] The perihilar distribution has been shown on CT to reflect the presence of consolidation mainly in the posterior segments of the upper lobes or superior segments of the lower lobes.[220] In uncomplicated

Table 16–7. ASPIRATION PNEUMONIA: RADIOLOGIC MANIFESTATIONS

Unilateral or bilateral air-space consolidation
Often basal and perihilar predominance
Anatomic distribution reflects position of patient
Often has segmental distribution
May be multicentric or diffuse
Frequently associated with loss of volume

cases, these abnormalities often worsen for several days and thereafter improve fairly rapidly. Progression of the radiographic abnormalities after initial improvement is associated with the development of bacterial pneumonia, adult respiratory distress syndrome, or thromboembolism.[219] The normal size of the heart and the absence of signs of pulmonary venous hypertension differentiate the edema from that of cardiac origin.

This form of aspiration pneumonia may not show an anatomic distribution, reflecting the influence of gravity. If the patient is lying in the prone or supine position at the time of aspiration, the highly irritative nature of the aspirate may result in widespread dissemination throughout the lungs (Fig. 16–32); however, predominant changes may be unilateral if the patient is lying on his or her side. If the patient survives, resolution is relatively rapid—averaging 7 to 10 days in our experience, about the same as for traumatic fat embolism but much slower than that for edema caused by acute cardiac decompensation.

In cases in which there is aspiration of oropharyngeal secretions or gastric contents containing an appreciable amount of admixed food, radiographic findings have a segmental distribution, often involving one or more of the posterior segments of the upper or lower lobes. The precise localization depends at least partly on the position of the patient at the time of aspiration.[219, 221] Some degree of atelectasis is present in almost all cases, and the picture can be typical of bacterial bronchopneumonia. With repeated aspiration, serial radiography over months or years shows much variation in the anatomic distribution of segments

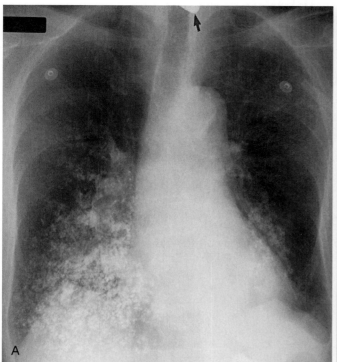

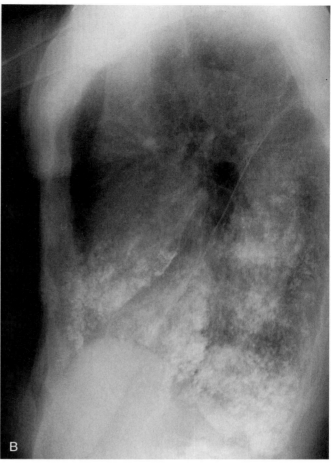

Figure 16–32. Aspiration of Oropharyngeal Contents and Barium. Posteroanterior *(A)* and lateral *(B)* chest radiographs in an 88-year-old woman show barium, mainly in the right middle and lower lobes and in the left lower lobe. Barium can be seen within the inferior margin of a Zenker's diverticulum *(arrow)*. The aspiration occurred shortly after a barium swallow.

involved, with disease clearing in one segment and appearing in another. A residuum of irregular accentuation of linear markings may remain, probably representing peribronchial scarring. Rarely, chest radiographs show reticulonodular[222] or miliary[223] patterns. Granulomatous pneumonitis associated with aspiration of leguminous vegetables, also known as *lentil aspiration pneumonia*, can be manifested as 1- to 5-mm diameter nodules on chest radiograph;[199] HRCT performed in two patients showed the nodules to have a centrilobular distribution.[199] A similar appearance may be seen with aspiration of psyllium, a medication used for treatment of chronic constipation.[286] Repeated aspiration of foreign particles into the bronchioles can result in diffuse aspiration bronchiolitis.[288] The HRCT findings consist of centrilobular nodules and branching linear opacities with a tree-in-bud appearance.[288]

Aspiration of Lipid

Lipid can accumulate in the lungs from endogenous or exogenous sources.[225] The former situation is seen in such conditions as obstructive pneumonitis, pulmonary alveolar proteinosis, and hereditary errors of lipid metabolism. These conditions are entirely different in nature from the exogenous form and are considered elsewhere in this book. The term *lipid (lipoid) pneumonia* is restricted here to disease caused by the aspiration of mineral oil or of the various vegetable or animal oils present in food.

Mineral oil is the most common agent to cause lipid pneumonia as defined. Disease occurs most frequently when the oil is used as a lubricant in infants who have feeding difficulties; in old people who are constipated; and in patients who have dysphagia caused by neurologic disease or intrinsic esophageal disease, such as hypopharyngeal (Zenker's) diverticulum, carcinoma, or achalasia.[226, 227] In these situations, there are presumably repeated subclinical episodes of aspiration, eventually resulting in sufficient accumulation of lipid to cause radiologic or clinical abnormalities.

The pathogenesis of mineral oil–related fibrosis is not well understood. The substance is a pure hydrocarbon and is believed to be inert, a feature that may explain the lack of airway-mediated cough reflex that follows aspiration. It has been suggested that release of lysosomal enzymes by injured or dead lipid-laden macrophages may be a factor in causing fibrosis.[228] Most patients are asymptomatic, the abnormality being discovered on screening chest radiograph. The diagnosis sometimes is made by histologic examination of tissue removed at thoracotomy performed on the basis of an erroneous diagnosis of pulmonary carcinoma.[229] Some patients complain of chronic, usually nonproductive cough or pleuritic pain.

Radiologic Manifestations

In the early stages, the typical pattern of disease is airspace consolidation (Table 16–8). Depending on the quan-

Table 16–8. LIPID PNEUMONIA: RADIOLOGIC MANIFESTATIONS

Air-space consolidation
Unifocal or multifocal
Segmental distribution
Predominantly lower lobes
May progress to masslike opacity simulating carcinoma
HRCT frequently shows foci of fat attenuation
MR imaging reflects the lipid content

HRCT, high-resolution computed tomography.

tity of oil aspirated, the resultant shadows can be confluent or discrete—isolated air-space nodules can form a distinctive feature during the early stages.[229] Although the radiographic pattern varies, its most common form is relatively homogeneous consolidation of one or more segments, often in precise segmental distribution (Fig. 16–33). In most cases, the lower lobes predominantly are affected, although in debilitated patients in a recumbent position, involvement is likely to occur in the superior segment of a lower lobe or the posterior segment of an upper lobe.[230, 231] The consolidated area may be several centimeters in diameter, with poorly defined or fairly sharply defined margins. Because the oil is transported from the alveoli into the interstitium, a predominantly interstitial pattern can develop in the later stages. Rarely, chronic lipid aspiration is sufficient to result in multiple masslike opacities. Withdrawal of the medication may be followed by slow but progressive radiographic resolution.

Another manifestation, occurring almost as commonly, is a peripheral mass, sometimes with fairly well-circumscribed margins, simulating pulmonary carcinoma (Fig. 16–34).[229] This abnormality develops chiefly in the dependent portions of the lung, although sometimes in the middle lobe or lingula. Linear shadows radiating from the periphery of such a mass result from the interlobular septal thickening caused by infiltration of lipid-laden macrophages and secondary chronic inflammation. Ossification is evident in some cases.[232] Rarely the acute phase of the process can be associated with cavitation, probably related to concomitant anaerobic infection.[225, 233]

The diagnosis of lipid pneumonia often can be made on CT by the presence of areas of low attenuation or fat attenuation (-90 HU) within the lesion (*see* Fig. 16–34).[227, 234, 288] In one investigation in which the radiographic and CT findings were compared in six patients—three who had a history of intake of shark liver oil as a restorative and three who had intake of mineral oil for constipation—chest radiography showed bilateral air-space consolidation in three, irregular masslike lesions in two, and a reticulonodular pattern in one.[234] In the three patients who had air-space consolidation, CT showed attenuation lower than that of chest wall musculature but slightly higher than that of subcutaneous fat. In the two patients who had masslike lesions, there were localized areas of consolidation containing fat; irregular lines and architectural distortion suggested fibrosis around the areas of consolidation. The patient who had a reticulonodular pattern on radiograph had no evidence of fat attenuation on CT scan. Occasionally, lipid pneumonia presents as multifocal areas of ground-glass attenuation associated with interlobular septal thickening, an appearance that resembles the *crazy-paving* pattern seen in alveolar proteinosis.[235]

The MR imaging findings of lipid pneumonia have been reported in a few patients.[236, 237] Using spin-echo imaging,

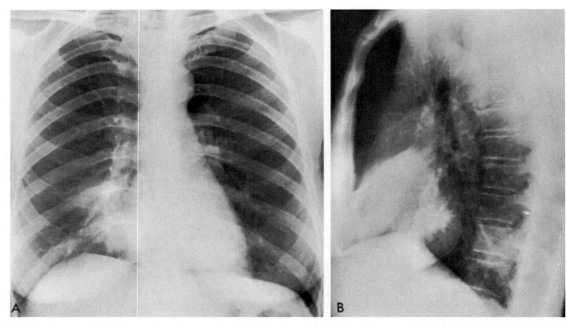

Figure 16–33. Exogenous Lipid Pneumonia. Posteroanterior *(A)* and lateral *(B)* radiographs of a 53-year-old symptom-free woman reveal poorly defined shadows of homogeneous density situated in the right middle lobe, the anterior segment of the right lower lobe, and the posterior basal segment of the left lower lobe. Thorough clinical and laboratory investigations failed to reveal the cause of these shadows. Ten years later, the patient died after rupture of a congenital berry aneurysm of the anterior cerebral artery. Autopsy revealed chronic lipid pneumonia of both lower lobes and the right middle lobe.

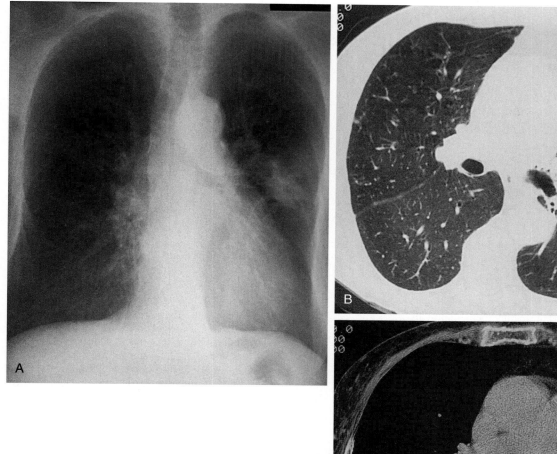

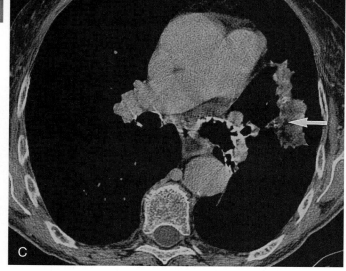

Figure 16–34. Lipid Pneumonia: Mass Lesion. Chest radiograph *(A)* in an 80-year-old woman shows consolidation in the left upper lobe and lingula. HRCT scan *(B and C)* shows focal area of consolidation with surrounding linear opacities and architectural distortion consistent with fibrosis. Localized areas of fat attenuation are present within the consolidation *(arrow)*, permitting the diagnosis of lipid pneumonia. The diagnosis was confirmed by fine-needle aspiration biopsy. The patient had a history of intake of mineral oil for constipation.

areas of consolidation have high signal intensity on T1-weighted and T2-weighted images, reflecting the lipid content of the aspirate.[236] A specific diagnosis can be made using chemical-shift MR imaging.[237]

Aspiration of Water (Drowning)

Drowning is defined as death caused by asphyxia as a result of submersion in liquid (usually water), provided that the victim succumbs within 24 hours of the submersion episode. Near-drowning is defined as survival (at least temporarily) after a submersion episode; the term *near-drowning* still has been used if the victim dies more than 24 hours after the submersion episode. Pathologic findings consist principally of air-space edema. The main mecha-

nism is increased capillary permeability. There is little clinical difference between victims of fresh water and salt water drowning.[239]

Radiologic Manifestations

The radiographic changes in patients who have experienced near-drowning from fresh water and seawater aspiration are similar.[238] The basic finding is air-space consolidation (Fig. 16–35), the severity presumably depending on the amount of aspirated water;[240–242] in the most severe cases, there is almost complete opacification of both lungs. Consolidation generally is bilateral and symmetric; however, in relatively mild disease, it can be predominantly parahilar and midzonal. An asymmetric distribution can

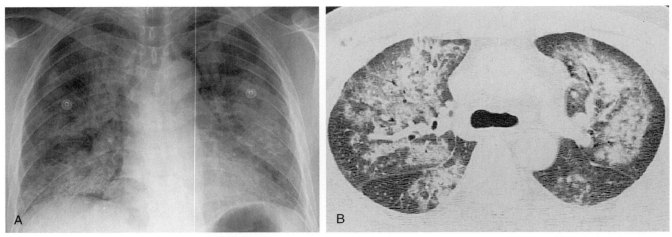

Figure 16–35. Near-Drowning in Seawater: Radiographic and CT Findings. Anteroposterior chest radiograph *(A)* in a 50-year-old man obtained within a few hours of near-drowning in seawater shows extensive, symmetric bilateral consolidation. HRCT scan *(B)* shows relative sparing of the peripheral lung, including the dependent lung regions. The consolidation resolved within 2 days.

occur (Fig. 16–36). There may be a delay in the radiographic appearance of edema, sometimes 24 to 48 hours.[242] Sand that is aspirated along with water can be radiopaque as a result of its calcium carbonate content and can cause a *sand bronchogram* on radiographs and CT scans;[243, 244] sand may be seen within the stomach. Pleural effusion occurs in some cases; in one study, it was found to be more likely in salt water than fresh water drowning and associated with a longer submersion time.[245]

The air-space consolidation generally improves in 3 to 5 days and resolves completely in 7 to 10 days.[241] In some patients, the radiographic changes persist or worsen, findings that may be the result of bacterial pneumonia or adult respiratory distress syndrome.[238]

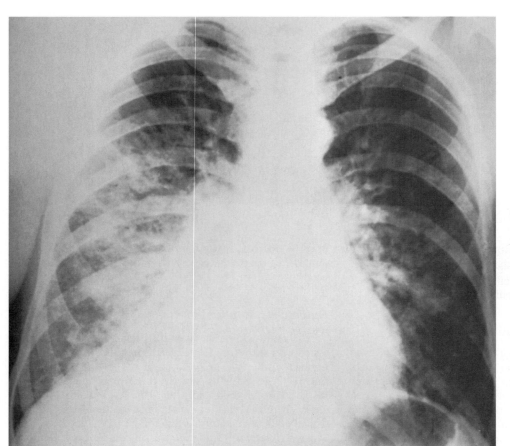

Figure 16–36. Near-Drowning in Seawater. A man was immersed for an indeterminate time in seawater. On radiograph, there is evidence of extensive bilateral air-space edema, more marked in the right than the left lung. The edema cleared in 3 days.

In one review of the clinical manifestations in 36 patients who experienced near-drowning (32 in salt water and 4 in chlorinated pools), 33 of the 36 survived.[238] Only 9 patients were unconscious on arrival to the hospital. Respiratory frequency was generally increased to 30 to 40 breaths per minute during the initial 24 hours; thereafter, it returned to normal levels.

INHALED TOXIC GASES, FUMES, AND AEROSOLS

Many gases and fumes as well as liquids in a finely dispersed state (aerosols) can cause acute and sometimes chronic damage to the pulmonary airways and parenchyma. The reaction depends to some extent on the chemical composition of the gas or aerosol. Some substances, particularly those that are highly soluble, such as sulfur dioxide, ammonia (NH_3), and chloride, are so irritating to the nasal mucosa that individuals may stop breathing on exposure and run away. Less soluble gases, such as phosgene, nitrogen dioxide (NO_2), ozone, and highly concentrated oxygen, may be inhaled deeply into the lungs before the irritating effect is perceived.

The manifestation of diseases that result from inhalation of these toxic substances is variable. In many instances, the underlying abnormality is alveolocapillary damage with resultant permeability pulmonary edema (Fig. 16–37). In others, the chemical injury appears to affect the airways predominantly,[246, 247] resulting in bronchitis and bronchiolitis, sometimes complicated by atelectasis and bacterial pneumonia. Patients who survive the acute insult may feel relatively well for several weeks, then undergo abrupt or insidious clinical deterioration, with cough, shortness of breath, and fever. This delayed form of disease is reflected pathologically by obliterative bronchiolitis.[248] The compli-

cation can occur in individuals who initially experience diffuse pulmonary edema.

An unusual form of aerosol injury results from inhalation of hydrocarbon-containing fluids in fire-eaters.[281] Fire-eaters blow out a mouthful of pyrofluid against a burning stick, creating an aerosol that ignites around the stick. This gives the spectators the illusion of flames emanating from the performer's mouth. Inhalation of the liquid hydrocarbons contained in the pyrofluid can result in acute and chronic airway and parenchymal abnormalities. The initial abnormalities consist of bronchial, interstitial and air-space inflammation and edema.[282] Chronic changes include proliferative bronchiolitis, pneumatocele formation, and fibrosis.[283] Radiographic manifestations in the acute stage show areas of air-space consolidation that may have a masslike appearance (Fig 16–38).[281, 284] CT shows coalescent areas of consolidation, cavitary lesions, and rapid development of pneumatoceles. The pneumatoceles usually resolve within a few days or weeks, leaving small residual scars.[281, 285]

Bronchopulmonary Disease Associated with Burns

Pulmonary complications occur in 20% to 30% of burn victims admitted to a hospital.[252–254] In addition to infection, shock, and the consequences of therapy, including overhydration,[249, 250] tracheobronchial and pulmonary disease can be caused by smoke and the materials it contains and by heat; assessment of the relative contribution of each of these mechanisms can be extremely difficult in an individual patient.[251] The incidence of these complications correlates with the severity of the burn and with a history of being in an enclosed space.[252, 254, 255]

During the first 24 hours, complications result from upper airway edema caused by direct heat injury or toxic products, usually in patients who have head and neck

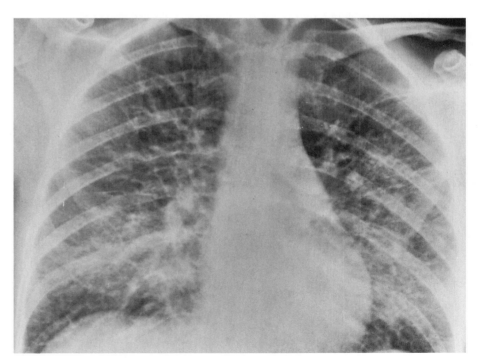

Figure 16–37. Acute Pulmonary Edema Caused by Inhalation of Mixed Fumes. Four days before this radiograph, a 34-year-old woman had sprayed a lampshade with a plastic substance containing dimethylsulfate and ethylene dichloride (a paint fixative), followed by gold paint. She had experienced an abrupt onset of severe dyspnea and nonproductive cough. The radiograph shows diffuse pulmonary edema that is predominantly interstitial in location. Prominent Kerley A and B lines are visible. The heart size is normal. Her recovery was uneventful; chest radiograph was normal 4 days later. (Courtesy of Dr. W. G. Brown, Regina Grey Nuns Hospital, Regina, Saskatchewan.)

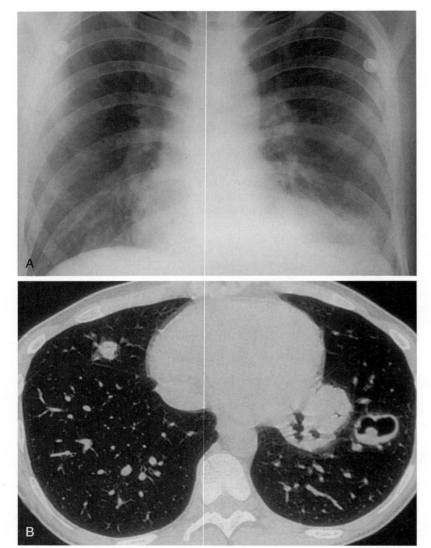

Figure 16–38. Pyrofluid Inhalation in Fire-Eater. Chest radiograph *(A)* shows focal areas of consolidation in the right middle and lower lobes and in the left lower lobe. CT scan performed 7 days later *(B)* shows cavitating lesions in the left lower lobe and soft tissue nodule in right middle lobe. The patient was a 21-year-old man who inhaled pyrofluids during a fire-eating performance. (Case courtesy of Dr. Tomás Franquet, Department of Radiology, Hospital de Sant Pau, Universidad Autónoma de Barcelona, Barcelona, Spain.)

burns.[256] After a latent period of 12 to 48 hours, symptoms and radiographic evidence of lower respiratory tract involvement may be evident.[257, 258] Pulmonary complications that become evident 2 to 5 days after the burn consist of atelectasis, edema, and pneumonia. Atelectasis may be caused by mucous plugging of large bronchi;[259] pneumonia occurs much more frequently in the presence of inhalation injury. In one review of the records of 1,058 burn patients treated at a single institution during a 5-year period, 373 (35%) suffered inhalation injury diagnosed by bronchoscopy, ventilation-perfusion scintigraphy, or both;[260] of these patients, 141 (38%) subsequently developed pneumonia. Among the 685 patients who did not have inhalation injury, pneumonia occurred in only 60 (9%). Complications that occur after 5 days include thromboembolism[252] and adult respiratory distress syndrome.[261]

The acute effects of smoke exposure among firefighters have been reported to be greater in current cigarette smokers than among nonsmokers similarly exposed to smoke.[262] Acute smoke exposure can cause transient bronchial hyperresponsiveness[263] or hypoxemia[264] and occasionally is complicated by the late development of bronchiectasis and obliterative bronchiolitis.[265]

Radiologic Manifestations

The radiographic findings of acute smoke inhalation unassociated with skin burns were described in one study of 21 patients;[266] in 6 patients, radiographs obtained 4 to 24 hours after the incident revealed focal opacities that were interpreted as atelectasis and that usually cleared within 3 days. In another study of 62 patients who required admission to a hospital after smoke inhalation, 35 (63%) developed radiographic evidence of pulmonary edema, in most cases within 24 hours after the injury (Fig. 16–39).[258] In a third study of 29 patients who required ventilatory support after acute smoke inhalation and burns, 13 had radiologic findings consistent with inhalation injury, including interstitial or air-space edema or linear atelectasis.[267] Based on these studies, chest radiograph is a relatively insensitive indicator of airway and parenchymal injury after acute smoke inhalation. Several groups of investigators have shown, however, that patients who have an abnormal radiograph within 48 hours after inhalation injuries are more likely to require ventilatory support and have a worse prognosis than those who have normal radiographs.[258, 268, 269]

The pattern of deposition and the rate of clearance of aerosolized technetium-99m DTPA has been used as a measure of the degree of acute inhalation injury in patients exposed to smoke; a pattern of inhomogeneous distribution and rapid uptake has been found to correlate with radiographic, lung function, and clinical markers of the severity of lung injury.[270]

Radiographic manifestations of large airway burns include subglottic edema and indistinctness of the trachea.[268, 271] Late manifestations include tracheal stenosis,[272]

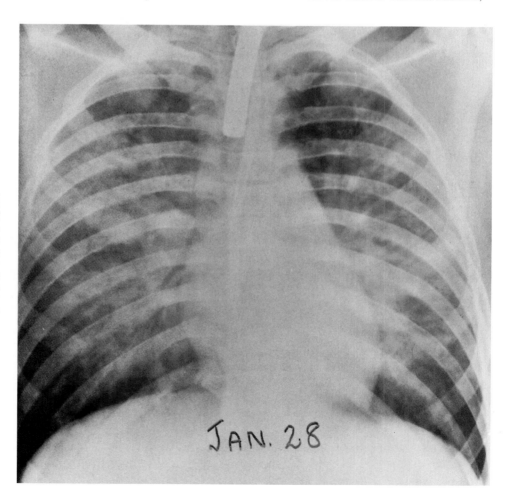

Figure 16–39. Acute Smoke Inhalation. A 30-year-old man was involved in a fire and inhaled large quantities of smoke before being rescued. He was brought to the emergency department in severe respiratory distress, and a tracheostomy was required. Anteroposterior radiograph shows massive consolidation of both lungs in a pattern characteristic of acute pulmonary edema. The patient had an uneventful recovery.

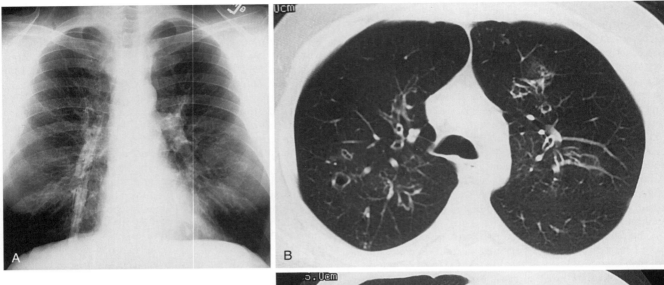

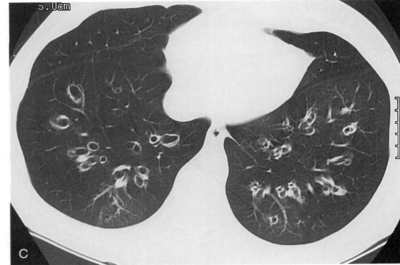

Figure 16–40. Bronchiectasis and Obliterative Bronchiolitis After Smoke Inhalation. Posteroanterior chest radiograph *(A)* in a 33-year-old man shows increased lung volume, bronchiectasis, and decreased peripheral vascular markings. HRCT scans *(B* and *C)* show extensive bronchiectasis and areas of decreased attenuation and vascularity as a result of obliterative bronchiolitis. The patient had experienced severe smoke inhalation several years earlier. (Courtesy of Dr. Christopher Griffin, Department of Radiology, Veterans Affairs Hospital, Portland, Oregon.)

bronchiectasis,[265, 273] and evidence of obliterative bronchiolitis (increased lung volumes and decreased vascularity in the peripheral lung regions).[265] Corresponding HRCT findings include bronchiectasis and areas of decreased attenuation and perfusion (Fig. 16–40).

References

1. Fink JN, Schlueter DP, Sosman AJ, et al: Clinical survey of pigeon breeders. Chest 62:277, 1972.
2. Channell S, Blyth W, Lloyd M, et al: Allergic alveolitis in maltworkers: A clinical, mycological, and immunological study. QJM 38:351, 1969.
3. Selman M, Chapela R, Raghu G: Hypersensitivity pneumonitis: Clinical manifestations, pathogenesis, diagnosis and therapeutic strategies. Semin Respir Med 14:353, 1993.
4. Kawanami O, Basset F, Barrios R, et al: Hypersensitivity pneumonitis in man: Light- and electron-microscopic studies of 18 lung biopsies. Am J Pathol 110:275, 1983.
5. Seal RME, Hapke EJ, Thomas GO, et al: The pathology of the acute and chronic stages of farmer's lung. Thorax 23:469, 1968.
6. Reyes CN, Wenzel FJ, Lawton BR, et al: The pulmonary pathology of farmers' lung disease. Chest 81:142, 1982.
7. Hogg JC: The histologic appearance of farmer's lung. Chest 81:133, 1982.
8. Hensley GT, Garancis JC, Cherayil GD, et al: Lung biopsies of pigeon breeders' disease. Arch Pathol 87:572, 1969.
9. Bankin J, Kobayashi M, Barbee RA, et al: Pulmonary granulomatoses due to inhaled organic antigens. Med Clin North Am 51:459, 1967.
10. Hargreave F, Hinson KF, Reid L, et al: The radiologic appearances of allergic alveolitis due to bird sensitivity (bird fancier's lung). Clin Radiol 23:1, 1972.
11. Mindell HJ: Roentgen findings in farmer's lung. Radiology 97:341, 1970.
12. Mönkäre S, Ikonen M, Haahtela T: Radiologic findings in farmer's lung: Prognosis and correlation to lung function. Chest 87:460, 1985.
13. Cook PG, Wells IP, McGavin CR: The distribution of pulmonary shadowing in farmer's lung. Clin Radiol 39:21, 1988.
14. Silver SF, Müller NL, Miller RR, et al: Hypersensitivity pneumonitis: Evaluation with CT. Radiology 173:441, 1989.
15. Hansell DM, Moskovic E: High-resolution computed tomography in extrinsic allergic alveolitis. Clin Radiol 43:8, 1991.
16. Stoltz JL, Arger PH, Benson JM: Mushroom worker's lung disease. Radiology 119:61, 1976.
17. Frank RC: Farmer's lung: A form of pneumoconiosis due to organic dusts. Am J Roentgenol 79:189, 1958.
18. Grenier P, Chevret S, Beigelman C, et al: Chronic diffuse infiltrative lung disease: Determination of the diagnostic value of clinical data, chest radiography, and CT with Bayesian analysis. Radiology 191:383, 1994.
19. Niimi H, Kang EY, Kwong JS, et al: CT of chronic infiltrative

lung disease: Prevalence of mediastinal lymphadenopathy. J Comput Assist Tomogr 20:305, 1996.

20. Remy-Jardin M, Remy J, Wallaert B, et al: Subacute and chronic bird breeder hypersensitivity pneumonitis: Sequential evaluation with CT and correlation with lung function tests and bronchoalveolar lavage. Radiology 189:111, 1993.

21. Mönkäre S: Clinical aspects of farmer's lung: Airway reactivity, treatment and prognosis. Eur J Respir Dis 137(Suppl):1, 1984.

22. Lynch DA, Rose CS, Way D, et al: Hypersensitivity pneumonitis: Sensitivity of high-resolution CT in a population-based study. Am J Roentgenol 159:469, 1992.

23. Gaensler EA, Carrington CB: Open biopsy for chronic diffuse infiltrative lung disease: Clinical, roentgenographic, and physiologic correlations in 502 patients. Ann Thorac Surg 30:411, 1980.

24. Dinda P, Chatterjee SS, Riding WD: Pulmonary function studies in bird breeder's lung. Thorax 24:374, 1969.

25. Moore VL, Pedersen GM, Hauser WC, et al: A study of lung lavage materials in patients with hypersensitivity pneumonitis: In vitro response to mitogen and antigen in pigeon breeders' disease. J Allergy Clin Immunol 65:365, 1980.

26. Cormier Y, Belanger J, Beaudoin J, et al: Abnormal bronchoalveolar lavage in asymptomatic dairy farmers: Study of lymphocytes. Am Rev Respir Dis 130:1046, 1984.

27. Adler BD, Padley SP, Müller NL, et al: Chronic hypersensitivity pneumonitis: High-resolution CT and radiographic features in 16 patients. Radiology 185:91, 1992.

28. Lynch DA, Newell JD, Logan PM, et al: Can CT distinguish hypersensitivity pneumonitis from idiopathic pulmonary fibrosis? Am J Roentgenol 165:807, 1995.

29. Akira M, Kita N, Higashihara T, et al: Summer-type hypersensitivity pneumonitis: Comparison of high-resolution CT and plain radiographic findings. Am J Roentgenol 158:1223, 1992.

30. Hansell DM, Wells AU, Padley SPG, et al: Hypersensitivity pneumonitis: Correlation of individual CT patterns with functional abnormalities. Radiology 199:123, 1996.

31. Fourth International Pneumoconiosis Conference: Working Party on the Definition of Pneumoconiosis Report. Geneva, 1971.

32. Vallyathan V, Mega JF, Shi X, et al: Enhanced generation of free radicals from phagocytes induced by mineral dusts. Am J Respir Cell Mol Biol 6:404, 1992.

33. Amandus HE, Reger RB, Pendergrass EP, et al: The pneumoconioses: Methods of measuring progression. Chest 63:736, 1973.

34. International Labour Office: Guidelines for the Use of ILO International Classification of Radiographs of Pneumoconioses. Geneva, ILO, 1980, pp 1–48.

35. Liddell FDK: An experiment in film reading. Br J Ind Med 20:300, 1963.

36. Liddell FDK, Lindars DC: An elaboration of the I.L.O. classification of simple pneumoconiosis. Br J Ind Med 26:89, 1969.

37. Middleton EL: The present position of silicosis in industry in Britain. BMJ 2:485, 1929.

38. Gong H Jr, Tashkin DP: Silicosis due to intentional inhalation of abrasive scouring powder: Case report with long-term survival and vasculitic sequelae. Am J Med 67:358, 1979.

39. Seaton A, Legge JS, Henderson J, et al: Accelerated silicosis in Scottish stonemasons. Lancet 337:341, 1991.

40. Bergin CJ, Müller NL, Vedall S, et al: CT in silicosis: Correlation with plain films and pulmonary function tests. Am J Roentgenol 146:477, 1986.

41. Theron CP, Walters LG, Webster I: The international classification of radiographs of the pneumoconioses: Based on the findings in 100 deceased white South African gold miners: An evaluation. Med Proc (Johannesburg) 10:352, 1964.

42. Greening RR, Heslep JH: The roentgenology of silicosis. Semin Roentgenol 2:265, 1967.

43. Pendergrass EP: Caldwell Lecture 1957: Silicosis and a few of the other pneumoconioses: Observations on certain aspects of the problem, with emphasis on the role of the radiologist. Am J Roentgenol 80:1, 1958.

44. Jacobson G, Felson B, Pendergrass EP, et al: Eggshell calcifications in coal and metal workers. Semin Roentgenol 2:276, 1967.

45. Bellini F, Ghislandi E: "Egg-shell" calcifications at extrahilar sites in a silicotuberculotic patient. Med Lav 51:600, 1960.

46. Jacobs LG, Gerstl B, Hollander AG, et al: Intra-abdominal egg-shell calcifications due to silicosis. Radiology 67:527, 1956.

47. Gross BH, Schneider HJ, Proto AV: Eggshell calcification of lymph nodes: An update. Am J Roentgenol 135:1265, 1980.

48. Tschopp JM, Rossini MJ, Richon CA, et al: Retroperitoneal silicosis mimicking pancreatic carcinoma in an Alpine miner with chronic lung silicosis. Thorax 47:480, 1992.

49. Cahill BC, Harmon KR, Shumway SJ, et al: Tracheobronchial obstruction due to silicosis. Am Rev Respir Dis 145:719, 1992.

50. Nicod J-L, Gardiol D: Silicose et paralysie du diaphragme. [Silicosis and paralysis of the diaphragm.] Schweiz Med Wochenschr 94:1461, 1964.

51. Paterson JF: Silicosis in hardrock miners in Ontario: The problem and its prevention. Can Med Assoc J 84:594, 1961.

52. Dee PM, Suratt P, Winn W: The radiographic findings in acute silicosis. Radiology 126:359, 1978.

53. Buechner HA, Ansari A: Acute silicoproteinosis: A new pathologic variant of acute silicosis in sandblasters, characterized by histologic features resembling alveolar proteinosis. Dis Chest 55:274, 1969.

54. Sluis-Cremer GK, Hessel PA, Hnizdo E, et al: Relationship between silicosis and rheumatoid arthritis. Thorax 41:596, 1986.

55. Maclaren WM, Soutar CA: Progressive massive fibrosis and simple pneumoconiosis in ex-miners. Br J Ind Med 42:734, 1985.

56. Bégin R, Bergeron D, Samson R, et al: CT assessment of silicosis in exposed workers. Am J Roentgenol 148:509, 1987.

57. Bégin R, Ostiguy G, Fillion R, et al: Computed tomography scan in the early detection of silicosis. Am Rev Respir Dis 144:697, 1991.

58. Akira M, Higashihara T, Yokoyama K, et al: Radiographic type p pneumoconiosis: High-resolution CT. Radiology 171:117, 1989.

59. Mathieson JR, Mayo JR, Staples CA, et al: Chronic diffuse infiltrative lung disease: Comparison of diagnostic accuracy of CT and chest radiography. Radiology 171:111, 1989.

60. Remy-Jardin M, Remy J, Farre I, et al: Computed tomographic evaluation of silicosis and coal worker's pneumoconiosis. Radiol Clin North Am 30:1155, 1992.

61. Kinsella M, Müller N, Vedal S, et al: Emphysema in silicosis. Am Rev Respir Dis 141:1497, 1990.

62. Nozaki S, Sawada Y: Progress of simple pulmonary silicosis in retired miners. Jpn J Clin Tuberc 18:154, 1959.

63. Oleru UG: Respiratory and nonrespiratory morbidity in a titanium oxide paint factory in Nigeria. Am J Ind Med 12:173, 1987.

64. Bailey WC, Brown M, Buechner HA, et al: Silico-mycobacterial disease in sandblasters. Am Rev Respir Dis 110:115, 1974.

65. Hughes JM, Jones RN, Gilson JC, et al: Determinants of progression in sandblasters' silicosis. Ann Occup Hyg 26:701, 1982.

66. Fisher ER, Watkins G, Lam NV, et al: Objective pathological diagnosis of coal workers' pneumoconiosis. JAMA 245:1829, 1981.

67. Morgan WKC: Respiratory disease in coal miners. JAMA 231:1347, 1975.

68. Caplan A: Certain unusual radiological appearances in the chest of coal-miners suffering from rheumatoid arthritis. Thorax 8:29, 1953.

69. Cockcroft AE, Wagner JC, Seal EM, et al: Irregular opacities in coalworkers' pneumoconiosis: Correlation with pulmonary function and pathology. Ann Occup Hyg 26:767, 1982.

70. Musk AW, Cotes JE, Bevan C, et al: Relationship between type of simple coalworkers pneumoconiosis and lung function: A 9-year follow-up study of subjects with small rounded opacities. Br J Ind Med 38:313, 1981.

71. Cockcroft A, Lyons JP, Andersson N, et al: Prevalence and relation to underground exposure of radiological irregular opacities in South Wales coal workers with pneumoconiosis. Br J Ind Med 40:169, 1983.

72. Gough J, James WRL, Wentworth JE: A comparison of the radiological and pathological changes in coalworkers' pneumoconiosis. J Fac Radiol 1:28, 1949.

73. Williams JL, Moller GA: Solitary mass in the lungs of coal miners. Am J Roentgenol 117:765, 1973.

74. Young RC Jr, Rachel RE, Carr PG, et al: Patterns of coal workers' pneumoconiosis in Appalachian former coalminers. J Natl Med Assoc 84:41, 1992.

75. Shennan DH, Washington JS, Thomas DJ, et al: Factors predisposing to the development of PMF in coal miners. Br J Ind Med 38:321, 1981.

76. Davies D: Disability and coal workers' pneumoconiosis. BMJ 2:652, 1974.

77. Seaton A, Soutar CA, Melville AWT: Radiological changes in coal-miners on leaving the industry. Br J Dis Chest 74:310, 1980.

78. Remy-Jardin M, Degreef JM, Beuscart R, et al: Coal worker's pneumoconiosis: CT assessment in exposed workers and correlation with radiographic findings. Radiology 177:363, 1990.

79. Gevenois PA, Pichot E, Dargent S, et al: Low grade coal worker's pneumoconiosis: Comparison of CT and chest radiography. Acta Radiol 35:351, 1994.

80. Remy-Jardin M, Beuscart R, Sault MC, et al: Subpleural micronodules in diffuse infiltrative lung diseases: Evaluation with thin-section CT scans. Radiology 177:133, 1990.

81. Rebstock-Bourgkard E, Chau N, Caillier I, et al: Respiratory symptoms of coal miners presenting radiological pulmonary abnormalities. Rev Epidemiol Sante Publique 42:533, 1994.

82. Ball J: The natural history and management of coal workers' pneumoconiosis. *In* King EJ, Fletcher CM (eds): Industrial Pulmonary Diseases: A Symposium held at the Postgraduate Medical School of London, 18–20 September 1957 and 25–27 March 1958. London, J & A Churchill, 1960, pp 241–254.

83. Cathcart RT, Theodos PA, Fraimow W: Anthracosilicosis: Selected aspects related to the evaluation of disability, cavitation, and the unusual x-ray. Arch Intern Med 106:368, 1960.

84. Mosquera JA: Massive melanoptysis: A serious unrecognized complication of coal worker's pneumoconiosis. Eur Respir J 1:766, 1988.

85. Bégin R, Dufresne A, Plante F, et al: Asbestos related disorders. Can Respir J 1:167, 1994.

86. Sluis-Cremer GK, Liddell FDK, Logan WPD, et al: The mortality of amphibole miners in South Africa, 1946–80. Br J Ind Med 49:566, 1992.

87. Oksa P, Koskinen H, Rinne JP, et al: Parenchymal and pleural fibrosis in construction workers. Am J Ind Med 21:561, 1992.

88. Rogan WJ, Gladen BC, Ragan ND, et al: U.S. prevalence of occupational pleural thickening: A look at chest x-rays from the first National Health and Nutrition Examination Survey. Am J Epidemiol 126:893, 1987.

89. Miller A, Teirstein AS, Selikoff IJ: Ventilatory failure due to asbestos pleurisy. Am J Med 75:911, 1983.

90. Murphy RLH Jr, Gaensler EA, Ferris BG, et al: Diagnosis of "asbestosis": Observations from a longitudinal survey of shipyard pipe coverers. Am J Med 65:488, 1978.

91. Kilburn KH, Warshaw R, Thornton JC: Asbestosis, pulmonary symptoms and functional impairment in shipyard workers. Chest 88:254, 1985.

92. Selikoff IJ, Lilis R, Levin G: Asbestotic radiological abnormalities among United States merchant marine seamen. Br J Ind Med 47:292, 1990.

93. Demers RY, Neale AV, Robins T, et al: Asbestos-related pulmonary disease in boilermakers. Am J Ind Med 17:327, 1990.

94. Oliver LC, Eisen EA, Greene RE, et al: Asbestos-related disease in railroad workers: A cross-sectional study. Am Rev Respir Dis 131:499, 1985.

95. McDonald AD, Fry JS, Woolley AJ, et al: Dust exposure and mortality in an American factory using chrysotile, amosite, and crocidolite in mainly textile manufacture. Br J Ind Med 40:368, 1983.

96. Sherson D, Maltbaek N, Olsen O: Small opacities among dental laboratory technicians in Copenhagen. Br J Ind Med 45:320, 1988.

97. Kern DG, Frumkin H: Asbestos-related disease in the jewelry industry: Report of two cases. Am J Ind Med 13:407, 1988.

98. Cordier S, Lazar P, Brochard P, et al: Epidemiologic investigation of respiratory effects related to asbestos inside insulated buildings. Arch Environ Health 42:303, 1987.

99. Sebastien P, Bignon J, Martin M: Indoor airborne asbestos pollution: From the ceiling and the floor. Science 216:1410, 1982.

100. Ganor E, Fischbein A, Brenner S, et al: Extreme airborne asbestos concentrations in a public building. Br J Ind Med 49:486, 1992.

101. Kiviluoto R: Pleural calcification as a roentgenologic sign of nonoccupational endemic anthophyllite asbestosis. Acta Radiol 194:1, 1960.

102. Lilis R, Miller A, Godbold J, et al: Radiographic abnormalities in asbestos insulators: Effects of duration from onset of exposure and smoking: Relationships of dyspnea with parenchymal and pleural fibrosis. Am J Ind Med 20:1, 1991.

103. Churg A: Asbestos fibers and pleural plaques in a general autopsy population. Am J Pathol 109:88, 1982.

104. Wain SL, Roggli VL, Foster WL Jr: Parietal pleural plaques, asbestos bodies, and neoplasia. Chest 86:707, 1984.

105. Churg A, Golden J: Current problems in the pathology of asbestos-related disease. Pathol Ann 17(Pt 2):33, 1982.

106. Roberts GH: The pathology of parietal pleural plaques. J Clin Pathol 24:348, 1971.

107. Hourihane DO, Lessof L, Richardson PC: Hyaline and calcified pleural plaques as an index of exposure to asbestos: A study of radiological and pathological features of 100 cases with a consideration of epidemiology. BMJ 1:1069, 1966.

108. Stephens M, Gibbs AR, Pooley FD, et al: Asbestos induced diffuse pleural fibrosis: Pathology and mineralogy. Thorax 42:583, 1987.

109. O'Brien CJ, Franks AJ: Paraplegia due to massive asbestos-related pleural and mediastinal fibrosis. Histopathology 11:541, 1987.

110. Churg A: Fiber counting and analysis in the diagnosis of asbestos-related disease. Hum Pathol 13:381, 1982.

111. Davis JMG: The pathology of asbestos-related disease. Thorax 39:801, 1984.

112. Tallroth K, Kiviranta K: Round atelectasis. Respiration 45:71, 1984.

113. Chung-Park M, Tomashefski JF Jr, Cohen AM, et al: Shrinking pleuritis with lobar atelectasis, a morphologic variant of "round atelectasis." Hum Pathol 20:382, 1989.

114. Hillerdal G: Rounded atelectasis: Clinical experience with 74 patients. Chest 95:836, 1989.

115. Freundlich IM, Greening RR: Asbestosis and associated medical problems. Radiology 89:224, 1967.

116. Fletcher DE, Edge JR: The early radiological changes in pulmonary and pleural asbestosis. Clin Radiol 21:355, 1970.

117. Anton HC: Multiple pleural plaques, part II. Br J Radiol 41:341, 1968.

118. Zitting A, Huuskonen MS, Alanko K, et al: Radiographic and physiological findings in patients with asbestosis. Scand J Work Environ Health 4:275, 1978.

119. Friedman AC, Fiel SB, Fisher MS, et al: Asbestos-related pleural disease and asbestosis: A comparison of CT and chest radiography. Am J Roentgenol 150:269, 1988.

120. Staples CA, Gamsu G, Ray CS, et al: High-resolution computed tomography and lung function in asbestos-exposed workers with normal chest radiographs. Am Rev Respir Dis 139:1502, 1989.

121. Gamsu G, Salmon CJ, Warnock ML, et al: CT quantification of interstitial fibrosis in patients with asbestosis: A comparison of two methods. Am J Roentgenol 164:63, 1995.

122. Sargent EN, Gordonson J, Jacobson G, et al: Bilateral pleural thickening: A manifestation of asbestos dust exposure. Am J Roentgenol 131:579, 1978.

123. Sprince NL, Oliver LC, McLoud TC: Asbestos-related disease in plumbers and pipefitters employed in building construction. J Occup Med 27:771, 1985.

124. Mackenzie FAF: The radiological investigation of the early manifestations of exposure to asbestos dust. Proc R Soc Med 64:834, 1971.

125. Bégin R, Boctor M, Bergeron D, et al: Radiographic assessment of pleuropulmonary disease in asbestos workers: Posteroanterior, four view films, and computed tomograms of the thorax. Br J Ind Med 41:373, 1984.

126. Fisher MS: Asymmetrical changes in asbestos-related disease. J Can Assoc Radiol 36:110, 1985.

127. Withers BF, Ducatman AM, Yang WN: Roentgenographic evidence for predominant left-sided location of unilateral pleural plaques. Chest 95:1262, 1984.

128. Hu H, Beckett L, Kelsey K, Christiani D: The left-sided predominance of asbestos-related pleural disease. Am Rev Respir Dis 148:981, 1993.

129. Gallego JC: Absence of left-sided predominance in asbestos-related pleural plaques: A CT study. Chest 113:1034, 1998.

130. Rockoff SD, Kagan E, Schwartz A, et al: Visceral pleural thickening in asbestos exposure: The occurrence and implications of thickened interlobar fissures. J Thorac Imaging 2:58, 1987.

131. Hillerdal G, Lindgren A: Pleural plaques: Correlation of autopsy findings to radiographic findings and occupational history. Eur J Respir Dis 61:315, 1980.

132. Sargent EN, Boswell WD Jr, Ralls PW, et al: Subpleural fat pads in patients exposed to asbestos: Distinction from noncalcified pleural plaques. Radiology 152:273, 1984.

133. Im JG, Webb WR, Rosen A, et al: Costal pleural: Appearance at high-resolution CT. Radiology 171:125, 1989.

134. Smith AR: Pleural calcification resulting from exposure to certain dusts. Am J Roentgenol 67:375, 1952.

135. Kleinfeld M: Pleural calcification as a sign of silicatosis. Am J Med Sci 251:215, 1966.
136. Krige L: Asbestosis—with special reference to the radiological diagnosis. S Afr J Radiol 4:13, 1966.
137. Solomon A: Radiology of asbestosis. Environ Res 3:320, 1970.
138. Sargent EN, Jacobson G, Wilkinson EE: Diaphragmatic pleural calcification following short occupational exposure to asbestos. Am J Roentgenol 115:473, 1972.
139. McLoud TC, Woods BO, Carrington CB, et al: Diffuse pleural thickening in an asbestos-exposed population: Prevalence and causes. Am J Roentgenol 144:9, 1985.
140. Lynch DA, Gamsu G, Aberle DR: Conventional and high resolution computed tomography in the diagnosis of asbestos-related diseases. Radiographics 9:523, 1989.
141. Hillerdal G, Malmberg P, Hemmingsson A: Asbestos-related lesions of the pleura: Parietal plaques compared to diffuse thickening studied with chest roentgenography, computed tomography, lung function, and gas exchange. Am J Ind Med 18:627, 1990.
142. Aberle DR, Gamsu G, Ray CS, et al: Asbestos-related pleural and parenchymal fibrosis: Detection with high-resolution CT. Radiology 166:729, 1988.
143. Leung AN, Müller NL, Miller RR: CT in differential diagnosis of diffuse pleural disease. Am J Roentgenol 154:487, 1990.
144. Friedman AC, Fiel SB, Radecki PD, et al: Computed tomography of benign pleural and pulmonary parenchymal abnormalities related to asbestos exposure. Semin Ultrasound CT MR 11:393, 1990.
145. Müller NL: Imaging of the pleura. Radiology 186:297, 1993.
146. Gaensler EA, Kaplan AI: Asbestos pleural effusion. Ann Intern Med 74:178, 1971.
147. Sluis-Cremer GK, Webster I: Acute pleurisy in asbestos exposed persons. Environ Res 5:380, 1972.
148. Epler GR, McLoud TC, Gaensler EA: Prevalence and incidence of benign asbestos pleural effusion in working population. JAMA 247:617, 1982.
149. Eisenstadt HB: Benign asbestos pleurisy. JAMA 192:419, 1965.
150. Adams VI, Unni KK, Muhm JR, et al: Diffuse malignant mesothelioma of pleura: Diagnosis and survival in 92 cases. Cancer 58:1540, 1986.
151. Grant DC, Seltzer SE, Antman KH, et al: Computed tomography of malignant pleural mesothelioma. J Comput Assist Tomogr 7:626, 1983.
152. Kawashima A, Libshitz HI: Malignant pleural mesothelioma: CT manifestations in 50 cases. Am J Roentgenol 155:965, 1990.
153. Goldstein B: Two malignant pleural mesotheliomas with unusual histological features. Thorax 34:375, 1979.
154. Nichols DM, Johnson MA: Calcification in a pleural mesothelioma. J Can Assoc Radiol 34:311, 1983.
155. Smith KW: Pulmonary disability in asbestos workers. AMA Arch Ind Health 12:198, 1955.
156. Sampson C, Hansell DM: The prevalence of enlarged mediastinal lymph nodes in asbestos-exposed individuals: A CT study. Clin Radiol 45:340, 1992.
157. Hillerdal G: Asbestos exposure and upper lobe involvement. Am J Roentgenol 139:1163, 1982.
158. Solomon A, Goldstein B, Webster I: Massive fibrosis in asbestosis. Environ Res 4:430, 1971.
159. Gefter WB, Conant EF: Issues and controversies in the plain-film diagnosis of asbestos-related disorders in the chest. J Thorac Imaging 3:11, 1988.
160. Epler GR, McLoud TC, Gaensler EA, et al: Normal chest roentgenograms in chronic diffuse infiltrative lung disease. N Engl J Med 298:934, 1978.
161. Kipen HM, Lilis R, Suzuki Y, et al: Pulmonary fibrosis in asbestos insulation workers with lung cancer: A radiological and histopathological evaluation. Br J Ind Med 44:96, 1987.
162. Akira M, Yokoyama K, Yamamoto S, et al: Early asbestosis: Evaluation with high-resolution CT. Radiology 178:409, 1991.
163. Yoshimura H, Hatakeyama M, Otsuji H, et al: Pulmonary asbestosis: CT study of subpleural curvilinear shadow. Radiology 158:653, 1986.
164. Akira M, Yamamoto S, Yokoyama K, et al: Asbestosis: High-resolution CT-pathologic correlation. Radiology 176:389, 1990.
165. Al-Jarad N, Strickland B, Pearson MC, et al: High-resolution computed tomographic assessment of asbestosis and cryptogenic fibrosing alveolitis: A comparative study. Thorax 47:645, 1992.
166. Primack SL, Hartman TE, Hansell DM, et al: End-stage lung disease: CT findings in 61 patients. Radiology 189:681, 1993.
167. Bergin CJ, Castellino RA, Blank N, et al: Specificity of high-resolution CT findings in pulmonary asbestosis: Do patients scanned for other indications have similar findings? Am J Roentgenol 163:551, 1994.
168. Murray KA, Gamsu G, Webb WR, et al: High-resolution computed tomography sampling for detection of asbestos-related lung disease. Acad Radiol 2:111, 1995.
169. Majurin ML, Varpula M, Kurki T, et al: High-resolution CT of the lung in asbestos-exposed subjects: Comparison of low-dose and high-dose HRCT. Acta Radiol 35:473, 1994.
170. Mintzer RA, Gore RM, Vogelzang RL, et al: Rounded atelectasis and its association with asbestos-induced pleural disease. Radiology 139:567, 1981.
171. Schneider HJ, Felson B, Gonzalez LL: Rounded atelectasis. Am J Roentgenol 134:225, 1980.
172. Franzblau A: Asbestos-associated round atelectasis: A case report and review of the literature. Mt Sinai J Med 56:321, 1989.
173. Lynch DA, Gamsu G, Ray CS, et al: Asbestos-related focal lung masses: Manifestations on conventional and high-resolution CT scans. Radiology 169:603, 1988.
174. McHugh K, Blaquiere RM: CT features of rounded atelectasis. Am J Roentgenol 153:257, 1989.
175. Carvalho PM, Carr DH: Computed tomography of folded lung. Clin Radiol 41:86, 1990.
176. Taylor PM: Dynamic contrast enhancement of asbestos-related pulmonary pseudotumours. Br J Radiol 61:1070, 1988.
177. Westcott JL, Hllisey MJ, Volpe JP: Dynamic CT of round atelectasis. Radiology 181:182, 1991.
178. Verschakelen JA, Demaerel P, Coolen J, et al: Rounded atelectasis of the lung: MR appearance. Am J Roentgenol 152:965, 1989.
179. McAdams HP, Erasmus JJ, Patz EF, et al: Evaluation of patients with round atelectasis using 2-[(18)F]fluoro-2-deoxy-D-glucose PET. J Comput Assist Tomogr 22:601, 1998.
180. Robinson BWS, Musk AW: Benign asbestos pleural effusion: Diagnosis and course. Thorax 36:896, 1981.
181. Hillerdal G: Non-malignant asbestos pleural disease. Thorax 36:669, 1981.
182. Hilt B, Lien JT, Lund-Larsen PG: Lung function and respiratory symptoms in subjects with asbestos-related disorders: A cross-sectional study. Am J Ind Med 11:517, 1987.
183. Schüler P, Maturana V, Cruz E, et al: Pulmonary asbestosis. Rev Chil Enferm Torax 25:37, 1959.
184. Kleinfeld M, Messite J, Shapiro J: Clinical, radiological, and physiological findings in asbestosis. Arch Intern Med 117:813, 1966.
185. McDonald JC: Asbestos and lung cancer: Has the case been proven? Chest 78(Suppl):374, 1980.
186. McDonald JC, McDonald AD: Epidemiology of asbestos-related lung cancer. In: Asbestos-Related Malignancy. Orlando, Grune & Stratton, 1986.
187. McDonald JC, Liddell FDK, Gibbs GW, et al: Dust exposure and mortality in chrysotile mining, 1910–75. Br J Ind Med 37:11, 1980.
188. McDonald JC, Liddell FDK, Dufresne A, et al: The 1891–1920 birth cohort of Quebec chrysotile miners and millers: Mortality 1976–88. Br J Ind Med 50:1073, 1993.
189. Selikoff IJ, Bader RA, Bader ME, et al: Asbestosis and neoplasia. Am J Med 42:487, 1967.
190. Keith FM, Charrette EJP, Lynn RB, et al: Inhalation of foreign bodies by children: A continuing challenge in management. Can Med Assoc J 122:52, 1980.
191. Mittleman RE: Fatal choking in infants and children. Am J Forensic Med Pathol 5:201, 1984.
192. Weissberg D, Schwartz I: Foreign bodies in the tracheobronchial tree. Chest 91:730, 1987.
193. Lan RS: Non-asphyxiating tracheobronchial foreign bodies in adults. Eur Respir J 7:510, 1994.
194. Limper AH, Prakash UB: Tracheobronchial foreign bodies in adults. Ann Intern Med 112:604, 1990.
195. Chen CH, Lai CL, Tsai TT, et al: Foreign body aspiration into the lower airway in Chinese adults. Chest 112:129, 1997.
196. Wager GC, Williams JH Jr: Flexible bronchoscopic removal of radioccult polyurethane foam, with pneumonitis in a hyperventilated lobe. Am Rev Respir Dis 142:1222, 1990.
197. Blazer S, Naveh Y, Friedman A: Foreign body in the airway: A review of 200 cases. Am J Dis Child 134:68, 1980.

198. Brown BS, Ma H, Dunbar JS, et al: Foreign bodies in the tracheo-bronchial tree in childhood. J Can Assoc Radiol 14:158, 1963.

199. Marom EM, McAdams HP, Sporn TA, et al: Lentil aspiration pneumonia: Radiographic and CT findings. J Comput Assist Tomogr 22:598, 1998.

200. Limper AH, Prakash UBS: Tracheobronchial foreign bodies in adults. Ann Intern Med 112:604, 1990.

201. Berger PE, Kuhn JP, Kuhns LR: Computed tomography and the occult tracheobronchial foreign body. Radiology 134:133, 1980.

202. Ikeda M, Kitahara S, Inouye T: Large radiolucent tracheal foreign body found by CT scan caused dyspnea: An admonition on flexible fiberscopic foreign body removal. Surg Endosc 10:164, 1996.

203. Kang EY, Miller RR, Müller NL: Bronchiectasis: Comparison of preoperative thin-section CT and pathologic findings in resected specimens. Radiology 195:649, 1995.

204. Kürklü EU, Williams MA, le Roux BT: Bronchiectasis consequent upon foreign body retention. Thorax 28:601, 1973.

205. Laks Y, Barzilay Z: Foreign body aspiration in childhood. Pediatr Emerg Care 4:102, 1988.

206. Miller GA, Gianturco C, Neucks HG: The asymptomatic period in retained foreign bodies of the bronchus. Am J Dis Child 95:282, 1958.

207. Cole MJ, Smith JT, Molnar C, et al: Aspiration after percutaneous gastrostomy: Assessment by Tc-99m labeling of the enteral feed. J Clin Gastroenterol 9:90, 1987.

208. Ben-Dov I, Aelony Y: Foreign body aspiration in the adult: An occult cause of chronic pulmonary symptoms. Postgrad Med J 65:299, 1989.

209. Lawes EG, Baskett PJ: Pulmonary aspiration during unsuccessful cardiopulmonary resuscitation. Intensive Care Med 13:379, 1987.

210. Chan TY, Critchley JA: Pulmonary aspiration following Dettol poisoning: The scope for prevention. Hum Exp Toxicol 15:843, 1996.

211. Schmidt J, Holas M, Halvorson K, et al: Videofluoroscopic evidence of aspiration predicts pneumonia and death but not dehydration following stroke. Dysphagia 9:7, 1994.

212. Nakagawa T, Sekizawa K, Arai H, et al: High incidence of pneumonia in elderly patients with basal ganglia infarction. Arch Intern Med 157:321, 1997.

213. Hughes RL, Freilich RA, Bytell DE, et al: Aspiration and occult esophageal disorders: Clinical conference in pulmonary disease from Northwestern University Medical School, Chicago. Chest 80:489, 1981.

214. Coelho CA, Ferrante R: Dysphagia in postpolio sequelae: Report of three cases. Arch Phys Med Rehabil 69:634, 1988.

215. Chen CT, Toung TJ, Haupt HM, et al: Evaluation of the efficacy of Alka-Seltzer Effervescent in gastric acid neutralization. Anesth Analg 63:325, 1984.

216. Schwartz DJ, Wynne JW, Gibbs CP, et al: The pulmonary consequences of aspiration of gastric contents at pH values greater than 2.5. Am Rev Respir Dis 121:119, 1980.

217. Bond VK, Stoelting RK, Gupta CD: Pulmonary aspiration syndrome after inhalation of gastric fluid containing antacids. Anesthesiology 51:452, 1979.

218. Wynne JW, Reynolds JC, Hood I, et al: Steroid therapy for pneumonitis induced in rabbits by aspiration of foodstuff. Anesthesiology 51:11, 1979.

219. Landay MJ, Christensen EE, Bynum LJ: Pulmonary manifestations of acute aspiration of gastric contents. Am J Roentgenol 131:587, 1978.

220. Müller NL: Aspiration pneumonia. *In* Siegel BA (ed): Chest Disease (fifth series): Test Syllabus. Reston, VA, American College of Radiology, 1996, p 378.

221. Brock RC, Hodgkiss F, Jones HO: Bronchial embolism and posture in relation to lung abscess. Guy's Hosp Rep 91:131, 1948.

222. Coriat P, Labrousse J, Vilde F, et al: Diffuse interstitial pneumonitis due to aspiration of gastric contents. Anaesthesia 39:703, 1984.

223. Ros PR: Lentil aspiration pneumonia (letter). JAMA 251:1277, 1984.

224. Campinos L, Duval G, Couturier M, et al: The value of early fibreoptic bronchoscopy after aspiration of gastric contents. Br J Anaesth 55:1103, 1983.

225. Genereux GP: Lipids in the lungs: Radiologic-pathologic correlation. J Can Assoc Radiol 21:2, 1970.

226. Spickard A, Hirschmann JV: Exogenous lipoid pneumonia. Arch Intern Med 154:686, 1994.

227. Gondouin A, Manzoni P, Ranfaing E, et al: Exogenous lipid pneumonia: A retrospective multicentre study of 44 cases in France. Eur Respir J 9:1463, 1996.

228. Scully RE, Galdabini JJ, McNeely BU: Case 19–1977: Lipoid pneumonia. N Engl J Med 296:1105, 1977.

229. Kennedy JD, Costello P, Balikian JP, et al: Exogenous lipoid pneumonia. Am J Roentgenol 136:1145, 1981.

230. Sundberg RH, Kirschner KE, Brown MJ: Evaluation of lipid pneumonia. Dis Chest 36:594, 1959.

231. Eyal Z, Borman JB, Milwidsky H: Solitary oil granuloma of the lung: A report of three cases. Br J Dis Chest 55:43, 1961.

232. Salm R, Hughes EW: A case of chronic paraffin pneumonitis. Thorax 25:762, 1970.

233. Borrie J, Gwynne JF: Paraffinoma of lung: Lipoid pneumonia: Report of two cases. Thorax 28:214, 1973.

234. Lee KS, Müller NL, Hale V, et al: Lipoid pneumonia: CT findings. J Comput Assist Tomogr 19:48, 1995.

235. Franquet T, Giménez A, Bordes R, et al: The crazy-paving pattern in exogenous lipoid pneumonia: CT-pathologic correlation. Am J Roentgenol 170:315, 1998.

236. Seo JW, Cho EO, Kim JS, et al: MR findings of lipoid pneumonia: Report of two cases. J Korean Radiol Soc 32:265, 1995.

237. Cox JE, Choplin RH, Chiles C, et al: Chemical-shift MRI of exogenous lipoid pneumonia. J Comput Assist Tomogr 20:465, 1996.

238. Hasan S, Avery WG, Fabian C, et al: Near drowning in humans: A report of 36 patients. Chest 59:191, 1971.

239. Bradley ME: Near-drowning: CPR is just the beginning. J Respir Dis 2:37, 1981.

240. Rosenbaum HT, Thompson WL, Fuller RH: Radiographic pulmonary changes in near drowning. Radiology 83:306, 1964.

241. Hunter TB, Whitehouse WM: Freshwater near-drowning: Radiological aspects. Radiology 112:51, 1974.

242. Putman CE, Tummillo AM, Myerson DA, et al: Drowning: Another plunge. Am J Roentgenol 125:543, 1975.

243. Dunagan DP, Cox JE, Chang MC, et al: Sand aspiration with near-drowning: Radiographic and bronchoscopic findings. Am J Respir Crit Care Med 156:292, 1997.

244. Bonilla-Santiago J, Fill WL: Sand aspiration in drowning and near drowning. Radiology 128:301, 1978.

245. Szpilman D: Near-drowning and drowning classification: A proposal to stratify mortality based on the analysis of 1,831 cases. Chest 112:660, 1997.

246. Kleinfeld M: Acute pulmonary edema of chemical origin. Arch Environ Health 10:942, 1965.

247. Conner E, Dubois A, Comroe J: Acute chemical injury of the airway and lungs. Anesthesiology 23:538, 1962.

248. Baar HS, Galindo J: Bronchiolitis fibrosa obliterans. Thorax 21:209, 1966.

249. The lung in burns (editorial). Lancet 2:673, 1981.

250. Moylan JA, Chan C-K: Inhalation injury: An increasing problem. Ann Surg 188:34, 1978.

251. Demling RH: Smoke inhalation injury. New Horiz 1:422, 1993.

252. Achauer BM, Allyn PA, Furnas DW, et al: Pulmonary complications of burns: The major threat to the burn patient. Ann Surg 177:311, 1973.

253. Whitener DR, Whitener LM, Robertson KJ, et al: Pulmonary function measurements in patients with thermal injury and smoke inhalation. Am Rev Respir Dis 122:731, 1980.

254. Teixidor HS, Novick G, Rubin E: Pulmonary complications in burn patients. J Can Assoc Radiol 34:264, 1983.

255. Peters WJ: Inhalation injury caused by the products of combustion. Can Med Assoc J 125:249, 1981.

256. Raman TK, Dobbins JR, Berte JB: Respiratory burns during oxygen therapy. Chest 57:485, 1970.

257. Crapo RO: Smoke-inhalation injuries. JAMA 246:1694, 1981.

258. Teixidor HS, Rubin E, Novick GS, et al: Smoke inhalation: Radiologic manifestations. Radiology 149:383, 1983.

259. Pietak SP, Delahaye DJ: Airway obstruction following smoke inhalation. Can Med Assoc J 115:329, 1976.

260. Shirani KZ, Pruitt BA Jr, Mason AD Jr: The influence of inhalation injury and pneumonia on burn mortality. Ann Surg 205:82, 1987.

261. Beachley MC, Ghahremani GG: The radiographic spectrum of pulmonary complications in burn victims. Am J Roentgenol 128:441, 1977.

262. Gu TL, Liou SH, Hsu CH, et al: Acute health hazards of firefighters after fighting a department store fire. Ind Health 34:13, 1996.

263. Kinsella J, Carter R, Reid WH, et al: Increased airways reactivity after smoke inhalation. Lancet 337:595, 1991.

264. Tashkin DP, Genovesi MG, Chopra S, et al: Respiratory status of Los Angeles firemen: One-month follow-up after inhalation of dense smoke. Chest 71:445, 1977.

265. Tasaka S, Kanazawa M, Mori M, et al: Long-term course of bronchiectasis and bronchiolitis obliterans as late complication of smoke inhalation. Respiration 62:40, 1995.

266. Putman CE, Loke J, Matthay RA, et al: Radiographic manifestations of acute smoke inhalation. Am J Roentgenol 129:865, 1977.

267. Wittram C, Kenny JB: The admission chest radiograph after acute inhalation injury and burns. Br J Radiol 67:51, 1994.

268. Lee MJ, O'Connell DJ: The plain chest radiograph after acute smoke inhalations. Clin Radiol 39:3, 1988.

269. Darling GE, Keresteci MA, Ibanez D, et al: Pulmonary complications in inhalation injuries with associated cutaneous burn. J Trauma 40:83, 1996.

270. Lin WY, Kao CH, Wang SJ: Detection of acute inhalation injury in fire victims by means of technetium-99m DTPA radioaerosol inhalation lung scintigraphy. Eur J Nucl Med 24:125, 1997.

271. Griglak MJ: Thermal injuries. Emerg Med Clin North Am 10:369, 1992.

272. Gaissert HA, Lofgren RH, Grillo HC, et al: Upper airway compromise after inhalation injury: Complex strictures of the larynx and trachea and their management. Ann Surg 218:672, 1993.

273. Slutzker AD, Kinn R, Said SI: Bronchiectasis and progressive respiratory failure following smoke inhalation. Chest 95:1349, 1989.

274. International Labour Office: Guidelines for the use of ILO international classification of radiographs for pneumoconioses. Occup Safety Health Series 22:1, 1980.

275. Welch LS, Hunting KL, Balmes J, et al: Variability in the classification of radiographs using the 1980 International Labor Organization classification for pneumoconioses. Chest 114:1740, 1998.

276. Attfield MD, Althouse R, Reger RB: An investigation of inter-reader variability among xray readers employed in the underground coal miner surveillance program. Ann Am Conf Gov Ind Hyg 4:401, 1986.

277. Ducatman AM: B-readers and asbestos medical surveillance. J Occup Med 30:644, 1988.

278. Fleiss JL, Cohen J: The equivalence of weighted kappa and the intraclass correlation coefficient as measures of reliability. Educ Psychol Meas 33:613, 1973.

279. Meyer JD, Islam SS, Ducatman AM, et al: Prevalence of small lung opacities in populations unexposed to dusts: A literature analysis. Chest 111:404, 1997.

280. Kavanagh PV, Mason AC, Müller NL: Thoracic foreign bodies in adults. Clin Radiol 54:353, 1999.

281. Bankier AA, Brunner C, Lomoschitz F, et al: Pyrofluid inhalation in "fire-eaters": Sequential findings on CT. J Thorac Imaging 14:303, 1999.

282. Beerman PG, Christensen T, Möller P, et al: A lipoid pneumonia: An occupational hazard in fire-eaters. BMJ 289:1728, 1984.

283. Truemper E, Reyes de la Rocha S, Atkinson SD: Clinical characteristics, pathophysiology, and management of hydrocarbon ingestion. Pediatr Emerg Care 3:187, 1987.

284. Brander PE, Taskinen E, Stenius-Aarniala B: Fire-eater's lung. Eur Respir J 5:112, 1992.

285. Ewert R, Lindemann I, Romberg B, et al: Accidental aspiration and ingestion of petroleum by a "fire-eater." Dtsch Med Wochenschr 1594, 1992.

286. Janoski MM, Raymond GS, Puttagunta L, et al: Psyllium aspiration causing bronchiolitis: Radiographic, high-resolution CT, and pathologic findings. Am J Roentgenol 174:799, 2000.

287. Grenier P, Chevret S, Beigelman C, et al: Chronic diffuse infiltrative lung disease: Determination of the diagnostic value of clinical data, chest radiography, and CT with Bayesian analysis. Radiology 191:383, 1994.

288. Franquet T, Gimenez A, Roson N, et al: Aspiration diseases: Findings, pitfalls, and differential diagnosis. Radiographics 20:673, 2000.

289. Patel S, Kazerooni EA: Case 31: Foreign body aspiration—Chicken vertebra. Radiology 218:523, 2001.

Drugs, Poisons, and Irradiation

Adverse drug reactions are an important cause of morbidity and mortality: It has been estimated that 5% of all hospitalizations are the result of untoward effects of drug therapy, and about 0.3% of deaths that occur in the hospital are believed to be drug related.[1] Early recognition of drug reactions is important; unrecognized, the process can be progressive and fatal, whereas cessation of the drug may be followed by prompt reversibility of toxicity.[2]

Most drug reactions affecting the lungs can be categorized into one of six well-defined types (although some drugs are capable of producing more than one response in different patients or simultaneously in the same patient, and other types of disease can occur):[1] (1) bronchospasm; (2) systemic lupus erythematosus–like syndrome; (3) eosinophilic reactions; (4) interstitial or air-space pneumonitis, which may be acute, subacute, or chronic and associated with a variable amount of fibrosis; and (5) increased permeability pulmonary edema (Table 17–1).

The identification of a drug-related etiology for a pa-

tient's disease may be difficult because of a lack of specific clinical, functional, or radiologic findings. This difficulty is compounded in some cases because of the use of concomitant radiation or oxygen therapy, each of which has its own toxicity. In most instances, the diagnosis is suspected because of the insidious onset of dyspnea and cough in a patient receiving a drug (or drugs) recognized as potentially damaging to the lungs. Onset with fever is common.

The toxicities of specific drugs vary; some are dose related, and others are not. Individual susceptibility may play a role in the severity of a drug reaction, even with agents known to cause cumulative, dose-related pulmonary damage.[4] In some cases, the simultaneous use of multiple drugs can make it difficult to be certain of identification of the specific agent responsible for the pulmonary disease.

If drugs causing lupus-like reactions and eosinophilic lung disease are included, more than 150 agents have been recognized to cause an adverse pulmonary reaction of some kind.[1] In this chapter, we discuss only the most common drugs known to cause lung injury.

CHEMOTHERAPEUTIC AND IMMUNOSUPPRESSIVE DRUGS

Bleomycin

Bleomycin is an antibiotic that has significant activity against a variety of cancers, including squamous cell carcinoma of the head and neck, cervix, and esophagus as well as germ cell tumors and Hodgkin's and non-Hodgkin's lymphoma.[5, 6] The reported incidence of lung toxicity ranges from 2%[7] to more than 40%.[5, 6] This wide variation is related partly to variations in the prevalence of associated risk factors in the populations studied and partly to the sensitivity of the tests used for diagnosis. In one study of 59 men who had testicular carcinoma and were treated with a bleomycin-containing regimen, 9 (15%) developed pulmonary symptoms considered to be the result of bleomycin toxicity, whereas 23 (39%) had significant changes on chest radiograph.[8]

The spectrum of bleomycin toxicity varies from mild (asymptomatic) disease to severe interstitial pneumonitis associated with a mortality rate of 60%;[9] however, most patients develop subacute to chronic interstitial pneumonitis with fibrosis.[5] In a few patients, acute toxicity appears to be primarily immunologic in origin and to consist of reversible eosinophilic pneumonia;[10, 11] rarely the drug causes pulmonary veno-occlusive disease.[12]

Table 17–1. DRUG-INDUCED LUNG DISEASE

Systemic Lupus Erythematosus–Like Syndrome

Common causes
    Procainamide, hydralazine, isoniazid, phenytoin
Main radiographic manifestations
    Pleural and pericardial effusions
    Basal areas of atelectasis

Eosinophilic Lung Reaction

Common causes
    Antibiotics, sulfasalazine, inhaled cocaine
Main radiographic manifestations
    Bilateral areas of consolidation
    Peripheral distribution

Interstitial or Air-Space Pneumonitis

Common causes
    Bleomycin, busulfan, cyclophosphamide, methotrexate,
    nitrofurantoin, amiodarone
Main radiographic manifestations
    Reticular pattern
    Bilateral air-space consolidation
    Lower lung zone predominance

Increased Permeability Pulmonary Edema

Common causes
    Chemotherapeutic drugs, acetylsalicylic acid, heroin, cocaine
Main radiographic manifestations
    Bilateral air-space consolidation
    Diffuse distribution

Radiographic abnormalities usually consist of bilateral bibasilar reticular, reticulonodular, or fine nodular opacities, often showing a striking peripheral distribution.[16, 17] In one study of 20 patients who had pulmonary complications associated with combination chemotherapy regimens containing bleomycin, the region of the costophrenic angles was involved in 90%; in 33%, the opacities were confined to this region.[17] With more severe disease, the abnormalities may extend into the middle and upper lung zones[17] or progress to patchy or massive air-space consolidation (Fig. 17–1).[18] The radiographic abnormalities appear 6 weeks to 3 months after the start of therapy[19] and may be seen before, synchronous with, or after the appearance of clinical symptoms.[15] An unusual manifestation is the development of multiple nodules, occasionally cavitary,[20] simulating metastases; in contrast to the latter, they tend to disappear on drug withdrawal.[21–23]

Several groups have assessed the conventional computed tomography (CT) and high-resolution computed tomography (HRCT) findings of bleomycin-induced lung disease.[24–26] In one series of 100 patients, parenchymal abnormalities were detected on conventional CT scan in 38% and on chest radiograph in 15%.[24] The findings consisted of bilateral irregular lines of attenuation or focal areas of consolidation. In patients who had mild disease, the abnormalities were pleural based and most marked in the posterior aspect of the lower lung zones; with more severe disease, the abnormalities became more diffuse throughout the lower lung zones and involved the middle and upper lung zones (*see* Fig. 17–1).[24] The findings on HRCT usually consist of bilateral irregular lines of attenuation, ground-glass attenuation, or focal areas of consolidation in a predominantly basal subpleural distribution.[26] Rarely the abnormalities affect predominantly or exclusively the upper lobes or are unilateral.[24, 26] Follow-up CT scans may show complete resolution of the parenchymal abnormalities within 9 months or less after cessation of therapy. In one study, 40% of patients who had mild to moderate parenchymal disease showed complete resolution on follow-up, and 60% showed no interval change;[24] persistent abnormalities were present in all patients who had severe disease, although some improvement was present in 50%.

Mitomycin

Mitomycin is an alkylating antibiotic that is used mainly in the treatment of patients who have gastrointestinal, breast, and cervical malignancies[7, 14] as well as in the therapy of non–small cell carcinoma of the lung.[27–29] In four series, clinically evident toxicity was identified in 3% to 6.5% of treated patients.[28–31] Although disease has been described with mitomycin alone,[32] most patients have been treated with other agents, usually the vinca alkaloids.[27, 28]

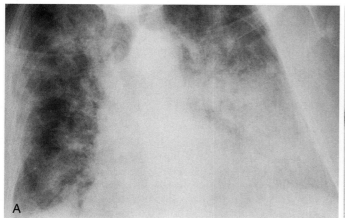
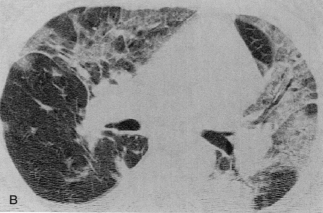

Figure 17–1. Bleomycin-Induced Pulmonary Disease. Anteroposterior chest radiograph *(A)* in a 36-year-old man shows extensive bilateral air-space consolidation with relative sparing of the right lower lobe. HRCT scan *(B)* shows bilateral areas of ground-glass attenuation, focal areas of consolidation, and a few linear areas of attenuation. Histologic assessment of a lung biopsy specimen showed diffuse alveolar damage, focal areas of bronchiolitis obliterans organizing pneumonia–like reaction, and mild veno-occlusive disease consistent with a drug reaction.

The radiologic manifestations of pulmonary damage have been described in a few patients.[29, 31] In one prospective study of 133 patients, 7 (5%) were considered to develop severe toxicity.[29] The radiographic findings consisted of bilateral reticular interstitial infiltrates that were diffuse but tended to have a lower lung zone predominance.[29] Rarely the radiographic and HRCT findings are those of adult respiratory distress syndrome (ARDS), with extensive bilateral areas of consolidation involving mainly the posterior aspects of the lungs (Fig. 17–2).[26, 29] Pleural effusion has been described in many patients and appears to be a more common feature of mitomycin toxicity than of other cytotoxic drug reactions.[29, 32]

Busulfan

Busulfan was the first drug to be identified as a cause of diffuse interstitial fibrosis.[34, 35] It is used in the treatment of myeloproliferative disorders, particularly chronic myelogenous leukemia, and in preparation for autologous or allogeneic bone marrow transplantation in patients who have hematologic and nonhematologic malignancies.[35,36] Although clinically recognized pulmonary toxicity occurs in only about 5% of patients,[3] some pathologic studies have found evidence of drug-induced damage in almost 50%.[37]

Clinically apparent pulmonary toxicity tends to occur only with long-term use, ranging from 8 months to 10 years in several studies (average, 3 to 4 years).[33, 34, 38] Prior use of other cytotoxic drugs or radiation therapy increases the risk.[39] The onset of disease usually is insidious, and the major complaints are dry cough, fever, weakness, weight loss, and dyspnea.[33, 41] Many patients eventually become severely disabled by shortness of breath.[42]

Chest radiograph usually shows a bilateral reticular or reticulonodular pattern, which may be diffuse or have a lower lung zone predominance (Fig. 17–3).[7] Less common radiographic and HRCT findings include patchy or widespread bilateral air-space consolidation.[7, 26] Pleural effusion has been reported occasionally.[40]

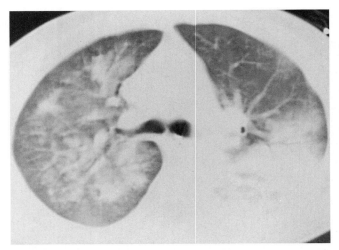

Figure 17–2. Acute Pulmonary Reaction to Mitomycin. Conventional CT scan in a 46-year-old woman shows bilateral areas of consolidation involving mainly the posterior lung regions. The patient developed the disease after mitomycin treatment. The diagnosis of adult respiratory distress syndrome was confirmed at autopsy.

Cyclophosphamide

Cyclophosphamide is used widely in the treatment of malignancies and autoimmune connective tissue disease. Because it often is combined with other agents, its contribution to lung toxicity may be difficult to assess.[13, 44] The incidence of pulmonary toxicity generally is considered to be low (probably <1%);[7] however, some authorities consider it likely that the incidence and the severity of toxicity have been underestimated.[1, 3] Chest radiograph usually shows a bilateral basilar reticular pattern, occasionally associated with focal areas of consolidation (Fig. 17–4).[7] In one review of five patients, pleural thickening accompanied the interstitial changes in all.[45]

Nitrosoureas

Nitrosoureas are used chiefly in the treatment of intracranial neoplasms, melanoma, breast carcinoma, and lymphoma.[7, 46, 47] Most adverse drug reactions have been caused by carmustine (BCNU);[48, 49] other agents, such as lomustine (CCNU)[27] and semustine (methyl-CCNU),[50] have been implicated rarely. The incidence of pulmonary toxicity after BCNU therapy as a single agent ranges from 1% to 20% in different series;[4, 52, 53] by contrast, the incidence is 40% to 60% of patients who have been treated with high-dose combination chemotherapy protocols before autologous bone marrow transplantation.[48, 56]

Chest radiograph becomes abnormal late in the course of pulmonary toxicity, typically after the onset of symptoms.[2] The most common manifestation is a bibasilar reticular pattern.[54] Less common findings include focal or patchy bilateral areas of consolidation, upper lobe reticular opacities, or pneumothorax.[2, 55] The radiograph may be normal in the presence of histologically proven pulmonary fibrosis,[51, 57] a feature that appears to be more common with nitrosoureas than with other cytotoxic agents.[7]

The findings on HRCT have been described in a few patients and consist of bilateral areas of ground-glass attenuation involving the lower lung zones.[26, 58] Although the early radiographic and CT abnormalities tend to involve mainly the lower lung zones, in six patients who had long-term follow-up (mean, 14 years), there was predominantly upper lobe fibrosis.[59, 177] The radiographic and CT findings consisted of irregular linear opacities involving mainly the subpleural lung regions; there was associated elevation of the hila.[60] Gallium scans in these patients were normal.[59]

ANTIMETABOLIC DRUGS

Methotrexate

Methotrexate is employed in the treatment of malignancy and, in lower doses, in a variety of nonmalignant diseases, including psoriasis, pemphigus, asthma, primary biliary cirrhosis, inflammatory bowel disease, and rheumatoid arthritis.[62–64] Use of the drug has been associated with pulmonary toxicity after oral, intravenous, or intrathecal administration. In contrast to other cytotoxic agents, methotrexate usually causes pulmonary disease that is reversible, presumably as a result of a hypersensitivity reaction;[61, 65] however, chronic interstitial fibrosis develops in some patients.[66]

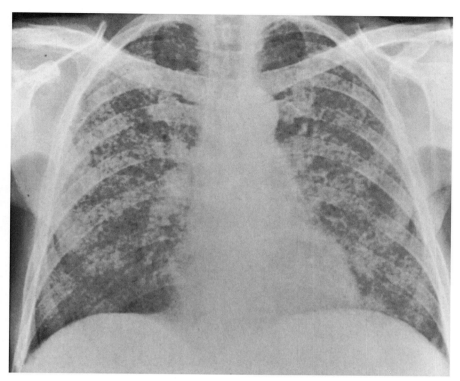

Figure 17–3. Busulfan Toxicity. At the time of the radiograph, this 61-year-old woman was being treated for chronic myeloid leukemia and was complaining of severe exertional dyspnea. Posteroanterior chest radiograph shows a widespread, coarse reticulonodular pattern throughout both lungs without anatomic predominance. The patient died about 1 year later; at autopsy, there was generalized alveolar wall interstitial fibrosis with preservation of lung architecture.

According to published reports, methotrexate pneumonitis is uncommon: In 1994, it was estimated that only 60 to 65 cases had been reported since the condition first was described 25 years previously.[61] In a retrospective cohort and literature review in 1997, only 37 cases were considered to satisfy criteria for definite methotrexate-induced lung injury.[75] Other workers have estimated, however, that the incidence of disease in patients receiving low-dose methotrexate for rheumatoid arthritis is about 2% to 5%;[61, 68] given the widespread use of such therapy, this constitutes a potentially serious health concern.

The duration of methotrexate therapy before symptoms

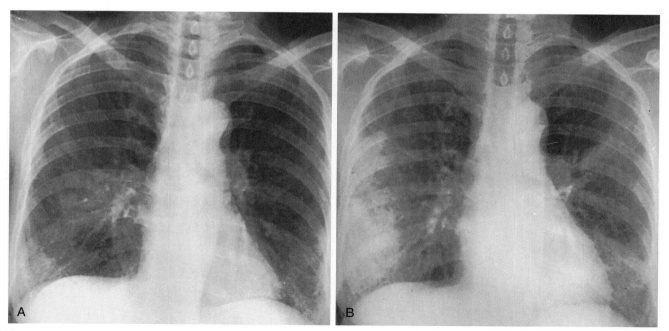

Figure 17–4. Cyclophosphamide Toxicity. Posteroanterior radiograph *(A)* shows ill-defined opacities in the midportion of the right lung and at both lung bases. The appearance suggests a combination of interstitial and air-space abnormalities. Seven months later *(B),* the opacities had become largely air space in character and, on the right side at least, showed considerable peripheral dominance. This middle-aged woman was being treated with cyclophosphamide for lymphoma.

and signs of toxicity become clinically apparent ranges from days to several years after initiation of therapy.[3, 13, 74] In most cases, the onset is acute to subacute and is characterized by fever, cough, dyspnea, and headache.[75, 76]

Radiographic changes are fairly characteristic and should suggest the diagnosis in the proper clinical setting. Initially, there is a basal or diffuse reticular or ground-glass pattern (Fig. 17–5).[67, 71] This pattern progresses rapidly to patchy air-space consolidation that in time reverts to an interstitial pattern followed by complete resolution (Fig. 17–6).[67, 69] Multiple nodules[70] and, in at least two patients, hilar lymph node enlargement have been reported.[70, 72] Radiographically demonstrable disease may be present for a few days[73] to 1 year or longer.[67] The HRCT findings described in one patient consisted of bilateral areas of ground-glass attenuation.[26]

Cytosine Arabinoside

Cytosine arabinoside is an antimetabolite that inhibits DNA synthesis. High-dose intravenous therapy is associated with a significant risk of pulmonary toxicity, having been reported in 15% to 30% of patients.[43, 77] Clinical findings are those of noncardiogenic pulmonary edema and fever developing 1 to 38 days after therapy.[78]

The radiographic manifestations consist of bilateral irregular linear opacities, air-space consolidation, or, more commonly, interstitial and air-space patterns.[79] In one review of 15 patients, the radiographs at the time of clinical presentation were abnormal in 13 and normal in the other 2 patients;[79] in 11 patients, the abnormalities were diffuse, and in 2 patients, they were limited to the lower or upper lobes. Two patients had pleural effusion.

ANTIMICROBIAL DRUGS

Nitrofurantoin

Although almost 1,000 cases of pulmonary toxicity caused by nitrofurantoin have been reported,[83, 84] overall, adverse pulmonary reactions are rare. In a review of records of 16,101 patients treated with the drug, pulmonary disease requiring hospitalization and possibly related to drug toxicity occurred only three times;[84] of 742 patients receiving long-term therapy, only 1 patient developed fatal lung fibrosis. There are two distinct presentations of nitrofurantoin-induced lung disease: (1) acute, developing hours to days after the onset of treatment, and (2) chronic and insidious, becoming manifest after weeks to years of continuous therapy. The former is the more common presentation.[83]

The radiographic manifestations of acute disease consist of a diffuse reticular pattern with some basilar predominance;[81, 85, 86] septal lines may be present (Fig. 17–7).[26] The pattern resembles interstitial pulmonary edema; the rapid clearing that occurs when the drug is withdrawn suggests that edema plays a considerable role in the production of the opacities.[87] Pleural effusions are relatively common and may be an isolated finding.[82, 88] One patient has been reported in whom all the clinical and radiographic features of ARDS developed after 2 weeks of therapy.[89]

The radiographic manifestations of the chronic form of nitrofurantoin lung toxicity consist of a bilateral reticular pattern usually involving mainly the lower lung zones.[54] HRCT may show a predominantly subpleural distribution of fibrosis.[26] A BOOP reaction may also be seen, with predominantly subpleural or peribronchial consolidation (Fig. 17–8).[267] Pleural effusions are uncommon.[54]

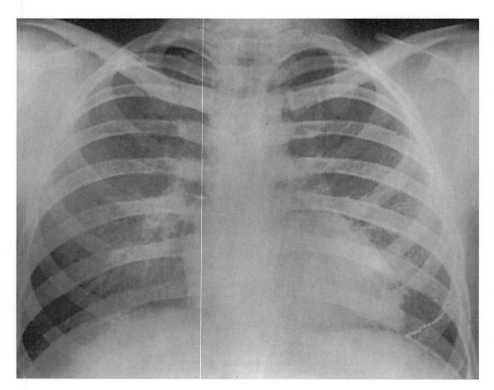

Figure 17–5. Methotrexate Toxicity. Posteroanterior chest radiograph shows a diffuse ground-glass pattern. Lung volume is reduced. This middle-aged man complained of mild dyspnea on effort. He was receiving methotrexate therapy for psoriasis.

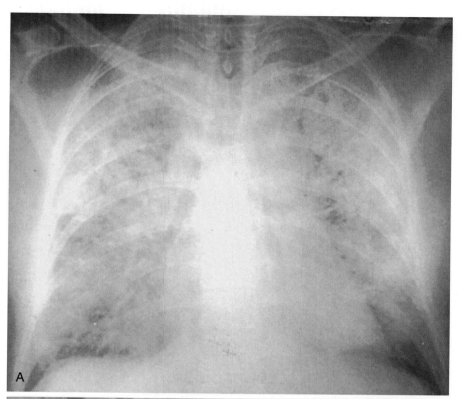

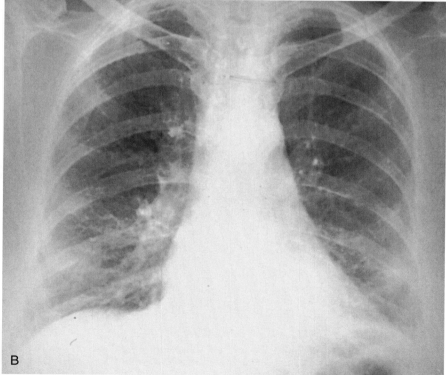

Figure 17–6. Methotrexate Toxicity. Posteroanterior radiograph *(A)* shows massive bilateral air-space consolidation containing a well-defined air bronchogram. The heart size is within normal limits. This appearance is highly suggestive of permeability pulmonary edema. Almost 2 weeks later, after cessation of methotrexate therapy for rheumatoid arthritis *(B)*, the consolidation had cleared almost completely.

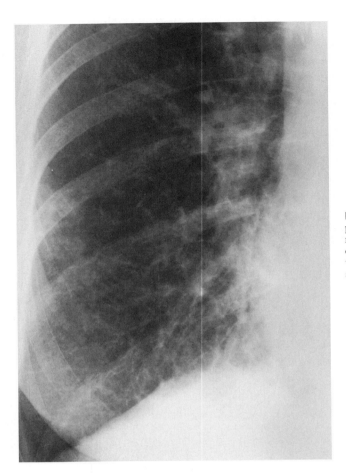

Figure 17–7. Acute Nitrofurantoin Toxicity. View of the right lung from posteroanterior chest radiograph shows a reticular pattern involving predominantly the lower lung zones. A few septal lines and a small right pleural effusion are evident. The patient was a 58-year-old woman who presented with progressive shortness of breath. The findings resolved within a few days after discontinuation of nitrofurantoin therapy.

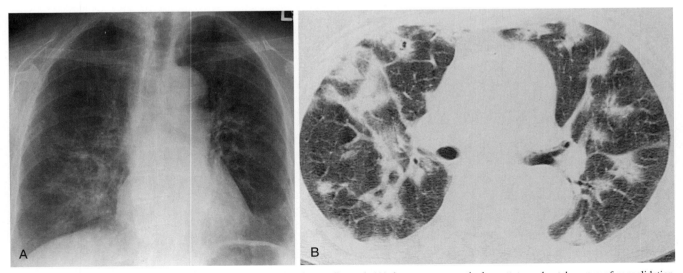

Figure 17–8. Chronic Nitrofurantoin Toxicity. Posteroanterior chest radiograph *(A)* shows a coarse reticular pattern and patchy areas of consolidation involving predominantly the middle and lower lung zones. HRCT scan *(B)* shows peribronchial distribution of the areas of consolidation and a few irregular linear opacities. The patient was an 81-year-old woman who presented with progressive shortness of breath. She had been on nitrofurantoin therapy for 2 years. Transbronchial biopsy specimen showed a bronchiolitis obliterans organizing pneumonia–like reaction. The radiologic findings improved within a few days after discontinuation of nitrofurantoin therapy; however, mild peribronchial reticulation still was present at 6-month follow-up.

Sulfasalazine

When used in the treatment of inflammatory bowel disease, sulfasalazine (salazosulfapyridine, salicylazosulfapyridine) is broken down into sulfapyridine and 5-aminosalicylate. Pulmonary toxicity has been reported in more than 24 patients.[80, 90] The complication probably represents a hypersensitivity reaction.

The radiographic manifestations typically consist of poorly defined bilateral areas of consolidation that commonly are peripheral in distribution and involve predominantly the upper lobes;[91] lower lobe involvement or diffuse infiltrates occur in a few cases.[92] In one patient we have seen, blood eosinophilia and radiographic resolution after withdrawal of therapy simulated Löffler's syndrome. Another case has been reported in which the clinical and radiologic features mimicked those of Wegener's granulomatosis;[93] chest radiograph showed bilateral nodular infiltrates, and CT scan showed bilateral peripheral wedge-shaped opacities and nodules, one of which had central cavitation. The opacities resolved after discontinuation of sulfasalazine therapy.

MISCELLANEOUS DRUGS

Amiodarone

Amiodarone hydrochloride is used in the treatment of cardiac arrhythmias. A conservative estimate of the number of cases of toxicity reported in the English language literature is more than 200.[97, 103] Most patients have received 400 mg/d or more of amiodarone before the appearance of pulmonary disease.[95, 96] It has been suggested that with current patterns of use, 5% to 7% of treated patients develop the complication, of whom 5% to 10% die as a consequence.[98]

Pulmonary damage has its onset months after the initiation of therapy.[80, 100] The drug is deposited in various organs and tissues throughout the body but particularly the lungs, where the concentration has been found to be four to seven times higher than in other organs.[101] It is eliminated slowly; the half-life has been estimated to be about 30 days.[80] The slow elimination may explain the interval of 1 month or longer after the cessation of therapy before complete radiographic and clinical resolution occurs.

Chest radiographs usually show a diffuse bilateral reticular pattern or bilateral areas of consolidation (Fig. 17–9).[54, 99, 102] The latter may be peripheral in distribution and may involve predominantly the upper lobes, resembling chronic eosinophilic pneumonia.[94, 99] Less common manifestations include focal consolidation and nodular opacities.[54] In one patient, cavitation occurred within one of the nodular infiltrates.[103] Pleural thickening has been described,[94] and one patient presented with bilateral exudative pleural effusions associated with toxic involvement of other organs.[104]

Because amiodarone contains about 37% iodine by weight, it has a high attenuation value on CT; as a result, this procedure allows confident recognition of drug deposition within pulmonary and other tissues (*see* Fig. 17–9).[105, 267] In one review of the CT findings in 11 patients who had symptoms of amiodarone pulmonary toxicity, high-attenuation (82 to 175 HU) pulmonary lesions were present in 8 (73%); increased liver or spleen attenuation, in 10 (91%); and increased myocardial attenuation, in 2 (18%).[105] Similar findings have been reported by others.[26, 106] The appearance of the parenchymal abnormalities is variable and may consist of bilateral areas of consolidation (frequently wedge shaped and pleural based), a reticular pattern, linear atelectasis, or (less commonly) focal round areas of consolidation.[26, 105, 106] Pleural effusions are seen on CT in about 50% of cases.[105] Visceral pleural thickening may be evident.[107] Distinction of amiodarone pneumonitis from congestive heart failure may be made by the documentation of increased uptake on gallium 67 radionuclide lung scans.[108, 109]

Acetylsalicylic Acid

Acetylsalicylic acid (aspirin) is a well-known cause of acute pulmonary edema, particularly in middle-aged and elderly people who habitually ingest large doses to alleviate chronic pain. Patients are dyspneic, lethargic, and confused; they tend to have proteinuria, perhaps reflecting increased capillary permeability in the systemic circulation. A history of long-term acetylsalicylic acid ingestion, usually in large quantities, is typical.[112–114] Chest radiographs show the typical diffuse air-space pattern of pulmonary edema.[110–112]

Penicillamine

Penicillamine is a derivative of penicillin that can chelate a variety of metals, including lead, copper, zinc, and mercury. It is used to treat lead poisoning, Wilson's disease, cystinuria, and connective tissue diseases, particularly progressive systemic sclerosis and rheumatoid arthritis. The variety of pulmonary complications caused by this drug is probably greater than that of any other and includes lupus-like[115] and myasthenia-like[118, 119] disease as well as alveolitis,[120, 122] obliterative bronchiolitis,[123–125] and diffuse alveolar hemorrhage.[116, 117] With the exception of bronchiolitis, the association of penicillamine with all these disorders appears to be causative. Because rheumatoid disease is a well-recognized cause of bronchiolitis and because most published cases of penicillamine-associated bronchiolitis have occurred in patients who have had rheumatoid arthritis, it is possible that some, if not all, reported cases of obliterative bronchiolitis have been a manifestation of the underlying disease rather than the drug.

Radiographic manifestations are of three types: (1) a reticular or reticulonodular pattern, with or without limited air-space opacities, indicating the presence of interstitial disease;[121] (2) overinflation unaccompanied by parenchymal abnormality, associated with obliterative bronchiolitis; and (3) diffuse air-space consolidation, typically seen in patients who have diffuse alveolar hemorrhage.[80, 126] In patients who have obliterative bronchiolitis, the HRCT findings consist of areas of decreased attenuation and perfusion (mosaic attenuation) and bronchial dilation.[125]

ILLICIT DRUGS

Although illicit drugs such as heroin and cocaine can induce a variety of specific pulmonary effects, their use may be associated with many nonspecific complications, the most important of which is infection.[128, 129] Opportunis-

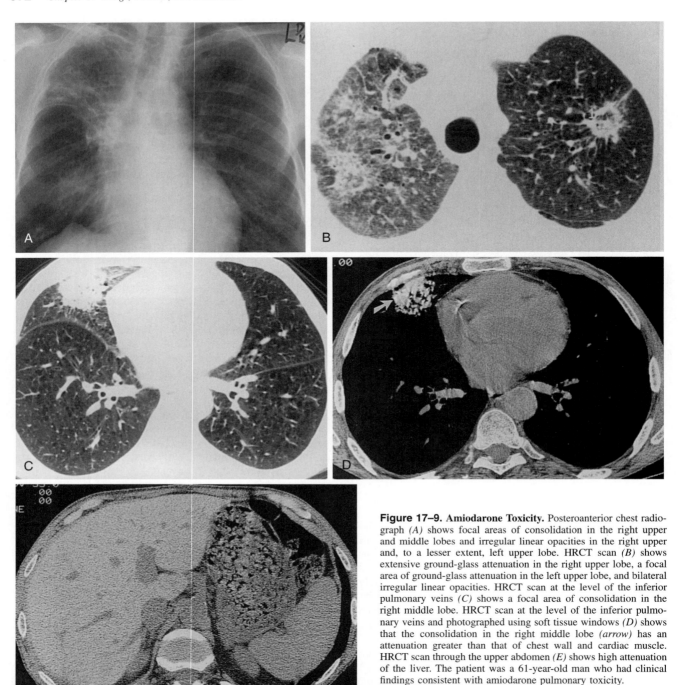

Figure 17–9. Amiodarone Toxicity. Posteroanterior chest radiograph *(A)* shows focal areas of consolidation in the right upper and middle lobes and irregular linear opacities in the right upper and, to a lesser extent, left upper lobe. HRCT scan *(B)* shows extensive ground-glass attenuation in the right upper lobe, a focal area of ground-glass attenuation in the left upper lobe, and bilateral irregular linear opacities. HRCT scan at the level of the inferior pulmonary veins *(C)* shows a focal area of consolidation in the right middle lobe. HRCT scan at the level of the inferior pulmonary veins and photographed using soft tissue windows *(D)* shows that the consolidation in the right middle lobe *(arrow)* has an attenuation greater than that of chest wall and cardiac muscle. HRCT scan through the upper abdomen *(E)* shows high attenuation of the liver. The patient was a 61-year-old man who had clinical findings consistent with amiodarone pulmonary toxicity.

tic infection associated with human immunodeficiency virus, including pneumonia caused by *Pneumocystis carinii*, *Mycobacterium tuberculosis*, and other bacteria,[128, 130] is now more common than septic pulmonary embolism and lung abscess among inner-city intravenous drug addicts. Aspiration pneumonia and atelectasis resulting from depressed levels of consciousness can occur in individuals using sedating drugs. Talcosis resulting from intravenous injection of drugs intended solely for oral use is discussed in Chapter 12.

Narcotic and Sedative Drugs

Opiates and related drugs are well-known causes of pulmonary edema. The incidence of the complication after heroin overdose ranges from 50% to 75%.[131, 132] The pathologic[133] and radiographic[134, 135] manifestations of the edema are indistinguishable from those of other etiologies (Fig. 17–10). The findings usually consist of bilateral and symmetric air-space consolidation, often with a predominantly perihilar distribution.[135] Less commonly, the edema is focal,

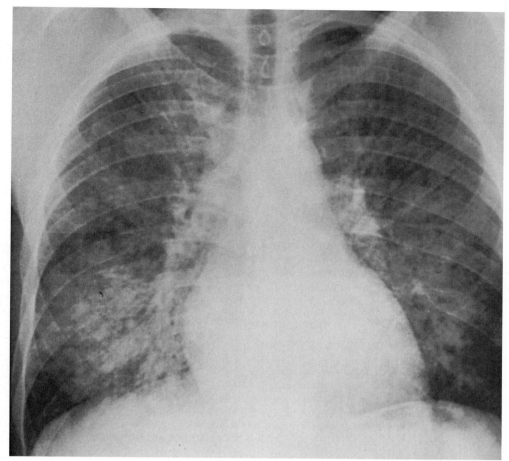

Figure 17–10. Acute Pulmonary Edema Caused by Drug Abuse. Posteroanterior chest radiograph shows air-space consolidation typical of acute pulmonary edema. Several hours previously, this 19-year-old man had injected a high dose of meperidine and methadone intravenously. He had an uneventful recovery.

is unilateral, or has an upper lobe distribution.[129, 135] The heart size is normal. The appearance of pulmonary edema may be delayed after admission to the hospital, sometimes for 6 to 10 hours;[136, 137] resolution characteristically occurs in 24 to 48 hours.[136, 138]

Cocaine

When smoked, the crystalline precipitate of free-base cocaine (crack) reaches the cerebral circulation within 6 to 8 seconds, causing virtually instantaneous euphoria. This property, along with its ease of administration, low price, and wide availability, has made the substance one of the most frequently abused controlled substances in the United States; it has been estimated that 6% of high school seniors in the United States have used cocaine, most commonly as crack.[130] Radiographic abnormalities have been reported in 13%[141] to 55%[139] of patients who have cardiopulmonary symptoms after drug inhalation.

A variety of pulmonary complications can occur. Radiographic manifestations of pulmonary edema consist of bilateral, symmetric, and predominantly perihilar interstitial or air-space opacities.[140, 141] These abnormalities usually resolve within 24 to 72 hours, regardless of treatment.[140, 141] Pulmonary hemorrhage may result in transient focal or diffuse bilateral air-space consolidation.[127, 142] Less commonly, fleeting areas of consolidation may result from a Löffler-like syndrome,[143] or diffuse consolidation associated with bronchiolitis obliterans organizing pneumonia.[130, 144] Barotrauma related to cocaine abuse may result in pneumomediastinum,[141, 145] pneumothorax,[141, 146] or (rarely) hemopneumothorax[141] or pneumopericardium.[147, 148]

CONTRAST MEDIA

Embolization of *ethiodized oil* used for lymphangiography can result in a *subacute* form of ARDS that possesses clinical features resembling fat embolism and that may have a similar pathogenesis. A significant decrease in diffusing capacity has been recorded after lymphangiography that is maximal in 48 hours and returns to normal in 1 month.[149, 160] Rarely, lymphangiography has been the cause of diffuse alveolar hemorrhage.[151]

Water-soluble contrast media occasionally have been reported to cause pulmonary edema. The pathogenesis of the complication has been debated.[152–155] Some investigators have suggested that it is a consequence of the high osmolarity of the solutions employed, particularly *sodium iothalamate* and *diatrizoate meglumine* (Gastrografin), the osmolarity of which is 5 to 10 times that of plasma.[153] In some patients who have underlying heart disease, hyperosmolality created by the contrast media causes an overloading of the circulation, which undoubtedly plays a role in the development of disease.[153, 156] Some affected patients are otherwise healthy, however, and the presence of a normal wedge pressure and a high protein content of the edema fluid indicates a permeability abnormality.[154, 155] Other observations supporting this mechanism are derived from experiments in rats, in which no difference in severity of edema has been identified between animals given low-osmolality or high-osmolality compounds,[157] and from reports of noncardiogenic pulmonary edema in patients given nonionic, low-osmolality contrast media intravenously.[158, 159]

Acute reactions to *ionic contrast medium* injected intravenously occur in 5% to 15% of patients who undergo the procedure.[160] These are usually mild; life-threatening reactions occur in only 0.05% to 0.1% of cases, with a mortality rate of about 1 in 75,000.[160, 161] Clinical manifestations of minor reactions include nausea, vomiting, urticaria, and diaphoresis; more severe disease is associated with faintness, severe vomiting, laryngeal edema, and bronchospasm. Severe reactions are characterized by pulmonary edema, hypotensive shock, convulsions, respiratory arrest, and cardiac arrest.[160]

Reactions to intravascular contrast media are classified into anaphylactoid (idiosyncratic) and chemotoxic.[160] The former are independent of dose, occur unpredictably, and account for most cases. Chemotoxic reactions are the result of specific physical and chemical effects of the contrast agent and are related to its concentration.[160] The risk of anaphylactoid reaction is increased in patients who have allergies, asthma, or previous reactions to the contrast medium. Chemotoxic effects are more likely to cause clinically significant complications in patients who are debilitated or who have renal dysfunction or severe cardiovascular disease.[160]

In a nationwide study of Japanese patients (about 170,000 who had received ionic contrast media and 170,000 who had received nonionic contrast media), the prevalence of adverse reactions was 12% for the former and 3% for the latter; the prevalence of severe reactions was 0.2% and 0.04%.[162] A meta-analysis of studies published before 1991 in which ionic and nonionic contrast media were used showed no difference in the fatality rate, however.[163] A review of the number and types of adverse drug reactions reported to the U.S. Food and Drug Administration between 1978 and 1994 showed no decrease in the number of nonfatal[164] and fatal[165] reactions to iodinated contrast media since the introduction of low-osmolality forms in 1986. The estimated 170 million contrast medium–enhanced studies performed in the United States between 1978 and 1994 produced 22,785 reports of mild or moderate adverse drug reactions, 2,639 reports of serious but nonfatal reactions, and 920 reports of death.[164] Excluding 22 myelography-related deaths, 42% more deaths were reported each year between 1987 and 1994 than between 1978 and 1986; most of this increase was associated with nonionic contrast media. In the period 1987 to 1994, 220 deaths were associated with the use of high-osmolality ionic contrast media alone, 32 with ionic low-osmolality contrast media alone, 214 with nonionic low-osmolality

contrast media alone, and 8 with combinations of contrast media.[165] The analysis of the data did not take into account the relative number of examinations performed using ionic versus nonionic agents during the study period, the increase in the number of examinations using contrast media since 1986, or trends in reporting adverse drug reactions. Although serious nonfatal and fatal reactions to contrast media are uncommon, they can occur with ionic and nonionic agents.

POISONS

Organophosphates

Poisoning with organophosphates occurs most commonly in agricultural workers during or shortly after the spraying of crops and less often in industrial workers during manufacture and transport; it also can happen accidentally in children and intentionally in suicide attempts.[166, 167] Parathion is the major cause of fatal poisoning; more than 50 deaths were reported during one 6-month period in Florida.[168] Symptoms and signs are attributable mainly to the accumulation of acetylcholine at cholinergic synapses, resulting in an initial stimulation and later inhibition of synaptic transmission. Miosis, diaphoresis, increased salivation, bronchorrhea, bronchoconstriction, bradycardia, and hyperperistalsis develop.

In one review of 13 cases, the radiographic findings consisted of bilateral interstitial or air-space pulmonary edema, usually associated with cardiomegaly (Fig. 17–11).[169] All patients presented with coma or depressed levels of consciousness; excessive lacrimation and salivation were seen 30 minutes to 9 hours after ingestion. In patients who survived, the radiographic findings cleared within 2 to 4 days.

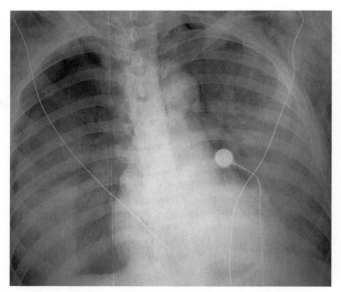

Figure 17–11. Organophosphate Poisoning. Chest radiograph in a 32-year-old man 4 days after ingestion of organophosphate pesticide shows extensive bilateral consolidation with associated bilateral pneumothoraces and subcutaneous emphysema. The findings essentially are those of increased permeability pulmonary edema. (Courtesy of Dr. Kyung-Soo Lee, Department of Radiology, Samsung Medical Center, Seoul, South Korea.)

Paraquat

Poisoning with the herbicide paraquat usually is associated with its ingestion, sometimes by mistake but more often for suicidal purposes; homicidal poisoning also has been described.[170] Large doses of the substance cause severe pulmonary edema and hemorrhage, resulting in rapid death.

The radiographic findings include extensive bilateral areas of consolidation (in about 60% of patients), pneumomediastinum with or without pneumothorax (in 40%), and cardiomegaly associated with widening of the superior mediastinum (in 20%).[171] Consolidation may be seen at presentation or may develop during several days in patients whose radiographs previously were normal or had a ground-glass opacity.[171, 172] In patients who survive, the consolidation may resolve completely or evolve into a chronic interstitial pattern consisting of irregular linear opacities or cystic spaces measuring 2 to 9 mm in diameter.[171]

The HRCT findings were reviewed in one study of 16 patients.[173] The most common pattern, seen 14 days after ingestion, consisted of diffuse bilateral areas of ground-glass attenuation. Associated areas of parenchymal consolidation involving mainly the lower lung zones were present in 40% of cases (Fig. 17–12). In some patients, the areas of ground-glass attenuation progressed to consolidation during several days. CT scans performed more than 14 days after ingestion in two patients showed consolidation in one and irregular lines consistent with fibrosis in the other.

IRRADIATION

Within the therapeutic range of doses usually administered, the pulmonary parenchyma can be assumed to react to ionizing radiation in virtually all patients. Many variables affect this reaction, however, and its clinical and radiologic manifestations, including the volume of lung tissue irradiated, the radiation dose administered, the time during which it is given, and the nature of the radiation.[174, 256] The lung can be affected by radiation in the absence of a demonstrable abnormality on conventional radiographs.[175, 176] There is some semantic confusion in the literature; the term *radiation pneumonitis* is used by some to denote a radiographic abnormality and by others to describe a clinical syndrome. For all these reasons, the incidence of pulmonary disease caused by radiotherapy varies considerably from series to series.

Pulmonary tissue usually is damaged by radiation aimed directly at the lungs; however, it also can be injured when the beam is directed elsewhere in the thorax, such as at the mediastinum or chest wall. In a review of 18 studies involving 5,534 patients reported before 1992, 7% of patients (range, 1% to 34%) developed symptomatic pneumonitis after radiation treatment for carcinoma of the lung, breast, or mesothelioma or for Hodgkin's disease;[177] 43% of patients (range, 13% to 100%) developed radiologic changes. In a more recent analysis of 24 series that included 1,911 patients, the incidence of radiation pneumonitis after combined modality therapy for pulmonary carcinoma was reported.[178] The total radiation dose used ranged from 25 to 63 Gy, with a median dose of 50 Gy (1 Gy = 100 rad). Symptomatic radiation pneumonitis occurred in 7.8% of patients. The risk was greater with higher total radiation dose, daily radiation fractions greater than 2.67 Gy, and use of once-daily as opposed to twice-daily irradiation (Table 17–2). Symptomatic radiation pneumonitis occurred in 6% of patients who received a total radiation dose lower than 45 Gy, in 9% who received doses between 45 and 54 Gy, and in 12% who had a total dose of 55 Gy or greater.

Focal radiation injury to the airways can occur after brachytherapy, a procedure that is used with increasing frequency for palliation of obstructing pulmonary carcinoma.[179–181] The technique consists of intraluminal endobronchial irradiation with a radioactive substance, usually iridium 192. Radiation injury to the lungs can follow inhalation of β-emitting radionuclides.[182–184] Rarely, it follows internal selective radiotherapy of the liver when radioactive

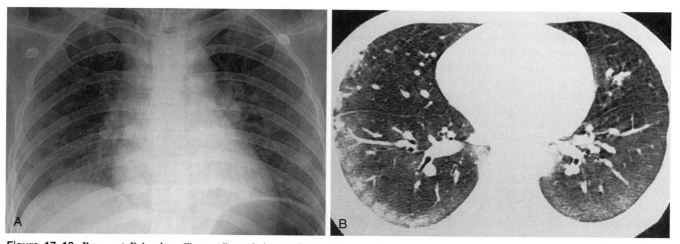

Figure 17–12. Paraquat Poisoning. Chest radiograph in an 18-year-old man with paraquat poisoning shows localized, poorly defined areas of increased opacity in the lower lung zones *(A)*. HRCT scan *(B)* shows extensive bilateral areas of ground-glass attenuation. Focal areas of consolidation are present, particularly in the subpleural lung regions in the right lower lobe, right middle lobe, and posterior basal segment of the left lower lobe. The patient recovered with complete resolution of the radiologic abnormalities. (Courtesy of Dr. Kyung-Soo Lee, Department of Radiology, Samsung Medical Center, Seoul, South Korea.)

Table 17–2. RADIATION LUNG INJURY

Risk Factors

Total radiation dose >30 Gy
Daily radiation fractions >2.7 Gy
Once-daily as compared with twice-daily radiation
Increased volume of irradiated lung
Previous or concurrent chemotherapy

Acute Radiation Pneumonitis

First evident on radiograph about 8 weeks after radiotherapy
Evident on HRCT 1–2 weeks before seen on radiograph
Most marked 3–4 months after radiotherapy
Radiologic manifestations
    Hazy, ground-glass opacities
    Areas of consolidation with air bronchograms
    Usually limited to the radiation ports

Radiation Fibrosis

Typically starts 3–4 months after radiotherapy
Usually stable 9–12 months after radiotherapy
Radiologic manifestations
    Irregular linear opacities, fibrotic strands
    Architectural distortion, traction bronchiectasis
    Loss of volume
    Limited to the radiation ports

HRCT, high-resolution computed tomography.

microspheres injected into the hepatic artery enter the pulmonary circulation through arterioportal shunts.[185] Pulmonary fibrosis associated with remote Thorotrast administration also has been reported.[186]

Risk Factors

Volume of Lung Irradiated. The likelihood of clinical symptoms and radiologic evidence of pulmonary injury is proportional to the volume of lung irradiated.[174] This variable is considered by some investigators to be the most important factor associated with lung damage.[187, 188] It has been estimated that a total dose of 30 Gy delivered in fractions to 25% of total lung volume may not produce any symptoms, whereas radiation delivered in the same manner to the entire volume of both lungs probably would prove fatal.[187]

Recognition of the importance of the volume of irradiated lung has led to the development of tangential ports to deliver radiotherapy, limiting radiation dose to normal structures. The prevalence of symptomatic radiation pneumonitis after treatment of breast carcinoma decreased from about 60% to 7% with the use of tangential ports rather than direct irradiation.[189, 190] Refinements in the tangential ports have led to further reduction. In one study of 1,624 patients treated for carcinoma of the breast with tangential field irradiation, only 17 (1%) developed symptomatic pneumonitis.[191] All 17 patients had radiographic changes that corresponded to the treatment portals; in 12, the radiographs became normal within 1 to 12 months after radiotherapy. Only 5 patients had radiation fibrosis, and none had late or persistent pulmonary symptoms. In another study, the incidence of symptomatic radiation pneumonitis after therapy for Hodgkin's disease was compared in patients receiving only mantle irradiation for mediastinal lymph nodes and patients receiving additional low-dose lung irradiation.[192] The mantle-field radiation dose ranged from 36 to 44 Gy, and the total-lung radiation dose was 15 Gy. Of 395 patients who received mantle irradiation alone, 12 (3%) developed radiation pneumonitis, as compared with 7 of 47 (15%) who received mantle-field plus total-lung irradiation.

Dose. Radiologic evidence of radiation pneumonitis seldom occurs with doses less than 30 Gy,[174, 193, 194] is variably present with doses between 30 and 40 Gy, and almost always is present with doses greater than 40 Gy.[174, 177, 194] There is, however, considerable individual variability in the pulmonary response, and it is impossible to predict which patients will develop radiologic changes or symptoms.[174, 190] Despite the fact that the average dose to patients in whom radiographically demonstrable changes develop is significantly higher than the average dose to those whose lungs remain normal, statistically significant differences between the doses that result in minimal, moderate, or severe pulmonary changes have not been found.[196]

Time and Dose Factor. Because fractionation permits time for repair of sublethal damage between fractions, the effect of radiation on the lung is related less to the total dose than to the rate at which it is delivered.[182] This variable biologic effect of equivalent doses of radiation is related to the total dose absorbed, the number of fractions, and the time elapsed between first and last treatments.[197–199] The severity of radiation effect increases with increased dose per fraction or when the same dose is given during a shorter period of time.[174]

Previous or Concurrent Therapy. The susceptibility to radiation pneumonitis is increased in patients who have had previous pulmonary irradiation[177, 190, 195] or previous or concurrent chemotherapy[174, 190] and in those in whom corticosteroid has been withdrawn.[200–202] Drugs known to enhance the effects of radiation include actinomycin D, doxorubicin, bleomycin, busulfan, cyclophosphamide, mitomycin C, methotrexate, and vincristine.[190, 203–207] In one study of 328 patients who had breast carcinoma and who received radiotherapy and chemotherapy, 11 (3%) developed symptomatic radiation pneumonitis, as compared with only 6 of 1,296 (0.5%) patients who received radiotherapy alone.[191] The risk of radiation pneumonitis is increased when irradiation and chemotherapy are administered simultaneously.[177, 191] In one investigation of 92 patients who had breast carcinoma treated concurrently with chemotherapy and radiotherapy, 8 (9%) developed symptomatic radiation pneumonitis, as compared with only 3 of 326 (1.3%) who were treated sequentially.[191] Radiation recall—the development of pneumonitis in a previously irradiated site after the administration of chemotherapeutic agents—can occur within hours to days of drug administration and can be seen from a few days up to 15 years after radiotherapy.[208–210]

Many patients who have radiographic evidence of radiation damage remain symptom-free.[196] When symptoms do develop, they usually appear between 2 and 3 months, and occasionally as late as 6 months, after the completion of therapy; rarely, symptoms arise during the first month. Discontinuation of corticosteroids in patients receiving combined steroid therapy and radiotherapy can precipitate severe symptomatic pneumonitis.[200–201] Symptoms generally have an insidious onset and consist of nonproductive cough, weakness, and shortness of breath on exertion.

Acute radiation pneumonitis may persist for 1 month

and can resolve completely or progress to fibrosis. With the onset of fibrosis, symptoms of the acute pneumonitis abate gradually. In a few patients, fibrosis develops insidiously without an acute phase being recognized. Death may be caused by respiratory insufficiency.

Radiologic Manifestations

Radiographic evidence of acute radiation pneumonitis usually becomes evident about 8 weeks after completion of radiotherapy with doses of 40 Gy and about 1 week earlier for every additional 10-Gy increment.[174, 194] Abnormalities are usually most marked 3 to 4 months after completion of radiotherapy;[174, 211] they are seen rarely immediately after its completion[212] and occasionally within 1 to 4 weeks (Fig. 17–13).[175, 195, 212]

The radiographic manifestations may be subtle, consisting of hazy ground-glass opacities with slight indistinctness of the pulmonary vessels, or more marked, consisting of patchy or homogeneous air-space consolidation (Fig. 17–14).[174, 190, 214] Air bronchograms commonly are present.[174, 213] The abnormalities usually have sharp boundaries, corresponding to the radiation portals, and cross normal anatomic structures without segmental or lobar distribution.[174, 214] Occasionally, mild abnormalities are seen beyond the radiation ports (Fig. 17–15).[175, 214] In a few patients, areas of consolidation initially limited to the radiation field have been shown to spread to involve both lungs.[257, 258] Lung biopsy performed in some of these patients has shown bronchiolitis obliterans organizing pneumonia (Table 17–3).[257, 258] Radiation-induced bronchiolitis obliterans organizing pneumonia usually occurs 6 weeks to 10 months after radiation therapy and has a migratory pattern and a predominantly subpleural and peribronchial

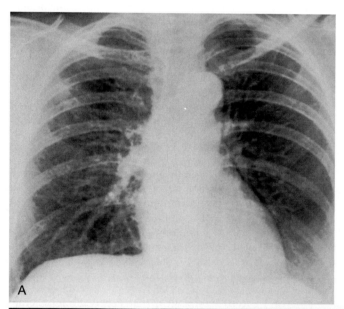

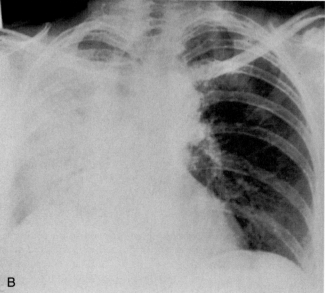

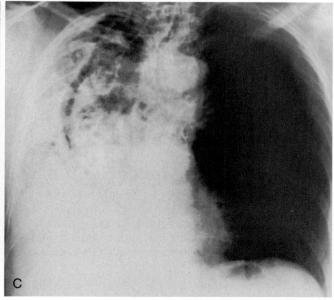

Figure 17–13. Acute Radiation Pneumonitis and Subsequent Fibrosis. This 52-year-old woman presented with a large carcinoma of the breast. She underwent mastectomy and postoperative radiotherapy administered to the right lung in a dosage of 51 Gy and to the mediastinum in a dose of 35 Gy. Posteroanterior radiograph *(A)* at the end of the radiotherapy showed no significant abnormalities. Three weeks later, however, a remarkable change had occurred in the appearance of the chest *(B):* The right lung had undergone severe loss of volume as evidenced by elevation of the hemidiaphragm and shift of the mediastinum. Posteroanterior radiograph taken about 1 month later *(C)* showed severe loss of volume of the right lung. The pattern observed earlier had changed to a coarse inhomogeneous pattern in which extensive bronchiectasis was readily apparent. In subsequent years, the radiographic appearance of the right hemithorax underwent no further change, and the patient's only complaint was shortness of breath on climbing stairs or walking rapidly on level ground.

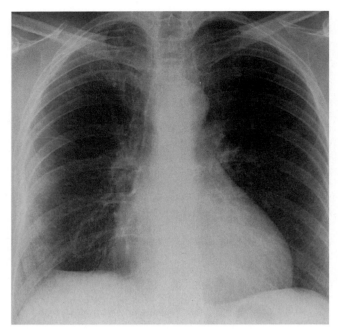

Figure 17–14. Acute Radiation Pneumonitis. Posteroanterior chest radiograph shows areas of consolidation with poorly defined margins in the axillary portion of the right lung. The patient was a 54-year-old woman who had undergone radiotherapy for carcinoma of the right breast 6 weeks previously. (Courtesy of Dr. Jackie Morgan-Parkes, British Columbia Cancer Agency, Vancouver, British Columbia.)

distribution.[258] Rarely, pneumonitis progresses rapidly to diffuse consolidation involving the entire lung[224, 227] or both lungs (ARDS).[216, 217]

Radiation pneumonitis usually is associated with considerable loss of volume, presumably as a result of a surfactant deficit and adhesive atelectasis.[213, 218] Atelectasis may occur

secondary to obstruction shortly after radiotherapy for an endobronchial lesion;[219] this is caused by radiation-induced edema of the bronchial wall that already is severely narrowed by the endobronchial lesion. A lung scan pattern suggesting pulmonary thromboembolism may result from vascular obliteration.[220] An uncommon but highly suggestive sign of previous mediastinal radiation consists of bilateral superomedial hilar displacement in the absence of radiographic evidence of parenchymal fibrosis.[221]

Evidence of acute radiation pneumonitis is seen more commonly and earlier on CT scans than on radiographs (Fig. 17–16)[175, 176, 222] and is seen better on HRCT scans than on conventional scans.[175, 223] In one review of 83 CT scans performed at relatively short intervals in 17 patients who had received 24 to 60 Gy, radiation-induced abnormalities were detected on CT scans in 15 (88%) of 17 patients and on chest radiographs in 12 (71%) patients.[175] In 13 patients, the earliest changes were evident on CT scan 1 to 4 weeks after completion of therapy; in the remaining 2 patients, the abnormalities became evident after 8 weeks and 13 weeks, respectively. In 3 of the 12 patients who developed radiographic abnormalities, these became evident 1 to 8 weeks after they first had been detected on CT; in the remaining 9 patients, the abnormalities were identified at the same time that they were first seen on CT.

A second group of investigators assessed the CT and radiographic findings in 18 patients who received 40 Gy of radiotherapy for Hodgkin's disease.[212] Parenchymal abnormalities were evident immediately after completion of radiotherapy on CT scan in 7 (39%) patients and on radiograph in 2 (11%) patients.[212] One month after completion of radiotherapy, radiation pneumonitis was visualized on CT scan in 78% of patients and on radiograph in 55%. Four months after irradiation, 17 of 18 patients (94%) had evidence of radiation pneumonitis on CT scan and radiograph.

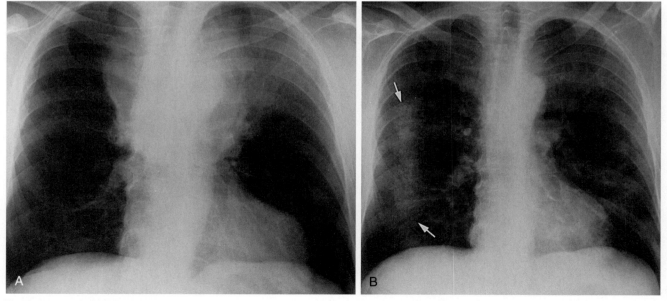

Figure 17–15. Acute Radiation Pneumonitis. Posteroanterior chest radiograph *(A)* before radiotherapy for Hodgkin's disease shows widening of the mediastinum. Chest radiograph 5 weeks later *(B)* shows consolidation in the right lung *(arrows)*. The consolidation resolved slowly over the following months. The diagnosis of radiation pneumonitis outside the radiation ports was made clinically. (Courtesy of Dr. Jackie Morgan-Parkes, British Columbia Cancer Agency, Vancouver, British Columbia.)

Table 17–3. COMPLICATIONS OF RADIATION THERAPY

Lung Parenchyma and Airways

Common
  Radiation pneumonitis, radiation fibrosis
Uncommon
  BOOP, ARDS, pulmonary necrosis and cavitation, unilateral hyperlucent lung, tracheal or bronchial stricture, necrosis of bronchial stump

Pleura

Common
  Pleural thickening
Uncommon
  Pleural effusion, pneumothorax, bronchopleural fistula, mesothelioma, fibrous tumor of the pleura

Cardiovascular

Relatively common
  Pericardial effusion
Uncommon
  Pericardial thickening, pericardial calcification, myocardial fibrosis, coronary artery disease, myocardial infarction, calcification of the aorta, stenosis of the subclavian or carotid arteries

Mediastinum

Relatively common
  Calcification of lymph nodes (in Hodgkin's disease)
Uncommon
  Thymic cysts, esophageal stricture

Chest Wall

Uncommon
  Dystrophic soft tissue calcification, bone demineralization, osteolysis, osteonecrosis, fractures of the ribs or clavicle, atypical callus formation, osteosarcoma, malignant fibrous histiocytoma, breast carcinoma

BOOP, bronchiolitis obliterans organizing pneumonia; ARDS, adult respiratory distress syndrome.

The CT manifestations of acute radiation pneumonitis consist of homogeneous areas of ground-glass attenuation or patchy or diffuse consolidation involving the radiated portions of the lungs; well-defined borders conforming to the shape of the radiation portals usually are present (Fig. 17–17).[175, 223, 224] In a few cases, areas of consolidation within the radiated lung are patchy in distribution and do not conform to the shape of the radiation portal;[224] occasionally, they extend beyond the radiation portals.[175, 225] Other characteristic findings include air bronchograms, loss of volume, and extension across normal anatomic boundaries.[214, 223]

The late or chronic stage of radiation damage is characterized by evidence of fibrosis (Fig. 17–18). Typically, fibrosis starts after 3 to 4 months, develops gradually, and becomes stable 9 to 12 months after completion of radiotherapy.[174, 211] The affected lung shows severe loss of volume, with obliteration of all normal architectural markings; the peripheral parenchyma is characteristically airless and opaque as a result of replacement by fibrous tissue. Dense fibrotic strands frequently extend from the hilum to the periphery. Radiation fibrosis develops in most patients who receive therapeutic doses of radiation and may be seen in patients who have no radiographic evidence of acute radiation pneumonitis.[174] The radiographic findings occasionally are subtle and consist only of mild elevation of one or both hila, mild retraction of pulmonary vessels, or mild pleural thickening.[174] The CT findings consist of dense consolidation or linear strands conforming to the radiation portals and associated with volume loss, architectural distortion, and bronchial dilation (traction bronchiectasis) (Fig. 17–19).[174, 222, 224]

Uncommon late complications include pulmonary or bronchial necrosis and hyperlucent lung (*see* Table 17–3).[214, 258] In a review of 1,000 patients with apical lung carcinoma who were treated with upper lobectomy followed by chemotherapy and adjuvant radiation therapy, 6 were identified who developed benign apical pleural or parenchymal necrosis.[258] Cavitation developed 1 to 7 years after radiation therapy.

Pleural effusions seldom are seen on chest radiograph during acute radiation pneumonitis,[196, 226, 227] although small effusions commonly are detected on CT.[174] Other pleural

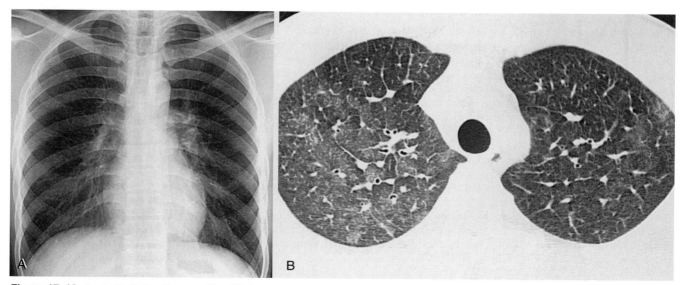

Figure 17–16. Acute Radiation Pneumonitis: CT Appearance. Posteroanterior chest radiograph *(A)* in a patient with acute radiation pneumonitis shows no definite abnormality. HRCT scan *(B)* performed the same day as chest radiograph shows extensive bilateral areas of ground-glass attenuation. (Courtesy of Dr. Kyung-Soo Lee, Samsung Medical Center, Seoul, South Korea.)

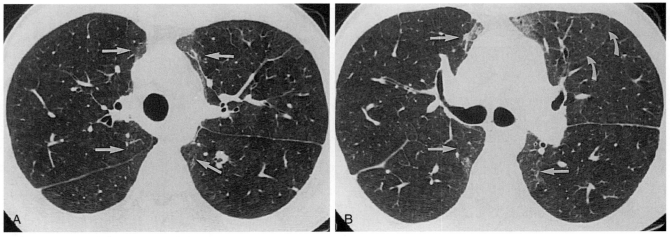

Figure 17–17. Acute Radiation Pneumonitis. HRCT scans *(A* and *B)* show areas of ground-glass attenuation *(straight arrows)* in the paramediastinal regions of both lungs. Mild focal extension of radiation pneumonitis outside of the radiation portal *(curved arrows in B)* is present in the anterior aspect of the left upper lobe. The patient was a 37-year-old man who had completed a course of radiotherapy for Hodgkin's disease 2 months previously.

complications include spontaneous pneumothorax (in patients with pulmonary carcinoma who develop thin-walled cavities)[231, 258] and bronchopleural fistula (related to necrosis of a postlobectomy or pneumonectomy stump) (*see* Table 17–3).[214, 232] Some degree of pleural thickening, occasionally extensive, develops in most patients in association with radiation-induced pulmonary fibrosis; it also is assessed more readily on CT scan than on radiograph.[176, 213] Rare pleural complications include mesothelioma[259] and fibrous tumor of the pleura.[260, 261]

Pericardial effusion after radiotherapy to the mediastinum is common; in one group of 31 patients who had a variety of malignancies and who developed pericarditis, 3 (10%) were considered to have radiation-induced pericarditis 2, 11, and 20 months after completion of radiotherapy;[228] 2 patients had pericardial effusion at echocardiography. The complication is seen most commonly after treatment of Hodgkin's disease.[258] Pericardial effusion usually appears 12 to 18 months after completion of radiation therapy[258] but may develop within a few months or be delayed for several years.[229, 230] Pericardial thickening and constriction, a complication observed in 15% to 20% of patients who have pericarditis, usually is manifested 4 years or more after radiation therapy.[258, 262] Occasionally the pericardium shows foci of calcification (Fig. 17–20).[235] Additional late complications within the radiation field include myocardial fibrosis, premature atherosclerosis (associated with an increased incidence of coronary artery disease and myocardial infarction) (*see* Table 17–3, Fig. 17–21),[233–235] calcification of the aorta,[236] stenosis of the subclavian and carotid arteries, and tracheal or bronchial stricture.[214, 235]

Bone changes within the radiation field include demineralization, small lytic areas, aseptic necrosis, and spontaneous fractures.[234, 237, 238] Pathologic fracture of the clavicle has been reported following radiotherapy for Hodgkin's disease, carcinoma of the breast, and carcinoma of the nasopharynx.[268] Fractures of the ribs or clavicle may be associated with nonunion or with atypical callus formation with irregular calcification mimicking radiation-induced osteosarcoma.[234] CT is superior to radiography in showing subtle fractures, changes in bone architecture, and dystro-

phic soft tissue calcification.[239] Osteonecrosis of the spine results in high signal intensity on T1-weighted MR images and intermediate intensity on T2-weighted images as a result of replacement of hematopoietic elements by fat.[239] Other chest wall complications include radiation-induced sarcoma and breast carcinoma.[258]

Radiation-induced sarcomas occur in 0.1% or less of patients who receive radiation therapy and survive 5 years or more.[263] Osteosarcoma is the most common; the most common soft tissue tumor is malignant fibrous histiocytoma.[237, 258] Another well-known complication of radiation therapy is breast carcinoma.[258] Patients at particularly high risk are those who receive radiation before the age of 30 years.[258] For example, women treated for Hodgkin's disease during childhood have been shown to have a risk of breast carcinoma 75 times greater than that of the general population.[264]

CT can be helpful in the detection of recurrent tumor within the irradiated field.[174] Findings suggestive of recurrent tumor include the presence of a mass lesion or development of a focal opacity not containing air bronchograms.[174, 240] Distinction of tumor recurrence from radiation fibrosis may be made using magnetic resonance (MR) imaging.[243] Radiation fibrosis has a low signal intensity on T2-weighted images, the signal being similar to or lower than that of muscle, whereas a neoplasm has greater signal intensity than muscle.[243] Persistence of an inflammatory process, infection, or hemorrhage also may lead to increased signal intensity on T2-weighted images, however.[241, 242] Persistent inflammation may result in enhancement in the affected area after intravenous administration of gadolinium-DTPA.[242]

Ventilation-perfusion scans frequently are abnormal after radiotherapy:[243–245] Perfusion abnormalities in the irradiated lung have been reported in 50% to 95% of patients and ventilation abnormalities in 35% to 45%.[245] The most common abnormality is ventilation of poorly perfused areas,[245, 246] in some cases mimicking thromboembolism.[247] Single-photon emission computed tomography (SPECT) ventilation-perfusion scans are more sensitive than conventional planar ventilation-perfusion scans and chest radio-

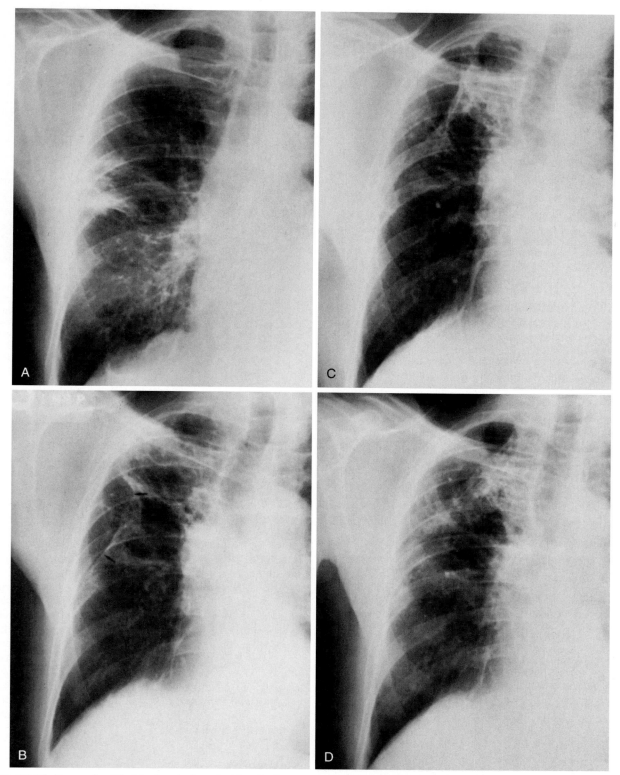

Figure 17–18. Progressive Cicatrization Atelectasis After Radiation Pneumonitis, Manifested by Migration of a Bulla. Several months after completion of a course of radiotherapy to the right hemithorax for inoperable pulmonary carcinoma, a radiograph *(A)* of this 66-year-old man shows some loss of volume of the right lung and a few patchy opacities in the axillary portion of the right upper lobe. Almost 1.5 years later *(B)*, the loss of volume was more severe, and a well-circumscribed cystic space had developed in the axillary portion of the right lung *(arrows)*, representing a bulla. Three months later *(C)*, the bulla had enlarged somewhat and had migrated superiorly in response to progressive fibrosis of the right upper lobe. A further 3 months later *(D)*, the bulla occupied the apical zone of the right hemithorax.

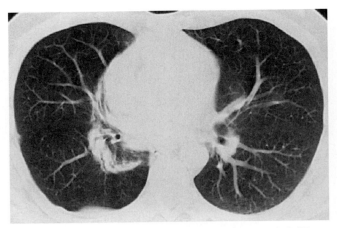

Figure 17–19. Radiation Fibrosis. A 7-mm collimation spiral CT scan shows a sharply marginated focal area of ground-glass attenuation with associated linear opacities and air bronchograms. Focal pleural thickening is evident. This 47-year-old man had undergone thymectomy and radiotherapy for invasive thymoma 4 years previously.

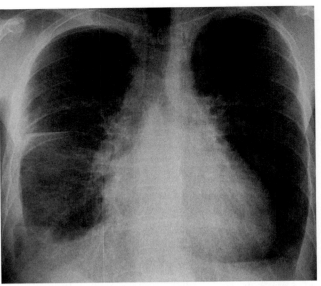

Figure 17–21. Congestive Cardiomyopathy After Radiotherapy. Anteroposterior chest radiograph in a 31-year-old man shows cardiomegaly, interstitial pulmonary edema, and small bilateral pleural effusions. The patient had experienced two myocardial infarcts and developed cardiomyopathy several years after radiotherapy for Hodgkin's disease. (Courtesy of Dr. Jackie Morgan-Parkes, British Columbia Cancer Agency, Vancouver, British Columbia.)

graphs in the detection of regional lung injury after radiotherapy.[176, 245, 248] There is evidence that gallium 67 scintigraphy may be superior to chest radiography in the demonstration of the spatial extent of radiation pneumonitis. In one study of 12 patients who developed radiation pneumonitis after radiotherapy for pulmonary carcinoma, gallium 67 uptake was confined to the radiated lung in 7 patients and was diffuse in 5;[249] pathologic assessment of the lung outside the radiated field in 4 of the 5 patients who had diffuse uptake revealed findings consistent with radiation pneumonitis. Evidence of radiation pneumonitis outside of the irradiated field was not apparent on chest radiographs.

Calcification of mediastinal lymph nodes[252, 253] and presternal soft tissue disease may be seen after radiotherapy for Hodgkin's disease.[254] Calcification of nonenlarged

nodes in Hodgkin's disease signifies a favorable response to therapy.[258, 265] Calcification of mediastinal lymph nodes may occur after radiotherapy for non-Hodgkin's lymphoma.[255] Thymic cysts, sometimes with a thin rim of calcification, may develop after radiotherapy for Hodgkin's disease; occasionally, they enlarge and simulate recurrent tumor.[250, 251] Esophageal complications of radiation therapy include abnormal peristalsis and, rarely, stricture.[258, 266]

Complications of brachytherapy include mucosal fibrosis with bronchostenosis, localized radiation pneumonitis, bronchoesophageal fistula, and hemoptysis.[179–181] In one study of 46 patients who had received endobronchial brachytherapy, 4 (9%) developed self-limited radiation pneumonitis, and 3 (7%) suffered fatal hemoptysis.[180]

In another study of 342 patients who had undergone brachytherapy (three fractions of 7.5 to 10 Gy at a calculated depth of 5 to 10 mm), 41 (12%) developed bronchitis and stenosis.[181] At bronchoscopy, predominantly inflammatory changes were seen at a mean of about 16 weeks from the date of first brachytherapy, and predominantly fibrotic changes were seen at 40 weeks. Twenty-five patients (9%) developed fatal hemoptysis. Variables associated with an increased risk of complications included large cell carcinoma, prior laser photo resection, and concurrent external-beam irradiation.

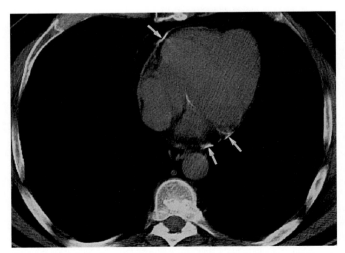

Figure 17–20. Pericardial Calcification After Radiotherapy. CT scan in a 51-year-old man shows focal areas of pericardial calcification *(arrows)*. The patient had undergone radiotherapy for Hodgkin's disease 21 years previously. Calcification was limited to the irradiation field. (Courtesy of Dr. Jackie Morgan-Parkes, British Columbia Cancer Agency, Vancouver, British Columbia.)

References

1. Rosenow EC III: Drug-induced pulmonary disease. Dis Mon 40:258, 1994.
2. Aronchick JM, Gefter WB: Drug-induced pulmonary disorders. Semin Roentgenol 30:18, 1995.
3. Rosenow EC III, Limper AH: Drug-induced pulmonary disease. Semin Respir Infect 10:86, 1995.
4. Demeter SL, Ahmad M, Tomashefski JF: Drug-induced pulmonary

disease: Part I. Patterns of response. Part II: Categories of drugs. Part III: Agents used to treat neoplasms or alter the immune system including a brief review of radiation therapy. Cleve Clin Q 46:89, 1979.

5. Jules-Elysee K, White DA: Bleomycin-induced pulmonary toxicity. Clin Chest Med 11:1, 1990.

6. Kreisman H, Wolkove N: Pulmonary toxicity of antineoplastic therapy. Semin Oncol 19:508, 1992.

7. Cooper JAD Jr, White DA, Matthay RA: Drug-induced pulmonary disease: Part 1. Cytotoxic drugs. Am Rev Respir Dis 133:321, 1986.

8. Wolkowicz J, Sturgeon J, Rawji M, et al: Bleomycin-induced pulmonary function abnormalities. Chest 101:97, 1992.

9. White DA, Stover DE: Severe bleomycin-induced pneumonitis: Clinical features and response to corticosteroids. Chest 86:723, 1984.

10. Holoye PY, Luna MA, MacKay B, et al: Bleomycin hypersensitivity pneumonitis. Ann Intern Med 88:47, 1978.

11. Yousem SA, Lifson JD, Colby TV: Chemotherapy-induced eosinophilic pneumonia: Relation to bleomycin. Chest 88:103, 1985.

12. Rose AG: Pulmonary veno-occlusive disease due to bleomycin therapy for lymphoma. S Afr Med J 64:636, 1983.

13. Batist G, Andrews JL Jr: Pulmonary toxicity of antineoplastic drugs. JAMA 246:1449, 1981.

14. Weiss RB, Muggia FM: Cytotoxic drug-induced pulmonary disease: Update 1980. Am J Med 68:259, 1980.

15. Samuels ML, Johnson DE, Holoye PY, et al: Large-dose bleomycin therapy and pulmonary toxicity: A possible role of prior radiotherapy. JAMA 235:1117, 1976.

16. Horowitz AL, Friedman M, Smith J, et al: The pulmonary changes of bleomycin toxicity. Radiology 106:65, 1973.

17. Balikian JP, Jochelson MS, Bauer KA, et al: Pulmonary complications of chemotherapy regimens containing bleomycin. Am J Roentgenol 139:455, 1982.

18. Iacovino JR, Leitner J, Abbas AK, et al: Fatal pulmonary reaction from low doses of bleomycin: An idiosyncratic tissue response. JAMA 235:1253, 1976.

19. Mills P, Husband J: Computed tomography of pulmonary bleomycin toxicity. Semin Ultrasound CT MR 11:417, 1990.

20. Talcott JA, Garnick MB, Stomper PC, et al: Cavitary lung nodules associated with combination chemotherapy containing bleomycin. J Urol 138:619, 1987.

21. Glasier CM, Siegel MJ: Multiple pulmonary nodules: Unusual manifestation of bleomycin toxicity. Am J Roentgenol 137:155, 1981.

22. McCrea ES, Diaconis JN, Wade JC, et al: Bleomycin toxicity simulating metastatic nodules to the lungs. Cancer 48:1096, 1981.

23. Dineen MK, Englander LS, Huben RP: Bleomycin-induced nodular pulmonary fibrosis masquerading as metastatic testicular cancer. J Urol 136:473, 1986.

24. Bellamy EA, Husband JE, Blaquiere RM, et al: Bleomycin-related lung damage: CT evidence. Radiology 156:155, 1985.

25. Rimmer MJ, Dixon AK, Flower CDR, et al: Bleomycin lung: Computed tomographic observations. Br J Radiol 58:1041, 1985.

26. Padley SPG, Adler B, Hansell DM, et al: High-resolution computed tomography of drug-induced lung disease. Clin Radiol 46:232, 1992.

27. Twohig KJ, Matthay RA: Pulmonary effects of cytotoxic agents other than bleomycin. Clin Chest Med 11:31, 1990.

28. Rivera MP, Kris MG, Gralla RJ, et al: Syndrome of acute dyspnea related to combined mitomycin plus vinca alkaloid chemotherapy. Am J Clin Oncol 18:245, 1995.

29. Castro M, Veeder MH, Mailliard JA, et al: A prospective study of pulmonary function in patients receiving mitomycin. Chest 109:939, 1996.

30. Gunstream SR, Seidenfeld JJ, Sobonya RE, et al: Mitomycin-associated lung disease. Cancer Treat Rep 67:301, 1983.

31. Budzar AU, Legha SS, Luna MA, et al: Pulmonary toxicity of mitomycin. Cancer 45:236, 1980.

32. Orwoll ES, Kiessling PJ, Patterson JR: Interstitial pneumonia from mitomycin. Ann Intern Med 89:352, 1978.

33. Oliner H, Schwartz R, Rubio F, et al: Interstitial pulmonary fibrosis following busulfan therapy. Am J Med 31:134, 1961.

34. Leake E, Smith WG, Woodliff HJ: Diffuse interstitial pulmonary fibrosis after busulphan therapy. Lancet 2:432, 1963.

35. Crilley P, Topolsky D, Styler MJ, et al: Extramedullary toxicity of a conditioning regimen containing busulfan, cyclophosphamide and etoposide in 84 patients undergoing autologous and allogenic bone marrow transplantation. Bone Marrow Transplant 15:361, 1995.

36. Lund MB, Kongerud J, Brinch L, et al: Decreased lung function in one year survivors of allogenic bone marrow transplantation conditioned with high-dose busulfan and cyclophosphamide. Eur Respir J 8:1269, 1995.

37. Heard BE, Cooke RA: Busulphan lung. Thorax 23:187, 1968.

38. Ginsberg SJ, Comis RL: The pulmonary toxicity of antineoplastic agents. Semin Oncol 9:34, 1982.

39. Soble AR, Perry H: Fatal radiation pneumonia following subclinical busulfan injury. Am J Roentgenol 128:15, 1977.

40. Smalley RV, Wall RL: Two cases of busulfan toxicity. Ann Intern Med 64:154, 1966.

41. Harrold BP: Syndrome resembling Addison's disease following prolonged treatment with busulphan. BMJ 1:463, 1966.

42. Podoll LN, Winkler SS: Busulfan lung: Report of two cases and review of the literature. Am J Roentgenol 120:151, 1974.

43. Rosenow EC, Myers J, Swensen SJ, et al: Drug-induced pulmonary disease. Chest 102:239, 1992.

44. Wilczynski SW, Erasmus JJ, Petros WP, et al: Delayed pulmonary toxicity syndrome following high-dose chemotherapy and bone marrow transplantation for breast cancer. Am J Respir Crit Care Med 157:565, 1998.

45. Malik SW, Myers JL, DeRemee RA, et al: Lung toxicity associated with cyclophosphamide use: Two distinct patterns. Am J Respir Crit Care Med 154:1851, 1996.

46. Cherniack RM, Abrams J, Kalica AR: Pulmonary disease associated with breast cancer therapy. Am J Respir Crit Care Med 150:1169, 1994.

47. Rubio C, Hill ME, Milan S, et al: Idiopathic pneumonia syndrome after high-dose chemotherapy for relapsed Hodgkin's disease. Br J Cancer 75:1044, 1997.

48. Massin F, Coudert B, Foucher P, et al: Nitrosourea-induced lung diseases. Rev Mal Respir 9:575, 1992.

49. Lena H, Desrues B, Le Coz A, et al: Severe diffuse interstitial pneumonitis induced by carmustine (BCNU). Chest 105:1602, 1994.

50. Lee W, Moore RP, Wampler GL: Interstitial pulmonary fibrosis as a complication of prolonged methyl-CCNU therapy. Cancer Treat Rep 62:1355, 1978.

51. Selker RG, Jacobs SA, Moore PB: BCNU (1,3-*bis*(2-chloroethyl)-1-nitrosourea–induced pulmonary fibrosis. Neurosurgery 7:560, 1980.

52. Wolff SN, Phillips GL, Herzig GP: High-dose carmustine with autologous bone marrow transplantation for the adjuvant treatment of high-grade gliomas of the central nervous system. Cancer Treat Rep 71:183, 1987.

53. Aronin PA, Mahalev MS Jr, Rudnick SA, et al: Prediction of BCNU pulmonary toxicity in patients with malignant gliomas: An assessment of risk factors. N Engl J Med 303:83, 1980.

54. Aronchick JM, Gefter WB: Drug-induced pulmonary disorders. Semin Roentgenol 30:18, 1995.

55. Holoye P, Jenkins DE, Greenberg SD, et al: Pulmonary toxicity in long-term administration of BCNU. Cancer Treat Rep 60:1691, 1976.

56. Chap L, Shpiner R, Levine M, et al: Pulmonary toxicity of high-dose chemotherapy for breast cancer: A non-invasive approach to diagnosis and treatment. Bone Marrow Transplant 20:1063, 1997.

57. Weiss RB, Muggia FM: Pulmonary effects of carmustine. Ann Intern Med 91:131, 1979.

58. Brown MJ, Miller RR, Muller NL: Acute lung disease in the immunocompromised host: CT and pathologic examination findings. Radiology 190:247, 1994.

59. O'Driscoll BR, Hasleton PS, Taylor PM, et al: Active lung fibrosis up to 17 years after chemotherapy with carmustine (BCNU) in childhood. N Engl J Med 323:378, 1990.

60. Taylor PM, O'Driscoll BR, Gattameneni HR, et al: Chronic lung fibrosis following carmustine (BCNU) chemotherapy: Radiological features. Clin Radiol 44:299, 1991.

61. Barrera P, Laan RF, van Riel PL, et al: Methotrexate-related pulmonary complications in rheumatoid arthritis. Ann Rheum Dis 53:434, 1994.

62. Goodman TA, Polusson RP: Methotrexate: Adverse reactions and major toxicities. Rheum Dis Clin North Am 20:513, 1994.

63. Tsai JJ, Shin JF, Chen CH, et al: Methotrexate pneumonitis in bronchial asthma. Int Arch Allergy Immunol 100:287, 1993.

64. Sharma A, Provenzale D, McKusick A, et al: Interstitial pneumonitis after low-dose methotrexate therapy in primary biliary cirrhosis. Gastroenterology 107:266, 1994.

65. White DA, Rankin JA, Stover DE, et al: Methotrexate pneumonitis: Bronchoalveolar lavage findings suggest an immunologic disorder. Am Rev Respir Dis 139:18, 1989.

66. Bedrossian CWM, Miller WC, Luna MA: Methotrexate-induced diffuse interstitial pulmonary fibrosis. South Med J 72:313, 1979.

67. Clarysse AM, Cathey WJ, Cartwright GE, et al: Pulmonary disease complicating intermittent therapy with methotrexate. JAMA 209:1861, 1969.

68. Salaffi F, Manganelli P, Carotti M, et al: Methotrexate-induced pneumonitis in patients with rheumatoid arthritis and psoriatic arthritis: Report of five cases and review of the literature. Clin Rheumatol 16:296, 1997.

69. Everts CS, Westcott JL, Bragg DG: Methotrexate therapy and pulmonary disease. Radiology 107:539, 1973.

70. Sostman HD, Matthay RA, Putman CE, et al: Methotrexate-induced pneumonitis. Medicine 55:371, 1976.

71. Case Records of the Massachusetts General Hospital. N Engl J Med 323:737, 1990.

72. Filip DJ, Logue GL, Harle TS, et al: Pulmonary and hepatic complications of methotrexate therapy of psoriasis. JAMA 216:881, 1971.

73. Schwartz IR, Kajani MK: Methotrexate therapy and pulmonary disease. JAMA 210:1924, 1969.

74. Whitcomb ME, Schwarz MI, Tormey DC: Methotrexate pneumonitis: Case report and review of the literature. Thorax 27:636, 1972.

75. Kremer JM, Alarcon GS, Weinblatt ME, et al: Clinical, laboratory, radiographic, and histopathologic features of methotrexate-associated lung injury in patients with rheumatoid arthritis: A multicenter study with literature review. Arthritis Rheum 40:1829, 1997.

76. Schnabel A, Dalhoff K, Bauerfeind S, et al: Sustained cough in methotrexate therapy for rheumatoid arthritis. Clin Rheumatol 15:277, 1996.

77. Hui KK, Keating MJ, McCredie KB: Fatal pulmonary failure complicating high-dose cytosine arabinoside therapy in acute leukemia. Cancer 65:1079, 1990.

78. Reed CR, Glauser FL: Drug-induced noncardiogenic pulmonary edema. Chest 100:1120, 1991.

79. Tjon A, Tham RTO, Peters WG, et al: Pulmonary complications of cytosine-arabinoside therapy: Radiographic findings. Am J Roentgenol 149:23, 1987.

80. Cooper JAD Jr, White DA, Matthay RA: Drug-induced pulmonary disease: Part 2. Noncytotoxic drugs. Am Rev Respir Dis 133:488, 1986.

81. Murray MJ, Kronenberg R: Pulmonary reactions simulating cardiac pulmonary edema caused by nitrofurantoin. N Engl J Med 273:1185, 1965.

82. Hailey FJ, Glascock HW Jr, Hewitt WF: Pleuropneumonic reactions to nitrofurantoin. N Engl J Med 281:1087, 1969.

83. Holmberg L, Boman G, Bottiger LE, et al: Adverse reactions to nitrofurantoin: Analysis of 921 reports. Am J Med 69:733, 1980.

84. Jick SS, Jick H, Walker AM, et al: Hospitalizations for pulmonary reactions following nitrofurantoin use. Chest 96:512, 1989.

85. Muir DCF, Stanton JA: Allergic pulmonary infiltration due to nitrofurantoin. BMJ 1:1072, 1963.

86. Nicklaus TM, Snyder AB: Nitrofurantoin pulmonary reaction: A unique syndrome. Arch Intern Med 121:151, 1968.

87. Ngan H, Millard RJ, Lant AF, et al: Nitrofurantoin lung. Br J Radiol 44:21, 1971.

88. Holmberg L, Boman G: Pulmonary reactions to nitrofurantoin: 447 cases reported to the Swedish Adverse Drug Reaction Committee 1966–1976. Eur J Respir Dis 62:180, 1981.

89. Israel RH, Gross RA, Bomba PA: Adult respiratory distress syndrome associated with acute nitrofurantoin toxicity: Successful treatment with continuous positive airway pressure. Respiration 39:318, 1980.

90. Kolbe J, Caughey D, Rainer S: Sulphasalazine-induced sub-acute hyper-sensitivity pneumonitis. Respir Med 88:149, 1994.

91. Cooper JAD Jr, Matthay RA: Drug-induced pulmonary disease. Dis Mon 33:61, 1987.

92. Camus P, Piard F, Ashcroft T, et al: The lung in inflammatory bowel disease. Medicine 72:151, 1993.

93. Salerno SM, Ormseth EJ, Roth BJ, et al: Sulfasalazine pulmonary toxicity in ulcerative colitis mimicking clinical features of Wegener's granulomatosis. Chest 110:556, 1996.

94. Marchlinski FE, Gansler TS, Waxman HL, et al: Amiodarone pulmonary toxicity. Ann Intern Med 97:839, 1982.

95. Rakita L, Sobol SM, Mostow N, et al: Amiodarone pulmonary toxicity. Am Heart J 106(4 pt 2):906, 1983.

96. Adams GD, Kehoe R, Lesch M, et al: Amiodarone-induced pneumonitis: Assessment of risk factors and possible risk reduction. Chest 93:253, 1988.

97. Coudert B, Bailly F, Lombard JN, et al: Amiodarone pneumonitis: Bronchoalveolar lavage findings in 15 patients and review of the literature. Chest 102:1005, 1992.

98. Martin WJ II, Rosenow EC III: Amiodarone pulmonary toxicity: Recognition and pathogenesis (Part 1). Chest 93:1067, 1988.

99. Gefter WB, Epstein DM, Pietra GG, et al: Lung disease caused by amiodarone, a new antiarrhythmia agent. Radiology 147:339, 1983.

100. Raeder EA, Podrid PJ, Lown B: Side effects and complications of amiodarone therapy. Am Heart J 109(5 pt 1):975, 1985.

101. Darmanata JI, van Zandwijk N, Duren DR, et al: Amiodarone pneumonitis: Three further cases with a review of published reports. Thorax 39:57, 1984.

102. Olson LK, Forrest JV, Friedman PJ, et al: Pneumonitis after amiodarone therapy. Radiology 150:327, 1984.

103. Pollak PT, Sami M: Acute necrotizing pneumonitis and hyperglycemia after amiodarone therapy. Am J Med 76:935, 1994.

104. Gonzalez-Rothi RJ, Hannan SE, Hood CI, et al: Amiodarone pulmonary toxicity presenting as bilateral exudative pleural effusions. Chest 92:179, 1987.

105. Kuhlman JE, Teigen C, Ren H, et al: Amiodarone pulmonary toxicity: CT findings in symptomatic patients. Radiology 177:121, 1990.

106. Nicholson AA, Hayward C: The value of computed tomography in the diagnosis of amiodarone-induced pulmonary toxicity. Clin Radiol 40:564, 1989.

107. Ren H, Kuhlman JE, Hruban RH, et al: CT-pathology correlation of amiodarone lung. J Comput Assist Tomogr 14:760, 1990.

108. Van Rooiji WJ, Vandermeer SC, Van Royen EA, et al: Pulmonary gallium-67 uptake in amiodarone pneumonitis. J Nucl Med 25:211, 1984.

109. Zhu YY, Botvinick E, Dae M, et al: Gallium lung scintigraphy in amiodarone pulmonary toxicity. Chest 93:1126, 1988.

110. Heffner JE, Sahn SA: Salicylate-induced pulmonary edema: Clinical features and prognosis. Ann Intern Med 95:405, 1981.

111. Walters JS, Woodring JH, Stelling CB, et al: Salicylate-induced pulmonary edema. Radiology 146:289, 1983.

112. Liebman RM, Katz HM: Pulmonary edema in a 52-year-old woman ingesting large amounts of aspirin. JAMA 246:2227, 1981.

113. Hormaechea E, Carlson RW, Rogove H, et al: Hypovolemia, pulmonary edema and protein changes in severe salicylate poisoning. Am J Med 66:1046, 1979.

114. Andersen R, Refstad S: Adult respiratory distress syndrome precipitated by massive salicylate poisoning. Intensive Care Med 4:211, 1978.

115. Gould DM, Daves ML: A review of roentgen findings in systemic lupus erythematosus (SLE). Am J Med Sci 235:596, 1958.

116. Ewan PW, Jones HA, Rhodes CG, et al: Detection of intrapulmonary hemorrhage with carbon monoxide uptake: Application in Goodpasture's syndrome. N Engl J Med 295:1391, 1976.

117. Macarron P, Garcia Diaz JE, Azofra JA, et al: D-penicillamine therapy associated with rapidly progressive glomerulonephritis. Nephrol Dial Transplant 7:161, 1992.

118. Bocanegra T, Espinoza LR, Vasey FB, et al: Myasthenia gravis and penicillamine therapy of rheumatoid arthritis. JAMA 244:1822, 1980.

119. Adelman HM, Winters PR, Mahan CS, et al: D-penicillamine-induced myasthenia gravis: Diagnosis obscured by coexisting chronic obstructive pulmonary disease. Am J Med Sci 309:191, 1995.

120. Eastmond CJ: Diffuse alveolitis as complication of penicillamine treatment for rheumatoid arthritis. BMJ 1:1506, 1976.

121. Davies D, Jones JKL: Pulmonary eosinophilia caused by penicillamine. Thorax 35:957, 1980.

122. Kumar A, Bhat A, Gupta DK, et al: D-penicillamine-induced acute hypersensitivity pneumonitis and cholestatic hepatitis in a patient with rheumatoid arthritis. Clin Exp Rheumatol 3:337, 1985.

123. Honda T, Hachiya T, Hayasaka M, et al: A case of rheumatoid arthritis with obstructive bronchiolitis appearing after D-penicillamine therapy. Nippon Kyobu Shikkan Gakkai Zasshi 31:1195, 1993.

124. Yam LY, Wong R: Bronchiolitis obliterans and rheumatoid arthritis: Report of a case in a Chinese patient on D-penicillamine and review of the literature. Ann Acad Med Singapore 22:365, 1993.

125. Padley SP, Adler BD, Hansell DM, et al: Bronchiolitis obliterans: High resolution CT findings and correlation with pulmonary function tests. Clin Radiol 47:236, 1993.

126. Zitnik RJ, Cooper JAD: Pulmonary disease due to antirheumatic agents. Clin Chest Med 11:139, 1990.

127. Cooke NT, Bamji AN: Gold and pulmonary function in rheumatoid arthritis. Br J Rheumatol 22:18, 1983.

128. O'Donnell AE, Selig J, Aravamuthan M, et al: Pulmonary complications associated with illicit drug use. Chest 108:460, 1995.

129. Heffner JE, Harley RA, Schabel SI: Pulmonary reactions from illicit substance abuse. Clin Chest Med 11:151, 1990.

130. Haim DY, Lippmann ML, Goldberg SK, et al: The pulmonary complications of crack cocaine. Chest 107:233, 1995.

131. Wilen SB, Ulreich S, Rabinowitz JG: Roentgenographic manifestations of methadone-induced pulmonary edema. Radiology 114:51, 1975.

132. Duberstein JL, Kaufman DM: A clinical study of an epidemic of heroin intoxication and heroin-induced pulmonary edema. Am J Med 51:704, 1971.

133. Siegel H: Human pulmonary pathology associated with narcotic and other addictive drugs. Hum Pathol 3:55, 1972.

134. Morrison WJ, Wetherill S, Zyroff J: The acute pulmonary edema of heroin intoxication. Radiology 97:347, 1970.

135. Stern WZ, Subbarao K: Pulmonary complications of drug addiction. Semin Roentgenol 18:183, 1983.

136. Steinberg AD, Karliner JS: The clinical spectrum of heroin pulmonary edema. Arch Intern Med 122:122, 1968.

137. Saba GP II, James AE Jr, Johnson BA, et al: Pulmonary complications of narcotic abuse. Am J Roentgenol 122:733, 1974.

138. Light RW, Dunham TR: Severe slowly resolving heroin-induced pulmonary edema. Chest 67:61, 1975.

139. McCarroll KA, Roszler MH: Lung disorders due to drug abuse. J Thorac Imaging 6:30, 1991.

140. Hoffman CK, Goodman PC: Pulmonary edema in cocaine smokers. Radiology 172:463, 1989.

141. Eurman DW, Potash HI, Eyler WR: Chest pain and dyspnea related to "crack" cocaine smoking: Value of chest radiography. Radiology 172:459, 1989.

142. Murray RJ, Albin RJ, Mergner W, et al: Diffuse alveolar hemorrhage temporally related to cocaine smoking. Chest 93:427, 1988.

143. Kissner DG, Lawrence DW, Selis JE, et al: Crack lung: Pulmonary disease caused by cocaine abuse. Am Rev Respir Dis 136:1250, 1987.

144. Patel RC, Dutta D, Schonfeld SA: Free-base cocaine use associated with bronchiolitis obliterans pneumonia. Ann Intern Med 107:186, 1987.

145. Goldberg REA, Lipuma JP, Cohen AM: Pneumomediastinum associated with cocaine abuse: Case report and review of the literature. J Thorac Imaging 2:88, 1987.

146. Cregler L, Mark H: Medical complications of cocaine abuse. N Engl J Med 315:1495, 1986.

147. Mundinger MO: Pneumopericardium from cocaine inhalation. N Engl J Med 313:46, 1985.

148. Leitman BS, Greengart A, Wasser HJ: Pneumomediastinum and pneumopericardium after cocaine abuse. Am J Roentgenol 151:614, 1988.

149. Fallat RJ, Powell MR, Youker JE, et al: Pulmonary deposition and clearance of (131)I-labeled oil after lymphography in man: Correlation with lung function. Radiology 97:511, 1970.

150. White RJ, Webb JAW, Tucker AK, et al: Pulmonary function after lymphography. BMJ 4:775, 1973.

151. Tapper DP, Taylor JR: Diffuse pulmonary infiltrates following lymphography. Chest 96:915, 1989.

152. Chiu CL, Gambach RR: Hypaque pulmonary edema: A case report. Radiology 111:91, 1974.

153. Malins AF: Pulmonary oedema after radiological investigation of peripheral occlusive vascular disease: Adverse reaction to contrast media. Lancet 1:413, 1978.

154. Greganti MA, Flowers WM Jr: Acute pulmonary edema after the intravenous administration of contrast media. Radiology 132:583, 1979.

155. Chamberlin WH, Stockman GD, Wray NP: Shock and noncardiogenic pulmonary edema following meglumine diatrizoate for intravenous pyelography. Am J Med 67:684, 1979.

156. Cameron JD: Pulmonary edema following drip-infusion urography. Radiology 111:89, 1974.

157. Hayashi H, Kumazaki T, Asano G: Pulmonary edema induced by intravenous administration of contrast media: Experimental study in rats. Radiat Med 12:47, 1994.

158. Goldsmith SR, Steinberg P: Noncardiogenic pulmonary edema induced by nonionic low-osmolality radiographic contrast media. J Allergy Clin Immunol 96:698, 1995.

159. Hudson ER, Smith TP, McDermott VG, et al: Pulmonary angiography performed with iopamidol: Complications in 1,434 patients. Radiology 198:61, 1996.

160. Bush WH, Swanson DP: Acute reactions to intravascular contrast media: Types, risk factors, recognition, and specific treatment. Am J Roentgenol 157:1153, 1991.

161. Hartman GW, Hattery RR, Witten DM, et al: Mortality during excretion urography: Mayo Clinic experience. Am J Roentgenol 139:919, 1982.

162. Katayama H, Yamaguchi K, Kozuka T, et al: Adverse reactions to ionic and nonionic contrast media: A report from the Japanese Committee on the Safety of Contrast Media. Radiology 175:621, 1990.

163. Caro JJ, Trindade E, McGregor M: The risks of death and of severe nonfatal reactions with high- versus low-osmolality contrast media: A meta-analysis. Am J Roentgenol 156:825, 1991.

164. Spring DB, Bettmann MA, Barkan HE: Nonfatal adverse reactions to iodinated contrast media: Spontaneous reporting to the U.S. Food and Drug Administration, 1978–1994. Radiology 204:325, 1997.

165. Spring DB, Bettmann MA, Barkan HE: Deaths related to iodinated contrast media reported spontaneously to the U.S. Food and Drug Administration, 1978–1994: Effect of the availability of low-osmolality contrast media. Radiology 204:333, 1997.

166. Namba T, Nolte CT, Jackrel J, et al: Poisoning due to organophosphate insecticides: Acute and chronic manifestations. Am J Med 50:475, 1971.

167. Bardin PG, van Eeden SF, Joubert JR: Intensive care management of acute organophosphate poisoning: A 7-year experience in the Western Cape. S Afr Med J 72:593, 1987.

168. Bledsoe FH, Seymour EQ: Acute pulmonary edema associated with parathion poisoning. Radiology 103:53, 1972.

169. Li C, Miller WT, Jiang J: Pulmonary edema due to ingestion of organophosphate insecticide. Am J Roentgenol 152:265, 1989.

170. Stephens BG, Moormeister SK: Homicidal poisoning by paraquat. Am J Forensic Med Pathol 18:33, 1997.

171. Im JG, Lee KS, Han MC, et al: Paraquat poisoning: Findings on chest radiography and CT in 42 patients. Am J Roentgenol 157:697, 1991.

172. Davidson JK, MacPherson P: Pulmonary changes in paraquat poisoning. Clin Radiol 23:18, 1972.

173. Lee SH, Lee KS, Ahn JM, et al: Paraquat poisoning of the lung: Thin-section CT findings. Radiology 195:271, 1995.

174. Libshitz HI: Radiation changes in the lung. Semin Roentgenol 28:303, 1993.

175. Ikezoe J, Takashima S, Morimoto S, et al: CT appearance of acute radiation-induced injury in the lung. Am J Roentgenol 150:765, 1988.

176. Bell D, McGivern J, Bullimore J, et al: Diagnostic imaging of post-irradiation changes in the chest. Clin Radiol 39:109, 1988.

177. Movas B, Raffin TA, Epstein AH, et al: Pulmonary radiation injury. Chest 111:1061, 1997.

178. Roach M III, Gandara DR, Yuo HS, et al: Radiation pneumonitis following combined modality therapy for lung cancer: Analysis of prognostic factors. J Clin Oncol 13:2606, 1995.

179. Khanavkar B, Stern P, Alberti W, et al: Complications associated with brachytherapy alone or with laser in lung cancer. Chest 99:1062, 1991.

180. Gustafson G, Vicini F, Freedman L, et al: High dose rate endobronchial brachytherapy in the management of primary and recurrent bronchogenic malignancies. Cancer 75:2345, 1995.

181. Speiser BL, Spratling L: Radiation bronchitis and stenosis secondary to high dose rate endobronchial irradiation. Int J Radiat Oncol Biol Phys 25:589, 1993.

182. Gross NJ: Pulmonary effects of radiation therapy. Ann Intern Med 86:81, 1977.

183. Pickrell JA, Harris DV, Mauderly JL, et al: Altered collagen metabolism in radiation-induced interstitial pulmonary fibrosis. Chest 69:311, 1976.

184. Case of acute radiation injury. BMJ 2:574, 1974.

185. Lin M: Radiation pneumonitis caused by yttrium-90 microspheres: Radiologic findings. Am J Roentgenol 162:1300, 1994.

186. de Vuyst P, Dumortier P, Ketelbant P, et al: Lung fibrosis induced by Thorotrast. Thorax 45:899, 1990.

187. Rubin P, Casarett GW: Clinical radiation pathology. Vol I. Philadelphia, WB Saunders, 1968.

188. Bloomer WD, Hellman S: Normal tissue responses to radiation therapy. N Engl J Med 293:80, 1975.

189. Chu FCH, Phillips R, Nickson JJ, et al: Pneumonitis following radiation therapy of cancer of the breast by tangential technique. Radiology 64:642, 1955.

190. Davis SD, Yankelevitz DF, Henschke CI: Radiation effects on the lung: Clinical features, pathology, and imaging findings. Am J Roentgenol 159:1157, 1992.

191. Lingos TI, Recht A, Vicini F, et al: Radiation pneumonitis in breast cancer patients treated with conservative surgery and radiation therapy. Int J Radiat Oncol Biol Phys 21:355, 1991.

192. Tarbell NJ, Thompson L, Mauch P: Thoracic irradiation in Hodgkin's disease: Disease control and long-term complications. Int J Radiat Oncol Biol Phys 18:275, 1990.

193. Jennings FL, Arden A: Development of radiation pneumonitis: Time and dose factors. Arch Pathol 74:351, 1962.

194. Libshitz HI, Brosof AB, Southard ME: Radiographic appearance of the chest following extended field radiation therapy for Hodgkin's disease: A consideration of time-dose relationships. Cancer 32:206, 1973.

195. Roswit B, White DC: Severe radiation injuries of the lung. Am J Roentgenol 129:127, 1977.

196. Lougheed MN, Maguire GH: Irradiation pneumonitis in the treatment of carcinoma of the breast. J Can Assoc Radiol 11:1, 1960.

197. Ellis F: Dose, time and fractionation: A clinical hypothesis. Clin Radiol 20:1, 1969.

198. Wara WM, Phillips TL, Margolis LW, et al: Radiation pneumonitis: A new approach to the derivation of time-dose factors. Cancer 32:547, 1973.

199. Gish JR, Coates EO, DuSault LA, et al: Pulmonary radiation reaction: A vital-capacity and time-dose study. Radiology 73:679, 1959.

200. Parris TM, Knight JG, Hess CE, et al: Severe radiation pneumonitis precipitated by withdrawal of corticosteroids: A diagnostic and therapeutic dilemma. Am J Roentgenol 132:284, 1979.

201. Pezner RD, Bertrand M, Cecchi GR, et al: Steroid-withdrawal radiation pneumonitis in cancer patients. Chest 85:816, 1984.

202. Gez E, Sulkes A, Isacson R, et al: Radiation pneumonitis: A complication resulting from combined radiation and chemotherapy for early breast cancer. J Surg Oncol 30:116, 1985.

203. Sostman HD, Putnam CE, Gamsu G: Diagnosis of chemotherapy lung. Am J Roentgenol 136:33, 1981.

204. Phillips TL: Effects of chemotherapy and irradiation on normal tissues. Front Radiat Ther Oncol 26:45, 1992.

205. Catane R, Schwade JG, Turrisi AT, et al: Pulmonary toxicity after radiation and bleomycin: A review. Int J Radiat Oncol Biol Phys 5:1513, 1979.

206. Mah K, Keane TJ, Van Dyk J, et al: Quantitative effect of combined chemotherapy and fractionated radiotherapy on the incidence of radiation-induced lung damage: A prospective clinical study. Int J Radiat Oncol Biol Phys 28:563, 1994.

207. Ma LD, Taylor GA, Wharam MD, et al: "Recall" pneumonitis: Adriamycin potentiation of radiation pneumonitis in two children. Radiology 187:465, 1993.

208. Burdon J, Bell R, Sullivan J, et al: Adriamycin-induced recall phenomenon 15 years after radiotherapy. JAMA 239:931, 1978.

209. McInerney DP: Reactivation of radiation pneumonitis by adriamycin. Br J Radiol 50:224, 1977.

210. Soh LT, Koo WH, Ang PT: Case report: Delayed radiation pneumonitis induced by chemotherapy. Clin Radiol 52:720, 1997.

211. Slanina J, Maschitzki R, Wannenmacher M: Die pulmonale strahlenreaktion im Röntgenbild des thorax nach megavolttherapie bei mammakarzinom. Radiologe 27:182, 1987.

212. Frija J, Fermé C, Baud L, et al: Radiation-induced lung injuries: A survey by computed tomography and pulmonary function tests in 18 cases of Hodgkin's disease. Eur J Radiol 8:18, 1988.

213. Fennessy JJ: Irradiation damage to the lung. J Thorac Imaging 1:68, 1987.

214. Logan PM: Thoracic manifestations of external beam radiotherapy. Am J Roentgenol 171:569, 1998.

215. DoPico GA, Wiley AL, Rao P, et al: Pulmonary reaction to upper mantle radiation therapy for Hodgkin's disease. Chest 75:688, 1979.

216. Fulkerson WJ, McLendon RE, Prosnitz LR: Adult respiratory distress syndrome after limited thoracic radiotherapy. Cancer 57:1941, 1986.

217. Byhardt RW, Abrams R, Almagro U: The association of adult respiratory distress syndrome (ARDS) with thoracic irradiation (RT). Int J Radiat Oncol Biol Phys 15:1441, 1988.

218. Gross NJ: The pathogenesis of radiation-induced lung damage. Lung 159:115, 1981.

219. Goldman AL, Enquist R: Hyperacute radiation pneumonitis. Chest 67:613, 1975.

220. Bateman NT, Croft DN: False-positive lung scans and radiotherapy. BMJ 1:807, 1976.

221. Harnsberger HR, Armstrong JD II: Bilateral superomedial hilar displacement: A unique sign of previous mediastinal radiation. Radiology 147:35, 1983.

222. Schratter-Sehn AU, Schurawitzki H, Zach M: High-resolution computed tomography of the lungs in irradiated breast cancer patients. Radiother Oncol 27:198, 1993.

223. Ikezoe J, Morimoto S, Takashima S, et al: Acute radiation-induced pulmonary injury: Computed tomography evaluation. Semin Ultrasound CT MR 11:409, 1990.

224. Libshitz HI, Shuman LS: Radiation-induced pulmonary change: CT findings. J Comput Assist Tomogr 8:15, 1984.

225. Mah K, Poon PY, Van Dyk J, et al: Assessment of acute radiation-induced pulmonary changes using computed tomography. J Comput Assist Tomogr 10:736, 1986.

226. Bachman AL, Macken K: Pleural effusions following supervoltage radiation for breast carcinoma. Radiology 72:699, 1959.

227. Whitcomb ME, Schwarz MI: Pleural effusion complicating intensive mediastinal radiation therapy. Am Rev Respir Dis 103:100, 1971.

228. Posner MR, Cohen GI, Skarin AT: Pericardial disease in patients with cancer: The differentiation of malignant from idiopathic and radiation-induced pericarditis. Am J Med 71:407, 1981.

229. Gomm SA, Stretton TB: Chronic pericardial effusion after mediastinal radiotherapy. Thorax 36:149, 1981.

230. Applefield MM, Cole JF, Pollock SH, et al: The late appearance of chronic pericardial disease in patients treated by radiotherapy for Hodgkin's disease. Ann Intern Med 94:338, 1981.

231. Okada M, Ebe K, Matsumoto T, et al: Case report: Ipsilateral spontaneous pneumothorax after rapid development of large thin-walled cavities in two patients who had undergone radiation therapy for lung cancer. Am J Roentgenol 170:932, 1998.

232. Deslauriers J, Ferraro P: Non-small cell lung cancer: Late complications. *In* Pearson FG, Deslauriers J, Ginsberg RJ, et al (eds): Thoracic Surgery. New York, Churchill Livingstone, 1995, pp 763–782.

233. Wallgren A: Late effects of radiotherapy in the treatment of breast cancer. Acta Oncol 31:237, 1992.

234. Iyer RB, Libshitz HI: Late sequelae after radiation therapy for breast cancer: Imaging findings. Am J Roentgenol 168:1335, 1997.

235. Schultz-Hector S, Kallfab P, Sund M: Strahlenfolgen an groben Arterien: Übersicht über klinische und experimentelle Daten. Strahlenther Onkol 171:427, 1995.

236. Coblentz C, Martin L, Tuttle R: Calcified ascending aorta after radiation therapy. Am J Roentgenol 147:477, 1986.

237. Libshitz HI: Radiation changes in bone. Semin Roentgenol 29:15, 1994.

238. Pierce SM, Recht A, Lingos TI, et al: Long-term radiation complications following conservative surgery (CS) and radiation therapy (RT) in patients with early stage breast cancer. Int J Radiat Oncol Biol Phys 23:915, 1992.

239. Mitchell MJ, Logan PM: Radiation-induced changes in bone. Radiographics 18:1125, 1998.

240. Bourgouin P, Cousineau G, Lemire P, et al: Differentiation of radiation-induced fibrosis from recurrent pulmonary neoplasm by CT. Can Assoc Radiol J 38:23, 1987.

241. Glazer HS, Lee JKT, Levitt RG, et al: Radiation fibrosis: Differentiation from recurrent tumor by MR imaging. Radiology 156:721, 1985.

242. Werthmuller WC, Schiebler ML, Whaley RA, et al: Gadolinium-DTPA enhancement of lung radiation fibrosis. J Comput Assist Tomogr 13:946, 1989.

243. Prato FS, Kurdyak R, Saibil EA, et al: Regional and total lung function in patients following pulmonary irradiation. Invest Radiol 12:224, 1977.

244. Prata FS, Kurdyak R, Saibil EA, et al: Physiological and radiographic assessment during the development of pulmonary radiation fibrosis. Radiology 122:389, 1977.

245. McDonald S, Rubin P, Phillips TL, et al: Injury to the lung from cancer therapy: Clinical syndromes, measurable endpoints, and potential scoring systems. Int J Radiat Oncol Biol Phys 31:1187, 1995.

246. Pezzulli F, Posner D, Mask K: Reverse V/P mismatch in radiation pneumonitis. Australas Radiol 38:135, 1994.

247. Slavin Jr JD, Friedman NC, Spencer RP: Radiation effects on pulmonary ventilation and perfusion. Clin Nucl Med 18:81, 1993.

248. Marks LB, Spencer DP, Bentel GC, et al: The utility of SPECT lung perfusion scans in minimizing and assessing the physiological consequences of thoracic irradiation. Int J Radiat Oncol Biol Phys 26:659, 1993.

249. Kataoka M, Kawamura M, Ueda N, et al: Diffuse gallium-67 uptake in radiation pneumonitis. Clin Nucl Med 15:707, 1990.

250. Baron RL, Sagel SS, Baglan RJ: Thymic cysts following radiation therapy for Hodgkin disease. Radiology 141:593, 1981.

251. Lindfors KK, Neyer JE, Dedrick CG, et al: Thymic cysts in mediastinal Hodgkin disease. Radiology 156:37, 1985.

252. Brereton HD, Johnson RE: Calcification in mediastinal lymph nodes after radiation therapy of Hodgkin's disease. Radiology 112:705, 1974.

253. Strickland B: Intrathoracic Hodgkin's disease: II. Peripheral manifestations of Hodgkin's disease in the chest. Br J Radiol 40:930, 1967.

254. Vainright JR, Diaconis JN, Haney PJ: Presternal soft tissue calcifications following mediastinal radiotherapy for Hodgkin's disease. Chest 91:136, 1987.

255. Fishman EK, Kuhlman JE, Jones RJ: CT of lymphoma: Spectrum of disease. Radiographics 11:647, 1991.

256. Park KJ, Chung JY, Chun MS, et al: Radiation-induced lung disease and the impact of radiation methods on imaging features. Radiographics 20:83, 2000.

257. Crestani B, Valeyre D, Roden S, et al: Bronchiolitis obliterans organizing pneumonia syndrome primed by radiation therapy to the breast. Am J Respir Crit Care Med 158:1929, 1998.

258. Mesurolle B, Qanadli SD, Merad M, et al: Unusual radiologic findings in the thorax after radiation therapy. Radiographics 20:67, 2000.

259. Shannon VR, Nesbitt JC, Libshitz HI: Malignant pleural mesothelioma after radiation therapy for breast cancer. Cancer 76:437, 1995.

260. Bilbey JH, Müller NL, Miller RR, et al: Localized fibrous mesothelioma of pleura following external ionizing radiation therapy. Chest 94:1291, 1988.

261. Hill JK, Heitmiller RF II, Askin FB, et al: Localized benign pleural mesothelioma arising in a radiation field. Clin Imaging 21:189, 1997.

262. Loyer EM, Despassand ES: Radiation-induced heart disease: Imaging features. Semin Roentgenol 28:321, 1993.

263. Taghian A, de Vathaire F, Terrier P, et al: Long-term risk of sarcoma following radiation treatment for breast cancer. Int J Radiat Oncol Biol Phys 21:361, 1991.

264. Bhatia S. Robison LL, Oberlin O, et al: Breast cancer and other neoplasms after childhood Hodgkin's disease. N Engl J Med 334:745, 1996.

265. Katz M, Piekarski JD, Bayle-Weisberger C, et al: Residual mediastinal mass following radiation therapy for Hodgkin's disease. Ann Radiol 20:667, 1977.

266. Coia LR, Myerson RJ, Tepper JE: Late effects of radiation therapy on the gastrointestinal tract. Int J Radiat Oncol Biol Phys 30:1213, 1995.

267. Ellis SJ, Cleverley JR, Müller NL: Drug-induced lung disease: High-resolution CT findings. Am J Roentgenol 175:1019, 2000.

268. To E, Pang P, Tsang W, et al: Pathologic fracture of the clavicle after radiotherapy. Am J Roentgenol 176:264, 2001.

CHAPTER *18*

Penetrating and Nonpenetrating Trauma

Trauma to the thorax can result in a wide variety of effects on the chest wall, diaphragm, mediastinum, trachea, and lungs.[1, 2] The results may be direct (e.g., fractures of the ribs, spine, or shoulder girdles; diaphragmatic hernia; esophageal rupture; and pulmonary contusion or laceration) or indirect (e.g., air embolism resulting from the escape of air into pulmonary veins subsequent to parenchymal laceration). Because the manifestations of such trauma are

dissimilar in different sites, each is considered separately. As might be anticipated, however, a great deal of overlap occurs. The effects of penetrating and nonpenetrating trauma may be different and require separate consideration. The consequences of iatrogenic trauma are considered in Chapter 19. Adult respiratory distress syndrome, one of the most ominous consequences of prolonged shock in the immediate post-traumatic period, is discussed in Chapter 14.

Although diagnosis of most traumatic abnormalities of the thorax can be established with reasonable confidence by conventional radiography, in some cases, significant abnormalities, such as fractures of the thoracic spine, pulmonary lacerations, pneumothorax, and hemothorax, may not be apparent on radiograph but may be seen on computed tomography (CT) scan.[4, 5, 9] Certain conditions, such as laceration of the aorta, often require special diagnostic procedures, including CT angiography or aortography, to confirm the injury and establish its extent.

EFFECTS ON THE LUNGS OF NONPENETRATING TRAUMA

Pulmonary Contusion

Pulmonary contusion consists of traumatic extravasation of blood into the parenchyma of the lung unaccompanied by substantial tissue disruption.[6] It is considered to be the most common pulmonary complication of chest trauma.[6] In a review of the findings in 515 patients who had blunt chest trauma, pulmonary contusion was identified radiographically in 134 (26%);[7] 35 of these 134 (26%) patients had no evidence of thoracic bone injury. The severity of the injury necessary to produce contusion varies from a trivial glancing blow to major trauma resulting from motor vehicle or aircraft accidents.[8]

Radiographically the pattern varies from irregular, patchy areas of air-space consolidation to diffuse and extensive homogeneous consolidation (Table 18–1; Fig. 18–1). As might be expected, the distribution of the contused areas does not conform to lobes or segments.[9, 10] Although the major change usually is in the lung directly deep to the traumatized areas, damage may occur also, sometimes predominantly, on the opposite side as a result of a contre-coup effect.[11] In blast injuries, the contusion typically is bilateral,[11] although the major change occurs in the thoracic

588

Table 18–1. PULMONARY CONTUSION

Patchy areas of consolidation
Nonsegmental distribution
Evident radiographically 0–6 hours after trauma
Improves within 24–48 hours after injury
Resolves within 3–10 days

area that faced the blast. Increase in the size and loss of definition of the vascular markings extending from the hila indicate the presence of hemorrhage and edema in the peribronchovascular interstitial tissue.[7, 10] Extensive bilateral contusion may lead to respiratory failure and adult respiratory distress syndrome.[6, 12]

The time between trauma and detection of the radiographic abnormality is important in diagnosis, particularly in the differentiation from fat embolism. In contusion, changes are apparent radiographically soon after trauma (almost invariably within 6 hours),[8, 9] whereas in fat embolism changes usually become manifest only 1 to 2 days or more after injury. Resolution of lung contusion typically occurs rapidly; improvement is noted within 24 to 48 hours,[9, 14] and clearing is complete within 3 to 10 days.[15]

The CT findings of pulmonary contusion consist of areas of consolidation, which may be patchy or homogeneous. They involve mainly the lung adjacent to the area of trauma.[9, 16, 17] Air bronchograms commonly are present.[6] Occasionally, CT scan shows contusion not apparent on radiograph.[17, 27] In an experimental study in dogs, 100% of pulmonary contusions were visible on CT scan immediately after trauma compared with only 37% on chest radiograph.[18] After 30 minutes, 75% of lesions were seen on radiograph.[18] Although contusion is by definition unassociated with radiographic evidence of pulmonary laceration, small lacerations—seen as small round or ovoid air collections with or without air-fluid level—commonly are evident on CT;[19] in one study, lacerations were detected in 95% of patients with a radiographic diagnosis of contusion.[3]

Pulmonary Laceration, Traumatic Pneumatocele, and Hematoma

Uncommonly, closed chest trauma results in the development of radiographically detectable lacerations within the lung that can remain air-filled (traumatic pneumatocele) or that can fill partly or completely with blood (hematoma). The trauma usually is blunt and often severe, as in automobile accidents. Children and young adults are particularly prone to the development of radiographically visible pulmonary lacerations, presumably because of the greater flexibility of their thoracic walls.[3]

Radiographically, traumatic pneumatoceles and hematomas (Table 18–2; Fig. 18–2) usually are not seen until a few hours or several days after trauma, often being initially masked by the surrounding contusion.[25, 27] They may be single or multiple, unilocular or multilocular, oval or spherical, and 2 to 14 cm in diameter.[23, 27] They typically are

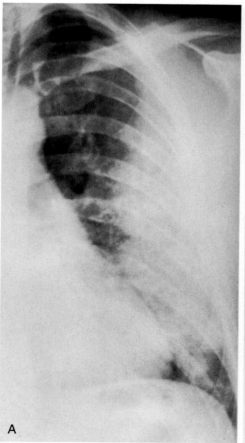 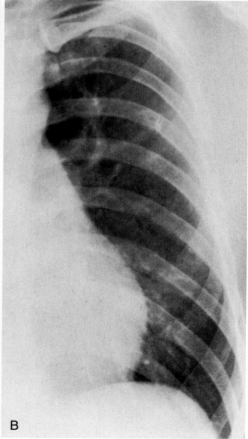

Figure 18–1. Pulmonary Contusion. Six hours before radiographic examination, this 33-year-old man was involved in a car accident in which he suffered severe trauma to the posterior portion of his left chest. View of the left hemithorax from anteroposterior radiograph *(A)* shows homogeneous consolidation of the posterolateral portion of the left lung in nonsegmental distribution. The margins of the consolidation are defined indistinctly, and there is no air bronchogram. No ribs were fractured. The right lung was clear. Six days later *(B)*, complete clearing had occurred.

A

B

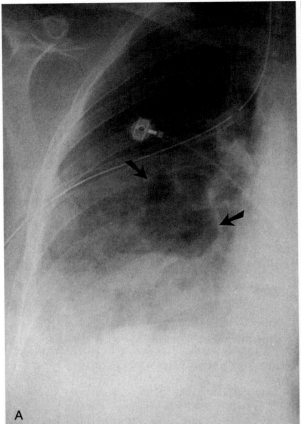

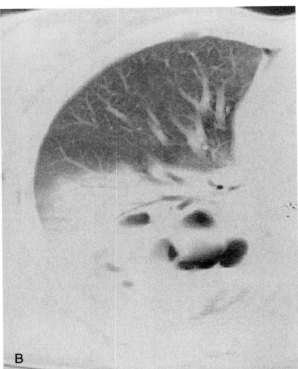

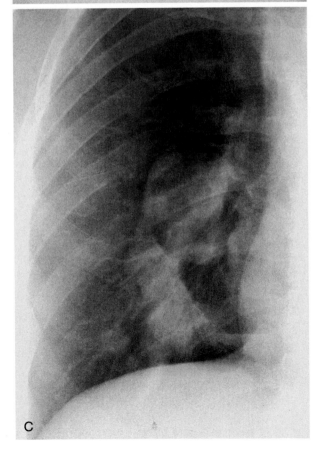

Figure 18–2. Traumatic Pneumatocele and Hematoma. View of the right lower chest from erect anteroposterior radiograph *(A)* in a 29-year-old woman after a motor vehicle accident shows extensive consolidation in the right lower lobe and an irregular area of increased radiolucency *(arrows)*. The patient initially had presented with a right hemopneumothorax and required chest tube drainage. CT scan *(B)* shows extensive consolidation with air bronchograms and several traumatic pneumatoceles. View from chest radiograph performed 3 weeks later *(C)* shows marked irregularity of the inner and outer walls of the traumatic pneumatoceles as a result of adjacent hematomas. An air-fluid level is evident.

Table 18–2. PULMONARY LACERATION

Often initially obscured by pulmonary contusion
May present as traumatic pneumatocele or hematoma
Pneumatoceles appear as thin-walled cystic spaces
With or without air-fluid levels
Unilocular or multilocular
Hematomas present as soft tissue masses
May persist for up to 1 year

located in the subpleural parenchyma.[8] In most cases, traumatic pneumatoceles and hematomas develop under the point of maximal injury; occasionally, they occur in a remote location as a result of a contrecoup effect.

The appearance of traumatic pneumatoceles and hematomas depends in large measure on whether hemorrhage has occurred into them. About half the lesions present as thin-walled, air-filled spaces with or without fluid levels (traumatic pneumatoceles) (Fig. 18–3);[24] the remainder appear as homogeneous, well-circumscribed masses of soft tissue density—pulmonary hematomas (Fig. 18–4).[177] Their presence should prompt confirmation of abdominal organ injury with spiral CT.[177] Traumatic pneumatoceles may enlarge rapidly in patients receiving high-pressure mechanical ventilation.[6] Occasionally, they have a markedly irregular contour. The development of a pneumatocele at the base of the left lung after trauma has been confused with a ruptured diaphragm;[21] however, identification of the diaphragmatic contour should prevent such misdiagnosis.

A characteristic of these lesions is their tendency to persist for a long time, frequently several months[3, 25] and occasionally 1 year (*see* Fig. 18–4).[19, 26] Rarely a traumatic hematoma increases in size, in which case it is termed *chronic expanding hematoma.*[19] More commonly, hematomas decrease in size progressively; if this is not apparent within 6 weeks, the possibility must be considered that trauma may have been coincidental with a solitary nodule of other etiology.[8]

CT is much more sensitive than chest radiography in the detection of pulmonary lacerations.[22] The CT findings of pulmonary laceration consist of one or more round, oval, or multiloculated air collections with or without air-fluid levels (*see* Fig. 18–3).[22, 27] Hemorrhage related to a pulmonary laceration may result in an air-fluid level, an air crescent sign, or, when the lacerated region is filled completely by blood, a round or oval soft tissue density.[26, 28] The appearance may be indistinguishable from pulmonary masses of other etiology.[26] Hematomas persisting for several months may have a central attenuation slightly greater than that of water and rim enhancement.[26]

Most patients do not have symptoms related to the pulmonary lesion itself. Hemoptysis occurs rarely and probably is attributable to the emptying of a pulmonary hematoma.[24]

Fractures of the Trachea and Bronchi

Fractures (rupture, transection) of the tracheobronchial tree as a result of nonpenetrating trauma usually are secondary to blunt injury of the anterior chest in a vehicular

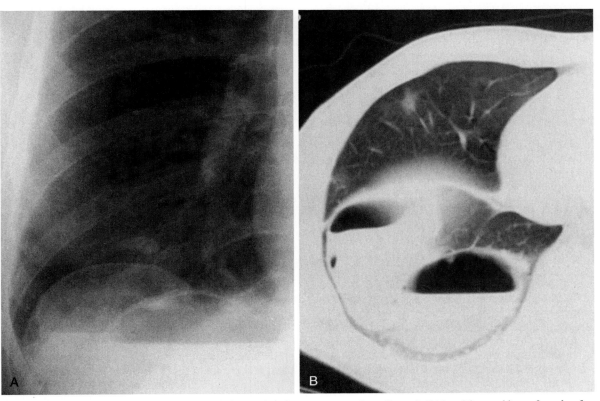

Figure 18–3. Traumatic Pneumatocele. View of the right lower chest from posteroanterior radiograph *(A)* in a 26-year-old man 2 weeks after a motor vehicle accident reveals thin-walled cystic lesions with air-fluid levels. CT scan *(B)* essentially confirms the radiographic findings. The appearance is characteristic of traumatic pneumatoceles.

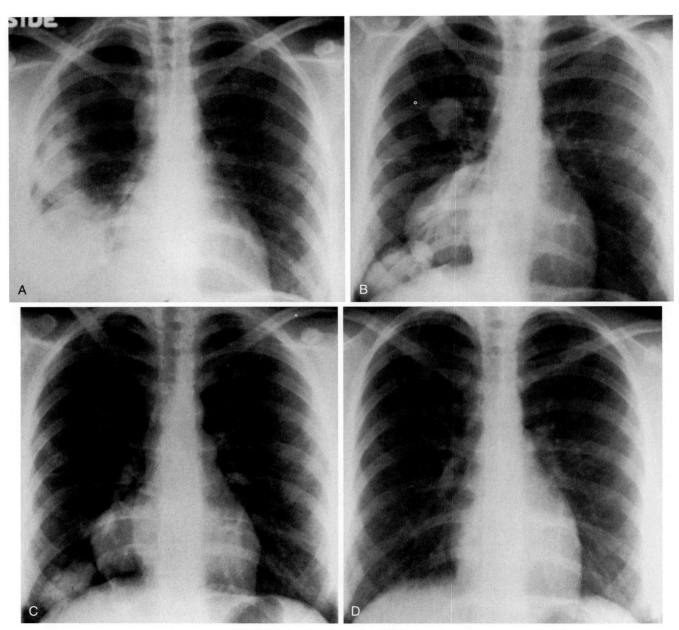

Figure 18–4. Multiple Unilateral Pulmonary Hematomas. This 17-year-old girl was involved in a two-car collision in which she sustained fractures of the right scapula and humerus. The day after admission, anteroposterior radiograph *(A)* showed extensive parenchymal consolidation in the lower two thirds of the right lung in nonsegmental distribution; the left lung was clear. There was some widening of the superior mediastinum from venous hemorrhage. Two months later, posteroanterior radiograph *(B)* showed multiple, sharply circumscribed homogeneous nodules in the right lung ranging from 1 to 6 cm in diameter (12 discrete nodules can be identified). No cavitation was present, and the left lung remained clear. Approximately 1 month later *(C)*, the nodules had diminished considerably in size, and several had disappeared altogether. Seven months after the injury, all signs of disease had disappeared, and the chest radiograph *(D)* was normal. (Courtesy of Dr. John D. Armstrong, Jr., University of Utah College of Medicine, Salt Lake City, Utah.)

accident;[29] occasionally, they occur as a result of a fall from height[30] or secondary to overdistention of the cuff of an endotracheal tube.[31] Most fractures associated with blunt trauma follow rapid anteroposterior compression of the chest.[37] This situation may result in a sudden increase in airway pressure causing *burst* tracheobronchial injury; alternatively the sudden lateral widening of the thorax may pull the lung apart, avulsing a bronchus.[37]

Although tracheobronchial fractures may occur in the absence of thoracic skeletal injury,[7] such injury often is

present. The incidence of rib fractures varies considerably in different series; they were observed in 53% of patients in one series,[32] in 91% in another,[33] and in only 2% in a third.[34] In another review of nine patients, four had fractures involving the clavicles, scapula, or sternum, but only two had rib fractures.[36]

Traumatic tracheobronchial fracture is uncommon; it has been estimated that only about 2% to 3% of patients who die as a result of trauma have the complication.[29] Its rarity probably contributes to the infrequency with which it is recognized early. In one series, 68% of cases were not diagnosed until obstructive pneumonitis had developed in the lung distal to the fracture.[33] Symptoms and signs include cyanosis, hemoptysis, shock, and cough; rarely, pain is caused by hemorrhage into the pleural space.[53] Air often is identifiable in the subcutaneous tissues, initially involving the neck and upper thorax and later becoming generalized.[38] Air may be seen to escape directly from a wound in the neck in cases of tracheal fracture.[29]

Fractures of the bronchi are more common than those of the trachea and constitute about 80% of all tracheobronchial injuries.[15, 37] They usually are parallel to the cartilage rings and involve the main bronchi 1 to 2 cm distal to the carina.[15, 37] The right side is affected more often than the left; pulmonary vessels rarely are damaged.[39] Fractures of the intrathoracic trachea are horizontal and usually occur just above the carina.[15, 50] Occasionally the proximal trachea ruptures as a result of blunt trauma to the throat, in which case other cervical structures usually are involved;[40] the tracheal tear tends to be vertical in the membranous portion and can be associated with vascular damage.[15, 41]

As might be expected, the most common radiographic findings are pneumomediastinum and pneumothorax (Table 18–3).[36] These findings are present in approximately 70% of patients with tracheobronchial tears.[35] In one review of nine patients who had tears or transection of the trachea or main bronchi after blunt trauma, seven had pneumomediastinum and subcutaneous emphysema, and six had pneumothorax;[36] in five patients, the pneumothorax was present on initial radiograph, and in one patient, it was not evident until the 13th day after admission. Tension pneumothorax occurred in four of the six patients. Four patients had upper thoracic fractures involving the clavicles, scapula, or sternum; only two had rib fractures. Certain combinations of findings related to pneumomediastinum and pneumothorax are highly suggestive of tracheobronchial fracture in a patient who has undergone trauma, including (1) a large pneumothorax that does not respond to chest tube drainage (because of the free communication between the fractured airway and the pleural space),[43, 44] (2) pneumothorax and pneumomediastinum in the absence of pleural effusion,[45] and (3) mediastinal and deep cervical emphysema in a trauma patient who is not receiving positive-pressure ventilation.[46]

Occasionally a small amount of air escapes from the airway and remains localized to the surrounding connective tissues, where it can be shown radiologically. This is an uncommon finding, however, having been seen in only one of nine patients in one study.[36] Sometimes, overdistention of the endotracheal balloon cuff is the only sign of tracheal

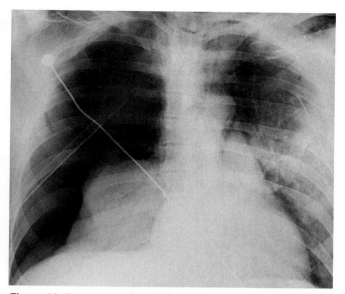

Figure 18–5. Fracture of the Right Main Bronchus. Anteroposterior chest radiograph in a 24-year-old man after a motor vehicle accident shows large right and small left pneumothoraces, extensive pneumomediastinum, and multiple rib fractures. Despite the presence of a chest tube, the right lung is collapsed and displaced inferior to the right hilum *(fallen-lung sign)*. A few air bronchograms still are visible within the collapsed lung. Complete transection of the right main bronchus was identified at surgery.

rupture; the overdistention results from herniation of the balloon through the tracheal tear into the mediastinum.[51]

Displacement of fracture ends can cause bronchial obstruction and atelectasis of an entire lung;[42] it is important to recognize that such atelectasis may be a late development, and the discovery of such a change some time after an accident should suggest the diagnosis. A diagnostic but uncommon sign of complete bronchial transection is the *fallen lung sign*, in which the collapsed lung falls away from the hilum toward the lateral and posterior chest wall or diaphragm (Fig. 18–5).[47–49] This sign may be more readily apparent on CT scan than on radiograph.[36] In one patient who had unsuspected rupture of the left main bronchus, we made a prospective diagnosis on CT scan based on discontinuity of the left bronchus and deviation of the trachea and right mainstem bronchus to the right.[50] The CT findings can be quite subtle, however, and may consist of only focal narrowing of the affected main bronchus (Fig. 18–6).[92] When tracheobronchial injury is suspected, bronchoscopy should be performed to confirm and locate the injury.

In about 10% of patients, tracheobronchial fracture is unassociated with any radiographically demonstrable abnormality or with much in the way of symptoms or signs.[15] In such cases, it is likely that the peribronchial connective tissue is preserved, preventing passage of air into the mediastinum or pleura. The consequence of the trauma may not become evident until the patient presents with atelectasis of a lobe or lung as a result of bronchial stenosis.[52] A review of 90 such cases showed that in one third of the patients, the condition was not diagnosed until 1 month to 19 years after the traumatic episode.[53]

Table 18–3. TRACHEOBRONCHIAL TEARS

Within 1–2 cm of tracheal carina
Common findings
  Pneumomediastinum and pneumothorax
Suggestive findings
  Large pneumothorax not responsive to chest tube drainage
  Pneumothorax in the absence of pleural effusion
  Pneumomediastinum in patient not being ventilated
Diagnostic finding
  Fallen lung sign

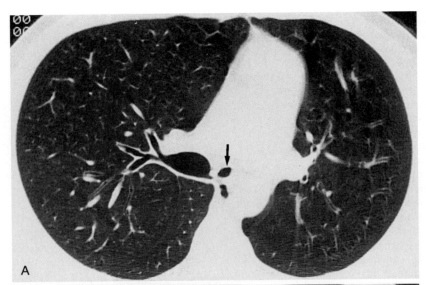

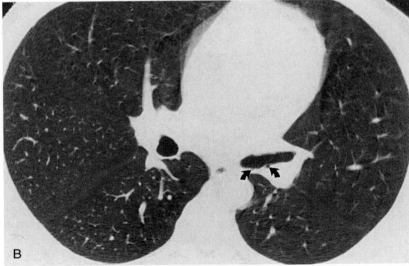

Figure 18–6. Fracture of the Left Main Bronchus. HRCT scan *(A)* in a 26-year-old man shows focal narrowing of the left main bronchus *(straight arrow).* HRCT scan at a more caudad level *(B)* shows focal collections of air within the wall of the left main and left upper lobe bronchus *(curved arrows).* The patient presented with a history of cough and progressive shortness of breath 1 month after a motor vehicle accident. The diagnosis of fracture of the left main bronchus was confirmed bronchoscopically.

EFFECTS ON THE PLEURA OF NONPENETRATING TRAUMA

Hemothorax and pneumothorax are common manifestations of nonpenetrating trauma, and each may develop from a variety of causes. Hemothorax occurs in 25% to 50% of patients who have had blunt chest trauma.[54] The complication usually is small and secondary to bleeding from lacerated pulmonary vessels.[54] Large hemothoraces usually are secondary to tears of large central pulmonary vessels or systemic arteries or veins.[54]

Pneumothorax occurs in 15% to 40% of patients who have blunt chest trauma.[54, 55] It usually follows alveolar rupture and dissection of gas into the adjacent interstitium and, eventually, pleural space; occasionally, it results from tracheobronchial fracture or esophageal rupture. Pneumothorax may occur without radiographic evidence of rib fracture; in one series of 15 survivors of attempted suicide who jumped into water from a considerable height (50 m), 10 developed a pneumothorax within 12 hours; an associated rib fracture was evident in only 4.[56] When fracture is present, the likely mechanism is laceration of the visceral pleura by rib fragments, and in such circumstances hemothorax may be expected as a concomitant finding.

Pneumothorax is detected more commonly on CT scan than on radiograph.[3] In one series of 85 patients who had pulmonary contusion, pneumothorax was detected on radiograph in 34 and on CT scan in 70.[3] In another review of abdominal CT scans performed for evaluation of blunt trauma, 35 patients had pneumothorax, 10 (29%) of which had not been diagnosed previously on chest radiograph;[57] 7 of the 10 patients required chest tube drainage. In all patients undergoing abdominal CT for blunt trauma, images should be obtained through the lung bases and viewed on lung settings to assess for the presence of pneumothorax.[28, 54]

EFFECTS ON THE MEDIASTINUM OF NONPENETRATING TRAUMA

Mediastinal Hemorrhage

Most cases of mediastinal hemorrhage result from trauma, usually of a severe nature, such as that associated with motor vehicle accidents or falls from a height.[58, 59] The source of bleeding in these cases is often the aorta; other origins include veins and smaller arteries. Mediastinal blood also may originate in traumatized retropharyngeal soft tissue. In some cases, the trauma is iatrogenic (e.g., after faulty placement of a central venous line[60, 61] or perforation of the superior vena cava[62]).

Radiographically, extensive hemorrhage typically results in uniform, symmetric widening of the mediastinum (Fig. 18–7). Local accumulation of blood in the form of a hematoma is manifested by a homogeneous focal opacity that may project to one or both sides of the mediastinum and may be situated in any compartment.[63, 64] The most important diagnostic consideration in patients who have radiographic evidence of mediastinal hemorrhage after trauma is aortic rupture. Only 10% to 20% of patients who have radiographic findings suggestive of mediastinal hemorrhage after trauma have an aortic injury, however.[5] Further diagnostic procedures, including contrast-enhanced CT, transesophageal ultrasound, and aortography, are required for a definitive diagnosis (*see* farther on).[58, 59, 65]

Symptoms and signs of mediastinal hemorrhage seldom are striking. Suspicion may be aroused when retrosternal pain that radiates into the back develops in a patient who suffered chest trauma recently.

Rupture of the Thoracic Aorta and Its Branches

Patients at risk for developing aortic injury after blunt trauma include those involved in high-speed (combined impact >30 mph [48 km/h]) motor vehicle accidents in which there is substantial vehicle deformity, pedestrians or cyclists struck by a vehicle, and individuals falling from a height greater than 10 feet (3 m).[94] One group of investiga-

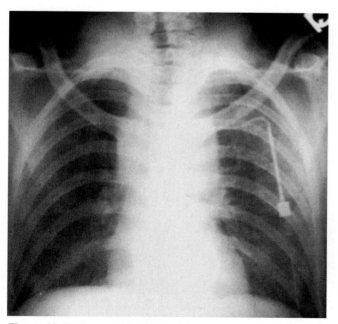

Figure 18–7. Traumatic Mediastinal Hemorrhage. Chest radiograph in anteroposterior projection, supine position, of a young man after severe closed chest trauma reveals moderate widening of the upper half of the mediastinum, roughly symmetric on both sides. The lungs are unremarkable.

tors assessed the risk factors using multivariate logistic regression and bayesian analysis.[95] The study included 31 patients who had traumatic aortic injury and 171 randomly selected control subjects who also had experienced major trauma. Predictors of aortic injury included head injury (odds ratio, 18), pelvic fracture (odds ratio, 27), pneumothorax (odds ratio, 27), and lack of seat belt use (odds ratio, 7).

The acute aortic injury almost always is a transverse tear that disrupts one or more structural layers of the aorta.[94] In about 60% of cases, the adventitia is intact.[94] About 90% of injuries diagnosed clinically and radiologically involve the region of the aortic isthmus immediately distal to the left subclavian artery;[5, 94] tears of the ascending aorta, the distal descending aorta, or abdominal aorta are much less common.[66, 94] Laceration is believed widely to be the result of a shearing force in which the relatively mobile anterior portion of the aortic arch joins the more fixed posterior arch and descending aorta.[94] It has been suggested that laceration may be caused by chest compression pinching the aorta between the anterior and posterior components of the bony thorax.[69, 70] According to this hypothesis, compressive forces depress the anterior thoracic osseous structures, causing them to rotate posteriorly and inferiorly about the posterior rib articulation, pinching and shearing the interposed vascular structures.

Laceration of the ascending aorta represents only about 5% of all thoracic aortic injuries identified clinically; however, the incidence of the injury at autopsy ranges from 8% to almost 25%.[68, 71] This disparity is caused by the association of severe and often fatal cardiac injury in roughly 80% of cases (compared with 25% when the laceration is at the isthmus).

Occasionally, mediastinal hemorrhage after severe chest trauma results from damage to one of the great vessels arising from the aortic arch. Avulsion of the innominate artery from the arch has been stated to be the second most common type of aortic injury in which the patient survives long enough for diagnostic evaluation.[72] The radiographic findings are similar to those of rupture of the aortic isthmus, with the possible exception that the outline of the descending aorta may be preserved.[72] Fractures of the upper thoracic spine also may cause radiographic findings similar to those of aortic rupture. In a retrospective analysis of the frontal chest radiographs of 54 patients who had traumatic fractures of at least one vertebral body from C6 to T8, 37 (69%) had signs generally considered to be consistent with aortic laceration;[73] spinal fracture could be identified on initial radiograph in about half of the 37 patients.

Radiographic Signs

A wide variety of radiographic signs have been described as being useful in the diagnosis of aortic rupture (Table 18–4). Some signs, particularly mediastinal widening and abnormal or indistinct contour of the aortic arch, have a relatively high sensitivity but a low specificity, whereas others, such as rightward deviation of the trachea, downward displacement of the left main bronchus, rightward displacement of a nasogastric tube, and thickening of the right paratracheal stripe, have greater specificity but lower sensitivity.[5, 94] The greatest value of chest

Table 18–4. RUPTURE OF THE AORTA: CHEST RADIOGRAPH

Signs with high sensitivity and low specificity
  Mediastinal widening
  Abnormal or indistinct contour of the aorta
Signs with relatively high specificity and low sensitivity
  Rightward deviation of trachea at level of T4
  Rightward deviation of nasogastric tube at level of T4
  Thickening of right paratracheal stripe
Negative predictive value of normal radiograph: 98%

radiograph is in excluding traumatic aortic injury; the negative predictive value of a normal erect frontal chest radiograph is approximately 98%.[66, 94] The positive predictive value of an abnormal chest radiograph is relatively low, however; only 10% to 20% of patients who have abnormalities suggestive of mediastinal hemorrhage have aortic injury.[5, 71]

Widening of the Upper Half of the Mediastinum

Plain chest radiographs frequently reveal widening of the superior mediastinum as a result of hemorrhage (Fig. 18–8), although the hemorrhage eventually may prove to be of venous origin resulting from either direct trauma or iatrogenic causes such as malpositioning of a central venous line.[74]

Assessment of mediastinal widening may be based solely on subjective criteria or on measurement of mediastinal diameter at the level of the aortic arch (>8 cm indicates pathologic widening).[5, 67] In a retrospective review of chest radiographs from 205 patients who had blunt chest trauma and who underwent aortography, a widened mediastinum, defined by subjective impression or width greater than 8 cm at the level of aortic arch, had a sensitivity of 36% and a specificity of 81% in the diagnosis of aortic rupture on erect anteroposterior chest radiographs and a sensitivity of 67% and specificity of 45% on radiographs performed with the patient supine.[66]

Compared with the appearance on upright radiograph, the mediastinum is widened and magnified on supine radiograph, decreasing the diagnostic usefulness of mediastinal widening. In one study of 123 patients radiographed in the supine position, mediastinal widening greater than 8 cm was present in 87% who had traumatic aortic rupture and in 69% who did not.[75]

Abnormal Contour of the Aortic Arch

Irregularity (Fig. 18–9) or obscuration of the contour of the aortic arch probably is the most reliable sign of aortic rupture. In a study of 205 patients who had blunt chest

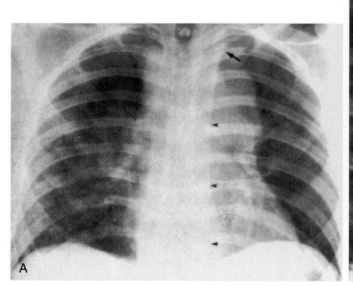

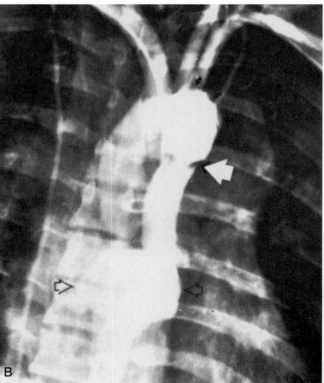

Figure 18–8. Traumatic Aneurysm and Rupture of the Thoracic Aorta. This 16-year-old boy crashed into a telephone pole in an automobile traveling at 85 mph. Shortly after his arrival in the emergency department, chest radiograph in anteroposterior projection *(A)* showed marked widening of the upper mediastinum and loss of visualization of the aortic arch. A wide paravertebral opacity *(arrowheads)* extends up to the apex, creating an extrapleural apical cap *(arrow)*. The suspicion of aortic rupture was confirmed by aortography *(B)*. The site of primary aortic laceration is indicated by a thick arrow, the irregular bulge immediately above *(small arrows)* representing dissection proximally. Several centimeters distally is a large, well-circumscribed collection of contrast medium *(open arrows)*, which represents an extra-aortic hematoma from a second rupture. The patient exsanguinated after section of the mediastinal pleura at thoracotomy.

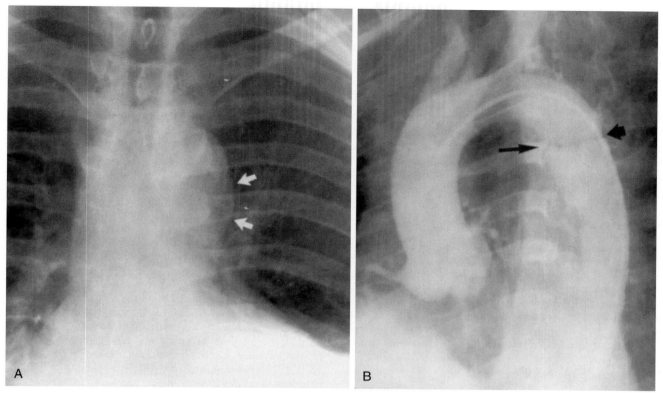

Figure 18–9. Traumatic Laceration of the Aorta. Detail view of the mediastinum in posteroanterior projection *(A)* reveals a small bulge on the descending arch of the aorta *(arrows);* there is a left pleural effusion of moderate size. Aortogram in right posterior oblique projection *(B)* shows a lucent defect in the descending arch *(arrows)*, representing the tear in the aortic wall.

trauma who underwent aortography, this sign had a sensitivity of 63% and a specificity of 62% on erect radiographs and a sensitivity of 81% and a specificity of 45% on radiographs performed with the patient supine.[66] Other related signs that have been found to be helpful include obscuration of the aortopulmonary window[66, 75] and obscuration of the proximal descending thoracic aorta.[66]

Deviation of the Trachea and Left Main Bronchus

As the amount of mediastinal blood increases, the left main bronchus may be deviated anteriorly, inferiorly, and to the right, and the trachea may be displaced to the right. Shift of the left tracheal wall to the right of the T4 spinous process has a specificity of greater than 90% in the detection of traumatic aortic laceration but has a low sensitivity, the finding being present on erect frontal views of the chest in only 15% of patients in some series.[66] Depression of the left main bronchus greater than 40 degrees below the horizontal in the absence of left lower lobe atelectasis also is suggestive of the diagnosis but is seen in only a few patients.[66]

Deviation of the Nasogastric Tube

Displacement of a nasogastric tube to the right of the T4 spinus process has a high specificity in the diagnosis of a traumatic tear of the aorta. The sensitivity is low, however; the finding was present in only approximately 10% of patients in one study.[66]

Displacement of the Right Paraspinous Interface

Displacement or widening of the right paraspinous interface is highly suggestive of the diagnosis;[66, 76] however, it is present in less than 10% of patients.[66]

Widening of the Right Paratracheal Stripe

Another sign that has been suggested as a possible indicator of aortic tear is widening of the right paratracheal stripe to a thickness greater than 5 mm *(see* Fig. 18–8).[77] In one investigation of 102 consecutive patients who had blunt chest trauma, all patients who had a right paratracheal stripe less than 5 mm in width had a normal aortogram;[77] by contrast, aortography revealed major arterial injury in 23% of patients whose right tracheal stripe measured 5 mm or greater. In another study of 87 patients, 83% who had aortic tear had widening of the right paratracheal stripe, compared with 29% without aortic injury.[75]

Left Apical Cap

A potential space exists between the isthmus of the aorta and the parietal pleura of the left lung. Provided that the parietal pleura is intact, extravasated blood can track cephalad along the course of the left subclavian artery between the parietal pleura and the extrapleural soft tissues, resulting in a homogeneous opacity over the apex of the left hemithorax—the extrapleural apical cap.[78] A left apical cap by itself constitutes an unreliable sign of acute aortic rupture.[66, 79] In one study in which angiograms were performed solely because of the presence of an apical cap, aortic ruptures were seen only in 2 of 12 patients;[79] in another series, the finding was present in only 10% of patients who had aortic rupture.[66]

Left Hemothorax

Hemothorax complicating acute aortic injury is almost invariably left-sided. In one investigation of 205 patients who had blunt chest trauma and underwent aortography, a left hemothorax was present in 5% of patients with traumatic aortic rupture.[81]

Summary

Many publications have attempted to assess the relative value of the many radiographic signs described previously.[66, 80, 81] The majority opinion, with which we agree, is that the most reliable features are mediastinal widening and an abnormal outline of the aortic arch. No single sign or combination of signs has sufficient sensitivity to avoid the performance of a large number of negative aortographic studies, however. As a result, the use of additional, noninvasive techniques—primarily CT—is indicated in most patients.

We believe any patient who has suffered severe chest trauma in whom conventional chest radiographs reveal upper mediastinal widening or loss of normal contour of the aortic arch should undergo further investigation by contrast-enhanced spiral CT, transesophageal echocardiography, or aortography to establish the diagnosis and reveal the anatomic extent of rupture. Patients who have equivocal radiographic findings or in whom only supine radiographs can be obtained should undergo contrast-enhanced spiral CT [58, 82, 83] or transesophageal echocardiography.[84, 136] Unstable patients who have obvious mediastinal abnormalities on chest radiograph should proceed directly to aortography or surgery.

Computed Tomography

CT permits ready distinction of mediastinal widening secondary to hemorrhage from that related to tortuous vessels, fat, or radiographic magnification. The findings include indirect and direct signs (Table 18–5).[86] Mediastinal hematoma abutting the aorta (Fig. 18–10) is an indirect sign, whereas irregularity of the wall (Fig. 18–11), presence of an aortic pseudoaneurysm, abrupt caliber change of the

Table 18–5. RUPTURE OF THE AORTA: SPIRAL CT

Direct signs
  Irregularity of the wall of the aorta
  Presence of pseudoaneurysm
  Abrupt caliber change of aorta
  Intimal flap
  Extravasation of contrast material
Indirect sign
  Periaortic hematoma
Negative predictive value of normal CT: 99.9%

aorta, and (less commonly) extravasation of contrast material from the aorta and presence of an intraluminal radiolucent filling defect (intimal flap) (Fig. 18–12) constitute direct signs.[58, 83, 86]

In a meta-analysis of the data from 3,334 cases published in the literature by 1996, in which the presence of mediastinal hematoma or direct signs of aortic injury was considered to be an indicator for a positive examination, the sensitivity of CT was 99.3%; the specificity, 87.1%; the positive predictive value, 19.9%; and the negative predictive value, 99.9%.[83] A cost-effectiveness analysis study published in 1995 compared six diagnostic strategies combining chest radiography, CT, and angiography in various sequences.[82] The authors concluded that selecting hemodynamically stable patients with suspected aortic injury after blunt chest trauma for angiography on the basis of CT scan findings is more effective than doing so based on chest radiograph findings.[82]

In most studies published before 1996, conventional CT was used for diagnosis. The relatively long time interval between each individual slice and the difference in inspiratory effort between slices often resulted in suboptimal contrast enhancement and interslice artefacts. The shortened scanning time of spiral CT resulted in greatly improved vascular contrast enhancement (*see* Figs. 18–11 and 18–12).[88] Rapid scanning of multiple levels during a single breath-hold eliminates interslice artefacts and allows CT angiography with excellent direct visualization of the aortic injury.[89]

The efficacy of spiral CT as a screening device to detect aortic injury was assessed in a prospective study of 1,518 consecutive patients who had nontrivial blunt chest trauma.[89] Chest radiograph was not used in the triage process. In 92% of patients, CT scans showed no evidence of mediastinal hematoma and no suggestion of aortic abnormality, and no further investigation was undertaken. On the basis of the 6-month clinical outcome, there were no false-negative CT scan interpretations. Of patients, 127 (about 8%) had abnormal or indeterminate CT scans and underwent aortography. In 89 (70%) patients, CT showed mediastinal hematoma and a normal aorta; no patients had evidence of aortic injury (in 85 patients, the aorta was normal at aortography; in 3 patients, aortography was indeterminate or falsely positive because of the presence of prominent atherosclerotic plaques; and in 1 patient, it was falsely positive because of a large ductus diverticulum proved at surgery). Of the 127 patients who had abnormal CT scans, 38 (21%) had direct evidence of thoracic injury (contour abnormality, localized area of narrowing, intimal flap, pseudoaneurysm, or contrast extravasation), indeterminate scans, or inadequate spiral CT scans; 17 of these patients had aortic injury shown at aortography, all of whom had direct signs of aortic injury on CT. In one patient, angiography was falsely negative—the presence of an intimal flap missed at aortography was confirmed by transesophageal echocardiography.

In this study, spiral CT was more sensitive than aortography (100% versus 94%) but less specific (82% versus 96%) in the detection of aortic injury. The main limitation of the study is the assumption that patients who had normal CT scans did not have traumatic aortic injury. Two branch vessel injuries were missed with direct CT visualization

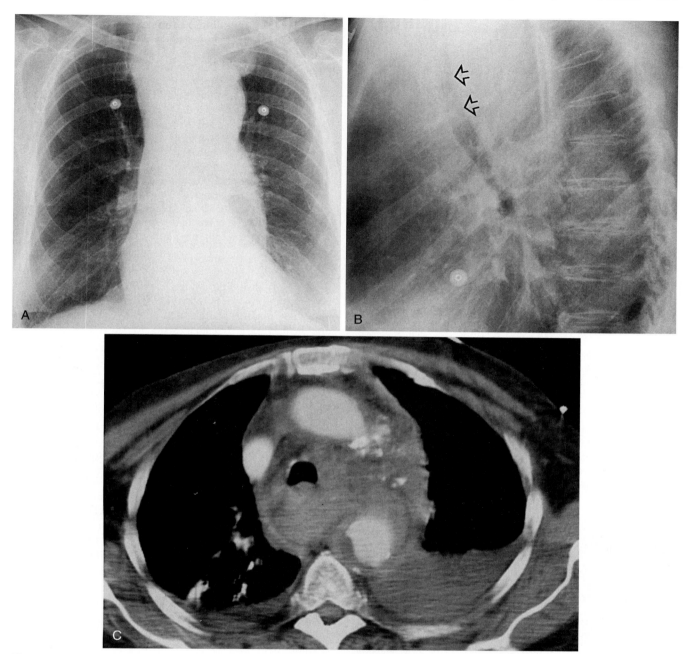

Figure 18–10. Aortic Rupture with Large Mediastinal Hematoma. Posteroanterior chest radiograph *(A)* in an 84-year-old man shows widening of the mediastinum. The lateral view *(B)* shows marked anterior displacement of the trachea *(arrows)*. Contrast-enhanced CT scan *(C)* shows extensive mediastinal hematoma with displacement of the trachea anteriorly and to the right. Bilateral pleural effusions are evident. The diagnosis of aortic rupture was confirmed at surgery.

(although adjacent hematoma suggested their presence); this is an important consideration because about 5% of aortic arch injuries involve major branch vessels.[88, 90] Because of cardiac motion artefact, ascending aortic injuries may be missed on spiral CT.[89, 90]

In a subsequent study from the same institution, investigators evaluated the use of spiral CT aortography in the assessment of thoracic aortic rupture.[91] This procedure consisted of two-dimensional multiplanar reconstructions and three-dimensional analysis based on maximum intensity projection or shaded-surface display reconstructions.[91] A

total of 38 injuries of the aorta and great vessels were detected in 36 of 3,229 patients who had nontrivial blunt chest trauma. The extent of injury was identified in 100% of cases on standard transverse spiral CT images, compared with 82% on two-dimensional reconstructions, 82% on three-dimensional maximal intensity projection reconstructions, 71% on three-dimensional surface shading reconstructions, and 88% on transcatheter thoracic aortograms.[91] All nondiagnostic images from transcatheter aortograms involved patients who had subtle intimal flaps. CT angiography accurately showed the presence and extent of aortic

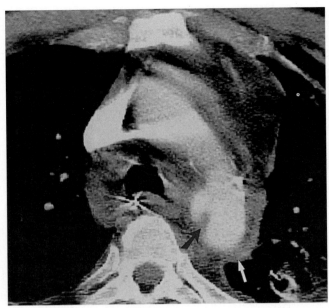

Figure 18–11. Traumatic Laceration of the Aorta on Spiral CT.
Contrast-enhanced 7-mm collimation spiral CT scan performed in a 53-year-old man after an automobile accident shows focal irregularity of the proximal descending thoracic aorta *(black arrow),* diagnostic of an aortic laceration. A small amount of blood can be seen adjacent to the aorta *(white arrow).*

injuries when these were greater than 15 mm long but was inferior to standard transverse CT images for small tears.

Some workers suggested that a normal aorta on spiral CT effectively excluded the possibility of aortic injury and that aortography was not necessary in this situation, even

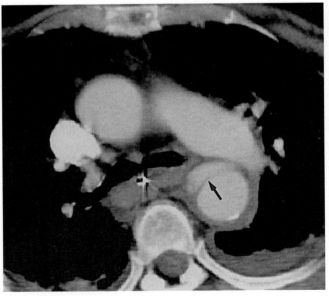

Figure 18–12. Traumatic Laceration of the Aorta with Intimal Flap.
Contrast-enhanced spiral CT scan shows irregularity of the lateral wall of the aorta and an intimal flap *(arrow).* A small amount of blood is evident around the proximal descending thoracic aorta, and there are small bilateral pleural effusions. The patient was a 79-year-old woman being assessed after a motor vehicle accident. The diagnosis of aortic laceration was confirmed at surgery.

when there was mediastinal hematoma.[91, 104] Most investigators consider that aortography is mandatory in patients who have periaortic hematoma, however.[92–94, 96] In one study of 21 patients who underwent spiral CT for the assessment of aortic injury, 8 of the 11 patients who had periaortic hematoma identified on CT had aortic injury proved at aortography;[93] the other 3 patients had normal angiograms. All 10 patients who did not have a periaortic hematoma had normal findings at angiography. The presence of periaortic hematoma had a sensitivity of 100%, a specificity of 77%, a negative predictive value of 100%, and a positive predictive value of 73% in predicting traumatic aortic rupture. Based on our review of the literature, we believe that the following recommendations are reasonable in a patient who has had blunt chest trauma:

1. Normal chest radiograph performed with the patient erect has a 98% negative predictive value for aortic injury; normal supine view has a 96% negative predictive value.[66] Because of these high values, further investigation seldom is warranted in these patients. Because it may provide important diagnostic information, however, spiral CT of the chest is indicated in patients who are undergoing CT of the abdomen and pelvis after trauma regardless of chest radiograph findings.[89]
2. Patients who have abnormal chest radiographs and are unstable should proceed directly to aortography or surgery.
3. Patients who are stable and who have suboptimal or abnormal chest radiographs should undergo spiral CT of the chest. Patients who have normal spiral CT scan need no further evaluation unless serial radiographs show progressive mediastinal widening.[87] Depending on the experience of the radiologist and surgeon, patients who have direct signs of aortic injury on CT scan may undergo transcatheter aortography or proceed directly to surgery. Patients who have a periaortic hematoma evident on CT scan or who have indeterminate or inadequate chest CT scans should undergo emergency aortography.

Assessment of traumatic aortic injury on spiral CT requires not only interpretive expertise, but also careful attention to technique.[92, 94] Intravenous contrast material (300 mg I/ml) is administered with a power injector at a rate of 2 to 3 ml per second for a total of 100 to 150 ml. Optimal scan delay can be determined by using a 20-ml test injection and obtaining images at a preselected level (such as the aortic arch) or by using a standard software package provided with the CT scanner. In most patients, a 30-second delay provides adequate visualization of the aorta. We currently perform spiral CT scans from 2 cm above the aortic arch to 2 cm below the tracheal carina using 3-mm collimation and reconstruct the images at 1-mm intervals.[92] The remainder of the chest is scanned using 7-mm collimation.

Transesophageal Echocardiography

The results of several studies have suggested that transesophageal echocardiography is a highly sensitive and specific method of detecting thoracic aortic injury.[84, 97, 98] In one investigation, the procedure was compared with aortography in 101 patients who had suspected traumatic aortic rupture.[85] It was performed successfully in 93 patients but could not be completed in 8 because of lack of cooperation or extensive maxillofacial trauma. Comparison of the results of transesophageal echocardiography with the results of aortography, surgery, or autopsy showed that echocardiography had detected all 11 cases of aortic injury (sensitivity 100%) and showed true-negative results in 82 patients and a false-positive result in 1 patient (specificity, 98%; positive predictive value, 99%).[85]

Other prospective studies have shown considerably lower sensitivity and specificity.[95, 99] In one investigation of 34 patients who had blunt chest trauma, transesophageal echocardiography and aortography were performed prospectively.[99] In five (15%) patients, echocardiography was unsuccessful; two of these five patients had aortic injury at aortography, and the unsuccessful echocardiography resulted in substantial delay in diagnosis. In the remaining patients, echocardiography had a 57% sensitivity and a 91% specificity for diagnosis of aortic injury.

Transesophageal echocardiography has many disadvantages. The procedure is more operator dependent and invasive than CT; takes an average of 30 minutes to complete; and, in patients who are awake, requires intravenous sedation.[85] Transesophageal echocardiography cannot be performed in patients who are uncooperative or who have maxillofacial trauma and should not be attempted in patients who have unstable neck and spine injuries.[85] The echocardiographic signs of aortic injury are complex and often are limited to a short section of the vessel.[100] Although the procedure yields detailed images of most of the thoracic aorta, a 3- to 5-cm portion of the ascending aorta cannot be assessed adequately;[101] injuries limited to this region, although rare, may be missed.[85] Finally, the procedure does not allow visualization of the great vessels coming off the aortic arch.

Aortography

Transfemoral aortography is the definitive imaging modality to diagnose the presence, location, and extent of aortic injury.[67, 82] At least two projections must be obtained, most commonly left anterior oblique and anteroposterior views.[67] The examination must include the entire thoracic aorta and great branch vessels.[82] Angiographic findings diagnostic of aortic injury include an intimal tear, extravasation of contrast material, dissection with an intimal flap, pseudoaneurysm, and pseudocoarctation (*see* Fig. 18–8).[82]

Although aortography is the gold standard imaging modality for the diagnosis of aortic injury, false-positive and false-negative interpretations may occur. The main reasons for false-positive interpretations are the presence of an atypical ductus diverticulum or an ulcerated atherosclerotic plaque.[102] In one study of 314 patients assessed for possible aortic trauma, the aortogram was falsely positive in 3 (1%) and equivocal in 9 (3%);[102] postoperative diagnoses in the false-positive cases were ductus diverticulum in 2 patients and ulcerating atherosclerotic plaque in 1 patient. A ductus diverticulum—defined as a focal bulge or convexity at the level of the aortic isthmus—was seen in 51 (26%) patients.[102] Distinction of a ductus diverticulum from an aortic injury usually can be made based on the absence of contrast material retention or intimal flap.[102] A diverticulum may

fold back against the aorta, however, creating an appearance of intimal radiolucency indistinguishable from an aortic tear.[102]

Aortography has a sensitivity of about 95% in the detection of aortic injuries and a negative predictive value of 99%.[89] Missed findings include the presence of a small traumatic intimal flap and a small localized rupture through the intima and media.[85, 89] The procedure is relatively safe; however, complications occur, including entry of the catheter into a false channel because of atherosclerotic or traumatic dissection and (rarely) rupture at the site of injury with subsequent exsanguination and death.[67, 103]

Perforation of the Esophagus

Rupture of the esophagus from closed chest trauma is rare and results in changes localized to the mediastinum and pleura.[35, 105] Manifestations include mediastinal widening related to acute mediastinitis, pneumomediastinum, pleural effusion, pneumothorax, and hydropneumothorax.[28, 35] In most cases, the site of rupture can be identified precisely—although sometimes with considerable difficulty—only by radiographic evidence of extravasation of ingested contrast material. CT scan may show pneumomediastinum not apparent on radiograph.[4] The area of greatest esophageal thickening on CT often represents the level of perforation.[35] In most cases, however, the perforation itself is obscured by edema or hemorrhage and is not seen on CT scan.[35] Occasionally the level of perforation can be identified by the presence of leakage of ingested contrast material into the mediastinum or pleural space (Fig. 18–13).[28]

Rupture of the Thoracic Duct

In addition to nonpenetrating injury, rupture of the thoracic duct may develop from surgical procedures or penetrating wounds from a bullet or knife.[106–108] The most common cause is iatrogenic; chylothorax is reported as a complication in about 0.2% of patients who have undergone thoracic surgery.[106] Thoracic duct injury from penetrating chest trauma usually is overshadowed by associated vascular or tracheoesophageal injuries;[107, 108] in a review of more than 13,000 patients treated for penetrating chest or neck trauma, only 8 were found to have isolated thoracic duct injury.[108] Thoracic duct injury from blunt trauma is rare; only 20 cases were reported by 1988.[109] It is thought to be secondary to hyperextension of the thoracic spine.[108]

The anatomic course of the thoracic duct and the site of damage establish on which side the chylothorax develops. As it enters the thorax, the duct lies slightly to the right of the midline so that rupture in its lower third—an unusual site in crushing injuries—leads to right-sided chylothorax. The duct crosses the midline to the left in the midthorax so that its disruption above this point tends to produce left-sided chylothorax. Although usually unilateral, chylothorax may be bilateral.[110]

Several days to weeks may elapse between the time of trauma and the development of radiographically demonstrable pleural fluid,[13, 111] a time lag that should suggest the diagnosis. It has been postulated that the delay occurs because the extravasated chyle initially is confined to the

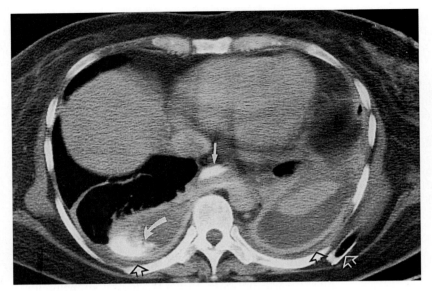

Figure 18–13. Bilateral Empyema after Esophageal Rupture. CT scan shows bilateral pleural effusions with associated smooth thickening of the pleura and increased attenuation of the extrapleural fat *(open black arrows)* consistent with empyema. A left chest tube lies outside the pleural space *(open white arrow)*. Orally administered contrast medium can be seen in the esophagus *(straight arrow)* and in the right pleural space *(curved arrow)* indicating the presence of an esophageal pleural fistula. The patient was a 41-year-old man who had developed a delayed diagnosis of esophageal rupture.

mediastinal space and ruptures into the pleural space only when the accumulation has acquired sufficient pressure.[13] Rarely the lymph collection remains contained within the mediastinum, where it is manifested as a rounded mass (lymphocele) on radiograph several weeks to months after injury.[112, 113]

The site of injury to the thoracic duct is shown best by lymphangiography. In a study of 12 patients who had chylous ascites or chylothorax after surgery, the site of injury was identified on lymphangiography in 7. The authors did not consider CT to have provided any additional information.[114] The CT appearance of chylous effusions is similar to that of other effusions. In one case, a traumatic mediastinal lymphocele was assessed by CT and magnetic resonance (MR) imaging, and the diagnosis was confirmed by CT-guided needle aspiration;[113] CT showed a homogeneous fluid collection that on MR imaging had the characteristics of proteinaceous fluid with increased signal intensity on T1-weighted spin-echo images and homogeneous high signal intensity on T2-weighted images. In another case, a traumatic lymphocele was shown by lymphoscintigraphy with modified technetium-99m sulfur colloid.[115]

EFFECTS ON THE CHEST WALL AND DIAPHRAGM OF NONPENETRATING TRAUMA

Rupture of the Diaphragm

Diaphragmatic rupture is diagnosed in 1% to 4% of patients admitted to the hospital with blunt trauma[7, 116] and in about 5% of patients undergoing laparotomy or thoracotomy for trauma.[116] Of penetrating injuries to the lower chest, about 15% of stab wounds and 45% of gunshot wounds are associated with this complication.[116, 117] In a review of 1,000 diaphragmatic injuries in 980 patients reported in the literature by 1995, 75% of ruptures were the result of blunt trauma, and 25% were the result of penetrating injury.[116]

Several mechanisms have been postulated for the development of diaphragmatic rupture during blunt trauma, including sudden increase in intrathoracic or intra-abdominal pressure against a fixed diaphragm, shearing stress on a stretched diaphragm, and avulsion of the diaphragm from its points of attachment;[116] the first of these is the most commonly accepted.[118, 119] The greater prevalence of left-sided ruptures has been ascribed to a variety of causes, including the buffer action of the liver, greater strength of the right hemidiaphragm (experimental studies in cadavers have shown a greater weakness of the left hemidiaphragm), and underdiagnosis of right-sided injuries.[116] Although ruptures may occur in any area, most develop through the weakest portion (posterolateral surface along the embryonic fusion lines).[7]

As might be expected, patients who have diaphragmatic rupture frequently have other serious injuries.[116, 120] In one review of 25 patients who had diaphragmatic rupture after blunt trauma, associated findings included rib fractures (52%), pelvic fractures (52%), splenic laceration or rupture (48%), closed head injury (32%), and liver laceration (16%).[120] In the same study, of 43 patients with penetrating diaphragmatic injuries, 44% had liver laceration, 30% had splenic laceration, and 30% had gastrointestinal injury.[120] These associated abnormalities often obscure the findings related to the diaphragmatic rupture. In a review of 1,000 diaphragmatic injuries, the diagnosis was made at the time of admission in 44% of cases and incidentally at thoracotomy, laparotomy, or autopsy in 41%;[116] in the remaining 15%, the diagnosis was delayed 24 hours or more.

After diaphragmatic rupture, intra-abdominal viscera may herniate into the chest. The hernial contents depend on the size and position of the rupture and can include the omentum, stomach, small and large intestines, spleen, kidney, and pancreas. Such traumatic herniated material frequently strangulates, particularly if the diagnosis is delayed beyond 24 hours. Although traumatic hernias account for only about 5% of diaphragmatic hernias,[121] 90% of strangulated diaphragmatic hernias are traumatic in origin.[116] Herniation of abdominal contents through a rent in the diaphragm may be delayed for several years or longer.[140] The true incidence of diaphragmatic injury that heals without coming to medical attention is unknown.

Radiologic Manifestations

The radiographic findings are influenced by mechanism of injury (blunt or penetrating), site of injury (left or right), presence of herniated viscera, and presence of concomitant pleural or pulmonary injury (which may be associated with obscuration of the diaphragm as a result of pleural effusion or atelectasis) (Table 18–6).[116, 120] Depending on these factors, a preoperative diagnosis based on the radiographic findings in various studies has been made in 4% to 63% of cases.[116, 123, 124] The likelihood of diagnosis is higher in patients who have left-sided perforation and blunt rather than perforating injury.[125, 126] In one study of 50 patients who had diaphragmatic rupture after blunt trauma, radiographic findings diagnostic or highly suggestive of rupture were present in 20 of 44 (46%) patients who had rupture on the left side and in only 1 of 6 (17%) patients who had rupture on the right.[125] The radiographic findings of penetrating diaphragmatic injury usually are normal or nonspecific and include hemothorax, pneumothorax, or apparent elevation of the hemidiaphragm.[126]

Diagnostic signs of diaphragmatic rupture include visualization of herniated stomach or bowel in the chest and cephalad extension of an intragastric tube above the level of the diaphragm (Fig. 18–14).[54, 116, 125] Suggestive findings include irregularity of the diaphragmatic contour, inability to visualize the diaphragm, a persistent basilar opacity (that may mimic atelectasis or a supradiaphragmatic mass), an elevated hemidiaphragm in the absence of atelectasis, and a contralateral shift of the mediastinum in the absence of a large pleural effusion or pneumothorax.[54, 116, 125]

When rupture occurs of the left hemidiaphragm, the stomach and the colon are the viscera that most commonly herniate into the thorax. The diagnosis can be confirmed by contrast-enhanced studies of these two organs, CT, or MR imaging.[54, 127, 128] A diagnostic finding is the presence of a focal constriction (*collar sign*) in the stomach or afferent and efferent loop of bowel where they traverse the orifice of the diaphragmatic rupture. This finding sometimes is seen on plain chest radiographs but is visualized more readily on contrast-enhanced stomach or colon studies or CT scans.[122, 128] When strangulation occurs, unilateral pleural effusion may be present.[129, 130]

When rupture of the right hemidiaphragm occurs, a portion of the liver may herniate through the rent and create a mushroom-like mass within the right hemithorax, with the herniated liver being constricted by the tear. In such circumstances, the diagnosis should be suspected by the high position of the lower border of the liver as indicated by the position of the hepatic flexure.[131, 132] The diagnosis can be confirmed by CT (Fig. 18–15), MR imaging (Fig. 18–16), ultrasound, or radionuclide liver scan.[126, 128, 133] The last-named may show nonspecific cephalad displacement of the liver or a diagnostic, relatively photopenic waist where the organ traverses the diaphragmatic orifice.[126] Scintigraphy has a low sensitivity, however, and seldom is used.[126]

Ultrasonography permits direct visualization of the hemidiaphragm and may show focal disruption or interruption of diaphragmatic echoes at the site of rupture.[133, 134] The procedure is helpful in the diagnosis of rupture of the right hemidiaphragm; however, it is of limited value in rupture of the left hemidiaphragm because the presence of gas within adjacent large bowel or stomach does not allow its visualization.

Several groups have assessed the use of CT in the diagnosis of diaphragmatic rupture.[128, 135, 136] Characteristic findings include sharp discontinuity of the diaphragm, intrathoracic visceral herniation, lack of visualization of a hemidiaphragm (*absent diaphragm sign*), and constriction of bowel or stomach at the site of herniation (collar sign) (Table 18–7).[128, 136]

Focal discontinuity of the diaphragm is seen on CT in 70% to 80% of patients who have diaphragmatic rupture (Fig. 18–17).[128, 136] It should be noted, however, that focal defects occasionally are seen in healthy people, particularly the elderly. In one review of CT scans in 120 patients without a history of trauma, localized diaphragmatic defects were seen in 13 (11%), all at least 40 years old;[137] the abnormality was seen in only 1 patient between 40 and

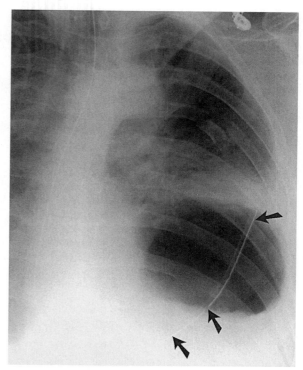

Figure 18–14. Traumatic Rupture of the Left Hemidiaphragm. View of the left chest from anteroposterior radiograph shows intrathoracic stomach with cephalad extension of the nasogastric tube *(arrows)*. Left rib fractures, areas of atelectasis in the left lung, and mediastinal shift to the right are visible. The patient was a 44-year-old man involved in a motor vehicle accident.

Table 18–6. RUPTURE OF THE DIAPHRAGM: RADIOGRAPH

Suggestive findings
    Visualization of herniated stomach or bowel in chest
    Cephalad extension of nasogastric tube above level of diaphragm
    Irregularity of diaphragmatic contour
    Elevated hemidiaphragm in the absence of atelectasis
    Contralateral shift of mediastinum
Suggestive findings present in 30–40% of cases

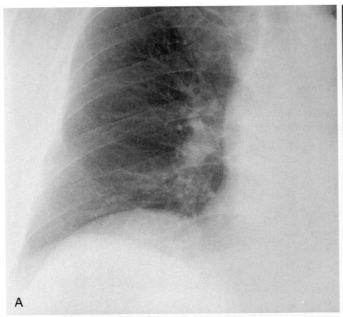

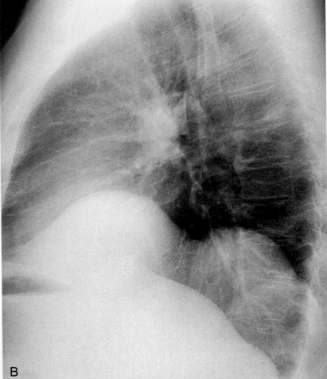

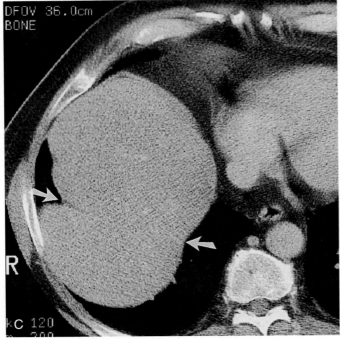

Figure 18–15. Traumatic Rupture of the Right Hemidiaphragm. A 53-year-old man was referred for further evaluation of an unusual diaphragmatic contour on radiograph. Views of the right chest from posterior anterior *(A)* and lateral *(B)* radiographs show apparent elevation of the right hemidiaphragm with a biconvex upper contour. CT scan *(C)* shows superior herniation of the liver and a focal constriction *(arrows)* characteristic of traumatic tear. The diagnosis was confirmed at surgery.

49 years but in 7 of 20 (35%) patients who were 70 years old or older. Most diaphragmatic ruptures occur in young adults,[123, 135] in whom discontinuity of the diaphragm normally is not seen. Regardless of age, the diagnosis of

Table 18–7. RUPTURE OF THE DIAPHRAGM: CT

Diagnostic findings
 Sharp discontinuity of hemidiaphragm
 Herniation of omental fat or abdominal viscera
 Waistlike narrowing of herniated viscera (collar sign)
 Lack of visualization of hemidiaphragm
Sensitivity of CT: 60–80%
Specificity of CT: 90%
Accuracy may be improved with multiplanar reconstructions

diaphragmatic rupture based solely on the presence of diaphragmatic discontinuity may result in a false-positive diagnosis and should be made with caution on this basis alone.[128, 136]

The diagnosis of diaphragmatic rupture can be made more confidently on CT when there is associated herniation of omental fat[138] or abdominal viscera;[128, 136] the latter includes bowel, liver, kidney, and spleen and is seen in 50% to 60% of cases (Fig. 18–18).[128, 136] Herniation of viscera may not be seen while patients are on positive-pressure ventilation and may develop only after discontinuation of ventilatory support.[123, 136] A waistlike narrowing of the stomach, bowel, or liver (*see* Fig. 18–15) at the site of herniation (collar sign) is seen on CT in 30% to 40% of cases;[128, 136] occasionally, it is the only CT abnormality.[128]

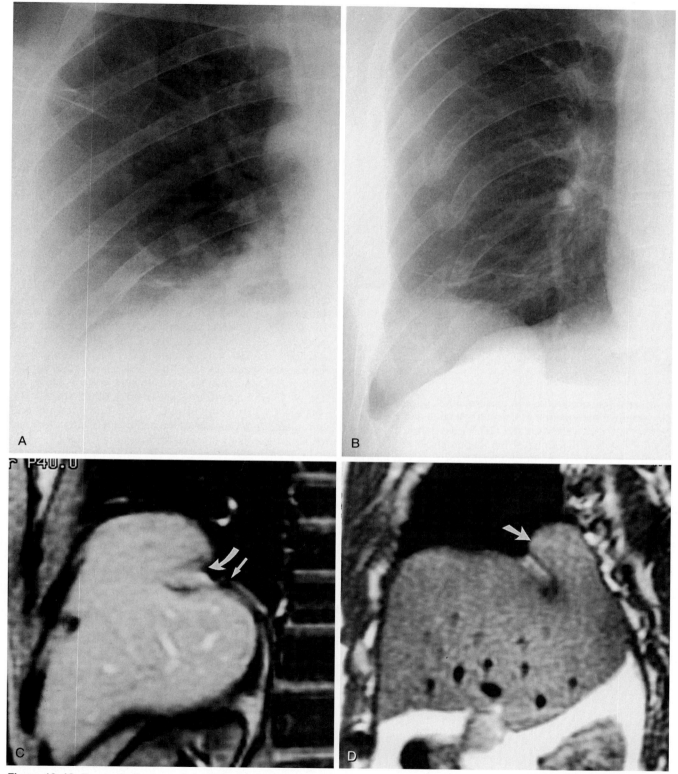

Figure 18–16. Traumatic Rupture of the Right Hemidiaphragm. View of the right chest from anteroposterior radiograph *(A)* performed after a motor vehicle accident in a 46-year-old man shows right rib fractures, a right pleural effusion, and apparent elevation of the right hemidiaphragm. The patient recovered and was discharged without further evaluation. Eleven months later, the patient presented with a 4-month history of right upper quadrant pain. View of the right chest from posteroanterior radiograph *(B)* shows mushroom-like mass in the right lower hemithorax. Several rib fractures and blunting of the right hemidiaphragm are evident. Coronal spin-echo T1-weighted MR image *(C)* shows discontinuity of the right hemidiaphragm *(straight arrow)* and waistlike constriction of the liver *(curved arrow)* where it traverses the diaphragmatic tear. Sagittal MR image *(D)* shows the posterior location of the herniated liver *(arrow)*.

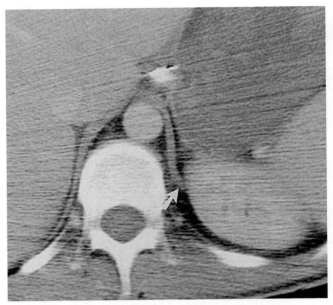

Figure 18–17. Traumatic Rupture of the Left Hemidiaphragm. Contrast-enhanced CT scan shows abrupt discontinuity of the left hemidiaphragm *(arrow)* at the level of the medial arcuate ligament. The patient was a 24-year-old man being assessed 10 days after a motor vehicle accident for unresolving pulmonary contusions. The diagnosis of traumatic tear of the hemidiaphragm was confirmed at surgery.

Most ruptures involve the posterolateral portion of the diaphragm at the junction of its central tendon and posterior leaves and are well seen on CT.[27] Less commonly the rupture involves the dome of the diaphragm, a region that is difficult to assess on conventional transverse CT images because it is tangential to the plane of section.[128] It may be difficult to distinguish a focal diaphragmatic injury in this region from a focal eventration or elevation of the diaphragm.[138] Optimal assessment of the diaphragmatic dome with detection of diaphragmatic ruptures that otherwise might be missed can be obtained using spiral CT with multiplanar coronal and sagittal reconstructions (Fig. 18–19).[92, 138, 139]

The results of initial studies suggested a poor sensitivity of CT in the detection of diaphragmatic injuries.[123, 135] Refinements in technology and the use of dynamic scanning of several levels during a single breath-hold or spiral CT have resulted in marked improvement, however.[128, 136, 139] In one study of 11 patients who had diaphragmatic rupture and 21 patients who had an intact diaphragm after blunt trauma, CT scans were reviewed independently by three observers who were unaware of the surgical findings.[136] Ten of the 11 patients who had diaphragmatic rupture were identified correctly on CT by at least one observer. The average sensitivity for the three observers in the detection of diaphragmatic ruptures was 61%, and the average specificity was 87%. False-negative results were due to hemothorax or hemoperitoneum that obscured the diaphragm; false-positive diagnosis occurred when the diagnosis was based solely on the presence of a diaphragmatic defect.

In a second study, investigators reviewed the spiral CT scans performed in 41 patients who had suspected diaphragmatic rupture.[139] Twenty-three patients had surgically confirmed diaphragmatic rupture (including 17 left, 5 right, and 1 bilateral rupture); 18 had an intact diaphragm. The CT images were assessed by three radiologists who reached a decision by consensus. The sensitivity of CT was 78% for left-sided rupture and 50% for right-sided rupture; the specificity was 100%. The most common CT finding of diaphragmatic rupture was the collar sign, identified in 15 of 23 patients (sensitivity 63%, specificity 100%).[139] Currently, spiral CT with thin sections and multiplanar re-formations is the imaging modality of choice for the diagnosis of diaphragmatic injuries.[9, 175]

Diaphragmatic rupture can be associated with several unusual complications, including concomitant involvement of the pericardial sac with passage of various organs into this space,[141, 142] herniation of the pancreas with the development of a bronchopancreatic fistula (an abnormality that occurs more frequently after acute pancreatitis),[143, 144] and splenosis (defined as the autotransplantation of splenic tissue). Splenosis usually occurs after splenic rupture and affects the peritoneum, omentum, and mesentery. Thoracic

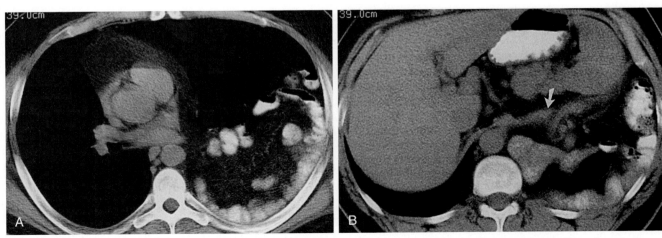

Figure 18–18. Traumatic Rupture of the Left Hemidiaphragm. Images from CT of the chest *(A)* and upper abdomen *(B)* performed after oral administration of contrast material show the torn end of the left hemidiaphragm *(arrow)* and intrathoracic herniation of bowel. The patient was a 28-year-old man who presented with a history of abdominal pain 1 year after trauma during wrestling.

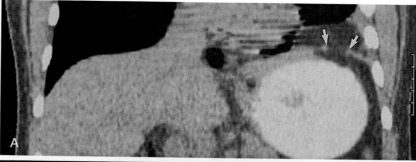

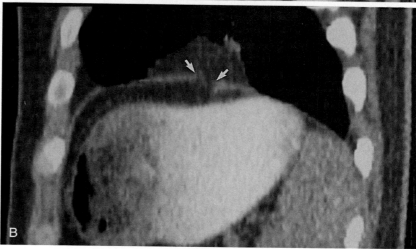

Figure 18–19. Spiral CT in the Diagnosis of Traumatic Rupture of the Left Hemidiaphragm. Coronal *(A)* and sagittal *(B)* reconstructions from a spiral CT scan obtained during a single breath-hold show focal defect in the left hemidiaphragm *(arrows)* with intrathoracic herniation of omental fat. (Case courtesy of Dr. Steven Primack, Department of Diagnostic Radiology, Oregon Health Sciences University.)

involvement may occur after combined diaphragmatic and splenic injury from blunt trauma[145, 146] or gunshot wounds.[147] Only 20 cases had been reported in the English literature by 1994.[146] It is likely that the incidence has been underestimated, however; in one study of 17 patients who had rupture of the spleen and left hemidiaphragm after motor vehicle accidents, 3 (18%) showed evidence of ectopic splenic activity in the left hemithorax on technetium-99m-tagged heated–red blood cell scintigraphy.[145]

In a review of the 20 cases published by 1994, thoracic splenosis was identified 6 to 42 years after injury.[146] All lesions were pleural based and involved the left hemithorax. Nodules were solitary in 10 patients and multiple in 10. They measured a few millimeters to 7.5 cm in diameter.[146] The implants may involve either the visceral or parietal pleura or the interlobar fissures.[145] They have not been described in the lung parenchyma. The nodules usually grow after implantation[146] but occasionally regress.[148]

The radiographic and CT findings include single or multiple pleural-based or paraspinal soft tissue nodules.[145, 146] Most are seen on the left side; rarely the disease is bilateral (Fig. 18–20). Findings such as healed fractures of a lower rib, diaphragmatic irregularity, or bullet fragments in the abdomen and left hemithorax provide helpful clues to the diagnosis.[149] The measured attenuation on CT may be similar to that of normal spleen (30 to 70 HU) or slightly lower.[145] The signal intensity on T1-weighted and T2-weighted MR images is comparable to that of the signal intensity of normal spleen.[145, 150] Also similar to the spleen, the foci of splenosis are isointense with respect to the paraspinal muscles on T1-weighted images and isointense

with respect to subcutaneous fat on T2-weighted images.[145, 150] Although these CT and MR imaging findings are characteristic of splenosis, confident radiologic diagnosis requires the use of radionuclide scintigraphy.[151] Ectopic splenic tissue is well delineated after intravenous administration of technetium-99m-tagged sulfur colloid[151] or heated red blood cells.[145, 152]

Fractures of the Ribs

Rib fractures occur in about half of all patients who have major blunt chest trauma.[153, 154] Most commonly, they involve the fourth to tenth ribs. The fractures often are missed on posteroanterior radiographs because the lateral portions of the ribs frequently are affected, and the fracture line is not tangential to the x-ray beam.[155, 156] The presence of fractures is easier to detect on oblique rib views.[157] The presence or not of rib fractures *per se* is of limited clinical significance,[157] however, the main value of the radiograph being the detection of associated pleural and pulmonary complications.[157] CT scan may show rib fractures not evident on radiograph as well as unsuspected associated complications, such as pneumothorax and hemothorax.[4, 153] Preliminary results suggest that sonography may also be superior to chest radiography in the detection of rib fractures.[176]

Fractures of certain ribs have specific clinical implications. Fractures of the 9th, 10th, or 11th ribs are apt to be associated with splenic or hepatic injury and sometimes with serious intra-abdominal hemorrhage.[20, 153] Their presence should prompt confirmation of abdominal organ injury

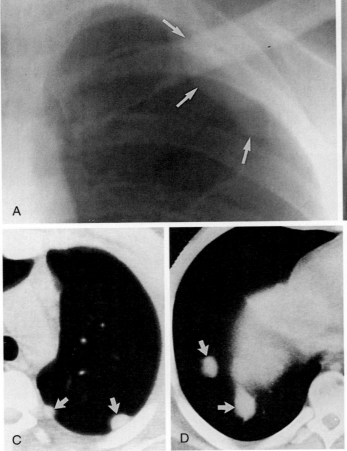

Figure 18–20. Thoracic Splenosis. Views of the left upper hemithorax *(A)* and right lower hemithorax *(B)* from postero-anterior chest radiograph in an asymptomatic 18-year-old man show pleural-based nodules *(arrows)*. The radiographic findings are confirmed by CT scans at the level of the aortic arch *(C)* and right hemidiaphragm *(D)*. The diagnosis was confirmed by technetium-99m-tagged heated–red blood cell scintigraphy. This case constitutes a rare example of bilateral thoracic splenosis that was secondary to splenic injury and bilateral diaphragmatic tears that the patient sustained when, at the age of 2 years, he was hit by a bus. (Courtesy of Dr. Robert Pugatch, University of Maryland Medical Center, Baltimore, Maryland.)

with spinal CT.[177] Because they are relatively protected, fractures of the first, second, and third ribs usually imply severe trauma.[155] In one study of 75 patients who had 90 first rib fractures, patients were considered in two groups. Group I consisted of 13 patients who had a fracture of one or both first ribs only, whereas group II (62 patients) had multiple rib fractures that included the first rib.[158] In group I, intrathoracic injuries were mild and did not involve major vessels, whereas in group II, many of the patients sustained severe intrathoracic injury, 58% involving the aorta.

Cough fractures of the ribs occur more often in women than in men[159, 160] and almost invariably involve the sixth to ninth ribs, most often the seventh and usually in the posterior axillary line.[159, 160] Unless special care is taken to obtain radiographs of superior quality that detail the involved ribs, these fractures may go undetected until evidenced by callus formation later.

Fractures of the Spine

Fractures of the thoracic spine account for 15% to 30% of all spine fractures.[161, 162, 177] They may result in extraosseous hemorrhage and the development of unilateral or bilateral paraspinal masses or diffuse widening of the mediastinum.[73, 163] The findings on chest radiograph may mimic those of aortic rupture.[73] About 70% to 90% of fractures

are visible on plain radiographs.[5] CT and MR imaging allow detection of otherwise occult fractures and assessment of the relationship between the fracture fragments and the spinal cord.[5, 161, 177]

Early recognition of thoracic spinal fractures is important because of the frequency with which they lead to neurologic deficits.[5] About 60% of patients who have fracture-dislocations of the thoracic spine have complete neurologic deficits, compared with 30% of patients who have similar injuries to the cervical spine and 2% with injury of the lumbar spine.[5]

Post-Traumatic Pulmonary Herniation

Protrusion of a portion of lung through an abnormal aperture of the chest wall may be congenital or acquired and may be cervical, thoracic, or (rarely) diaphragmatic in location.[164] The protrusion is covered by parietal and visceral pleura. Congenital hernias occur most frequently in the supraclavicular fossa and less often at the costochondral junction. Traumatic hernias may follow chest trauma or surgery or chest tube drainage.[164] In a few cases, the weakened area is the result of inflammatory or neoplastic damage to the chest wall.[166]

The most common location of post-traumatic herniation is the parasternal region just medial to the costochondral junction, where the intercostal musculature is thinnest. The

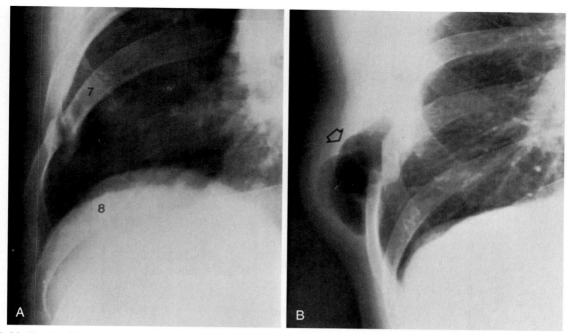

Figure 18–21. Hernia of the Lung. About 1 year before the radiographs illustrated, this 46-year-old man suffered comminuted fractures of the axillary portions of ribs 6, 7, and 8 on the right in a crush injury to the chest. Healing of the rib fractures had occurred such that there was considerable separation between ribs 7 and 8 *(A)*. The patient noted a soft, fluctuant bulge in the axillary region of the chest on coughing and straining. Radiography of the chest in full inspiration during the Valsalva maneuver *(B)* showed herniation of a sizable portion of lung through the defect in the rib cage into the contiguous soft tissues of the axilla *(arrow)*. The first radiograph *(A)* was exposed at full expiration and shows no evidence of lung herniation. The defect was repaired surgically.

patient usually complains of a bulge appearing during coughing and straining. In most cases, the diagnosis can be made by the observation of a soft crepitant mass that develops under these conditions and disappears during expiration or rest. Chest radiographs show pulmonary herniation through an obvious defect in the rib cage (Fig. 18–21) or through the supraclavicular fossa.[167] Optimal visualization requires the performance of a Valsalva maneuver or CT.[164, 168]

EFFECTS ON THE THORAX OF PENETRATING TRAUMA

The usual radiographic appearance of the path of a bullet through lung parenchyma is a poorly defined homogeneous shadow, which, as might be expected, is more or less circular when viewed in the direction in which the bullet passed and longitudinal when viewed in perpendicular projection (Fig. 18–22). The indistinct definition is caused by hemorrhage and edema into the parenchyma surrounding the bullet track; both usually resolve within 3 to 8 days, permitting clear visualization of the bullet track, which now contains blood and is seen as a soft tissue density that is circular when seen *en face* or tubular when seen in profile.[165] The hematoma in the bullet track slowly decreases in size from its periphery.[165] In a few cases, a central radiolucency may be apparent along the bullet's course and reveal communication between the central core of blood and the bronchial tree.[165, 169] In such circumstances, a history of hemoptysis usually can be elicited. In most cases, the bullet track resolves completely within a few months. Delay or failure in resolution should suggest the possibility of superimposed infection.[165, 168] Usually, bullets

follow straight paths through the chest. Occasionally, bullets ricochet off body structures, particularly vertebrae and ribs. Rarely, bullets move along an artery, vein, or the tracheobronchial tree.[170]

Penetrating wounds of the thorax from a knife or bullet

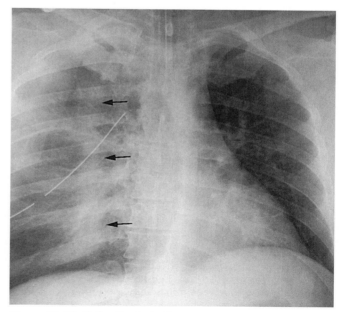

Figure 18–22. Bullet Track. A 40-year-old man was shot in the back of the neck. The bullet traversed the pleura, lung, diaphragm, and anterior aspect of the liver. Anteroposterior chest radiograph shows the bullet track in the lung *(arrows)* as well as a right hemopneumothorax. A chest tube is in place.

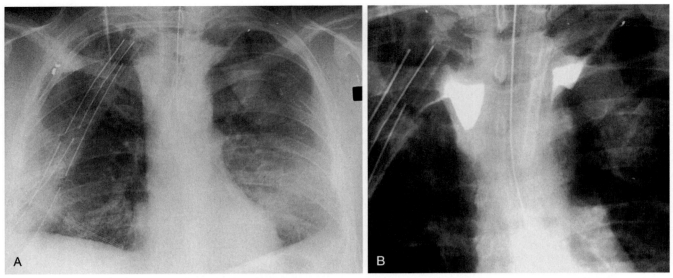

Figure 18–23. Gunshot Wound to the Esophagus. A 30-year-old man presented with a large right hemopneumothorax after a gunshot wound. The hemopneumothorax required three chest tubes for appropriate drainage. Anteroposterior chest radiograph *(A)* shows widening of the superior mediastinum. Metallic fragments from the gunshot can be seen over the upper chest and left axilla. View from chest radiograph performed after oral administration of contrast material *(B)* shows extravasation into the mediastinum and communication with the pleural spaces. The esophageal perforation was corrected surgically.

may induce traumatic pneumothorax or hemopneumothorax, although the searing effect of a bullet as it passes through the pleura may cauterize the tissues sufficiently to prevent escape of air into the pleural space. In one series of 250 consecutive patients who had gunshot wounds involving the thorax, 90% presented with hemothorax or hemopneumothorax, and only 3% presented with pneumothorax alone.[173]

Chest radiograph with radiopaque markers placed at entrance and exit wounds plays an important role in the evaluation of patients with penetrating chest injuries.[171] Patients with normal radiograph at presentation should have a repeat radiograph after 3 to 6 hours to rule out a delayed pneumothorax.[171, 172]

Penetrating injury to the lungs may be associated with damage to other intrathoracic structures with corresponding radiologic and clinical manifestations. For example, laceration of the esophagus may result in pneumomediastinum, mediastinitis, and pleural effusion (Fig. 18–23). The diaphragm can be damaged without evidence of visceral injury and with normal radiographic findings;[174] patients usually complain of abdominal pain, and examination reveals tenderness and rigidity of the abdominal wall. When present, the radiographic abnormalities associated with penetrating diaphragmatic injury are nonspecific and consist of hemothorax, pneumothorax, or apparent elevation of the hemidiaphragm.[126]

References

1. Boyd AD, Glassman LR: Trauma to the lung. Chest Surg Clin North Am 7:263, 1997.
2. Mayberry JC: Imaging in thoracic trauma: The trauma surgeon's perspective. J Thorac Imaging 15:76, 2000.
3. Wagner RB, Crawford WO Jr, Schimpf PP: Classification of parenchymal injuries of the lung. Radiology 167:77, 1988.
4. Kerns SR, Gay SB: CT of blunt chest trauma. Am J Roentgenol 154:55, 1990.
5. Groskin SA: Selected topics in chest trauma. Semin Ultrasound CT MR 17:119, 1996.
6. Greene R: Lung alterations in thoracic trauma. J Thorac Imaging 2:1, 1987.
7. Shorr RM, Crittenden M, Indeck M, et al: Blunt thoracic trauma: Analysis of 515 patients. Ann Surg 206:200, 1987.
8. Errion AR, Houk VN, Kettering DL: Pulmonary hematoma due to blunt, nonpenetrating thoracic trauma. Am Rev Respir Dis 88:384, 1963.
9. Zinck SE, Primack SL: Radiographic and CT findings in blunt chest trauma. J Thorac Imaging 15:87, 2000.
10. Stevens E, Templeton AW: Traumatic nonpenetrating lung contusion. Radiology 85:247, 1965.
11. Williams JR, Stembridge VA: Pulmonary contusion secondary to nonpenetrating chest trauma. Am J Roentgenol 91:284, 1964.
12. Kollmorgen DR, Murray KA, Sullivan JJ, et al: Predictors of mortality in pulmonary contusion. Am J Surg 168:659, 1994.
13. Reynolds J, Davis JT: Injuries of the chest wall, pleura, pericardium, lungs, bronchi and esophagus. Radiol Clin North Am 4:383, 1966.
14. Ting YM: Pulmonary parenchymal findings in blunt trauma to the chest. Am J Roentgenol 98:343, 1966.
15. Wiot JF: The radiologic manifestations of blunt chest trauma. JAMA 231:500, 1975.
16. Toombs BD, Sandler CM, Lester RG: Computed tomography of chest trauma. Radiology 140:733, 1981.
17. Smejkal R, O'Malley KF, David E, et al: Routine initial computed tomography of the chest in blunt torso trauma. Chest 100:667, 1991.
18. Schild HH, Strunk H, Weber W, et al: Pulmonary contusion: CT vs plain radiograms. J Comput Assist Tomogr 13:417, 1989.
19. Reid JD, Kommareddi S, Lankerani M, et al: Chronic expanding hematomas: A clinicopathologic entity. JAMA 244:2441, 1980.
20. Wilson RF, Murray C, Antonenko DR: Nonpenetrating thoracic injuries. Surg Clin North Am 57:17, 1977.
21. Chochlin DL, Shaw MRP: Traumatic lung cysts following minor blunt chest trauma. Clin Radiol 29:151, 1978.
22. Kuhlman JE, Pozniak MA, Collins J, et al: Radiographic and CT findings of blunt chest trauma: Aortic injuries and looking beyond them. Radiographics 18:1085, 1998.
23. Fagan CJ: Traumatic lung cyst. Am J Roentgenol 97:186, 1966.
24. Santos GH, Mahendra T: Traumatic pulmonary pseudocysts. Ann Thorac Surg 27:359, 1979.
25. Hollister M, Stern EJ, Steinberg KP: Type 2 pulmonary laceration: A marker of blunt high-energy injury to the lung. Am J Roentgenol 165:1126, 1995.

26. Takahashi N, Murakami J, Murayama S, et al: MR evaluation of intrapulmonary hematoma. J Comput Assist Tomogr 19:125, 1995.

27. Kang EY, Müller NL: CT in blunt chest trauma: Pulmonary, tracheobronchial, and diaphragmatic injuries. Semin Ultrasound CT MR 17:114, 1996.

28. Mirvis SE, Templeton P: Imaging in acute thoracic trauma. Semin Roentgenol 27:184, 1992.

29. Rossbach MM, Johnson SB, Gomez MA, et al: Management of major tracheobronchial injuries: A 28-year experience. Ann Thorac Surg 65:182, 1998.

30. Song JK, Beaty CD: Diagnosis of pulmonary contusions and a bronchial laceration after a fall. Am J Roentgenol 167:1510, 1996.

31. Roxburgh JC: Rupture of the tracheobronchial tree. Thorax 42:681, 1987.

32. Chesterman JT, Satsangi PN: Rupture of the trachea and bronchi by closed injury. Thorax 21:21, 1966.

33. Burke JF: Early diagnosis of traumatic rupture of the bronchus. JAMA 181:682, 1962.

34. Woodring JH, Fried AM, Hatfield DR, et al: Fractures of first and second ribs: Predictive value for arterial and bronchial injury. Am J Roentgenol 138:211, 1982.

35. Ketai L, Brandt MM, Schermer C: Nonaortic mediastinal injuries from blunt chest trauma. J Thorac Imaging 15:120, 2000.

36. Unger JM, Schuchmann GG, Grossman JE, et al: Tears of the trachea and main bronchi caused by blunt trauma: Radiologic findings. Am J Roentgenol 153:1175, 1989.

37. Barmada H, Gibbons JR: Tracheobronchial injury in blunt and penetrating chest trauma. Chest 106:74, 1994.

38. Larizadeh R: Rupture of the bronchus. Thorax 21:28, 1966.

39. Collins JP, Ketharanathan V, McConchie I: Rupture of major bronchi resulting from closed chest injuries. Thorax 28:371, 1973.

40. Bertelsen S, Howitz P: Injuries of the trachea and bronchi. Thorax 27:188, 1972.

41. Hecceta WG, Torpoco J, Richardson RL: Extensive linear "blowout" of the thoracic membranous trachea with innominate artery avulsion secondary to blunt chest trauma. Chest 67:247, 1975.

42. Silbiger ML, Kushner LN: Tracheobronchial perforation: Its diagnosis and treatment. Radiology 85:242, 1965.

43. Harvey-Smith W, Bush W, Northrop C: Traumatic bronchial rupture. Am J Roentgenol 134:1189, 1980.

44. Travis SP, Layer GT: Traumatic transection of the thoracic trachea. Ann R Coll Surg Engl 65:240, 1983.

45. Döpper TH: Zur Röntgendiagnostik stumpfer Thoraxtrauman. [Roentgen diagnosis of injuries of the thorax due to blunt trauma.] Fortschr Roentgenstr 95:524, 1960.

46. Lotz PR, Martel W, Rohwedder JJ, et al: Significance of pneumomediastinum in blunt trauma to the thorax. Am J Roentgenol 132:817, 1979.

47. Oh KS, Fleishner FG, Wyman SM: Characteristic pulmonary finding in traumatic complete transection of a mainstem bronchus. Radiology 92:371, 1969.

48. Kumpe DA, Oh KS, Wyman SM: A characteristic pulmonary finding in unilateral complete bronchial transection. Am J Roentgenol 110:704, 1970.

49. Peterson C, Deslauriers J, McClish A: A classic image of complete right main bronchus avulsion. Chest 96:1415, 1989.

50. Weir IH, Müller NL, Connell DG: CT diagnosis of bronchial rupture. J Comput Assist Tomogr 12:1035, 1988.

51. Rollins RJ, Tocino I: Early radiographic signs of tracheal rupture. Am J Roentgenol 148:695, 1987.

52. Vidinel I: Displacement of the mediastinum. Chest 62:215, 1972.

53. Hood RM, Sloan HE: Injuries to the trachea and major bronchi. J Thorac Cardiovasc Surg 38:458, 1959.

54. Groskin SA: Selected topics in chest trauma. Radiology 183:605, 1992.

55. Ashbaugh DG, Peters GN, Halgrimson CG, et al: Chest trauma: Analysis of 685 patients. Arch Surg 95:546, 1967.

56. Robertson HT, Lakshminarayan S, Hudson LD: Lung injury following a 50-metre fall into water. Thorax 33:175, 1978.

57. Wall SD, Federle MP, Jeffry RB, et al: CT diagnosis of unsuspected pneumothorax after blunt abdominal trauma. Am J Roentgenol 141:919, 1983.

58. Raptopoulos V, Sheiman RG, Phillips DA, et al: Traumatic aortic tear: Screening with chest CT. Radiology 182:667, 1992.

59. Fisher RG, Chasen MH, Lamki N: Diagnosis of injuries of the aorta and brachiocephalic arteries caused by blunt chest trauma: CT vs aortography. Am J Roentgenol 162:1047, 1994.

60. Langston CS: The aberrant central venous catheter and its complications. Radiology 100:55, 1971.

61. Mitchell SE, Clark RA: Complications of central venous catheterization. Am J Roentgenol 133:467, 1979.

62. Tocino IM, Watanabe A: Impending catheter perforation of superior vena cava: Radiographic recognition. Am J Roentgenol 146:487, 1986.

63. Raphael MJ: Mediastinal haematoma: A description of some radiologic appearances. Br J Radiol 36:921, 1963.

64. Leigh TF: Mass lesions of the mediastinum. Radiol Clin North Am 1:377, 1963.

65. Kearney PA, Smith W, Johnson SB, et al: Use of transesophageal echocardiography in the evaluation of traumatic aortic injury. J Trauma 34:696, 1993.

66. Mirvis SE, Bidwell JK, Buddemeyer EU, et al: Value of chest radiography in excluding traumatic aortic rupture. Radiology 163:487, 1987.

67. Creasy JD, Chiles C, Routh WD, et al: Overview of traumatic injury of the thoracic aorta. Radiographics 17:27, 1997.

68. Williams JS, Graff JA, Uku JM, et al: Aortic injury in vehicular trauma. Ann Thorac Surg 57:726, 1994.

69. Crass JR, Cohen AM, Motta AO, et al: A proposed new mechanism of traumatic aortic rupture: The osseous pinch. Radiology 176:645, 1990.

70. Cohen AM, Crass JR, Thomas HA, et al: CT evidence for the "osseous pinch" mechanism of traumatic aortic injury. Am J Roentgenol 159:271, 1992.

71. Pretre R, Chilcott M: Blunt trauma to the heart and great vessels. N Engl J Med 336:626, 1997.

72. Eller JL, Ziter FMH Jr: Avulsion of the innominate artery from the aortic arch: An evaluation of roentgenographic findings. Radiology 94:75, 1970.

73. Dennis LN, Rogers LF: Superior mediastinal widening from spine fractures mimicking aortic rupture on chest radiographs. Am J Roentgenol 152:27, 1989.

74. Hewes RC, Smith DC, Lavine MH: Iatrogenic hydromediastinum simulating aortic laceration. Am J Roentgenol 133:817, 1979.

75. Heystraten FM, Rosenbusch G, Kingma LM, et al: Chest radiography in acute traumatic rupture of the thoracic aorta. Acta Radiol 29:411, 1988.

76. Peters DR, Gamsu G: Displacement of the right paraspinous interface: A radiographic sign of acute traumatic rupture of the thoracic aorta. Radiology 134:599, 1980.

77. Woodring JH, Pulmano CM, Stevens RK: The right paratracheal stripe in blunt chest trauma. Radiology 143:605, 1982.

78. Simeone JF, Minagi H, Putman CE: Traumatic disruption of the thoracic aorta: Significance of the left apical extrapleural cap. Radiology 117:265, 1975.

79. Simeone JF, Deren MM, Cagle F: The value of the left apical cap in the diagnosis of aortic rupture: A prospective and retrospective study. Radiology 139:35, 1981.

80. Marnocha KE, Maglinte DDT: Plain-film criteria for excluding aortic rupture in blunt chest trauma. Am J Roentgenol 144:19, 1985.

81. Mirvis SE, Bidwell JK, Buddemeyer EU, et al: Imaging diagnosis of traumatic aortic rupture: A review and experience at a major trauma center. Invest Radiol 22:187, 1987.

82. Hunink MGM, Bos JJ: Triage of patients to angiography for detection of aortic rupture after blunt chest trauma: Cost-effectiveness analysis of using CT. Am J Roentgenol 165:27, 1995.

83. Mirvis SE, Shanmuganathan K, Miller BH, et al: Traumatic aortic injury: Diagnosis with contrast-enhanced thoracic CT: Five-year experience at a major trauma center. Radiology 200:413, 1996.

84. Braithwaite CE, Cilley JM, O'Connor WH, et al: The pivotal role of transeosophageal echocardiography in the management of traumatic thoracic aortic rupture with associated intra-abdominal hemorrhage. Chest 105:1899, 1994.

85. Smith MD, Cassidy JM, Souther S, et al: Transesophageal echocardiography in the diagnosis of traumatic rupture of the aorta. N Engl J Med 332:356, 1995.

86. Marotta R, Franchetto AA: The CT appearance of aortic transection. Am J Roentgenol 166:647, 1996.

87. Morgan PW, Goodman LR, Aprahamian C, et al: Evaluation of traumatic aortic injury: Does dynamic contrast-enhanced CT play a role? Radiology 182:661, 1992.

88. Rigauts H, Marchal G, Baert AL, et al: Initial experience with volume CT scanning. J Comput Assist Tomogr 14:675, 1990.

89. Gavant ML, Menke PG, Fabian T, et al: Blunt traumatic aortic rupture: Detection with helical CT of the chest. Radiology 197:125, 1995.

90. Trerotola SO: Can helical CT replace aortography in thoracic trauma? Radiology 197:13, 1995.

91. Gavant ML, Flick P, Menke P, et al: CT aortography of thoracic aortic rupture. Am J Roentgenol 166:955, 1996.

92. Van Hise ML, Primack SL, Israel RS, et al: CT in blunt chest trauma: Indications and limitations. Radiographics 18:1071, 1998.

93. Wong Y-C, Wang L-J, Lim K-E, et al: Periaortic hematoma on helical CT of the chest: A criterion for predicting blunt traumatic aortic rupture. Am J Roentgenol 170:1523, 1998.

94. Patel NH, Stephens KE Jr, Mirvis SE, et al: Imaging of acute thoracic aortic injury due to blunt trauma: A review. Radiology 209:335, 1998.

95. Blackmore CC, Zweibel A, Mann FA: Determining risk of traumatic aortic injury: How to optimize imaging strategy. Am J Roentgenol 174:343, 2000.

96. Dyer DS, Moore EE, Mestek MF, et al: Can chest CT be used to exclude aortic injury? Radiology 213:195, 1999.

97. Shapiro MJ, Yanofsky SD, Trapp J, et al: Cardiovascular evaluation in blunt chest trauma using transesophageal echocardiography. J Trauma 31:835, 1991.

98. Brooks SW, Young JC, Cmolik B, et al: The use of transesophageal echocardiography in the evaluation of chest trauma. J Trauma 32:761, 1992.

99. Minard G, Schurr MJ, Croce MA, et al: A prospective analysis of transesophageal echocardiography in the diagnosis of traumatic disruption of the aorta. J Trauma 40:225, 1996.

100. Goarin JP, Catoire P, Jacquens Y, et al: Use of transesophageal echocardiography for diagnosis of traumatic aortic injury. Chest 112:71, 1997.

101. Seward JB, Khandheria BK, Edwards WD, et al: Biplanar transesophageal echocardiography: Anatomic correlations, image orientation, and clinical applications. Mayo Clin Proc 65:1193, 1990.

102. Morse SS, Glickman MG, Greenwood LH, et al: Traumatic aortic rupture: False-positive aortographic diagnosis due to atypical ductus diverticulum. Am J Roentgenol 150:793, 1988.

103. LaBerge JM, Jeffrey RB: Aortic lacerations: Fatal complications of thoracic aortography. Radiology 165:36, 1987.

104. Zeiger MA, Clark DE, Morton JR: Reappraisal of surgical treatment of traumatic transection of the thoracic aorta. J Cardiovasc Surg 31:607, 1990.

105. Stanbridge RD: Tracheo-oesophageal fistula and bilateral recurrent laryngeal nerve palsies after blunt chest trauma. Thorax 37:548, 1982.

106. Cevese PG, Vecchioni R, D'Amico DF, et al: Postoperative chylothorax: Six cases in 2,500 operations, with a survey of the world literature. J Thorac Cardiovasc Surg 89:966, 1975.

107. Grant PW, Brown SW: Traumatic chylothorax: A case report. Aust N Z J Surg 61:798, 1991.

108. Worthington MG, de Groot M, Gunning AJ, et al: Isolated thoracic duct injury after penetrating chest trauma. Ann Thorac Surg 60:272, 1995.

109. Dulchavsky SA, Ledgerwood AM, Lucas CE: Management of chylothorax after blunt chest trauma. J Trauma 28:1400, 1988.

110. Brook MP, Dupree DW: Bilateral traumatic chylothorax. Ann Emerg Med 17:69, 1988.

111. Rea D: Traumatic chylothorax in a closed chest injury: Report of a case. Br J Dis Chest 54:82, 1960.

112. Thorne PS: Traumatic chylothorax. Tubercle 39:29, 1958.

113. Hom M, Jolles H: Traumatic mediastinal lymphocele mimicking other thoracic injuries: Case report. J Thorac Imaging 7:78, 1992.

114. Sachs PB, Zelch MG, Rice TW, et al: Diagnosis and localization of laceration of the thoracic duct: Usefulness of lymphangiography and CT. Am J Roentgenol 157:703, 1991.

115. Ellis MC, Gordon L, Gobien RP, et al: Traumatic lymphocele: Demonstration by lymphoscintigraphy with modified 99mTc sulfur colloid. Am J Roentgenol 140:973, 1983.

116. Shah R, Sabanathan S, Mearns AJ, et al: Traumatic rupture of diaphragm. Ann Thorac Surg 60:1444, 1995.

117. Broos PLO, Rommens PM, Carlier H, et al: Traumatic rupture of the diaphragm: Review of 62 successive cases. Int Surg 74:88, 1989

118. de la Rocha AG, Creel RJ, Mulligan GWN, et al: Diaphragmatic rupture due to blunt abdominal trauma. Surg Gynecol Obstet 154:175, 1982.

119. Leaman PL: Rupture of the right hemidiaphragm due to blunt trauma. Ann Emerg Med 12:351, 1983.

120. Meyers BF, McCabe CJ: Traumatic diaphragmatic hernia: Occult marker of serious injury. Ann Surg 218:783, 1993.

121. Marchand P: Traumatic hiatus hernia. BMJ 1:754, 1962.

122. Carter BN, Giuseffi J, Felson B: Traumatic diaphragmatic hernia. Am J Roentgenol 65:56, 1951.

123. Miller LW, Bennett EV, Root DH, et al: Management of blunt and penetrating diaphragmatic injury. J Trauma 24:403, 1984.

124. Beauchamp G, Khalfallah A, Girard R, et al: Blunt diaphragmatic rupture. Am J Surg 148:292, 1984.

125. Gelman R, Mirvis SE, Gens D: Diaphragmatic rupture due to blunt trauma: Sensitivity of plain chest radiographs. Am J Roentgenol 156:51, 1991.

126. Shackleton KL, Stewart ET, Taylor AJ: Traumatic diaphragmatic injuries: Spectrum of radiographic findings. Radiographics 18:49, 1998.

127. Shanmuganathan K, Mirvis SE, White CS, et al: MR imaging evaluation of hemidiaphragms in acute blunt trauma: Experience with 16 patients. Am J Roentgenol 167:397, 1996.

128. Worthy SA, Kang EY, Hartman TE, et al: Diaphragmatic rupture: CT findings in 11 patients. Radiology 194:885, 1995.

129. Aronchick JM, Epstein DM, Gefter WB, et al: Chronic traumatic diaphragmatic hernia: The significance of pleural effusion. Radiology 168:675, 1988.

130. Radin DR, Ray MJ, Halls JM: Strangulated diaphragmatic hernia with pneumothorax due to colopleural fistula. Am J Roentgenol 146:321, 1986.

131. Laws HL, Waldschmidt ML: Rupture of diaphragm (letter). JAMA 243:32, 1980.

132. Salomon NW, Zukoski CF: Rupture of the right hemidiaphragm with eventration of the liver. JAMA 241:1929, 1979.

133. Somers JM, Gleeson FV, Flower CD: Rupture of the right hemidiaphragm following blunt trauma: The use of ultrasound in diagnosis. Clin Radiol 42:97, 1990.

134. Ammann A, Brewer W, Maull K, et al: Traumatic rupture of the diaphragm: Real-time sonographic diagnosis. Am J Roentgenol 140:915, 1983.

135. Voeller GR, Reisser JR, Fabian TC, et al: Blunt diaphragm injuries. Am Surg 56:28, 1990.

136. Murray JG, Caoili E, Gruden JF, et al: Acute rupture of the diaphragm due to blunt trauma: Diagnostic sensitivity and specificity of CT. Am J Roentgenol 166:1035, 1996.

137. Caskey CI, Zerhouni EA, Fishman EK, et al: Aging of the diaphragm: A CT study. Radiology 171:385, 1989.

138. Israel RS, Mayberry JC, Primack SL: Diaphragmatic rupture: Use of helical CT scanning with multiplanar reformations. Am J Roentgenol 167:1201, 1996.

139. Killeen KL, Mirvis SE, Shanmuganathan K: Helical CT of diaphragmatic rupture caused by blunt trauma. Am J Roentgenol 173:1611, 1999.

140. Root HD, Harmen PK: Injury to the diaphragm. *In* Moore EE, Mattox KL, Feliciano DV (eds): Trauma. 2nd ed. Norwalk, CT, Appleton & Lange, 1991.

141. Fagan CJ, Schreiber MH, Amparo EG, et al: Traumatic diaphragmatic hernia into the pericardium: Verification of diagnosis by computed tomography: Case report. J Comput Assist Tomogr 3:405, 1979.

142. Glasser DL, Shanmuganathan K, Mirvis SE: General case of the day. Radiographics 18:799, 1998.

143. Bell JW: Pancreatic-bronchial fistula. Am Rev Respir Dis 106:97, 1972.

144. Cox CL Jr, Anderson JN, Guest JL Jr: Bronchopancreatic fistula following traumatic rupture of the diaphragm. JAMA 237:1461, 1977.

145. Normand JP, Rioux M, Dumont M, et al: Thoracic splenosis after blunt trauma: Frequency and imaging findings. Am J Roentgenol 161:739, 1993.

146. Madjar S, Weissberg D. Thoracic splenosis. Thorax 49:1020, 1994.

147. Dalton ML Jr, Strange WH, Downs EA: Intrathoracic splenosis: Case report and review of the literature. Am Rev Respir Dis 103:827, 1971.

148. Dalton ML Jr, Strange WH, Downs EA: Intrathoracic splenosis. Am Rev Respir Dis 103:827, 1971.

149. Bordlee RP, Eshaghi N, Oz O: Thoracic splenosis: MR demonstration. J Thorac Imaging 10:146, 1995.

150. Mirowitz SA, Brown JJ, Lee JKT, et al: Dynamic gadolinium-enhanced MR imaging of the spleen: Normal enhancement patterns and evaluation of splenic lesions. Radiology 179:681, 1991.

151. Fidvi SA, Kroop SA, Klein SA: Posttraumatic thoracic splenosis and chronic aortic pseudoaneurysm. J Thorac Imaging 14:300, 1999.

152. Bidet AC, Dreyfus-Schmidt G, Combe J, et al: Diagnosis of splenosis: The advantages of splenic scintiscanning with Tc99m heat damaged red blood cells. Eur J Nucl Med 12:357, 1986.

153. Tocino I, Miller MH: Computed tomography in blunt chest trauma. J Thorac Imaging 2:45, 1987.

154. Dougall AM, Paul ME, Finley RJ, et al: Chest trauma: Current morbidity and mortality. J Trauma 17:547, 1977.

155. Stark P: Radiology of thoracic trauma. Invest Radiol 25:1265, 1990.

156. Shulman HS, Samuels TH: The radiology of blunt chest trauma. J Can Assoc Radiol 34:204, 1983.

157. DeLuca SA, Rhea JT, O'Malley T: Radiographic evaluation of rib fractures. Am J Roentgenol 138:91, 1982.

158. Albers JE, Rath RK, Glaser RS, et al: Severity of intrathoracic injuries associated with 1st rib fractures. Ann Thorac Surg 33:614, 1982.

159. Wynn-Williams N, Young RD: Cough fracture of the ribs: Including one complicated by pneumothorax. Tubercle 40:47, 1959.

160. Pearson JEG: Cough fracture of the ribs. Br J Tuberc 51:251, 1957.

161. Meyer S: Thoracic spine trauma. Semin Roentgenol 27:254, 1992.

162. Pal J, Mulder D, Brown R, et al: Assessing multiple trauma: Is the cervical spine enough? J Trauma 28:1282, 1988.

163. Bolesta MJ, Bohlman HH: Mediastinal widening associated with fractures of the upper thoracic spine. J Bone Joint Surg Am 73:447, 1991.

164. Bhalla M, Leitman BS, Forcade C, et al: Lung hernia: Radiographic features. Am J Roentgenol 154:51, 1990.

165. George PY, Goodman P: Radiographic appearance of bullet tracks in the lung. Am J Roentgenol 159:967, 1992.

166. Bidstrup P, Nordentoft JM, Petersen B: Hernia of the lung: Brief survey and report of two cases. Acta Radiol Diagn (Stockh) 4:490, 1966.

167. Taylor DA, Jacobson HG: Posttraumatic herniation of the lung. Am J Roentgenol 87:896, 1962.

168. Spees EK, Strevey TE, Geiger JP, et al: Persistent traumatic lung cavities resulting from medium- and high-velocity missiles. Ann Thorac Surg 4:133, 1967.

169. Larose JH: Cavitation of missile tracks in the lung. Radiology 90:995, 1968.

170. Hollerman JJ, Fackler ML: Gunshot wounds: Radiology and wound ballistics. Emerg Radiol 2:171, 1995.

171. LeBlang SD, Dolich MO: Imaging of penetrating thoracic trauma. J Thorac Imaging 15:128, 2000.

172. Kiev J, Kerstein MD: Role of three hour roentgenogram of the chest in penetrating and nonpenetrating injuries of the chest. Surg Gynecol Obstet 75:249, 1992.

173. Oparah SS, Mandal AK: Penetrating gunshot wounds of the chest in civilian practice: Experience with 250 consecutive cases. Br J Surg 65:45, 1978.

174. Sandrasagra FA: Penetrating thoracoabdominal injuries. Br J Surg 64:638, 1977.

175. Shanmuganathan K, Killeen K, Mirvis SE, White CS: Imaging of diaphragmatic injuries. J Thorac Imaging 15:104, 2000.

176. Griffith JF, Rainer TH, Ching ASC, et al: Sonography compared to radiography in revealing acute rib fracture. Am J Roentgenol 173:1603, 1999.

177. Collins J: Chest wall trauma. J Thorac Imaging 15:112, 2000.

Complications of Therapeutic and Monitoring Procedures

COMPLICATIONS OF THORACIC SURGERY

Most complications related to thoracic surgery occur in the immediate postoperative period (up to day 10), although certain manifestations may not become apparent for several weeks or months postoperatively. Although radiographic changes observed in the chest wall, pleura, mediastinum, diaphragm, and lungs are in many ways interdependent and should be considered together in interpretation, it is convenient to deal with them separately. The complica-

tions of median sternotomy and of lung surgery are summarized in Tables 19–1 and 19–2.

Chest Wall

Thoracotomy. Soft tissue swelling caused by hemorrhage and edema in the vicinity of the incision is common but seldom leads to difficulty in radiologic interpretation; it is often not radiographically apparent. Subcutaneous emphysema, manifested by linear streaks of gas density in the lateral chest wall and frequently in the neck, almost invariably is apparent for 2 or 3 days postoperatively. It need cause concern only when it is present in exceptionally large quantities, in which case it may be the result of ongoing leak from the surgical anastomosis; such an event is rare.

The absence of a rib, usually the fifth or sixth, is an occasional finding after thoracotomy. Nowadays the ribs usually are spread, however, rather than resected in pulmonary and cardiac procedures so that an intact rib cage is compatible with prior thoracotomy. Ribs that have been spread may be fractured.

Median Sternotomy. This procedure has become the principal surgical approach to the heart and great vessels and to a variety of mediastinal abnormalities. Although the incidence of complications after median sternotomy is low (<5%), the overall mortality rate of three of the major events (sternal dehiscence, mediastinitis, and osteomyelitis) approaches 50%.[1, 2] Complications usually become manifest 1 to 2 weeks postoperatively. Conventional radiography plays a limited role in the assessment of these abnormalities, and computed tomography (CT) is required for adequate evaluation, particularly when the presence of retrosternal collections or mediastinitis is suspected clinically.

Normal postoperative findings that may persist on CT for 2 to 3 weeks after sternotomy include minimal presternal and retrosternal soft tissue infiltration with edema fluid and blood, localized hematoma, postincisional bone defect, minor sternal irregularities such as slight misalignment, and minimal pericardial thickening.[3] Small localized collections of air may be present in the immediate postoperative period but usually resolve by 7 days after surgery.[1, 3] Presternal complications, including draining sinus tracts and frank abscess formation, can be identified readily using CT. The presence and extent of mediastinal communication of draining sinus tracts can be documented with CT contrast sinography.[3] Although retrosternal complications, such as

Table 19–1. COMPLICATIONS OF MEDIAN STERNOTOMY

Hematoma	Empyema
Abscess formation	Sternal osteomyelitis
Mediastinitis	Sternal dehiscence
Pericardial effusion	Fracture of first rib

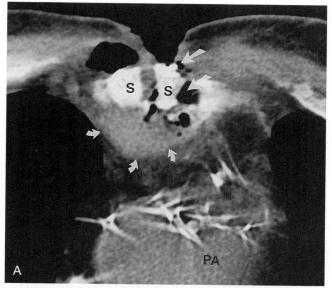

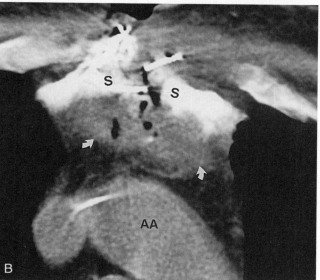

Figure 19–1. Retrosternal Abscess After Sternotomy. A 64-year-old patient had persistent wound infection 5 weeks after coronary artery bypass surgery. CT scan at the level of the main pulmonary artery (PA) *(A)* shows a draining sinus *(straight arrows)* communicating with a retrosternal collection *(curved arrows)*. The collection extended cephalad to the level of the aortic arch (AA) *(B)*. Note sternal (S) dehiscence and broken sternal wires. The presence of a retrosternal abscess was confirmed at surgery. Cultures grew *Staphylococcus aureus*.

hematoma, abscess formation, mediastinitis, pericardial effusion, and empyema, can be diagnosed with CT (Fig. 19–1),[3] the procedure is of limited value in the early detection of sternal osteomyelitis. When the latter is suspected clinically and the CT findings are equivocal, technetium-99m phosphate or gallium 67 scintigraphy can be helpful in establishing the diagnosis.[3]

A 2- to 4-mm gap at the sternotomy site (the *midsternal stripe*) can be recognized in 30% to 60% of patients sometime during the postoperative period and is of no diagnostic or prognostic significance.[4] Of much greater importance in establishing sternal separation is migration or reorientation of the sternal wires. In one investigation of 19 patients who had sternal dehiscence, 17 (89%) had sternal wire abnormalities evident on radiograph, including displacement in 16 (84%), rotation in 10 (53%), and disruption in 4 (21%).[178] In most, the radiographic abnormalities preceded the clinical diagnosis.

The only evidence of previous sternotomy may be the presence of wire sutures. Fracture of the first rib is seen occasionally after midline sternotomy; in a review of 50 randomly selected patients in one study, such fractures were visualized on chest radiograph in 3 (6%).[5] On radionuclide bone scans, first-rib fractures are identified in about 50% of patients who have undergone sternal retraction.[6]

Pleura

After pneumonectomy, fluid gradually fills the empty hemithorax. The rate of accumulation is variable. In most cases, about one half to two thirds of the hemithorax fills with fluid within the first week; complete filling usually occurs within 2 to 4 months, although occasionally it takes 6 months.[7] Long-term follow-up of postpneumonectomy patients has shown partial or complete resorption of the pleural fluid. In one series of patients examined by CT, this outcome was observed in about one third.[8] In these patients, there was marked ipsilateral shift of the mediasti-

Table 19–2. COMPLICATIONS OF LUNG SURGERY

Atelectasis
Pneumonia
Pulmonary thromboembolism
Pulmonary edema
Pneumothorax
Hemothorax
Bronchopleural fistula
Empyema
Chylothorax
Bronchial obstruction (Postpneumonectomy syndrome)
Lung herniation
Lung torsion

num, elevation of the hemidiaphragm, and overinflation of the contralateral lung. In the other two thirds, a variable amount of fluid still was evident several years after pneumonectomy; this was associated with less marked shift of the mediastinum.

On spin-echo magnetic resonance (MR) imaging, the postpneumonectomy space has a heterogeneous signal intensity regardless of the interval between pneumonectomy and the MR examination.[9] The contents of the space have a low to medium signal intensity on T1-weighted images (the signal intensity is usually less than that of muscle) and medium to high signal intensity on T2-weighted images.

MR imaging is comparable to CT in the assessment of tumor recurrence after pneumonectomy.[10] Usually, tumor can be identified by its inhomogeneous appearance and its mass effect;[10] tumor has a relatively low signal intensity on T1-weighted images and high intensity on T2-weighted images.

In patients who have not undergone pneumonectomy, little or no fluid is evident during the first 2 or 3 days after thoracotomy because the pleural space effectively is drained. After removal of the drainage tube, however, a small amount of fluid often appears, only to disappear quickly during convalescence. Minimal residual pleural thickening may remain, particularly over the lung base.

The accumulation of fluid in larger-than-expected amounts may result from a variety of causes, including poor positioning of the drainage tube, hemorrhage from an intercostal vessel, or infection (empyema). In the presence of pleural adhesions, fluid may loculate in areas that are not in communication with the drainage tube, a finding that is particularly common after pleural decortication. In this circumstance, absorption of the fluid may be prolonged, sometimes requiring several weeks. Such local intrapleural collections may be simulated by an extrapleural hematoma secondary to the thoracotomy incision; however, in either event, the finding is not important, unless the accumulation is large or infected. Extrapleural hematomas are particularly common after surgery over the lung apex and sometimes create an ominous-looking shadow (Fig. 19–2), which actually is of little or no clinical significance.

In contrast to the small amount of fluid that often accumulates, gas seldom is visible in the pleural space after removal of the drainage tube, even on radiographs exposed with the patient erect. Postoperative pneumothorax also has a variety of causes. Lack of communication with the drainage tube is probably the most common, particularly if the gas is loculated or the tube is positioned incorrectly (e.g., in the major fissure). Other causes include leakage into the pleural space from a *blown* bronchial stump (bronchopleural fistula) or from a bare area of lung after wedge or segmental resection of lung (Fig. 19–3). In the presence of pleural adhesions, a loculated collection of gas may remain for a considerable period of time because of lack of communication with the drainage tube; it may be associated with a collection of fluid in the form of hydropneumothorax.

The incidence of bronchopleural fistula as a complication of pulmonary resection is about 2%;[11, 12] the reported mortality rate ranges from 30% to 70%.[11-13] The complication occurs as a result of necrosis of bronchial stump tissue or dehiscence of sutures. It is most common after right pneumonectomy and occurs rarely after lower lobectomy on either side. In one investigation of 2,359 pulmonary resections, multivariate analysis showed an increased risk in association with more extensive surgery (e.g., pneumonectomy), residual carcinoma at the bronchial stump, preoperative radiation, and diabetes.[12] Characteristically the development of a fistula is heralded by the sudden onset of dyspnea and expectoration of bloody fluid during the first 10 days postoperatively; dehiscence is uncommon greater than 90 days after resection.[13] Chest radiograph may show an unexpected disappearance of fluid as a result of emptying of the pleural space by way of the tracheobron-

chial tree.[14] Radiologic evaluation of this complication can be facilitated by CT,[15] particularly with the use of thin sections (2-mm collimation) and spiral technique.[16, 17]

Esophageal-pleural fistulas may develop after esophagectomy, anterior fusion of the cervical spine, or esophageal dilation.[18] Radiographic findings include mediastinal widening, pleural effusion, pneumothorax, and hydropneumothorax.[18, 19] Mediastinal widening may be absent because of drainage of the esophageal contents into the pleural space.[18] The diagnosis is made readily by demonstration of orally administered contrast material in the pleural space by fluoroscopically guided esophagography or CT.[19, 20] The latter procedure is superior to esophagography because it requires little cooperation of the patient, allows evaluation of the pleura and the mediastinum, and may show a fistula in a patient who has a normal esophagogram.[18, 20]

Mediastinum

The two major radiologic abnormalities of the mediastinum that occur in the postoperative period are enlargement and displacement. Enlargement results from the accumulation of gas or fluid. Pneumomediastinum is a frequent finding after mediastinotomy and should not occasion alarm; however, its persistence in the absence of other potential causes (such as tracheostomy) should raise the suspicion of interstitial pulmonary emphysema associated with some form of pulmonary disease.[21] Venous hemorrhage and edema are common after mediastinotomy and should not be considered serious unless widening is excessive or progressive. Severe bleeding should be suspected when there is an abrupt increase in the mediastinal width or change in contour after sternotomy.[22] Although the radiographic findings may be helpful in diagnosis, in most cases, it is made based on excessive bloody mediastinal tube drainage.[23] In one series of 100 patients, 7 required re-exploration for mediastinal bleeding after cardiac surgery;[23] only 1 of the 7 patients had mediastinal widening. In this patient, the diagnosis first was suggested because of a rapid increase in mediastinal width in the early postoperative period; mediastinal tube drainage was deceptively normal as a result of partial blockage of the tube.

Other causes of mediastinal widening after cardiac surgery include aortic dissection and traumatic venous catheter insertion.[23] Rarely, focal mediastinal widening or an anterior mediastinal mass after coronary artery bypass surgery represents a saphenous vein graft aneurysm[24] or intrathoracic fat from an internal mammary artery pedicle.[25] Distinction of mediastinal hemorrhage from these two abnormalities can be made with contrast-enhanced CT.[24, 25] A sponge rarely is retained in the pericardial cavity[26] or mediastinum[190] after cardiac surgery. Detection is difficult on standard anteroposterior chest radiographs because of exposure factors but can be made on the lateral view or on CT.[26]

Alterations in contour of the mediastinum after thoracic surgery may be caused by transposed muscle or by omental or pericardial fat used to obliterate spaces, to promote repair and healing, to cover a bronchial stump, or to reinforce airway and esophageal anastomosis.[27, 28] Blood supply to these *surgical flaps* is maintained by keeping their vascular pedicle intact. On CT, the flaps are visualized as vascu-

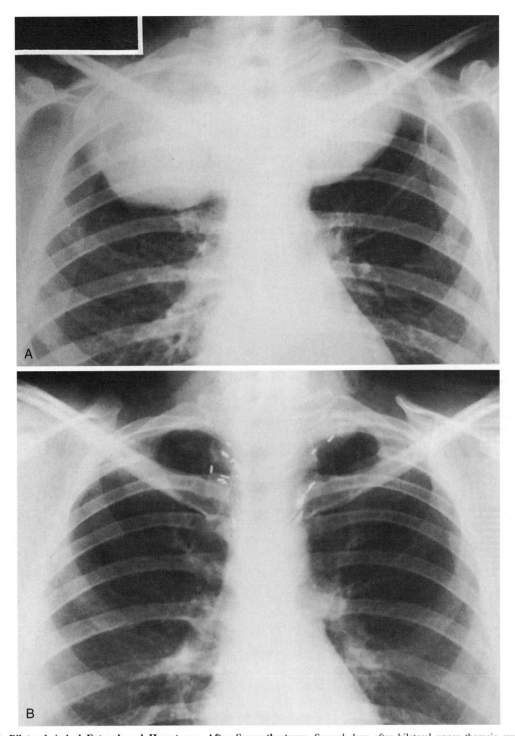

Figure 19–2. Bilateral Apical Extrapleural Hematomas After Sympathectomy. Several days after bilateral upper thoracic sympathectomy, a radiograph *(A)* shows sharply defined homogeneous masses occupying the apical portion of both hemithoraces (preoperative radiograph was normal). Three months later *(B)*, the hematomas had resolved completely.

larized structures that, depending on their nature, have soft tissue or adipose tissue attenuation.[27, 28]

Position of the mediastinum is one of the most important indicators of pulmonary abnormality during the postoperative period. Displacement may occur toward or away from the side of the thoracotomy. Ipsilateral displacement is an expected finding after lobectomy or pneumonectomy. In the former situation, it is temporary, and the normal midline position is regained as the remainder of the lung undergoes compensatory overinflation. Excessive displacement toward the operated side may be a sign of atelectasis in the ipsilateral lung. In the case of pneumonectomy, ipsilateral mediastinal displacement is progressive and permanent (*see* farther on). Mediastinal displacement away from the oper-

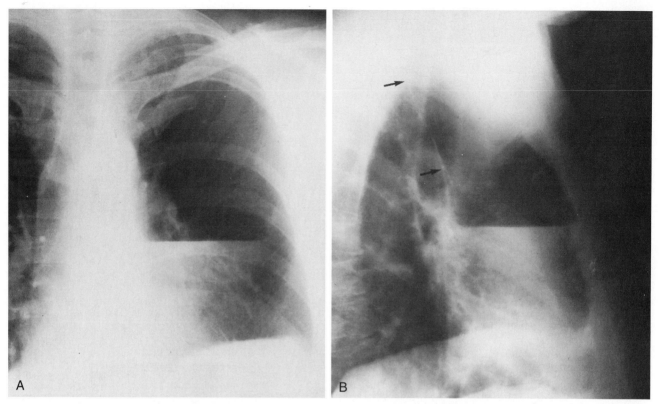

Figure 19–3. Loculated Hydropneumothorax After Lobectomy. Posteroanterior *(A)* and lateral *(B)* radiographs show a large loculated collection of gas and fluid in the anterior portion of the left hemithorax (the upper half of the lower lobe major fissure is indicated by *arrows* in *B*). These films were made about 2 weeks after left upper lobectomy; the persistence of pneumothorax was caused by an air leak from lower lobe parenchyma. Several weeks were required for spontaneous absorption.

ated side may occur as a result of atelectasis in the contralateral lung or an accumulation of excessive fluid or gas in the ipsilateral pleural space.

The changes on chest radiograph after pneumonectomy were assessed in one review of 110 cases.[8] Within 24 hours of the procedure, the ipsilateral pleural space is air containing, the mediastinum is shifted slightly to the ipsilateral side, and the hemidiaphragm is elevated slightly (Fig. 19–4). The postpneumonectomy space begins to fill with fluid in a progressive and predictable manner at a rate of about two rib spaces per day. In most cases, there is 80% to 90% obliteration of the space at the end of 2 weeks and complete obliteration by 2 to 4 months. Such obliteration occurs as a result of fluid accumulation as well as by progressive ipsilateral displacement of the mediastinum and elevation of the hemidiaphragm. Mediastinal displacement is an almost invariable finding and constitutes the most reliable indicator of a normal postoperative course. It generally requires 6 to 8 months to reach its maximum. Failure of the mediastinum to shift in the postoperative period almost always indicates an abnormality in the postpneumonectomy space, regardless of the character or level of the air-fluid interface.

The postpneumonectomy space tends to fill more rapidly on the left than on the right and when the pneumonectomy is extrapleural (i.e., when it includes the parietal pleura).[8] In one study, the character of the fluid level was found to have little or no diagnostic or prognostic significance; the contour of the air-fluid interface was less important than the appearance of bubbles or a drop in the level of fluid

by more than 2 cm. The hallmark of a normal course of events after pneumonectomy was progressive shift of the mediastinum to the operative side, associated with compensatory overinflation of the contralateral lung (*see* Fig. 19–4). The absence of such a shift in the immediate postoperative period indicated the presence of bronchopleural fistula, empyema (Fig. 19–5), hemorrhage, or (occasionally) chylothorax.

The most sensitive indicator of late complications was a return to the midline of a previously shifted mediastinum, particularly the tracheal air column.[8] This movement indicated the presence within the postpneumonectomy space of recurrent neoplasm, bronchopleural fistula, hemorrhage, chylothorax, or empyema. In some patients who have recurrent carcinoma after pneumonectomy, conventional radiographs do not manifest signs of such an expanding process within the ipsilateral hemithorax. In these cases, CT can be of great value in documenting tumor recurrence, either as enlarged mediastinal lymph nodes or as a soft tissue mass projecting into the near–water density postpneumonectomy space.[29]

CT is helpful in the assessment of patients who have suspected postpneumonectomy empyema. Although a shift of the trachea and mediastinal contents back to midline and a sudden appearance of an air-fluid level on radiograph are helpful clues to the diagnosis, they are present in only a few cases. For example, in one series of nine patients who had late-onset postpneumonectomy empyema, only one had shift of the trachea toward the remaining lung.[30] On CT scan, the mediastinal border of the postpneumonec-

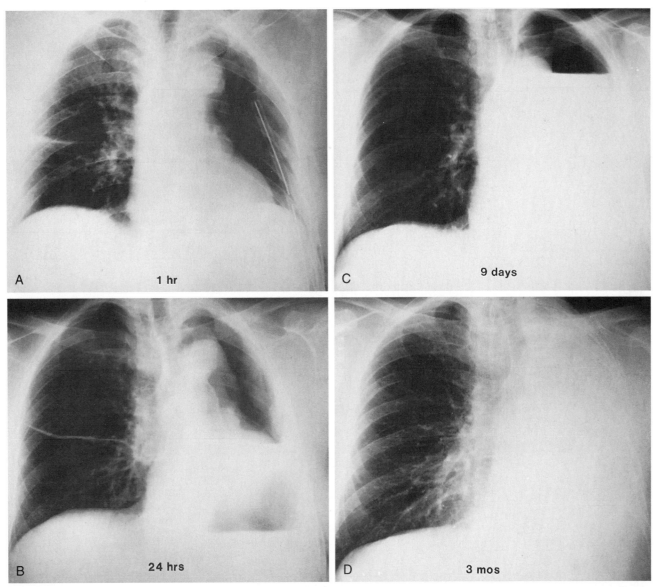

Figure 19–4. Postpneumonectomy Course: Normal. Anteroposterior radiograph obtained in the supine position at the bedside 1 hour after left pneumonectomy *(A)* shows a slight reduction in the volume of the left hemithorax. The space is air-filled, and the mediastinum is in the midline. After 24 hours, radiograph in the erect position *(B)* shows moderate elevation of the left hemidiaphragm (as indicated by the gastric air bubble), a moderate shift of the mediastinum to the left, and a prominent air-fluid level in the plane of the third interspace anteriorly. By 9 days *(C)*, fluid has filled about two thirds of the cavity of the left hemithorax, but the mediastinum still is displaced to the left (note the curvature of the tracheal air column). By 3 months *(D)*, the left hemithorax has become completely airless. Note the persistent shift of the mediastinum to the left and the prominent curve of the air column of the trachea.

tomy space normally has a concave margin;[15] loss of this margin with development of convex expansion of the post-pneumonectomy space has been described as a characteristic finding of empyema.[15]

A rare but potentially catastrophic event is herniation of the heart through a pericardial defect after radical pneumonectomy in which partial pericardiectomy has been carried out or in which intrapericardial ligation of pulmonary vessels has been performed.[31, 179] Only 50 cases had been reported by 1997.[7] The herniation occurs at the end of the surgical procedure or in the immediate postoperative period.[7] It may occur on either side and frequently is associated with the abrupt onset of circulatory collapse or superior vena cava obstruction. Radiologically the appearance

varies with the side on which the pneumonectomy has been performed: If on the right, the heart is dextrorotated into the right hemithorax, producing an unmistakable appearance;[32, 33] when on the left, the heart may rotate posteriorly or laterally, and herniation usually is less evident, particularly if there is a sizable accumulation of pleural fluid. On the left side, an indentation or notch may become apparent between the great vessels and the heart, simulating the appearance of congenital absence of the left side of the pericardium. An early sign of right cardiac herniation is a focal convex bulge in the right heart border (*snow cone sign*), which represents herniation of a portion of the right atrium through a pericardial defect.[179, 180] In the correct clinical setting, this grave complication should be readily

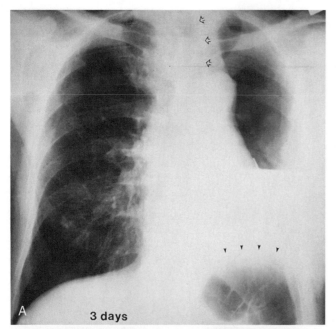

3 days

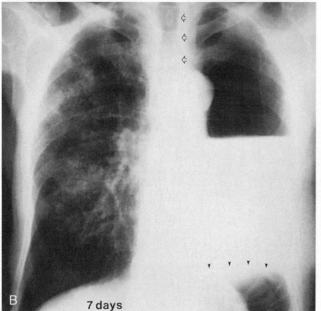

7 days

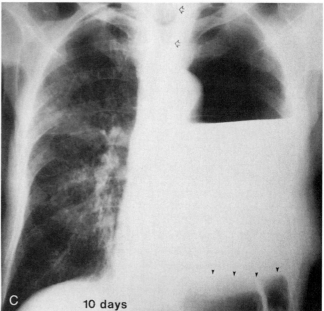

10 days

Figure 19–5. Postpneumonectomy Course Complicated by Empyema. Three days after left pneumonectomy *(A)*, the amount of fluid that has accumulated, the position of the left hemidiaphragm *(arrowheads)*, and the shift of the tracheal air column to the left *(open arrows)* all are consistent with a normal postoperative course (compare with Fig. 19–4). At 7 days *(B)*, the left hemidiaphragm *(arrowheads)* has undergone some depression, and the tracheal air column *(open arrows)* has returned to the midline. Such a change should suggest empyema, bronchopleural fistula, pleural hemorrhage, or (possibly) chylothorax. By 10 days *(C)*, the left hemidiaphragm *(arrowheads)* has become concave superiorly, and the mediastinum and tracheal air column *(open arrows)* have shifted farther to the right.

recognizable radiologically, leading to life-saving thoracotomy.[34] The diagnosis can be confirmed by thoracoscopy.[35]

Another rare complication of pneumonectomy is proximal bronchial obstruction resulting from excessive mediastinal shift and rotation, a condition known as *postpneumonectomy syndrome* (Fig. 19–6).[37, 181] This complication tends to occur a long time after surgery (often <12 months but occasionally 37 years[36]).[37] The condition typically follows right pneumonectomy and is seen most commonly in children and adolescents.[181] Radiographic manifestations after right pneumonectomy include marked rightward and posterior displacement of the mediastinum, clockwise rotation of the heart and great vessels, and displacement of the overinflated left lung into the anterior portion of the right hemithorax. As a result of the rotation of the heart and

great vessels, the distal trachea and left main bronchus become compressed between the aorta and pulmonary artery, with resulting dyspnea and recurrent left-sided pneumonia. Another radiographic manifestation is hyperinflation as a result of air-trapping.[181] Rarely, postpneumonectomy syndrome develops after left pneumonectomy.[37–39] Marked rotation of the mediastinal structures to the left and herniation of the right lung into the left hemithorax in these cases is associated with narrowing of the right upper lobe and right middle lobe bronchi or the bronchus intermedius as they are splayed anterior to the spine.[39] The bronchus intermedius may be compressed between the right pulmonary artery anteriorly and the vertebral body posteriorly.[39] CT can facilitate identification of the syndrome.[36, 39] CT shows the extent and severity of bronchial narrowing and extrinsic compression.[181]

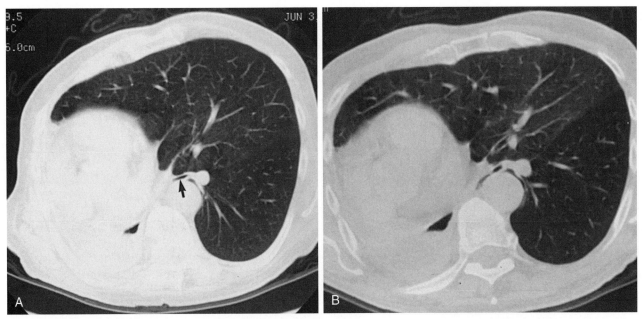

Figure 19–6. Postpneumonectomy Syndrome. CT scan performed at end-inspiration *(A)* shows narrowing of the left lower lobe bronchus *(arrow)*. Expiratory CT scan *(B)* shows decreased attenuation and vascularity in the left lower lobe as a result of air-trapping. (Case courtesy of Dr. Fred Matzinger, Department of Radiology, The Ottawa Civic Hospital, Ottawa, Canada.)

Diaphragm

The value of diaphragmatic position in the assessment of postoperative chest radiograph depends largely on the position of the patient at the time of radiography. In the supine position, the normally higher position of the right hemidiaphragm is accentuated, presumably because of the mass of the liver; this must not be mistaken for evidence of intrathoracic abnormality. With the patient erect, the usual rules regarding diaphragmatic position pertain.

After pneumonectomy or lobectomy, the ipsilateral hemidiaphragm almost invariably is elevated during the first few days. With pneumonectomy, this elevation persists along with ipsilateral mediastinal shift, despite accumulation of fluid in the pleural space; with lobectomy, elevation and mediastinal displacement disappear during a period of several days or weeks as the remainder of the ipsilateral lung undergoes compensatory overinflation. Marked elevation of a hemidiaphragm can result from injury to the phrenic nerve sustained during surgery. Elevation can be caused by many pathologic states within the lungs, including atelectasis, bronchopneumonia, and thromboembolism. Depression of one hemidiaphragm is an uncommon postoperative abnormality and invariably is caused by a massive pneumothorax or hydrothorax.

Lungs

The radiographic changes in the lungs that can be anticipated after thoracotomy depend on the nature of the surgical procedure. For example, after lobectomy, there is a predictable pattern of reorientation of the remaining lobe or lobes that rotate and hyperinflate to occupy the residual space.[40] The rearrangement of fissures resulting from reorientation of lobes should not be misinterpreted as evidence of atelectasis. Similarly the vascular markings become more widely spaced, and lung density is reduced as a result of compensatory overinflation, signs that must not be confused with signs resulting from atelectasis or from reduced perfusion as a result of thromboembolism. Hematoma formation is common after wedge or segmental resection and results from hemorrhage at the site of excision (Fig. 19–7). Provided that the radiologist is aware of the type of surgical procedure carried out, these ominous-looking, yet clinically insignificant, opacities should present little difficulty in diagnosis.

Any local pulmonary opacity identified in the postoperative period must be regarded as one of the *big four*—atelectasis, pneumonia, infarction, or edema. The manifestations of these complications are no different from those that develop in a nonsurgical setting. As might be anticipated, diffuse pulmonary edema is much more common in patients who have undergone cardiac surgery. Additional rare complications of thoracic surgery include pulmonary herniation and torsion.

Atelectasis

The most common pulmonary complication of surgical procedures is atelectasis, whether the surgery is thoracic or abdominal.[23] The abnormality varies widely in extent, in some cases affecting an entire lobe and in others many lobular units, whose airlessness causes insufficient density to be appreciated radiographically. In the latter circumstance, atelectasis may be evidenced only by alterations in lung function and gas exchange.[41] The mechanisms by which postoperative atelectasis develops also vary considerably. The most common cause is probably mucous plugging, which occurs chiefly as a result of diminished diaphragmatic excursion (caused by splinting as a result of pain).[41] Disruption of mucociliary clearance has been documented after major surgery.[42]

Atelectasis is the most common complication after lo-

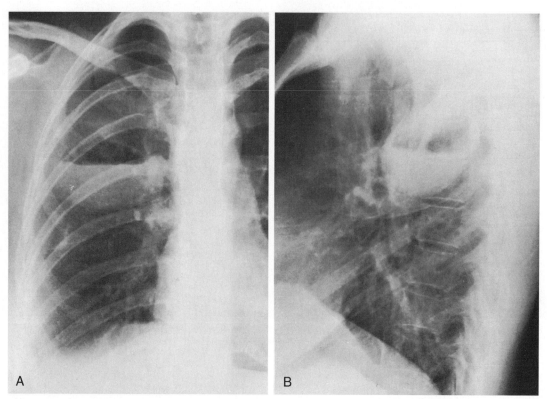

Figure 19–7. Postoperative Pulmonary Hematoma. Views of the right hemithorax from posteroanterior *(A)* and lateral *(B)* radiographs show a large, well-defined circular shadow in the upper portion of the right lung, possessing a prominent air-fluid level. It is thin walled. These radiographs were made about 3 days after wedge resection of a bulla of the right upper lobe. The shadow represents an accumulation of blood and gas in the bare area after resection. During a period of 4 weeks, the hematoma underwent slow but progressive resolution and left no significant residuum. The patient was a 39-year-old woman.

bectomy, and various degrees are present in 60% of cases.[43] In one review of radiographic findings in 218 patients undergoing lobectomy or bilobectomy, 8% were found to have developed complete ipsilateral lobar or bilobar collapse with whiteout of the involved lobe or lobes and mediastinal shift.[43] Patients who had severe atelectasis had significantly longer intensive care unit and hospital stays than patients who did not have complications. Right upper lobectomy, alone or in combination with middle lobectomy, was associated with a fivefold greater incidence of severe atelectasis than all other types of resection.

A common abnormality that occurs postoperatively in patients who have undergone cardiopulmonary bypass for open heart surgical procedures is left lower lobe atelectasis, usually seen as a homogeneous opacity behind the heart and often associated with an air bronchogram (Fig. 19–8). Right lower lobe atelectasis may occur but is less common and less severe. In one review of radiographs from 99 patients, atelectasis was identified in 84;[23] the abnormality involved the left lower lobe in 40, both lower lobes in 43, and only the right lower lobe in one. In another series of 57 patients who had undergone coronary artery bypass surgery, review of daily chest radiographs showed evidence of left lower lobe atelectasis at some time between surgery and discharge in about 90% and right lower lobe atelectasis in 60%.[44] The atelectasis increased progressively until the fourth postoperative day, then gradually improved; it was more severe in the left lower lobe than the right on all postoperative days.

The left and right lower lobe atelectasis appear to cause little clinical disability and are such a frequent finding after bypass surgery that they can be regarded as an expected part of a satisfactory postoperative appearance. Small pleural effusions are seen in most of these patients.

Edema

Pulmonary edema, usually mild, is seen in most patients immediately after cardiac surgery.[22] It may be caused by fluid overload, intrinsic left ventricular dysfunction, or increased capillary permeability related to cardiopulmonary bypass.[22] The edema usually resolves within 24 to 48 hours. Pulmonary edema may occur after lung surgery as a result of fluid overload, congestive heart failure, thromboembolism, or adult respiratory distress syndrome (ARDS) secondary to aspiration, pneumonia, or sepsis.[45] Occasionally, no cause is apparent. The latter situation is known as *postpneumonectomy pulmonary edema* and has a high mortality rate.[45]

Miscellaneous Complications

An uncommon complication of thoracotomy, video-assisted thoracoscopic surgery, or chest tube drainage is herniation of lung through the surgical defect.[46, 47, 182] Such hernias may not be detectable on conventional chest radiographs performed at end-inspiration but usually are shown readily on radiographs performed at end-expiration, during

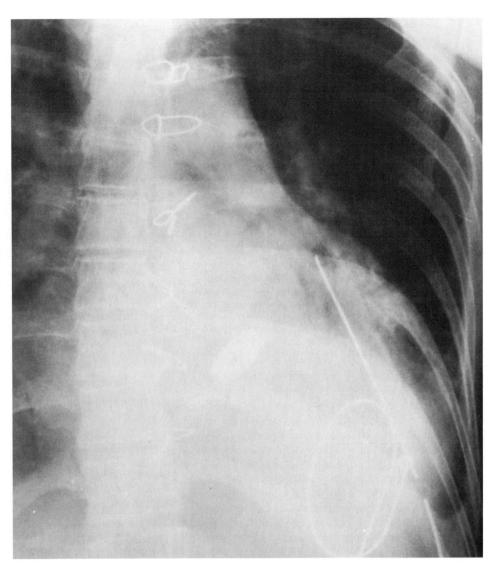

Figure 19–8. Adhesive Atelectasis of the Left Lower Lobe After Open Heart Surgery. View of the left lung from anteroposterior radiograph exposed at the patient's bedside shows airlessness and loss of volume of much of the left lower lobe associated with a prominent air bronchogram. Such an appearance is so common after open heart surgery that it represents an expected finding.

cough, or during a Valsalva maneuver or on CT scan (Fig. 19–9). Lung hernias may be congenital or result from direct trauma, lifting heavy weights, or playing wind instruments.[46]

Another rare complication of thoracotomy is torsion of a lobe or lung.[48, 49] Early recognition is essential because complete 180-degree torsion leads to infarction.[49] Lobar torsion occurs most commonly after lobectomy but may be seen after wedge resection, severance of pleural adhesions, pleurectomy, or lung transplantation.[49–51] The radiologic findings consist of atelectasis resulting from airway obstruction, abnormal positioning and orientation of pulmonary vessels and bronchi within the atelectatic lobe, abnormal position of the hilum in relation to the atelectatic lobe, and rapid expansion of an abnormally located consolidated lobe.[49–51] CT shows twisting and narrowing or occlusion of the bronchus as well as abnormal orientation of the pulmonary vessels and delayed opacification after intravenous administration of contrast material.[51, 52] Fusiform tapering of the pulmonary artery is particularly well seen on angiography.[52]

Occasionally a surgical swab or sponge is left in the chest accidentally after thoracotomy.[183, 184] Radiologic diagnosis is facilitated by the incorporation of radiopaque markers (Fig. 19–10). The marker may be misinterpreted as an area of calcification, however.[183] The radiographic and CT appearance is variable depending on the site of the retained sponge and chronicity.[53, 184] Rarely, it serves as a focus for the development of infection. Retained pleural sponges may result in infolding of the lung and a masslike lesion or cavity that can resemble an intrapulmonary abscess on CT scan.[183]

The pulmonary artery or bronchial stumps left after pneumonectomy can be the site of a process that leads to subsequent intrathoracic disease. Thrombosis of the artery stump is common and usually innocuous; rarely, however, it may embolize to the residual lung and lead to radiologic and clinical findings (Fig. 19–11). *Aspergillus* species can colonize the bronchial stump and grow into a fungus ball;[54, 55] extension of the organism across the wall into the adjacent pleural space has been followed by empyema.

COMPLICATIONS OF NONTHORACIC SURGERY

The major thoracic complications of abdominal surgery are atelectasis, pneumonia, thromboembolism, subphrenic

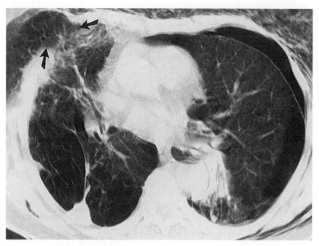

Figure 19–9. Lung Hernia. CT scan in a 74-year-old man shows herniation of a portion of the right lung *(arrows)* through a defect in the chest wall. The patient had undergone right thoracotomy and bullectomy several years previously and was being evaluated for recurrent left pneumothorax. Emphysema and scarring in both lungs, left lower lobe atelectasis, left pneumothorax, and subcutaneous emphysema are evident.

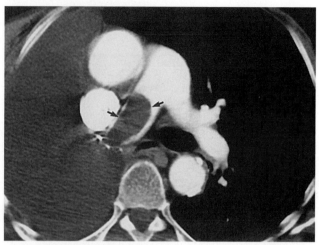

Figure 19–11. Thrombus in Pulmonary Artery Stump. A 79-year-old woman presented with a history of recurrent episodes of dyspnea after right pneumonectomy. Confirmation of the clinical diagnosis of recurrent pulmonary thromboembolism was made by ventilation-perfusion scintigraphy. Contrast-enhanced spiral CT scan shows thrombus *(arrows)* within the right pulmonary artery stump, presumed to be the site of origin of the recurrent emboli. (Courtesy of Dr. J. Stephen Kwong, Richmond General Hospital, Richmond, British Columbia.)

abscess, cardiogenic pulmonary edema, and ARDS.[56–58] The reported incidence of such complications has varied from about 20% to 75%;[59] series associated with the higher figures undoubtedly have included patients who had radiographic abnormalities of little clinical significance.

As discussed previously, atelectasis is the most common complication of surgery and in most patients is related to airway mucous plugging. The process may be complicated by infection;[59] with and without such infection, the separation of atelectasis from pneumonia in the postoperative setting can be difficult because symptoms of cough, sputum production, and fever do not permit an accurate distinction of one from the other.[59] The radiographic and clinical features of acute pneumonia and pulmonary thromboembo-

lism are no different from those observed in other clinical settings. Subphrenic abscess, although uncommon, almost always is a complication of abdominal surgery; its clinical signs (pain in the hypochondrium, limitation of respiratory motion, and fever), timing (10 days after surgery), and radiographic manifestations (pleural effusion and diaphragmatic elevation) do not allow its easy distinction from thromboembolism.

COMPLICATIONS OF THERAPEUTIC PROCEDURES

Tracheostomy

Tracheal stenosis, tracheomalacia, and tracheal perforation are well-recognized complications of tracheostomy. The first of these is the most common and can occur at the level of the stoma or at the site at which an endotracheal tube impinged on the mucosa. The radiologic manifestations are discussed in Chapter 15.

Airway and Vascular Stents

Expandable metal or silicone stents have been used in the definitive or (more often) palliative therapy of many intrathoracic diseases.[60] The most common has been carcinoma, usually pulmonary[61, 62] and occasionally esophageal.[63] Benign conditions causing airway stenosis, including airway compression secondary to congenital pulmonary artery aneurysm,[64] relapsing polychondritis,[65] tuberculosis,[66] postpneumonectomy syndrome,[67] and lung transplantation,[68] also have been treated in this manner. Stenting of vascular stenoses that have resulted from congenital cardiovascular disease,[69, 70] thromboemboli,[71] or lung transplantation[72] has been used.

The incidence of complications associated with these stents is low. In one study of four patients who had wire

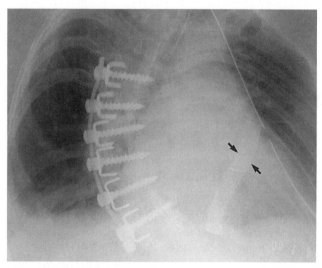

Figure 19–10. Retained Sponge. Anteroposterior chest radiograph in a 42-year-old woman who had fever 3 days after left thoracotomy and extensive thoracic spine surgery shows a radiopaque sponge *(arrows)* in left pleural space. The patient recovered uneventfully after removal of the sponge.

stents inserted into the trachea or main bronchi for the control of tracheobronchial malacia, strut fracture and progressive airway widening were observed and suggested the possibility of airway perforation.[73] The formation of obstructing granulation tissue or mucous webs has been reported by some investigators.[74] Erosion of an esophageal stent into a bronchus has been associated with the development of recurrent pneumonia.[75] Recurrent vascular stenosis secondary to intimal fibrosis at the stent site has been reported in a few patients.[69] Focal pulmonary edema has been documented during stent insertion into a stenotic pulmonary artery.[76]

Pulmonary hemorrhage after coronary artery stent placement has been reported. In one study of 88 patients, the complication was diagnosed in 4 (5%);[77] the authors speculated it was related to anticoagulation therapy given to prevent stent thrombosis.

Brachytherapy

Complications of brachytherapy include mucosal fibrosis with bronchostenosis, localized radiation pneumonitis, bronchoesophageal fistula, and hemoptysis (*see* Chapter 17).[78, 79]

Esophageal Procedures

Esophageal rupture occurs most commonly as a complication of esophagoscopy or gastroscopy[80] but also follows a variety of therapeutic procedures, such as dilation of a stricture or achalasia, esophageal resection and anastomosis (followed by disruption of the suture line), variceal sclerotherapy, or (rarely) passage of an esophageal obturator airway by paramedical personnel during cardiopulmonary resuscitation.[81, 185] About 75% of esophageal ruptures are the result of such iatrogenic interventions; perforation occurs in 0.1% of all esophageal endoscopies, 5% of esophageal dilations, and 10% to 35% of Sengstaken-Blakemore tube placements.[82, 83] The most common sites of perforation are below the cricopharyngeal muscle, at the level of the left main bronchus, and immediately above the gastroesophageal junction.[82] Rupture can be associated with fistulas from the esophagus to the pleura, mediastinum, or bronchi, with corresponding consequences.

The usual result of esophageal rupture is acute mediastinitis, manifested radiographically by mediastinal widening that typically possesses a smooth, sharply defined margin. Other manifestations include pneumomediastinum, left pleural effusion, pneumothorax, hydropneumothorax, and chylothorax (Fig. 19–12).[84]

COMPLICATIONS OF INTUBATION AND MONITORING APPARATUS

Chest Drainage Tubes

Complications of chest drainage tubes are uncommon and usually are readily apparent clinically.[85, 89] They include

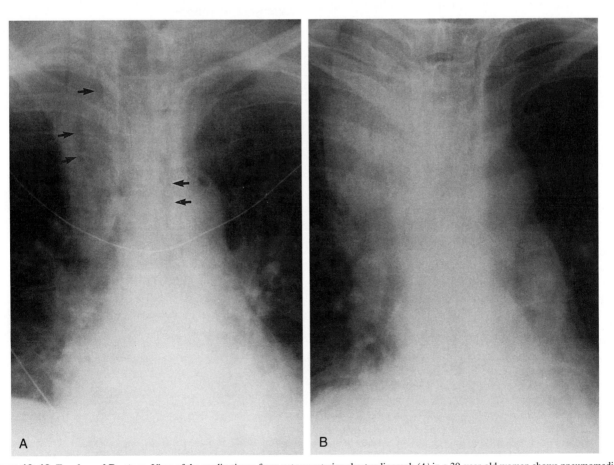

Figure 19–12. Esophageal Rupture. View of the mediastinum from anteroposterior chest radiograph *(A)* in a 39-year-old woman shows pneumomediastinum *(arrows)* and mild mediastinal widening. Radiograph taken 5 days later *(B)* shows increased mediastinal widening. Esophageal rupture at the level of the T1 vertebral body, which occurred during attempted endotracheal intubation, was confirmed by Gastrografin swallow.

Table 19–3. COMPLICATIONS OF CHEST DRAINAGE TUBES

Laceration of intercostal artery or vein
Laceration of diaphragm, liver, spleen, or stomach
Pulmonary perforation
Empyema
Systemic-to-pulmonary artery shunt
Perforation of right ventricle

laceration of an intercostal artery or vein; laceration of the diaphragm, liver, spleen, or stomach; malposition of the tube (such as in the chest wall, abdomen, or interlobar fissure); pulmonary perforation; infection (predominantly empyema); formation of a systemic artery-to-pulmonary artery shunt; and perforation of the right ventricle (Table 19–3).[86, 87, 186]

Hemorrhage from a lacerated intercostal vessel can be avoided by insertion of the tube in the intercostal space as close as possible to the superior surface of a rib; however, intercostal vessels may be tortuous, especially in the elderly, and insertion elsewhere carries a risk.[86] Laceration of an intercostal vessel can occur during insertion of a needle into the chest.

Malposition of the chest tube can occur within the pleural space, in which case the complication is one of inadequate drainage. Such malposition can occur in several ways. For example, a tube inserted anterolaterally and directed posteriorly drains the posterior pleural space but, with the patient lying in a supine position, does not drain a pneumothorax situated anteriorly. A drainage tube in any position would not drain a loculated accumulation of fluid or gas in an area not in communication with the tube's holes. The incidence of malposition of a chest tube within a major fissure probably is higher than generally believed.[88–90] Such malposition often cannot be recognized convincingly on a single anteroposterior radiograph; however, when drainage of a pneumothorax or hydrothorax is not occurring satisfactorily, the abnormal position can be confirmed, if necessary, by lateral radiography. In some cases, suboptimal tube positioning may be unrecognized even when frontal and lateral radiographs are obtained.[91] CT may show unexpected tube malplacement, including extrapleural location, intraparenchymal course, transdiaphragmatic course, trans-splenic course, and impingement on the trachea or posterior mediastinum.[92]

Although drainage of chest tubes placed within interlobar fissures may be suboptimal,[90] there is evidence that it is adequate in most cases. In one prospective study of 58 consecutive patients who presented to the emergency department with chest trauma requiring tube thoracostomy, assessment of frontal and lateral radiographs showed 58% of tubes to be within an interlobar fissure;[93] no significant difference was found in the duration of thoracoscopy drainage, need for further tubes, or need for surgical intervention between patients whose tubes were located within a fissure and other patients. As the authors pointed out, however, these observations would be applicable to patients who have trauma or transudate and would not be relevant for patients who have empyema. In the latter situation, adhesions and loculation develop rapidly, and precise tube

placement is important. Although only frontal radiographs are required for assessment of chest tube location in most patients, frontal and lateral radiographs are recommended after every tube insertion for empyema unless the tube was placed under CT or ultrasound guidance.[93]

Pulmonary perforation rarely is recognized radiographically as a complication of tube insertion[85, 189] but can be detected on CT.[92] CT shows the intraparenchymal location of the tube as well as the presence of associated laceration and hematoma (Fig. 19–13).[92] Care must be taken, however, in assessing the lung periphery, particularly near the lung apex and diaphragm, where partial volume averaging and indentation of the lung by a chest tube in the pleural space may mimic perforation.[92]

Abdominal Drainage Tubes

Potentially serious complications can follow transgression of the pleural space during placement of interventional drainage catheters into the liver and upper abdomen.[94, 95] Two groups of investigators have emphasized the importance of not puncturing the ninth intercostal space in the midaxillary line because needles inserted through this interspace have traversed the pleura in virtually all cadaver studies.[94, 95] Complications of percutaneous catheter drainage of an abdominal abscess through the intercostal space include hemothorax, pneumothorax, and empyema.[95, 96]

Nasogastric Tubes

Because most nasogastric tubes are opaque, any malposition should be readily apparent radiographically. The two most common abnormalities are coiling within the esophagus and incomplete insertion; in each situation, the function of the nasogastric tube is not being served. Of far greater clinical importance is the faulty insertion of the nasogastric tube into the tracheobronchial tree rather than into the esophagus. This complication that has been reported in about 0.2% to 0.3% of feeding tube placements[97–99] and

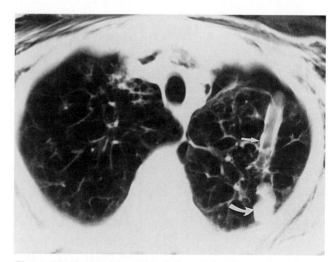

Figure 19–13. Intraparenchymal Chest Tube. CT scan in a 69-year-old patient shows a left chest tube *(straight arrow)* with its tip in the left upper lobe; a small hematoma *(curved arrow)* is present. Severe emphysema, a small left pneumothorax, pneumomediastinum, and subcutaneous emphysema are evident.

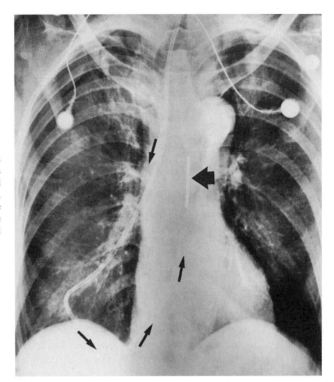

Figure 19–14. Faulty Insertion of a Feeding Tube. The circuitous course taken by this feeding tube can be established only partly from this anteroposterior radiograph. It passed into the right lower lobe. As it turned to the left, it presumably penetrated the visceral pleura covering this lobe, then passed superiorly either within the mediastinum or in the pleural space adjacent to the azygoesophageal recess to a point where its tip overlies the region of the tracheal carina *(large arrow).* The patient suffered no ill effects after removal of the tube.

can lead to intrabronchial infusion of feedings, pneumonia, lung abscess, pneumothorax, hydropneumothorax, and empyema.[100–102] In these cases, the tip of the tube sometimes ends up in an unusual location, such as the mediastinum (Fig. 19–14) or abdomen. Such malposition can be particularly hazardous if the tube is meant for hyperalimentation, in which case fluid is injected into the lungs or pleural cavity, rather than the stomach (Fig. 19–15).

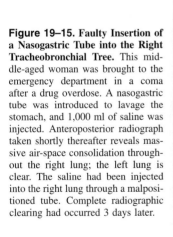

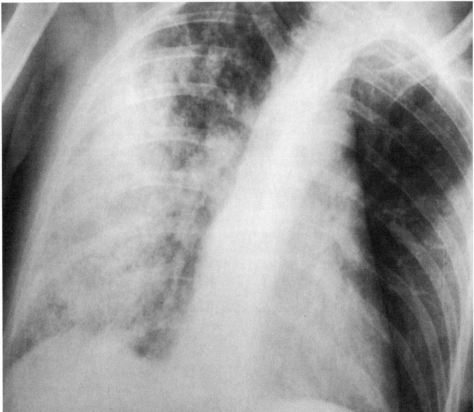

Figure 19–15. Faulty Insertion of a Nasogastric Tube into the Right Tracheobronchial Tree. This middle-aged woman was brought to the emergency department in a coma after a drug overdose. A nasogastric tube was introduced to lavage the stomach, and 1,000 ml of saline was injected. Anteroposterior radiograph taken shortly thereafter reveals massive air-space consolidation throughout the right lung; the left lung is clear. The saline had been injected into the right lung through a malpositioned tube. Complete radiographic clearing had occurred 3 days later.

Despite the presence of inflatable cuffs on endotracheal tubes, the low pressure within them does not prevent passage of the tube into the distal airways.[103] A patient receiving mechanical ventilation in whom a feeding tube has been placed inadvertently in the tracheobronchial tree close to the pleural surface is in danger of developing a large pneumothorax on removal of the tube.[104] In this situation, the attending physician or surgeon should be warned that the feeding tube may be acting as a *finger in the dike* and that insertion of a thoracostomy tube into the pleural space may be advisable before the feeding tube is withdrawn. Inadvertent placement of feeding tubes into the tracheobronchial tree, with subsequent insertion into the pleural space, appears to be a particular complication of the use of the narrow-bore nasogastric tube with stylet[101, 105] and is most apt to occur in patients with impaired mental status or diminished gag, cough, or swallowing reflexes.[106]

Endotracheal Tubes

During the first few days after insertion of an endotracheal tube, serious complications are infrequent; they occur more often in association with emergency resuscitation than with more routine interventions.[107] The chief complication is large airway obstruction resulting from placement of the tube too low in the trachea or in the proximal bronchi. In most instances, the tube enters the right main bronchus (in 27 of 28 cases in one series[107]), and the orifice of the left main bronchus is occluded by the balloon cuff of the endotracheal tube, resulting in complete obstruction and atelectasis of the left lung. If the tube is advanced sufficiently into the right main bronchus, the right upper lobe bronchus also may be occluded, resulting in atelectasis of this lobe as well as the left lung or of the right upper lobe alone.[107] Occasionally the tube enters the left rather than the right main bronchus, leading to atelectasis of the right lung.

The rate at which atelectasis occurs depends on the gas content of the lung at the moment of occlusion. Total collapse requires 18 to 24 hours if the parenchyma is air-containing but may occur in a matter of minutes if the lung contains 100% oxygen (often the case in acute respiratory emergencies). Withdrawal of the tube typically results in rapid re-expansion of the collapsed lung or lobe.

With the head and neck in a neutral position, the ideal distance between the tip of the endotracheal tube and the carina is 5 $\pm$ 2 cm.[108] Flexion and extension of the neck cause a 2-cm descent and ascent of the tip of the endotracheal tube; if the position of the neck can be established from radiograph (through visualization of the mandible), the ideal distance between the tip of the endotracheal tube and the carina should be 3 $\pm$ 2 cm with the neck flexed and 7 $\pm$ 2 cm with the neck extended.[108] When the carina is not visualized, it is sufficient to establish the relationship of the tip of the endotracheal tube to the fifth, sixth, or seventh thoracic vertebral bodies; this relationship pertained in 92 of 100 patients whose bedside chest radiographs were reviewed in one study.[109]

Malpositioning of an endotracheal tube in the esophagus is uncommon and usually is evident clinically. Because the trachea and esophagus are superimposed on anteroposterior radiograph, such malpositioning is seldom apparent radiographically; when present, findings include projection of the tip of the endotracheal tube lateral to the trachea, gaseous distention of the distal esophagus or stomach, and (rarely) deviation of the trachea by an overinflated balloon cuff (Fig. 19–16).[110] Complications that result from prolonged inflation of the cuff of an endotracheal tube, such as tracheal stenosis, are discussed in Chapter 15.

Transtracheal Catheters

The use of long-term indwelling transtracheal catheters to administer oxygen to patients who have chronic obstructive pulmonary disease was developed in the 1980s to cut the cost and increase the ease of home oxygen care.[112] The catheters may be inserted directly into the trachea through the skin of the neck (percutaneous catheters) or may be implanted through an incision in the suprasternal notch, stitched to the tracheal wall, and tunneled under the skin to exit in the upper abdomen (tunneled catheters).[111]

Complications associated with these catheters include subcutaneous emphysema, localized skin infection or hemorrhage, abnormal tracheal mucus production, breakage of catheter parts into the trachea, and formation of partly occlusive mucous or mucopurulent plugs around the catheter tip.[112, 113] Increase in the size or dislodgment of such a plug may result in tracheal or bronchial obstruction that can compromise air flow significantly.[113, 114]

Percutaneous Central Venous Catheters

Several reviews of the literature have been published on the complications of central venous catheterization,[115, 116, 187] highlighting their great variety and potentially serious consequences. Some complications pertain to the catheterization procedure itself and relate to abnormalities within or around the catheterized vein; others, perhaps most, arise from incorrect positioning of the tip of the catheter.

Faulty Insertion

Central venous catheters can be inserted through an arm vein, a subclavian vein (by either an infraclavicular or supraclavicular route), or an external or internal jugular vein. Most faulty placements occur in arm and infraclavicular subclavian approaches. Only about 65% to 75% of catheters reach their proper location after arm vein insertion; the results through external jugular placement are less satisfactory.[118] Supraclavicular, subclavian, and internal jugular approaches result in a relatively small percentage of improper placements. In one review, only 186 (62%) of 300 central venous lines were positioned in the subclavian or innominate veins or superior vena cava at the time of initial chest radiograph obtained immediately after catheterization.[119] Of the remainder, 48 (16%) were in the internal jugular vein (Fig. 19–17), 39 (13%) in the right atrium or right ventricle, 2 in the azygous vein, 1 in a left-sided superior vena cava that drained into the coronary sinus, and 2 coiled in the subclavian vein; 22 were in extrathoracic sites other than the internal jugular vein. In none of these cases was the incorrect position recognized clinically.

Phlebothrombosis

Phlebothrombosis is probably the most common complication of venous catheterization and can be manifested

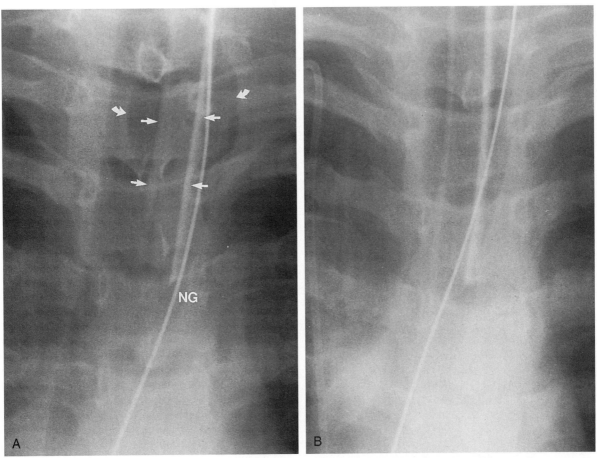

Figure 19–16. Esophageal Intubation. View of the thoracic inlet from anteroposterior chest radiograph *(A)* in a 22-year-old patient after a motor vehicle accident shows an endotracheal tube *(straight arrows)* lying lateral to the trachea and in close proximity to the nasogastric tube (NG); the appearance is consistent with esophageal intubation. Note the inflated cuff of endotracheal tube *(curved arrows)*. View after reintubation *(B)* shows a normal endotracheal position.

in two ways: sleeve thrombosis and mural thrombosis.[115] Autopsy studies have shown that circumferential fibrin sleeves develop around indwelling venous catheters 24 hours after insertion in 80% to 100% of cases.[120, 121] Although this condition seldom gives rise to complications, parts of the thrombus may embolize to the lungs, particularly as the catheter is removed.[115, 121, 122]

Mural thrombosis can lead to partial or complete venous obstruction.[121] It has been estimated that venous catheters account for 30% to 40% of axillary and subclavian venous obstructions in the United States.[123, 124] In an autopsy series of 139 burn patients who had thoracic venous catheters, 37% had central venous thrombosis.[125] In another investigation of 204 patients in the intensive care unit who had internal jugular or subclavian catheters, color Doppler ultrasound examination performed just before or within 24 hours of catheter removal showed thrombosis at the catheter site in 33%. The thrombus was limited (2 to 4 mm) in 8%, large (≥4 mm) in 22%, and occlusive in 3%. The risk of catheter-associated sepsis was 2.6-fold greater when thrombus was present. The prevalence of venous obstruction is related to the duration the catheter is left in place; 75% of thoracic venous catheters cause mural thrombosis after 14 days.[122] Complications of the thrombosis include loss of central venous access, superior vena cava syndrome,

septic thrombophlebitis, and pulmonary thromboembolism.[121, 123, 124]

The radiographic findings are neither sensitive nor specific and include enlargement of the vena cava, pleural effusion, and dilated collateral vessels (including the arch of the azygous vein or left superior intercostal vein).[121] The diagnosis can be confirmed by venography, color-flow Doppler ultrasonography, CT, or MR imaging.[126–128] All these modalities have limitations, and the technique of choice is influenced by the suspected localization of the thrombosis, cost, and local experience. Venography allows diagnosis of partial and complete obstruction but does not permit confident distinction of intrinsic from extrinsic compression. This distinction can be made on CT or MR imaging; however, both procedures may fail to show small nonocclusive thrombi that are seen on phlebography.[115] Color-flow Doppler has been shown to be an accurate noninvasive method;[115, 126] its major limitation is inability to image the midportion of the subclavian veins and superior vena cava.[115]

Although most venous thromboses are sterile, catheter-related septic thrombosis may occur, particularly in patients who have long-term indwelling central venous catheters.[116] Other infectious complications include mediastinitis, osteomyelitis of the clavicle, and exit site or tunnel infections.[116]

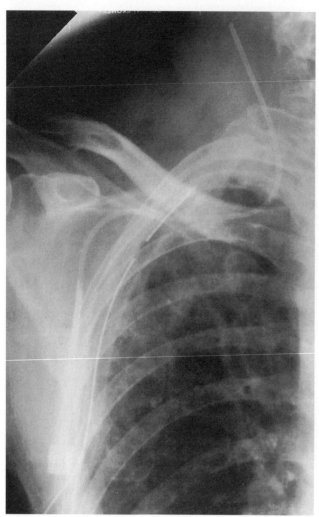

Figure 19–17. Malpositioning of a Subclavian Catheter in the Jugular Vein. The catheter occupies a correct position in the subclavian vein, but then ascends the jugular vein. Central venous pressure cannot be recorded properly with a catheter in this position.

Perforation of a Vein

A vein can be perforated at the time of catheter insertion[129] or some time later;[131] late perforation is caused by gradual erosion of a relatively thin-walled intrathoracic vessel by the catheter, partly as a result of cardiac and respiratory movements affecting the catheter tip.[132] Most perforations occur after introduction of catheters for pressure measurements and hyperalimentation; they occur less often with electrode insertion for cardiac pacing[133] and with catheter insertion for plasmapheresis and hemodialysis.[134]

Depending on the vein involved, perforation can result in pneumothorax, hemothorax, hydrothorax, mediastinal hemorrhage (Fig. 19–18), bronchopulmonary-venous fistula, or extrapleural hematoma.[117, 130, 136] Unilateral pneumothorax is the most common of these. A particularly serious consequence is bilateral pneumothorax,[129] a complication that arises when an unsuspected perforation with consequent pneumothorax occurs in an unsuccessful attempt on one side followed by induction of a pneumothorax with a catheter insertion on the contralateral side. Rarely, pleural effusion is bilateral and massive.[137, 138]

Vascular erosion by central venous catheters usually affects the superior vena cava and is considerably more common with left-sided catheters: In one review of 61 patients who had catheter-induced hydrothorax, the route of catheterization was left-sided in 74% and right-sided in 26%.[117] It has been postulated that the predisposition of left-sided catheters to perforate derives from the more horizontal orientation of the left brachiocephalic vein compared with the right. As a consequence, the tip of a left-sided catheter inserted an insufficient length tends to abut against the right lateral wall of the superior vena cava within 45 degrees of perpendicular.[117] An early sign of impending perforation of the superior vena cava is a gentle curvature of the distal portion of the catheter with the tip directed toward the right lateral vein wall.[132] Venous erosion may occur when a catheter tip is located in the right or left brachiocephalic vein.[117]

Air embolism has been reported as a complication of subclavian vein catheterization, during either insertion or withdrawal of the catheter.[139–141] Asymptomatic air embolism is probably a common complication after central or peripheral vein injection of any kind (Fig. 19–19).[142] In one study of 100 patients who underwent contrast-enhanced CT (contrast material was injected through a 19-gauge needle inserted into a hand or forearm vein), venous air embolism was detected in 23%.[142] In 20 patients, the amount of air was minimal, consisting of small bubbles of air within the blood; however, the amount was sufficient to form air-fluid levels in the other 3 patients. The amount of air in all cases was considered to be only a few milliliters, and no patients had symptoms.

Perforation of the Myocardium

It is common for the tip of a central venous catheter to reside in one of the right heart chambers; for example, in one investigation of 300 patients, it was identified in the right atrium or right ventricle in 40 (13%).[119] This is a potentially hazardous position, particularly if the catheter has a firm or sharp tip; perforation of the atrium or ventricle may result in fatal pericardial tamponade (from blood or infused fluid),[143] and irritation of the myocardium may cause arrhythmias.

Catheter Coiling, Knotting, and Breaking

Coiled catheters traumatize the vein and are much more likely to perforate, break, and embolize. They also show a much greater tendency to twist into knots; although these sometimes can be manipulated free, this is not always possible, and thoracotomy occasionally is required for removal.[144]

Miscellaneous Complications

Other complications of percutaneous central venous catheter insertion include sepsis;[135, 145] embolization of catheter fragments to the lungs (Fig. 19–20);[135, 146] thoracic duct laceration;[135] entanglement in an intravenous filter inserted to prevent pulmonary thromboemboli;[147] and damage to the brachial plexus, sympathetic chain, or phrenic, recurrent laryngeal, or ninth to twelfth cranial nerves.[135, 148]

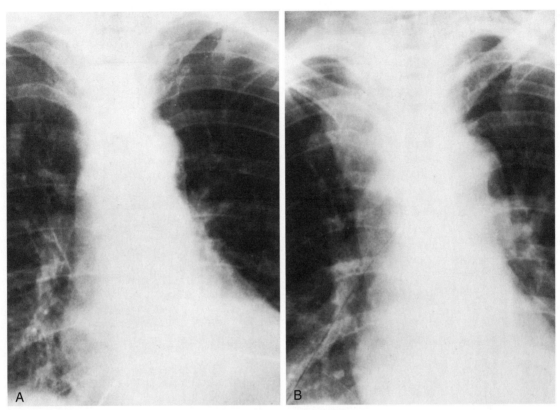

Figure 19–18. Mediastinal Hemorrhage After Faulty Insertion of a Subclavian Catheter. Radiograph *(A)* shows a normal appearance of the upper mediastinum. Three days later *(B),* after attempted insertion of a right subclavian line, moderate widening of the superior mediastinum has occurred as a result of venous hemorrhage secondary to perforation of a vein by the catheter.

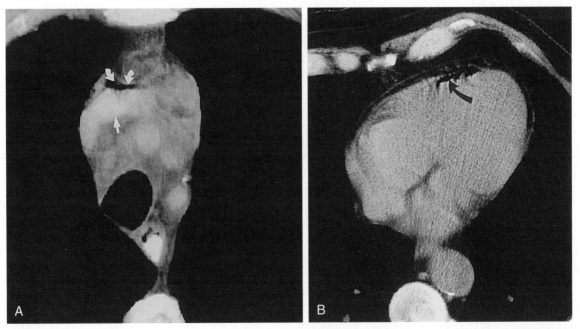

Figure 19–19. Venous Air Embolism. CT scan in a 65-year-old patient *(A)* shows intravenous contrast material *(straight arrow)* and air *(curved arrows)* within the left brachiocephalic vein. Injection of air presumably occurred concomitantly with injection of contrast material. CT scan in another patient *(B)* shows air *(curved arrow)* within the right ventricle. In this patient, the scan was performed after starting an intravenous infusion of saline. Neither patient developed symptoms.

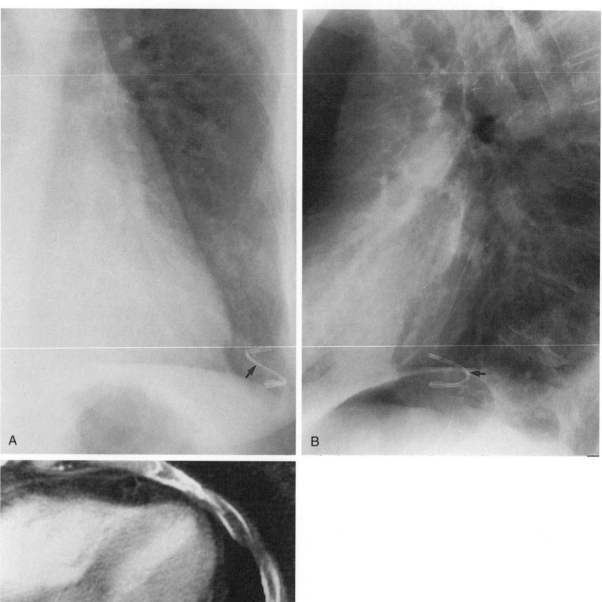

Figure 19–20. Embolization of Broken Central Venous Catheter. Views of the left lung from posteroanterior *(A)* and lateral *(B)* chest radiographs and CT scan *(C)* show the broken distal portion of an intravenous catheter *(arrows)* in the left lower lobe. The tip presumably lies within a pulmonary artery. The patient did not have symptoms, and the catheter was left in place; no associated symptoms were observed during a 4-year follow-up.

Indwelling Balloon-Tipped Pulmonary Arterial Catheters

Flow-directed balloon-tipped (Swan-Ganz) catheters are used to monitor circulatory hemodynamics in critically ill patients. Complications associated with their use include atrial and ventricular arrhythmias, rupture of the balloon, knotting of the catheter, perforation of the pulmonary artery, perforation of the visceral pleura (resulting in pneumothorax or hemothorax), false aneurysms of the pulmonary artery, pulmonary artery occlusion with pulmonary infarction, and air embolism.[150, 152, 153] The catheters can act as a nidus for bacterial colonization[154] and platelet consumption,[155] with the potential of causing sepsis or contributing to hemorrhage. As a group, these events are not rare; in one prospective study of 528 catheterizations, serious complications were considered to have occurred in 23 (4.4%).[156]

Pulmonary artery occlusion, with or without infarction, is probably the most common pulmonary complication (Fig. 19–21). In one series of 125 patients undergoing catheterization, some sort of ischemic lesion was identified in 9 (7.2%);[149] in another review of 391 patients, evidence of thromboembolism was found in 16 (4%).[150] Although it has been estimated that the pulmonary artery is perforated in only about 0.001% to 0.5% of all cases of catheter insertion,[157] there is evidence that it may be a more common event. In one autopsy review, 4 such cases were identified in a consecutive series of 270 cases (1.5%);[158] in only 1 case was the perforation suspected clinically.

As might be expected, the usual result of pulmonary artery perforation is hemorrhage, generally into pulmonary

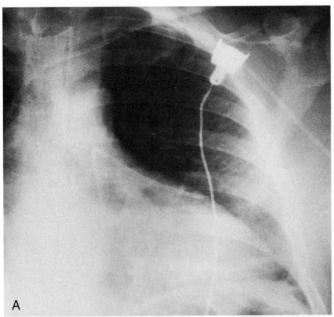

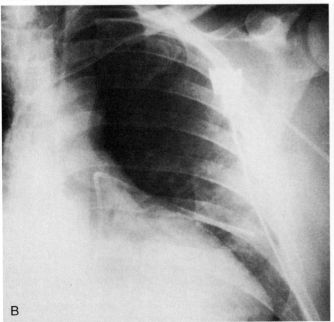

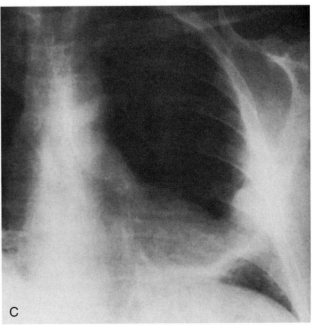

Figure 19–21. Pulmonary Infarction Associated with a Swan-Ganz Catheter. Anteroposterior radiograph *(A)* shows a Swan-Ganz catheter in position in the left lower lobe, its tip in a position consistent with a subsegmental artery. Twenty-four hours later *(B)*, the intrapulmonary extent of the catheter had increased considerably, such that its tip now lies less than 2 cm from the visceral pleural surface. Several days later *(C)*, a wedge-shaped opacity had appeared in the left axillary lung zone, which was highly suggestive of a pulmonary infarct; its position corresponds precisely to what was undoubtedly an impacted Swan-Ganz catheter tip.

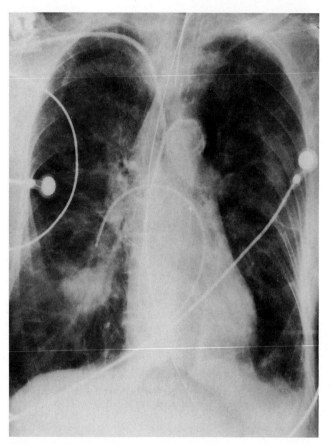

Figure 19–22. Pulmonary Artery Perforation by a Swan-Ganz Catheter. Posteroanterior radiograph shows the tip of a Swan-Ganz catheter in the region of the right interlobar artery. Distal to it is a fairly well-defined opacity that could be situated in either the middle or the lower lobe. Shortly thereafter, this 83-year-old woman coughed up a small amount of blood and died. At autopsy, the right middle lobe showed extensive airspace hemorrhage and a defect in a subsegmental pulmonary artery associated with an irregularly shaped intraparenchymal hematoma.

parenchyma but on occasion predominantly into the bronchovascular interstitium or pleural space.[159] Only a few cases have been examined pathologically;[158] in many, the site of rupture has been undetected, whereas in others, a localized intraparenchymal hematoma or nodule of intraparenchymal thrombus (false aneurysm) reveals the location.

Shortly after pulmonary artery perforation, the chest radiograph may show localized areas of consolidation with hazy margins (Fig. 19–22).[152, 160] The consolidation is replaced within 1 to 3 weeks by a round, well-circumscribed nodule or mass ranging from 2 to 8 cm in diameter, corresponding to the development of a false aneurysm.[152, 160] Contrast-enhanced CT shows the latter as an enhancing mass associated with a vessel and sometimes containing a partially thrombosed lumen.[152, 161, 162] The mass may be surrounded by a halo of ground-glass attenuation as a result of recent hemorrhage.[152, 163] Chest radiograph may be unremarkable or show nonspecific findings: In one review of seven false aneurysms in five patients, chest radiographs were unremarkable in two and showed focal consolidation in one and a pulmonary mass consistent with false aneurysm in two.[152] The diagnosis can be confirmed with pulmonary angiography.[152]

Perforation should be suspected whenever a new airspace opacity develops in association with hemoptysis,[151, 164] which can be massive.[165, 166] The mortality rate associated with clinically evident pulmonary artery perforation has been estimated to be 45% to 65%.[167] Patients who develop false aneurysms can have recurrent life-threatening hemorrhage; the rate of this complication has been estimated to be about 30% to 40% and the mortality rate 40% to 70%.[152, 168]

Intra-Aortic Counterpulsation Balloons

The intra-aortic counterpulsation balloon catheter has been used in conditions characterized by low-output cardiac decompensation and cardiogenic shock. This catheter provides augmentation of diastolic coronary artery perfusion as well as reduced impedance to ventricular ejection.[169, 170] Reported complications resulting from its use include aortic dissection, laceration, and subadventitial hematoma formation; red blood cell destruction; embolic phenomena, such as vascular insufficiency of the catheterized limb; and balloon rupture with secondary gas embolism.[170, 171] The most common complication observed by radiologists is improper positioning.[102] The ideal position

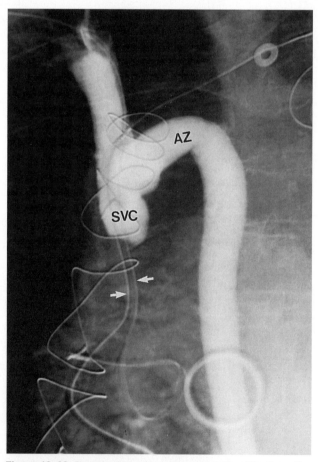

Figure 19–23. Superior Vena Cava Thrombosis Resulting from Cardiac Pacemaker Leads. View of a digital venogram shows complete obstruction of the superior vena cava (SVC) and collateral flow through the azygos vein (AZ). The patient had undergone insertion of sequential atrioventricular pacemaker leads *(arrows)* 11 years previously and subsequently had developed SVC syndrome.

of the tip is just distal to the origin of the left subclavian artery. A more proximally located tip can occlude the left subclavian artery, and one more distal can result in decreased effectiveness of diastolic counterpulsation. Angulation of the catheter tip suggests incorrect positioning within the transverse portion of the aortic arch.[102]

Cardiac Pacemakers

The impact that radiology can make in determining the cause of pacemaker malfunction and in the evaluation of lead position and integrity can be considerable and has been reviewed.[172–174] Complications include electrode malposition, redundant or taut leads, infection of the subcutaneous pacemaker pouch or along the lead, myocardial perforation, pneumothorax, pleural effusion, and fracture of the lead.[173, 174] Wire fracture causes loss of pacing and the potential risk of embolism of the distal segment to the pulmonary artery.[102] Venous thrombosis may lead to partial or complete occlusion of the subclavian and brachiocephalic veins or superior vena cava (Fig. 19–23).[173, 174] The complications from automatic implantable cardioverter defibrillators have been reviewed[175] and include hemoptysis as a result of erosion of the ventricular patch into a bronchus.[176, 177] Bronchopericardial fistula may develop after placement of an automatic implantable cardioverter defibrillator using pericardial or epicardial defibrillator patches.[188] Patients present with hemoptysis. The diagnosis can be confirmed by showing the presence of air between the defibrillator patch and the heart on chest radiograph or CT scan.[188]

References

1. Goodman LR, Kay HR, Teplick SK, et al: Complications of median sternotomy: Computed tomographic evaluation. Am J Roentgenol 141:225, 1983.
2. Carrol CL, Jeffrey RB Jr, Federle MP, et al: CT evaluation of mediastinal infections. J Comput Assist Tomogr 11:449, 1987.
3. Templeton PA, Fishman EK: CT evaluation of poststernotomy complications. Am J Roentgenol 159:45, 1992.
4. Goodman LR: Review: Postoperative chest radiograph: II. Alterations after major intrathoracic surgery. Am J Roentgenol 134:803, 1980.
5. Curtis JA, Libshitz HI, Dalinka MK: Fracture of the first rib as a complication of midline sternotomy. Radiology 115:63, 1975.
6. Greenwald LV, Baisden CE, Symbas PN: Rib fractures in coronary artery bypass patients: Radionuclide detection. Radiology 48:553, 1983.
7. Tsukada G, Start P: Postpneumonectomy complications. Am J Roentgenol 169:1363, 1997.
8. Hansen RE, Kloiber R, Lesperance RR, et al: Unpublished data.
9. Laissy JP, Rebibo G, Iba-Zizen MT, et al: MR appearance of the normal chest after pneumonectomy. J Comput Assist Tomogr 13:248, 1989.
10. Heelan RT, Panicek DM, Burt ME, et al: Magnetic resonance imaging of the postpneumonectomy chest: Normal and abnormal findings. J Thorac Imaging 12:200, 1997.
11. Williams NS, Lewis CT: Bronchopleural fistula: A review of 86 cases. Br J Surg 63:520, 1976.
12. Asamura H, Naruke T, Tsuchiya R, et al: Bronchopleural fistulas associated with lung cancer operations: Univariate and multivariate analysis of risk factors, management, and outcome. J Thorac Cardiovasc Surg 104:1456, 1992.
13. Hollaus PH, Lax F, el-Nashef BB, et al: Natural history of bron-

14. chopleural fistula after pneumonectomy: A review of 96 cases. Ann Thorac Surg 63:1391, 1997.
14. Leading article: Bronchopleural fistula. BMJ 2:1093, 1976.
15. Heater K, Revzani L, Rubin JM: CT evaluation of empyema in the postpneumonectomy space. Am J Roentgenol 145:39, 1985.
16. Westcott JL, Volpe JP: Peripheral bronchopleural fistula: CT evaluation in 20 patients with pneumonia, empyema, or postoperative air leak. Radiology 196:175, 1995.
17. Stern EJ, Sun H, Haramati LB: Peripheral bronchopleural fistulas: CT imaging features. Am J Roentgenol 167:117, 1996.
18. Wechsler RJ: CT of esophageal-pleural fistulae. Am J Roentgenol 147:907, 1986.
19. Wechsler RJ, Steiner RM, Goodman LR, et al: Iatrogenic esophageal-pleural fistula: Subtlety of diagnosis in the absence of mediastinitis. Radiology 144:239, 1982.
20. Heiken JP, Balfe DM, Roper CL: CT evaluation after esophagogastrectomy. Am J Roentgenol 143:555, 1984.
21. Westcott JL, Cole SR: Interstitial pulmonary emphysema in children and adults: Roentgenographic features. Radiology 111:367, 1974.
22. Henry DA, Jolles H, Berberich JJ, et al: The post-cardiac surgery chest radiograph: A clinically integrated approach. J Thorac Imaging 4:20, 1989.
23. Carter AR, Sostman HD, Curtis AM, et al: Thoracic alterations after cardiac surgery. Am J Roentgenol 140:475, 1983.
24. Doyle MT, Spizarny DL, Baker DE: Saphenous vein graft aneurysm after coronary artery bypass surgery. Am J Roentgenol 168:747, 1997.
25. Benya EC, Joseph AE, Nemcek AA: Mediastinal mass after coronary artery bypass surgery with internal mammary artery grafts. J Thorac Imaging 6:40, 1991.
26. Scott WW, Beall DP, Wheeler PS: The retained intrapericardial sponge: Value of the lateral chest radiograph. Am J Roentgenol 171:595, 1998.
27. Bhalla M, Wain JC, Shepard JAO, et al: Surgical flaps in the chest: Anatomic considerations, applications, and radiologic appearance. Radiology 192:825, 1994.
28. Coppage L, Jolles H, Wornom IL III: Computed tomography findings in patients who have undergone muscle flap and omental transposition procedures in the treatment of poststernotomy mediastinitis. J Thorac Imaging 9:14, 1994.
29. Peters JC, Desai KK: CT demonstration of postpneumonectomy tumor recurrence. Am J Roentgenol 141:259, 1983.
30. Kerr WF: Late-onset post-pneumonectomy empyema. Thorax 32:149, 1977.
31. Tschersich HU, Skopara V Jr, Fleming WH: Acute cardiac herniation following pneumonectomy. Radiology 120:546, 1976.
32. Brady MB, Brogdon BG: Cardiac herniation and volvulus: Radiographic findings. Radiology 161:657, 1986.
33. Castillo M, Oldham S: Cardiac volvulus: Plain film recognition of an often fatal condition. Am J Roentgenol 145:271, 1985.
34. Arndt RD, Frank CG, Schmitz AL, et al: Cardiac herniation with volvulus after pneumonectomy. Am J Roentgenol 130:155, 1978.
35. Rodgers BM, Moulder PV, DeLaney A: Thoracoscopy: New method of early diagnosis of cardiac herniation. J Thorac Cardiovasc Surg 78:623, 1979.
36. Shepard JO, Grillo HC, McLoud TC, et al: Right-pneumonectomy syndrome: Radiologic finding and CT correlation. Radiology 151:661, 1986.
37. Grillo HC, Shepard JO, Mathisen DJ, et al: Postpneumonectomy syndrome: Diagnosis, management, and results. Ann Thorac Surg 54:638, 1992.
38. Quillin SP, Shackelford GD: Postpneumonectomy syndrome after left lung resection. Radiology 179:100, 1991.
39. Boiselle PM, Shepard JAO, McLoud TC, et al: Postpneumonectomy syndrome: Another twist. J Thorac Imaging 12:209, 1997.
40. Holbert JM, Libshitz HI, Chasen MH, et al: The postlobectomy chest: Anatomic considerations. Radiographics 7:889, 1987.
41. Hamilton W: Atelectasis, pneumothorax, and aspiration as postoperative complications. Anesthesiology 22:708, 1961.
42. Gamsu G, Singer MM, Vincent HH, et al: Postoperative impairment of mucous transport in the lung. Am Rev Respir Dis 114:673, 1976.
43. Korst RJ, Humphrey CB: Complete lobar collapse following pulmonary lobectomy: Its incidence, predisposing factors, and clinical ramifications. Chest 111:1285, 1997.
44. Wilcox P, Baile EM, Hards J, et al: Phrenic nerve function and its

relationship to atelectasis after coronary artery bypass surgery. Chest 93:693, 1988.

45. van der Werff YD, van der Houwen HK, Heijmans PJM, et al: Postpneumonectomy pulmonary edema: A retrospective analysis of incidence and possible risk factors. Chest 111:1278, 1997.

46. Bhalla M, Leitman BS, Forcade C, et al: Lung hernia: Radiographic features. Am J Roentgenol 154:51, 1990.

47. DiMarco AF, Oca O, Renston JP: Lung herniation: A cause of chronic chest pain following thoracotomy. Chest 107:877, 1995.

48. Kelly MV II, Kyger ER, Miller WC: Postoperative lobar torsion and gangrene. Thorax 32:501, 1977.

49. Moser ES Jr, Proto AV: Lung torsion: Case report and literature review. Radiology 162:639, 1987.

50. Felson B: Lung torsion: Radiographic findings in nine cases. Radiology 162:631, 1987.

51. Collins J, Love RB: Pulmonary torsion: Complication of lung transplantation. Clin Pulmonary Med 3:297, 1996.

52. Munk PL, Vellet AD, Zwirewich C: Torsion of the upper lobe of the lung after surgery: Findings on pulmonary angiography. Am J Roentgenol 157:471, 1991.

53. Taylor FH, Zollinger RW II, Edgerton TA, et al: Intrapulmonary foreign body: Sponge retained for 43 years. J Thorac Imaging 9:56, 1994.

54. Sawasaki H, Horie K, Yamada M, et al: Bronchial stump aspergillosis: Experimental and clinical study. J Thorac Cardiovasc Surg 58:198, 1969.

55. Parry MF, Coughlin FR, Zambetti FX: Aspergillus empyema. Chest 81:768, 1982.

56. Goodman LR: Review: Postoperative chest radiograph: I. Alterations after abdominal surgery. Am J Roentgenol 134:533, 1980.

57. Harman E, Lillington G: Pulmonary risk factors in surgery. Med Clin North Am 63:1289, 1979.

58. Kroenke K, Lawrence VA, Theroux JF, et al: Postoperative complications after thoracic and major abdominal surgery in patients with and without obstructive lung disease. Chest 104:1445, 1993.

59. Hall JC, Tarala RA, Hall JL, et al: A multivariate analysis of the risk of pulmonary complications after laparotomy. Chest 99:923, 1991.

60. Nesbitt JC, Carrasco H: Expandable stents. Chest Surg Clin North Am 6:305, 1996.

61. Wilson GE, Walshaw MJ, Hind CR: Treatment of large airway obstruction in lung cancer using expandable metal stents inserted under direct vision via the fibreoptic bronchoscope. Thorax 51:248, 1996.

62. Hauck RW, Lembeck RM, Emslander HP, et al: Implantation of Accuflex and Strecker stents in malignant bronchial stenoses by flexible bronchoscopy. Chest 112:134, 1997.

63. Takamori S, Fujita H, Hayashi A, et al: Expandable metallic stents for tracheobronchial stenoses in esophageal cancer. Ann Thorac Surg 62:844, 1996.

64. Subramanian V, Anstead M, Cottrill CM, et al: Tetralogy of Fallot with absent pulmonary valve and bronchial compression: Treatment with endobronchial stents. Pediatr Cardiol 18:237, 1997.

65. Sacco O, Fregonese B, Oddone M, et al: Severe endobronchial obstruction in a girl with relapsing polychondritis: Treatment with Nd YAG laser and endobronchial silicon stent. Eur Respir J 10:494, 1997.

66. Watanabe Y, Murakami S, Oda M, et al: Treatment of bronchial stricture due to endobronchial tuberculosis. World J Surg 21:480, 1997.

67. Moser NJ, Woodring JH, Wolf KM, et al: Management of postpneumonectomy syndrome with a bronchoscopically placed endobronchial stent. South Med J 87:1156, 1994.

68. Higgins R, McNeil K, Dennis C, et al: Airway stenoses after lung transplantation: Management with expanding metal stents. J Heart Lung Transplant 13:774, 1994.

69. Hijazi ZM, al-Fadley F, Geggel RL, et al: Stent implantation for relief of pulmonary artery stenosis: Immediate and short-term results. Cathet Cardiovasc Diagn 38:16, 1996.

70. Abdulhamed JM, Alyousef SA, Mullins C: Endovascular stent placement for pulmonary venous obstruction after Mustard operation for transposition of the great arteries. Heart 75:210, 1996.

71. Haskal ZJ, Soulen MC, Huettl EA, et al: Life-threatening pulmonary emboli and cor pulmonale: Treatment with percutaneous pulmonary artery stent placement. Radiology 191:473, 1994.

72. Clark SC, Levine AJ, Hasan A, et al: Vascular complications of lung transplantation. Ann Thorac Surg 61:1079, 1996.

73. Hramiec JE, Haasler GB: Tracheal wire stent complications in malacia: Implications of position and design. Ann Thorac Surg 63:209, 1997.

74. Remacle M, Lawson G, Minet M, et al: Endoscopic treatment of tracheal stenosis using the carbon dioxide laser and the Gianturco stent: Indications and results. Laryngoscope 106:306, 1996.

75. Hendra KP, Saukkonen JJ: Erosion of the right mainstem bronchus by an esophageal stent. Chest 110:857, 1996.

76. Erasmus JJ, Goodman PC: Focal pulmonary edema: A complication of endovascular stent dilatation of pulmonary artery stenoses. Am J Roentgenol 165:821, 1995.

77. Brown DL, MacIsaac AI, Topol EJ: Pulmonary hemorrhage after intracoronary stent placement. J Am Coll Cardiol 24:91, 1994.

78. Khanavkar B, Stern P, Alberti W, et al: Complications associated with brachytherapy alone or with laser in lung cancer. Chest 99:1062, 1991.

79. Gustafson G, Vicini F, Freedman L, et al: High dose rate endobronchial brachytherapy in the management of primary and recurrent bronchogenic malignancies. Cancer 75:2345, 1995.

80. Leading article: Traumatic perforation of oesophagus. BMJ 1:524, 1972.

81. Scholl DG, Tsai SH: Esophageal perforation following the use of the esophageal obturator airway. Radiology 122:315, 1977.

82. Stark P: Radiology of thoracic trauma. Invest Radiol 25:1265, 1990.

83. Stark P, Phillips JM: Rupture of the esophagus as a complication of Sengstaken-Blakemore tube. Radiology 25:76, 1985.

84. Nygaard SD, Berger HA, Fick RB: Chylothorax as a complication of oesophageal sclerotherapy. Thorax 47:134, 1992.

85. Daly RC, Mucha P, Pairolero PC, et al: The risk of percutaneous chest tube thoracostomy for blunt thoracic trauma. Ann Emerg Med 14:865, 1985.

86. Miller KS, Sahn SA: Chest tubes: Indications, technique, management and complications. Chest 91:258, 1987.

87. Dalbec DL, Krome RL: Thoracostomy. Emerg Med Clin North Am 4:441, 1986.

88. Maurer JR, Friedman PJ, Wing VW: Thoracostomy tube in an interlobar fissure: Radiologic recognition of a potential problem. Am J Roentgenol 139:1155, 1982.

89. Stark DD, Federle MP, Goodman PC: CT and radiographic assessment of tube thoracostomy. Am J Roentgenol 141:253, 1983.

90. Webb WR, LaBerge JM: Radiographic recognition of chest tube malposition in the major fissure. Chest 85:81, 1984.

91. Mirvis SE, Tobin KD, Kostrubiak I, et al: Thoracic CT in detecting occult disease in critically ill patients. Am J Roentgenol 148:685, 1987.

92. Cameron EW, Mirvis SE, Shanmuganathan K, et al: Computed tomography of malpositioned thoracostomy drains: A pictorial essay. Clin Radiol 52:187, 1997.

93. Curtin JJ, Goodman LR, Quebbeman EJ, et al: Thoracostomy tubes after acute chest injury: Relationship between location in a pleural fissure and function. Am J Roentgenol 163:1339, 1994.

94. Neff CC, Mueller PR, Ferrucci JT Jr, et al: Serious complications following transgression of the pleural space in drainage procedures. Radiology 152:335, 1984.

95. Nichols DM, Cooperberg PL, Golding RH, et al: The safe intercostal approach? Pleural complications in abdominal interventional radiology. Am J Roentgenol 141:1013, 1984.

96. Samelson SL, Ferguson MK: Empyema following percutaneous catheter drainage of upper abdominal abscess. Chest 102:1612, 1992.

97. Valentine RJ, Turner WW: Pleural complications of nasoenteric feeding tubes. J Parenter Enteral Nutr 8:450, 1984.

98. Hendry PJ, Akyurekl Y, McIntyre R, et al: Bronchopleural complications of nasogastric feeding tubes. Crit Care Med 14:892, 1986.

99. Ghahremani GG, Gould RJ: Nasoenteric feeding tubes: Radiographic detection of complications. Dig Dis Sci 31:574, 1986.

100. Miller KS, Tomlinson JR, Sahn SA: Pleuropulmonary complications of enteral tube feedings: Two reports, review of the literature and recommendations. Chest 86:230, 1985.

101. Woodall BH, Winfield DF, Bisset GS: Inadvertent tracheobronchial placement of feeding tubes. Radiology 165:727, 1987.

102. Wiener MD, Garay SM, Leitman BS, et al: Imaging of the intensive care unit patient. Clin Chest Med 12:169, 1991.

103. Stark P: Inadvertent nasogastric tube insertion into the tracheobronchial tree: A hazard of new high-residual volume cuffs. Radiology 142:239, 1982.

104. Miller WT: Inadvertent tracheobronchial placement of feeding tubes (letter to the editor). Radiology 167:875, 1988.

105. Hand RW, Kempster M, Levy JH, et al: Inadvertent transbronchial insertion of narrow-bore feeding tubes into the pleural space. JAMA 251:2396, 1984.

106. Roubenoff R, Ravich WJ: Pneumothorax due to nasogastric feeding tubes: Report of four cases, review of the literature, and recommendations for prevention. Arch Intern Med 149:184, 1989.

107. Twigg HL, Buckley CE: Complications of endotracheal intubation. Am J Roentgenol 109:452, 1970.

108. Conrardy PA, Goodman LR, Laing F, et al: Alteration of endotracheal tube position: Flexion and extension of the neck. Crit Care Med 4:7, 1976.

109. Goodman LR, Conrardy PA, Laing F, et al: Radiographic evaluation of endotracheal tube position. Am J Roentgenol 127:433, 1976.

110. Smith GM, Reed JC, Choplin RH: Radiographic detection of esophageal malpositioning of endotracheal tubes. Am J Roentgenol 154:23, 1990.

111. Shneerson J: Transtracheal oxygen delivery. Thorax 47:57, 1992.

112. Heimlich HJ, Carr GC: Transtracheal catheter technique for pulmonary rehabilitation. Ann Otol Rhinol Laryngol 94:502, 1985.

113. Fletcher EC, Nickeson D, Costarangos-Galarza C: Endotracheal mass resulting from a transtracheal oxygen catheter. Chest 93:438, 1988.

114. Borer H, Frey M, Keller R: Ulcerous tracheitis and mucus ball formation: A nearly fatal complication of a transtracheal oxygen catheter. Respiration 63:400, 1996.

115. Wechsler RJ, Spirn PW, Conant EF, et al: Thrombosis and infection caused by thoracic venous catheters: Pathogenesis and imaging findings. Am J Roentgenol 160:467, 1993.

116. Clarke DE, Raffin TA: Infectious complications of indwelling long-term central venous catheters. Chest 97:966, 1990.

117. Duntley P, Siever J, Korwes ML, et al: Vascular erosion by central venous catheters: Clinical features and outcome. Chest 101:1633, 1992.

118. Dunbar RD, Mitchell R, Lavine M: Aberrant locations of central venous catheters. Lancet 1:711, 1981.

119. Langston CS: The aberrant central venous catheter and its complications. Radiology 100:55, 1971.

120. Hoshal VL Jr, Ause RG, Hoskins PA: Fibrin sleeve formation on indwelling subclavian central venous catheters. Arch Surg 102:353, 1971.

121. Ahmed N, Payne RF: Thrombosis after central venous cannulation. Med J Aust 1:217, 1976.

122. Brismar B, Hardstedt C, Jacobson S: Diagnosis of thrombosis by catheter phlebography after prolonged central venous catheterization. Ann Surg 194:779, 1981.

123. Horattas MC, Wright DJ, Fenton AH, et al: Changing concepts of deep venous thrombosis of upper extremity: Report of a series and review of the literature. Surgery 104:561, 1988.

124. Hill SL, Berry RE: Subclavian vein thrombosis: A continuing challenge. Surgery 108:1, 1990.

125. Warden GD, Wilmore DW, Pruitt BA Jr: Central venous thrombosis: Hazard of medical process. J Trauma 13:620, 1973.

126. Falk RL, Smith DF: Thrombosis of upper extremity thoracic inlet veins: Diagnosis with duplex Doppler sonography. Am J Roentgenol 149:677, 1987.

127. Yedlicka JW Jr, Cormier MG, Gray R, et al: Computed tomography of superior vena cava obstruction. J Thorac Imaging 2:72, 1987.

128. Hansen ME, Spritzer CE, Sostman HD: Assessing the patency of mediastinal and thoracic inlet veins: Value of MR imaging. Am J Roentgenol 155:1177, 1990.

129. Maggs PR, Schwaber JR: Fatal bilateral pneumothoraces complicating subclavian vein catheterization. Chest 71:552, 1977.

130. Shiloni E, Meretyk S, Weiss Y: Tension haemothorax: An unusual complication of central vein catheterization. Injury 16:385, 1985.

131. Chute E, Cerrs FB: Late development of hydrothorax and hydromediastinum in patients with central venous catheters. Crit Care Med 10:868, 1982.

132. Tocino IM, Watanabe A: Impending catheter perforation of superior vena cava: Radiographic recognition. Am J Roentgenol 146:487, 1986.

133. Topaz O, Sharon M, Rechavia E, et al: Traumatic internal jugular vein cannulation. Ann Emerg Med 16:1394, 1987.

134. Tapson JS, Uldall PR: Fatal hemothorax caused by a subclavian hemodialysis catheter: Thoughts on prevention. Arch Intern Med 144:1685, 1984.

135. McGoon MD, Benedetto PW, Greene BM: Complications of percutaneous central venous catheterization: A report of two cases and review of the literature. Johns Hopkins Med 145:1, 1979.

136. Kotozoglou T, Mambo N: Fatal retropleural hematoma complicating internal jugular vein catheterization: A case report. Am J Forensic Med Pathol 4:125, 1983.

137. Molinari PS, Belani KG, Buckley JJ: Delayed hydrothorax following percutaneous central venous cannulation. Acta Anaesthesiol Scand 28:493, 1984.

138. Usselman JA, Seat SG: Superior caval catheter displacement causing bilateral pleural effusions. Am J Roentgenol 133:738, 1979.

139. Paskin DL, Hoffman WS, Tuddenham WJ: A new complication of subclavian vein catheterization. Ann Surg 179:266, 1974.

140. Johnson CL, Lazarchick J, Lynn HB: Subclavian venipuncture: Preventable complications: Report of two cases. Mayo Clin Proc 45:712, 1970.

141. Flanagan JP, Gradisar IA, Gross RJ, et al: Air embolus: A lethal complication of subclavian venipuncture. N Engl J Med 281:488, 1969.

142. Woodring JH, Fried AM: Nonfatal venous air embolism after contrast-enhanced CT. Radiology 167:405, 1988.

143. Hunt R, Hunter TB: Cardiac tamponade and death from perforation of the right atrium by a central venous catheter (letter to the editor). Am J Roentgenol 151:1250, 1988.

144. Rossleigh MA: Unusual complication of intravenous catheterisation. Med J Aust 1:236, 1982.

145. Kappes S, Towne J, Adams M, et al: Perforation of the superior vena cava: A complication of subclavian dialysis. JAMA 249:2232, 1983.

146. Weiner P, Sznajder I, Plavnick L, et al: Unusual complications of subclavian vein catheterization. Crit Care Med 12:538, 1984.

147. Amesbury S, Vargish T, Hall J: An unusual complication of central venous catheterization. Chest 105:905, 1994.

148. Milam MG, Sahn SA: Horner's syndrome secondary to hydromediastinum: A complication of extravascular migration of a central venous catheter. Chest 94:1093, 1988.

149. Foote GA, Schabel SI, Hodges M: Pulmonary complications of the flow-directed balloon-tipped catheter. N Engl J Med 290:927, 1974.

150. Katz JD, Cronau LH, Barash PG, et al: Pulmonary artery flow-guided catheters in the perioperative period: Indications and complications. JAMA 237:2832, 1977.

151. Hannan AT, Brown M, Bigman O: Pulmonary artery catheter-induced hemorrhage. Chest 85:128, 1984.

152. Ferretti GR, Thony F, Link KM, et al: False aneurysm of the pulmonary artery induced by a Swan-Ganz catheter: Clinical presentation and radiologic management. Am J Roentgenol 167:941, 1996.

153. Hartung EJ, Ender J, Sgouropoulou S, et al: Severe air embolism caused by a pulmonary artery introducer sheath. Anesthesiology 80:1402, 1994.

154. Michel L, Marsh HM, McMichan JC, et al: Infection of pulmonary artery catheters in critically ill patients. JAMA 245:1032, 1981.

155. Vicente Rull JR, Loza Aquirre J, de la Puerta E: Thrombocytopenia induced by pulmonary artery flotation catheters: A prospective study. Intensive Care Med 10:29, 1984.

156. Boyd KD, Thomas SJ, Gold J, et al: A prospective study of complications of pulmonary artery catheterizations in 500 consecutive patients. Chest 84:245, 1983.

157. Kearney TJ, Shabot MM: Pulmonary artery rupture associated with the Swan-Ganz catheter. Chest 108:1349, 1995.

158. Fraser RS: Catheter-induced pulmonary artery perforation: Pathologic and pathogenic features. Hum Pathol 18:1246, 1987.

159. Rosenblum SE, Ratliff NB, Shirey EK, et al: Pulmonary artery dissection induced by a Swan-Ganz catheter. Cleve Clin Q 51:671, 1984.

160. Dieden JD, Friloux LA III, Renner JW: Pulmonary artery false aneurysms secondary to Swan-Ganz pulmonary artery catheters. Am J Roentgenol 149:901, 1987.

161. Davis SD, Neithamer CD, Schreiber TS, et al: False pulmonary artery aneurysm induced by Swan-Ganz catheter: Diagnosis and embolotherapy. Radiology 164:741, 1987.

162. Cooper JP, Jackson J, Walker JM: False aneurysm of the pulmonary artery associated with cardiac catheterisation. Br Heart J 69:188, 1993.

163. Guttentag AR, Shepard J-AO, McLoud TC: Catheter-induced pul-

monary artery pseudoaneurysm: The halo sign on CT. Am J Roentgenol 158:637, 1992.

164. Pellegrini RV, Marcelli GD, DiMarco RF, et al: Swan-Ganz catheter induced pulmonary hemorrhage. J Cardiovasc Surg 28:646, 1987.

165. Rubin SA, Puckett RP: Pulmonary artery-bronchial fistula: A new complication of Swan-Ganz catheterization. Chest 75:515, 1979.

166. Kron IL, Piepgrass W, Carabello B, et al: False aneurysm of the pulmonary artery: A complication of pulmonary artery catheterization. Ann Thorac Surg 33:629, 1982.

167. Urschel JD, Myerowitz PD: Catheter-induced pulmonary artery rupture in the setting of cardiopulmonary bypass. Ann Thorac Surg 56:585, 1993.

168. Kirton OC, Varon AJ, Henry RP, et al: Flow-directed, pulmonary artery catheter-induced pseudoaneurysm: Urgent diagnosis and endovascular obliteration. Crit Care Med 20:1178, 1992.

169. Brown BG, Goldfarb D, Topaz SR, et al: Diastolic augmentation by intra-aortic balloon: Circulatory hemodynamics and treatment of severe acute left ventricular failure in dogs. J Thorac Cardiovasc Surg 53:789, 1967.

170. Hyson EA, Ravin CE, Kelley MJ, et al: Intra-aortic counterpulsation balloon: Radiographic considerations. Am J Roentgenol 128:915, 1977.

171. Ravin CE, Putman CE, McLoud TC: Hazards of the intensive care unit. Am J Roentgenol 126:423, 1976.

172. Steiner RM, Tegtmeyer CJ, Morse D, et al: The radiology of cardiac pacemakers. Radiographics 6:373, 1986.

173. Grier D, Cook PG, Hartnell GG: Chest radiographs after permanent pacing: Are they really necessary? Clin Radiol 42:244, 1990.

174. Bejvan SM, Ephron JH, Takasugi JE, et al: Imaging of cardiac pacemakers. Am J Roentgenol 169:1371, 1997.

175. Goodman LR, Almassi GH, Troup PJ, et al: Complications of automatic implantable cardioverter defibrillators: Radiographic CT and echocardiographic evaluation. Radiology 170:447, 1989.

176. Verheyden CN, Price L, Lynch DJ, et al: Implantable cardioverter defibrillator patch erosion presenting as hemoptysis. J Cardiovasc Electrophysiol 5:961, 1994.

177. Dasgupta A, Mehta AC, Rick TW, et al: Erosion of implantable cardioverter defibrillator patch electrode into airways: An unusual cause of recurrent hemoptysis. Chest 113:252, 1998.

178. Boiselle PM, Mansilla AV, Fisher MS, et al: Wandering wires: Frequency of sternal wire abnormalities in patients with sternal dehiscence. Am J Roentgenol 173:777, 1999.

179. Ouellette H, Matzinger F, Dennie C, et al: Cardiac herniation with torsion. Can Assoc Radiol J 50:51, 1999.

180. Gurney JW, Arnold S, Goodman LR: Impending cardiac herniation: The snow cone sign. Radiology 161:653, 1986.

181. Valji MDCM, Maziak DE, Shamji FM, et al: Postpneumonectomy syndrome: Recognition and management. Chest 114:1766, 1998.

182. Bousson V, Arrivé L: Lung herniation occurring after video-assisted thoracic surgery. Am J Roentgenol 172:1145, 1999.

183. Kopka L, Fischder U, Gross AJ, et al: CT of retained surgical sponges (textilomas): Pitfalls in detection and evaluation. J Comput Assist Tomogr 20:919, 1996.

184. Sheehan RE, Sheppard MN, Hansell DM: Retained intrathoracic surgical swab: CT appearances. J Thorac Imaging 15:61, 2000.

185. Kang S-G, Song H-Y, Lim M-K, et al: Esophageal rupture during balloon dilation of strictures of benign or malignant causes: Prevalence and clinical importance. Radiology 209:741, 1998.

186. Kopec SE, Conlan AA, Irwin RS: Perforation of the right ventricle: A complication of blind placement of a chest tube into the postpneumonectomy space. Chest 114:1213, 1998.

187. Kidney DD, Nguyen DT, Deutsch L-S: Radiologic evaluation and management of malfunctioning long-term central vein catheters. Am J Roentgenol 171:1251, 1998.

188. Nolan RL, McAdams HP: Bronchopericardial fistula after placement of an automatic implantable cardioverter defibrillator: Radiographic and CT findings. Am J Roentgenol 172:365, 1999.

189. Millikan JS, Moore EE, Steiner E, et al: Complications of tube thoracostomy for acute trauma. Am J Surg 140:738, 1980.

190. Wolfson KA, Seeger LL, Kadell BM, Eckardt JJ: Imaging of surgical paraphernalia: What belongs in the patient and what does not. RadioGraphics 20:1665, 2000.

CHAPTER 20

Metabolic Pulmonary Disease

METASTATIC PULMONARY CALCIFICATION
PULMONARY ALVEOLAR PROTEINOSIS
  Radiologic Manifestations
AMYLOIDOSIS
  Radiologic Manifestations
PULMONARY ALVEOLAR MICROLITHIASIS
  Radiologic Manifestations

The diseases covered in this chapter comprise a heterogeneous group based on their generally accepted, or suspected, metabolic pathogenesis. They are rare and often associated with no or only mild clinical and functional abnormalities.

METASTATIC PULMONARY CALCIFICATION

Metastatic calcification typically occurs in patients who have hypercalcemia, usually associated with chronic renal failure and secondary hyperparathyroidism[1, 2] and less often with multiple myeloma.[3, 4] The complication has been reported after kidney[5] and liver[6, 7] transplantation. It is especially common in patients undergoing maintenance hemodialysis.[8] In one prospective study of 31 patients undergoing maintenance hemodialysis, of whom 15 died, 9 (60%) had histologic evidence of calcification at autopsy.[2] Metastatic calcification seldom causes any clinical symptoms.

On radiographs and high-resolution computed tomography (HRCT) scans (Fig. 20–1), metastatic pulmonary calcification may be manifested as numerous 3- to 10-mm-diameter calcified nodules or, more commonly, as fluffy, poorly defined nodular opacities mimicking air-space nodules (Table 20–1).[10, 11] When coalescent, the nodular opacities seen on radiograph may be misdiagnosed as pulmonary edema or pneumonia.[12] The calcific nature of the opacities in these situations can be confirmed by scanning with bone imaging agents, such as technetium-99m diphosphonate,[13] or by HRCT.[9, 10] HRCT may show calcification of arteries in the chest wall or, less commonly, of the pulmonary arteries, superior vena cava, or myocardium (see Fig. 20–1).[9–11]

The abnormality shows a predilection for apical and subapical lung zones, a feature attributable to regional differences in pulmonary physiology.[14] Because there is a much higher ventilation-perfusion ratio at the apex than at the base of the lung, the local milieu at the former site has a higher partial pressure of oxygen, a lower partial pressure of carbon dioxide, and a higher pH; it has been estimated that the pH at the apex of the normal lung is roughly 7.50 versus 7.39 at the base.[15] The relative alkalinity favors the precipitation of calcium salts.

Few patients in whom metastatic calcification is demonstrable pathologically show evidence of its presence on radiographs.[2, 16] In a study of nine patients who had metastatic calcification at autopsy, only one had positive findings on chest radiograph;[2] this patient had extremely high tissue levels of calcium. In another review of chest radiographs and computed tomography (CT) scans of seven patients who had biopsy-proven disease, calcification was evident on radiographs in only two cases and on CT scans in four.[10]

PULMONARY ALVEOLAR PROTEINOSIS

Pulmonary alveolar proteinosis is characterized by the accumulation of abundant protein-rich and lipid-rich material resembling surfactant within the parenchymal air spaces.[18] Pulmonary alveolar proteinosis is uncommon; only about 330 patients were reported by 1998.[83] Although the disease occurs predominantly in patients between the ages of 20 and 50 years, very young children constitute a subgroup at increased risk.[20, 21] There is a male-to-female predominance of about 2 to 4:1.[18]

The etiology and pathogenesis of pulmonary alveolar proteinosis are poorly understood. The bulk of evidence suggests an abnormality of surfactant production, metabolism, or clearance by type II alveolar cells and macrophages. Histologically, alveoli are filled with finely granular material that shows a positive reaction to periodic acid–Schiff stain. Ultrastructural,[23] immunochemical,[24] and

Table 20–1. METASTATIC PULMONARY CALCIFICATION

Etiology
  Most commonly chronic renal failure
Clinical symptoms
  Usually asymptomatic
Radiologic manifestations
  Poorly defined nodular opacities
  Upper lobe predominance
  Calcification commonly evident on HRCT
  Calcification of chest wall arteries on HRCT
  Lung uptake on bone scintigraphy

HRCT = high-resolution computed tomography.

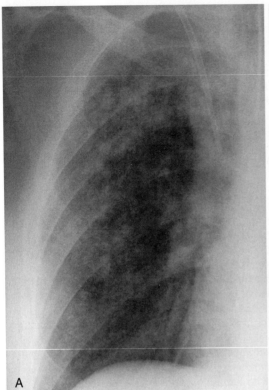

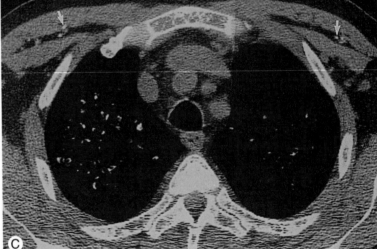

Figure 20–1. Metastatic Pulmonary Calcification. Close-up view of the right lung from posteroanterior chest radiograph *(A)* in a 42-year-old patient who had chronic renal failure shows poorly defined nodular opacities involving mainly the upper lobe. Similar findings were present in the left lung. A hemodialysis catheter is in place. HRCT scan through the lung apices *(B)* shows nodular areas of increased attenuation. Soft tissue windows *(C)* show the presence of calcification within the opacities. Vascular calcification in the chest wall also is evident *(arrows).*

biochemical[25] investigations have shown that the intra-alveolar material resembles surfactant or a component thereof.

Approximately one third of patients are asymptomatic. The remainder manifest a variety of symptoms, the most frequent being shortness of breath on exertion that usually is slowly progressive in severity; rarely, disease is fulminant.[34] Cough, usually nonproductive, often is present.

Radiologic Manifestations

The characteristic radiographic pattern of pulmonary alveolar proteinosis consists of bilateral and symmetric areas of air-space consolidation that have a vaguely nodular appearance and a predominantly perihilar or lower lobe distribution (Fig. 20–2).[18, 26, 83] In patients who have less severe disease, the appearance may be one of ground-glass opacities rather than consolidation (Table 20–2).[27] Differentiation from edema of cardiac origin can be made by the absence of cardiac enlargement and the lack of upper lobe vessel distention, Kerley B lines, or pleural effusions. Occasionally the parenchymal involvement is asymmetric or unilateral.[17, 26, 29] In some patients, a linear interstitial pattern can be seen superimposed on the areas

of consolidation or ground-glass opacities; rarely, it is the predominant or only abnormality seen on radiograph.[26, 30]

Conventional 7- to 10-mm-collimation CT scans show bilateral areas of consolidation with poorly defined margins.[26] HRCT is superior to conventional CT and chest radiography in the assessment of the pattern and distribution of abnormalities[26, 28] and may show lesions even when radiography is normal.[29] The predominant abnormality consists of areas of ground-glass attenuation, although consoli-

Table 20–2. PULMONARY ALVEOLAR PROTEINOSIS

Etiology
    Unknown
Clinical symptoms
    Cough and shortness of breath
Radiologic manifestations
    Ground-glass opacities or consolidation
    Granular appearance
    Diffuse or perihilar distribution
    HRCT shows septal thickening in areas of ground-glass opacities
    HRCT frequently shows geographic distribution

HRCT = high-resolution computed tomography.

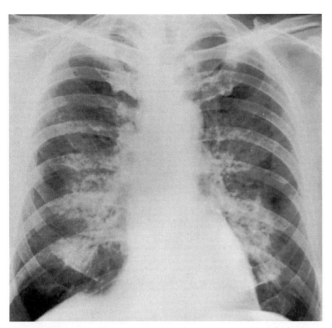

Figure 20–2. Pulmonary Alveolar Proteinosis. Posteroanterior chest radiograph reveals air-space consolidation with a vaguely nodular appearance involving the middle and lower lung zones. The disease possesses a *butterfly* pattern of distribution, with the peripheral zones of the lungs being spared. The patient was a 65-year-old man who had a 5-month history of dry cough and dyspnea.

dation also may be present (particularly in the dorsal lung regions).[18, 26, 28] The distribution of disease is variable; most commonly, it is random, but sometimes it is predominantly central or peripheral.[26, 28] The areas of ground-glass attenuation often have sharply defined straight and angulated margins, giving them a geographic appearance.[28] The sharp margination usually reflects lobular or lobar boundaries.

In most cases, a fine linear pattern forming polygonal shapes measuring 3 to 10 mm in diameter can be seen superimposed on the areas of ground-glass attenuation (Fig. 20–3).[27, 28] This combination gives an appearance that has been described as *crazy-paving*; in one study, this pattern was seen in all six patients.[28] The linear pattern was seen only in the areas of ground-glass attenuation or consolidation and was not apparent on chest radiograph;[28] histologic assessment of open-lung biopsy specimens showed septal edema. Apparent thickening of interlobular septa may be seen at HRCT in patients who have normal septa pathologically, an effect that presumably is related to accumulation of lipoprotein in the air spaces adjacent to the septa.[31] The crazy-paving appearance is not a specific finding; it can be seen in a variety of other conditions, including bronchioloalveolar carcinoma, lipid pneumonia, pulmonary hemorrhage, hydrostatic and permeability pulmonary edema, and bacterial pneumonia.[22, 32, 33]

AMYLOIDOSIS

Although originally considered to represent a single substance, amyloid now is known to consist of several proteins, each of which resembles the others morphologically but is distinctive biochemically.[35] Because of its great variety of clinical and pathologic manifestations, amy-

loidosis has been classified in several ways.[36] The traditional division has been into four major forms depending on the underlying clinical features: (1) *primary amyloidosis*, in which no associated disease is recognized or in which there is an underlying plasma cell disorder (most commonly multiple myeloma); (2) *secondary amyloidosis*, in which there is an identifiable underlying chronic inflammatory abnormality, such as tuberculosis, bronchiectasis, rheumatoid disease, or certain neoplasms such as Hodgkin's disease; (3) *familial amyloidosis*, a relatively uncommon form that may be localized to a specific tissue, such as nerve; and (4) so-called *senile amyloidosis*, which affects many organs and tissues and usually is seen in persons older than age 70 years. A subdivision of amyloidosis into localized (i.e., within a single organ or tissue) and generalized forms is common.

Although these classifications are helpful in understanding the underlying nature of amyloidosis, from the point of view of diagnosis and the clinical consequences of thoracic involvement, it is more useful to consider the anatomic location of disease. According to this concept, three major patterns of amyloid deposition can be seen: (1) tracheobronchial, (2) nodular parenchymal, and (3) diffuse parenchymal (interstitial) (Table 20–3).

Airway involvement occurs most commonly in the trachea and proximal bronchi. Although there is overlap, it usually is manifested in one of two ways:[37, 39] a localized tumor-like nodule or (more commonly) multiple discrete or confluent plaques that cause distortion of the airway wall and stenosis of its lumen. Calcification, ossification, and foreign body giant cell reaction may be present but probably are less common than in the nodular form of parenchymal disease;[38] however, ossification is so severe in some patients that the disease can be confused with tracheobronchopathia osteochondroplastica.[40] The plaque-like form of disease can cause progressive dyspnea or symptoms that simulate asthma;[54] hemoptysis[46] and recurrent bronchitis and pneumonia are common.[46] Discrete tracheal and endobronchial *tumors* seldom cause symptoms and usually are discovered incidentally at bronchoscopy;

Table 20–3. AMYLOIDOSIS

Etiology
    Usually idiopathic
Clinical manifestations
    Often asymptomatic
    Can present with cough and shortness of breath
Radiologic manifestations
    Tracheobronchial amyloidosis
        Focal or diffuse thickening of the trachea
        Foci of calcification common
        Atelectasis and obstructive pneumonitis
    Nodular parenchymal amyloidosis
        Single or multiple nodules
        Foci of calcification common
    Diffuse interstitial amyloidosis
        Diffuse linear interstitial pattern
        Air-space consolidation
        Ground-glass opacities on HRCT
        Interlobular septal thickening on HRCT
        Foci of calcification common

HRCT = high-resolution computed tomography.

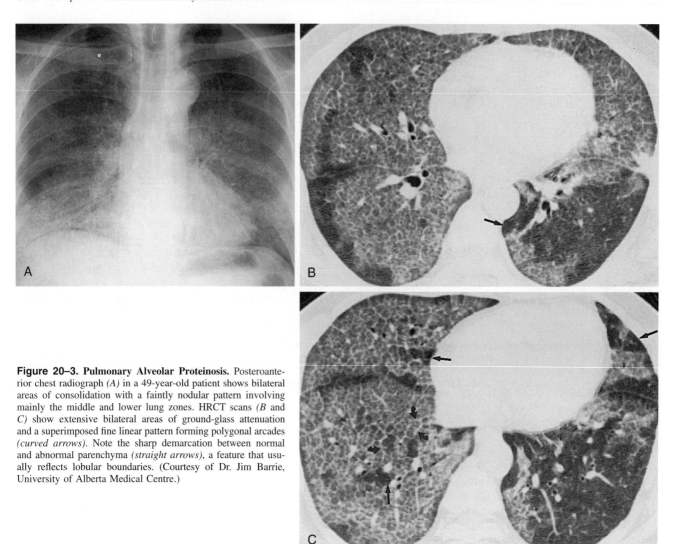

Figure 20–3. Pulmonary Alveolar Proteinosis. Posteroanterior chest radiograph *(A)* in a 49-year-old patient shows bilateral areas of consolidation with a faintly nodular pattern involving mainly the middle and lower lung zones. HRCT scans *(B and C)* show extensive bilateral areas of ground-glass attenuation and a superimposed fine linear pattern forming polygonal arcades *(curved arrows)*. Note the sharp demarcation between normal and abnormal parenchyma *(straight arrows)*, a feature that usually reflects lobular boundaries. (Courtesy of Dr. Jim Barrie, University of Alberta Medical Centre.)

however, they can be large enough to cause airway obstruction, atelectasis, and bronchiectasis.[55, 56]

The parenchymal nodules of localized pulmonary amyloidosis can be solitary or multiple and usually are fairly well defined. Patients usually are asymptomatic,[38] with the lesion being discovered on screening chest radiograph; rarely the nodules are extensive and large enough to cause respiratory symptoms and respiratory failure.[57] In diffuse interstitial disease, amyloid is present in the media of small (and occasionally medium-sized) blood vessels and in the parenchymal interstitium. This variant commonly is accompanied by dyspnea and may be associated with respiratory insufficiency.[38]

Radiologic Manifestations

Tracheobronchial amyloidosis results in focal or diffuse (Fig. 20–4) thickening of the airway wall or, rarely, a localized intraluminal nodule.[41–43] The involvement generally is confined to the trachea. CT may show submucosal foci of calcification.[41, 84]

Nodular parenchymal amyloidosis is manifested by solitary or, less commonly, multiple nodules usually ranging from 0.5 to 5 cm in diameter (Fig. 20–5).[38, 43, 47] Calcifica-

tion seldom is evident on radiograph[48] but is seen in 20% to 50% of nodules on CT scans.[42, 47] Rarely the nodules are cavitated.[37, 49] Occasionally, cystic changes are seen adjacent to the nodules *(see* Fig. 20–5). The nodules occur most commonly in the lower lobes and typically are located peripherally.[38, 47] Disease usually progresses slowly over several years, with a slight increase in size of the nodules and the development of additional nodules.[49, 50] Obstructive bronchial amyloidosis and nodular parenchymal disease occasionally occur concomitantly.[44, 45] A combination of lymphoid interstitial pneumonitis and amyloid nodules that had irregular margins and cystic changes on HRCT has been reported.[51]

Diffuse interstitial disease rarely is seen in primary pulmonary amyloidosis, being present in only 6 of 48 cases in one study[38] and in none of 55 in another.[43] The radiographic findings consist of a diffuse, linear interstitial pattern or, less commonly, air-space consolidation or a small nodular pattern.[38, 52, 53] HRCT in one case showed a linear interstitial pattern, small nodules, and patchy areas of consolidation involving mainly the subpleural regions of the lower lung zones;[52] several of the small nodules contained calcific foci.

In patients who have systemic amyloidosis associated

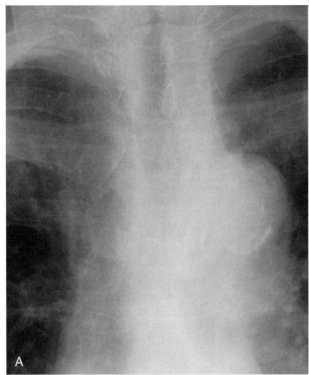
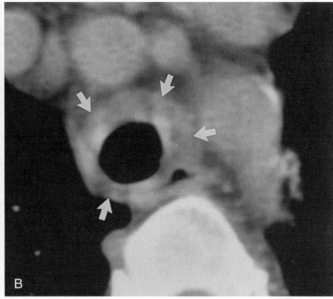

Figure 20–4. Diffuse Tracheal Amyloidosis. View from posteroanterior chest radiograph *(A)* shows irregular narrowing of the trachea. CT scan immediately above the level of the aortic arch *(B)* shows marked circumferential thickening of the trachea *(arrows)*. On CT and at bronchoscopy, the entire trachea was abnormal. The diagnosis of diffuse tracheal amyloidosis was proved by endoscopic biopsy.

with pulmonary parenchymal involvement, the radiographic findings consist of a reticular, nodular, or reticulonodular pattern that may be diffuse or involve mainly the lower lobes.[43] The nodules may be small, mimicking miliary tuberculosis, or measure 2.5 cm in diameter.[47] Unilateral or bilateral pleural effusions may be seen and occasionally constitute the only abnormality evident on chest radiograph.[43] In a review of the HRCT findings in 12 patients who had systemic amyloidosis with thoracic involvement, the most common abnormality was hilar and mediastinal lymph node enlargement, present in 9 patients (75%).[47] Punctate calcifications were present within the enlarged nodes in three of the nine patients. Diffuse lung involvement was present in eight patients (66%). The parenchymal abnormalities consisted of multiple small nodules, interlobular septal thickening, irregular lines giving a reticular pattern, and areas of ground-glass attenuation or consolidation. Punctate calcification was seen in some of the nodules and areas of consolidation. The abnormalities frequently had a predominantly basilar and peripheral distribution.

PULMONARY ALVEOLAR MICROLITHIASIS

Pulmonary alveolar microlithiasis is a rare disease characterized by the presence of innumerable tiny calculi *(calcispherytes)* within alveolar air spaces. Although the disease can occur at any age, having been identified in premature stillborn twins[62] and in an 80-year-old woman,[63] most reported cases have been in patients between the ages of 20 and 50 years.[61] A familial occurrence has been noted in approximately half the reported cases.[60, 71] The etiology and pathogenesis are unknown.

On histologic examination, microliths range in size from about 250 to 750 μm in diameter and are located almost invariably within alveolar air spaces.[59, 65] Nevertheless, evidence suggests that they are formed in the alveolar walls,

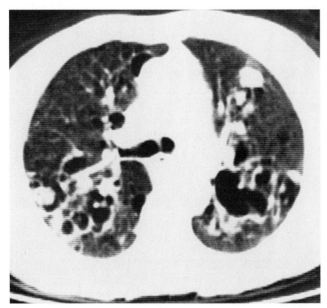

Figure 20–5. Amyloidosis: Nodular Parenchymal. CT scan at the level of the carina shows multiple nodules and cystic spaces. The patient was an elderly woman who complained of dyspnea.

possibly in association with type II cells,[62] and subsequently are extruded into the air spaces.[68] Occasionally, microliths are present outside the alveolar lumen in bronchial wall or fibrotic interstitium;[72] rarely, they are found in extrapulmonary sites.[66, 69] In the early stages of the disease, the alveolar walls are histologically normal;[58] eventually, interstitial fibrosis develops, sometimes associated with multinucleated giant cell formation.[69]

Many patients are asymptomatic when the disease first is discovered,[58] and the diagnosis is made on the basis of the typical radiographic pattern on screening chest radiograph or on a film obtained in an individual whose sibling is known to have the disease. The most common symptom is dyspnea on exertion.[58] Cough develops in some patients;[81] although it is typically nonproductive, some patients have been reported to expectorate microliths.[67] Microliths can be identified in sputum, bronchoalveolar lavage fluid,[85] and transbronchial biopsy specimens.[82]

Radiologic Manifestations

The diagnosis of pulmonary alveolar microlithiasis usually can be made with confidence from the classic radiographic pattern and the striking radiologic-clinical dissociation. The pattern is one of a fine micronodulation diffusely involving both lungs (Fig. 20–6).[72, 73] Regardless of the effect of superimposition or summation of shadows, individual deposits usually are identifiable as sharply defined nodules measuring less than 1 mm in diameter (Table 20–4). The overall density is greater over the lower than the upper zones. The opacities may be so numerous as to appear confluent, in which circumstance a normally exposed chest radiograph shows the lungs as almost uniformly white, often with total obliteration of the mediastinal and diaphragmatic contours; however, use of an overexposed radiographic technique usually reveals the underlying pattern to better advantage. In most cases, chest

Table 20–4. PULMONARY ALVEOLAR MICROLITHIASIS

Etiology
  Unknown
Symptoms
  Progressive shortness of breath
Radiologic manifestations
  Innumerable sandlike nodules
  <1 mm in diameter
  Lower lobe predominance
  HRCT shows innumerable calcific nodules
  HRCT often shows calcified septal lines

HRCT = high-resolution computed tomography.

radiographs obtained 20 to 30 years previously, sometimes in early childhood, are abnormal.[59, 71] Radiographs from asymptomatic relatives of an index patient may show characteristic manifestations of the disease.[72]

Occasionally, radiographic changes consist of a reticular pattern or septal lines superimposed on the characteristic *sandstorm* appearance.[73] Other findings that may be seen include bullae in the lung apices, a zone of increased lucency between the lung parenchyma and the ribs (known as a *black pleural line*), and pleural calcification.[64, 74, 75]

The HRCT manifestations consist of calcific nodules measuring 1 mm or less in diameter, sometimes confluent, and distributed predominantly along the cardiac borders and dorsal portions of the lower lung zones (Fig. 20–7).[76–78] The higher attenuation in the dorsal portion of the lungs persists when scans are obtained with the patient in the prone position.[77] Calcific interlobular septal thickening commonly is seen (*see* Fig. 20–7).[31, 76, 78] Correlation of HRCT findings with pathologic specimens has shown that this apparent thickening is the result of a high concentration of microliths in the periphery of the secondary lobules, rather than calcification of the septa themselves.[31, 76] Other

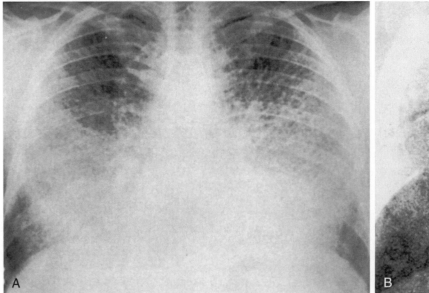
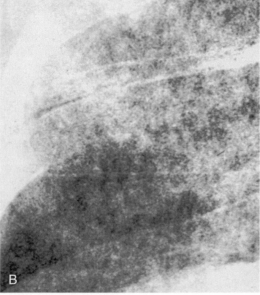

Figure 20–6. Alveolar Microlithiasis. Posteroanterior radiograph *(A)* of this 40-year-old asymptomatic man reveals a remarkably uniform opacification of both lungs. On close scrutiny *(B)*, a multitude of tiny, discrete opacities of calcific density can be seen. Pulmonary function test results were normal except for a reduction in residual volume of 800 ml, representing the displacement of pulmonary volume by the calcispherytes.

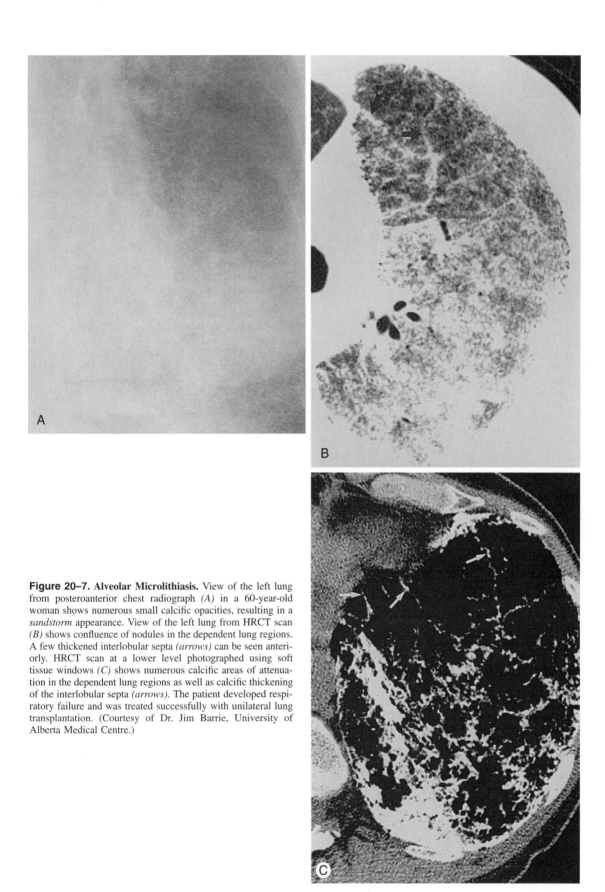

Figure 20–7. Alveolar Microlithiasis. View of the left lung from posteroanterior chest radiograph *(A)* in a 60-year-old woman shows numerous small calcific opacities, resulting in a *sandstorm* appearance. View of the left lung from HRCT scan *(B)* shows confluence of nodules in the dependent lung regions. A few thickened interlobular septa *(arrows)* can be seen anteriorly. HRCT scan at a lower level photographed using soft tissue windows *(C)* shows numerous calcific areas of attenuation in the dependent lung regions as well as calcific thickening of the interlobular septa *(arrows)*. The patient developed respiratory failure and was treated successfully with unilateral lung transplantation. (Courtesy of Dr. Jim Barrie, University of Alberta Medical Centre.)

features seen on HRCT scans include apical bullae and thin-walled subpleural cysts.[77] Correlation of HRCT with radiographic findings has shown that the black pleural line mentioned previously can be caused by subpleural cysts along the costal and mediastinal pleura[77] or by a layer of extrapleural fat.[70] The cysts and apical bullae presumably are the cause of the recurrent pneumothoraces that occur in some patients.[77, 79, 80]

References

1. Faubert PF, Shapiro WB, Porush JG, et al: Pulmonary calcification in hemodialyzed patients detected by technetium-99m diphosphate scanning. Kidney Int 18:95, 1980.
2. Conger JD, Hammond WS, Alfrey AC, et al: Pulmonary calcification in chronic dialysis patients. Ann Intern Med 83:330, 1975.
3. Kempf K, Capesius P, Mugel JL: Un cas de calcinose pulmonaire au cours d'une myélomatose diffuse. J Radiol Electrol Med Nucl 53:861, 1972.
4. Weber CK, Friedrich JM, Merkle E, et al: Reversible metastatic pulmonary calcification in a patient with multiple myeloma. Ann Hematol 72:329, 1996.
5. Breitz HB, Sirotta PS, Nelp WB, et al: Progressive pulmonary calcification complicating successful renal transplantation. Am Rev Respir Dis 136:1480, 1987.
6. Munoz SJ, Nagelberg SB, Green PJ, et al: Ectopic soft tissue calcium deposition following liver transplantation. Hepatology 8:476, 1988.
7. Raisis IP, Park CH, Yang SL, et al: Lung uptake of technetium-99m phosphate compounds after liver transplantation. Clin Nucl Med 13:188, 1988.
8. Parfitt AM, Massry SG, Winfield AC, et al: Disordered calcium and phosphorus metabolism during maintenance hemodialysis: Correlation of clinical, roentgenographic and biochemical changes. Am J Med 51:319, 1971.
9. Johkoh T, Ikezoe J, Nagareda T, et al: Case report: Metastatic pulmonary calcification: Early detection by high-resolution CT. J Comput Assist Tomogr 17:471, 1993.
10. Hartman TE, Müller NL, Primack SL, et al: Metastatic pulmonary calcification in patients with hypercalcemia: Findings on chest radiographs and CT scans. Am J Roentgenol 162:799, 1994.
11. Greenberg S, Suster B: Metastatic pulmonary calcification: Appearance on high resolution CT. J Comput Assist Tomogr 18:497, 1994.
12. Firooznia H, Pudlowski R, Golimbu C, et al: Diffuse interstitial calcification of the lungs in chronic renal failure mimicking pulmonary edema. Am J Roentgenol 129:1103, 1977.
13. Rosenthal DI, Chandler HL, Azizi F, et al: Uptake of bone imaging agents by diffuse pulmonary metastatic calcification. Am J Roentgenol 129:871, 1977.
14. Jost RG, Sagel SS: Metastatic calcification in the lung apex. Am J Roentgenol 133:1188, 1979.
15. West JB: Regional Differences in the Lung. New York, Academic Press, 1977.
16. Murris-Espin M, Lacassagne L, Didier A, et al: Metastatic pulmonary calcification after renal transplantation. Eur Respir J 10:1925, 1997.
17. Prakash USB, Barham SS, Carpenter HA, et al: Pulmonary alveolar phospholipoproteinosis: Experience with 34 cases and a review. Mayo Clin Proc 62:499, 1987.
18. Wang BM, Stern EJ, Schmidt RA, et al: Diagnosing pulmonary alveolar proteinosis: A review and an update. Chest 111:460, 1997.
19. McCook TA, Kirks DR, Merton DF, et al: Pulmonary alveolar proteinosis in children. Am J Roentgenol 137:1023, 1981.
20. Kariman K, Kylstra JA, Spook A: Pulmonary alveolar proteinosis: Prospective clinical experience in 23 patients for 15 years. Lung 162:223, 1984.
21. Mahut B, Delacourt C, Scheinmann P, et al: Pulmonary alveolar proteinosis: Experience with eight pediatric cases and a review. Pediatrics 97:117, 1996.
22. Johkoh T, Itoh H, Müller NL, et al: Crazy-paving appearance at thin-section CT: Spectrum of disease and pathologic findings. Radiology 211:155, 1999.
23. Gilmore LB, Talley FA, Hook GE: Classification and morphometric quantitation of insoluble materials from the lungs of patients with alveolar proteinosis. Am J Pathol 133:252, 1988.
24. Singh G, Katyal SL: Surfactant apoprotein in nonmalignant pulmonary disorders. Am J Pathol 101:51, 1980.
25. Bell DY, Hook GER: Pulmonary alveolar proteinosis: Analysis of airway and alveolar proteins. Am Rev Respir Dis 119:979, 1979.
26. Godwin JD, Müller NL, Takasugi JE: Pulmonary alveolar proteinosis: CT findings. Radiology 169:609, 1988.
27. Lee KN, Levin DL, Webb WR, et al: Pulmonary alveolar proteinosis: High-resolution CT, chest radiographic, and functional correlations. Chest 111:989, 1997.
28. Murch CR, Carr DH: Computed tomography appearances of pulmonary alveolar proteinosis. Clin Radiol 40:240, 1989.
29. Zimmer WE, Chew FS: Pulmonary alveolar proteinosis. Am J Roentgenol 161:26, 1993.
30. Miller PA, Ravin CE, Smith GJW, et al: Pulmonary alveolar proteinosis with interstitial involvement. Am J Roentgenol 137:1069, 1981.
31. Kang EY, Grenier P, Laurent F, Müller NL: Interlobular septal thickening: Patterns at high-resolution computed tomography. J Thorac Imaging 11:260, 1996.
32. Tan RT, Kuzo RS: High-resolution CT findings of mucinous bronchioloalveolar carcinoma: A case of pseudopulmonary alveolar proteinosis. Am J Roentgenol 168:99, 1997.
33. Franquet T, Giménez A, Bordes R, et al: The crazy-paving pattern in exogenous lipoid pneumonia: CT-pathologic correlation. Am J Roentgenol 170:315, 1998.
34. Ito K, Iwabe K, Okai T, et al: Rapidly progressive pulmonary alveolar proteinosis in a patient with chronic myelogenous leukemia. Intern Med 33:710, 1994.
35. Westermark P: The pathogenesis of amyloidosis: Understanding general principles. Am J Pathol 152:1125, 1998.
36. Editorial: Amyloid and the lower respiratory tract. Thorax 38:84, 1983.
37. Cordier JF, Loire R, Brune J: Amyloidosis of the lower respiratory tract: Clinical and pathologic features in a series of 21 patients. Chest 90:827, 1986.
38. Hui AN, Koss MN, Hochholzer L, et al: Amyloidosis presenting in the lower respiratory tract: Clinicopathologic, radiologic, immunohistochemical, and histochemical studies on 48 cases. Arch Pathol Lab Med 110:212, 1986.
39. Toyoda M, Ebihara Y, Kato H, et al: Tracheobronchial amyloidosis: Histologic, immunohistochemical, ultrastructural, and immunoelectron microscopic observations. Hum Pathol 24:970, 1993.
40. Jones AW, Chatterji AN: Primary tracheobronchial amyloidosis with tracheobronchopathia osteoplastica. Br J Dis Chest 71:268, 1977.
41. Kwong JS, Müller NL, Miller RR: Diseases of the trachea and mainstem bronchi: Correlation of CT with pathologic findings. Radiographics 12:645, 1992.
42. Urban BA, Fishman EK, Goldman SM, et al: CT evaluation of amyloidosis: Spectrum of disease. Radiographics 13:1295, 1993.
43. Utz JP, Swensen SJ, Gertz MA: Pulmonary amyloidosis: The Mayo Clinic experience from 1980 to 1993. Ann Intern Med 124:407, 1996.
44. Cotton RE, Jackson JW: Localized amyloid "tumours" of the lung simulating malignant neoplasms. Thorax 19:97, 1964.
45. Mosetitsch W: Amyloid "tumoren" der lungen. [Amyloid tumors of the lungs.] Fortschr Roentgenstr 94:579, 1961.
46. Rubinow A, Celli BR, Cohen AS, et al: Localized amyloidosis of the lower respiratory tract. Am Rev Respir Dis 118:603, 1978.
47. Pickford HA, Swensen SJ, Utz JP: Thoracic cross-sectional imaging of amyloidosis. Am J Roentgenol 168:351, 1997.
48. Bhate DV: Case of the spring season: Diffuse primary amyloidosis with nodular calcified lung lesions. Semin Roentgenol 14:81, 1979.
49. Gross BH, Felson B, Birnberg FA: The respiratory tract in amyloidosis and the plasma cell dyscrasias. Semin Roentgenol 21:113, 1986.
50. Tamura K, Nakajima N, Makino S, et al: Primary pulmonary amyloidosis with multiple nodules. Eur J Radiol 8:128, 1988.
51. Desai SR, Nicholson AG, Stewart S, et al: Benign pulmonary lymphocytic infiltration and amyloidosis: Computed tomographic and pathological features in three cases. J Thorac Imaging 12:215, 1997.
52. Graham CM, Stern EJ, Finkbeiner WE, et al: High-resolution CT appearance of diffuse alveolar septal amyloidosis. Am J Roentgenol 158:265, 1992.
53. Morgan RA, Ring NJ, Marshall AJ: Pulmonary alveolar-septal amyloidosis—an unusual radiographic presentation. Respir Med 86:345, 1992.

54. Brown J: Primary amyloidosis. Clin Radiol 15:358, 1964.

55. Simpson GT 2nd, Strong MS, Skinner M, et al: Localized amyloidosis of the head and neck and upper aerodigestive and lower respiratory tracts. Ann Otol Rhinol Laryngol 93:374, 1984.

56. Flemming AFS, Fairfax AJ, Arnold AG, et al: Treatment of endobronchial amyloidosis by intermittent bronchoscopic resection. Br J Dis Chest 74:183, 1980.

57. Laden SA, Cohen ML, Harley RA: Nodular pulmonary amyloidosis with extrapulmonary involvement. Hum Pathol 15:594, 1984.

58. Sosman MC, Dodd GD, Jones WD, et al: The familial occurrence of pulmonary alveolar microlithiasis. Am J Roentgenol 77:947, 1957.

59. Prakash UBS, Barham SS, Rosenow EC III, et al: Pulmonary alveolar microlithiasis: A review including ultrastructural and pulmonary function studies. Mayo Clin Proc 58:290, 1983.

60. Mariotta S, Guidi L, Papale M, et al: Pulmonary alveolar microlithiasis: Review of Italian reports. Eur J Epidemiol 13:587, 1997.

61. Ucan ES, Keyf AI, Aydilek R, et al: Pulmonary alveolar microlithiasis: Review of Turkish reports. Thorax 48:171, 1993.

62. Caffrey PR, Altman RS: Pulmonary alveolar microlithiasis occurring in premature twins. J Pediatr 66:758, 1965.

63. Sears MR, Chang AR, Taylor AJ: Pulmonary alveolar microlithiasis. Thorax 26:704, 1971.

64. Gómez GE, Lichtemberger E, Santamaria A, et al: Familial pulmonary alveolar microlithiasis: Four cases from Colombia, S.A.: Is microlithiasis also an environmental disease? Radiology 72:550, 1959.

65. Moran CA, Hochholzer L, Hasleton PS, et al: Pulmonary alveolar microlithiasis: A clinicopathologic and chemical analysis of seven cases. Arch Pathol Lab Med 121:607, 1997.

66. Coetzee T: Pulmonary alveolar microlithiasis with involvement of the sympathetic nervous system and gonads. Thorax 25:637, 1970.

67. Brown ML, Swee RG, Olson RJ, et al: Pulmonary uptake of ^{99m}Tc-diphosphonate in alveolar microlithiasis. Am J Roentgenol 131:703, 1978.

68. Bab I, Rosenmann E, Ne'eman Z, et al: The occurrence of extracellular matrix vesicles in pulmonary alveolar microlithiasis. Virchows Arch [Pathol Anat] 391:357, 1981.

69. Barnard NJ, Crocker PR, Blainey AD, et al: Pulmonary alveolar microlithiasis: A new analytical approach. Histopathology 11:639, 1987.

70. Hoshino H, Koba H, Inomata S-I, et al: Pulmonary alveolar microlithiasis: High-resolution CT and MR findings. J Comput Assist Tomogr 22:245, 1998.

71. Thind GS, Bhatia JL: Pulmonary alveolar microlithiasis. Br J Dis Chest 72:151, 1978.

72. Helbich TH, Wojnarovsky C, Wunderbaldinger P, et al: Pulmonary alveolar microlithiasis in children: Radiographic and high-resolution CT findings. Am J Roentgenol 168:63, 1997.

73. Balikian JP, Fuleihan FJD, Nucho CN: Pulmonary alveolar microlithiasis: Report on 5 cases with special reference to roentgen manifestations. Am J Roentgenol 103:509, 1968.

74. Cheong WY, Wang YT, Tan LKA, et al: Pulmonary alveolar microlithiasis. Australas Radiol 32:401, 1988.

75. Felson B: The roentgen diagnosis of disseminated pulmonary alveolar diseases. Semin Roentgenol 2:3, 1967.

76. Cluzel P, Grenier P, Bernadac P, et al: Pulmonary alveolar microlithiasis: CT findings. J Comput Assist Tomogr 15:938, 1991.

77. Korn MA, Schurawitzki H, Klepetko W, et al: Pulmonary alveolar microlithiasis: Findings on high-resolution CT. Am J Roentgenol 158:981, 1992.

78. Melamed JW, Sostman HD, Ravin CE: Interstitial thickening in pulmonary alveolar microlithiasis: An underappreciated finding. J Thorac Imaging 9:126, 1994.

79. Waters MH: Microlithiasis alveolaris pulmonum. Tubercle 41:276, 1960.

80. Winzelberg GG, Boller M, Sachs M, et al: CT evaluation of pulmonary alveolar microlithiasis. J Comput Assist Tomogr 8:1029, 1984.

81. Turktas I, Saribas S, Balkanci F: Pulmonary alveolar microlithiasis presenting with chronic cough. Postgrad Med J 69:70, 1993.

82. Cale WF, Petsonk EL, Boyd CB: Transbronchial biopsy of pulmonary alveolar microlithiasis. Arch Intern Med 143:358, 1983.

83. Goldstein LS, Kavuru MS, Curtis-McCarthy P, et al: Pulmonary alveolar proteinosis: Clinical features and outcomes. Chest 114:1357, 1998.

84. Webb EM, Elicker BM, Webb WR: Using CT to diagnose nonneoplastic tracheal abnormalities: Appearance of the tracheal wall. Am J Roentgenol 174:1315, 2000.

85. Chalmers AG, Wyatt J, Robinson PJ: Computed tomographic and pathological findings in pulmonary alveolar micolithiasis. Br J Radiol 59:408, 1986.

CHAPTER 21

Pleural Disease

PLEURAL EFFUSION

General Features of Pleural Effusion

Pleural effusion is an accumulation of fluid in the pleural space that results when homeostatic forces that control the flow in and out of the space are disrupted.[1] The character of fluid in the pleural space—transudate, exudate, pus, blood, chyle, or any combination of these—seldom is discernible radiographically; *increase in pleural fluid* and not *pleural effusion* should be the correct term for reporting these radiographic appearances. Because it is in common usage, however, the term *effusion* is used here. Where appropriate, the precise terms *hydrothorax* (for serous effusions, either transudate or exudate), *pyothorax, hemothorax,* and *chylothorax* are employed. Although the precise incidence of pleural effusion is unknown, it has been estimated that approximately 1 million people develop the abnormality each year in the United States.[2]

This chapter is concerned with the diagnosis and differential diagnosis of diseases of the pleura. The radiographic signs of pleural disease and the use of imaging in the detection of loculated effusion are discussed in Chapter 3. Before reviewing the specific causes of pleural effusion—of which there are many (Table 21–1)—the general features of clinical disturbances, the findings on biochemical analysis of pleural fluid, and the means of investigation are summarized briefly.

Clinical Manifestations

Pleural pain that is sharp, localized, and exacerbated by inspiration is a frequent manifestation of *dry* pleurisy but often diminishes when effusion develops. In some cases, the pain is not accentuated by breathing and is felt as a dull ache. Dry cough may be seen and can become productive if there is associated pneumonia. Dyspnea is common and may be severe, as a result of compromise of respiratory reserve by the effusion or concomitant pulmonary parenchymal or vascular disease. Approximately 15% of patients who have pleural effusions are asymptomatic.[3] Many conditions are associated with pleural effusions in the absence of chest-related symptoms, including recent childbirth or abdominal surgery, asbestos-related effusion, uremia, malignancy, and tuberculosis.

Thoracentesis, Thoracoscopy, and Pleural Biopsy

Thoracentesis often is the first diagnostic test performed in patients who have pleural effusion of unknown etiology;[4] it also serves to drain pleural fluid for the relief of dyspnea. When performed by relatively inexperienced operators, complications are common.[5] Although many of these complications are minor, pneumothorax developed in 15 of 129

Table 21–1. PLEURAL EFFUSION—ETIOLOGY

Etiology	Selected References
Pleuropulmonary infection	See text
Mycobacterium tuberculosis	
Nontuberculous mycobacteria	
Actinomyces and *Nocardia* species	
Fungi	
Parasites	
Viruses, *Mycoplasma,* and Rickettsiae	
Pleuropulmonary malignancy	See text
Pulmonary carcinoma	
Metastatic neoplasm to pleura and mediastinal lymph nodes	
Lymphoma	
Leukemia	
Connective tissue disease	See text
Systemic lupus erythematosus	
Rheumatoid disease	
Others	
Asbestos	46
Drugs (see Table 21–2)	
Heart failure	See text
Trauma	
Penetrating and nonpenetrating injury	
Coronary artery bypass graft procedures	
Pulmonary resection	
Esophageal rupture	
Intravascular therapeutic or monitoring devices	
Abdominal surgery	87
Subarachnoid–pleural fistula	138
Metabolic and endocrine disease	
Myxedema	102
Diabetes mellitus	139
Amyloidosis	140, 141
Skeletal disease	
Neoplasms	
Langerhans' cell histiocytosis	142
Spondylitis	143, 183
Gorham's disease	144
Liver disease	
Cirrhosis	85, 86
Biliary tract fistula	88
Transplantation	89
Kidney disease	
Dialysis	90
Urinoma	91
Nephrotic syndrome	92
Acute glomerulonephritis	93
Uremia	94
Pancreatic disease	
Acute pancreatitis	95
Chronic pancreatitis with pleuropancreatic fistula	96
Gynecologic tumors	
Ovary, uterus, fallopian tube	97, 98
Gastrointestinal tract	
Gastric/duodenal-pleural fistula	99
Diaphragmatic hernia	84
Idiopathic inflammatory bowel disease	100
Miscellaneous causes	
Ovarian hyperstimulation syndrome	184
Endometriosis	109
Subphrenic abscess	101
Lymphatic hypoplasia	103
Dressler's syndrome	104
Familial paroxysmal polyserositis	108
Rupture of silicon gel mammoplasty device	145
Systemic cholesterol embolization	146
Extramedullary hematopoiesis	185
Idiopathic	147

patients (12%) in one series;[5] pain at the site of thoracentesis was experienced by many of the patients.

Although an appreciation of clinical, radiologic, and laboratory findings results in an etiologic diagnosis in many patients who have pleural effusion, sometimes this remains unclear even after extensive diagnostic evaluation, including thoracentesis. In this situation, invasive diagnostic procedures often are necessary; the usual sequence of events after thoracentesis is closed biopsy, followed (if necessary) by thoracoscopic or open biopsy.

Pleural Effusion Caused by Infection

Pleural infection invariably produces an exudative effusion. The most common etiologic agents are bacteria.

Mycobacteria

As with pulmonary disease, most cases of pleural mycobacterial infection are caused by *Mycobacterium tuberculosis*; only occasional cases are related to nontuberculous mycobacteria, either as a manifestation of primary disease or in association with reactivation.[7, 8] Tuberculous pleural effusion is believed to result from rupture of subpleural foci of necrosis into the adjacent pleural space.[12] Although such foci usually cannot be seen on conventional chest radiographs, they have been documented pathologically[12] and on computed tomography (CT) scans.[14]

In regions where exposure to tuberculosis is common, tuberculous effusion occurs most often in young people.[10] In regions where tuberculosis is less prevalent, infection and associated pleural disease develop more commonly in middle-aged or elderly patients.[11] In one investigation from Alabama, the median age of 70 patients who had tuberculous pleurisy was 47 years;[11] half had evidence of simultaneous parenchymal disease on chest radiograph. Other workers have estimated that 80% of patients who have tuberculous pleural effusion have concomitant pulmonary tuberculosis.[10]

The clinical presentation of tuberculous pleural effusion is acute in about two thirds of patients and relatively indolent in the remainder.[9, 15] Symptoms of chest pain, cough, breathlessness, fever, and prostration may suggest the diagnosis of acute pneumonia.[16] The effusion almost invariably is unilateral and seldom massive.

Bacteria Other than Mycobacteria

It has been estimated that parapneumonic pleural effusion occurs in approximately 40% of the 1.2 million cases of bacterial pneumonia annually in the United States;[331] of these, tube thoracostomy is required for drainage in about 10%. A parapneumonic effusion is a pleural effusion associated with pneumonia; it may be infected or uninfected. Although some investigators have considered any infection in the pleural space to be empyema,[17] we and others believe the term is reserved better for cases in which infection is associated with frank pus in the pleural space.[18, 19] It is likely that the complication is more common than these figures suggest because its presence frequently is unrecognized as a result of the small amount of fluid (i.e., the recorded incidence of parapneumonic effusion would increase sharply if radiographs were obtained in the lateral decubitus position in all cases, Fig. 21–1). This supposition was borne out by the results of a prospective evaluation of 203 patients who had acute bacterial pneumonia on whom bilateral decubitus radiographs were obtained within 72 hours of the onset of the pneumonia;[20] 90 patients (44%) were found to have radiographically demonstrable pleural

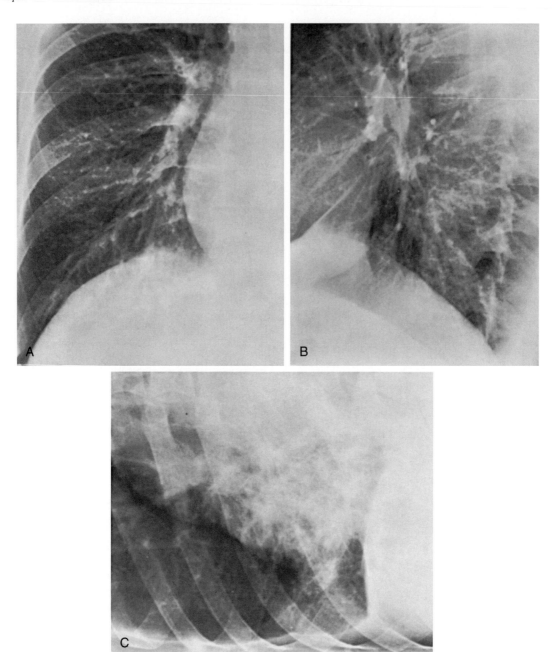

Figure 21–1. Pleural Effusion Associated with Acute Bronchopneumonia. Detail views of the lower half of the right lung from posteroanterior *(A)* and lateral *(B)* radiographs reveal inhomogeneous consolidation of all basal segments of the right lower lobe. The parenchymal abnormality extends from the hilum to the diaphragmatic pleural surface in strict segmental distribution. Although no pleural effusion is evident on these radiographs exposed in the erect position, lateral decubitus view *(C)* shows a small free pleural effusion extending along the lateral chest wall.

effusion. Parapneumonic effusions usually are serous exudates that resolve spontaneously.[20]

The incidence of empyema is about 0.5 to 0.8 per 1,000 hospital admissions;[17] the complication is acquired in the hospital in about one third of these cases. In an acutely ill but debilitated group of New York City patients hospitalized for pneumonia, the incidence of nontuberculous bacterial empyema was almost 7%.[21]

As in the bacterial pneumonias, the organisms responsible for empyema vary with the host's state of health. In developed countries, about two thirds of cases generally are attributed to aerobic bacteria;[23, 24] anaerobic bacteria with or without associated aerobic infection are responsible

for the remainder.[26, 27] Among the aerobic organisms, *Staphylococcus aureus* and enteric gram-negative bacilli are important pathogens,[22, 28] particularly in the post-trauma setting. The same organisms as well as anaerobic bacteria are a common cause of empyema in human immunodeficiency virus (HIV)–positive drug abusers.[25] *Streptococcus pneumoniae* is an important cause in some series.[28, 29]

Although most patients who have empyema are febrile and have blood neutrophilia, the compromised host[21] and patients receiving corticosteroid therapy[30] can be afebrile and have a normal white blood cell count. Patients who have aerobic bacterial pneumonia and effusion usually have an acute onset of chest pain, fever, cough, and sputum, whereas symptoms are more indolent in patients who have anaerobic infection.[2]

In most cases of empyema, there are no radiologic findings that suggest a specific cause, and the diagnosis is made by isolation of the organism from the pleural fluid. A rare exception is infection by the gas-forming bacteria *Clostridium perfringens* and *Bacteroides fragilis*, in which pneumonia and pleural effusion may be associated with gas in the soft tissues of the chest wall or in the pleural space (pyopneumothorax).

Pleural Effusion Caused by Immunologic Disease

Among the connective tissue diseases, systemic lupus erythematosus and rheumatoid disease are the most important causes of pleural effusion. In patients who have other disorders, such as progressive systemic sclerosis,[31] dermatomyositis, and Sjögren's syndrome, effusion more commonly results from other causes (e.g., heart failure) than from the primary disease.

Systemic Lupus Erythematosus

Clinical involvement of the pleura occurs during the course of systemic lupus erythematosus in 70% of patients and is the presenting manifestation in 5% to 10%.[325, 326] Patients typically have pleuritic pain accompanied by dyspnea, cough, and fever.[32] Effusions generally are bilateral and small to moderate in size but may be unilateral, massive, or both.[325]

Effusions related to lupus pleuritis generally are serous or serosanguineous and invariably exudative.[327] The most common associated radiologic finding is enlargement of the cardiopericardial silhouette, which has been reported to occur in 50% of patients.[328] This enlargement usually is nonspecific in character and minimal to moderate in degree. It has been ascribed to pericardial effusion, endocarditis, or myocarditis or to the effects of hypertension, renal disease, or anemia. Pericarditis is seen at presentation in approximately 10% of patients who have systemic lupus erythematosus[325] and occurs at some time during the course of disease in 20% to 30% of patients.[328] Variation in size of the cardiopericardial silhouette usually takes place during a period of weeks but may occur with startling abruptness; in the latter situation, pericardial effusion is the most likely cause. When enlargement of the cardiopericardial silhouette is associated with bilateral pleural effusion, the diagnosis of lupus serositis should be considered, particularly in young women. Echocardiography is the imaging method of choice to confirm the presence of pericardial effusion.[328]

Rheumatoid Disease

Pleural abnormalities are probably the most frequent manifestation of rheumatoid disease in the thorax;[33] pleuritis and pleural effusion are the most common of these. For unknown reasons, pleural effusion in association with rheumatoid disease has a strong predilection for men,[35] despite the fact that rheumatoid arthritis occurs predominantly in women. It is also much more likely to occur in patients who have subcutaneous nodules than in those who do not[36] and has a tendency to remain relatively unchanged

radiographically for many months or years.[37] In one review of 25 cases, 23 were unilateral (14 on the right and 9 on the left).[34]

The effusion may be entirely unsuspected because of lack of symptoms,[37] as was the case in approximately 50% of patients in one series.[34] Occasionally, effusion develops abruptly and is associated with pain and fever.[38] As the amount of fluid increases, so does the likelihood of dyspnea; rarely the effusion is so massive that it is associated with respiratory failure.[39] The effusion may antedate clinical evidence of rheumatoid arthritis[36] or may occur when joint disease is only mild;[40] in many cases, it is associated with episodic exacerbations of arthritis[34] and in some with pericarditis. The effusion can be transient, persisting, or relapsing.[325] When chronic, it may lead to fibrothorax requiring decortication.[325]

Empyema occurs with increased frequency in patients who have rheumatoid disease.[41] The most plausible explanation is impaired host defense, perhaps most commonly related to corticosteroid therapy.[41] The complication should be distinguished from the sterile effusion that results from the exudation of white blood cells and debris into the pleural space after rupture of rheumatoid nodules located in the subpleural parenchyma.[332]

Pleural Effusion Caused by Asbestos

Benign asbestos pleural effusion is probably more common than generally is recognized.[42, 43] Estimates of its prevalence and incidence in an asbestos-exposed population have been derived from a study of 1,134 exposed workers and 717 control subjects.[43] The abnormality was defined by (1) a history of exposure to asbestos, (2) confirmation of the presence of effusion by radiographs or thoracentesis, (3) lack of other disease associated with pleural effusion, and (4) absence of malignant tumor within 3 years. Among the exposed workers, 34 (3%) benign effusions were found compared with no unexplained effusions among the control subjects; this contrasts with a reported history of symptomatic benign pleural effusion in only 20 (0.7%) of 2,815 insulation workers.[44]

The pathogenesis of benign asbestos effusion is uncertain. Its development appears to be dose related, the latency period being shorter than that for other asbestos-related disorders;[43] it is probably the most common abnormality during the first 20 years after exposure. Most patients are asymptomatic;[45, 46] however, chest pain has been found to occur in about one third in some studies.[43] Persistent pleuritic pain associated with intermittent pleural friction rubs has been described in some patients.[47] Others have fever suggesting infection.[43] Effusions usually are smaller than 500 ml and persist 2 weeks to 6 months;[45, 51] they are recurrent in 15% to 30% of cases.[42, 48] Occasional cases are associated with the development of round atelectasis.[49]

In most patients, the fluid is a sterile serous or blood-tinged exudate. The differential diagnosis includes tuberculosis and mesothelioma. Large effusions are more likely to be caused by mesothelioma;[50] a bloody effusion, although typical of malignancy, may be benign in the setting of asbestos exposure. Differentiation from tuberculosis can be made with confidence only if biopsy and culture results are negative. Follow-up has shown that some workers are left with blunting of the costophrenic angle and diffuse pleural thickening, with consequent deleterious effects on lung function.[44]

Pleural Effusion Caused by Drugs

Many drugs have been reported to cause pleural effusion (Table 21–2).[51] Some, such as bromocriptine, methysergide, and dantrolene sodium, appear to affect the pleura almost selectively.[52]

Pleural Effusion Caused by Neoplasms

The most common cause of exudative pleural effusion is malignancy.[6, 9] In one series of 83 patients who had pleural exudates, malignancy was the cause in 64 (77%).[6] Although most common in patients who have clinical features indicating a primary extrapleural tumor, effusion may

Table 21–2. DRUG CAUSES OF PLEURAL EFFUSION

Drug	Selected References
Drug-Induced Lupus Syndrome	148, 149
Hydralazine	
Procainamide	
Isoniazid	
Phenytoin and other anticonvulsants	
Quinidine	
Methyldopa	
Chlorpromazine	
Sulfasalazine	
β-adrenoreceptor blocking agents (acebutolol, labetalol, pindolol, propranolol)	
Drugs that Affect the Pleural Space Selectively	52
Bromocriptine	
Methysergide	
Dantrolene sodium	
Drugs that Affect the Pleural Space Nonselectively	
Chemotherapeutic Agents	
Bleomycin	150
Mitomycin C	151, 152
Busulfan	153
Mephalan	154
Cystosine arabinoside	155
Methotrexate	157, 158
Biologic response modifiers	
Interleukin-2	159
Granulocyte-macrophage colony–stimulating factor	160
Antibiotics	
Nitrofurantoin	161
Minocycline	162, 163
Metronidazole	
Antiarrhythmia drugs	
Amiodarone	164
Miscellaneous drugs	
Acyclovir	165
Prophylthiouracil	166
Minoxidil	156
Ergotamine	2
Ethchlorvynol	2

be the first manifestation of malignancy or the first evidence of disease recurrence. In one series of 96 patients who had neoplastic involvement of the pleura, effusion was the abnormality that led to the diagnosis of carcinoma in 44 (46%).[53]

The results of several reviews indicate that the major causes of malignant pleural effusion are pulmonary, breast, ovarian, and gastric carcinoma and lymphoma;[54–56] pulmonary carcinoma, breast carcinoma, and lymphoma account for 75% of all malignant pleural effusions.[57] In one series, malignancies manifesting with pleural effusion represented 32 of 459 (7%) carcinomas of the lung, 20 of 645 (3%) neoplasms of the breast, 9 of 303 (3%) carcinomas of the ovary, and 7 of 195 (4%) carcinomas of the stomach.[53] Approximately 90% of the lung, breast, and ovarian malignant effusions were on the same side as the primary lesions.[53] An additional important, although relatively infrequent, cause of malignant pleural effusion is mesothelioma. Regardless of primary site, bilateral pleural involvement in metastatic carcinoma frequently is associated with hepatic metastases.[58]

The pathogenesis of pleural effusion in malignancy is multifactorial.[9, 59] Possible mechanisms include (1) tumor invasion of the pleura, stimulating an inflammatory reaction associated with capillary fluid leak; (2) tumor invasion of the pulmonary or pleural lymphatics and bronchopulmonary, hilar, or mediastinal lymph nodes, hindering the return of lymphatic fluid to the circulation; (3) bronchial obstruction by a carcinoma, creating an increased negative intrapleural pressure, increasing transudation; (4) hypoproteinemia in debilitated patients, leading to increased transudation; (5) infection resulting in a parapneumonic effusion; and (6) drug reaction, radiation therapy, or deposition of immune complexes related to circulating tumor antigens, causing increased pleural capillary permeability.[60] The most common mechanism is lymphatic obstruction.[9]

Pleural involvement by carcinoma does not necessarily result in effusion; in a detailed autopsy report of 52 patients who had pleural metastases (29 from the lung, 9 from the breast, 4 from the pancreas, 5 from the stomach, and 5 miscellaneous), effusions were found in only 31 patients (60%).[58] The effusions bore no relation to the extent of pleural involvement by metastases; fluid appeared to accumulate principally as a result of neoplastic infiltration of mediastinal lymph nodes.

The diagnosis of carcinoma as the cause of pleural effusion may be suspected from chest radiograph, the manifestation being one of either primary pulmonary carcinoma or nodular or reticulonodular opacities characteristic of metastatic carcinoma. Tension hydrothorax has been reported as a result of extensive neoplastic involvement of the pleura, apparently related to impaired lymphatic drainage and hypoproteinemia;[61] in the case reported, the clinical picture was similar to that of tension pneumothorax, and the fluid was found to be under high pressure on thoracentesis. Radiologically, tension hydrothorax may be diagnosed by the presence of marked contralateral shift of the mediastinum and inversion of the diaphragm (Fig. 21–2). It can be confirmed by ultrasonography, CT, or magnetic resonance (MR) imaging.[62, 63, 259]

The incidence of a positive cytologic examination in patients who have malignant pleural effusion ranges from

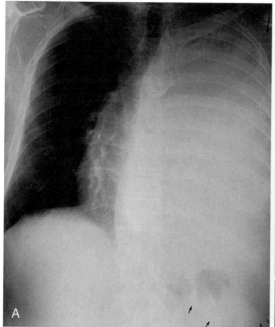

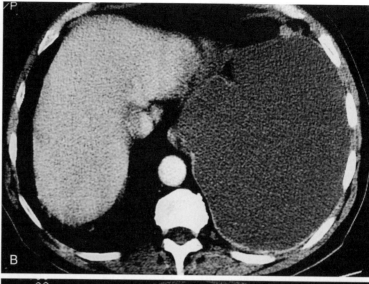

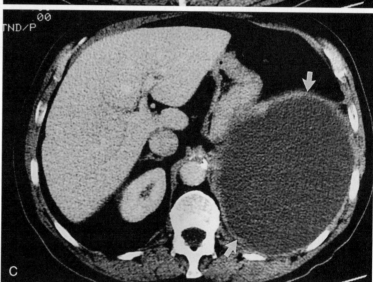

Figure 21–2. Tension Pleural Effusion. Posteroanterior chest radiograph *(A)* in a 69-year-old man shows opacification of the left hemithorax as a result of a large pleural effusion. The effusion is associated with considerable contralateral shift of the mediastinum, widening of the spaces between the ribs, and inversion of the posterior aspect of the left hemidiaphragm *(arrows)*, indicating that it is under tension. (The inversion was easier to visualize on the original radiograph than on the figure.) CT scan at the level of the dome of the right hemidiaphragm *(B)* shows a large left pleural effusion. CT scan at a more caudad level *(C)* shows pleural fluid central to the left hemidiaphragm *(arrows)*, a characteristic finding of inversion. The presence of abundant intraperitoneal fat anterior to the inverted left hemidiaphragm provides the soft tissue contrast that allows visualization of the inverted posterior aspect of the hemidiaphragm on chest radiograph. Cytologic examination of the pleural fluid revealed adenocarcinoma. The primary tumor was in the left lung.

about 35% to 85%, with most investigators reporting a value of about 50%. As a diagnostic procedure, cytologic examination of pleural fluid gives a higher yield than closed pleural biopsy, although data gained from these procedures are complementary.[54, 64]

Pleural Effusion Caused by Thromboemboli

As a radiographic manifestation of thromboembolic disease, pleural effusion is as common as parenchymal consolidation.[66, 67] In a review of the radiographic findings of 1,063 patients who underwent pulmonary angiography for suspected pulmonary thromboembolism in the PIOPED trial, 35% of 383 patients who were diagnosed as having pulmonary thromboembolism had pleural effusion on the side of the embolism.[68] Pleural effusions were present in 74% of patients who had pleural-based areas of increased opacity. The prevalence of effusions or of pleural-based areas of increased opacity was not significantly different from that in the 680 patients who did not have pulmonary thromboembolism, however.[68] In a prospective study of 62 patients who had pulmonary thromboembolism and effu-

sion, radiographic evidence of infarction was found in only half.[69]

Pleural Effusion Caused by Cardiac Failure

One of the most common forms of pleural effusion is that associated with an increase in hydrostatic pressure in the pulmonary venous circulation.[70] Although it occurs most commonly with cardiac decompensation, it also has been documented in about 60% of patients who have constrictive pericarditis, for which it may be the presenting clinical finding.[71] The fluid is usually a transudate.

Hydrothorax in congestive heart failure is most often bilateral; almost 90% of patients in one autopsy study were found to have bilateral effusions.[72] For unknown reasons, unilateral effusion is more prone to be right-sided than left-sided; if an effusion is confined to the left hemithorax, a cause other than heart failure should be sought.[70] Associated clinical and radiologic evidence of cardiac enlargement, with or without pulmonary venous hypertension, makes the diagnosis obvious in most cases. A radiologic finding peculiar to hydrothorax associated with congestive heart failure is the so-called phantom tumor, in which fluid tends to localize (not loculate) in an interlobar pleural fissure (Fig. 21–3). For unknown reasons, these *disappearing tumors* occur most frequently in the minor fissure.

Pleural Effusion Caused by Trauma

As might be expected, pleural effusion secondary to trauma most often is caused by an accumulation of blood; occasionally, it is chyle (after rupture of the thoracic duct) or cerebrospinal fluid or is serosanguineous in nature. Although hemorrhage may result from laceration of the parietal or visceral pleura by fractured ribs, it also can occur (with or without associated pneumothorax) in closed chest trauma without fracture. Hemothorax commonly complicates traumatic rupture of the aorta and almost invariably is left-sided;[329] as a result, care should be taken not to attribute effusion erroneously to left-sided rib fracture.

Rupture of the esophagus after closed chest trauma is rare and results in changes localized to the mediastinum and pleura.[73] Of considerably greater frequency is the rupture that occurs spontaneously after severe vomiting (Boerhaave's syndrome) or as a complication of esophagoscopy or gastroscopy,[74] overzealous dilation of a stricture or achalasia, disruption of the suture line after esophageal resection and anastomosis, or passage of an esophageal obturator airway by paramedical personnel during cardiopulmonary resuscitation.[75] Although almost always left-sided, rare cases of right-sided effusion have been documented.[76] In most patients, the site of rupture can be identified precisely (although sometimes with considerable difficulty) by ingestion of radiographic contrast material.

The most common pleural effusion of traumatic etiology is that caused by thoracotomy. Chest radiographs 2 or 3 days after thoracotomy usually show no fluid because the pleural space is drained effectively. After removal of the drainage tube, however, a small amount of fluid often appears, only to disappear quite quickly during convalescence. Minimal pleural thickening may remain.

Pleural effusion is common after myocardial revascularization procedures, occurring in 90% of patients.[77, 78] The accumulation of fluid in larger than expected amounts may be attributable to a variety of causes, including poor positioning of the drainage tube, hemorrhage from an intercostal vessel, or infection (empyema). Hemorrhage from intercostal vessels occasionally is an important complication in patients undergoing heart-lung transplantation.[79]

Malpositioning of percutaneous central venous and Swan-Ganz catheters can cause perforation of a vessel, either at the time of insertion or some time later as a result of gradual erosion of a relatively thin-walled intrathoracic vessel by the catheter tip.[80] Depending on the vessel involved and on the reason for catheter insertion (monitoring of pressure or hyperalimentation), the result may be mediastinal hemorrhage, hemothorax,[81] pneumothorax, massive hydrothorax,[82] or extrapleural hematoma.[83]

Pleural Effusion Related to Disease of Abdominal Organs

A variety of intra-abdominal or pelvic disorders are associated with pleural effusion (*see* Table 21–1). The pathogenesis is complex and varies according to the particular disease examined; it can be related to secondary effects

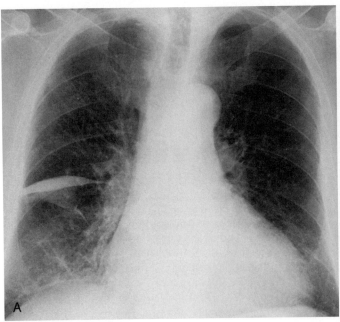

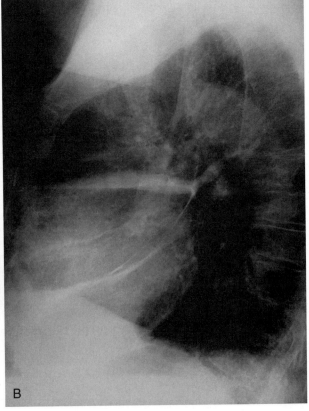

Figure 21–3. Focal Interlobar Pleural Effusions in Cardiac Decompensation. Posteroanterior *(A)* and lateral *(B)* chest radiographs show localized effusions within the right major and minor interlobar fissures. This 75-year-old patient had left ventricular failure and pulmonary edema secondary to myocardial infarction.

on cardiac function, changes in plasma oncotic pressure, or production of ascites or secretions that are transferred through diaphragmatic lymphatics or defects into the pleural space.

Miscellaneous Causes of Pleural Effusion

Dressler's Syndrome

The postpericardiectomy or post–myocardial infarction syndrome, known eponymously as *Dressler's syndrome*, is characterized by chest pain, fever, and pericardial and pleural effusion. Dressler[104] estimated the incidence to be 3% to 4% of patients after myocardial infarction, and it is probable that the incidence is higher after surgical procedures that affect the pericardium.[13] In the era of thrombolytic therapy, the incidence after myocardial infarction seems to be decreasing; in one study of 210 patients who were given thrombolytic therapy for this reason, only 1 developed the syndrome in the following 3 weeks.[105] In patients who have infarction, the syndrome is particularly apt to occur in the presence of transmural myocardial damage with epicardial extension.[106] The pathogenesis is unknown but is suspected to be the result of an immunologic reaction.

In one retrospective study of 35 patients who had the syndrome (21 after cardiac surgery and 14 after myocardial infarction), the onset of symptoms occurred, on average, 20 days after the injury.[107] The major clinical findings were chest pain (91%), fever (66%), pericardial rub (63%), and dyspnea (57%). Chest radiograph was abnormal in 94% of the patients. Pleural effusion was present in 83% of patients, parenchymal opacities were present in 74%, and an enlarged cardiopericardial silhouette was present in 49%.

Endometriosis

The presence of endometrial tissue within the thorax is uncommon; only about 110 cases were documented in the English literature by 1996.[109] In most, the abnormal tissue is located in the visceral or parietal pleura and is discovered after the development of pneumothorax or hemothorax; approximately 15% of patients present with recurrent hemoptysis or are found to have a nodule on screening chest radiograph, indicating involvement of the pulmonary parenchyma.[109]

Although metaplasia of pleural mesothelial and submesothelial connective tissue into endometrial tissue has been hypothesized to be a mechanism for the development of thoracic endometriosis,[110] more widely believed theories involve embolization of endometrial tissue via the pulmonary arteries and migration of tissue from the peritoneum across the diaphragm.[109]

Most women who have thoracic endometriosis are between 20 and 40 years old, the mean age at diagnosis in one literature review being 35.[109] Pleural involvement usually manifests itself as catamenial pneumothorax (about 75% of cases) or hemothorax (about 15%).[109] The main symptoms are shoulder or chest pain and dyspnea.[110] These symptoms appear within 72 hours of the onset of menses and typically are recurrent; in 63 cases in one review, the number of episodes of pneumothorax ranged from 2 to 42 (average, 14).[110]

Grossly, pleural endometriosis appears as multiple (occasionally single) bluish purple nodules 1 mm to several centimeters in diameter. The right pleural cavity is affected in most cases.

The radiographic manifestations are those of pneumothorax or hemothorax; pleural nodules are only rarely visible.[111, 112] In one case, CT and ultrasound showed soft tissue nodules in the pleural and peritoneal cavities as well as localized defects in the right hemidiaphragm.[113]

CHYLOTHORAX

Chylothorax is the presence of lymphatic fluid in the pleural space resulting from obstruction or disruption of the thoracic duct or one of its major divisions.[114] (The lymphatic drainage of the small intestine, chyle, is carried entirely by the thoracic duct; chylothorax can occur only with obstruction or laceration of this duct. Lesions that obstruct the right lymphatic duct or pulmonary lymphatics can cause pleural effusion but never chylothorax.[115]) The fluid is characteristically *milky* in appearance, although not all milky effusions are chylous in nature,[65, 116] and not all chylous effusions are milky.[117] A *chyliform* effusion results from degeneration of malignant and other cells in pleural fluid. This *pseudochylous* effusion results from the presence of cholesterol crystals and occurs most commonly in tuberculosis, rheumatoid disease, and nephrotic syndrome. Because the separation of pseudochylous and chyliform effusions serves little useful purpose, we designate them both as chyliform.

There are numerous causes of chylothorax (Table 21–3). In a review of 143 cases derived from five series, the most common were neoplasm and trauma, the former being responsible twice as often as the latter.[13] Lymphoma is the most common neoplasm,[119] being the cause in about 75% of patients who have malignancy.[13, 120] Pulmonary carcinoma and metastatic cancer from virtually every organ in the body have been reported to obstruct the thoracic duct and cause chylothorax. In the presence of cancer, the effusion often is bilateral and usually is accompanied by chylous ascites.[121, 122]

Trauma is the second most common cause of chylothorax, most episodes being related to surgery and some to penetrating or nonpenetrating thoracic injury.[123, 124] Because the thoracic duct crosses to the left of the spine between the fifth and the seventh thoracic vertebrae, disruption tends to cause right-sided chylothorax when the lower portion is affected and left-sided disease when the upper half is involved. Once the duct has been disrupted, chyle can leak into the mediastinum and into the pleural cavity, either because of damage to the parietal pleura by the initial trauma or because the pleura ruptures under the pressure of the mediastinal fluid collection. Because of its anatomic course, the thoracic duct is particularly vulnerable to traumatic injury during surgery on the vertebral column.[125, 126]

Radiographic findings are no different from those of pleural effusion of nonchylous etiology. Occasionally the abnormality can be diagnosed on CT scan by the presence of attenuation values as low as −17 HU as a result of the presence of fat; however, in most patients the high protein content leads to higher attenuation values that are indistinguishable from those of pleural effusions of other etiol-

Table 21–3. CHYLOTHORAX—ETIOLOGY

Etiology	Selected References
Neoplasia	
Metastatic carcinoma	121
Lymphoma/leukemia	118, 120
Kaposi's sarcoma	
Penetrating or nonpenetrating thoracic injury	123, 134
Surgery	
Sclerotherapy of esophageal varices	335
Thoracic	124, 167
Abdominal	127, 128
Neck	129, 130
Congenital anomalies	
Congenital lymphangiectasis	131
Noonan's syndrome	132
Jaffe-Campanacci syndrome	168
Adams-Oliver syndrome	169
46 XY/46 XX mosaicism	170
Miscellaneous	
Pancreatitis	171
Tuberculous spondylitis or lymphadenitis	172, 173
Chronic sclerosing mediastinitis	174
Subclavian vein thrombosis	175
Sarcoidosis	176, 177
Severe heart failure	178
Retrosternal goiter	179
Behçet's syndrome	180
Gorham's syndrome	181
Lymphangioleiomyomatosis	337
Thoracic aortic aneurysm	182
Castleman's disease	186
Cirrhosis	187

ogy.[133] A fat-fluid level may occasionally be seen on CT in patients with nonchylous lipid accumulation (pseudochylous effusion).[389] In one report of six patients with pseudochylous pleural effusion with fat-fluid levels, in five the effusion was due to tuberculosis.[389] Although usually free fluid, loculated collections may result in a masslike appearance (chyloma).[134] Lymphangiography has an important role in the investigation,[135, 136] and has been shown to be superior to CT.[137] The abnormalities that can be identified with this examination have been described in detail.[115]

PNEUMOTHORAX

The presence of air within the pleural space, or pneumothorax, is one of the more common forms of thoracic disease. It is caused most often by trauma, either accidental or iatrogenic. In the absence of such a history, pneumothorax traditionally is referred to as spontaneous: In this situation, it can be primary (unassociated with clinical or radiographic evidence of significant pulmonary disease) or secondary (in which significant pulmonary disease is present). The primary form occurs most commonly in men in their twenties or thirties.[189–191] Although the male-to-female predominance varies in different studies, from 2:1[192] to 15:1,[193] most investigators have found a ratio of about 4:1 or 5:1.[194–197]

Pneumothorax can occur secondary to pneumomediastinum, air tracking from that location into the pleural space through the mediastinal pleura. In this situation, there is evidence that the most likely sites of rupture are small areas just above the root of the left lung and at the junction with the pericardium.[188] This section is concerned predominantly with the epidemiology, etiology, pathogenesis, and clinical manifestations of pneumothorax; radiologic signs are discussed in detail in Chapter 3.

Primary Spontaneous Pneumothorax

The primary form of spontaneous pneumothorax appears to be caused by rupture of an air-containing space within or immediately deep to the visceral pleura. These spaces may be a *bulla* (defined as a sharply demarcated region of emphysema >1 cm in diameter[198]) or a *bleb* (a focal gas-containing space situated entirely within the pleura). Although often referred to as blebs, it is likely that most of the air-containing spaces associated with pneumothorax are bullae. CT scans show focal areas of emphysema in more than 80% of patients who have spontaneous pneumothorax, even those who are lifelong nonsmokers.[194–196] These areas are situated predominantly in the peripheral regions of the apex of upper lobes and are seen as localized areas of low attenuation measuring 3 mm or more in diameter that may or may not be delineated by thin walls (Fig. 21–4).[195]

At surgery or pathologic examination emphysema is evident in more than 90% of patients with pneumothorax.[195, 199] In one study of 116 consecutive patients who had undergone thoracotomy for recurrent or persistent primary or secondary pneumothorax, emphysema with bulla formation was identified histologically in 93 (80%); emphysema without bulla formation, in 13 (11%); isolated bullae or blebs, in 2 patients each; and other pulmonary or pleural abnormalities, in 6 (5%).[199] Seventy-four patients had irregular emphysema, 26 had paraseptal emphysema, 4 had mixed irregular and centrilobular or paraseptal emphysema, and 2 had unclassifiable emphysema.[199] In lifelong nonsmokers, the areas of emphysema often measure less than 1 cm in diameter.

Bullae can be recognized on radiograph as localized areas of radiolucency measuring 1 cm or more in diameter. They are more likely to be identified when they cause an irregular outline of the visceral pleura, a finding most easily appreciated in the presence of pneumothorax (Fig. 21–5). Even in the latter situation, however, bullae often are not identifiable on conventional chest radiographs.[204, 205] By contrast, bullae can be seen on CT scan in most patients.[194, 195, 199] In one study, evidence of emphysema was seen on CT scan in 16 of 20 (80%) patients who had spontaneous pneumothorax.[194] In another investigation in which the conventional CT findings in 27 lifelong nonsmokers who had previous spontaneous pneumothorax were compared with the findings in 10 nonsmoking controls, localized areas of emphysema were identified in 22 (81%) of the patients and in none of the controls.[195] The emphysema involved mainly the upper lobes and the peripheral rather than the central lung region; in patients who had unilateral pneumothorax, the ipsilateral lung was affected predominantly or exclusively. In none of the patients was the emphysema evident on chest radiograph.[195]

In a third study, conventional 10-mm collimation CT was compared with chest radiography in 35 patients who

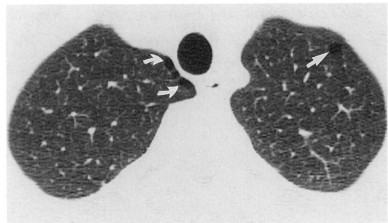

Figure 21–4. Localized Emphysema in a Nonsmoker.
HRCT scan in an 18-year-old man shows small subpleural bullae in the right lung apex *(curved arrows)* and a localized area of emphysema in the left lung apex *(straight arrow)*. The patient was a lifelong nonsmoker who previously had undergone chest tube drainage for recurrent right pneumothorax. The emphysema and bullae could not be visualized on chest radiograph even in retrospect.

had primary spontaneous pneumothorax.[206] Localized emphysema with or without bulla formation was identified on CT scan in 31 patients (89%) and on radiograph in 15 (43%). Abnormalities were detected in the lung ipsilateral to the pneumothorax on 28 (80%) CT scans and on 11 (31%) chest radiographs and in the contralateral lung on 23 (66%) CT scans and on 4 (11%) chest radiographs. In most cases, the abnormalities consisted of a few localized areas of emphysema (n < 5) measuring less than 2 cm in diameter.

The immediate cause of rupture of a bleb or bulla often is unknown. It is not related to exertional effort because

most patients are at rest when the pneumothorax occurs.[207] Localized areas of emphysema distend with decrease in atmospheric pressure (e.g., with increasing altitude during flight[208] and with rapid surfacing after diving[209, 210]), and this mechanism may be important in some cases.

Secondary Spontaneous Pneumothorax

The pathogenesis of secondary spontaneous pneumothorax is multifactorial. Many cases are associated with the formation of subpleural cystic spaces related to diffuse interstitial fibrosis or emphysema; rupture of one of these is likely the immediate cause of pneumothorax in many cases. The most common concurrent condition in patients who have secondary spontaneous pneumothorax is chronic obstructive pulmonary disease (COPD); presumably reflecting this association, the incidence of pneumothorax increases with age.[200]

Numerous conditions have been associated with secondary spontaneous pneumothorax; the list given in Table 21–4 is incomplete. In some cases, the pneumothorax is the first manifestation of the disease. Examples of the complication associated with emphysema (Fig. 21–6) and lymphangioleiomyomatosis (Fig. 21–7) are given for illustrative purposes.

The prevalence of the various causes of pneumothorax has been assessed in two studies of 116 and 120 patients.[199, 211] In the first study, emphysema with or without bullae was identified in the resected specimens in 106 of the 116 patients (91%); isolated bullae or blebs, in 2 patients each; and other etiologies, in 6 (5%).[199] The pathologic diagnoses in the patients without emphysema, bullae, or blebs included mesothelioma (in two patients) and metastatic angiosarcoma from the breast, subpleural fibrosis, interstitial fibrosis with honeycombing, and congenital cystic adenomatoid malformation (in one patient each).

In a second retrospective study of 120 patients who had spontaneous pneumothorax and were admitted to the hospital, 31 (26%) had localized areas of emphysema, bullae, or blebs; 12 (10%) had COPD; 32 (27%) had acquired immunodeficiency syndrome (AIDS); and 45 (37%) had other underlying lung diseases.[211] Of the patients who had AIDS, 25 (78%) had *Pneumocystis carinii* pneumonia, and the remaining 7 had infection by *M. tuberculo-*

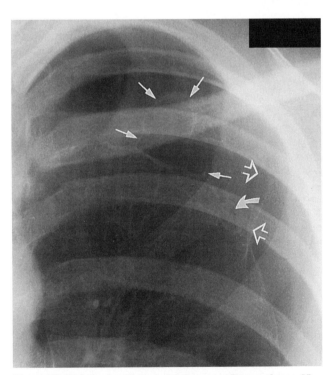

Figure 21–5. Bullae in a Patient with Recurrent Pneumothorax. View of the left upper chest from posteroanterior radiograph in a 17-year-old man who had recurrent pneumothorax shows large bullae *(straight arrows)*. Irregularity of the margins of the visceral pleura as a result of subpleural bullae *(curved arrow)* and adhesions between the visceral and parietal pleura *(open arrows)* are evident. The patient was a 3-pack-per-year smoker.

Table 21–4. SECONDARY SPONTANEOUS PNEUMOTHORAX

Etiology	Selected References
Developmental disease	
Congenital cystic adenomatoid malformation	199
Connective tissue disease	
Lymphangioleiomyomatosis	336, 337
Tuberous sclerosis	338, 339
Neurofibromatosis	340
Marfan's syndrome	201, 202
Ehlers-Danlos syndrome	211
Mitral valve prolapse	203
Infection	
Fungal pneumonia (particularly *Pneumocystis carinii* pneumonia patients who have AIDS	342, 343
Hydatid disease	344
Bacterial pneumonia	211
Neoplasms	
Primary pulmonary carcinoma	345
Carcinoid tumor	346
Mesothelioma	199, 211
Metastatic carcinoma	347
Metastatic sarcoma	348
Metastatic germ cell tumors	349
Drugs and toxins	
Chemotherapy for malignancy	211, 350
Paraquat poisoning	351
Hyperbaric oxygen therapy	352
Radiation therapy	353, 354
Aerosolized pentamidine therapy in patients with AIDS	355
Immunologic disease	
Wegener's granulomatosis	356
Idiopathic pulmonary hemorrhage	357
Idiopathic pulmonary fibrosis	211
Langerhans' cell histiocytosis	211, 358
Sarcoidosis	211, 359
Chronic obstructive pulmonary disease	
Asthma	211, 360
Emphysema	194, 361
Cystic fibrosis	362
Pneumoconiosis	
Silicoproteinosis	363
Berylliosis	364
Bauxite pneumoconiosis	365
Vascular disease	
Pulmonary infarction	366, 367
Metabolic disease	
Pulmonary alveolar proteinosis	368
Intra-abdominal disease	
Gastropleural fistula	369, 370
Colopleural fistula	371

AIDS = acquired immunodeficiency syndrome.

sis or nontuberculous mycobacteria. The diagnoses in the 45 patients who had underlying disease other than AIDS, emphysema, or COPD included pneumonia, carcinoma, asthma, tuberculosis, Langerhans' cell histiocytosis, sarcoidosis, idiopathic pulmonary fibrosis, Job's syndrome, drug-induced lung disease, and immunologically mediated connective tissue disease. In addition to the numerous diseases associated with pneumothorax listed in Table 21–4, several specific disease processes and forms of pneumothorax deserve more detailed comment.

Catamenial Pneumothorax

The term *catamenial pneumothorax* refers to the development of pneumothorax at the time of menstruation. The complication probably can develop by several mechanisms. It is likely that some cases are the result of migration of air directly through the vagina, uterus, and fallopian tubes into the peritoneal cavity and through diaphragmatic fenestrations into the pleural space.[212] Another, probably more frequent, mechanism is related to pleural endometriosis. Clinical or pathologic evidence of pelvic endometriosis is present in 20% to 60% of patients who have catamenial pneumothorax,[213, 214] and diaphragmatic or pleural endometrial implants have been shown at thoracotomy in about 25% to 35% of patients.[215, 216]

The main symptoms are shoulder or chest pain and dyspnea.[110] They usually appear within 72 hours of the onset of menses and typically are recurrent. In 63 cases in one review, the number of episodes of pneumothorax ranged from 2 to 42 (average, 14).[110] Symptoms are absent between menstruations.[213, 215]

The radiologic manifestations typically are those of pneumothorax, hemothorax, or pleural effusion;[213, 217] pleural nodules are visible rarely.[111–113] About 85% to 90% of cases occur on the right side, 5% on the left, and 5% bilaterally.[213] One patient has been described in whom pleural endometriosis was shown by CT and ultrasonography;[113] the abnormal tissue extended into the pleural space through defects in the diaphragm.

Traumatic Pneumothorax

As indicated previously, trauma probably is the most common cause of pneumothorax. Of the 318 cases described in one series, it was the responsible mechanism in 177 (56%);[200] the trauma was iatrogenic in 102 cases and noniatrogenic in 75. In a second study of 196 patients seen during a 5-year period, iatrogenic pneumothorax was seen in 106 (54%) and spontaneous pneumothorax in 90.[218] Traumatic pneumothorax can be caused by direct communication of the pleural space with the atmosphere through chest wall puncture or by disruption of the proximal tracheobronchial tree or the visceral pleura.

A variety of investigative and biopsy procedures can be complicated by pneumothorax (Table 21–5). In a review of 106 cases of iatrogenic pneumothorax, 35 (33%) were related to transthoracic needle aspiration biopsy, 30 (28%) to thoracentesis, 23 (22%) to subclavian vein catheterization, 7 (7%) to positive-pressure ventilation, and 11 (10%) to miscellaneous causes.[218] Two of the 106 patients died as a result of pneumothorax.

PLEURAL FIBROSIS

After effusion, fibrosis is the most common pleural abnormality. As with pleural effusion, fibrosis has numerous etiologies and is the outcome of many primary pleural diseases as well as a potential complication of virtually every inflammatory condition that affects the lungs. In most cases, the fibrosis is patchy or is localized to a single, relatively small area; in these circumstances, clinical and

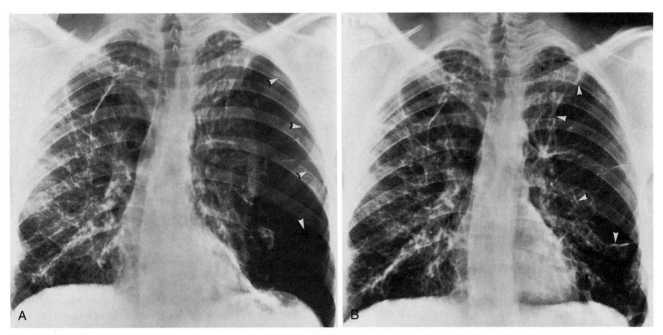

Figure 21–6. Spontaneous Pneumothorax Associated with Diffuse Bullae. Posteroanterior radiograph *(A)* reveals a left pneumothorax. Both lungs contain a multitude of small and large thin-walled bullae, several of which have failed to collapse because of air-trapping *(arrowheads).* A chest tube was inserted promptly, and the pneumothorax was evacuated. After removal of the chest tube 4 days later *(B),* the pneumothorax is no longer evident. The bullae that failed to collapse at the time of the pneumothorax are indicated by *arrowheads.*

functional abnormalities are absent, and the condition is recognized on screening radiograph or CT scan during the investigation of other intrathoracic disease or at autopsy. Less commonly the fibrosis is more or less diffuse in one or both pleural cavities, in which case functional abnormalities may be apparent. Because of this important difference, the two forms are discussed separately.

Local Pleural Fibrosis

Healed Pleuritis

The most common cause of localized pleural fibrosis is organized fibrinous or fibrinopurulent pleuritis secondary to pneumonia. Because pleural effusions of infectious etiology almost invariably are basal, it is not surprising that this is the anatomic location of most pleural thickening related to this etiology. The usual radiographic abnormality is partial obliteration or blunting of the posterior and lateral costophrenic sulci, in some cases associated with line shadows. Thickening of the pleural line may extend for a variable distance up the lateral and posterior thoracic walls, diminishing gradually toward the apex and seldom amounting to more than 1 to 2 mm in width. Obliteration of the costophrenic sulci sometimes has a radiographic appearance difficult to differentiate from that of a small

Figure 21–7. Pneumothorax Associated with Lymphangioleiomyomatosis. HRCT scan in a 40-year-old woman shows a small right pneumothorax and numerous cystic lesions with well-defined walls, characteristic of lymphangioleiomyomatosis. Pleural adhesions *(arrows)* related to recurrent pneumothorax can be seen on the right.

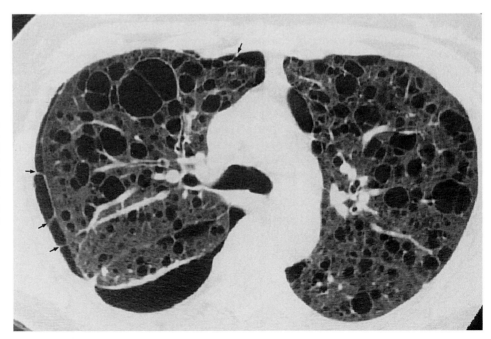

Table 21–5. IATROGENIC CAUSES OF PNEUMOTHORAX

Procedure	Selected References
Biopsy Procedures	
Transthoracic needle aspiration	372, 373
Transbronchial biopsy	374
Transtracheal biopsy	218
Colonoscopy	375
Liver biopsy	218
Fine-needle aspiration of breast	376
Therapeutic Procedures	
Thoracentesis	218
Central venous catheterization	377, 378
Feeding tube insertion	379, 380
Positive–pressure ventilation	218
Tracheal intubation	381, 382
Pacemaker insertion	218
Electromyographic electrode insertion	383
Acupuncture	384, 388
Percutaneous nephrolithotomy	385, 386
Use of a voice box prosthesis	387

pleural effusion, in which case radiography in the lateral decubitus position, ultrasound, or CT is required for clarification.

Apical Cap

An *apical cap* is defined radiographically as a curved soft tissue opacity at the apex of one or both hemithoraces (Fig. 21–8).[219, 220] Although the abnormality can have many causes, in most cases a specific cause is not identified. Such idiopathic caps usually measure less than 5 mm in height and have a sharply marginated smooth or undulating lower margin.[219, 220] In a review of chest radiographs of 258 patients, a unilateral cap was seen in 11% and bilateral caps in 12%.[219] The prevalence increased with age, being identified in 6% of patients younger than 45 years and 16% of patients older than 45.[219] The prevalence is similar in men and women.[219]

As indicated, a specific cause for a cap is identified only occasionally. The abnormality commonly is present in patients who have upper lobe fibrosis secondary to tuberculosis.[221] In this situation, the cap often is larger than in the idiopathic variety, commonly measuring several centimeters in thickness (Fig. 21–9).[221] In one high-resolution computed tomography (HRCT) study of 18 patients who had long-standing tuberculosis, most of the apical cap

was the result of an accumulation of extrapleural fat.[221] Where the fat and lung came in contact, a 1- to 3-mm-thick rim of soft tissue was evident, presumably representing the thickened visceral and parietal pleural layers. The lung adjacent to the cap showed evidence of scarring and traction bronchiectasis. Apical caps may be the result of pleural and subpleural fibrosis after radiation therapy for carcinoma of the breast, lung, or neck.[220, 222]

An apical cap may be confused radiologically with the companion shadows of the first and second ribs. Of greater importance from a differential diagnostic point of view is the early stage of an apical pulmonary carcinoma (Pancoast's tumor, Fig. 21–10). Suspicion of Pancoast's tumor should be aroused when the apical abnormality is predominantly unilateral, when there is a greater than 5 mm difference in height between right and left apical caps, when there is a focal convexity, or when sequential radiographs show progressive enlargement. Other uncommon causes of an increased apical opacity include extrapleural extension of tumor in patients who have lymphoma or mesothelioma and dilation of the subclavian veins.[220] Apical caps that develop acutely usually are the result of the extrapleural accumulation of blood after trauma to the chest wall or thoracic aorta.[223, 224] A similar process may occur as a complication of placement of internal jugular or subclavian venous catheters.[220]

Pleural Plaques

Pleural plaques are well-circumscribed foci of dense fibrous tissue that typically are located on the parietal pleura. The lesion is common: of 7,085 autopsies in the general population reported in 16 separate studies, they were identified in 857 (12%).[225] Because the cause of the fibrosis is asbestos in most cases, the prevalence is influenced by the population studied and is especially high if there has been contact with an increased level of asbestos particles in the ambient air. The prevalence has been found to be approximately 4% in 381 autopsies in a general urban population,[226] 8% in 862 autopsies in a general population in an asbestos-industrial region,[227] and 39% in a population in an asbestos-mining region.[228]

Pleural plaques are evident on chest radiograph in 20% to 60% of workers exposed to high concentrations of asbestos.[225] The latency period between exposure to asbestos and development of radiologically visible plaques is approximately 15 years; for radiologically visible calcified plaques, the latency period is at least 20 years.[225, 230]

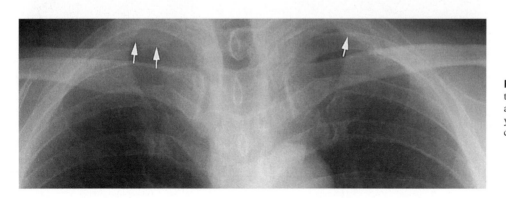

Figure 21–8. Apical Cap. View of the upper hemithorax from posteroanterior chest radiograph in a 72-year-old man shows normal apical caps *(arrows)*.

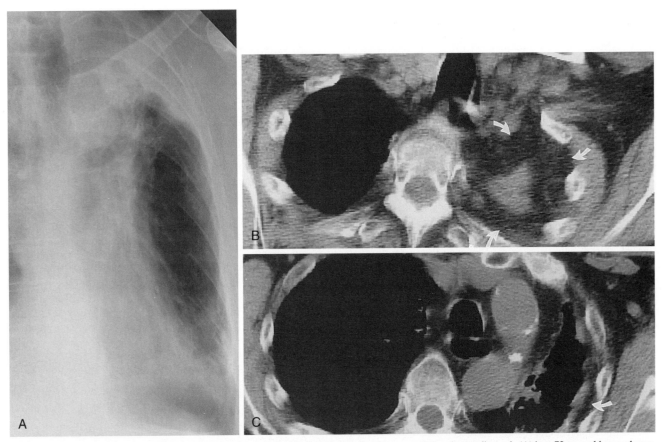

Figure 21–9. Apical Cap: Previous Tuberculosis. View of the left hemithorax from posteroanterior chest radiograph *(A)* in a 72-year-old man shows marked loss of volume of the left upper lobe with superior retraction of the hilum. A large left apical cap is present. HRCT scans *(B and C)* show that most of the apparent pleural thickening is due to the accumulation of extrapleural fat *(arrows)*. The patient had been treated for tuberculosis 20 years previously.

Radiologic Manifestations

Radiographically the earliest manifestation of a pleural plaque is a thin line of soft tissue density under a rib in the axillary region, usually the seventh or eighth, on one or both sides. The plaques may be difficult to visualize, particularly when viewed *en face*, and tangential radiographs or CT scans may be necessary. Although the value of 45-degree oblique projections has been stressed by some researchers,[230, 234] others have concluded that these views add little to the detection of asbestos-induced disease in exposed workers: in a series of 489 male pipefitters examined in a screening program, the oblique views represented the sole evidence of an asbestos-related radiographic abnormality in only 8 (1.6%).[235] A comparison of radiographic findings during life with observations at autopsy indicates that many pleural plaques are missed on premortem radiographs.[236]

Pleural plaques are usually, but not invariably, bilateral. In a review of radiographs of 105,064 civilian and military employees of the U.S. Navy, 1,914 (1.8%) were interpreted as definitely showing pleural plaques.[237] Of these radio-

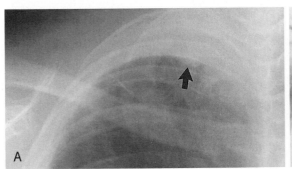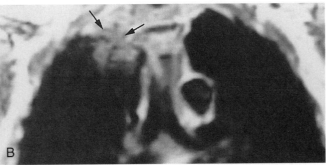

Figure 21–10. Pancoast's Tumor. View of the right upper hemithorax from posteroanterior chest radiograph *(A)* in a 44-year-old woman shows a poorly defined right apical opacity with a focal inferior convexity *(arrow)*. Localized areas of scarring in the right upper lobe are evident. Cardiac-gated T1-weighted (TR/TE, 706/20) spin-echo coronal MR image *(B)* shows tumor in the right lung apex with focal infiltration of the pleura and extrapleural soft tissues *(arrows)*. At surgery, the lesion proved to be a pulmonary carcinoma with focal chest wall invasion.

graphs, 1,545 (81%) showed bilateral pleural plaques, 287 (15%) showed only left-sided plaques, and 82 (4%) showed only right-sided. This unexplained left-sided predominance has been reported by others.[238, 239] The width and extent of pleural thickening and the extent of pleural plaque calcification frequently are greater on the left than on the right (Fig. 21–11). In one review of 408 patients who had asbestos-related pleural disease, the subjects were shown to be approximately 1.5 times as likely to have more severe localized pleural thickening and costal pleural calcification on the left than on the right;[239] diaphragmatic calcification was 2.5 times as likely to be more severe on the left than on the right.

The greatest problem in the diagnosis of early plaque formation lies in distinguishing plaques from normal companion shadows of the chest wall—not those that are associated with the first three ribs (because this area rarely is involved in asbestos-related disease) but muscle and fat shadows that may be identified in 75% of normal postero-anterior radiographs along the convexity of the thorax inferiorly. It sometimes is impossible to differentiate

plaques from such companion shadows with conviction. In one study of 30 asbestos-exposed patients in whom CT scans were performed because of uncertainty as to whether the pleural changes observed on chest radiographs were due to plaques or extrapleural fat, the radiographic findings in 14 of the 30 patients (47%) were shown on CT scan to be related to extrapleural fat (Fig. 21–12).[240] Noncalcified pleural plaques may be difficult to differentiate from normal diaphragmatic undulations and from focal postinfectious pleural thickening.

The accuracy in the diagnosis of pleural plaques on chest radiography depends on the disease prevalence in the sample population and the presence or absence of calcification.[229, 241, 242] In a study in which radiographic findings were correlated with those at autopsy, the combination of bilateral abnormalities and posterolateral pleural-based opacities at least 5 mm thick or bilateral calcified diaphragmatic plaques had a 100% positive predictive value for pathologically confirmed asbestos-related plaques;[229] however, these criteria allowed detection of only 3 of 24 (12%) plaques found at autopsy. Using less strict

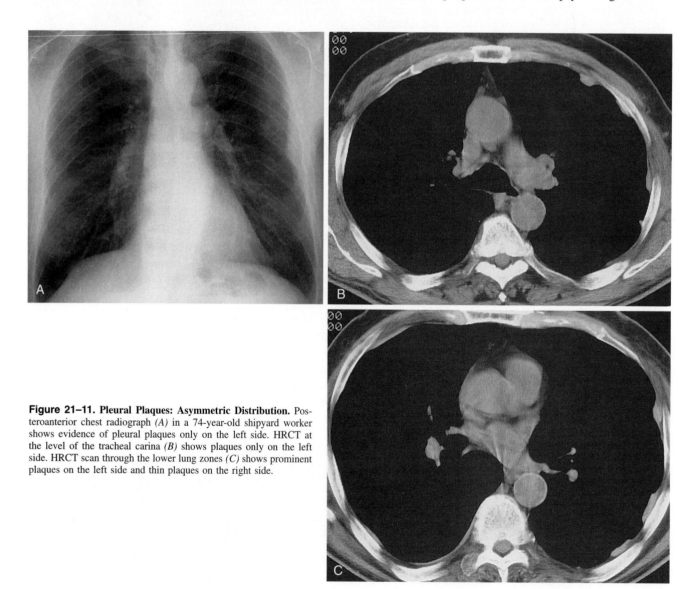

Figure 21–11. Pleural Plaques: Asymmetric Distribution. Posteroanterior chest radiograph *(A)* in a 74-year-old shipyard worker shows evidence of pleural plaques only on the left side. HRCT at the level of the tracheal carina *(B)* shows plaques only on the left side. HRCT scan through the lower lung zones *(C)* shows prominent plaques on the left side and thin plaques on the right side.

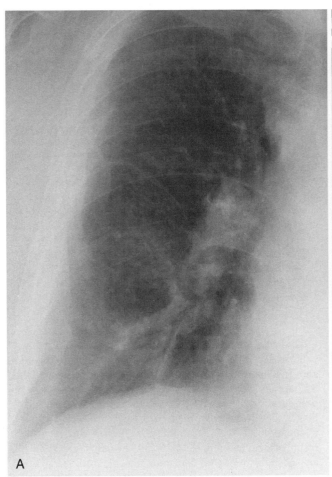

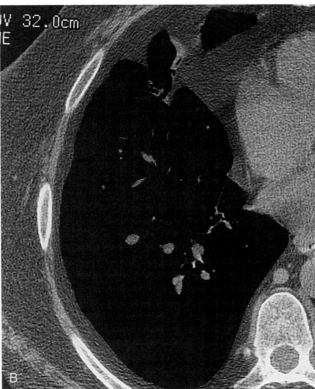

Figure 21–12. Extrapleural Fat Mimicking Pleural Thickening. View of the right chest from posteroanterior radiograph *(A)* in a 50-year-old woman shows apparent diffuse right pleural thickening and pleural plaques. View from HRCT scan *(B)* shows that the apparent pleural thickening is the result of an accumulation of extrapleural fat.

criteria, similar to those recommended by the International Labour Office,[243] 11 of 24 (46%) cases were identified; however, there were 15 (8.4%) false-positive diagnoses.[229]

The detection of noncalcified pleural plaques on chest radiograph is determined mainly by plaque thickness.[236] In one study of 402 patients from a general urban and rural industrial region, 70 (17%) had pleural plaques at autopsy;[236] 27 (39%) of these were detected by chest radiography. None of the plaques measuring less than 3 mm in thickness at autopsy was detected radiographically. Overall the sensitivity of radiography in the detection of pleural plaques in various studies ranges from about 30% to 80% and the specificity from 60% to 80%.[226, 229, 244]

Several groups of investigators have shown that CT is superior to chest radiography in the detection of pleural plaques *(see* Fig. 21–11).[245–247] Normally a 1- to 2-mm-thick stripe of soft tissue attenuation is visible on HRCT in the intercostal spaces at the point of contact between the lung and the chest wall.[249] This stripe (the *intercostal stripe*) corresponds to the visceral and parietal pleura, the endothoracic fascia, and the innermost intercostal muscle. Normally, no soft tissue attenuation is seen internal to a rib or in the paravertebral regions because the intercostal muscles do not pass internally to these bones and because the pleura normally is not thick enough to be seen in these locations. Pleural plaques are identified as circumscribed areas of pleural thickening, usually separated from the underlying rib and extrapleural soft tissues by a thin layer

of fat. Most plaques are seen along the posterolateral surface of the parietal pleura in the lower thorax, with sparing of the lung apex and costophrenic angles. Occasionally, visceral pleural plaques can be identified within the interlobar fissures (Fig. 21–13).[231–233]

It is controversial whether HRCT is superior to conventional CT in the detection of pleural plaques.[245, 248, 250] In one study in which HRCT, conventional CT, and chest radiographic findings were analyzed prospectively in 100 asbestos-exposed workers, plaques were evident on chest radiographs in 49 individuals, on conventional CT in 56, and on HRCT in 64.[245] In a second study in which HRCT was compared with conventional CT findings in 159 asbestos-exposed workers who had normal chest radiographs, plaques were identified by both techniques in 48 patients, by HRCT alone in 1 patient, and by conventional CT alone in 10 patients.[248]

The frequency of radiologically detectable calcification in pleural plaques is variable (Fig. 21–14); some investigators found calcified and noncalcified plaques in roughly equal numbers,[251] and others observed calcification in only about 20% of patients.[252] In one survey of 261 American workers exposed to asbestos in industry, none had evidence of pleural calcification,[253] whereas in Finland calcification was common;[254] this difference may be related to the variety of asbestos to which the individuals were exposed. Radiologically, calcified plaques vary from small linear or circular shadows usually situated over the diaphragmatic

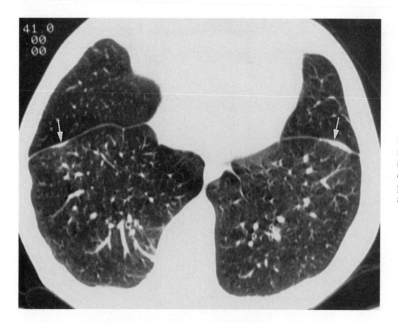

Figure 21–13. Plaques Within Interlobar Fissures. HRCT scan shows pleural plaques in the right and left major fissures *(arrows)*. Curvilinear opacities in the right paravertebral region can be seen to extend to an area of pleural thickening. The patient was a 71-year-old man who previously had worked in a shipyard.

domes[255] to large shadows that completely encircle the lower portion of the lungs.[256] When calcification is minimal, a radiograph overexposed at maximal inspiration facilitates visibility.[257] When extensive and viewed *en face*, the calcified plaques may obscure or be confused with interstitial lung disease.

Diffuse Pleural Fibrosis

Radiographically, diffuse pleural thickening (fibrothorax) is considered to be present when a smooth, uninterrupted pleural opacity is seen extending over at least one fourth of the chest wall with or without obliteration of the costophrenic sulci.[258, 259] The thickness of the pleural *peel* may be 2 cm or more but usually is less than 1 cm.[260]

Pleural thickening is diagnosed as diffuse on CT when it extends for more than 8 cm in a craniocaudad direction and 5 cm in a lateral direction and the pleura is more than 3 mm thick.[259, 261] Depending to some extent on the severity and duration of the fibrosis, calcification may or may not be evident. Although focal or diffuse areas of increased attenuation of the pleura in fibrothorax usually are the result of calcification, occasionally a similar appearance is caused by clusters of talc after talc pleurodesis.[262] Long-standing fibrothorax frequently is associated with accumulation of extrapleural fat (Fig. 21–15).

Fibrothorax seldom affects the mediastinal pleura (Fig. 21–16).[259, 260] (The latter is defined as the pleura that abuts the mediastinum, the posterior extent of which is demarcated by the anterior aspect of the vertebrae; the paraverte-

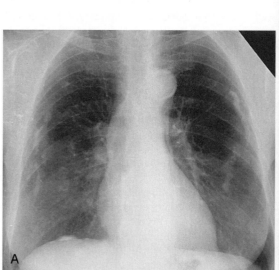
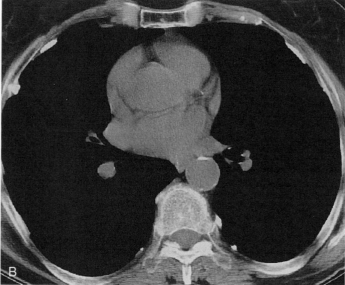

Figure 21–14. Calcified Asbestos-Related Pleural Plaques. Posteroanterior chest radiograph *(A)* and CT scan *(B)* reveal multiple bilateral discrete calcified pleural plaques involving the costal, diaphragmatic, and paravertebral pleura. The patient was a 79-year-old man who had had previous occupational asbestos exposure.

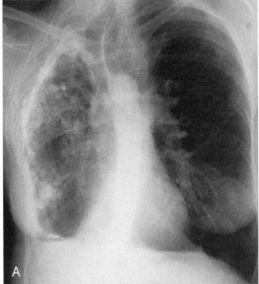

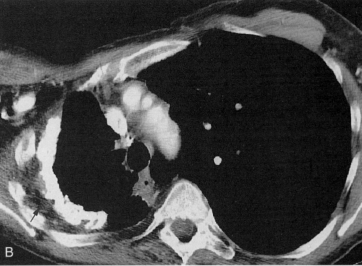

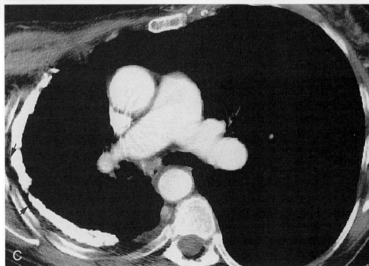

Figure 21–15. Calcified Fibrothorax. View of the right chest from posteroanterior chest radiograph *(A)* shows extensive right pleural calcification associated with loss of volume. Increased thickness of the extrapleural soft tissues is evident. Contrast-enhanced CT scans *(B and C)* show marked calcification of the right costal pleura. On this examination, the increased thickness of the extrapleural tissues is related mainly to accumulation of extrapleural fat *(arrows)*. The patient was a 71-year-old woman who had long-standing calcification as a result of previous tuberculosis.

bral pleura is considered part of the costal pleura.[249, 260]) In one study of 16 patients who had diffuse pleural thickening related to asbestos exposure and 8 who had fibrothorax owing to other causes, only 1 in each group (6% and 12.5%) had thickening of the mediastinal pleura evident on CT.[260] By comparison, thickening of the mediastinal pleura was seen on CT in 8 of 11 (73%) patients who had mesothelioma and in 13 of 24 (54%) patients who had pleural metastases.

Fibrous obliteration of the pleural space develops most often after tuberculosis, empyema associated with nontuberculous bacteria, hemorrhagic effusion, and benign asbestos-related effusion (Table 21–6). Less common causes include connective tissue diseases (particularly rheumatoid disease) and uremia.[263] The abnormality is a less common sequela of asbestos exposure than circumscribed plaques (*see* Fig. 21–16);[245, 258] in a prospective study of 100 asbestos-exposed workers, plaques were identified on HRCT in 64 and diffuse pleural thickening in only 7.[245] Four patients were reported who had disabling bilateral pleural effusions that progressed to diffuse pleural thickening; all four were human leukocyte antigen (HLA)-B44 positive, and none gave a history of asbestos exposure. The authors referred to this disorder as *cryptogenic bilateral fibrosing pleuritis.*[147]

The distribution and character of the fibrosis may yield clues to its cause. Fibrothorax secondary to tuberculosis, nontuberculous bacterial empyema, and hemorrhagic effusion is most often unilateral, whereas asbestos disease is usually bilateral pleural (manifested either as diffuse pleural thickening or as plaques).[259–261] Extensive calcification in fibrothorax is seen most commonly in patients who have had previous tuberculosis, empyema, or hemothorax and is uncommon in asbestos-related thickening.[232] Assessment of

Table 21–6. FIBROTHORAX

Chest radiograph
   Pleural thickening extending over at least one fourth of chest wall
CT
   >8 cm craniocaudad and 5 cm lateral extension
Etiology
   Tuberculosis
   Pyogenic empyema
   Hemorrhagic effusion
   Asbestos-related pleurisy
   Rheumatoid arthritis
   Progressive systemic sclerosis
   Uremia

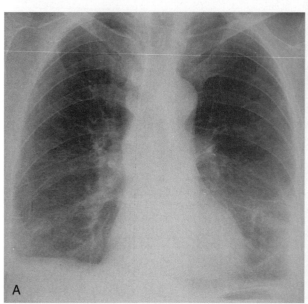
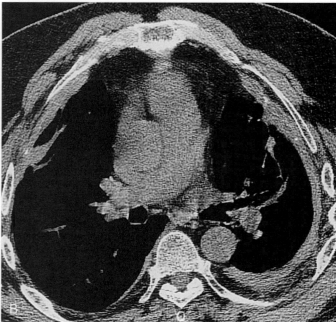

Figure 21–16. Diffuse Pleural Fibrosis. Posteroanterior chest radiograph *(A)* shows extensive bilateral pleural thickening. The blunted costophrenic angles are angulated sharply rather than meniscus-shaped, a finding helpful in distinguishing pleural thickening from effusion. Curved bands of increased opacity can be seen to extend from the left lung to the pleural thickening. This feature is seen most commonly with pleural thickening related to asbestos. CT scan *(B)* shows marked bilateral pleural thickening with small areas of calcification. Although there is marked thickening of the costal and paravertebral pleura, the mediastinal pleura is not affected. The patient was a 53-year-old man who had a history of exposure to asbestos.

the underlying lungs may be helpful in assessing etiology. If the lung appears relatively normal, the antecedent abnormality was most likely traumatic hemothorax. If there is local scarring and loss of volume, the pleural change probably was the result of a remote empyema secondary to *M. tuberculosis* or a pyogenic organism.

PLEURAL NEOPLASMS

Mesothelioma

Diffuse mesothelioma is an uncommon but increasingly recognized malignant neoplasm derived from mesothelial cells of the pericardium, peritoneum, or pleura; of all these sites, the pleura is the most common. The neoplasm is important not only because of its dismal prognosis but also because of the potential economic impact of litigation and workers' compensation.[264] Most tumors are associated with a history of asbestos exposure.[270] There are some patients, however, in whom the lung asbestos burden is relatively slight[266] or overlaps that of the general population.[267] The tumor was recognized at the turn of the twentieth century when little asbestos was being used[268] and sporadic cases occurred in children too young to have had significant asbestos exposure within the usually accepted latent period.[269]

The most common clinical manifestations consist of vague chest or shoulder ache or true pleuritic pain;[286, 390] however, a substantial number (one third of patients in some series[390]) have pleural effusion unassociated with pain. As the disease progresses, shortness of breath and a dry, sometimes hacking, cough can develop; fatigue and weight loss are common.

The prognosis of diffuse pleural mesothelioma is ex-

tremely poor: Most patients die within the first year of the onset of symptoms, and long-term survival is rare. In two series of 167[295] and 114[287] patients, only 7 (2.5%) lived more than 5 years. In another review of 80 patients, the overall 2- and 5-year survival rates were 23% and 0%.[296] As with most other cancers, prognosis is related to the extent of local or distant tumor spread.[294, 297] Several staging systems have been described,[298] the most detailed and recent being that of the International Mesothelioma Interest Group.[294]

Radiologic Manifestations

The most common radiographic manifestation of malignant mesothelioma is unilateral sheetlike or lobulated pleural thickening encasing the entire lung (Table 21–7, Fig. 21–17).[259, 272] In one review of the radiographic findings in 25 patients, this thickening was seen in 22 (88%);[271] additional findings included volume loss of the ipsilateral hemithorax (in 64%), extension of tumor into the major fissure

Table 21–7. MESOTHELIOMA: RADIOLOGIC MANIFESTATIONS

Common
    Nodular pleural thickening
    Diffuse sheetlike pleural thickening
    Extension into interlobar fissures
    Pleural effusion
    Ipsilateral mediastinal shift
    Lymphadenopathy (on CT)
Uncommon
    Contralateral mediastinal shift (10% cases)
    Bilateral pleural plaques (8% cases)

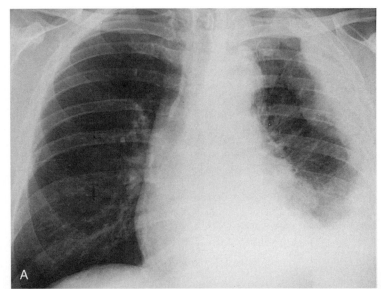

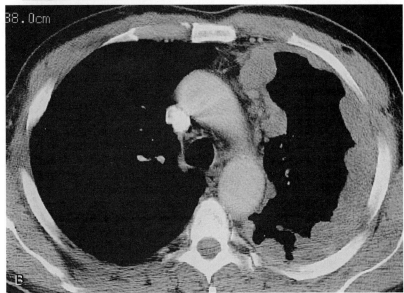

Figure 21–17. Mesothelioma. Posteroanterior chest radiograph *(A)* in a 70-year-old man shows marked, lobulated left pleural thickening encasing the entire lung. Contrast-enhanced CT scan *(B)* shows a nodular pleural rind. The diagnosis of mesothelioma was confirmed by pleural biopsy.

(in 44%), and extension into the minor fissure (in 16%). Less commonly, the tumor is manifested as multiple masses; rarely, it presents as a solitary mass.[272] Unilateral pleural effusion is identified at presentation in 30% to 80% of cases[271, 272] and often obscures the underlying neoplasm (Fig. 21–18).

In advanced tumors, chest wall invasion may be identified on radiograph by the presence of periosteal reaction along the ribs, rib erosion, or rib destruction.[272] Occasionally, hematogenous metastases to the lung may be seen as lung nodules or masses;[288] rarely a miliary pattern is identified.[273, 274] In two cases, the predominant radiographic finding consisted of an interstitial pattern secondary to lymphangitic spread.[275, 276]

CT is superior to conventional radiography in the determination of the presence and extent of mesothelioma and in the assessment of invasion of mediastinum, chest wall, and upper abdomen.[271, 277, 278] In a review of the CT manifestations in 70 patients, the most common findings consisted of pleural thickening (seen in 94%) and pleural effusion

(seen in 76%).[330] The pleural thickening was nodular in 72% of patients and uniform in 28% (Fig. 21–19). Extension of tumor into the minor or major interlobar fissure, manifested as thickening, nodularity, or both, was seen in 84% of patients, and evidence of diaphragm invasion was seen in 80%. Less common findings included loss of volume of the ipsilateral hemithorax in 27%, contralateral shift of the mediastinum in 10%, lymph node enlargement in 34%, chest wall invasion in 16%, and rib involvement in 9%.

Calcification within mesothelioma is seen in approximately 10% of cases and usually represents engulfment of calcified plaques;[279] rarely, it is the result of an osteosarcomatous component (Fig. 21–20).[280] Findings suggestive of chest wall invasion include obscuration of fat planes, infiltration of intercostal muscles, periosteal reaction, and bone destruction. Features of mediastinal invasion include obliteration of fat planes, nodular pericardial thickening, and direct soft tissue extension.

Diffuse sheetlike or nodular pleural thickening identical

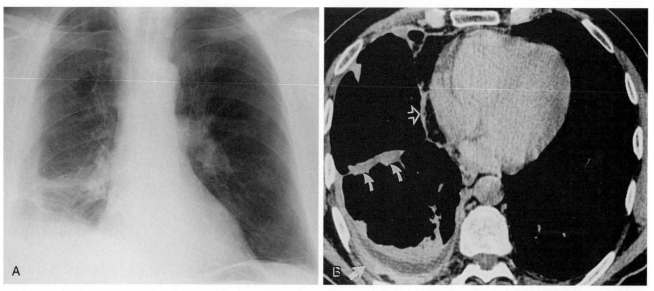

Figure 21–18. Mesothelioma. Posteroanterior chest radiograph *(A)* in a 59-year-old man shows a right pleural effusion, linear areas of atelectasis in the right lower lobe, and loss of volume of the right hemithorax. The appearance on radiograph would be consistent with either a benign or a malignant process. CT scan *(B)* shows nodular thickening of the right parietal *(straight arrow)* and visceral pleura associated with extension of tumor into the right major fissure *(curved arrows)*. Mild thickening of the mediastinal pleura *(open arrow)* is evident. The diagnosis of mesothelioma was proved by open pleural biopsy. The patient had been a shipyard worker.

to that of mesothelioma may be seen on CT with pleural metastasis or lymphoma but rarely is present with benign processes.[259, 260] In one CT study of 74 consecutive patients who had diffuse pleural disease, including 39 who had malignancy (11 mesothelioma) and 35 who had benign thickening, findings most helpful in distinguishing malignant from benign disease included circumferential, mediastinal, and nodular pleural thickening (seen in 73%, 73%, and 55% of patients who had malignant mesothelioma as compared with 0%, 12%, and 25% of patients who had fibrothorax, Fig. 21–21).[260] Loss of volume of the ipsilateral

hemithorax, pleural plaques, and effusion were not helpful in distinguishing the two. The combination of mesothelioma and bilateral pleural plaques is seen only in a small percentage of cases. In one review of the CT findings in 50 patients who had mesothelioma, bilateral pleural plaques were seen in 4 (8%).[279]

In another study in which the CT findings were evaluated in 34 consecutive patients who underwent surgery for mesothelioma, 10 had surgically unresectable tumors (2 with diaphragmatic invasion, 4 with chest wall invasion, and 4 with mediastinal invasion), and 24 underwent com-

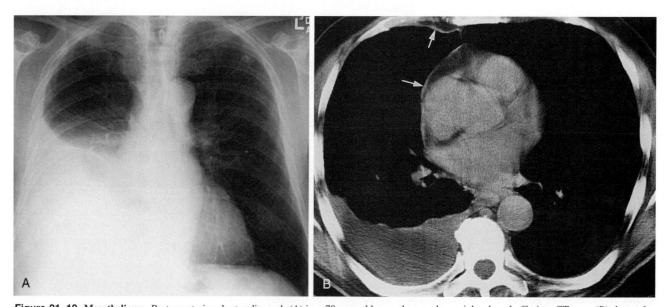

Figure 21–19. Mesothelioma. Posteroanterior chest radiograph *(A)* in a 79-year-old man shows a large right pleural effusion. CT scan *(B)* shows the effusion and focal plaquelike areas of thickening involving the anterior costal and mediastinal pleura *(arrows)*. Initial biopsy of the posterior costal pleura was negative. Repeat CT-guided surgical biopsy of the anterior costal pleura was diagnostic of mesothelioma. The patient had been a shipyard worker.

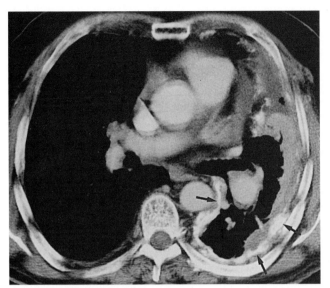

Figure 21–20. Mesothelioma. Contrast-enhanced CT scan in a 63-year-old man shows extensive left pleural thickening associated with loss of volume of the left hemithorax. A loculated pleural effusion is present anteriorly. Extensive calcification of the thickened left pleura is present *(arrows)*. At biopsy, this was shown to be a mesothelioma with an osteosarcomatous component. The patient was a construction worker.

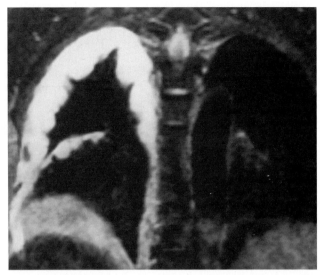

Figure 21–22. Mesothelioma. Coronal T2-weighted (TR/TE, 2118/100) spin-echo MR image shows diffuse nodular thickening of the right pleura associated with extension of tumor into the mediastinal pleura and right major interlobar fissure. The patient was a 37-year-old man without a history of asbestos exposure.

plete extrapleural pneumonectomy.[281] The sensitivity of CT was 93% for excluding chest wall involvement, 94% for excluding transdiaphragmatic extension, and 100% for excluding mediastinal involvement. The most helpful findings in assessing resectability included preservation of normal extrapleural fat for excluding chest wall invasion, a clear fat plane between the inferior diaphragmatic surface and the adjacent abdominal organs for excluding transdiaphragmatic extension, and preservation of normal mediastinal fat for exclusion of mediastinal invasion. The application of

the proposed international TNM staging system for the CT evaluation of malignant pleural mesothelioma has been reviewed.[282]

MR imaging is comparable or slightly superior to CT in the assessment of the morphologic features and tumor extent.[281, 283, 284] Mesothelioma has slightly greater signal intensity than the intercostal muscles on T1-weighted imaging but considerably greater signal intensity on proton-density and T2-weighted images (Fig. 21–22). In one study, all six mesotheliomas had a hyperintense signal relative to intercostal muscle on proton-density and T2-weighted

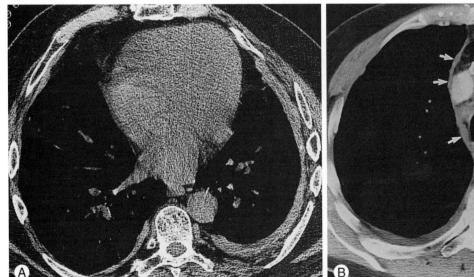

Figure 21–21. Benign Versus Malignant Pleural Thickening. CT scan in a 53-year-old man *(A)* shows extensive left pleural thickening associated with loss of volume. Localized pleural plaques are present on the right side. Despite the diffuse involvement of the costal pleura, the thickening does not involve the mediastinal pleura. The diagnosis was considered to be benign asbestos-related pleural thickening; no change was seen on follow-up during 2 years. CT scan in a 64-year-old woman *(B)* shows a small right pleural effusion and thickening of the mediastinal pleura *(arrows)*. At biopsy, this was shown to represent a mesothelioma. The patient had no known history of asbestos exposure.

images, whereas 14 of 16 benign causes of pleural thickening, including all pleural plaques and cases of fibrothorax, were isointense or hypointense.[283] The two exceptions were a case of tuberculous pleurisy and one of acute pleurisy. MR imaging is comparable to CT in predicting tumor resectability.[281]

Preliminary results suggest that positron emission tomography (PET) imaging with 2-(^{18}F)-fluoro-2-deoxy-d-glucose (FDG) may be helpful in the assessment of patients who have suspected mesothelioma. In one investigation of 28 such patients, the uptake of FDG was significantly higher in the 24 who had biopsy-proven malignant disease (22 mesothelioma, 2 metastatic adenocarcinoma) than in the 4 who had benign disease (2 pleuritis, 1 angiolipoma, and 1 asbestos-related pleural fibrosis).[285] Two patients who had mesothelioma had mildly increased FDG uptake, and one patient who had pleuritis had markedly increased FDG uptake. FDG-PET imaging had a sensitivity of 92% (22 of 24) and a specificity of 75% (3 of 4) in detecting the presence of malignant pleural disease.

Although metastases outside the thorax are common at autopsy[286, 288] and may be widespread,[289] they infrequently are detected clinically.[290, 291] Rarely, they are the initial manifestation of disease, usually in cervical[292] or axillary lymph nodes.[293]

Mesenchymal Neoplasms

Solitary Fibrous Tumor

The solitary fibrous tumor has been given a variety of names, including local, fibrous, or benign mesothelioma; localized or solitary fibrous tumor; subpleural, submesothelial, or pleural fibroma; and fibrosarcoma. Among these, the relatively nonspecific *solitary fibrous tumor* is preferred for several reasons: (1) Although the neoplasm is usually histologically and biologically benign, malignant forms exist, and in some cases the histologic distinction between the two is difficult, if not impossible; (2) the neoplasm often shows evidence of fibroblastic differentiation; and (3) the results of ultrastructural, immunohistochemical, and experimental studies suggest that the tumor originates in submesothelial connective tissue of the pleura rather than the mesothelium itself. For these reasons, use of the term *mesothelioma* and of specific modifiers implying a definite benign or malignant behavior is inappropriate.

The solitary fibrous tumor is uncommon; approximately 350 cases had been documented in the literature by 1980,[299] and an additional 223 cases were reported from the files of the Armed Forces Institute of Pathology (AFIP) in 1989.[300] It occurs slightly more often in women than in men. Although it can be seen at any age,[265] the mean age at presentation is about 50 years.[299] The cause is unknown in most cases, although occasional tumors have developed after radiation therapy to the chest wall.[301, 302] There is no association with cigarette smoking or asbestos exposure.[299, 300]

Of solitary fibrous tumors, 65% to 80% arise in relation to the visceral pleura.[299, 300] Most project into the pleural space and compress the adjacent lung to a variable degree. Occasionally, tumors arising in the medial pleura extend into the mediastinum,[303] and those in a fissure extend into

the pulmonary parenchyma.[299, 300] Most are spherical or oval and well circumscribed; many are attached to the pleura by a short vascular pedicle. They can grow to a huge size, with tumors 36 cm in diameter having been reported.[299]

Most patients are asymptomatic;[300] cough, chest pain, and dyspnea occur occasionally,[299] especially in association with larger tumors.[318] One particularly common finding is hypertrophic osteoarthropathy, which was seen in about one third of 350 patients identified in a literature review to 1981.[299] The association of this abnormality with solitary fibrous tumor is much stronger than with pulmonary carcinoma, and its presence in a patient who has a large intrathoracic mass should suggest the diagnosis. Surgical removal of the tumor relieves the symptoms of arthropathy in most cases.[319] Symptomatic hypoglycemia (Doege-Potter syndrome) has been documented in about 5% of patients;[318, 320] in the AFIP series, it was more common in malignant than in benign tumors (11% versus 3%) and three times more frequent in women than in men.[300]

Most solitary fibrous tumors behave in a benign fashion, with intrathoracic growth resulting in compression but not invasion of contiguous structures. Most tumors grow slowly; in one case, a 12-cm tumor was excised 20 years after it first was identified radiographically.[333] Surgical excision usually results in complete cure, particularly when the tumor possesses a well-defined pedicle; however, local recurrence can occur if initial surgery is inadequate. Tumor-related death was documented in 13% of the 350 patients reported in the literature by 1981.[299] Patients who have unresectable primary or recurrent disease usually die within 2 years as a result of extensive intrathoracic disease;[299] extrathoracic metastases are rare.

Radiologic Manifestations

Radiographically, solitary fibrous tumors are sharply defined, smooth, or lobulated masses of homogeneous density ranging in diameter from 1 to almost 40 cm (Table 21–8, Fig. 21–23).[305, 306] They may be located in an interlobar fissure or adjacent to the diaphragm, mediastinum, or chest wall.[307] Small lesions (≤4 cm) typically have tapering margins and form obtuse angles with the chest wall or mediastinum, important findings in establishing the extrapulmonary nature of a thoracic mass (Fig. 21–24).[307] When a tumor is large, however, its site of origin frequently is difficult or impossible to determine on radiography or CT

Table 21–8. SOLITARY FIBROUS TUMOR OF THE PLEURA

No relation to asbestos exposure
Most arise in visceral pleura
Most are benign
One third are associated with hypertrophic osteoarthropathy
5% are associated with hypoglycemia
Radiologic manifestations
    Sharply defined, smooth margins
    Pleural based
    1–40 cm diameter
    Foci of calcification in 5–10%
    Pleural effusion in 15–20%

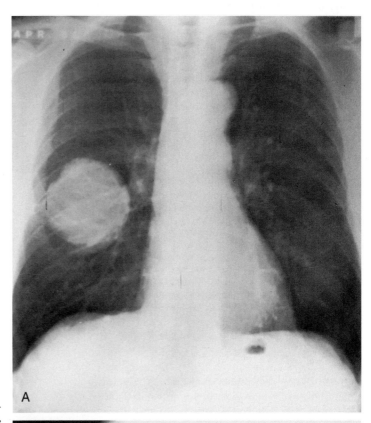

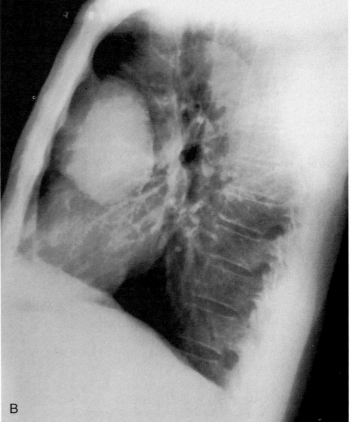

Figure 21–23. Solitary Fibrous Tumor of the Pleura. Postero-anterior *(A)* and lateral *(B)* radiographs reveal a homogeneous, somewhat lobulated mass in the anterior aspect of the right hemi-thorax. The relationship of the mass to the visceral pleura cannot be established from these two projections. The patient was an asymptomatic 50-year-old man.

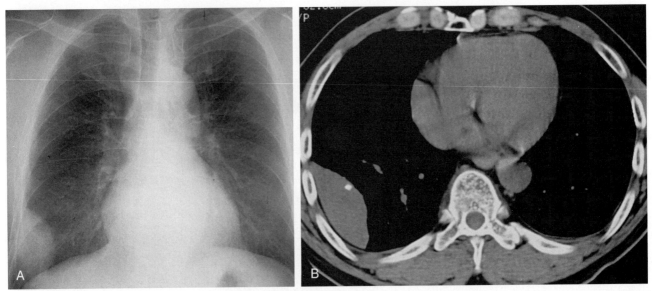

Figure 21–24. Solitary Fibrous Tumor of the Pleura. Posteroanterior chest radiograph *(A)* in a 62-year-old man shows a well-defined, pleural-based tumor in the right lower hemithorax. The cephalad border of the tumor tapers smoothly and forms an obtuse angle with the chest wall. CT scan *(B)* without intravenous contrast medium enhancement shows a smoothly marginated pleural-based soft tissue lesion with a focal area of calcification. The diagnosis of fibrous tumor was proved at surgical resection.

(Fig. 21–25);[306, 308] in one series of six patients who had tumors 5 to 17 cm in diameter, none formed obtuse angles with the pleura with either procedure.[308] Calcification or pleural effusion was evident in 4 (7%) and 10 (17%) of 58 cases reviewed in the AFIP series.[300] The latter complication occurs more commonly in malignant than in benign tumors.[305]

A finding of considerable diagnostic value is a change in position of a pedunculated tumor with respiration, needling, or change in body position.[306, 309] If the tumor originates in the visceral pleura, movement is detected by relating the position of the tumor to contiguous ribs or mediastinal structures; if origin is in the parietal pleura, movement may be related to the presence of a pedicle. Occasionally the pedicle becomes twisted, resulting in detachment of the tumor from the pleura and the formation of a free intrapleural body.[310, 311]

Several authors described the CT findings of fibrous pleural tumors.[308, 312, 313] Most tumors larger than 5 cm in diameter have been shown to form acute or straight angles with the chest wall.[308, 312, 313] Helpful signs in determining the extrapulmonary nature of the lesion include the presence of tapering margins and displacement of adjacent lung parenchyma *(see Fig. 21–24)*.[313]

In one review of the CT manifestations in 16 patients who had tumors ranging from 4 to 17 cm in diameter, all showed enhancement equal to or greater than that of muscle after intravenous administration of contrast medium.[312] Enhancement was homogeneous in 10 patients and heterogeneous in 6. A pedicle was identified in four patients, areas of low attenuation in four, and calcification in two. In another study of nine patients, all tumors showed enhancement with intravenous contrast medium;[304] tumors less than 6 cm in diameter showed homogeneous enhancement, whereas larger tumors had inhomogeneous enhancement, with round or tubular areas of fluid attenuation within

the mass *(see Fig. 21–25)*. Correlation with the pathologic specimens revealed that enhancement could be explained by the vascularity of the tumor, whereas the localized round or tubular areas of low attenuation were related to myxoid or cystic degeneration or hemorrhage. In a third review of five patients who had malignant tumors, large areas of low attenuation resulting from necrosis were present in all patients, and calcification was noted in three.[313]

MR imaging is superior to CT in determining the tissue characteristics of these tumors. With this technique, benign variants usually have low signal intensity on T1-weighted and T2-weighted images, consistent with the presence of fibrous tissue.[314, 315] These characteristics allow distinction from pulmonary carcinoma, which usually has increased signal intensity on T2-weighted images. Although the low signal intensity is not pathognomonic for fibrous tumor, it allows a presumptive diagnosis and may obviate the need for transthoracic needle biopsy. One case has been reported of a benign fibrous tumor of the pleura that had high signal intensity on T2-weighted images, presumably related to the presence of foci of necrosis and hemorrhage.[316] High signal intensity on T2-weighted images may be the result of myxoid degeneration.[305] Fibrous tumors show marked increase in signal intensity after intravenous injection of gadolinium.[305, 317] MR imaging may be helpful in determining the exact location and extent of large lesions, which may be misdiagnosed occasionally on CT as invading the mediastinum or liver *(see Fig. 21–25)*.[313]

Lipoma

Lipomas related to the pleura are seen on chest radiograph as soft tissue masses that have well-defined margins where they abut the lung and poorly defined margins where they abut the chest wall. When small, they often have tapering margins and form obtuse angles with the chest

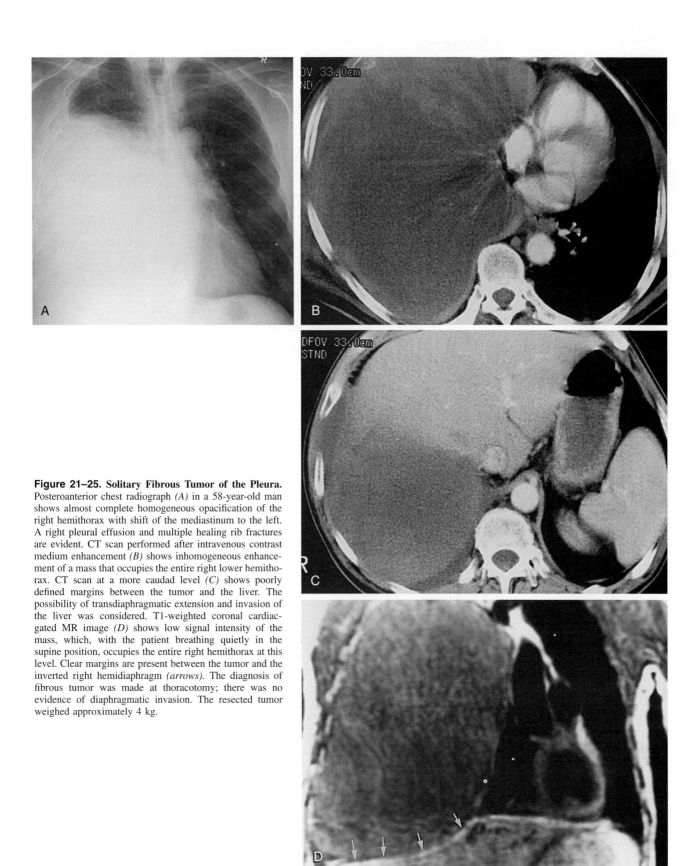

Figure 21–25. Solitary Fibrous Tumor of the Pleura. Posteroanterior chest radiograph *(A)* in a 58-year-old man shows almost complete homogeneous opacification of the right hemithorax with shift of the mediastinum to the left. A right pleural effusion and multiple healing rib fractures are evident. CT scan performed after intravenous contrast medium enhancement *(B)* shows inhomogeneous enhancement of a mass that occupies the entire right lower hemithorax. CT scan at a more caudad level *(C)* shows poorly defined margins between the tumor and the liver. The possibility of transdiaphragmatic extension and invasion of the liver was considered. T1-weighted coronal cardiac-gated MR image *(D)* shows low signal intensity of the mass, which, with the patient breathing quietly in the supine position, occupies the entire right hemithorax at this level. Clear margins are present between the tumor and the inverted right hemidiaphragm *(arrows)*. The diagnosis of fibrous tumor was made at thoracotomy; there was no evidence of diaphragmatic invasion. The resected tumor weighed approximately 4 kg.

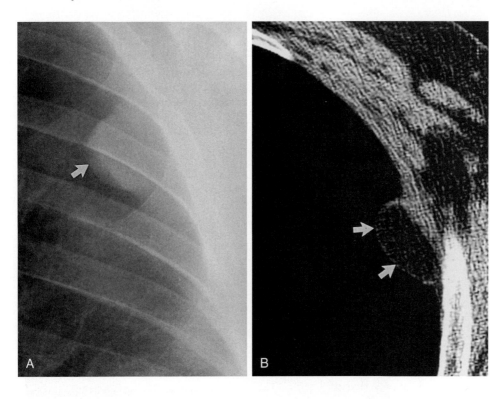

Figure 21–26. Pleural Lipoma. View of the left upper chest from posteroanterior radiograph *(A)* shows homogeneous opacity *(arrow)* with smooth margins, sharply defined medial edge, and ill-defined lateral border characteristic of a pleural-based lesion. View from HRCT scan *(B)* shows characteristic homogeneous fat attenuation of a pleural lipoma *(arrows)*. The patient was a 55-year-old man.

wall.[321, 322] CT allows a specific diagnosis by showing a uniform attenuation (-50 to -100 HU) similar to that of subcutaneous fat (Fig. 21–26). A few linear strands of soft tissue attenuation may be seen related to their fibrous stroma;[322] however, when the lesion has a heterogeneous appearance with attenuation values greater than -50 HU, liposarcoma should be suspected (Fig. 21–27).[323, 334]

Lymphoma

Pleural lymphoma usually occurs as part of disseminated disease and can be seen with virtually any histologic subtype;[324] rarely, it is primary in this site. In most cases, the tumor appears as a more or less diffuse or focal plaquelike thickening, rather than a localized tumor. Radiographic and

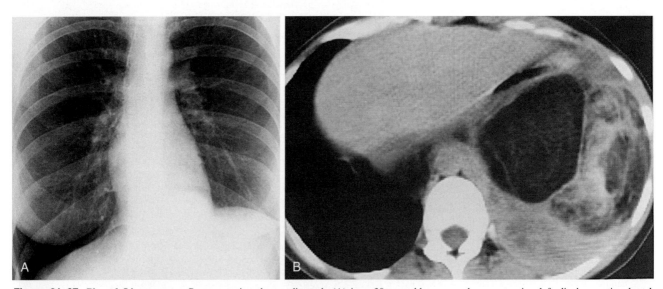

Figure 21–27. Pleural Liposarcoma. Posteroanterior chest radiograph *(A)* in a 30-year-old woman shows extensive left diaphragmatic pleural thickening. No further investigation was performed at that time. CT scan 2 years later *(B)*, at which time chest radiograph showed considerable increase in size of the tumor, shows an inhomogeneous soft tissue mass in the left lower hemithorax. The tumor contains areas with attenuation similar to that of subcutaneous fat and areas of soft tissue attenuation. The diagnosis of pleural liposarcoma was proved at thoracotomy.

CT findings consist of pleural effusion with or without pleural thickening.[260] The radiologic manifestations of lymphoma and Hodgkin's disease are discussed in greater detail in Chapter 7.

References

1. Andrews CO, Gora ML: Pleural effusions: Pathophysiology and management. Ann Pharmacother 28:894, 1994.
2. Light RW: Pleural diseases. Dis Mon 38:261, 1992.
3. Smyrnios NA, Jederlinic PJ, Irwin RS: Pleural effusion in an asymptomatic patient: Spectrum and frequency of causes and management considerations. Chest 97:192, 1990.
4. Sokolowski JW, Burgher LW, Jones FL Jr, et al: American Thoracic Society: Guidelines for thoracentesis and needle biopsy of the pleura. Am Rev Respir Dis 140:257, 1989.
5. Collins TR, Sahn SA: Thoracentesis: Clinical value, complications, technical problems, and patient experience. Chest 91:817, 1987.
6. Storey DD, Dines DE, Coles DT: Pleural effusion: A diagnostic dilemma. JAMA 236:2183, 1976.
7. Okada Y, Ichinose Y, Yamaguchi K, et al: *Mycobacterium avium-intracellulare* pleuritis with massive pleural effusion. Eur Respir J 8:1428, 1995.
8. Igari H, Kikuchi N: Nontuberculous mycobacterium pulmonary infection with pleural effusion caused by *Mycobacterium kansasii.* Kekkaku 68:527, 1993.
9. Sahn SA: The pleura. Am Rev Respir Dis 138:184, 1988.
10. Ellner JJ, Barnes PF, Wallis RS, et al: The immunology of tuberculous pleurisy. Semin Respir Infect 3:335, 1988.
11. Seibert AF, Haynes J Jr, Middleton R, et al: Tuberculous pleural effusion. Chest 99:883, 1991.
12. Stead WW, Eichenholz A, Stauss HK: Operative and pathologic findings in twenty-four patients with syndrome of idiopathic pleurisy with effusion, presumably tuberculous. Am Rev Respir Dis 71:473, 1955.
13. Light RW: Pleural Diseases. Philadelphia, Lea & Febiger, 1983.
14. Hulnick DH, Naidich DP, McCauley DI: Pleural tuberculosis evaluated by computed tomography. Radiology 149:759, 1983.
15. Levine H, Szanto PB, Cugell DW: Tuberculous pleurisy—an acute illness. Arch Intern Med 122:329, 1968.
16. Korzeniewska-Kosela M, Krysl J, Muller N, et al: Tuberculosis in young adults and the elderly: A prospective comparison study. Chest 106:28, 1994.
17. Bartlett JG: Bacterial infections of the pleural space. Semin Respir Infect 3:308, 1988.
18. Sahn SA: Management of complicated parapneumonic effusions. Am Rev Respir Dis 148:813, 1993.
19. Light RW: A new classification of parapneumonic effusions and empyema. Chest 108:299, 1995.
20. Light RW, Girard WM, Jenkinson SG, et al: Parapneumonic effusions. Am J Med 69:507, 1980.
21. Vianna NJ: Nontuberculous bacterial empyema in patients with and without underlying diseases. JAMA 215:69, 1971.
22. Smith JA, Mullerworth MH, Westlake GW, et al: Empyema thoracis: 14 year experience in a teaching center. Ann Thorac Surg 51:39, 1991.
23. Ali I, Unruh H: Management of empyema thoracis. Ann Thorac Surg 50:355, 1990.
24. Alfageme I, Mûnoz F, Pêna N, et al: Empyema of the thorax in adults: Etiology, microbiologic findings and management. Chest 103:839, 1993.
25. Borge JH, Michavila IA, Mendez JM, et al: Thoracic empyema in HIV-infected patients. Chest 113:732, 1998.
26. Varkey B, Rose HD, Kutty CPK, et al: Empyema thoracis during a 10-year period: Analysis of 72 cases and comparison to a previous study (1952 to 1967). Arch Intern Med 141:1771, 1981.
27. Caplan ES, Hoyt NJ, Rodriguez A, et al: Empyema occurring in the multiple traumatized patient. J Trauma 24:785, 1984.
28. Brook I, Frazier EH: Aerobic and anaerobic microbiology of empyema: A retrospective review in two military hospitals. Chest 103:1502, 1993.
29. Ashbaugh DG: Empyema thoracis: Factors influencing morbidity and mortality. Chest 99:1162, 1991.
30. Sahn SA, Lakshminarayan S, Char DC: "Silent" empyema in patients receiving corticosteroids. Am Rev Respir Dis 107:873, 1973.
31. Lee YH, Ji JD, Shim JJ, et al: Exudative pleural effusion and pleural leukocytoclastic vasculitis in limited scleroderma. J Rheumatol 25:1006, 1998.
32. Good JT Jr, King TE, Antony VB, et al: Lupus pleuritis: Clinical features and pleural fluid characteristics with special references to pleural fluid antinuclear antibodies. Chest 84:714, 1983.
33. Wiedemann HP, Matthay RA: Pulmonary manifestations of the collagen vascular diseases. Clin Chest Med 10:677, 1989.
34. Carr DT, Mayne JG: Pleurisy with effusion in rheumatoid arthritis, with reference to the low concentration of glucose in pleural fluid. Am Rev Respir Dis 85:345, 1962.
35. Petty TL, Wilkins M: The five manifestations of rheumatoid lung. Dis Chest 49:75, 1966.
36. Pleurisy and rheumatoid arthritis. BMJ 2:1, 1968.
37. Locke CB: Rheumatoid lung. Clin Radiol 14:43, 1963.
38. Torrington KG: Rapid appearance of rheumatoid pleural effusion. Chest 73:409, 1978.
39. Pritikin JD, Jensen WA, Yenokida GG, et al: Respiratory failure due to a massive rheumatoid pleural effusion. J Rheumatol 17:673, 1990.
40. Schools GS, Mikkelsen WM: Rheumatoid pleuritis. Arthritis Rheum 5:369, 1962.
41. Jones FL Jr, Blodgett RC Jr: Empyema in rheumatic pleuropulmonary disease. Ann Intern Med 74:665, 1971.
42. Robinson BWS, Musk AW: Benign asbestos pleural effusion: Diagnosis and course. Thorax 36:896, 1981.
43. Epler GR, McCloud TC, Gaensler EA: Prevalence and incidence of benign asbestos pleural effusion in a working population. JAMA 247:617, 1982.
44. Lilis R, Lerman Y, Selikoff IJ: Symptomatic benign pleural effusions among asbestos insulation workers: Residual radiographic abnormalities. Br J Ind Med 45:443, 1988.
45. Smith KW: Pulmonary disability in asbestos workers. AMA Arch Ind Health 12:198, 1955.
46. Gaenslor EA, Kaplan AI: Asbestos pleural effusion. Ann Intern Med 74:178, 1971.
47. Miller A: Chronic pleuritic pain in four patients with asbestos induced pleural fibrosis. Br J Ind Med 47:147, 1990.
48. Hillerdal G: Non-malignant asbestos pleural disease. Thorax 36:669, 1981.
49. Smith LS, Schillaci RF: Rounded atelectasis due to acute exudative effusion: Spontaneous resolution. Chest 85:830, 1984.
50. Mysterious pleural effusion (editorial). Lancet 1:1226, 1982.
51. Antony VB: Drug-induced pleural disease. Clin Chest Med 19:331, 1998.
52. Jurivich DA: Iatrogenic pleural effusions. South Med J 81:1417, 1988.
53. Chernow B, Sahn SA: Carcinomatous involvement of the pleura: An analysis of 96 patients. Am J Med 63:695, 1977.
54. Hsu C: Cytologic detection of malignancy in pleural effusion: A review of 5,255 samples from 3,811 patients. Diagn Cytopathol 3:8, 1987.
55. Johnston WW: The malignant pleural effusion: A review of cytopathologic diagnoses of 584 specimens from 472 consecutive patients. Cancer 56:905, 1985.
56. Ruckdeschel JC: Management of malignant pleural effusions. Semin Oncol 22:58, 1995.
57. Vargas FS, Teixeira LR: Pleural malignancies. Curr Opin Pulm Med 2:335, 1996.
58. Meyer PC: Metastatic carcinoma of the pleura. Thorax 21:437, 1966.
59. Treatment of malignant effusions (editorial). Lancet 1:198, 1981.
60. Andrews BS, Arora NS, Shadforth MF, et al: The role of immune complexes in the pathogenesis of pleural effusions. Am Rev Respir Dis 124:115, 1981.
61. Rabinov K, Stein M, Frank H: Tension hydrothorax—an unrecognized danger. Thorax 21:465, 1966.
62. Subramanyam BR, Raghavendra BN, Lefleur RS: Sonography of the inverted right hemidiaphragm. Am J Roentgenol 136:1004, 1981.
63. Halvorsen RA, Redyshin PJ, Korobkin M, et al: Ascites or pleural effusion? CT differentiation: Four useful criteria. Radiographics 6:135, 1986.
64. Irani DR, Underwood RD, Johnson EH, et al: Malignant pleural effusions: A clinical cytopathologic study. Arch Intern Med 147:1133, 1987.

65. Bruneau R, Rubin P: The management of pleural effusions and chylothorax in lymphoma. Radiology 85:1085, 1965.

66. Williams JR, Wilcox WC: Pulmonary embolism: Roentgenographic and angiographic considerations. Am J Roentgenol 89:333, 1963.

67. Wiener SN, Edelstein J, Charms BL: Observations on pulmonary embolism and the pulmonary angiogram. Am J Roentgenol 98:859, 1966.

68. Worsley DF, Alavi A, Aronchick JM, et al: Chest radiographic findings in patients with acute pulmonary embolism: Observations from the PIOPED study. Radiology 189:133, 1993.

69. Bynum LJ, Wilson JE III: Radiographic features of pleural effusions in pulmonary embolism. Am Rev Respir Dis 117:829, 1978.

70. Logue RB, Rogers JV Jr, Gay BB Jr: Subtle roentgenographic signs of left heart failure. Am Heart J 65:464, 1963.

71. Tomaselli G, Gamsu G, Stulbarg MS: Constrictive pericarditis presenting as pleural effusion of unknown origin. Arch Intern Med 149:201, 1989.

72. Race GA, Scheifley CH, Edwards JE: Hydrothorax in congestive heart failure. Am J Med 22:83, 1957.

73. Williams JR, Bonte FJ: The Roentgenologic Aspect of Nonpenetrating Chest Injuries. Springfield, IL, Charles C Thomas, 1961.

74. Traumatic perforation of oesophagus. BMJ 1:524, 1972.

75. Scholl DG, Tsai SH: Esophageal perforation following the use of the esophageal obturator airway. Radiology 122:315, 1977.

76. Levy F, Mysko WK, Kelen GD: Spontaneous esophageal perforation presenting with right-sided pleural effusion. J Emerg Med 13:321, 1995.

77. Vargas FS, Cukier A, Hueb W, et al: Relationship between pleural effusion and pericardial involvement after myocardial revascularization. Chest 105:1748, 1994.

78. Peng MJ, Vargas FS, Cukier A, et al: Postoperative pleural changes after coronary revascularization. Chest 101:327, 1992.

79. Tazelaar HD, Yousem SA: The pathology of combined heart-lung transplantation: An autopsy study. Hum Pathol 19:1403, 1988.

80. Hart U, Ward DR, Gillilian R, et al: Fatal pulmonary hemorrhage complicating Swan-Ganz catheterization. Surgery 91:24, 1982.

81. Carbone K, Gimenez LF, Rogers WH, et al: Hemothorax due to vena caval erosion by a subclavian dual-lumen dialysis catheter. South Med J 80:795, 1987.

82. Rudge CJ, Bewick M, McColl I: Hydrothorax after central venous catheterization. BMJ 3:23, 1973.

83. Holt S, Kirkham N, Myrescough E: Haemothorax after subclavian vein cannulation. Thorax 32:101, 1977.

84. Aronchick JM, Epstein DM, Gefter WB, et al: Chronic traumatic diaphragmatic hernia: The significance of pleural effusion. Radiology 168:675, 1988.

85. Johnston RF, Loo RV: Hepatic hydrothorax: Studies to determine the source of the fluid and report of thirteen cases. Ann Intern Med 61:385, 1964.

86. Alberts WM, Salem AJ, Solomon DA, et al: Hepatic hydrothorax—cause and management. Arch Intern Med 151:2383, 1991.

87. Light RW, George RB: Incidence and significance of pleural effusion after abdominal surgery. Chest 69:621, 1976.

88. Pisani RJ, Zeller FA: Bilious pleural effusion following liver biopsy. Chest 98:1535, 1990.

89. Olutola PS, Hutton L, Wall WJ: Pleural effusion following liver transplantation. Radiology 157:594, 1985.

90. Lepage S, Bisson G, Verreault J, et al: Massive hydrothorax complicating peritoneal dialysis: Isotopic investigation (peritoneopleural scintigraphy). Clin Nucl Med 18:498, 1993.

91. Nusser RA, Culhane RH: Recurrent transudative effusion with an abdominal mass: Urinothorax. Chest 90:263, 1986.

92. Cavina C, Vichi G: Radiological aspects of pleural effusions in medical nephropathy in children. Ann Radiol Diagn 31:163, 1958.

93. Kirkpatrick JA Jr, Fleisher DS: The roentgenographic appearance of the chest in acute glomerulonephritis in children. J Pediatr 64:492, 1964.

94. Hopps HC, Wissler RW: Uremic pneumonitis. Am J Pathol 31:261, 1955.

95. Maringhini A, Ciambra M, Patti R, et al: Ascites, pleural, and pericardial effusions in acute pancreatitis: A prospective study of incidence, natural history, and prognostic role. Dig Dis Sci 41:848, 1996.

96. Uchiyama T, Suzuki T, Adachi A, et al: Pancreatic pleural effusion: Case report and review of 113 cases in Japan. Am J Gastroenterol 87:387, 1992.

97. Mokrohisky JF: So-called "Meigs' syndrome" associated with benign and malignant ovarian tumors. Radiology 70:578, 1958.

98. Terada S, Suzuki N, Uchide K, et al: Uterine leiomyoma associated with ascites and hydrothorax. Gynecol Obstet Invest 33:54, 1992.

99. Brandstetter RD, Klass SC, Gutherz P, et al: Pleural effusion due to communicating gastric ulcer. N Y State J Med 85:706, 1985.

100. Patwardhan RV, Heilpern RJ, Brewster AC, et al: Pleuropericarditis: An extraintestinal complication of inflammatory bowel disease: Report of three cases and review of literature. Arch Intern Med 143:94, 1983.

101. Miller WT, Talman EA: Subphrenic abscess. Am J Roentgenol 101:961, 1967.

102. Schneierson SJ, Katz M: Solitary pleural effusion due to myxedema. JAMA 168:1003, 1958.

103. Morandi U, Golinelli M, Brandi L, et al: "Yellow nail syndrome" associated with chronic recurrent pericardial and pleural effusions. Eur J Cardiothorac Surg 9:42, 1995.

104. Dressler W: The post-myocardial infarction syndrome. Arch Intern Med 103:28, 1959.

105. Shahar A, Hod H, Barabash GM, et al: Disappearance of a syndrome: Dressler's syndrome in the era of thrombolysis. Cardiology 85:255, 1994.

106. Wen JY, Baughman KL: The Dressler syndrome. Johns Hopkins Med J 148:179, 1981.

107. Stelzner TJ, King TE Jr, Antony VB, et al: The pleuropulmonary manifestations of the postcardiac injury syndrome. Chest 84:383, 1983.

108. Barakat MH, Karnik AM, Majeed HW, et al: Familial Mediterranean fever (recurrent hereditary polyserositis) in Arabs—a study of 175 patients and review of the literature. QJM 60:837, 1986.

109. Joseph J, Sahn SA: Thoracic endometriosis syndrome: New observations from an analysis of 110 cases. Am J Med 100:164, 1996.

110. Karpel JP, Appel D, Merav A: Pulmonary endometriosis. Lung 163:151, 1985.

111. Foster DC, Stern JL, Buscema J, et al: Pleural and parenchymal pulmonary endometriosis. Obstet Gynecol 58:552, 1981.

112. Yamazaki S, Ogawa J, Koide S, et al: Catamenial pneumothorax associated with endometriosis of the diaphragm. Chest 77:107, 1980.

113. Im J-G, Kang HS, Choi BI, et al: Pleural endometriosis: CT and sonographic findings. Am J Roentgenol 148:523, 1987.

114. Miller JI Jr: Diagnosis and management of chylothorax. Chest Surg Clin N Am 6:139, 1996.

115. Schulman A, Fataar S, Dalrymple R, et al: The lymphographic anatomy of chylothorax. Br J Radiol 51:420, 1978.

116. Latner AL: Cantarow and Trumper Clinical Biochemistry. 7th ed. Philadelphia, WB Saunders, 1975.

117. Staats BA, Ellefson RD, Budahn LL, et al: The lipoprotein profile of chylous and nonchylous pleural effusions. Mayo Clin Proc 55:700, 1980.

118. Mares DC, Mathur PN: Medical thoracoscopic talc pleurodesis for chylothorax due to lymphoma. Chest 114:731, 1998.

119. Strausser JL, Flye MW: Management of nontraumatic chylothorax. Ann Thorac Surg 31:520, 1981.

120. Ampil FL, Burton GV, Hardjasudarma M, et al: Chylous effusion complicating chronic lymphocytic leukemia. Leuk Lymphoma 10:507, 1993.

121. Quinonez A, Halabe J, Avelar F, et al: Chylothorax due to metastatic prostatic carcinoma. Br J Urol 63:325, 1989.

122. Tani K, Ogushi F, Sone S, et al: Chylothorax and chylous ascites in a patient with uterine cancer. Jpn J Clin Oncol 18:175, 1988.

123. Dulchavsky SA, Ledgerwood AM, Lucas CE: Management of chylothorax after blunt chest trauma. J Trauma 28:1400, 1988.

124. Haniuda M, Nishimura H, Kobayashi O, et al: Management of chylothorax after pulmonary resection. J Am Coll Surg 180:537, 1995.

125. Fine PG, Bubela C: Chylothorax following celiac plexus block. Anesthesiology 63:454, 1985.

126. Nakai S, Zielke K: Chylothorax—a rare complication after anterior and posterior spinal correction: Report of six cases. Spine 11:830, 1986.

127. Muns G, Rennard SI, Floreani AA: Combined occurrence of chyloperitoneum and chylothorax after retroperitoneal surgery. Eur Respir J 8:185, 1995.

128. Cespedes RD, Peretsman SJ, Harris MJ: Chylothorax as a complication of radical nephrectomy. J Urol 150:1895, 1993.
129. Jabbar AS, al-Abdulkareem A: Bilateral chylothorax following neck dissection. Head Neck 17:69, 1995.
130. La Hei ER, Menzie SJ, Thompson JF: Right chylothorax following left radical neck dissection. Aust N Z J Surg 63:77, 1993.
131. Canil K, Fitzgerald P, Lau G: Massive chylothorax associated with lymphangiomatosis of the bone. J Pediatr Surg 29:1186, 1994.
132. Sailer M, Unsinn K, Fink C, et al: Pulmonary lymphangiectasis with spontaneous chylothorax bei Noonan-syndrome. Klin Padiatr 207:302, 1995.
133. Sullivan KL, Steiner RM, Wexler RJ: Lymphaticopleural fistula: Diagnosis by computed tomography. J Comput Assist Tomogr 8:1005, 1984.
134. Milano S, Maroldi R, Vezzoli G, et al: Chylothorax after blunt chest trauma: An unusual case with a long latent period. Thorac Cardiovasc Surg 42:187, 1994.
135. Freundlich IM: The role of lymphangiography in chylothorax: A report of six nontraumatic cases. Am J Roentgenol 125:617, 1975.
136. Ngan H, Fok M, Wong J: The role of lymphography in chylothorax following thoracic surgery. Br J Radiol 61:1032, 1988.
137. Sachs PB, Zelch MG, Rice TW, et al: Diagnosis and localization of laceration of the thoracic duct: Usefulness of lymphangiography and CT. Am J Roentgenol 157:703, 1991.
138. Sarwal V, Suri RK, Sharma OP, et al: Traumatic subarachnoid-pleural fistula. Ann Thorac Surg 62:1622, 1996.
139. Chertow BS, Kadzielawa R, Burger AJ: Benign pleural effusions in long-standing diabetes mellitus. Chest 99:1108, 1991.
140. Kavuru MS, Adamo JP, Ahmad M, et al: Amyloidosis and pleural disease. Chest 98:20, 1990.
141. Graham DR, Ahmad D: Amyloidosis with pleural involvement. Eur Respir J 1:571, 1988.
142. Pappas CA, Rheinlander HF, Stadecker MJ: Pleural effusion as a complication of solitary eosinophilic granuloma of the rib. Hum Pathol 11:675, 1980.
143. Horn BR, Byrd RB: Simulation of pleural disease by disk space infection. Chest 74:575, 1978.
144. Feigl D, Seidel L, Marmor A: Gorham's disease of the clavicle with bilateral pleural effusions. Chest 79:242, 1981.
145. Hirmand H, Hoffman LA, Smith JP: Silicone migration to the pleural space associated with silicone-gel augmentation mammaplasty. Ann Plast Surg 32:645, 1994.
146. Kolef MH, McCormack MT, Kristo DA, et al: Pleural effusion in patients with systemic cholesterol embolization. Chest 103:792, 1993.
147. Buchanan DR, Johnston IDA, Kerr IH, et al: Cryptogenic bilateral fibrosing pleuritis. Br J Dis Chest 82:186, 1988.
148. Hughes GRV: Hypotensive agents, beta-blockers, and drug-induced lupus. BMJ 284:1358, 1982.
149. Price EJ, Venables PJ: Drug-induced lupus. Drug Saf 112:283, 1995.
150. Yousem S, Lifson J, Colby T: Chemotherapy-induced eosinophilic pneumonia: Relation to bleomycin. Chest 88:103, 1985.
151. Orwoll ES, Kiessling PJ, Patterson JR: Interstitial pneumonia from mitomycin. Ann Intern Med 89:352, 1978.
152. Castro M, Veeder MH, Mailliard JA, et al: A prospective study of pulmonary function in patients receiving mitomycin. Chest 109:939, 1996.
153. Smalley RV, Wall RL: Two cases of busulfan toxicity. Ann Intern Med 64:154, 1966.
154. Major PP, Laurin S, Bettez P: Pulmonary fibrosis following therapy with melphalan: Report of two cases. Can Med Assoc J 123:197, 1980.
155. Tjon A, Tham RTO, Peters WG, et al: Pulmonary complications of cytosine-arabinoside therapy: Radiographic findings. Am J Roentgenol 149:23, 1987.
156. Thompson J, Chengappa KN, Good CB, et al: Hepatitis, hyperglycemia, pleural effusion, eosinophilia, hematuria and proteinuria occurring early in clozapine treatment. Int Clin Psychopharmacol 13:95, 1998.
157. Kreisman H, Wolkove N: Pulmonary toxicity of antineoplastic therapy. Semin Oncol 19:508, 1992.
158. Twohig KJ, Matthay RA: Pulmonary effects of cytotoxic agents other than bleomycin. Clin Chest Med 11:31, 1990.
159. Vogelzang PJ, Bloom SM, Mier JW, et al: Chest roentgenographic abnormalities in IL-2 recipients. Chest 101:746, 1992.
160. Seebach J, Speich R, Fehr J, et al: GM-CSF-induced eosinophilic pneumonia. Br J Haematol 90:963, 1995.
161. Murray MJ, Kronenberg R: Pulmonary reactions simulating cardiac pulmonary edema caused by nitrofurantoin. N Engl J Med 273:1185, 1965.
162. Bando T, Fujimura M, Noda Y, et al: Minocycline-induced pneumonitis with bilateral hilar lymphadenopathy and pleural effusion. Intern Med 33:177, 1994.
163. Osanai S, Fukuzawa J, Akiba Y, et al: Minocycline-induced pneumonia and pleurisy—a case report. Nippon Kyobu Shikkan Gakkai Zasshi 30:322, 1992.
164. McNeil KD, Firouz-Abadi A, Oliver W, et al: Amiodarone pulmonary toxicity—three unusual manifestations. Aust N Z J Med 22:14, 1992.
165. Pusateri DW, Muder RR: Fever, pulmonary infiltrates and pleural effusion following acyclovir therapy for herpes zoster ophthalmicus. Chest 98:754, 1990.
166. Middleton KL, Santella R, Couser JI Jr: Eosinophilic pleuritis due to propylthiouracil. Chest 103:955, 1993.
167. Zaidenstein R, Cohen N, Dishi V, et al: Chylothorax following median sternotomy. Clin Cardiol 19:910, 1996.
168. Kotzot D, Stoss H, Wagner H, et al: Jaffe-Campanacci syndrome: Case report and review of literature. Clin Dysmorphol 3:328, 1994.
169. Farrell SA, Warda LJ, LaFlair P, et al: Adams-Oliver syndrome: A case with juvenile chronic myelogenous leukemia and chylothorax. Am J Med Genet 47:1175, 1993.
170. Fryns JP, Moerman P: 46,XY/46XX mosaicism and congenital pulmonary lymphangiectasis with chylothorax. Am J Med Genet 47:934, 1993.
171. Goldfarb JP: Chylous effusions secondary to pancreatitis: Case report and review of the literature. Am J Gastroenterol 79:133, 1984.
172. Menzies R, Hidvegi R: Chylothorax associated with tuberculous spondylitis. J Can Assoc Radiol 39:238, 1988.
173. Anton PA, Rubio S, Casan P, et al: Chylothorax due to *Mycobacterium tuberculosis*. Thorax 50:1019, 1995.
174. Bristo LD, Mandal AK, Oparah SS, et al: Bilateral chylothorax associated with sclerosing mediastinitis. Int Surg 68:273, 1983.
175. Van Veldhuizen PJ, Taylor S: Chylothorax: A complication of a left subclavian vein thrombosis. Am J Clin Oncol 19:99, 1996.
176. Lengyel RJ, Shanley DJ: Recurrent chylothorax associated with sarcoidosis. Hawaii Med J 54:817, 1995.
177. Jarman PR, Whyte MK, Sabroe I, et al: Sarcoidosis presenting with chylothorax. Thorax 50:1324, 1995.
178. Villena V, De Pablo A, Martin-Escribano P: Chylothorax and chylous ascites due to heart failure. Eur Respir J 8:1235, 1995.
179. Delgado C, Martin M, de la Portilla F: Retrosternal goiter associated with chylothorax. Chest 106:1924, 1994.
180. Cöplu L, Emri S, Selcuk ZT, et al: Life threatening chylous pleural and pericardial effusion in a patient with Behçet's syndrome. Thorax 47:64, 1992.
181. Tie MLH, Poland GA, Rossenow EC III: Chylothorax in Gorhams' syndrome: A common complication of a rare disease. Chest 105:208, 1994.
182. Gil-Suay V, Martinez-Moragon E, de Diego A, et al: Chylothorax complicating a thoracic aortic aneurysm. Eur Respir J 10:737, 1997.
183. Bass SN, Ailani RK, Shekar R, et al: Pyogenic vertebral osteomyelitis presenting as exudative pleural effusion: A series of five cases. Chest 114:642, 1998.
184. Wood N, Edozien L, Lieberman B: Symptomatic unilateral pleural effusion as a presentation of ovarian hyperstimulation syndrome. Hum Reprod 13:571, 1998.
185. Garcia-Riego A, Cuinas C. Vilanova JJ, et al: Extramedullary hematopoietic effusions. Acta Cytol 42:1116, 1998.
186. Blankenship ME, Rowlett J, Timby JW, et al: Giant lymph node hyperplasia (Castleman's disease) presenting with chylous pleural effusion. Chest 112:1132, 1997.
187. Romero S, Martin C, Hernandez L, et al: Chylothorax in cirrhosis of the liver: Analysis of its frequency and clinical characteristics. Chest 114:154, 1998.
188. Riemann R, Jakse R: Pneumothorax nach mediastinalemphysem: Uber den ort und den mechanismus der pleuraruptur. Acta Anat 128:115, 1986.
189. Smith WG, Rothwell PPG: Treatment of spontaneous pneumothorax. Thorax 17:342, 1962.
190. Hyde L: Benign spontaneous pneumothorax. Ann Intern Med 56:746, 1962.

191. Lindskog GE, Halasz NA: Spontaneous pneumothorax: A consideration of pathogenesis and management with review of seventy-two hospitalized cases. Arch Surg 75:693, 1957.

192. Primrose WR: Spontaneous pneumothorax: A retrospective review of aetiology, pathogenesis and management. Scott Med J 29:15, 1984.

193. Chan TB, Tan WC, Tech PC: Spontaneous pneumothorax in medical practise in a general hospital. Ann Acad Med Singapore 14:457, 1985.

194. Lesur O, Delorme N, Fromaget JM, et al: Computed tomography in the etiologic assessment of idiopathic spontaneous pneumothorax. Chest 98:341, 1990.

195. Bense L, Lewander R, Eklund G, et al: Nonsmoking, non-alpha$_1$-antitrypsin deficiency-induced emphysema in nonsmokers with healed spontaneous pneumothorax, identified by computed tomography of the lungs. Chest 103:433, 1993.

196. Andrivet P, Kjedaini K, Teboul JL, et al: Spontaneous pneumothorax: Comparison of thoracic drainage vs immediate or delayed needle aspiration. Chest 108:335, 1995.

197. Melton LJ III, Hepper NGG, Offord KP: Incidence of spontaneous pneumothorax in Olmsted County, Minnesota: 1950 to 1974. Am Rev Respir Dis 120:1379, 1979.

198. Lichter I, Gwynne JF: Spontaneous pneumothorax in young subjects. Thorax 26:409, 1971.

199. Jordan KG, Kwong JS, Flint J, Müller NL: Surgically treated pneumothorax: Radiologic and pathologic findings. Chest 111:280, 1997.

200. Melton LJ III, Hepper NGG, Offord KP: Influence of height on the risk of spontaneous pneumothorax. Mayo Clin Proc 56:678, 1981.

201. Hall JR, Pyeritz RE, Dudgeon DL, et al: Pneumothorax in the Marfan syndrome: Prevalence and therapy. Ann Thorac Surg 37:500, 1984.

202. Lipton RA, Greenwald RA, Seriff NS: Pneumothorax and bilateral honeycombed lung in Marfan syndrome: Report of a case and review of the pulmonary abnormalities in this disorder. Am Rev Respir Dis 104:924, 1971.

203. Margaliot SZ, Barzilay J, Bar-David M, et al: Spontaneous pneumothorax and mitral valve prolapse. Chest 89:93, 1986.

204. Inouye WY, Berggren RB, Johnson J: Spontaneous pneumothorax: Treatment and mortality. Dis Chest 51:67, 1967.

205. Ruckley CV, McCormack RJM: The management of spontaneous pneumothorax. Thorax 21:139, 1966.

206. Mitlehner W, Friedrich M, Dissmann W: Value of computer tomography in the detection of bullae and blebs in patients with primary spontaneous pneumothorax. Respiration 59:221, 1992.

207. Bense L, Wiman LG, Hedenstierna G: Onset of symptoms in spontaneous pneumothorax: Correlations to physical activity. Eur J Respir Dis 71:181, 1987.

208. Dermksian G, Lamb LE: Spontaneous pneumothorax in apparently healthy flying personnel. Ann Intern Med 51:39, 1959.

209. Rose DM, Jarczyk PA: Spontaneous pneumoperitoneum after scuba diving. JAMA 239:223, 1978.

210. Saywell WR: Submarine escape training, lung cysts and tension pneumothorax. Br J Radiol 62:276, 1989.

211. Wait MA, Estrera A: Changing clinical spectrum of spontaneous pneumothorax. Am J Surg 164:528, 1992.

212. Maurer ER, Schaal JA, Mendez FL: Chronic recurrent spontaneous pneumothorax due to endometriosis of the diaphragm. JAMA 168:2013, 1958.

213. Shiraishi T: Catamenial pneumothorax: A report of a case and review of the Japanese and non-Japanese literature. Thorac Cardiovasc Surg 39:304, 1991.

214. Balasingham S, Arulkumaran S, Nadarajah K, et al: Catamenial pneumothorax. Aust N Z J Obstet Gynaecol 26:88, 1986.

215. Schoenfeld A, Ziv E, Zeelel Y, et al: Catamenial pneumothorax: A literature review and report of an unusual case. Obstet Gynecol Surv 41:20, 1986.

216. Carter EJ, Ettensohn DB: Catamenial pneumothorax. Chest 98:713, 1990.

217. Van Schil PE, Vercauteren SR, Vermeire PA, et al: Catamenial pneumothorax caused by thoracic endometriosis. Ann Thorac Surg 62:585, 1996.

218. Despars JA, Sassoon CSH, Light RW: Significance of iatrogenic pneumothoraces. Chest 105:1147, 1994.

219. Renner RR, Markarian B, Pernice NJ, et al: The apical cap. Radiology 110:569, 1974.

220. McLoud TC, Isler RJ, Novelline RA, et al: The apical cap. Am J Roentgenol 137:299, 1981.

221. Im JG, Webb WR, Han MC, et al: Apical opacity associated with pulmonary tuberculosis: High-resolution CT findings. Radiology 178:727, 1991.

222. Fennessy JJ: Irradiation damage to the lung. J Thorac Imaging 2:68, 1987.

223. Marnocha KE, Maglinte DDT: Plain-film criteria for excluding aortic rupture in blunt chest trauma. Am J Roentgenol 144:19, 1985.

224. Mirvis SE, Bidwell JK, Buddemeyer EU, et al: Value of chest radiography in excluding traumatic aortic rupture. Radiology 163:487, 1987.

225. Schwartz DA: New developments in asbestos-induced pleural disease. Chest 99:191, 1991.

226. Hourihane DO, Lessof L, Richardson PC: Hyaline and calcified pleural plaques as an index of exposure to asbestos: A study of radiological and pathological features of 100 cases with a consideration of epidemiology. BMJ 1:1069, 1966.

227. Rubino GF, Scansetti G, Pira E, et al: Pleural plaques and lung asbestos bodies in the general population: An autopical and clinical-radiological survey. *In* Wagner JC (ed): Biological Effects of Mineral Fibres. Lyon, France, International Agency for Research on Cancer, 1980.

228. Meurman L: Asbestos bodies and pleural plaques in a Finnish series of autopsy cases. Acta Pathol Microbiol Scand 181(Suppl):1, 1966.

229. Hillerdal G, Lindgren A: Pleural plaques: Correlation of autopsy findings to radiographic findings and occupational history. Eur J Respir Dis 61:315, 1980.

230. Fletcher DE, Edge JR: The early radiological changes in pulmonary and pleural asbestosis. Clin Radiol 21:355, 1970.

231. Rockoff SD, Kagan E, Schwartz A, et al: Visceral pleural thickening in asbestos exposure: The occurrence and implications of thickening interlobar fissures. J Thorac Imaging 2:58, 1987.

232. Friedman AC, Fiel SB, Radecki PD, et al: Computed tomography of benign pleural and pulmonary parenchymal abnormalities related to asbestos exposure. Semin Ultrasound CT MR 11:393, 1990.

233. Solomon A: Radiological features of asbestos-related visceral pleural changes. Am J Ind Med 19:339, 1991.

234. MacKenzie FAF: The radiological investigation of the early manifestations of exposure to asbestos dust. Proc R Soc Med 64:834, 1971.

235. Sherman CB, Barnhart S, Rosenstock L: Use of oblique chest roentgenograms in detecting pleural disease in asbestos-exposed workers. J Occup Med 30:681, 1988.

236. Svenes KB, Borgersen A, Haaversen O, et al: Parietal pleural plaques: A comparison between autopsy and x-ray findings. Eur J Respir Dis 69:10, 1986.

237. Withers BF, Ducatman AM, Yang WN: Roentgenographic evidence for predominant left-sided location of unilateral pleural plaques. Chest 95:1262, 1989.

238. Fisher MS: Asymmetrical changes in asbestos-related disease. J Can Assoc Radiol 36:110, 1985.

239. Hu H, Beckett L, Kelsey K, et al: The left-sided predominance of asbestos-related pleural disease. Am Rev Respir Dis 148:981, 1993.

240. Sargent EN, Boswell WD Jr, Ralls PW, et al: Subpleural fat pads in patients exposed to asbestos: Distinction from non-calcified pleural plaques. Radiology 152:273, 1984.

241. Greene R, Boggis C, Jantsch H: Asbestos-related pleural thickening: Effect of threshold criteria on interpretation. Radiology 152:569, 1984.

242. Gefter WB, Conant EF: Issues and controversies in the plain-film diagnosis of asbestos-related disorders in the chest. J Thorac Imaging 3:11, 1988.

243. Bourbeau J, Ernst P: Between- and within-reader variability in the assessment of pleural abnormality using the ILO 1980 international classification of pneumoconiosis. Am J Ind Med 14:537, 1988.

244. Wain SL, Roggli VL, Foster WL: Parietal pleural plaques, asbestos bodies, and neoplasia: A clinical, pathologic, and roentgenographic correlation of 25 consecutive cases. Chest 86:707, 1984.

245. Aberle DR, Gamsu G, Ray CS: High-resolution CT of benign asbestos-related diseases: Clinical and radiographic correlation. Am J Roentgenol 151:883, 1988.

246. Friedman AC, Fiel SB, Fisher MS, et al: Asbestos-related pleural disease and asbestosis: A comparison of CT and chest radiography. Am J Roentgenol 150:269, 1988.

247. Staples CA, Gamsu G, Ray CS, et al: High resolution computed

tomography and lung function in asbestos-exposed workers with normal chest radiographs. Am Rev Respir Dis 139:1502, 1989.

248. Gevenois PA, de Vuyst P, Dedeire S, et al: Conventional and high-resolution CT in asymptomatic asbestos-exposed workers. Acta Radiol 35:226, 1994.

249. Im JG, Webb WR, Rosen A, et al: Costal pleura: Appearances at high-resolution CT. Radiology 171:125, 1989.

250. Aberle DR, Gamsu G, Ray CS, et al: Asbestos-related pleural and parenchymal fibrosis: Detection with high-resolution CT. Radiology 166:729, 1988.

251. Anton HC: Multiple pleural plaques, part II. Br J Radiol 41:341, 1968.

252. Freundlich IM, Greening RR: Asbestosis and associated medical problems. Radiology 89:224, 1967.

253. Smith AR: Pleural calcification resulting from exposure to certain dusts. Am J Roentgenol 67:375, 1952.

254. Kiviluoto R: Pleural calcification as a roentgenologic sign of nonoccupational endemic anthophyllite-asbestosis. Acta Radiol (Suppl)194, 1960.

255. Solomon A: Radiology of asbestosis. Environ Res 3:320, 1970.

256. Kleinfeld M: Pleural calcification as a sign of silicatosis. Am J Med Sci 251:215, 1966.

257. Krige L: Asbestosis—with special reference to the radiological diagnosis. S Afr J Radiol 4:13, 1966.

258. McLoud TC, Woods BO, Carrington CB, et al: Diffuse pleural thickening in an asbestos-exposed population. Am J Roentgenol 144:9, 1985.

259. Müller NL: Imaging of the pleura. Radiology 186:297, 1993.

260. Leung AN, Müller NL, Miller RR: CT in differential diagnosis of diffuse pleural disease. Am J Roentgenol 154:487, 1990.

261. Lynch DA, Gamsu G, Aberle DR: Conventional and high resolution computed tomography in the diagnosis of asbestos-related diseases. Radiographics 9:523, 1989.

262. Murray JG, Patz EF Jr, Erasmus JJ, et al: CT appearance of the pleural space after talc pleurodesis. Am J Roentgenol 169:89, 1997.

263. Gilbert L, Ribot S, Frankel H, et al: Fibrinous uremic pleuritis—surgical entity. Chest 67:53, 1975.

264. Hoogsteden HC, Langerak AW, van der Kwast TH, et al: Malignant pleural mesothelioma. Crit Rev Oncol Hematol 25:97, 1997.

265. Coffin CM, Dehner LP: Mesothelial and related neoplasms in children and adolescents: A clinicopathologic and immunohistochemical analysis of eight cases. Pediatr Pathol 12:333, 1992.

266. Roggli VL, McGavran MH, Subach J, et al: Pulmonary asbestos body counts and electron probe analysis of asbestos body cores in patients with mesothelioma: A study of 25 cases. Cancer 50:2423, 1982.

267. Mowé G, Gylseth B, Hartveit F, et al: Occupational asbestos exposure, lung-fiber concentration and latency time in malignant mesothelioma. Scand J Work Environ Health 10:293, 1984.

268. Davies D: Are all mesotheliomas due to asbestos (editorial)? BMJ 289:1164, 1984.

269. Lin-Chu M, Lee Y-J, Ho MY: Malignant mesothelioma in infancy. Arch Pathol Lab Med 113:409, 1989.

270. McDonald JC, McDonald AD: The epidemiology of mesothelioma in historical context. Eur Respir J 9:1932, 1996.

271. Alexander E, Clark RA, Colley DP, et al: CT of malignant pleural mesothelioma. Am J Roentgenol 137:287, 1981.

272. Miller BH, Rosado-de-Christenson ML, Mason AC, et al: Malignant pleural mesothelioma: Radiologic-pathologic correlation. Radiographics 16:613, 1996.

273. Wechsler RJ, Rao VM, Steiner RM: The radiology of thoracic malignant mesothelioma. Crit Rev Diagn Imaging 20:283, 1983.

274. Huncharek M: Miliary mesothelioma. Chest 106:605, 1994.

275. Solomons K, Polakow R, Marchand P: Diffuse malignant mesothelioma presenting as bilateral malignant lymphangitis. Thorax 40:682, 1985.

276. Ohishi N, Oka T, Fukuhara T, et al: Extensive pulmonary metastases in malignant pleural mesothelioma: A rare clinical and radiographic presentation. Chest 110:296, 1996.

277. Rabinowitz JG, Efremidis SC, Cohen B, et al: A comparative study of mesothelioma and asbestosis using computed tomography and conventional chest radiography. Radiology 144:453, 1982.

278. Rusch VW, Godwin JD, Shuman WP: The role of computed tomography scanning in the initial assessment and the follow-up of malignant pleural mesothelioma. J Thorac Cardiovasc Surg 96:171, 1988.

279. Kawashima A, Libshitz HI: Malignant pleural mesothelioma: CT manifestations in 50 cases. Am J Roentgenol 155:965, 1990.

280. Raizon A, Schwartz A, Hix W, et al: Calcification as a sign of sarcomatous degeneration of malignant pleural mesotheliomas: A new CT finding. J Comput Assist Tomogr 20:42, 1996.

281. Patz EF Jr, Shaffer K, Piwnica-Worms DR, et al: Malignant pleural mesothelioma: Value of CT and MR imaging in predicting resectability. Am J Roentgenol 159:961, 1992.

282. Patz EF Jr, Rusch VW, Heelan R: The proposed new international TNM staging system for malignant pleural mesothelioma: Application to imaging. Am J Roentgenol 166:323, 1996.

283. Falaschi F, Battolla L, Mascalchi M, et al: Usefulness of MR signal intensity in distinguishing benign from malignant pleural disease. Am J Roentgenol 166:963, 1996.

284. Lorigan JG, Libshitz HI: MR imaging of malignant pleural mesothelioma. J Comput Assist Tomogr 13:617, 1989.

285. Bénard F, Sterman D, Smith RJ, et al: Metabolic imaging of malignant pleural mesothelioma with fluorodeoxyglucose positron emission tomography. Chest 114:713, 1998.

286. Tammilehto L, Maasilta P, Kostiainen S, et al: Diagnosis and prognostic factors in malignant pleural mesothelioma: A retrospective analysis of sixty-five patients. Respiration 59:129, 1992.

287. Brenner J, Sordillo PP, Magill GB, et al: Malignant mesothelioma of the pleura: Review of 123 patients. Cancer 49:2431, 1982.

288. Krumhaar D, Lange S, Hartmann C, et al: Follow-up study of 100 malignant pleural mesotheliomas. J Thorac Cardiovasc Surg 33:272, 1985.

289. Grellner W, Staak M: Multiple skeletal muscle metastases from malignant pleural mesothelioma. Pathol Res Pract 191:456, 1995.

290. Kim SB, Varkey B, Choi H: Diagnosis of malignant pleural mesothelioma by axillary lymph node biopsy. Chest 91:279, 1987.

291. Kaye JA, Wang AM, Joachim CL, et al: Malignant mesothelioma with brain metastases. Am J Med 80:95, 1986.

292. Wills EJ: Pleural mesothelioma with initial presentation as cervical lymphadenopathy. Ultrastruct Pathol 19:389, 1995.

293. Lloreta J, Serrano S: Pleural mesothelioma presenting as an axillary lymph node metastasis with anemone cell appearance. Ultrastruct Pathol 18:293, 1994.

294. Rusch VW, Venkatraman E: The importance of surgical staging in the treatment of malignant pleural mesothelioma. J Thorac Cardiovasc Surg 111:815, 1996.

295. Chailleux E, Dabouis G, Pioche D, et al: Prognostic factors in diffuse malignant pleural mesothelioma: A study of 167 patients. Chest 93:159, 1988.

296. De Pangher Manzini V, Brollo A, Franceschi S, et al: Prognostic factors of malignant mesothelioma of the pleura. Cancer 72:410, 1993.

297. Tammilehto L, Kivisaari L, Salminen US, et al: Evaluation of the clinical TNM staging system for malignant pleural mesothelioma: An assessment in 88 patients. Lung Cancer 12:25, 1995.

298. Rusch VW: A proposed new international TNM staging system for malignant pleural mesothelioma. From the International Mesothelioma Interest Group. Chest 108:1122, 1995.

299. Briselli M, Mark EJ, Dickerson GR: Solitary fibrous tumors of the pleura: Eight new cases and review of 360 cases in the literature. Cancer 47:2678, 1981.

300. England DM, Hochholzer L, McCarthy MJ: Localized benign and malignant fibrous tumors of the pleura: A clinicopathologic review of 223 cases. Am J Surg Pathol 13:640, 1989.

301. Bilbey JH, Müller NL, Miller RR, et al: Localized fibrous mesothelioma of pleura following external ionizing radiation therapy. Chest 94:1291, 1988.

302. Hill JK, Heitmiller RF II, Askin FB, et al: Localized benign pleural mesothelioma arising in a radiation field. Clin Imaging 21:189, 1997.

303. Witkin GB, Rosai J: Solitary fibrous tumor of the mediastinum: A report of 14 cases. Am J Surg Pathol 13:547, 1989.

304. Lee KS, Im JG, Choe KO, et al: CT findings in benign fibrous mesothelioma of the pleura: Pathologic correlation in nine patients. Am J Roentgenol 158:983, 1992.

305. Ferretti GR, Chiles C, Choplin RH, et al: Localized benign fibrous tumors of the pleura. Am J Roentgenol 169:683, 1997.

306. Desser TS, Stark P: Pictorial essay: Solitary fibrous tumor of the pleura. J Thorac Imaging 13:27, 1998.

307. Hutchinson WB, Friedenberg MJ: Intrathoracic mesothelioma. Radiology 80:937, 1963.

308. Dedrick CG, McLoud TC, Shepard JO, et al: Computed tomography of localized pleural mesothelioma. Am J Roentgenol 144:275, 1985.

309. Soulen MC, Greco-Hunt VT, Templeton P: Migratory chest mass. Invest Radiol 25:209, 1990.

310. Zamperlin A, Drigo R, Famulare CI, et al: A vagabond pleural pebble. Respiration 51:155, 1987.

311. Mengeot PM, Gailly CH: Spontaneous detachment of benign mesothelioma into the pleural space and removal during pleuroscopy. Eur J Respir Dis 68:141, 1986.

312. Mendelson DS, Meary E, Buy JN, et al: Localized fibrous pleural mesothelioma: CT findings. Clin Imaging 15:105, 1991.

313. Saifuddin A, Da Costa P, Chalmers AG, et al: Primary malignant localized fibrous tumours of the pleura: Clinical, radiological and pathological features. Clin Radiol 45:13, 1992.

314. Harris GN, Rozenshtein A, Schiff MJ: Benign fibrous mesothelioma of the pleura: MR imaging findings. Am J Roentgenol 165:1143, 1995.

315. Ferretti GR, Chiles C, Cox JE, et al: Localized benign fibrous tumors of the pleura: MR appearance. J Comput Assist Tomogr 21:115, 1997.

316. Versluis PJ, Lamers RJS: Localized pleural fibroma: Radiological features. Eur J Radiol 18:124, 1994.

317. Padovani B, Mouroux J, Raffaelli C, et al: Benign fibrous mesothelioma of the pleura: MR study and pathologic correlation. Eur Radiol 6:425, 1996.

318. Kniznik DO, Roncoroni AJ, Rosenberg M, et al: Giant fibrous pleural mesothelioma associated with myocardial restriction and hypoglycemia: Respiration 37:346, 1979.

319. Okike N, Bernatz PE, Woolner LB: Localized mesothelioma of the pleura: Benign and malignant variants. J Thorac Cardiovasc Surg 75:363, 1978.

320. Mandal AK, Rozer MA, Salem FA, et al: Localized benign mesothelioma of the pleura associated with a hypoglycemic episode. Arch Intern Med 143:1608, 1983.

321. Epler GR, McLoud TC, Munn CS, et al: Pleural lipoma: Diagnosis by computed tomography. Chest 90:265, 1986.

322. Buxton RC, Tan CS, Khine NM, et al: Atypical transmural thoracic lipoma: CT diagnosis. J Comput Assist Tomogr 12:196, 1988.

323. Munk PL, Müller NL: Pleural liposarcoma: CT diagnosis. J Comput Assist Tomogr 12:709, 1988.

324. Szalay F, Szathmari M, Paloczi K, et al: Immunologic and molecular biologic characterization of pleural involvement in a case of T-chronic lymphocytic leukemia. Chest 106:1283, 1994.

325. Joseph J, Sahn SA: Connective tissue diseases and the pleura. Chest 104:262, 1993.

326. Pistiner M, Wallace DJ, Nessim S, et al: Lupus erythematosus in the 1980s: A survey of 570 patients. Semin Arthritis Rheum 21:55, 1991.

327. Wiedemann HP, Matthay RA: Pulmonary manifestations of systemic lupus erythematosus. J Thorac Imaging 7:1, 1992.

328. Chang RW: Cardiac manifestations of SLE. Clin Rheum Dis 8:197, 1982.

329. Creasy JD, Chiles C, Routh WD, et al: Overview of traumatic injury of the thoracic aorta. Radiographics 17:27, 1997.

330. Ng CS, Munden RF, Libshitz HI: Malignant pleural mesothelioma: The spectrum of manifestations on CT in 70 cases. Clin Radiol 54:415, 1999.

331. Light RW: Management of parapneumonic effusions. Arch Intern Med 141:1339, 1981.

332. Joseph JJ, Sahn SA: Connective tissue disease and the pleura. Chest 104:262, 1993.

333. Sharifker D, Kaneko M: Localized fibrous "mesothelioma" of pleura (submesothelial fibroma): A clinicopathologic study of 18 cases. Cancer 43:627, 1979.

334. Müller NL: Imaging of the pleura. Radiology 186:297, 1993.

335. Nygaard SD, Berger HA, Fick RB: Chylothorax as a complication of oesophageal sclerotherapy. Thorax 47:134, 1992.

336. Graham ML, Spelsberg TC, Dines DE, et al: Pulmonary lymphangiomyomatosis: With particular reference to steroid-receptor assay studies and pathologic correlation. Mayo Clin Proc 59:3, 1984.

337. Müller NL, Chiles C, Kullnig P: Pulmonary lymphangiomyomatosis: Correlation of CT with radiographic and functional findings. Radiology 175:335, 1990.

338. Babcock TL, Snyder BA: Spontaneous pneumothorax associated with tuberous sclerosis. J Thorac Cardiovasc Surg 83:100, 1982.

339. Castro M, Shepherd CW, Gomez MR, et al: Pulmonary tuberous sclerosis. Chest 107:189, 1995.

340. Torrington KG, Ashbaugh DG, Stackle EG: Recklinghausen's disease: Occurrence with intrathoracic vagal neurofibroma and contralateral spontaneous pneumothorax. Arch Intern Med 143:568, 1983.

341. Cohen S, Hossain MS-A: Primary carcinoma of the lung: A review of 417 histologically proved cases. Dis Chest 49:67, 1966.

342. Torre D, Martegani R, Speranza F, et al: Pulmonary cryptococcosis presenting as pneumothorax in a patient with AIDS. Clin Infect Dis 21:1524, 1995.

343. McClellan MD, Miller SB, Pasons PE, et al: Pneumothorax with *Pneumocystis carinii* pneumonia in AIDS: Incidence and clinical characteristics. Chest 100:1224, 1991.

344. Bakir F, Al-Omeri MM: Echinococcal tension pneumothorax. Thorax 24:547, 1969.

345. Khan F, Seriff NS: Pneumothorax: A rare presenting manifestation of lung cancer. Am Rev Respir Dis 108:1397, 1973.

346. Wagner RB, Knox GS: Pneumothorax: An unusual manifestation of a bronchial carcinoid. Md Med J 39:263, 1990.

347. Michelassi PL, Sbragia S: Clinicoradiological considerations in 2 cases of spontaneous pneumothorax, apparently idiopathic, secondary to pulmonary metastases. Ann Radio Diagn 33:39, 1960.

348. Smevik B, Klepp O: The risk of spontaneous pneumothorax in patients with osteogenic sarcoma and testicular cancer. Cancer 49:1734, 1982.

349. Slasky BS, Deutsch M: Germ cell tumors complicated by pneumothorax. Urology 22:39, 1983.

350. Lesser JE, Carr D: Fatal pneumothorax following bleomycin and other cytotoxic drugs. Cancer Treat REp 69:344, 1985.

351. Chen KW, Wu MH, Huang JJ, et al: Bilateral spontaneous pneumothoraces, pneumopericardium, pneumomediastinum, and subcutaneous emphysema: A rare presentation of paraquat intoxication. Ann Emerg Med 23:1132, 1994.

352. Murphy DG, Sloan EP, Hart RG, et al: Tension pneumothorax associated with hyperbaric oxygen therapy. Am J Emerg Med 9:176, 1991.

353. Pezner RD, Horak DA, Sayegh HO, et al: Spontaneous pneumothorax in patients irradiated for Hodgkin's disease and other malignant lymphomas. Int J Radiat Oncol Biol Phys 18:193, 1990.

354. Okada M, Ebe K, Matsumoto T, et al: Ipsilateral spontaneous pneumothorax after rapid development of large thin-walled cavities in two patients who had undergone radiation therapy for lung cancer. Am J Roentgenol 170:932, 1998.

355. Metersky ML, Colt HG, Olson LK, et al: AIDS-related spontaneous pneumothorax: Risk factors and treatment. Chest 109:946, 1995.

356. Epstein DM, Geften WB, Miller WT, et al: Spontaneous pneumothorax: An uncommon manifestation of Wegener granulomatosis. Radiology 135:327, 1980.

357. Nickol KH: Idiopathic pulmonary haemosiderosis presenting with spontaneous pneumothorax. Tubercle 41:216, 1960.

358. Moore ADA, Godwin JD, Müller NL, et al: Pulmonary histiocytosis X: Comparison of radiographic and CT findings. Radiology 172:249, 1989.

359. Froudarakis ME, Bouros D, Voloudaki A, et al: Pneumothorax as a first manifestation of sarcoidosis. Chest 112:278, 1997.

360. Bierman CW: Pneumomediastinum and pneumothorax complicating asthma in children. Am J Dis Child 114:42, 1967.

361. Bense L, Eklund G, Wiman LG: Smoking and the increased risk of contracting spontaneous pneumothorax. Chest 92:1009, 1987.

362. Spector ML, Stern RC: Pneumothorax in cystic fibrosis: A 26-year experience. Ann Thorac Surg 47:204, 1989.

363. Bailey WC, Brown M, Buechner HA, et al: Silico-mycobacterial disease in sandblasters. Am Rev Respir Dis 110:115, 1974.

364. Weber AL, Stoeckle JD, Hardy HL: Roentgenologic patterns in long-standing beryllium disease: Report of 8 cases. Am J Roentgenol 93:879, 1965.

365. Shaver CG, Riddell AR: Lung changes associated with the manifestation of alumina abrasives. J Industr Hyg Toxicol 29:145, 1947.

366. Blundell JE: Pneumothorax complicating pulmonary infarction. Br J Radio 40:226, 1967.

367. Hall FM, Salzman EW, Ellis BI, et al: Pneumothorax complicating septic cavitating pulmonary infarction. Chest 72:232, 1977.

368. Anton HC, Gray B: Pulmonaory alveolar proteinosis presenting with pneumothorax. Clin Radiol 18:428, 1967.

369. McDonald CF, Walbaum PR, Sircus W, et al: Intrapleural perforation

of peptic ulcer in association with diaphragmatic hernia. Br J Dis Chest 79:196, 1985.

370. Rotstein OD, Pruett TL, Simmons RL: Gastropleural fistula: Report of three cases and review of the literature. Am J Surg 150:392, 1985.

371. Price BA, Elliott MJ, Featherstone G, et al: Perforation of intrathoracic colon causing acute pneumothorax. Thorax 38:959, 1983.

372. Kazerooni EA, Lim FT, Mikhail A, et al: Risk of pneumothorax in CT-guided transthoracic needle aspiration biopsy of the lung. Radiology 198:371, 1996.

373. Westcott JL, Rao N, Colley DP: Thoracic needle biopsy of small pulmonary nodules. Radiology 202:97, 1997.

374. Anders GT, Johnson JE, Bush BA, et al: Transbronchial biopsy without fluoroscopy: A seven-year perspective. Chest 94:557, 1988.

375. Schmidt G, Börsch G, Wegener M: Subcutaneous emphysema and pneumothorax complicating diagnostic colonoscopy. Dis Colon Rectum 29:136, 1986.

376. Catania S, Boccato P, Bono A, et al: Pneumothorax: A rare complication of fine needle aspiration of the breast. Acta Cytol 33:140, 1989.

377. Maggs PR, Schwaber JR: Fatal bilateral pneumothoraces complicating subclavian vein catheterization. Chest 71:552, 1977.

378. Slezak FA, Williams GB: Delayed pneumothorax: A complication of subclavian vein catheterization. J Parenter Enteral Nutr 8:571, 1984.

379. Sheffner SE, Gross BH, Birnberg FA, et al: Iatrogenic bronchopleural fistula caused by feeding tube insertion. J Can Assoc Radiol 36:52, 1985.

380. Scholten DJ, Wood TL, Thompson DR: Pneumothorax from nasoenteric feeding tube insertion: A report of five cases. Am Surg 52:381, 1986.

381. Padovan IF, Dawson CA, Henschel EO, et al: Pathogenesis of mediastinal emphysema and pneumothorax following tracheotomy (experimental approaches). Chest 66:553, 1974.

382. Biswas C, Jana N, Maitra S: Bilateral pneumothorax following tracheal intubation. Br J Anaesth 62:338, 1989.

383. Honet JE, Honet JC, Cascade P: Pneumothorax after electromyographic electrode insertion in the paracervical muscles: Case report and radiographic analysis. Arch Phys Med Rehabil 67:601, 1986.

384. Ritter HG, Tarala R: Pneumothorax after acupuncture. BMJ 2:602, 1978.

385. Munshi CA, Bardeen-Henschel A: Hydropneumothorax after percutaneous nephrolithotomy. Anesth Analg 64:840, 1985.

386. O'Donnell A, Schoenberger C, Weiner J, et al: Pulmonary complications of percutaneous nephrostomy and kidney stone extraction. South Med J 81:1002, 1988.

387. Odland R, Adams G: Pneumothorax as a complication of tracheoesophageal voice prosthesis use. Ann Otol Rhinol Laryngol 97:537, 1988.

388. Nakamura H, Konishiike J, Sugamura A, et al: Epidemiology of spontaneous pneumothorax in women. Chest 89:378, 1986.

389. Song J-W, Im J-G, Goo JM, et al: Pseudochylous pleural effusion with fat-fluid levels: report of six cases. Radiology 216:478, 2000.

390. Yates DH, Corrin B, Stidolph PN, et al: Malignant mesothelioma in southeast England: Clinicopathological experience of 272 cases. Thorax 52:507, 1997.

CHAPTER 22

Mediastinal Disease

MEDIASTINITIS, PNEUMOMEDIASTINUM, AND MEDIASTINAL HEMORRHAGE

Mediastinitis

Infections of the mediastinum can be acute or chronic. Acute infections usually are caused by bacteria and sometimes progress to abscess formation; they often are associated with signs and symptoms (especially retrosternal pain and fever), and many are fulminating and lethal. By contrast, chronic disease is most often the result of tuberculous or fungal infection; although these characteristically are

682

insidious in onset and unassociated with clinical manifestations, some patients have symptoms or signs related to obstruction or compression of one or more mediastinal structures. In addition to cases of chronic mediastinitis of infectious origin, there is a group of mediastinopathies of unknown cause characterized by the accumulation of dense fibrous tissue, sometimes associated with similar deposits elsewhere in the body (fibrosing mediastinitis).

Acute Mediastinitis

Acute infections of the mediastinum are relatively uncommon. Most infections are associated with esophageal perforation[1, 2] or with esophageal[3] or cardiac[4] surgery; less common causes include direct extension of infection from adjacent tissues, such as the retropharyngeal space;[5] bones and sternoclavicular or costochondral joints;[6] lymph nodes;[8] pericardium, lungs, or pleura;[3, 9] and tracheal or bronchial perforation after intubation, bronchoscopy, or penetrating trauma.[3, 9]

Greater than 75% of cases of esophageal rupture follow diagnostic and therapeutic endoscopic procedures.[10] Such perforation most commonly results from esophagoscopy and balloon dilation.[2, 11] Spontaneous perforation after a sudden rise in intraesophageal pressure (Boerhaave's syndrome) occurs most frequently after episodes of severe vomiting,[2, 12] but this also can develop during labor, a severe asthmatic attack, or strenuous exercise and, rarely, with no apparent cause.[7] Spontaneous rupture of the esophagus is second only to instrumentation as a cause of esophageal perforation.[2, 10] The usual site of rupture is the lower 8 cm, often adjacent to the gastroesophageal junction; typically the tear is vertical and involves the left posterolateral wall.[12, 13] The principal symptom is retrosternal pain, often severe and abrupt in onset; radiation to the neck may occur. Chills and high fever are common, and the effects of obstruction of the superior vena cava may be seen. The prognosis for patients who have acute mediastinitis resulting from esophageal rupture is poor;[24] in one series of 16 patients, 6 (38%) died, all of polymicrobial sepsis.[1]

Radiologic Manifestations

The main radiographic manifestation of acute mediastinitis is widening of the mediastinum, usually more evident superiorly; typically the abnormal region possesses a smooth, sharply defined margin (Fig. 22–1). Air may be visible within the mediastinum as well as in the soft tissues of the neck.[14, 15] Pneumothorax or hydropneumothorax may be evident.[15] In one study of 24 patients, distal esophageal perforation usually resulted in left hydrothorax or hydropneumothorax, whereas midesophageal perforation tended to cause pleural changes on the right.[16] Multiple abscesses may develop.

The diagnosis can be confirmed by showing extravasation of ingested contrast material into the mediastinum or pleural space (Fig. 22–2). Esophagography can be performed safely with barium.[17] Some authors have recommended the use of water-soluble contrast agents in patients who have suspected or known esophageal perforation;[17, 18] however, small leaks may be missed, and aspiration of this material may result in pulmonary edema.[17, 19]

Computed tomography (CT) can be helpful in diagnosis and in guiding percutaneous aspiration and drainage of mediastinal abscesses.[7, 20] Manifestations include esophageal thickening, obliteration of the normal fat planes, periesophageal areas of soft tissue or fluid attenuation, single or multiple abscesses, extraluminal gas, and extraluminal contrast (Fig. 22–3).[21–23] In one series of 12 patients who had esophageal perforation, esophageal thickening was seen on CT scan in 11 patients, extraluminal gas was seen in 11, and pleural effusion was seen in 9;[22] the site of perforation was visible in only 2 patients. Because esophageal thickening, obliteration of fat planes, and small fluid collections often are present after surgery, it may be difficult to distinguish normal postoperative findings from those of early mediastinitis.

Fibrosing Mediastinitis

Fibrosing mediastinitis is a rare condition characterized by chronic inflammation and fibrosis of mediastinal soft tissues. The process often is progressive and can occur either focally or more or less diffusely throughout the mediastinum. It can cause compression and sometimes obliteration of vessels, airways, and esophagus and result in a variety of functional and radiologic manifestations and, occasionally, death.

The cause is probably multifactorial. The most frequently implicated process is infection, of which the most common cause is *Histoplasma capsulatum*.[40] In one review of 33 patients who had fibrosing mediastinitis, a localized pattern of disease was seen in 27 (82%) and a diffuse pattern in 6 (18%).[25] Necrotizing granulomatous inflammation was seen in 10 patients, microorganisms consistent with *H. capsulatum* were identified in 2 patients, and both abnormalities were seen in 2 patients. Nine patients had presumed histoplasmosis based on positive results of serologic or skin tests or on the presence of calcified granulomas or lymph nodes and negative results of skin tests for tuberculosis. Three patients had retroperitoneal fibrosis, a history of methysergide therapy, and orbital pseudotumor, and seven patients had no associated abnormality or evident causative factor.[25] Evidence of histoplasmosis was seen mostly in the patients who had localized disease, whereas the diffuse pattern was usually idiopathic.[25]

In geographic regions in which histoplasmosis is not endemic, tuberculosis is likely to be a more important cause of the disease. In a review of the pathologic files of the Royal Brompton Hospital in London, only 18 cases of fibrosing mediastinitis were identified between 1970 and 1993.[27] Although no organisms or positive cultures were identified in any case, nine patients had a history of tuberculosis; three had previous mediastinal malignancy treated with chemotherapy and radiotherapy; two had autoimmune disease (rheumatoid arthritis in one and systemic lupus erythematosus in the other); one, who had previously lived in the United States, had positive serology for *Histoplasma*; and the remaining three patients had no known predisposing factors.[27]

By definition, idiopathic disease shows no cultural or histologic evidence of an infectious origin. This group can be substantial in size; in one review of 77 patients, an infectious cause was established positively in only 3 (histo-

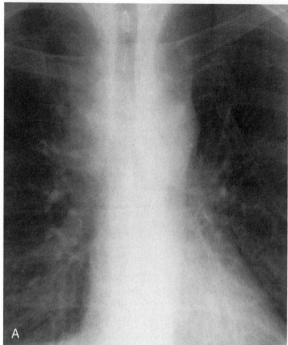

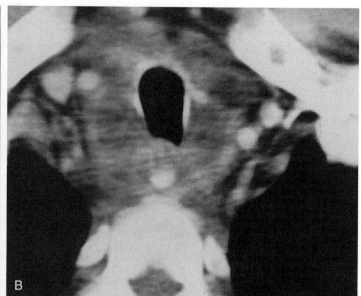

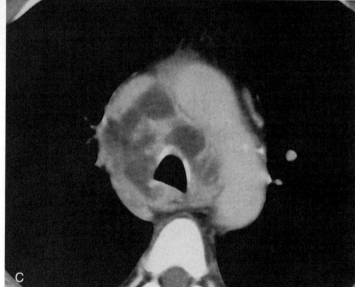

Figure 22–1. Acute Mediastinitis Secondary to Retropharyngeal Abscess. A 47-year-old man presented with acute dysphagia and high fever. Clinical examination showed a retropharyngeal abscess. Close-up view from posteroanterior chest radiograph *(A)* shows smooth widening of the upper mediastinum. Intravenous contrast–enhanced CT scan at the level of the thoracic inlet *(B)* shows inhomogeneous areas of attenuation surrounding the trachea. CT scan at the level of the aortic arch *(C)* shows localized areas of low attenuation consistent with abscess formation anterior and lateral to the trachea.

plasmosis in 2 and tuberculosis in 1).[26] Although some of these cases (perhaps most) may represent the end stage of chronic infection in which the organism is difficult to identify, in others the cause and pathogenesis are undoubtedly noninfectious. Evidence for this supposition derives from the occasional patient in whom a similar fibrotic process can be identified elsewhere,[28] including the retroperitoneal space (retroperitoneal fibrosis), the orbit (pseudotumor of the orbit), the thyroid (Riedel's struma), and the cecum (ligneous perityphlitis).

Symptoms and signs of fibrosing mediastinitis are variable depending on the extent of the fibrosis and the particular structures within the mediastinum that are affected.[40] Involvement of the superior vena cava is probably the most common cause of clinical abnormalities and results in manifestations of the superior vena cava syndrome, including headache; cyanosis; and puffiness of the face, neck, and arms.[26] The severity of these symptoms can lessen with time as collateral venous channels develop.

Radiologic Manifestations

As indicated previously, fibrosing mediastinitis can present as a focal mediastinal soft tissue mass or as diffuse mediastinal widening.[25] Focal lesions involve the right paratracheal region most commonly (Fig. 22–4); less often the left paratracheal, subcarinal, or posterior mediastinal regions are affected.[25, 30, 33] Because most of these lesions are the result of histoplasmosis or tuberculosis, areas of calcification may be evident, particularly on CT scans, on which this feature has been identified in 60% to 90% of cases.[25, 31] In a few patients, parenchymal disease or bronchopulmonary lymph node enlargement suggests a pulmonary origin for the mediastinal disease. The diffuse form of disease results in extensive widening of the mediastinum, most commonly involving its upper portion; the mediastinal outline may be smooth or lobulated.[25, 30] In contrast to the findings reported in patients who have localized disease, calcification is rare in the diffuse form, even when it is associated with histoplasmosis.[25]

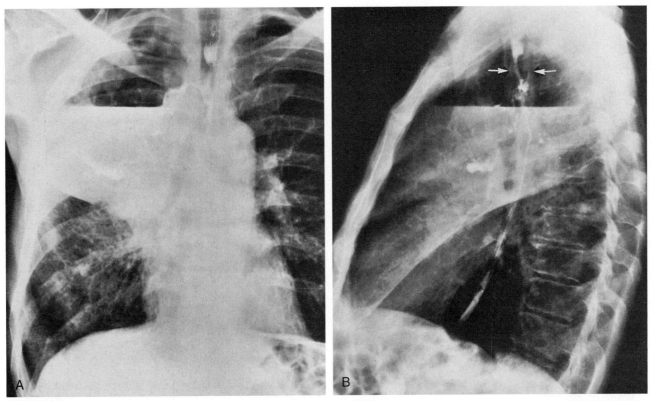

Figure 22–2. Carcinoma of the Esophagus with Perforation into the Right Lung and Abscess Formation. Posteroanterior *(A)* and lateral *(B)* radiographs reveal a large ragged cavity in the upper half of the right lung. Barium administered by mouth shows deformity of the esophageal lumen characteristic of primary carcinoma *(arrows in B)*. Barium has passed from the esophagus into the large lung abscess.

In some cases of focal or diffuse disease, the mediastinal silhouette is normal, and the radiographic manifestations result from narrowing of the trachea or major bronchi, obstruction of pulmonary veins or arteries, or narrowing of the esophagus.[25, 33, 34] In the series of 33 patients cited previously, bronchial narrowing was evident on radiograph or CT scan in 11 (33%), obstruction or narrowing of the superior vena cava in 13 (39%), and narrowing or obstruction of the pulmonary artery in 6 (18%).[25] Bronchial narrowing most commonly affected the right main bronchus,

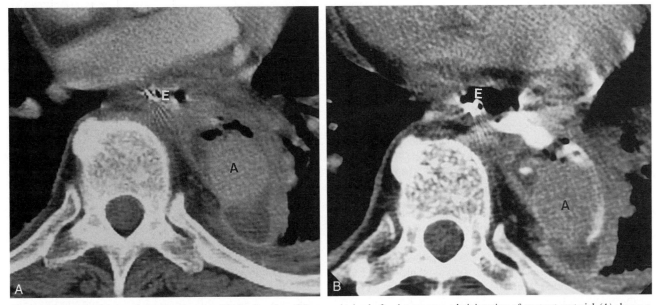

Figure 22–3. Carcinoma of the Esophagus with Perforation. CT scan obtained after intravenous administration of contrast material *(A)* shows a nasogastric tube within the esophagus (E), increased soft tissue between the esophagus and the aorta (A), and localized collections of gas and fluid consistent with abscess formation. A small left pleural effusion also is visible. CT scan obtained after oral administration of contrast material *(B)* shows extravasation of contrast material, confirming the presence of esophageal perforation and communication with the periaortic fluid and air collections.

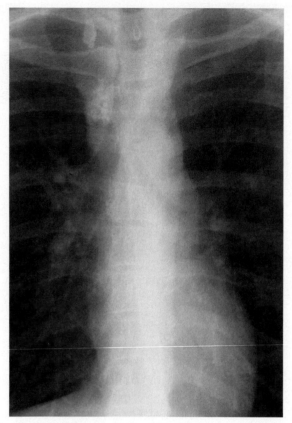

Figure 22–4. Fibrosing Mediastinitis Related to Histoplasmosis. Close-up view of the chest from posteroanterior radiograph shows enlarged and calcified right paratracheal lymph nodes. The patient presented with superior vena cava syndrome. (Courtesy of Dr. Robert Tarver, Indiana University Medical Center, Indianapolis, IN.)

followed in decreasing frequency by the left main bronchus, bronchus intermedius, right upper lobe bronchus, left upper lobe bronchus, and right middle lobe bronchus. Bronchial obstruction frequently was associated with obstructive pneumonitis, atelectasis, or both.

Involvement of the superior vena cava frequently results in a prominent aortic nipple as a result of a dilated left superior intercostal vein.[25] Obstruction or narrowing of a pulmonary artery may result in localized areas of decreased opacification and vascularity, volume loss, or thrombosis.[25, 34] We have seen one patient in whom there was a combination of total occlusion of the left interlobar artery and compression of multiple pulmonary veins leading to interstitial pulmonary edema in all regions except the left lower lobe (Fig. 22–5). Pulmonary infarction is seen occasionally.[29, 35] A case has been described in which fibrosing mediastinitis presented initially as a predominantly posterior mediastinal mass that subsequently extended into continuous lung parenchyma and the retroperitoneal space.[32]

CT is performed almost routinely in the assessment of patients suspected of having fibrosing mediastinitis (Fig. 22–6).[25, 27] CT allows excellent evaluation of the extent of mediastinal soft tissue infiltration and calcification and can identify the degree of narrowing of the tracheobronchial tree. With the use of intravenous contrast material, involvement of the pulmonary arteries, veins, and superior vena cava can be appreciated (Fig. 22–7).[25, 27, 31] In the appropriate clinical context, the presence of a localized mediastinal soft tissue mass with calcification is virtually diagnostic of the disease and obviates the need for tissue sampling.[25, 31] If the mass is not calcified or if there is clinical or radiologic evidence of disease progression, biopsy may be required to exclude a neoplasm.[25] Fibrosing mediastinitis associated with Riedel's struma can be recognized on CT scan by the continuity of fibrous tissue of the thyroid with the mediastinum.[490]

Many other studies may be helpful in selected patients. Esophagography (barium swallow) is indicated for the assessment of esophageal obstruction. Extrinsic compression of the esophagus usually involves its supracarinal portion.[493] In one series of 29 patients, esophageal obstruction was present in 4;[30] in all cases, the radiographic appearance was distinguishable from that of carcinoma by the smooth, tapering, and funnel-shaped upper and lower borders on barium swallow. CT angiography or conventional pulmonary angiography may be performed to assess the extent of pulmonary artery narrowing or the presence of pulmonary venous obstruction.[33] Scintigraphy may show decreased perfusion or, rarely, nonvisualization of one lung.[36]

Magnetic resonance (MR) imaging allows assessment of tracheal or bronchial involvement and vascular involvement; it has the advantage over CT of not requiring the use of intravenous contrast material.[37, 38] On MR studies, fibrosing mediastinitis has heterogeneous signal intensity on T1-weighted images and, because of its fibrous content, low signal intensity on T2-weighted images.[38, 39] Because MR imaging does not allow confident identification of calcification, however, it plays a limited role in diagnostic evaluation.

Pneumomediastinum

Pneumomediastinum (mediastinal emphysema) connotes the presence of gas in the mediastinal space. The gas can originate from five sites: (1) the lung, (2) the mediastinal airways, (3) the esophagus, (4) the neck, and (5) the abdominal cavity.[42]

Lung Parenchyma. The most common pathogenesis is extension of gas from the air spaces of the pulmonary parenchyma into the interstitial tissues and into the mediastinum. In most patients, the initial event probably is related to an incident that causes a sudden increase in alveolar pressure, often accompanied by airway narrowing. This increase in pressure results in rupture of alveoli adjacent to airways or to pulmonary arteries or veins; gas then passes into the perivascular or peribronchial interstitium and tracks through the interstitial tissue to the hilum and the mediastinum.[43, 44]

In addition to tracking proximally into the mediastinum, gas can extend peripherally in the interstitial tissue toward the visceral pleura and rupture into the pleural space to cause pneumothorax. This complication can result directly from rupture of the mediastinal pleura when sufficient gas accumulates in this compartment. Mediastinal gas may track into the neck, subcutaneous tissues, retroperitoneum, and, rarely, peritoneal space[45] or spinal canal.[46, 47]

In some patients, a precipitating event for pneumomediastinum cannot be identified, and the diagnosis is made

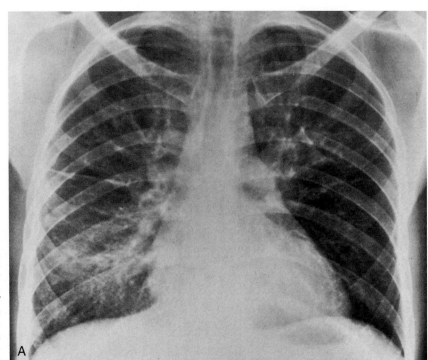

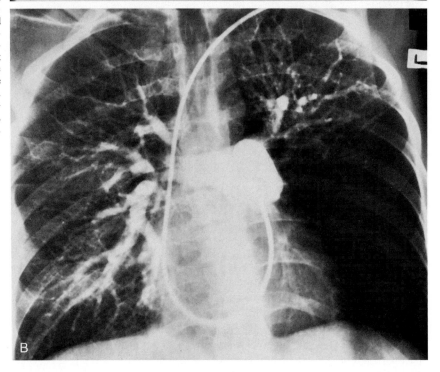

Figure 22–5. Fibrosing Mediastinitis with Encasement of Pulmonary Arteries and Veins. Posteroanterior radiograph *(A)* reveals interstitial edema throughout the right lung and left upper zone. Septal lines are present in the right costophrenic angle. A striking disparity in density of the lower half of the two lungs is observed, the left being radiolucent and oligemic. Pulmonary arteriogram *(B)* shows almost complete occlusion of the left interlobar artery with virtually no perfusion of the left lower lobe and lingula. Although there appears to be good opacification of the arteries of the right lung, the truncus anterior and interlobar arteries show concentric narrowing medial to the hilum. The venous phase of the angiogram is not available, but it is almost certain that the pulmonary veins were affected in the same manner, resulting in venous hypertension and the interstitial edema apparent on plain radiograph. The cause of the fibrosis was *Histoplasma capsulatum* infection. (Courtesy Dr. M. J. Palayew, Jewish General Hospital, Montreal, Quebec, Canada.)

after the discovery of subcutaneous emphysema in the soft tissues of the neck or from a chest radiograph obtained because of retrosternal discomfort.[49] In most patients, however, the development of pneumomediastinum can be related to an incident that results in a sudden rise in alveolar pressure or to a disease process in which such an incident is likely to occur. These include the following:

- Deep respiratory maneuvers, such as those that occur during strenuous exercise[50] or forced vital capacity breaths[51]

- Valsalva maneuvers, such as those that occur during parturition[52]—a particularly common event associated with pneumomediastinum—or weightlifting[53] or during the smoking of marijuana[54] or cocaine[55]
- Asthma, particularly in children[49] but also in adults[56]
- Vomiting of any cause (e.g., diabetic acidosis)[57]
- Mechanical ventilation, particularly in patients who have obstructive pulmonary disease[58] and in patients being maintained on positive end-expiratory pressure,[59] in whom the risk of barotrauma is influenced by the maximal distending pressures, mean airway pressure, duration

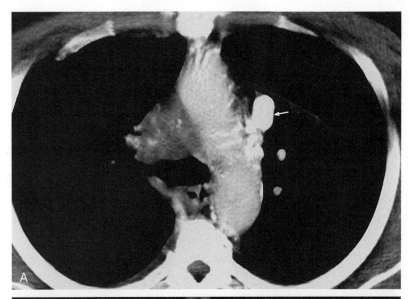

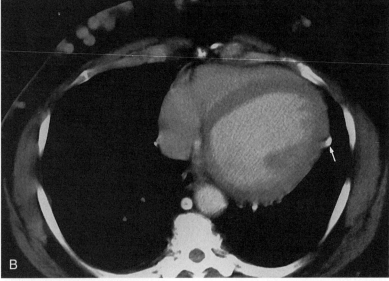

Figure 22–6. Fibrosing Mediastinitis Related to Histoplasmosis. Contrast-enhanced CT scan at the level of the aortic arch *(A)* shows complete obstruction of the superior vena cava and collateral venous circulation through the left superior intercostal vein *(arrow)*. Note foci of calcification within the right paratracheal mass consistent with previous histoplasmosis. Calcified mediastinal lymph nodes were present at several levels. CT scan at a more caudad level *(B)* shows extensive collateral circulation through the left pericardiophrenic vein *(arrow)*, azygos vein, and chest wall veins. (Courtesy of Dr. Robert Tarver, Indiana University Medical Center, Indianapolis, IN.)

of ventilation, tissue fragility, surfactant depletion, secretion retention, and shear forces[60]

- Closed chest trauma, in which shear forces directly disrupt alveolar walls
- A sudden drop in atmospheric pressure, such as occurs during the rapid ascent of a scuba diver or pilot

Mediastinal Airways. Rupture of the trachea or the proximal main bronchi inevitably results in pneumomediastinum. Such rupture most often is caused by trauma, usually accidental but occasionally after diagnostic instrumentation, such as bronchoscopic biopsy.

Esophagus. As discussed previously, rupture of the esophagus occurs most frequently during episodes of severe vomiting[12] but can also develop as a result of trauma or during labor, a severe asthmatic attack, or strenuous exercise.

Neck. Air can track into the mediastinum along deep fascial planes as a result of trauma to the neck or after surgical procedures or dental extraction.[496]

Abdominal Cavity. Pneumomediastinum is caused rarely by extension of gas from below the diaphragm, most often from the retroperitoneal space after perforation of a hollow abdominal viscus.[61]

Clinical Manifestations

Symptoms and signs of pneumomediastinum depend largely on the amount of air in the mediastinal space and on the presence or absence of associated infection. The diagnosis may be suggested by a history of abrupt onset of retrosternal pain radiating to the shoulders and down both arms, usually preceded by an event that resulted in excessive increase in intrathoracic pressure, such as a spasm of coughing, sneezing, or vomiting. The pain usually is aggravated by respiration and sometimes is worsened by swallowing. Dyspnea may be severe. Physical examination generally reveals the presence of air in the subcutaneous tissues of the neck or over the thoracic wall.

Radiologic Manifestations

The radiographic manifestations of pneumomediastinum consist of lucent streaks or focal bubble-like or larger

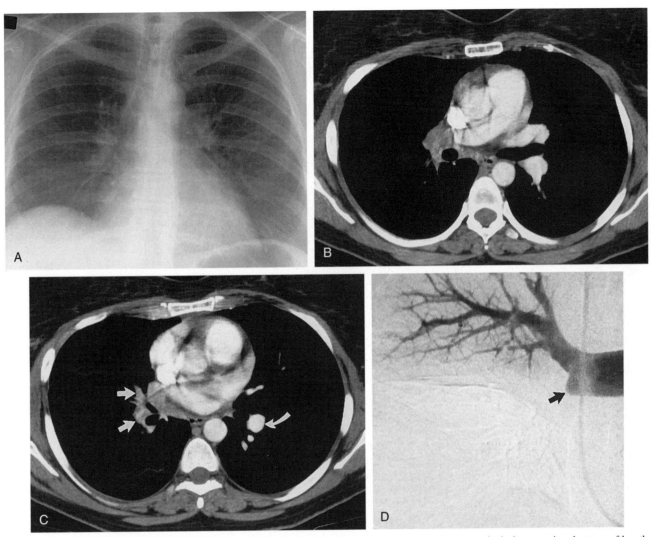

Figure 22–7. Focal Fibrosing Mediastinitis. Posteroanterior chest radiograph *(A)* from a 43-year-old woman who had progressive shortness of breath shows mild enlargement of the right hilum and slightly reduced vascularity of the right lung. Images from CT scans (5-mm collimation) with intravenous contrast enhancement *(B, C)* show a focal soft tissue mass in the right perihilar region resulting in obstruction of the right interlobular pulmonary artery. There is lack of enhancement of the right lower and middle lobe pulmonary arteries *(straight arrows)* compared with the left lower lobe artery *(curved arrow)*, indicating complete vascular occlusion. Selected view of right pulmonary angiogram *(D)* shows complete obstruction of the right interlobar artery *(arrow)* and normal flow to the right upper lobe. The diagnosis of fibrosing mediastinitis was made at thoracotomy. Extensive fibrosis around the hilum and mediastinum precluded surgical treatment. No etiologic agent was identified.

collections of gas outlining the mediastinal structures.[53] In posteroanterior projection, the mediastinal pleura is seen to be displaced laterally, creating a longitudinal line shadow parallel to the heart border and separated from the heart by gas. This shadow usually is more evident on the left side (Fig. 22–8). A longitudinal gas shadow also may be identified adjacent to the thoracic aorta and around the pulmonary artery *(ring-around-the-artery sign)*.[62] A thin line of radiolucency frequently can be identified along the border of the heart and aortic arch. This line should not be confused with pneumomediastinum: The lateral margin of this radiolucency consists of pulmonary parenchyma rather than displaced pleura and represents a Mach band rather than pneumomediastinum.[63]

In some cases, pneumomediastinum is identified more readily on lateral radiograph as lucent streaks that outline the ascending aorta, aortic arch, and pulmonary arteries.[53] Gas may outline the sternal insertions of the diaphragm,

the thymus, and the brachiocephalic veins.[42] Occasionally the only radiographic manifestation consists of substernal gas anterior to the heart, a finding that can be seen only on lateral radiograph.[53]

In some cases, gas from the mediastinum extends between the parietal pleura and the diaphragm or between the parietal pleura and the extrapleural tissues at the lung apex.[41, 53] Although such extrapleural gas can resemble a pneumothorax, it does not shift on radiographs exposed with the patient in different body positions.[53] The pleural line in this situation is not smooth, as in pneumothorax but tends to be irregular as a result of tethering of the parietal pleural by overlying fascia.[53] This tethering is detected more readily on CT scan than on radiograph.[53] When the gas extends between the parietal pleura and the medial portion of the left hemidiaphragm and outlines the descending aorta, it has a configuration that resembles a V—a finding known as the *V sign of Naclerio*.[53, 64]

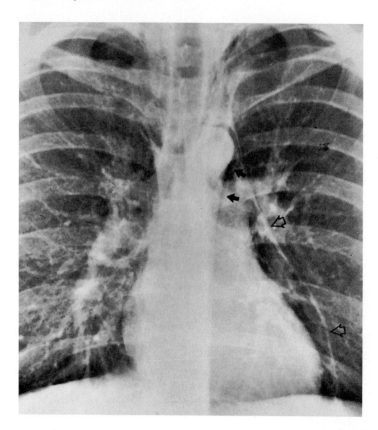

Figure 22–8. Spontaneous Pneumomediastinum. A 20-year-old man noted an abrupt onset of severe retrosternal pain. Posteroanterior chest radiograph shows a long linear opacity roughly paralleling the left heart border *(open arrows)*, representing the laterally displaced mediastinal pleura. Considerable gas is present around the aortic arch and proximal descending thoracic aorta *(solid arrows)*.

When gas becomes interposed between the heart and diaphragm, it permits identification of the central portion of the diaphragm in continuity with the lateral portions, a finding known as the *continuous diaphragm sign* (Fig. 22–9).[65] In theory, gas within the pericardial sac should permit visualization of the central portion of the diaphragm; however, pneumopericardium almost always is associated with pericardial fluid, leading to obliteration of the central portion of the diaphragm, at least on radiographs exposed with the patient in the erect position.[65] When it is not

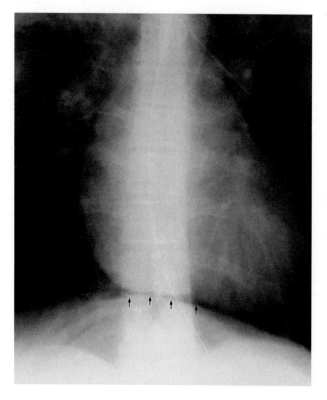

Figure 22–9. Pneumomediastinum with Continuous Diaphragm Sign. Anteroposterior chest radiograph in a 58-year-old woman shows pneumomediastinum outlining the central portion of the diaphragm *(arrows)*, a finding known as the *continuous diaphragm sign.* The pneumomediastinum was secondary to barotrauma related to mechanical ventilation instituted for adult respiratory distress syndrome.

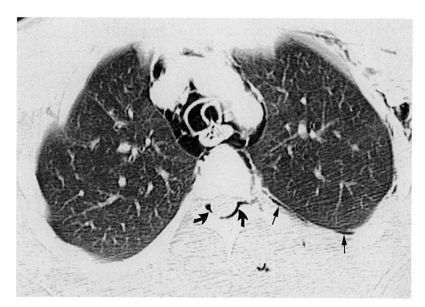

Figure 22–10. Pneumorrhachis Associated with Traumatic Pneumomediastinum. An 18-year-old man developed extensive pneumomediastinum after a snowmobile accident. CT scan shows extrapleural extension *(straight arrows)* of the pneumomediastinum and extension into the spinal canal *(curved arrows)*. Subcutaneous emphysema also is evident.

certain whether a collection of gas is within the pericardial sac or the mediastinal space, differentiation is established by showing a change in the position of the gas in the pericardial sac on radiographs exposed with the patient in different body positions.[66] Occasionally, gas extends from the mediastinum into the extrapleural interstitial tissue in the paravertebral space or into the spinal canal (pneumorachis), leading to spinal epidural emphysema (Fig. 22–10).[67, 68]

Sometimes, air within the interstitial tissues of the lung (interstitial emphysema) can be detected radiographically. Because gas in the interstitial tissues of otherwise normal lung should not be apparent owing to lack of contrast, its identification requires the presence of disease in contiguous parenchyma, a feature of particular note in patients who have adult respiratory distress syndrome. The radiographic findings include focal lucent areas giving a mottled or stippled appearance to the parenchyma, lucent bands, perivascular lucencies, and subpleural and parenchymal cysts.[69] Although these findings often are difficult to identify on radiographs, they can be seen on CT scans.[70] On CT scans, air may be seen to extend along the peribronchovascular interstitium into the mediastinum (Fig. 22–11). Pneumomediastinum resulting from traumatic or spontaneous rupture of the esophagus is associated in many cases with hydrothorax or hydropneumothorax, usually on the left[13] but sometimes bilaterally or on the right.[14]

Mediastinal Hemorrhage

Most cases of mediastinal hemorrhage result from trauma, usually of a severe nature such as that associated with an automobile accident[72] or vigorous cardiopulmonary resuscitation (see Chapter 18). Most bleeding probably originates in veins.[71, 74] Less common causes of mediastinal hemorrhage include perforation of a vein by faulty insertion of a central venous line and migration of a central venous catheter,[10] rupture of an aortic aneurysm,[48] and spontaneous hemorrhage in patients who have mediastinal tumors or a coagulopathy[75] or who are undergoing long-term hemodialysis.[77] Rare causes include a sudden increase in intratho-

racic pressure from sneezing, vomiting, or severe cough;[78, 79] radiation therapy;[76] and intracoronary infusion of streptokinase for coronary thrombosis.[80]

Radiologically, hemorrhage typically results in uniform, symmetric widening of the mediastinum.[81] Local accumulation of blood in the form of a hematoma is manifested by a homogeneous mass that can project to one or both sides of the mediastinum and may be situated in any compartment (Fig. 22–12).[10, 81] Hemorrhage resulting from nontraumatic rupture of the aorta often results in obscuration or a convex appearance of the aortopulmonary window and displacement of the left paraspinal interface.[48] Dissection of blood from the mediastinum in the peribronchovascular interstitial tissue can result in a radiographic pattern that simulates interstitial edema.[82] When mediastinal hemorrhage is caused by a ruptured aorta, the blood may extend into a pleural space, usually the left only but sometimes the right as well.[73, 83]

CT is superior to plain radiography in showing the presence of mediastinal hemorrhage and the underlying cause.[72–74] Approximately 90% of acute hematomas are associated with localized areas of high attenuation as a result of the high attenuation of clotted blood (Fig. 22–13).[84, 85] These areas persist for about 72 hours; the high attenuation then decreases gradually to values similar to those for fluid secondary to lysis of the hemoglobin.[85]

MEDIASTINAL MASSES

A wide variety of lesions can present as a localized tumor or mass in the mediastinum.[86, 87] Because many of these arise in a specific tissue or structure that is situated in a particular site within the mediastinum, it is logical to classify these lesions on the basis of their anatomic location. One of the most widely used of such classification schemes divides the mediastinum into three compartments: (1) an *anterior* compartment, comprising the tissues in front of the heart, aorta, and brachiocephalic vessels, including the thymus, adipose tissue, and lymph nodes; (2) a *middle* mediastinal compartment, comprising the heart, pericardium, all the major vessels leaving and entering

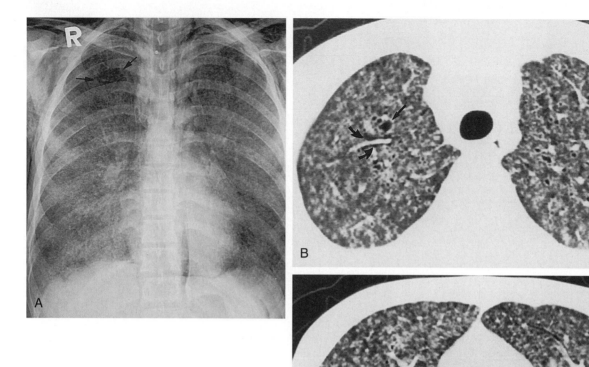

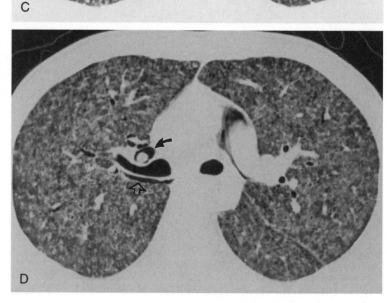

Figure 22–11. Interstitial Emphysema and Pneumomediastinum in Miliary Tuberculosis. Anteroposterior chest radiograph *(A)* in a 21-year-old man who had miliary tuberculosis shows focal lucencies in the right upper lobe *(arrows)*, pneumomediastinum, and subcutaneous emphysema. HRCT scan in the region of the apical segment of the right upper lobe *(B)* shows focal lucency *(straight arrow)* and perivascular dissection of gas *(curved arrows)*. HRCT scan at a more caudad level *(C)* shows perivascular gas *(curved arrows)* and pneumomediastinum. HRCT scan at the level of the right upper lobe bronchus *(D)* shows peribronchial *(open arrow)* and perivascular gas *(curved arrow)* and pneumomediastinum. (Courtesy of Dr. Kun-Il Kim, Pusan National University Hospital, Pusan, Korea.)

this organ, trachea and main bronchi, paratracheal and tracheobronchial lymph nodes, phrenic nerves, and upper portions of the vagus nerves; and (3) a *posterior* compartment, comprising the descending thoracic aorta, esophagus, thoracic duct, lower portion of the vagus nerves, posterior group of mediastinal lymph nodes, and (usually) the para-

vertebral tissue between the anterior vertebral bodies and the chest wall.

There are many practical and conceptual difficulties with this division, including the following: (1) The tissue adjacent to the vertebral bodies is not in the mediastinum; (2) the distinction between the middle and the posterior

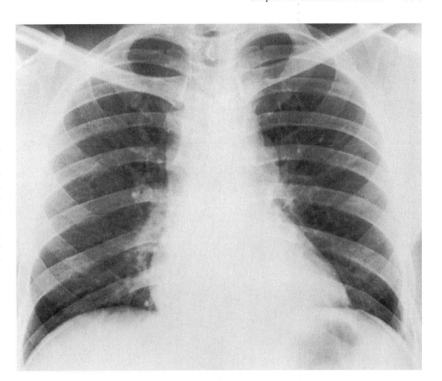

Figure 22–12. Spontaneous Mediastinal Hemorrhage. A 35-year-old hemophiliac was admitted to the hospital with evidence of recent extrathoracic hemorrhage. He had no symptoms referable to the thorax. Posteroanterior radiograph shows bilateral widening of the mediastinum by a process whose lateral margins are lobulated. Involvement appears to be chiefly of the middle mediastinal compartment. (Lateral radiograph was not helpful in localizing the abnormality.) The lesion resolved completely in 10 days without residua and was assumed to represent a spontaneous hematoma.

mediastinal compartments is artificial because it is often difficult to decide whether a lesion is in one or the other, and because many masses actually affect both compartments; (3) the anterior margin of the brachiocephalic vessels and ascending aorta often is difficult to identify on chest radiograph;[88] and (4) anterior mediastinal masses often project over the heart.[89] For these reasons, we prefer to consider the various masses that affect these anatomic regions in the following three groups: (1) the *anterior mediastinum*, when a mass is situated predominantly in the region in front of a line drawn along the anterior border of the trachea and the posterior border of the heart (Fig. 22–14);[89] (2) the *middle-posterior mediastinum*, when a mass is located predominantly between this line and the

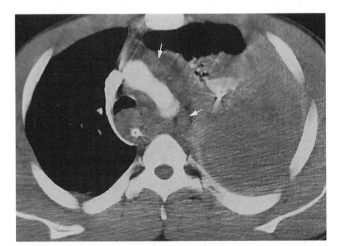

Figure 22–13. Acute Mediastinal Hemorrhage. Contrast-enhanced CT scan in a 30-year-old man shows inhomogeneous areas of increased attenuation *(arrows)* in the mediastinum as a result of hemorrhage. A large left hemothorax with shift of the mediastinum to the right also is evident. A left chest tube is in place. The findings were related to traumatic tear of the aorta after a motor vehicle accident.

anterior aspect of the vertebral bodies; and (3) the *paravertebral region*, when a mass is situated predominantly in the potential space adjacent to a vertebral body.

Overlap is bound to occur; all that this classification implies is that a lesion is present *predominantly* in one or another compartment. Aortic aneurysms may be situated in any of the three compartments, as may certain neoplasms, such as leiomyoma and neurofibroma; in addition, lymph node enlargement in lymphoma occurs almost as frequently in the anterior as in the middle-posterior compartment, although it is most likely to be massive at the former site. Such overlap is inevitable because the anatomic structures in which many masses arise are situated in more than one compartment. Nevertheless, separation into these three groups is helpful in suggesting a diagnosis of many mediastinal and paravertebral tumors, particularly if this information is combined with a knowledge of the patient's clinical manifestations and the radiologic characteristics of the mass.

Most mediastinal abnormalities initially are suspected after chest radiography; the need for further investigation and the optimal imaging modality or other test by which it should be conducted are dictated largely by the tentative diagnosis made on this examination. CT and MR imaging allow visualization of the exact location of the lesions and, in some cases, identification of the structures from which they arise; one or both of these techniques are indicated in almost all cases. Because of their anatomic precision, it is preferable to describe the exact location of a lesion in relation to the adjacent mediastinal structures with both of these techniques, rather than limiting the description to a particular mediastinal compartment.

MASSES SITUATED PREDOMINANTLY IN THE ANTERIOR MEDIASTINAL COMPARTMENT

The anterior mediastinum is the site of most clinically important primary mediastinal masses, including thymoma

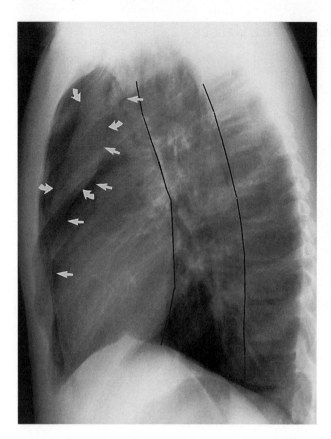

Figure 22–14. Mediastinal Compartments. The presence of a pneumomediastinum in this patient allows identification of the anterior border of the heart, ascending aorta, and brachiocephalic vessels *(straight arrows)*. The anatomic anterior mediastinum is composed of the tissue anterior to these structures and includes the thymus *(curved arrows)*, adipose tissue, and lymph nodes. Normally the anterior margins of the ascending aorta and brachiocephalic vessels are difficult to visualize. Anterior mediastinal masses often project over the heart. On lateral chest radiograph, a mass can be considered probably to lie in the anterior mediastinum if it is situated predominantly in the region in front of a line drawn along the anterior border of the trachea and the posterior border of the heart. A mass probably lies in the middle-posterior mediastinum if it is situated between this line and a line drawn along the anterior aspect of the vertebral bodies. Extrapulmonary masses located posterior to this line lie outside of the mediastinum and should be considered paravertebral in location.

and a variety of other thymic abnormalities, lymphoma, germ cell tumors, and hyperplastic and neoplastic abnormalities of thyroid and ectopic parathyroid tissue (Table 22–1). Abnormalities involving the ascending aorta can mimic an anterior mediastinal mass.

Tumors and Tumor-Like Conditions of the Thymus

Thymic Hyperplasia

True thymic hyperplasia, as opposed to lymphoid hyperplasia that is associated with myasthenia gravis (*see* farther on), is an increase in the size of the thymus gland associated with a more or less normal gross architecture and histologic appearance.[92, 93] The pathogenesis is variable. Most commonly, it appears to be a rebound phenomenon secondary to atrophy caused by chemotherapy for malignancy (usually lymphoma or a germ cell tumor[94, 96]) or by hypercortisolism;[97] a similar process has been reported after treatment of Cushing's syndrome.[99] Such rebound enlargement is common; in one CT study of 120 patients treated for testicular carcinoma, evidence of thymic enlargement was found in 14 (12%) after therapy.[95] In another investigation in which serial CT scans were performed in 20 patients who were 2 to 35 years of age and who had various malignancies, the thymic volume decreased an average of 43% after chemotherapy.[101] On further follow-up, rebound hyperplasia occurred in 25% of patients, the volume of the thymus exceeding the baseline volume by 50% (Fig. 22–15).[101] For unexplained reasons, some cases of hyperplasia have been found in association with testicular carcinoma before the induction of chemotherapy.[102] A second

relatively common group of patients with thymic hyperplasia has hyperthyroidism (Graves' disease);[104, 105] rare cases of hyperplasia associated with Hodgkin's disease also have been reported.[106]

Thymic hyperplasia seldom is apparent on chest radiograph in adults.[107] On CT, the most helpful measurement for determining an increase in the size of the thymus is its thickness (Fig. 22–16):[108, 109] The maximal normal thickness in individuals younger than 20 years old is 1.8 cm;[108] in individuals older than 20, it is 1.3 cm. Measurements greater than these are consistent with hyperplasia. In patients who have Hodgkin's disease or non-Hodgkin's lymphoma, rebound thymic hyperplasia must be distinguished from residual or recurrent tumor.[104] Although this distinction cannot be made reliably by CT or MR imaging, it is often possible using gallium scintigraphy,[110, 111] with gallium uptake being seen in residual tumor but not in fibrotic or necrotic tissue. Although such increased uptake is relatively common in children who have rebound thymic hyperplasia,[110, 111] it is rare in adults.[112]

Thymic Lymphoid Hyperplasia

The term *thymic hyperplasia* has been used to describe a distinctive histologic reaction in the thymus of patients who have myasthenia gravis. In approximately two thirds of individuals with the latter condition, the thymic cortex is the site of multiple well-defined lymphoid follicles, many containing germinal centers. Because the weight of the thymus gland in these cases usually is within normal limits,[103, 113] the designation *thymic hyperplasia* is, strictly speaking, incorrect; it has been suggested that the terms

Table 22–1. ANTERIOR MEDIASTINAL MASSES

Etiology	Radiographic Manifestations	CT Findings
Developmental		
Mesothelial cyst (pericardial and pleuropericardial cysts)	Usually round, oval, or "tear-drop" in appearance. Smooth margins	Usually of homogeneous water density
Neoplastic		
Tumors of the thymus		
Thymolipoma	Smooth or lobulated contour	Pliable mass of predominantly fat attenuation originating from thymus
Thymic cysts	Smooth contour	Homogeneous water density
Thymoma	Smooth or lobulated; well-defined contour	Homogeneous or heterogeneous attenuation; can contain cystic areas and calcification
Thymic carcinoma	Irregular, poorly defined margins	Homogeneous or heterogeneous attenuation: frequent invasion of adjacent structures
Germ cell neoplasms	Smooth or lobulated contour. Calcification, bone, teeth, or fat may be identified in teratomas	Mature cystic teratomas often contain areas of fat attenuation and may contain fluid and foci of calcification; malignant germ cell tumors may have homogeneous or heterogeneous soft tissue attenuation
Thyroid goiter and tumors	Smooth or lobulated contour. Extend above thoracic inlet. Calcification fairly common	Lesion can be seen to arise from thyroid gland; goiters typically have high attenuation and marked enhancement with intraveous contrast material; neoplasms may have homogeneous or heterogeneous soft tissue attenuation
Hodgkin's disease and non-Hodgkin's lymphoma	Symmetrically widened mediastinum, lobulated contour	Mediastinal lymph node enlargement; may have homogeneous or heterogeneous attenuation and contain cystic areas
Metastatic carcinoma	Lobulated paratracheal or hilar lymph node enlargement common	Mediastinal lymph node enlargement
Cardiovascular		
Aortic aneurysm	Fusiform or saccular contour. Calcification may be present in wall	CT and MR imaging are diagnostic
Traumatic		
Mediastinal hemorrhage or hematoma	May be local or diffuse, commonly in upper mediastinum	Contrast-enhanced CT diagnostic for aortic dissection; angiography may be required to diagnose traumatic tear of the aorta or great vessels
Miscellaneous causes		
Herniation through foramen of Morgagni	Round or oval; usually to right of pericardium	CT diagnostic; shows discontinuity of the diaphragm and herniation of omental fat and, less commonly, colon

lymphoid or *follicular* hyperplasia might be more appropriate to describe the abnormality.[103]

Thymic lymphoid hyperplasia seldom leads to radiographically apparent abnormalities.[98, 107] Although it may be associated with a normal-appearing thymus on CT scan, a diffusely enlarged thymus (Fig. 22–17) or a focal mass is common.[109] In a retrospective study of 45 patients who had myasthenia gravis, 22 had histologically proven lymphoid hyperplasia.[109] On CT, 10 (45%) of the 22 patients had a normal-appearing thymus, 7 (32%) had a diffusely enlarged thymus, and 5 (23%) had a focal mass. All 7 patients who had a diffusely enlarged thymus had lymphoid hyperplasia; of the 26 patients who had a normal-appearing thymus, 10 (38%) had lymphoid hyperplasia, and 16 (62%) had normal histologic findings. Of 12 patients who had a focal mass, 5 (42%) had lymphoid hyperplasia, and 7 (58%) had thymoma.[109] These findings, which have been replicated by other investigators,[115, 116] indicate the limitations of CT in the diagnosis of thymic lymphoid hyperplasia. MR imaging is also of limited value in diagnosis.[115]

Thymolipoma

Thymolipomas are uncommon anterior mediastinal tumors consisting of an admixture of fat and thymic epithelial and lymphoid tissue. By 1990, approximately 90 cases had been reported;[118] in a review from the Armed Forces Institute of Pathology in 1995, an additional 33 cases were documented.[119] The tumors characteristically cause few or no symptoms even when large; the lesion usually is discovered on a screening radiograph. The behavior is typically benign.

The characteristic radiographic appearance consists of an anterior mediastinal mass that droops into the lower chest (Fig. 22–18);[86, 117, 120] extension into one or both hemithoraces may be seen. The tumor typically conforms to the adjacent structures and may mimic cardiomegaly or elevation of one or both hemidiaphragms.[100, 117, 120] When small, it is round or oval in shape, mimicking other mediastinal masses.[117] In a review of the radiographic manifestations in 27 patients, 14 masses occupied the entire anteroposterior diameter of the chest;[120] in 14, the low density of the tumor could be appreciated on radiograph, and in 7, a change of shape or position of the mass was seen when the patient assumed a decubitus position.

CT scans characteristically show predominant fat attenuation or equivalent fat and soft tissue attenuation (Fig. 22–19).[120] The soft tissue may appear as linear whorls intermixed with fat or, less commonly, as small rounded opacities embedded within it.[121, 122] The mass often can be seen to be connected to the thymus. MR imaging shows high signal intensity on T1-weighted spin-echo images as a result of fat and areas of intermediate signal intensity related to soft tissue.[120, 123, 124] The characteristic features of thymolipoma on radiograph and CT allow distinction from other mediastinal masses in most cases. In one study of 128 patients who had anterior mediastinal masses, three of which were thymolipomas, two independent observers made a correct first-choice diagnosis of thymolipoma based

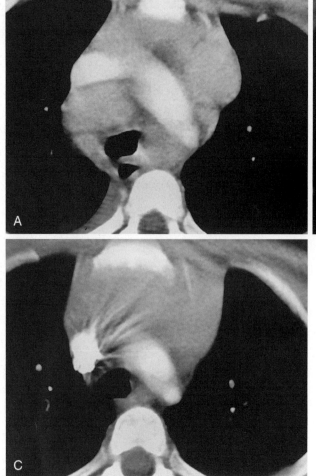

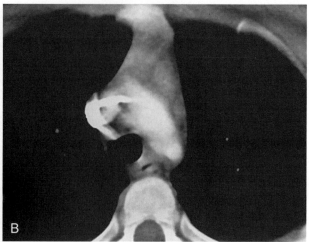

Figure 22–15. Thymic Rebound: Hyperplasia. Contrast-enhanced CT scan in a 9-year-old child *(A)* shows extensive mediastinal lymphadenopathy (proved to be due to Hodgkin's disease). The patient underwent successful treatment. CT scan performed 6 months later *(B)* shows a small residual thymus. CT scan performed 1 year after the initial scan *(C)* shows a significant increase in thymic size, representing *rebound* hyperplasia. There was no evidence of tumor recurrence. (Courtesy of Dr. Ella Kazerooni, Department of Radiology, University of Michigan Hospital, Ann Arbor, MI.)

on chest radiographic findings in two cases and on CT in all three.[125]

Thymic Cysts

Thymic cysts are uncommon mediastinal lesions that account for only 1% to 2% of all tumors in the anterior

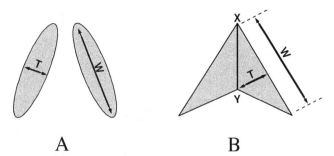

Figure 22–16. Measurement of Thymic Size on CT. The two thymic lobes are measured separately. The width (W) corresponds to the long axis of the lobe as seen on the transverse CT image, and the thickness (T) corresponds to the short-axis diameter *(A)*. When the two lobes are confluent, the thymus has a triangular or arrowhead shape *(B)*. The thymus is divided in half by a line through the anterior apex of the gland and perpendicular to it (X-Y). The width (W) and thickness (T) of each lobe then are measured. (Measurement described by Baron RL, et al: Radiology 142:121, 1982.)

compartment.[126, 127] Most probably are derived from remnants of the fetal thymopharyngeal duct. Occasional cysts have been reported after thoracic surgery[129] or chemotherapy for a malignant neoplasm,[130] suggesting a relationship to trauma or to drug-related involution of the thymus gland. An association with human immunodeficiency virus (HIV) infection also has been documented in some cases.[131, 132] Pathologically the cysts are unilocular or multilocular and range in size from microscopic to 18 cm in maximal diameter.[128] Most patients are asymptomatic.

The appearance on chest radiograph consists of a smoothly marginated anterior mediastinal mass.[86, 133] When large, the cyst may obscure the margins of the adjacent structures and simulate cardiomegaly (Fig. 22–20). On CT, cysts typically have water density (0 HU) and thin walls.[133] Occasionally, soft tissue septa, ringlike calcifications, or foci of linear calcification in the cyst wall are seen, presumably as a result of previous hemorrhage.[90, 133] Bleeding into the cyst may be manifested by a density measurement greater than water.[133] Thymic cysts have low signal intensity on T1-weighted MR images and high signal intensity on T2-weighted images.[124] Hemorrhage results in increased signal on T1-weighted images as a result of the T1 shortening effect of methemoglobin.[133] Cysts that develop after radiation or chemotherapy usually have a predominant soft tissue component; occasionally, however, they may resemble congenital cysts.[133]

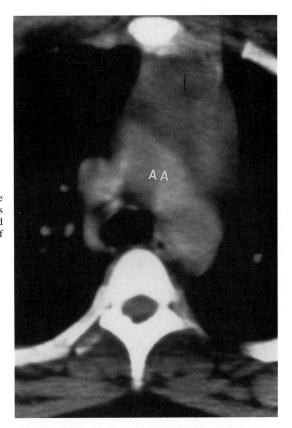

Figure 22–17. Thymic Lymphoid Hyperplasia. Contrast-enhanced CT scan at the level of the aortic arch (AA) in a 29-year-old woman who had myasthenia gravis shows a diffusely enlarged thymus. Diffuse lymphoid follicular hyperplasia was proved surgically. (Courtesy of Dr. Ella Kazerooni, Department of Radiology, University of Michigan Hospital, Ann Arbor, MI.)

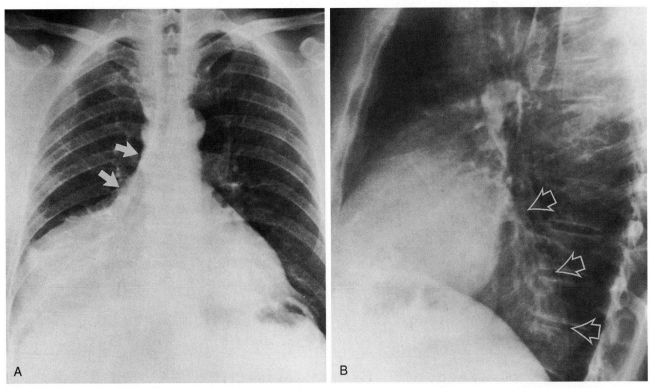

Figure 22–18. Thymolipoma. Posteroanterior *(A)* and lateral *(B)* radiographs show a large mass situated in the lower half of the right hemithorax. The obtuse angle the mass creates with the mediastinum *(arrows* in *A)* indicates its origin from that structure. In lateral projection, the mass extends almost the whole anteroposterior depth of the thorax, obscuring most of the right hemidiaphragm (the posterior margin of the mass is indicated by *open arrows* in *B).* The anterior mediastinum looks *empty.* (Courtesy of Dr. R. Hedvigi, Montreal Chest Institute.)

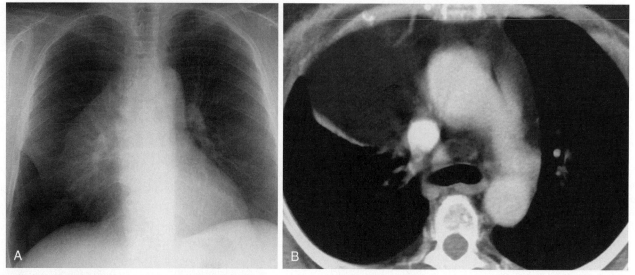

Figure 22–19. Thymolipoma. Posteroanterior chest radiograph *(A)* in a 61-year-old woman shows a mediastinal mass that has lower density than the adjacent soft tissues, consistent with fat. Contrast-enhanced CT scan *(B)* shows that the mass lies in the region of the right lobe of the thymus and that it is made up almost exclusively of fat. The findings are characteristic of thymolipoma. (Courtesy of Dr. Ella Kazerooni, Department of Radiology, University of Michigan Hospital, Ann Arbor, MI.)

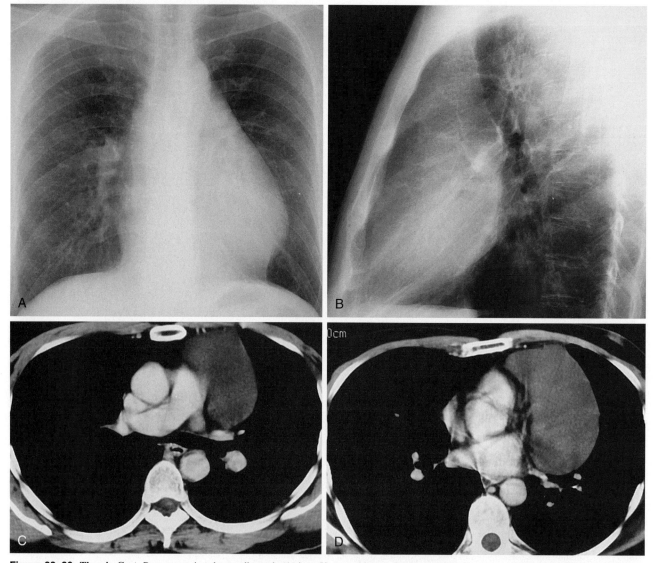

Figure 22–20. Thymic Cyst. Posteroanterior chest radiograph *(A)* in a 53-year-old man shows an unusual contour of the mediastinum and apparent cardiomegaly. Lateral radiograph *(B)* shows poorly defined increased opacity in the anterior mediastinum and normal heart size. Contrast-enhanced CT scans *(C* and *D)* show a thin-walled, fluid-filled cyst. The presence of a thymic cyst was confirmed surgically.

Thymoma

Thymomas are neoplasms of thymic epithelium that characteristically consist of uniform cells with a variable amount of admixed lymphocytes; although cytologically bland, they can behave in either a benign or a malignant fashion. Thymic epithelial neoplasms composed of cells that have significant cytologic atypia and a high mitotic rate are more appropriately termed *thymic carcinoma* and are discussed separately (*see* farther on).

Thymoma is the most common primary neoplasm to affect the anterior mediastinum; it constitutes approximately 20% of all mediastinal tumors.[134] Most are discovered in middle-aged adults; the average age at diagnosis is 45 to 50 years.[135, 136] Most patients manifest symptoms related to local compression or invasion of thoracic structures or to systemic paraneoplastic disease. The effects of local compression or invasion are seen in about one third of patients, the most frequent being chest pain, shortness of breath, dysphagia, and cough;[136] hoarseness, evidence of pericarditis (rarely, with cardiac tamponade),[156, 157] and the superior vena cava syndrome[158] (sometimes with intravascular tumor extension[159]) can be seen.

Myasthenia gravis is the most common paraneoplastic disease associated with thymoma. Approximately 10% to 15% of patients who have myasthenia have the tumor,[136] and about 35% to 40% of all patients who have thymoma have myasthenia.[136–138]

A variety of hematologic abnormalities are associated with thymoma. Pure red blood cell aplasia (hypoplasia) is probably the most common;[161] of all patients who have this disorder, approximately 10% to 15% have a thymoma.[114] Other hematologic conditions associated with thymoma—at least some of which probably represent paraneoplastic phenomena—include aplastic anemia,[163] agranulocytosis,[164] cryoglobulinemia,[165] hypogammaglobulinemia[166] (sometimes associated with persistent candidiasis),[160] hypergammaglobulinemia,[162] T-cell lymphocytosis,[167] and leukemia.[168]

Most thymomas are slow-growing, encapsulated neoplasms whose excision results in cure; however, some are locally aggressive tumors that are unresectable or that recur after apparent complete excision. Recurrence or local invasion at the time of initial diagnosis occurs most commonly in the anterior mediastinal soft tissue, pericardium, or pleura. The most common sites of metastasis are the lung; pleura; thoracic skeleton; and mediastinal, supraclavicular, or cervical lymph nodes. Extrathoracic metastases are uncommon.[169] There is little question that the best predictor of a malignant or benign behavior (apart from metastasis) is the presence or absence of local invasion, a finding that usually is established by the surgeon at the time of thoracotomy.

Radiologic Manifestations

Most thymomas are situated near the junction of the heart and great vessels. Radiographically, they are round or oval in shape, and their margins are usually smooth or lobulated (Fig. 22–21).[86, 139] They can protrude to one or both sides of the mediastinum and can displace the heart and great vessels posteriorly. In some cases, calcification is apparent at the periphery of the lesion or throughout its substance (Fig. 22–22).[139] Occasionally a tumor simulates cardiac enlargement[133, 139] or is located in an unusual site, such as the cardiophrenic angle[139] or posterior mediastinum.[139, 140] The radiographic appearances of invasive and noninvasive tumors usually are indistinguishable.[139] Sometimes an invasive tumor spreads to the pleural space and leads to focal or diffuse pleural thickening.[139, 142] Such pleural involvement usually is unilateral; when extensive, it may mimic malignant mesothelioma (Fig. 22–23).[139, 141]

Several investigators have shown that CT is superior to chest radiography in diagnosis and assessment of tumor extent.[143–145] With this procedure, most thymomas present as round or oval soft tissue masses that have sharply demarcated margins. Typically, they are located in the region of the thymus anterior to the aortic root and main pulmonary artery and project to one side of the mediastinum (*see* Fig. 22–21).[86, 109, 139, 142] Tumors usually have homogeneous attenuation; less commonly and usually in large tumors, the presence of hemorrhage, necrosis, or cyst formation leads to focal areas of low attenuation.[86, 133, 139] Rarely, such areas are the predominant feature.[125, 139] Foci of calcification may be seen in the capsule or throughout the tumor (*see* Fig. 22–22).[133, 139]

CT does not allow reliable distinction of invasive from noninvasive thymoma. Although preservation of fat planes between the tumor and adjacent structures is most suggestive of a noninvasive tumor, limited invasion cannot be excluded.[86, 139] Similarly, although obliteration of the fat planes is suggestive of invasion (Fig. 22–24), this may be seen with noninvasive tumors.[142, 146] In one investigation of 15 thymomas, partial obliteration of fat planes was present in 8 invasive tumors and 7 noninvasive ones;[116] it was also evident in one thymic cyst. Despite these observations, certain findings on CT are highly suggestive of tumor invasion, including complete obliteration of fat planes,[116] pericardial thickening,[146] encasement of mediastinal vessels,[86, 139] an irregular interface with the adjacent lung,[139, 147] and focal or diffuse pleural thickening.[139, 146, 148] Pleural implants, when present, usually are unilateral and result in focal or diffuse thickening; associated effusions are uncommon.[86, 149] Because invasive thymomas can extend into the posterior mediastinum, retrocrural space, and retroperitoneum,[139, 147, 150] CT performed for assessment of thymoma should include the upper abdomen.

Thymomas have intermediate signal intensity (equal to that of skeletal muscle) on T1-weighted MR images and increased signal intensity (approaching that of fat) on T2-weighted images (*see* Fig. 22–24).[120, 139, 151] The capsule has low signal intensity. Cystic regions and areas of hemorrhage have low signal intensity on T1-weighted images and high signal intensity on T2-weighted images.[86, 139] Inhomogeneous areas of signal intensity on T2-weighted images are seen more commonly in invasive than in noninvasive tumors. In one investigation of 12 invasive thymomas, 11 showed this feature compared with none of five benign tumors;[151] 6 of the invasive thymomas had a lobulated internal architecture on T2-weighted images, internal lobules being separated by low-intensity septations.

Because of the relatively high prevalence of abnormalities in the thymus,[109, 152] CT is indicated in the investigation of patients who have myasthenia gravis.[109, 154, 155] In one

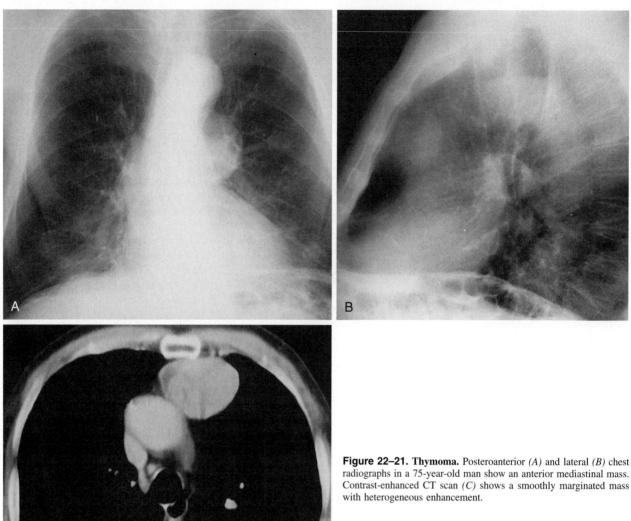

Figure 22–21. Thymoma. Posteroanterior *(A)* and lateral *(B)* chest radiographs in a 75-year-old man show an anterior mediastinal mass. Contrast-enhanced CT scan *(C)* shows a smoothly marginated mass with heterogeneous enhancement.

study of 57 patients who had this disorder, chest radiographs and CT scans were correlated with pathologic findings after thymectomy;[153] 14 of 16 cases of thymoma were either suspected or definitely diagnosed on CT. In another investigation of 19 patients who had myasthenia gravis and who underwent thymectomy, CT was accurate in detecting the nine thymic masses;[154] however, it could not distinguish thymomas from nonthymomatous masses, including cysts.

In an investigation of 45 patients who had myasthenia gravis and who underwent thymectomy, 26 had normal CT findings, 7 had a diffusely enlarged thymus, and 12 had a focal mass.[109] Pathologic assessment showed that 16 of 26 patients who had normal CT findings had normal thymic tissue, and 10 had lymphoid hyperplasia; all 7 patients who had a diffusely enlarged thymus had lymphoid hyperplasia. Five of 12 patients who had a focal mass at CT had lymphoid hyperplasia, and 7 had thymoma. On the basis

of these results, one can conclude that the presence of a diffusely enlarged thymus or a focal mass on CT scan in a patient who has myasthenia gravis indicates the presence of an abnormality, either lymphoid hyperplasia or thymoma; however, CT is of limited value in distinguishing lymphoid hyperplasia from a normal thymus or from thymoma.[109]

Thymic Carcinoma

The nosology of malignant thymic epithelial tumors is confusing. As discussed in the previous section, some thymomas that show histologic features suggestive of a benign neoplasm invade adjacent mediastinal tissues and lung and occasionally metastasize. Although this behavior indicates that such tumors are malignant and might be called carcinomas, the term *carcinoma* usually is reserved for neoplasms that possess the traditional histologic and

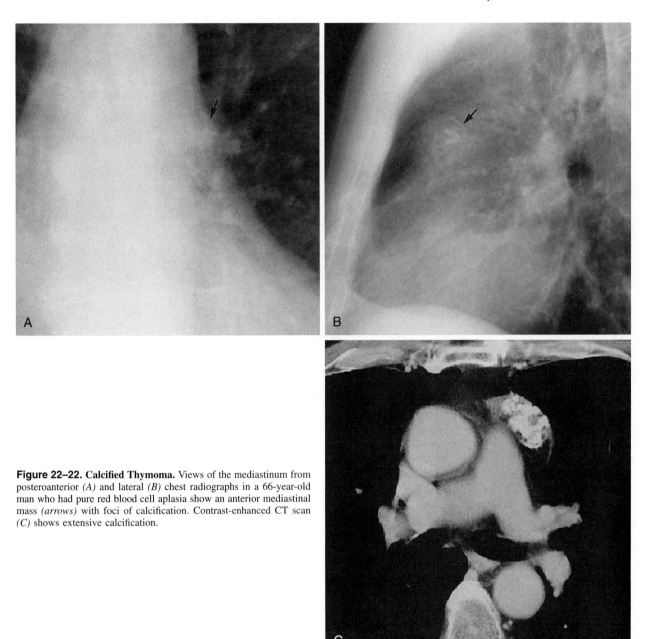

Figure 22–22. Calcified Thymoma. Views of the mediastinum from posteroanterior *(A)* and lateral *(B)* chest radiographs in a 66-year-old man who had pure red blood cell aplasia show an anterior mediastinal mass *(arrows)* with foci of calcification. Contrast-enhanced CT scan *(C)* shows extensive calcification.

cytologic features of malignancy, such as nuclear atypia, significant mitotic activity, and necrosis.[170] A wide variety of histologic patterns has been reported, the most common being squamous cell carcinoma (some well differentiated and others resembling lymphoepithelioma of the nasopharynx).

Similar to thymoma, well-differentiated thymic carcinoma has been found to occur predominantly in adults (the average age in one series was 50 years[171]). Clinically, most patients are symptomatic at the time of diagnosis, the most common complaints being chest pain and cough; systemic findings, such as fever, weight loss, fatigue, and night sweats, are common.[174] Compared with thymoma, the presence of a paraneoplastic syndrome is uncommon;[172, 175, 176] an association with myasthenia gravis was identified in only four cases in one report published in 1993.[177] Rare

cases have been associated with hypercalcemia[178] and hypertrophic osteoarthropathy.[179]

Radiologically, thymic carcinomas usually present as large anterior mediastinal masses that have lobulated or poorly defined margins (Fig. 22–25).[86, 125, 148] On CT, they can have homogeneous soft tissue attenuation or heterogeneous attenuation as a result of necrosis; foci of calcification are present in 10% to 40% of cases.[148, 177] Focal or diffuse obliteration of the adjacent fat planes and evidence of extension into the pericardium or pleura are present in most.[148, 173] Although local pleural extension and associated effusion are common, distal pleural implants seldom are seen.[148] Mediastinal lymphadenopathy is present in 40% of cases.[148, 173] Invasion of the great vessels, lymph node enlargement, extrathymic metastases, and phrenic nerve palsy are seen more commonly in patients with thymic

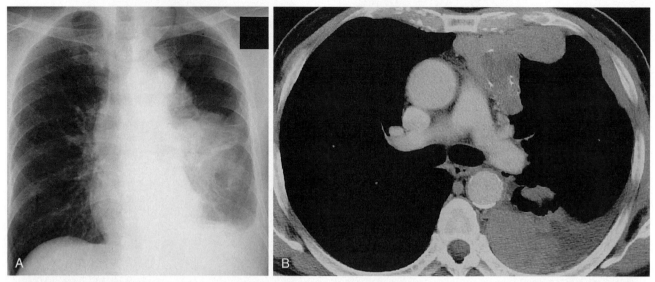

Figure 22–23. Thymoma with Pleural Involvement. Posteroanterior chest radiograph in a 65-year-old man *(A)* shows extensive left pleural thickening and a small left pleural effusion. Contrast-enhanced CT scan *(B)* shows an inhomogeneous anterior mediastinal mass with focal areas of calcification, nodular left pleural thickening, and a small left pleural effusion. The diagnosis of invasive thymoma with left pleural seeding was proved at thoracotomy.

carcinoma than in those with invasive thymoma.[500] In a review of the CT manifestations in 18 patients with thymic carcinoma, CT findings suggestive of invasion of the great vessels were present in 7 (39%), mediastinal lymph node enlargement was found in 8 (44%), metastases to the lung or liver were seen in 5 (28%), and phrenic nerve palsy was present in one patient.[500] The prognosis for thymic carcinoma is poor, with progressive intrathoracic growth and extrathoracic metastases developing in most patients.[172]

Thymic Neuroendocrine Neoplasms

The term *thymic neuroendocrine neoplasms* encompasses several varieties of thymic neoplasm, all of which have in common histologic, ultrastructural, immunohistochemical, and, occasionally, clinical features of neuroendocrine function.[180] Although specific names have been given to the several histologic varieties, it is possible that they represent a spectrum of differentiation rather than specific entities. These tumors are uncommon.[182] They may occur at any age;[183] the average age at the time of diagnosis is about 45 years. There is a 3:1 male-to-female predominance.[182]

Pathologically the most common histologic subtype is carcinoid tumor; as with their pulmonary counterparts, these may be well differentiated (typical carcinoid tumor) or may show features suggestive of a more aggressive nature (atypical carcinoid). Clinical findings of paraneoplastic disease are present in about one third of patients, reflecting the neuroendocrine nature of these neoplasms.[180] Cushing's syndrome is the most common manifestation,[185] being seen in approximately 25% of cases;[182] other syndromes, including inappropriate secretion of antidiuretic hormone[181] and carcinoid syndrome,[188, 189] are rare. Cushing's syndrome may be related to the production of adrenocorticotropic hormone or corticotropin-releasing hormone.[190] Many mediastinal carcinoid tumors produce no symptoms and are discovered on screening chest radiography.

Chest radiograph can be normal, a feature that is particularly likely in patients who have corticotropin-producing carcinoid tumors;[184, 185] in one investigation of five patients who presented with Cushing's syndrome, four had normal chest radiographs.[184] Nonsecreting tumors or tumors associated with multiple endocrine neoplasia syndromes more commonly manifest as large anterior mediastinal masses.[186] On CT, the tumors are 1 to 25 cm in diameter[185, 186] and have homogeneous attenuation (Fig. 22–26) or heterogeneous attenuation as a result of necrosis or calcification (Fig. 22–27).[86, 184, 185] Evidence of invasion of adjacent structures and metastases to the regional lymph nodes or lungs is common.[186, 187] Skeletal metastases are typically osteoblastic.[133, 184]

Germ Cell Neoplasms

The group of germ cell neoplasms consists of tumors that are histologically identical to certain testicular and ovarian neoplasms, all of which are believed to be derived from primitive germ cell elements. Tumors include mature (benign) and malignant teratoma, seminoma, endodermal sinus tumor, choriocarcinoma, and embryonal carcinoma.[191] Most of these mediastinal tumors are located in the anterior compartment:[192, 193] In a review of 86 benign and 20 malignant tumors from the Mayo Clinic, 100 (94%) were located at this site;[91] the remaining 6 tumors (4 benign and 2 malignant) were found in the posterior mediastinum.

In most cases, tumors become manifest in early adulthood; the mean age at diagnosis is 20 to 40 years.[191, 195] For unexplained reasons, benign lesions are more common in women, and malignant tumors are more frequent in men.[195, 196] The most common form of mediastinal germ cell tumor is mature teratoma, constituting almost 75% of tumors in two series of 133 cases[91, 192] and 45% in another.[195] The most common malignant tumor is seminoma.[194]

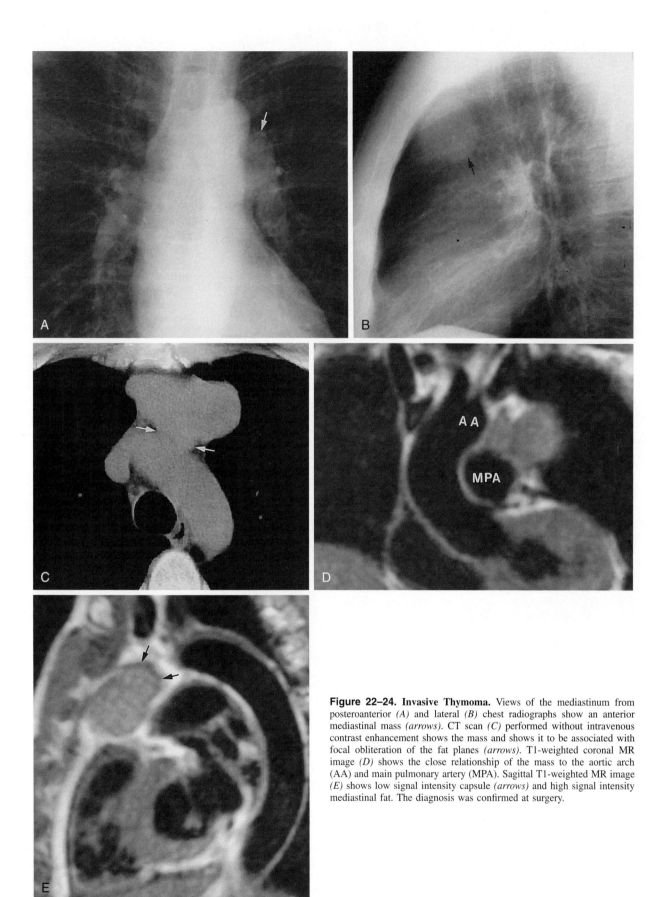

Figure 22–24. Invasive Thymoma. Views of the mediastinum from posteroanterior *(A)* and lateral *(B)* chest radiographs show an anterior mediastinal mass *(arrows)*. CT scan *(C)* performed without intravenous contrast enhancement shows the mass and shows it to be associated with focal obliteration of the fat planes *(arrows)*. T1-weighted coronal MR image *(D)* shows the close relationship of the mass to the aortic arch (AA) and main pulmonary artery (MPA). Sagittal T1-weighted MR image *(E)* shows low signal intensity capsule *(arrows)* and high signal intensity mediastinal fat. The diagnosis was confirmed at surgery.

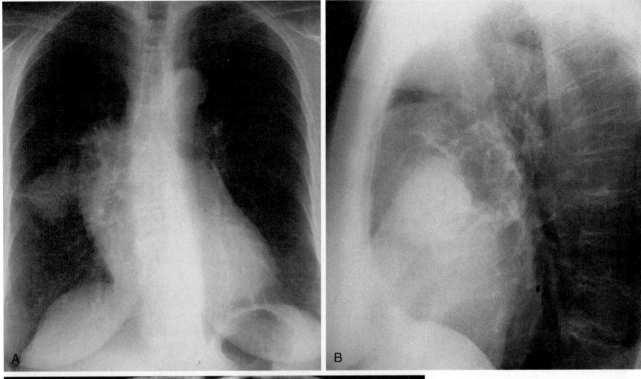

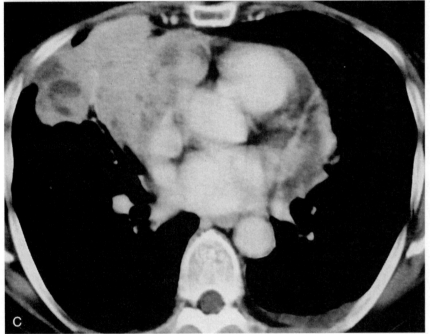

Figure 22–25. Thymic Carcinoma. Posteroanterior *(A)* and lateral *(B)* chest radiographs in a 69-year-old woman show a large, lobulated anterior mediastinal mass. A soft tissue component projects into the right midlung zone. Contrast-enhanced CT scan *(C)* shows a lobulated anterior mediastinal mass with inhomogeneous attenuation and obliteration of the adjacent fat planes. The mass can be seen extending into the right middle lobe. At surgery, this was shown to be a thymic carcinoma with pericardial, pleural, and right middle lobe involvement.

Teratoma

A teratoma is a neoplasm consisting of one or more types of tissue, usually derived from more than one germ cell layer, at least some of which are not native to the area in which the tumor arises. In the mediastinum, most lesions are cystic and benign; solid neoplasms are uncommon and usually malignant.[199, 200] The tumor is recognized most often in adolescence or early adulthood, although occasional series consisting of older individuals have been reported.[201] Most mature teratomas do not produce symptoms and are discovered on screening chest radiograph. Teratomas that

grow to a large size can cause shortness of breath, cough, and a sensation of pressure or pain in the retrosternal area.

Radiologic Manifestations

Most mediastinal teratomas are seen on radiograph as a localized mass in the anterior compartment close to the origin of the major vessels from the heart (Fig. 22–28).[86, 197, 202] In one investigation of 66 cases, 54 (82%) were found in the anterior mediastinum, 3 (4%) in the middle-posterior mediastinum, and 9 (14%) in multiple compartments;[202] findings included a focal mediastinal mass (in

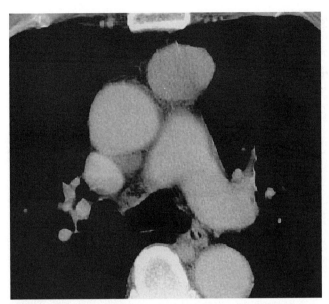

Figure 22–26. Thymic Carcinoid Tumor. CT scan in a 67-year-old man shows a 3-cm-diameter anterior mediastinal mass with homogeneous enhancement. At surgery, this was shown to be a *typical* carcinoid tumor.

(mean, 10 cm). Calcification was evident on radiograph in 14 mature teratomas (21%) and was classified as amorphous in 6 and as peripheral and curvilinear in 5; in 4 cases, it appeared to represent teeth or bone.

On CT, 59 tumors (89%) had well-defined margins that were smooth or lobulated.[202] Twenty-six mature teratomas (39%) had heterogeneous attenuation with soft tissue, fluid, fat, and calcium attenuation components (Fig. 22–29). Other common combinations included soft tissue, fluid, and fat (in 24% of cases) and soft tissue and fluid (15%). Although soft tissue attenuation was present in all mature cystic teratomas, it was the dominant component (occupying >50% of the total volume of the mass) in only two tumors (3%). Fifty-eight teratomas had fluid attenuation on CT, 50 had fat attenuation, and 35 had foci of calcification. MR imaging, performed in eight mature cystic teratomas, showed areas that had soft tissue signal intensity in all cases, signal intensity consistent with fluid in seven (88%), and signal intensity consistent with fat in five (63%). Sonography, performed in six cases, showed heterogeneous echogenicity with a predominant fluid component (hypoechoic regions and increased through transmission).

Occasionally a fat-fluid level is seen on radiograph and CT scan.[197, 203] The combination of fat, fluid, and soft tissue allows diagnosis of most mature cystic teratomas. In one study of 128 patients who had anterior mediastinal masses, of whom 16 had teratoma, a confident, correct diagnosis of the tumor was made on chest radiograph in 2 (13%) and on CT scan in 10 (63%).[125]

92% of cases), diffuse mediastinal widening (3%), a mediastinal mass partially obscured by adjacent pulmonary consolidation (3%), and cardiomegaly in 1 case (2%). The tumors ranged from 5 to 17 cm in longest dimension

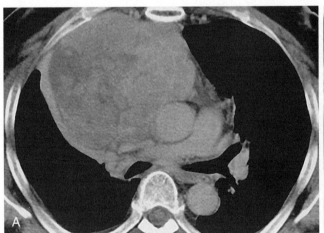
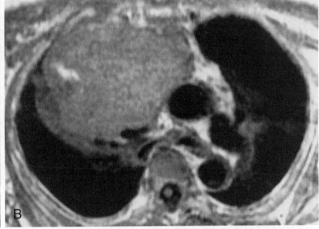
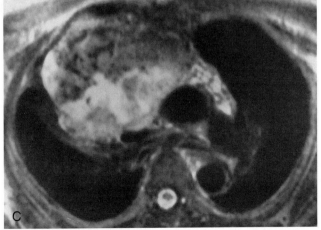

Figure 22–27. Thymic Carcinoid Tumor. CT scan *(A)* in a 64-year-old man shows a large anterior mediastinal mass with inhomogeneous attenuation. Note the obscuring of the adjacent fat planes. T1-weighted *(B)* and T2-weighted *(C)* MR images show inhomogeneous signal intensity of the tumor. *Atypical* carcinoid of the thymus with mediastinal invasion was proved surgically.

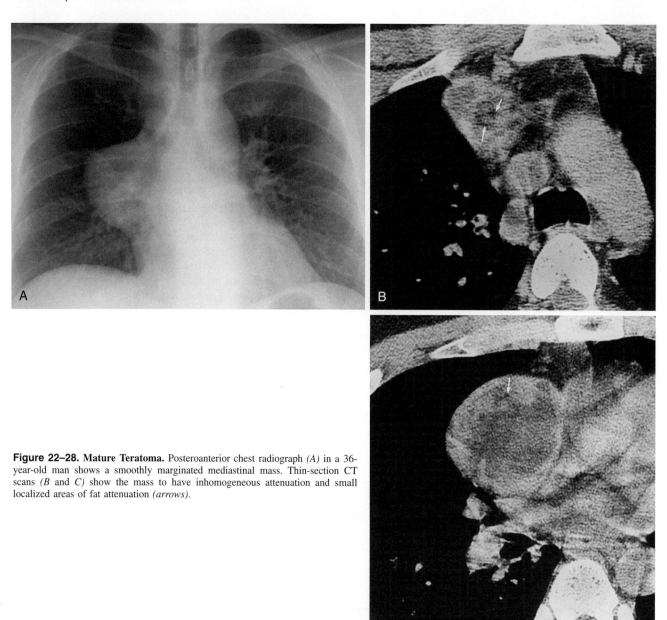

Figure 22–28. Mature Teratoma. Posteroanterior chest radiograph *(A)* in a 36-year-old man shows a smoothly marginated mediastinal mass. Thin-section CT scans *(B* and *C)* show the mass to have inhomogeneous attenuation and small localized areas of fat attenuation *(arrows).*

Complications of teratoma that may be evident on radiograph or CT scan include atelectasis and obstructive pneumonitis (as a result of airway compression),[197, 202, 204] pneumonitis (after rupture into the lung),[204, 207] and effusion (secondary to rupture into the pleural space or pericardium).[202, 204] Occasionally an effusion has a fat-fluid level;[205] rarely the accumulated fluid is sufficient to cause cardiac tamponade.[197] Perforation of the aorta and superior vena cava are additional rare complications.[204]

Seminoma

Seminoma (germinoma) is the most frequent mediastinal germ cell neoplasm after teratoma and is the most common form of histologically pure malignant tumor. Approximately 20% to 30% of patients are asymptomatic at the time of initial diagnosis. When present, symptoms usually derive from pressure or invasion of mediastinal vessels or

the major airways and include chest pain and shortness of breath.[206]

Radiographically, seminomas usually manifest as large masses that may project into one or both sides of the anterior mediastinum.[197, 208] They typically have homogeneous attenuation on CT scan and enhance only slightly after intravenous administration of contrast material.[197] Occasionally a few localized areas of low attenuation[198] or ringlike and stippled foci of calcification are seen.[197, 209] Evidence of invasion of adjacent structures is seldom apparent.[86, 198] Metastases may result in regional lymph node enlargement or bone destruction.[86, 208]

Endodermal Sinus Tumor

Endodermal sinus tumors are highly malignant neoplasms believed to show differentiation toward yolk sac endoderm. Origin in the mediastinum is rare; only 38 cases

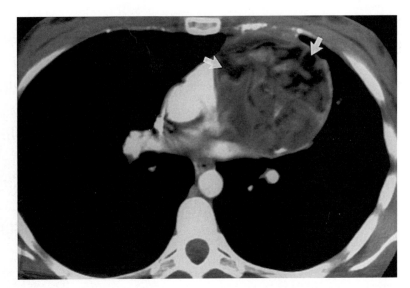

Figure 22–29. Anterior Mediastinal Mass: Mature Cystic Teratoma. Intravenous contrast–enhanced CT scan in a 29-year-old woman shows a heterogeneous anterior mediastinal mass, which contains areas of fat attenuation *(arrows)*. The diagnosis of teratoma was confirmed at surgery.

of the pure form had been reported in the English language literature by 1986.[210] Most tumors appear in young adults, the mean age in the 1986 review cited previously being about 23 years;[210] most occur in men. Radiographic and CT findings are similar to those of other malignant mediastinal germ cell tumors (Fig. 22–30).[197, 198]

Choriocarcinoma

Choriocarcinoma is a rare variety of mediastinal germ cell neoplasm that usually is seen in combination with other forms, especially embryonal carcinoma.[211, 212] Similar to other malignant germ cell tumors, the incidence peaks between 20 and 30 years of age, and most occur in men.[213] The radiographic and CT findings are similar to those of other malignant nonseminomatous germ cell tumors.[86, 197]

Primary Mediastinal Lymphoma

Lymphoma is one of the most common causes of mediastinal abnormality: It has been estimated that lymphoma constitutes about 20% of all mediastinal neoplasms in adults and 50% in children.[214] Most often, mediastinal involvement occurs in association with clinical or radiographic evidence of extrathoracic lymphoma; in about 5% of cases, the mediastinum is the sole site of abnormality,[215] in which case differentiation from other mediastinal abnormalities can be difficult on the basis of radiologic findings alone. The most common causes of such primary disease are Hodgkin's disease, large cell lymphoma, and lymphoblastic lymphoma; other forms are infrequent.[216–218]

Hodgkin's disease is the most common lymphoma to manifest in the mediastinum; lymph node enlargement is evident on the initial radiograph of approximately 50% of

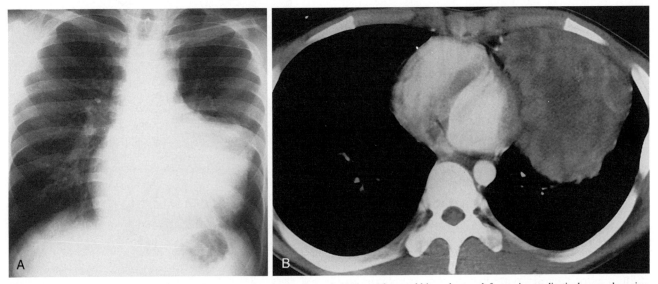

Figure 22–30. Endodermal Sinus Tumor. Posteroanterior chest radiograph *(A)* in a 16-year-old boy shows a left anterior mediastinal mass obscuring the heart border. Contrast-enhanced CT scan *(B)* shows inhomogeneous soft tissue attenuation and focal central areas of decreased attenuation. (Courtesy of Dr. Ella Kazerooni, Department of Radiology, University of Michigan Hospital, Ann Arbor, MI.)

patients.[219, 220] An anterior mediastinal mass involving the thymus is common.[221, 222] Nodular sclerosis is the most frequent histologic subtype; the disease is seen most often in young women. The radiologic features of Hodgkin's and non-Hodgkin's lymphoma are discussed in Chapter 7.

Tumors and Tumor-Like Conditions of Endocrine Organs

Thyroid Tumors

Although extension of thyroid tissue into the thorax is seen in only 1% to 3% of patients subjected to thyroidectomy,[223] such tissue nevertheless constitutes a significant percentage of anterior mediastinal masses. The most frequent pathologic finding is multinodular goiter,[224] a condition that occurs most commonly in women in their forties;[225] occasionally the abnormality is due to acute[226, 227] or chronic[228] thyroiditis or thyroid carcinoma.[225]

Of mediastinal thyroid tumors, 75% to 80% arise from a lower pole or the isthmus and extend into the anterior or middle mediastinum. Most of the remainder arise from the posterior aspect of either thyroid lobe and extend into the posterior mediastinum behind the trachea, innominate or brachiocephalic vein, and innominate or subclavian arteries;[229, 230] in the last-mentioned location, they are situated almost exclusively on the right.[229] In a few cases (probably <1%), there is no evident connection between the cervical and intrathoracic thyroid tissue;[225] in these cases, it is assumed that the intrathoracic tumor arises from ectopic thyroid tissue displaced during fetal development.[231] As might be expected from this discussion, the abnormal thyroid tissue is located in the uppermost portion of the mediastinum in most patients; however, occasionally, growth extends from the neck to the diaphragm.[225]

Many patients who have intrathoracic goiter are asymptomatic,[225] with the abnormality being discovered on screening chest radiograph. When present, symptoms include respiratory distress (which can be worsened by certain movements of the neck) and hoarseness. The latter usually is caused by compression of the recurrent laryngeal nerve;[497] however, its presence should raise the possibility of extracapsular invasion and malignancy.

Radiologic Manifestations

Radiographically the characteristic appearance of a retrosternal goiter is that of a sharply defined, smooth or lobulated mass that causes displacement and narrowing of the trachea (Fig. 22–31).[133, 232] Anterior and middle mediastinal goiters displace the trachea posteriorly and laterally, whereas those in the posterior mediastinum displace it anteriorly.

Because CT allows accurate assessment of the position of an intrathoracic goiter and its relationship to adjacent structures as well as the diagnosis of other masses that may mimic the abnormality on chest radiograph, it is currently the imaging modality of choice in the assessment of these tumors. Characteristic features include continuity with the cervical thyroid, focal calcification, relatively high attenuation, and marked and prolonged enhancement after bolus administration of iodinated contrast material (Fig.

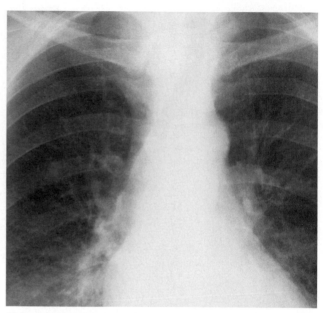

Figure 22–31. Retrosternal Multinodular Goiter. View from posteroanterior chest radiograph in a 64-year-old woman shows extrinsic compression and smooth displacement of the trachea by a soft tissue mass extending from the lower neck into the thoracic inlet.

22–32).[233] The attenuation value of the thyroid is often greater than 100 HU before administration of contrast material; because the gland concentrates iodine, it enhances intensely and for a prolonged period (>2 minutes) after intravenous injection.[233, 234] The attenuation of the intrathoracic component of a goiter is usually greater than that of muscle but less than that of the cervical thyroid gland. Focal nonenhancing areas of low attenuation as a result of hemorrhage or cyst formation are common.[86, 232] The connection between the intrathoracic thyroid tissue and the thyroid gland is usually readily apparent on CT scan; rarely

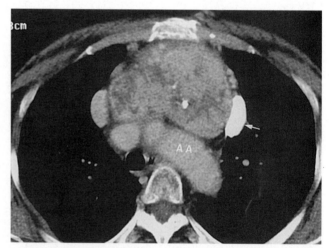

Figure 22–32. Multinodular Goiter. CT scan performed during intravenous administration of contrast material shows a large anterior mediastinal mass that has inhomogeneous attenuation and contains small foci of calcification. The mass lies anterior to the aortic arch (AA) and innominate artery and displaces the left brachiocephalic vein *(arrow)*. The patient was a 67-year-old woman with long-standing multinodular goiter.

the only connection is a narrow fibrous or vascular pedicle that may not be apparent.[232]

Thyroid carcinoma usually manifests as a mass of inhomogeneous attenuation in the lower neck, which may extend into the thorax.[85, 236] The distinction between carcinoma and a goiter can be made on CT when there is evidence of spread into the adjacent tissue or lymph node enlargement.[234, 236] In many cases, however, the borders of a carcinoma are well defined.[234] Localized areas of low attenuation and foci of calcification can be seen in benign and malignant masses.[234, 235]

MR imaging, particularly in the coronal and sagittal planes, can show the extent of intrathoracic thyroid tissue and its relationship to adjacent structures. Multinodular goiters have heterogeneous signal characteristics on T1-weighted and T2-weighted images.[237, 238] Because of its low sensitivity in the detection of calcification and its high cost, MR imaging has a limited, if any, role in the assessment of the intrathoracic thyroid.

Most intrathoracic goiters show evidence of function on radionuclide imaging.[239–241] Radionuclides used include iodine 123, technetium 99m, and iodine 131,[239] the last-named being the agent of choice.[241] In one investigation of 54 consecutive patients in whom chest radiographs suggested the presence of an upper mediastinal mass, scintigraphy detected 39 of 42 intrathoracic goiters (sensitivity 93%) and correctly excluded goiter in 12 patients (specificity 100%).[239] *False-positive* uptake can be seen, however, in association with hiatal hernia[242, 243] and in the thymus,[244] the latter possibly as a result of binding of iodine to protein in Hassall's corpuscles.

Parathyroid Tumors

Parathyroid tumors constitute a rare cause of an anterior mediastinal mass. Their presence within the mediastinum is explained best on the basis of the migration of parathyroid glands with the thymus during embryonic development. Most abnormal glands contain an adenoma or are hyperplastic; occasionally a tumor is malignant (parathyroid carcinoma).[245] In contrast to most other mediastinal masses, parathyroid tumors usually can be diagnosed on the basis of clinical and laboratory findings. Because most are functioning, patients present with signs and symptoms of hyperparathyroidism, including anorexia, weakness, fatigue, nausea, vomiting, constipation, and hypotonicity of muscles.

Radiologic Manifestations

Most mediastinal parathyroid lesions are so small as to be invisible radiographically. Occasionally a tumor is sufficiently large to widen the mediastinal silhouette, usually unilaterally.[247, 248] Calcification may be apparent.[249] On CT, mediastinal parathyroid adenomas usually present as small nodules that show minimal, if any, enhancement after intravenous administration of contrast material (Fig. 22–33).[250, 251] The appearance may be similar to that of lymph nodes.[250, 251] Most tumors occur in the upper portion of the anterior mediastinum;[250, 251] they are seen less commonly in the paraesophageal regions[252] and rarely in the

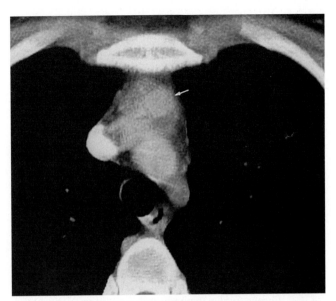

Figure 22–33. Mediastinal Parathyroid Adenoma. CT scan performed during intravenous administration of contrast material shows a poorly defined nodule *(arrow)* immediately anterior to the lower margin of the left brachiocephalic vein. (Contrast material can be seen in the right brachiocephalic vein.) The patient was a 30-year-old woman who had hyperparathyroidism. Surgical excision confirmed the lesion to be a parathyroid adenoma.

aortopulmonary window.[253] Tracheal compression has been seen in association with parathyroid cysts.[254]

On MR imaging, adenomas have signal intensity that is hypointense or isointense relative to muscle on T1-weighted images and high signal intensity on T2-weighted images.[252, 253, 255] Hemorrhage can result in high signal intensity on T1-weighted and T2-weighted images.[255] The signal intensity may be altered by the presence of fat or fibrous tissue.[256] Tumors usually enhance after intravenous administration of gadolinium-based contrast agents.[257] In one investigation of 25 patients, MR imaging had a higher sensitivity (22 of 25 cases [88%]) than did scintigraphy (11 of 19 cases [58%]) or ultrasound (3 of 24 cases [12%]) in detecting tumors.[254]

Radionuclide imaging of mediastinal parathyroid glands can be performed using double-tracer radionuclide imaging (thallium 201 and technetium-99m pertechnetate)[252] or technetium-99m sestamibi. Several groups of investigators have shown technetium-99m sestamibi to be associated with the greatest sensitivity and specificity.[253, 258, 259] Optimal assessment is obtained by using technetium-99m sestamibi combined with single-photon emission computed tomography (SPECT) imaging.[253, 260] In one investigation of nine patients who had ectopic parathyroid tissue (eight adenomas, one hyperplastic gland) in the aortopulmonary window, the abnormal glands were identified on the sestamibi SPECT scans in all six patients in whom the procedure was performed compared with eight of nine patients (89%) on CT and five of eight patients (63%) on MR imaging.[253] Because of the limited spatial resolution of scintigraphy, it has been suggested that the combination of sestamibi SPECT scintigraphy and fast-spin-echo MR imaging provides the best overall assessment of the presence and anatomic location of hyperfunctioning glands.[256, 261]

Mediastinal parathyroid glands can be identified using selective arteriography;[262, 263] however, the technique is invasive and has limited sensitivity for the detection of adenomas. Preliminary results suggest that localization of adenomas can be improved by serial measurement of parathyroid hormone in the superior vena cava during selective arteriography with nonionic contrast media. In one investigation, a 1.4-fold increase in parathyroid hormone level in the superior vena cava within 20 to 120 seconds after arteriography allowed correct prediction of the site of an adenoma in 13 of 20 patients (65%);[264] 8 of 9 patients who had positive arteriograms and 5 of 11 patients who had negative arteriograms had positive results of venous sampling.

Soft Tissue Tumors and Tumor-Like Conditions

Soft tissue tumors account for about 5% of all mediastinal masses[265] and include benign and malignant neoplasms of fat, fibrous tissue, smooth and striated muscle, blood and lymphatic vessels, bone, and neural tissue.[266] Several developmental and acquired abnormalities composed predominantly of mesenchymal tissue (e.g., hemangioma and lipomatosis) can present as mediastinal masses. Each of these can occur in any mediastinal compartment; however, tumors of neural tissue are most common in the paravertebral region, whereas most of the others more frequently are located anteriorly. Probably the most common soft tissue tumors to occur in the mediastinum are lipoma and lymphangioma.

Lipoma

Although uncommon compared with other neoplasms, extrathymic lipoma is probably the most common nonneurogenic mesenchymal tumor to occur in the mediastinum; in one series of 396 mediastinal neoplasms, it constituted 2.3% of the total.[267] Perhaps because of their pliability, the tumors usually do not cause symptoms, even when massive.[267]

Certain radiographic features aid in diagnosis. Because the density of fat is lower than that of other soft tissues, the radiographic density of lipomas is often, although not always, less than that of other mediastinal masses. This is particularly true if the mass happens to be surrounded by mediastinal tissue of unit density (Fig. 22–34).[268] Most

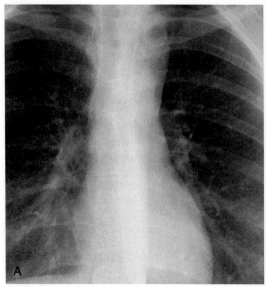
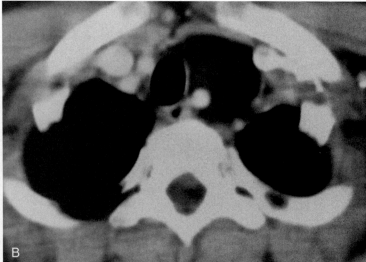
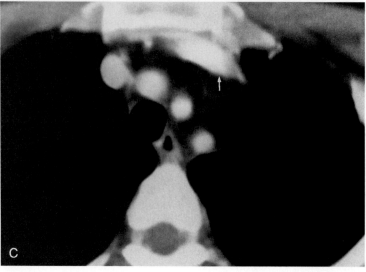
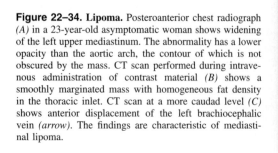

Figure 22–34. Lipoma. Posteroanterior chest radiograph *(A)* in a 23-year-old asymptomatic woman shows widening of the left upper mediastinum. The abnormality has a lower opacity than the aortic arch, the contour of which is not obscured by the mass. CT scan performed during intravenous administration of contrast material *(B)* shows a smoothly marginated mass with homogeneous fat density in the thoracic inlet. CT scan at a more caudad level *(C)* shows anterior displacement of the left brachiocephalic vein *(arrow)*. The findings are characteristic of mediastinal lipoma.

tumors project from only one side of the mediastinum.[246] CT usually is diagnostic, the characteristic finding consisting of a mass that has homogeneous fat attenuation.[269] The presence of heterogeneous attenuation with soft tissue components should raise the possibility of a liposarcoma. Mediastinal liposarcomas are rare. Their appearance on CT ranges from predominantly fat attenuation to homogeneous soft tissue attenuation.[491, 492]

Lipomatosis

Lipomatosis is an unusual non-neoplastic abnormality of mediastinal adipose tissue characterized by the excessive accumulation of fat in its normal locations. The abnormality is seen most commonly in conditions associated with hypercortisolism, such as Cushing's syndrome,[270] ectopic adrenocorticotropic hormone syndrome,[498] and long-term corticosteroid therapy.[272] In all these situations, there is a redistribution of normal adipose tissue with excessive deposition in the upper mediastinum and in the pleuropericardial angles. The abnormality has been described in obese individuals not receiving corticosteroid therapy (Fig. 22–35).[274] Typically, patients do not have symptoms from the fat deposits.

Radiologically, mediastinal widening tends to be smooth and symmetric, although the margins can be lobulated if the accumulation is large. The widening usually extends from the thoracic inlet to the hila bilaterally (see Fig. 22–35); occasionally the accumulation is predominantly paraspinal and symmetric.[275] Increasing size of the pleuro-pericardial fat pads may be evident on serial radio-graphs.[271, 273] In cases in which doubt exists on conventional radiographs, CT is invariably diagnostic.[275, 276]

Lymphangioma

Mediastinal lymphangiomas have two clinicopathologic forms: (1) a form in which the lesion extends from the neck into the mediastinum and usually occurs in infants (cystic hygroma)[277] and (2) a more or less well-circumscribed tumor that usually is discovered in adults and is located in the lower anterior mediastinum remote from the neck.[278] Lymphangiomas probably represent developmental anomalies rather than true neoplasms. Pathologically, they consist of thin-walled, usually multilocular cysts containing numerous vascular spaces lined by endothelial cells. The wall is composed of connective tissue with a variable amount of lymphoid tissue.[91] Because of their soft consistency, the lesions seldom cause symptoms, even when large.[283]

The radiographic findings are nonspecific and consist of a sharply defined, smoothly marginated mediastinal mass, which frequently displaces adjacent mediastinal structures.[279] One case was associated with adjacent rib and clavicle erosion.[280] In one investigation of 19 adult patients, seven (37%) tumors were located in the anterior mediastinum, five (26%) in the middle mediastinum, three (16%) in the posterior mediastinum, three (16%) in the thoracic inlet, and one in the lung.[281]

The most common CT appearance, seen in about 60% of patients, consists of a smoothly marginated cystic mass with homogeneous water density (Fig. 22–36).[281, 282] Multiple loculations can be seen within the mass in approxi-

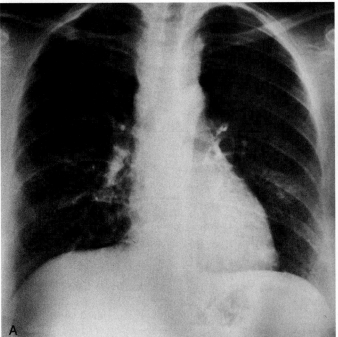
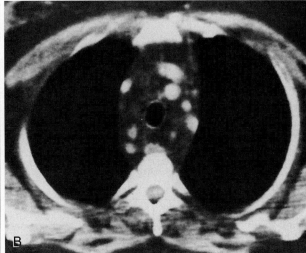

Figure 22–35. Mediastinal Lipomatosis. Posteroanterior radiograph (A) shows widening of the upper mediastinum to an equal extent on both sides. The contour is smooth. No other abnormalities are apparent other than thickening of bronchial walls consistent with chronic bronchitis. CT scan at the level of the left brachiocephalic vein (B) shows wide separation of vessels as a result of an accumulation of a large amount of fat. This 58-year-old woman was receiving no therapy, and she did not have any underlying condition to which the lipomatosis could be attributed: She was simply obese. The widened mediastinum returned to normal after a 40-lb weight loss.

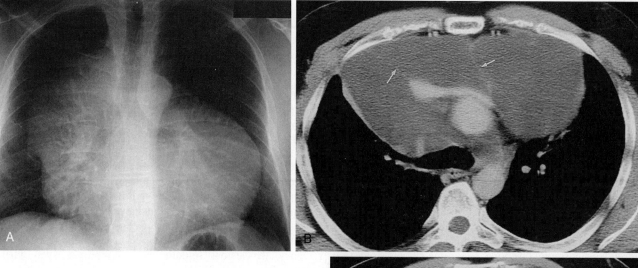

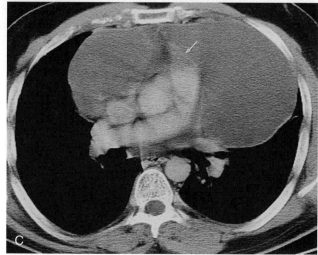

Figure 22–36. Lymphangioma. Posteroanterior chest radiograph *(A)* in a 37-year-old man shows diffuse mediastinal widening. Contrast-enhanced CT scans *(B* and *C)* show a predominantly anterior mediastinal cystic mass. The mass has homogeneous water attenuation and contains a few soft tissue septations *(arrows).*

mately one third.[281, 282] The mass can displace or surround adjacent vessels.[281, 282] Less common findings include foci of calcification, homogeneous soft tissue density, and spiculated margins.[281] Hemorrhage results in an increase in the size of the mass and an increase in the attenuation values on CT.[282] The findings on MR imaging in three patients were variable and nonspecific.[281]

Tumors Situated in the Anterior Cardiophrenic Angle

Although masses in the vicinity of the cardiophrenic angle on either side originate in the middle mediastinum, they project into the anterior compartment and so are discussed at this point. The differential diagnosis of such masses is extensive and includes lesions arising in the lung parenchyma, in the visceral or parietal pleura or pleural space, in the pericardium or contiguous myocardium, and in or beneath the diaphragm. Although lesions arising in any of these anatomic regions can produce similar radiographic findings, specific diagnoses usually can be made on CT.[125, 232] Only three lesions are considered in detail at this point—pleuropericardial fat, mesothelial cysts, and enlargement of diaphragmatic lymph nodes. Although hernia through the foramina of Morgagni appears radiographi-

cally as a homogeneous shadow usually indistinguishable from a large pleuropericardial fat pad, for convenience these lesions are discussed in Chapter 23.

Pleuropericardial Fat

Accumulations of fat that normally occupy the cardiophrenic angles can attain a considerable size. Although such pleuropericardial fat pads always are bilateral, they may be asymmetric. Fat pads can increase substantially in size over time, as a result of obesity or hyperadrenocorticism (e.g., Cushing's syndrome); as such, they can cause a potentially confusing radiographic opacity. The diagnosis can be made on CT[125, 284] or MR imaging.[285]

Mesothelial (Pericardial) Cysts

Most mesothelial (pericardial, pleuropericardial) cysts are congenital and result from aberrations in the formation of the coelomic cavities. Rarely an otherwise typical *congenital* cyst develops years after an episode of acute pericarditis,[286] suggesting that some cysts may be acquired. The cysts are spherical or oval in shape, thin walled, and often translucent; most are unilocular and contain clear or straw-colored fluid.[91] Symptoms almost invariably are

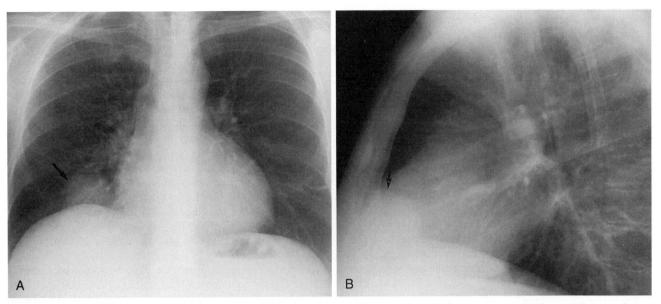

Figure 22–37. Mesothelial (Pericardial) Cyst. Posteroanterior *(A)* and lateral *(B)* chest radiographs in an asymptomatic 47-year-old woman show a smoothly marginated mass in the right anterior cardiophrenic angle *(arrows)*.

absent; most cysts are discovered on screening chest radiograph.

Radiographically, most cysts are located in the cardiophrenic angles (Fig. 22–37). In one study of 72 cases, 54 were identified at this site and 18 at a higher level;[91] 11 of the latter extended into the superior aspect of the mediastinum. Most—almost 75% of cases in the study cited[91]—are located on the right side.[287] Typically the cysts are smooth in contour and round or oval in shape. Most are between 3 and 8 cm in diameter; rare examples have been reported to be 1 cm or 28 cm.[288–290]

The benign cystic nature of these masses usually can be confirmed by CT (Fig. 22–38),[234, 291] MR imaging,[293] or ultrasonography,[294] even when their location is atypical, such as the superior portion of the mediastinum.[292, 295] The characteristic CT appearance consists of a smooth, round, or oval cystic water density lesion abutting the pericardium. Occasional cysts have soft tissue attenuation, presumably as a result of the presence of viscous material;[287, 296] such lesions cannot be distinguished reliably from a neoplasm.[125] Cysts typically have low echogenicity and increased through transmission on ultrasound.

Enlargement of Diaphragmatic Lymph Nodes

The superior diaphragmatic lymph nodes are distributed in three clusters: anterior (prepericardiac), middle (lateral pericardiac), and posterior.[297, 298] They can be affected by tumors developing above the diaphragm—most commonly lymphoma and Hodgkin's disease and less commonly carci-

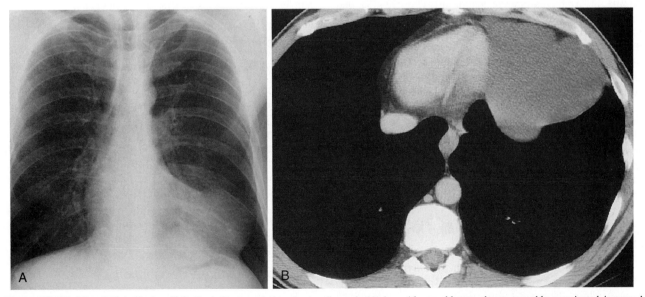

Figure 22–38. Mesothelial (Pericardial) Cyst. Posteroanterior chest radiograph *(A)* in a 46-year-old man shows smoothly marginated increased opacity in the left cardiophrenic angle. Contrast-enhanced CT scan *(B)* shows a water density cyst. The diagnosis was confirmed at thoracotomy.

noma of the breast and lung—or by tumors developing below the diaphragm, particularly carcinoma of the colon and ovary.[298, 299]

The nodes normally are not visible on chest radiographs because of their small size and their investment with fat and other connective tissue adjacent to the pleura. When enlarged, the nodes displace the pleura laterally and produce a smooth or lobulated mass projecting out of the cardiophrenic angle, an appearance that can simulate pleuropericardial fat pads. Although such enlargement may be apparent on conventional radiographs, CT is a superior method of assessment.[299, 300] In one investigation of 274 CT scans obtained on 209 patients who had lymphoma (153 Hodgkin's disease and 56 non-Hodgkin's lymphoma), evidence of enlargement of cardiophrenic angle lymph nodes was found in 14 (7%);[300] in only 3 of these was node enlargement evident on conventional radiographs. Although node enlargement can occur as the initial presentation in patients who have Hodgkin's disease,[301, 302] it is more common during a relapse.[301] It is important to compare the cardiophrenic angles on serial chest radiographs.

MASSES SITUATED PREDOMINANTLY IN THE MIDDLE-POSTERIOR MEDIASTINAL COMPARTMENT

For practical purposes, a tumor can be considered to lie in the middle-posterior mediastinal compartment when, on lateral chest radiograph, it is situated between a line drawn along the anterior border of the trachea and the posterior border of the heart and one drawn along the anterior aspect of the vertebral bodies (*see* Fig. 22–14). The most common abnormalities of this region are lymph node enlargement and aortic aneurysms;[87] esophageal lesions and congenital cysts are less frequent, and most other lesions are rare (Table 22–2).

Lymph Node Enlargement

Lymph node enlargement is caused most often by lymphoma, metastatic carcinoma, sarcoidosis (Fig. 22–39), and infection (either directly by organisms such as *H. capsulatum* and *Mycobacterium tuberculosis* or as a hyperplastic reaction to the presence of infection within the lungs). Most of these and other less common conditions are discussed elsewhere in this book; only giant lymph node hyperplasia (Castleman's disease) is considered in detail here.

Clinicopathologic effects of enlarged lymph nodes in the middle-posterior mediastinum usually are minimal or absent altogether. Because of their intimate association with the airways and vessels that course through this region, however, stenosis or obstruction may ensue and result in signs and symptoms, sometimes associated with life-threatening consequences.[304]

Castleman's Disease (Giant Lymph Node Hyperplasia)

Castleman's disease (giant lymph node hyperplasia, angiofollicular lymph node hyperplasia) is an unusual condition of which there are two distinct histologic variants.[306] The *hyaline vascular type* is more common and is charac-

terized by the presence of numerous germinal centers interspersed in a population of mononuclear cells (predominantly lymphocytes) and numerous capillaries. This form of disease usually is unassociated with symptoms. The *plasma cell type* is characterized histologically by the presence of numerous plasma cells between the germinal centers, which often are larger than those in the hyaline vascular type; relatively few capillaries are present. In contrast to patients who have the hyaline vascular type, patients who have the plasma cell type tend to have systemic manifestations of disease, most often nonspecific findings such as fever, anemia, weight loss, and hypergammaglobulinemia.[306] Most lesions are solitary, usually involving only the mediastinum or hilum.[305, 306] Patients have been identified who have multifocal disease that tends to affect superficial lymph node groups with or without involvement of the mediastinum.[307]

The radiographic appearance of the localized form of giant lymph node hyperplasia is that of a solitary, smooth or lobulated mass situated most commonly in the left or right hilum or middle-posterior mediastinum; less commonly the anterior mediastinum is affected (Fig. 22–40).[310–312] In multicentric disease, the lymphadenopathy often involves multiple mediastinal compartments (Fig. 22–41).[308, 309] The latter form can be associated with pulmonary parenchymal involvement, consisting on CT scans of areas of ground-glass attenuation, poorly defined centrilobular nodules, thickening of the bronchoarterial bundles, and interlobular septal thickening (Fig. 22–42).[309, 310] The enlarged nodes typically show marked homogeneous enhancement after intravenous administration of contrast material;[311, 312] such enhancement is less marked in the plasma cell type than in the hyaline vascular type of disease.[309] Focal calcification can be seen.[308, 310, 311]

MR studies show a signal that is hypointense compared with that characteristic of mediastinal fat but hyperintense compared with that of skeletal muscle on T1-weighted images and high signal intensity on T2-weighted images.[313, 314] The lesions enhance after administration of gadolinium-based contrast medium.[312] Foci of calcification result in localized areas of low signal intensity.[313]

Tumors and Tumor-Like Conditions

Primary Tracheal Neoplasms

Although pulmonary carcinoma usually is manifested in the mediastinum in the form of metastases to lymph nodes from a primary lesion in the lung, rarely the carcinoma arises in the trachea or main bronchi just distal to the carina and is situated within the middle mediastinum. If the neoplasm extends outward into the paratracheal space, it may widen the mediastinum to either side. An irregular, shaggy mass usually is evident within the tracheal air column on standard radiographs or CT scans. A similar appearance can be caused by other primary tracheal neoplasms and by endotracheal metastases.

Aorticopulmonary Paraganglioma

Paragangliomas (chemodectomas) arise from small collections of neuroendocrine cells (paraganglia) in intimate

Table 22–2. MIDDLE-POSTERIOR MEDIASTINAL MASSES

Etiology	Radiographic Manifestations	CT Findings
Developmental		
Bronchogenic cyst	Round or oval, well-defined contour	Approximately 50% of cysts have water density and 50% have soft tissue attenuation. MR imaging shows homogeneous high signal intensity on T2-weighted images
Diverticula of the pharynx	Cystlike structure	Often have heterogeneous attenuation owing to the presence of air, food, and secretions
Infectious		
Fibrosing mediastinitis	Lobulated contour. May show calcification	May show compression of superior vena cava and collateral circulation; calcification highly suggestive of previous histoplasmosis
Acute mediastinitis	Symmetric or localized widening	Obliteration of fat planes; areas of low attenuation suggest abscess formation
Neoplastic		
Thyroid goiter and neoplasms	Smooth or lobulated contour. Extend above thoracic inlet. Calcification fairly common	Lesion can be seen to arise from thyroid gland; goiters typically have high attenuation and marked enhancement with intraveanous contrast material; often with calcification; malignant tumors may have homogeneous or heterogeneous soft tissue attenuation
Primary tracheal neoplasms	Smooth or lobulated contour	Airway narrowing and peritracheal tumor extension
Hodgkin's disease and non-Hodgkin's lymphoma	Symmetrically widened mediastinum, lobulated contour	Mediastinal lymph node enlargement; may have homogeneous or heterogeneous attenuation and contain cystic areas
Metastatic carcinoma	Lobulated contour	Mediastinal lymph node enlargement
Esophageal neoplasms	Smooth, rounded margin	Abnormalities can include focal esophageal thickening, extensive soft tissue infiltration, or, less commonly, a large focal mass
Cardiovascular		
Aortic aneurysm	Fusiform or saccular contour. Calcification may be present in wall	CT and MR imaging are diagnostic
Buckling or aneurysm of the innominate artery	Smooth, lateral bulging, convex laterally from level of aortic arch upward	CT and MR imaging are diagnostic
Superior vena cava dilation	Smooth contour extending along right paramediastinal border	CT and MR imaging are diagnostic
Azygos dilation	Smooth, round, or oval mass at tracheobronchial angle	CT and MR imaging are diagnostic
Dilation of pulmonary artery	Smooth contour	CT and MR imaging are diagnostic
Traumatic		
Mediastinal hemorrhage or hematoma	Focal or diffuse mediastinal widening	Contrast-enhanced CT diagnostic for aortic dissection; angiography may be required to diagnose traumatic tear of the aorta or great vessels
Miscellaneous causes		
Mediastinal lipomatosis	Smooth and symmetric widening of mediastinum. Enlargement of pleuropericardial fat pads	Fatty infiltration of the mediastinum; CT diagnostic but seldom required
Esophageal hiatus hernia	Retrocardiac mass of variable size containing air	CT diagnostic but seldom required
Megaesophagus	Broad vertical opacity on the right side of the mediastinum. Air in lumen with fluid level at varying distance from diaphragm	CT diagnostic but seldom required
Bochdalek's hernia	Round or oval retrocardiac or paravertebral density	CT diagnostic; shows discontinuity of diaphragm and herniation of omental fat and, less commonly in the adult, abdominal viscera

association with the autonomic nervous system. In the thorax, they generally develop in one of two locations:[315] (1) the perivascular adventitial tissue bounded by the aorta superiorly, the pulmonary artery inferiorly, and the ligamentum arteriosum and right pulmonary artery on either side (aorticopulmonary paragangliomas), and (2) in association with the ganglia of the sympathetic chain in the paravertebral region adjacent to the posterior aspects of the ribs (paravertebral paragangliomas). Tumors are occasionally multiple within and outside the thorax. Clinically, most aorticopulmonary paragangliomas do not induce symptoms and are discovered on screening chest radiograph.

Radiographic features of aorticopulmonary paragangliomas are those of a mass in the mediastinum in close relation to the base of the heart and aortic arch.[316] Occasional tumors are located in the subcarinal region[317, 318] or

extend into the paratracheal soft tissue (Fig. 22–43). CT shows a soft tissue mass that can have homogeneous attenuation or can contain large central areas of low attenuation as a result of necrosis.[317, 318, 320] Tumors usually show marked enhancement after intravenous administration of contrast material.[318–320] Use of contrast agents is essential in the identification of these tumors, particularly when they are located within the pericardium; in one investigation of eight such tumors, six were missed on unenhanced CT scans, whereas all eight were evident after intravenous administration of contrast material.[318]

On MR studies, paragangliomas have signal intensity that is hypointense or isointense to muscle on T1-weighted images and hyperintense on T2-weighted images.[318] Areas of signal void may be seen on T1-weighted images as a result of flowing blood.[317] Angiography shows multiple

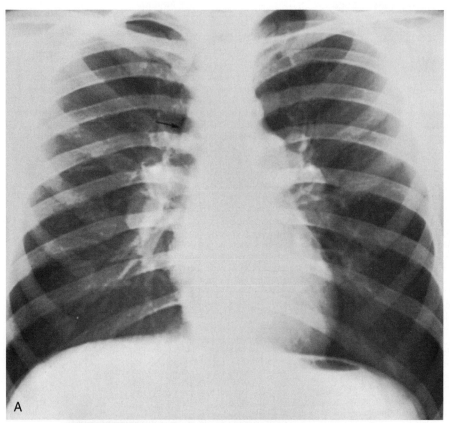

A

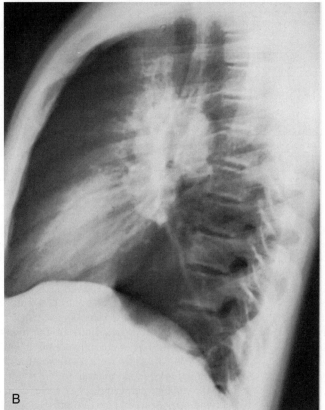

B

Figure 22–39. Hilar and Mediastinal Lymph Node Enlargement: Sarcoidosis. Posteroanterior *(A)* and lateral *(B)* chest radiographs show enlargement of both hila as a result of enlarged lymph nodes; the lobulated contour is particularly well shown in lateral projection. Bilateral paratracheal (middle mediastinal) and tracheobronchial lymph node enlargement is present; the azygos lymph node is clearly visible in posteroanterior projection *(arrow)*. The lungs are clear.

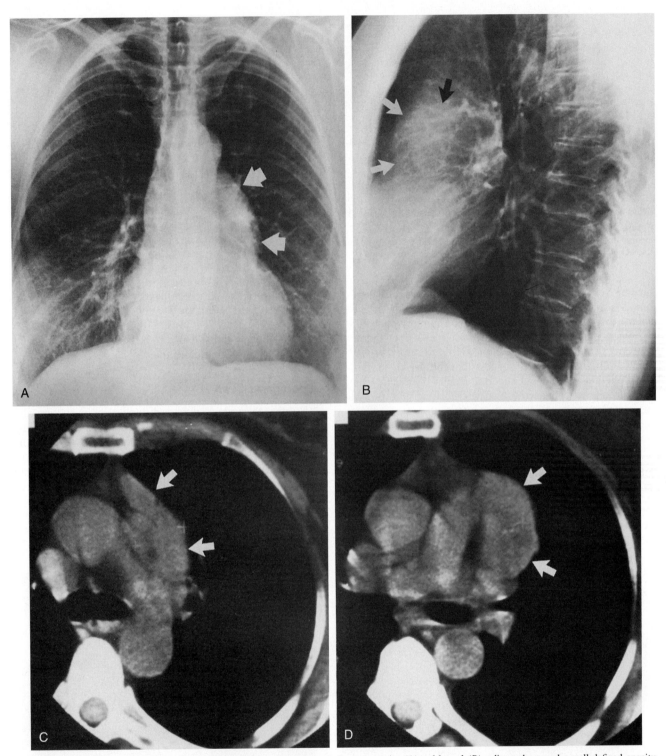

Figure 22–40. Giant Lymph Node Hyperplasia (Castleman's Disease). Posteroanterior *(A)* and lateral *(B)* radiographs reveal a well-defined opacity protruding to the left from the region of the main pulmonary artery *(arrows in A)*. In the lateral projection, an ill-defined opacity can be identified in the anterior mediastinum *(arrows)*. CT scans at the level of the aortopulmonary window *(C)* and main pulmonary artery *(D)* show a well-defined, homogeneous mass *(arrows)* contiguous with the left side of the mediastinum and protruding into the left hemithorax. The patient was a 63-year-old woman who had no symptoms referable to the chest.

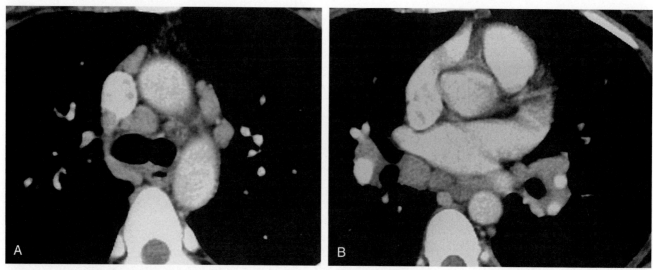

Figure 22–41. Multicentric Castleman's Disease. Contrast-enhanced CT scans *(A and B)* from a 44-year-old woman show enlarged mediastinal and bilateral hilar lymph nodes. The diagnosis of Castleman's disease was proved by lymph node biopsy. (Courtesy of Dr. Takeshi Johkoh, Department of Radiology, Osaka University Medical School, Osaka, Japan.)

feeding vessels, hypervascularity, and homogeneous capillary blush.[320] Scintigraphy is the imaging modality of choice to confirm the diagnosis.[318, 321] Approximately 90% of tumors show abnormal uptake on iodine-131 or iodine-123 metaiodobenzylguanidine (MIBG) scintigraphy.[318, 321, 322] Preliminary reports suggest that the use of indium-111 octreotide may yield superior results.[323, 324] The main role of contrast-enhanced CT or MR imaging is in providing detailed assessment of the extent of tumor and its relationship to adjacent structures before surgical resection.[318]

Cysts

Bronchogenic Cyst

Congenital bronchogenic cysts of the mediastinum are described in detail in Chapter 4 and are reviewed only

briefly here. Although these cysts can occur anywhere in the mediastinum, most are located in the paratracheal or subcarinal region.[303] They usually are discovered in children or young adults but can be seen as an incidental finding at autopsy in elderly individuals.

Esophageal Cyst

Esophageal cysts (esophageal duplication cysts) are distinguished from bronchogenic cysts pathologically by the presence of a double layer of smooth muscle in the walls and a lack of cartilage. They usually are located within or adjacent to the wall of the esophagus. Many patients are asymptomatic, the abnormality sometimes being discovered incidentally at an advanced age.[328]

The CT findings consist of a round mass of homogeneous water density or soft tissue density that does not

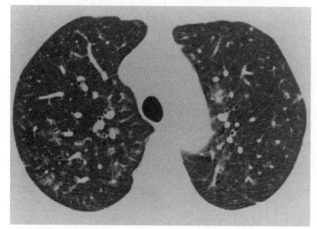

Figure 22–42. Multicentric Castleman's Disease. HRCT scan from a 43-year-old woman with multicentric Castleman's disease shows mild bilateral peribronchial and perivascular interstitial thickening and poorly defined centrilobular nodular opacities. Open-lung biopsy showed an extensive infiltrate of plasma cells localized predominantly in the peribronchovascular interstitial tissue. A scalene lymph node excised 2 years previously had shown plasma cell–type giant lymph node hyperplasia.

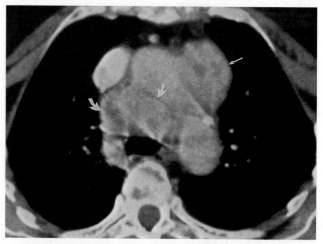

Figure 22–43. Aorticopulmonary Paraganglioma. Contrast-enhanced CT scan shows an inhomogeneous soft tissue mass involving the aortopulmonary window *(straight arrow)* and paratracheal region *(curved arrows)*. The patient was a 68-year-old woman who had surgically proven middle mediastinal paraganglioma.

enhance after intravenous administration of contrast material (Fig. 22–44).[87, 325] On MR studies, the cysts can have low or high signal intensity on T1-weighted images but characteristically have homogeneous high signal intensity on T2-weighted images.[87, 327] The CT findings and MR signal characteristics are indistinguishable from those of bronchogenic cysts (Fig. 22–45). Transesophageal ultrasonography has been used successfully in diagnosis.[328]

Pancreatic Pseudocyst

Pancreatic pseudocysts are encapsulated collections of pancreatic secretions often containing blood and necrotic

material.[326] Most occur in patients who have acute or chronic pancreatitis and are located in the peripancreatic tissue. Occasionally a lesion extends into the posterior mediastinum through the esophageal or aortic hiatus.[326, 329, 501] Usually the cysts are of water density on CT scans (Fig. 22–46); however, hemorrhage or infection can result in areas of soft tissue attenuation.[326] The diagnosis usually can be made on CT by showing continuity with pancreatic or peripancreatic fluid collections.[326, 501]

Thoracic Duct Cyst

Thoracic duct cyst is a rare type of middle-posterior mediastinal mass that can occur anywhere from the thoracic

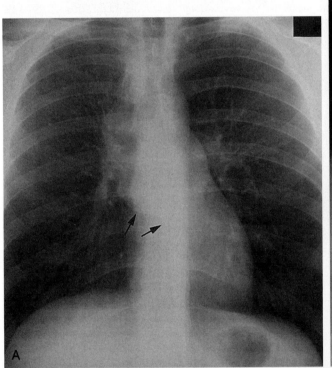
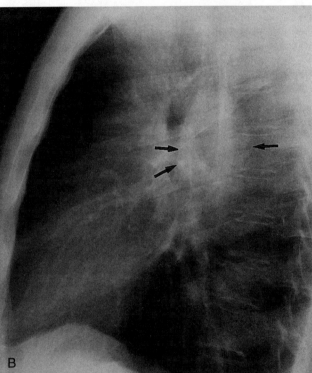
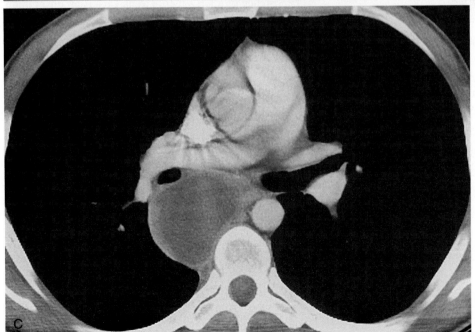

Figure 22–44. Esophageal Duplication Cyst. Posteroanterior chest radiograph *(A)* from a 22-year-old man shows a subcarinal mass displacing the azygoesophageal recess interface *(arrows)*. Lateral radiograph *(B)* shows the mass posterior to the bronchus intermedius *(arrows)*. CT scan obtained after intravenous administration of contrast material *(C)* shows a nonenhancing cystic mass adjacent to the esophagus. The lesion was proved surgically to be an esophageal duplication cyst.

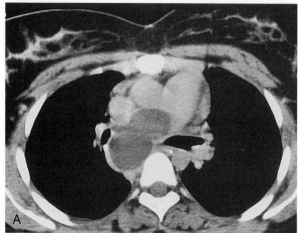
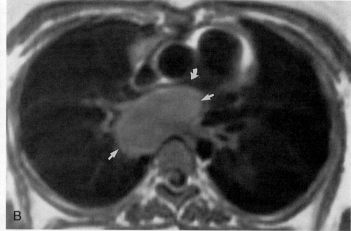
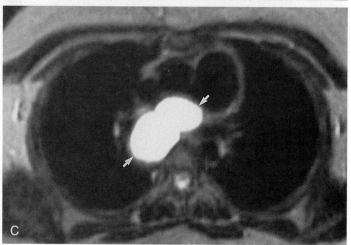

Figure 22–45. Middle and Posterior Mediastinal Bronchogenic Cyst. Contrast-enhanced CT scan from a 26-year-old woman *(A)* shows a dumbbell-shaped mass with inhomogeneous low attenuation in the subcarinal region. The lesion has middle and posterior mediastinal components and compresses the proximal right pulmonary artery. The attenuation values within the mass were greater than 20 HU. A transverse T1-weighted (TR/TE, 645/20) MR image *(B)* shows a slightly inhomogeneous mass *(straight arrows)* with a signal intensity similar to that of chest wall muscle. There is marked narrowing of the right pulmonary artery *(curved arrow)*. Transverse T2-weighted (TR/TE, 2,581/90) spin-echo MR image *(C)* shows homogeneous high signal intensity *(arrows)* characteristic of fluid. At surgery, this was shown to be a mediastinal bronchogenic cyst associated with a partial pericardial defect.

inlet to the diaphragm and can communicate with the thoracic duct superiorly or inferiorly.[330, 331] The diagnosis can be suggested by appearance on lymphangiography[331, 332] and by analysis of fluid obtained by fluoroscopically or CT-guided needle aspiration.[333, 335]

Vascular Abnormalities

Dilation of the Main Pulmonary Artery

Dilation of the main pulmonary artery may be of sufficient degree to suggest a mediastinal mass.[334] Most cases are associated with pulmonary arterial hypertension or left-to-right shunt; some are related to pulmonary valve stenosis,[334] pulmonary artery banding,[334] infection, or vasculitis (typically Behçet's disease) *(see page 302)*.

On posteroanterior chest radiograph, dilation of the main pulmonary artery results in a focal convexity caudad to the aortic arch and cephalad to the left main bronchus (Fig. 22–47). It usually is accompanied by dilation of the pulmonary trunk and enlargement of the right ventricle, findings that are apparent most readily on lateral radiograph.

Dilation of the Mediastinal Veins

Superior Vena Cava

Most cases of dilation of the superior vena cava are the result of raised central venous pressure, most commonly

from cardiac decompensation; rare causes include tricuspid valvular stenosis and cardiac tamponade secondary to pericardial effusion or constrictive pericarditis. The radiographic appearance is distinctive, consisting of a smooth, well-defined widening of the right side of the mediastinum.

Persistence of a left superior vena cava is an uncommon anomaly that occurs in about 0.3% of normal individuals and in 4.4% of patients who have congenital heart disease. Radiographically it results in a straight-edged shadow on the left side of the mediastinum that overlies the aortic arch and proximal descending aorta;[336] drainage is usually via the coronary sinus. The diagnosis can be confirmed by CT,[338–340] MR imaging,[337] or transesophageal echocardiography.[341] The right superior vena cava often is decreased in size;[337, 342] in approximately 15% of cases, it is absent.[337, 338]

Superior Vena Cava Syndrome

Superior vena cava syndrome is characterized clinically by edema of the face, neck, upper extremities, and thorax, often associated with prominent, dilated chest wall veins. It is caused by external compression or intraluminal thrombosis or neoplastic infiltration of the vena cava; frequently a combination of all three processes is involved.[343] In most published series, the cause is malignancy in 95% or more of cases;[344–346] pulmonary carcinoma is the cause in 80% to 85% and lymphoma and metastatic carcinoma of nonpulmonary origin in 5% to 10%.

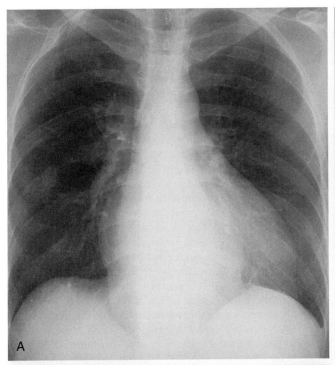

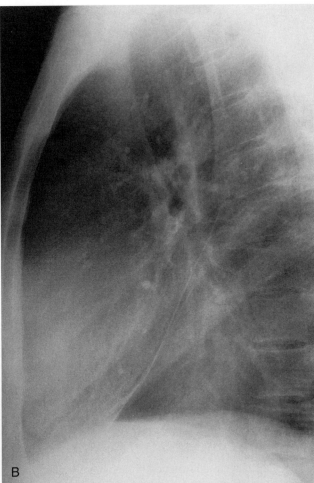

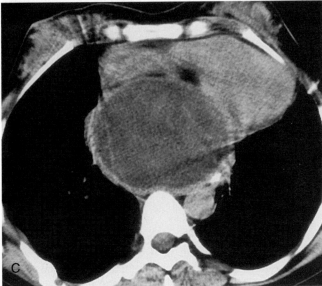

Figure 22–46. Pancreatic Pseudocyst. Posteroanterior *(A)* and lateral *(B)* chest radiographs from a 34-year-old woman show widening of the posterior mediastinum. CT scan *(C)* shows a large cystic mass with smooth walls. The lesion subsequently was shown to be a pancreatic pseudocyst. (Courtesy of Dr. Michael Lefcoe, Department of Radiology, Victoria Hospital, London, Ontario, Canada.)

Although precise figures are not available, it is possible that the most common benign abnormality causing superior vena cava syndrome today is the insertion of intravenous devices such as cardiac pacemakers[347, 348] and Hickman catheters.[349] The pathogenesis of the obstruction in these cases presumably is thrombosis and (after thrombus organization) fibrosis. The most common noniatrogenic benign disorder causing superior vena cava syndrome is probably fibrosing mediastinitis.[345, 350]

In most cases, chest radiograph shows a mass widening the mediastinum on the right; a prominent azygos vein may be evident (Fig. 22–48). In patients who develop superior vena cava thrombosis related to indwelling central venous catheters, radiographs commonly show lateral displacement of the catheter.[351] The diagnosis can be confirmed by CT,[352–354] MR imaging,[355, 493] or venography.[346]

With CT, it is based on decreased or absent opacification of the superior vena cava and the presence of opacification of collateral veins after the intravenous administration of contrast agents (Fig. 22–49).[352, 353] Both findings need to be present to make a definitive diagnosis because opacification of collateral vessels is seen in about 5% of patients who do not have superior vena cava obstruction.[353]

Azygos and Hemiazygos Veins

Dilation of the azygos and hemiazygos veins usually results from elevated central venous pressure secondary to cardiac decompensation. Other causes of elevated right-sided pressure, such as tricuspid stenosis, acute pericardial tamponade, or constrictive pericarditis, are less frequent. Additional causes of dilation include intrahepatic and extra-

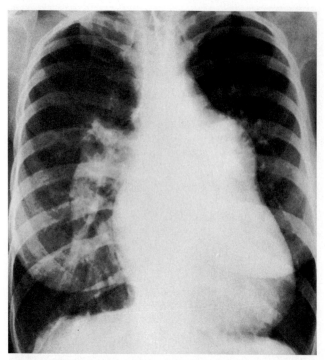

Figure 22–47. Dilation of Main Pulmonary Artery. Posteroanterior chest radiograph shows dilation of the hilar and peripheral pulmonary arteries, indicating pulmonary pleonemia. The main pulmonary artery is greatly dilated, creating a smooth protuberance of the left border of the cardiovascular silhouette. The patient was known to have a patent ductus arteriosus.

hepatic portal vein obstruction,[448] anomalous pulmonary venous drainage, acquired occlusion of the inferior or superior vena cava,[449] and azygos continuation (infrahepatic interruption) of the inferior vena cava.[450]

Radiographically, dilation of the azygos vein is manifested by a round or oval shadow in the right tracheobronchial angle greater than 10 mm in diameter on radiographs exposed with the patient in the erect position (*see* Fig. 22–48).[89] In one study of 54 patients 23 to 77 years old, a vein diameter greater than 15 mm as measured on anteroposterior chest radiograph obtained with the patient in the supine position corresponded to a central venous pressure greater than 10 cm H$_2$O.[356] In another investigation in 48 patients, none of whom had any lesion known to cause azygos vein enlargement, the mean diameter of the vein was 14 mm when the patient was in the supine position.[357] Measurements exceeding 10 mm on radiographs obtained when the patient was in the erect position or exceeding 15 mm when the patient was in the supine position indicated increase in either pressure or flow. A dilated azygos vein can be differentiated from an enlarged azygos lymph node fairly easily by comparing the diameters of the shadow on radiographs exposed in the erect and supine positions: When the shadow is the vein, there is a noticeable difference in size.

Dilation of the posterior portions of the azygos or hemiazygos vein may result in widening and irregularity of the paraspinal line on the right or left side.[358, 359] Extreme tortuosity of a dilated azygos arch may simulate a pulmonary mass on lateral chest radiograph.[360] The normal anatomy of the azygos and hemiazygos veins and their abnormalities are well visualized by CT (see Fig. 22–48)[354, 361, 362] and MR imaging.[337, 355]

Left Superior Intercostal Vein

Dilation of the left superior intercostal vein has the same causes as those associated with dilation of the azygos vein, although visibility of this vein radiographically is not as frequent as that of the azygos vein. The normal left superior intercostal vein originates from a confluence of the second, third, and fourth left intercostal veins. As it passes anteriorly from the spine, it relates intimately to some portion of the aortic arch and in this location is seen end-on as the *aortic nipple*, a local protuberance in the contour of the arch that is identifiable in about 10% of normal individuals.[363] On posteroanterior radiograph taken with the patient in an erect position, the maximum normal diameter of the aortic nipple is 4.5 mm.[364] A diameter greater than 4.5 mm is a useful sign of circulatory abnormalities, the most common of which are azygos continuation of the inferior vena cava, hypoplasia of the left innominate vein, cardiac decompensation, portal hypertension, Budd-Chiari syndrome, obstruction of the superior or inferior vena cava (Fig. 22-50),[364] and congenital absence of the azygos vein.[365]

Abnormalities of the Aorta and Its Branches

Aneurysms of the Thoracic Aorta

The normal diameter of the aorta is 3.7 ± 0.3 cm at the level of its root, 3.3 ± 0.6 cm at the ascending portion, and 2.4 ± 0.3 cm at the descending portion.[366] An aneurysm is considered to be present when the diameter is 5 cm or greater. Aneurysms can be classified according to the composition of their wall, their location, or their shape. The wall of a true aneurysm is composed of intima, media, and adventitia, whereas the wall of a false aneurysm (pseudoaneurysm) is composed of fibrous tissue, compressed blood clot, or both.

Most true thoracic aortic aneurysms are the result of atherosclerosis and occur in the descending portion.[367, 370] They usually are fusiform, start immediately distal to the takeoff of the left subclavian artery, and often extend into the abdomen.[369, 370] Such aneurysms typically are seen in elderly persons and are more common in men.[370, 371] Aneurysms of the ascending aorta are less common and can be the result of atherosclerosis, cystic medial degeneration (cystic medial necrosis), or, rarely, infection (mycotic aneurysm).[368, 370] Cystic medial degeneration is the most common pathologic finding associated with aneurysms of the ascending aorta.[368, 372] The abnormality can be idiopathic or associated with a connective tissue disorder, such as Marfan's syndrome or Ehlers-Danlos syndrome.[370, 372] Most mycotic aneurysms are true aneurysms;[370] predisposing conditions include bacterial endocarditis, drug abuse, atherosclerosis, and immunosuppression.[370, 373]

False aneurysms most often are the result of blunt trauma and usually are eccentric or saccular in shape.[369, 370] Such aneurysms typically are located in the proximal descending thoracic aorta just beyond the origin of the left subclavian artery. Occasionally a false aneurysm follows

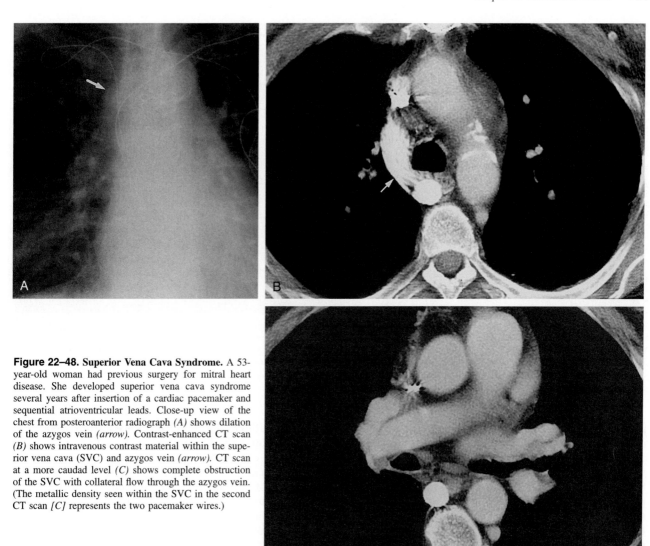

Figure 22–48. Superior Vena Cava Syndrome. A 53-year-old woman had previous surgery for mitral heart disease. She developed superior vena cava syndrome several years after insertion of a cardiac pacemaker and sequential atrioventricular leads. Close-up view of the chest from posteroanterior radiograph *(A)* shows dilation of the azygos vein *(arrow)*. Contrast-enhanced CT scan *(B)* shows intravenous contrast material within the superior vena cava (SVC) and azygos vein *(arrow)*. CT scan at a more caudad level *(C)* shows complete obstruction of the SVC with collateral flow through the azygos vein. (The metallic density seen within the SVC in the second CT scan *[C]* represents the two pacemaker wires.)

Figure 22–49. Superior Vena Cava Syndrome. Contrast-enhanced CT scan shows extensive mediastinal lymphadenopathy, lack of opacification of the superior vena cava, and extensive collateral venous circulation in the chest wall *(arrows)* and mediastinum. The patient was a 61-year-old man who had extensive mediastinal metastases from pulmonary carcinoma.

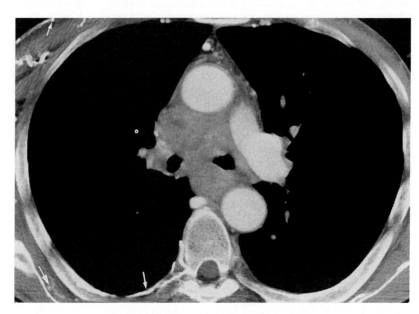

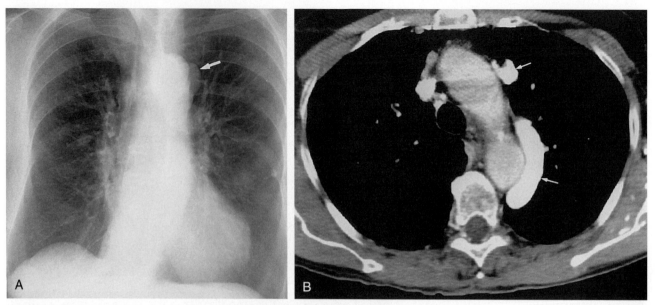

Figure 22–50. Enlarged Left Superior Intercostal Vein. Posteroanterior chest radiograph *(A)* shows a prominent aortic nipple *(arrow)*. (Incidental note is made of a calcified granuloma in the left lung.) Contrast-enhanced CT scan *(B)* shows a dilated left superior intercostal vein *(arrows)* resulting from collateral blood flow from the left brachiocephalic vein into the hemiazygos and azygos veins. Collateral blood flow in the left axilla is visible. The patient was a 77-year-old woman who had long-standing superior vena cava obstruction related to fibrosing mediastinitis (presumed to be due to histoplasmosis). Note calcified paratracheal lymph nodes.

penetrating trauma or iatrogenic injury; rarely, it is associated with tuberculosis.[369, 370, 374]

Many patients are asymptomatic. Clinical manifestations vary according to the size and location of the aneurysm. Symptoms caused by aneurysms of the transverse arch are particularly notable and result from compression of the superior vena cava, recurrent laryngeal nerve, or tracheobronchial tree. Symptoms include a brassy cough, hemoptysis, and hoarseness.

On chest radiograph, aneurysms of the ascending aorta and proximal aortic arch usually project anteriorly and to the right, whereas those of the distal arch and descending aorta project posteriorly and to the left (Fig. 22–51). Aortic aneurysms should be considered in the differential diagnosis for any abnormal opacity that is contiguous with any part of the aorta. Calcification of the aneurysm wall is relatively common.

The diagnosis can be confirmed using CT (Fig. 22–52),[375, 376] MR imaging (Fig. 22–53),[377, 378, 502] transesophageal echocardiography,[379] or angiography. Contrast-enhanced CT currently is the most commonly used technique. Spiral CT, particularly with multidetector arrays, allows excellent visualization of the aorta with relatively small doses of iodinated contrast material.[502] CT allows accurate assessment of the presence and extent of the aneurysm; its relationship to adjacent structures; and the presence of complications such as compression of the trachea, bronchi, or pulmonary arteries or veins and superior vena cava.[370, 380, 381] Foci of intimal calcification are seen on CT scans in approximately 75% of patients. Mural thrombus also frequently is evident, particularly in patients who have large aneurysms (Fig. 22–54).[370, 382]

Excellent anatomic assessment of the aorta is obtained by using spin-echo MR imaging with T1 weighting and electrocardiographic gating.[378] Spin-echo sequences are prone to artifacts, however, secondary to slow blood flow, and alternative techniques, such as cine gradient-echo and cine phase-contrast MR imaging, may be required to distinguish such artifacts from mural thrombus.[378] Optimal visualization of the aorta on MR imaging is obtained using intravenous contrast material, three-dimensional reconstructions, and cardiac gating and by performing the scan during breath-hold.[494, 502]

Aortic Dissection

Aortic dissection occurs when blood collects in the media and divides it into two distinct layers. In most patients, the primary event is an intimal tear.[383, 384] Because it is under high pressure, the blood cleaves a channel in the media, resulting in the formation of a second (false) lumen for blood flow.[385] Such dissection can proceed proximal and distal to the entry site. As it progresses, it may be associated with multiple tears in the intima, leading to additional entry and exit sites. Occasionally, dissection occurs as a result of bleeding from the vasa vasorum into the media and is followed by a tear of the intima.[384] In a few cases, rupture of the vasa vasorum results in thickening of the aortic wall without intimal rupture.[386]

The most widely accepted classification of aortic dissection is the Stanford system, which designates dissections involving the ascending aorta as type A, regardless of the distal extension of the dissection, and all other types of dissection as type B. Depending on the series, about 55% to 90% of dissections are type A.[387–389] They can extend into the perivalvular region and result in aortic insufficiency,[390] extend to and occlude the branches of the aortic arch,[390] or rupture into the pericardial sac and cause tamponade.[391]

Aortic dissection is seen most commonly in patients

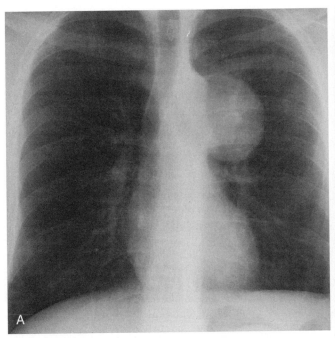

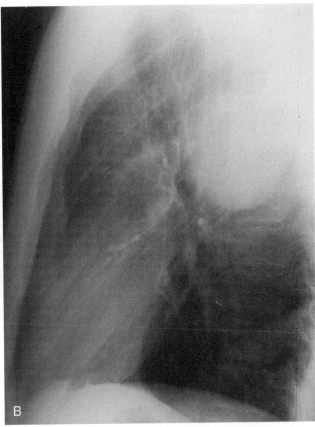

Figure 22–51. Mycotic Aneurysm of the Proximal Descending Thoracic Aorta. Posteroanterior *(A)* and lateral *(B)* radiographs from a 22-year-old man show a well-circumscribed mass abutting the aorta and projecting posteriorly and to the left. The lesion was proved surgically to be mycotic aneurysm.

who have systemic arterial hypertension; less common causes include Ehlers-Danlos syndrome, Marfan's syndrome, aortitis, and vascular catheterization.[383, 392] In many cases, cystic medial degeneration is evident in the aortic wall. Because most patients are older, atherosclerosis often is present; however, it is more likely to be a coincidental finding than a significant contributing factor in the dissec-

tion. Dissection most commonly involves the ascending aorta, in which atherosclerosis tends to be relatively mild, and dissections rarely begin in the lower abdominal aorta, where arteriosclerosis is common and often severe.[393]

The diagnosis of aortic dissection usually is suggested by the clinical history.[403] Typically the onset is sudden and associated with severe pain, which may be described as

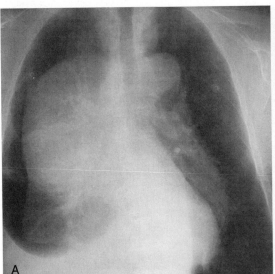

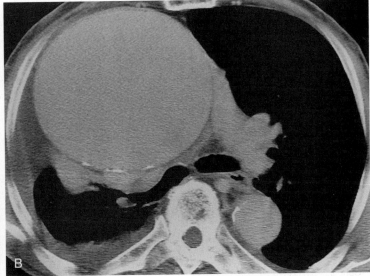

Figure 22–52. Aneurysm of the Aorta. Posteroanterior chest radiograph *(A)* from an 86-year-old man shows a large homogeneous opacity in the right upper mediastinum. CT scan performed without intravenous contrast material *(B)* shows an aneurysm of the ascending thoracic aorta measuring 11 cm in diameter. Note focal intimal calcification in the ascending and descending thoracic aorta and the presence of small bilateral pleural effusions.

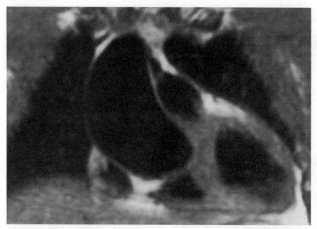

Figure 22–53. Aneurysm of the Ascending Aorta. Coronal cardiac-gated MR image shows a 5-cm-diameter ascending aortic aneurysm that showed cystic medial *necrosis* on histologic examination. The patient was a 28-year-old man.

tearing or ripping in nature and often radiates to the throat, jaw, back, or abdomen as the dissection extends from its point of origin.

The most common radiographic manifestations are widening of the superior mediastinum and aorta, a double contour of the aortic arch, increase in size of the aorta or change in configuration on serial chest radiographs, and displacement of a calcified plaque by 10 mm or more.[369, 384] Enlargement of the aorta is a nonspecific finding seen in many patients who have systemic arterial hypertension or atherosclerosis. Acute enlargement on serial chest radiographs should raise the possibility of dissection, however.[385] A normal configuration of the aorta does not exclude the diagnosis because it is seen in approximately 25% of patients.[384, 394] Displacement of intimal calcification also is not a reliable diagnostic finding:[384, 391] The lateral border of the visualized aorta may not be at the same level as that of the calcified plaque, mimicking displacement of the calcification;[384, 391] in addition, other processes, such as accumulation of fat or a neoplasm, can simulate the appearance of aortic wall thickening.[391] Because of the equivocal significance of these features, plain chest radiograph is of limited value in the diagnosis of aortic dissection. In one investigation of 75 patients, the diagnosis of aortic dissection or thoracic aortic aneurysm was suggested prospectively based on the findings on chest radiograph in only 19 (25%);[395] retrospective analysis of chest radiographs showed that only 36 patients (48%) had abnormalities suggestive of dissection.

CT is a rapid and relatively noninvasive method for diagnosing acute aortic dissection. The diagnostic accuracy using dynamic or spiral CT technique after intravenous administration of contrast material in various studies ranged from 88% to 100%.[389, 396, 397] The accuracy of CT is influenced by technique and the type of scanner used. In one investigation of 110 patients who had clinically suspected dissection and in whom the final diagnosis was proved by contrast angiography, intraoperative inspection, or autopsy, conventional CT had a sensitivity of 94% and a specificity of 87%.[389] In another investigation of 49 patients, spiral CT had an accuracy of 100%.[397] Current spiral CT technology, particularly with multidetector array scanners, should have an accuracy approaching 100% in detecting aortic dissection.[502]

The characteristic CT findings consist of a linear filling defect (intimal flap) and the presence of a false lumen (Fig. 22–55). The true and false lumens have differential enhancement on CT scans, the former showing greater enhancement than the latter. Another sign of dissection is increased attenuation of the thrombosed false lumen or of the aortic wall.[384, 391] Such increased attenuation is present in the acute phase and decreases gradually as the hematoma resolves.[391] Although acute dissection characteristically is associated with central displacement of intimal calcification, this finding is not diagnostic. In one study of 136

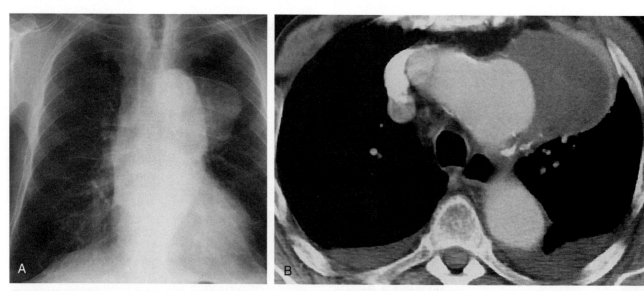

Figure 22–54. Aneurysm of the Aorta. Posteroanterior chest radiograph *(A)* from an 87-year-old man shows a homogeneous soft tissue opacity abutting the proximal descending thoracic aorta. Contrast-enhanced CT scan *(B)* shows a focal saccular aneurysm involving the proximal descending thoracic aorta and containing a large mural thrombus. Small bilateral pleural effusions are evident. The aneurysm was proved to be secondary to atherosclerosis.

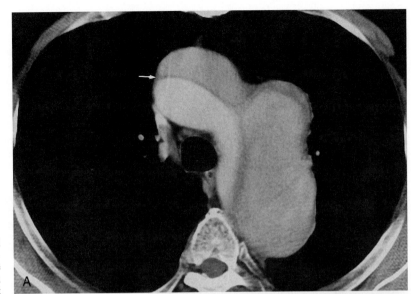

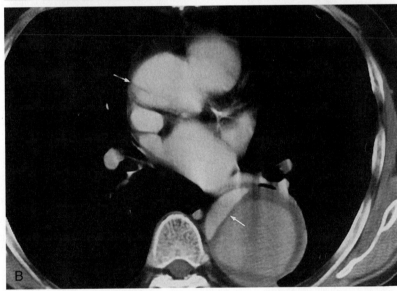

Figure 22–55. Aortic Dissection. Contrast-enhanced CT scan at the level of the aortic arch *(A)* from a 57-year-old man shows marked enhancement of the true aortic lumen and poor enhancement of the false lumen of the dissection. The presence of a linear filling defect (intimal flap) *(arrows)* separates the true from the false lumen. CT scan at a more caudad level *(B)* shows that the dissection involves the ascending aorta (type A), which is of normal caliber; the descending thoracic aorta shows aneurysmal dilation. The patient had systemic arterial hypertension.

patients, it was seen in 33 (24%) who had an aortic aneurysm unassociated with dissection;[398] the abnormality in such cases is the result of calcification of thrombus within the aneurysm. False-negative or false-positive diagnoses based on CT appearance can result from insufficient contrast enhancement or from motion artifacts.[384, 391, 502]

MR imaging is comparable to CT in the evaluation of patients who have suspected aortic dissection (Fig. 22–56).[389, 391, 397] The diagnosis usually can be made using conventional spin-echo MR technique with electrocardiographic gating and T1 weighting; however, slow flow of blood within the false lumen may mimic intramural thrombus on spin-echo MR imaging.[378] The distinction can be made using gradient-echo MR imaging, cine phase-contrast imaging, or gadolinium-enhanced MR angiography.[378]

Transthoracic echocardiography is a rapid, noninvasive method for assessment of the ascending aorta but does not provide adequate visualization of the aortic arch and descending aorta. Better assessment of these regions can be obtained using transesophageal echocardiography. In

one study of 110 patients who had clinically suspected dissection of the thoracic aorta, the sensitivity for detecting dissection was similar for CT, MR imaging, and transesophageal echocardiography (98%, 98%, and 94%) but was considerably lower for transthoracic echocardiography (59%).[389] The specificity for transthoracic (83%) and transesophageal echocardiography (77%) was lower than that for contrast-enhanced CT (87%) or MR imaging (98%). Echocardiography should be limited to the assessment of patients who are too unstable to be moved.

For many years, angiography was considered the imaging modality of choice in the diagnosis of aortic dissection.[399, 400] The procedure has several limitations, however, including the time required to assemble the angiography team, its invasiveness, and its relatively low sensitivity (about 80% to 90%).[400–402] False-negative angiograms can result from lack of visualization of the intimal flap, poor opacification of the false lumen, or thrombosis of the false lumen.[391, 400] Because of these limitations, angiography has been replaced by CT and MRI.

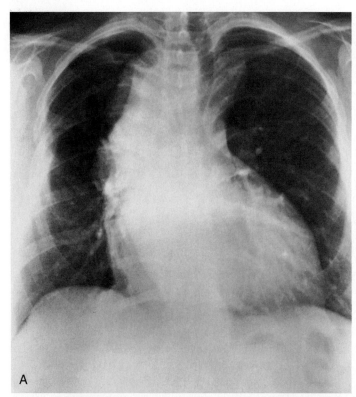

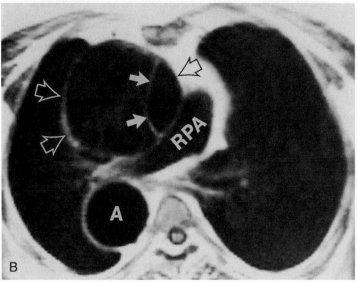

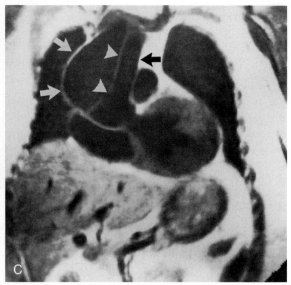

Figure 22–56. Dissection of the Ascending Aorta in a Patient with a Right Aortic Arch. Posteroanterior radiograph *(A)* reveals evidence of a former right thoracotomy that had been performed many years previously for repair of a coarctation and aortic valvotomy. The trachea is deviated markedly to the left by a right-sided aortic arch. The width of the aorta at the point of maximal tracheal displacement is greater than normal. T1-weighted MR image in transverse section *(B)* at the level of the right pulmonary artery (RPA) shows a markedly dilated ascending aorta *(open arrows)*. Situated within it is a curvilinear shadow *(arrows)* representing the intimal flap; the smaller area to the left of the flap is the true lumen, and the larger area to the right is the false lumen. The descending aorta *(A)* at this level is still on the right side. Coronal reconstruction *(C)* reveals the markedly dilated ascending aorta *(arrows)* containing the intimal flap *(arrowheads)*; the true lumen is on the left, and the false lumen is on the right. The patient was a 27-year-old woman who had Turner's syndrome.

Buckling and Aneurysm of the Innominate Artery

Buckling and aneurysm of the innominate artery are manifested radiographically as a smooth, well-defined opacity in the right superior paramediastinal area, extending upward from the aortic arch. It is a relatively common condition that occurs in about 15% of patients who have hypertension, atherosclerosis, or both (Fig. 22–57).[404] Aneurysms are much less common.

Congenital Anomalies of the Aorta

Although most congenital malformations of the aortic arch become evident during the first year of life,[405] occa-

sional examples are not recognized until adulthood.[406, 407] A congenital aortic vascular ring results from persistence of the two aortic arches or of the right aortic arch and left ductus arteriosus; in a few patients, the right subclavian artery, also of anomalous origin, arises from the descending aorta.[408] The diagnosis can be made radiographically by the demonstration of a double aortic arch and of a vessel posterior to the esophagus. On frontal view, the trachea is midline; on lateral radiograph, the trachea is displaced posteriorly by the larger anterior arch. A specific diagnosis can be made using CT or MR imaging.[376, 378, 409] Symptoms result from compression of the trachea or esophagus and include shortness of breath, dysphagia, and those secondary to recurrent respiratory infections.

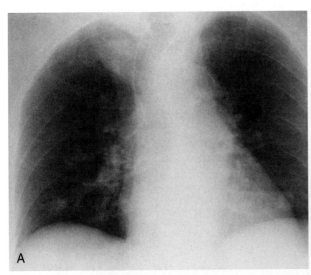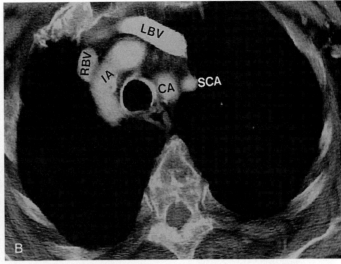

Figure 22–57. Buckling of the Innominate Artery. Anteroposterior chest radiograph *(A)* from an 86-year-old woman shows a focal opacity in the right superior paramediastinal area. Contrast-enhanced CT scan *(B)* shows that the opacity is the result of buckling of the innominate artery (IA). Contrast material is present in the left brachiocephalic vein (LBV), right brachiocephalic vein (RBV), left carotid artery (CA), and left subclavian artery (SCA).

Other congenital anomalies of the aorta that result in abnormalities of mediastinal contour include (1) pseudocoarctation of the aorta (Fig. 22–58), in which a left paramediastinal mass is visible just above the aortic arch as a result of elongation and buckling of the aorta;[410] (2) a cervical aortic arch, in which the aortic arch extends into the soft tissues of the neck before turning downward on itself to become the descending aorta;[411] (3) aortic diverticula;[412] and (4) the most common, a right aortic arch (Fig. 22–59).[413] The last-named is present in about 0.1% to 0.2% of the general population.[414] In approximately 70% of cases, there is an aberrant left subclavian artery.[414] Occasionally the abnormal arch compresses the trachea sufficiently to result in upper airway obstruction and a clinical picture that can be confused with asthma.[415]

In approximately 0.5% of individuals, a normal left aortic arch is associated with an aberrant right subclavian artery.[414] Occasionally, this vessel can be visualized as a soft tissue opacity, typically having an oblique course from left to right and extending cephalad from the aortic arch.[416] The proximal portion of the aberrant artery frequently is dilated, a finding known as a diverticulum of Kommerell (Fig. 22–60).[414, 417] The diagnosis can be confirmed using contrast-enhanced CT, MR imaging, or angiography.[409, 414]

Diseases of the Esophagus

Esophageal lesions that may present radiographically as mediastinal masses or as diffuse mediastinal widening include neoplasms, diverticula, hiatal hernia, and megaesophagus.

Neoplasms

Carcinoma. Although barium examination and esophagoscopy are the two definitive procedures in the diagnosis of primary carcinoma of the esophagus, conventional radiographs of the chest can provide clues to its presence.[418, 422]

In a review of 103 patients, significant abnormalities were found in 49.[418] The most frequent abnormalities included an abnormal azygoesophageal recess interface (27%), a widened mediastinum (18%), a posterior tracheal indentation or mass (16%), a widened retrotracheal stripe (11%), and tracheal deviation (10%). Less common abnormalities included deformity of the gastric air bubble, a retrocardiac mass, an esophageal fluid level, and a retrohilar mass. In another plain film study of 102 patients who had carcinoma of the middle third of the esophagus, 63 (62%) had thickening of the retrotracheal stripe, anterior bowing of the posterior wall of the trachea, or a combination of these findings.[419] Progressive thickening of the retrotracheal stripe has been shown to be a useful marker for recurrent esophageal carcinoma after surgery or radiation therapy.[420]

CT manifestations include esophageal wall thickening, proximal dilation, obscuration of the periesophageal fat planes, and periesophageal lymph node enlargement.[421, 422, 424] Although esophageal wall thickening is the earliest manifestation of carcinoma, it is not diagnostic. In one study of 200 consecutive CT examinations in which thickened esophageal walls (>3 mm) were found in 35%, esophageal carcinoma was identified as the cause in only half;[423] other causes included esophagitis, varices, and postirradiation scarring.

CT is helpful in the staging of esophageal carcinoma.[426, 427] The tumor may invade the adjacent mediastinal soft tissue, aorta, trachea, or bronchi and metastasize to mediastinal and upper abdominal lymph nodes, the lungs, and extrathoracic organs, most commonly the liver. Extension into mediastinal fat can be detected by the presence of increased periesophageal soft tissue density, often ill defined.[421] The assessment of aortic invasion using CT is based on the evaluation of the arc of contact between the esophageal mass and the aorta (in turn based on a 360-degree aortic circumference).[421] Some authors have considered an interface arc of less than 45 degrees as reliably excluding aortic invasion, an arc between 45 and 90 de-

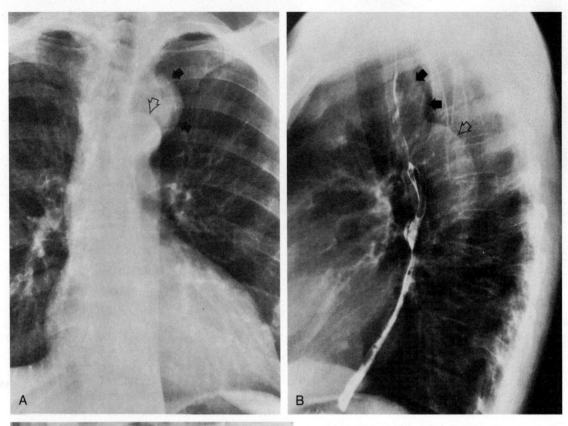

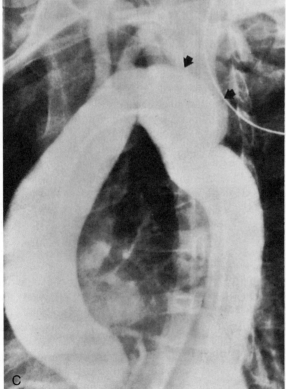

Figure 22–58. Pseudocoarctation of the Aorta. Posteroanterior view *(A)* of the chest of a 63-year-old asymptomatic woman reveals a homogeneous soft tissue opacity *(solid arrows)* that projects above the shadow of the aortic arch *(open arrow)*. In lateral projection *(B)*, the posterior aspect of the mass is identified by *solid arrows* and the posterior portion of the aortic arch by an *open arrow*. On the basis of this plain film evidence, the findings were thought to be compatible with pseudocoarctation of the aorta; however, an aortogram was performed for confirmation. In oblique projection *(C)*, this study confirms the fact that the abnormal opacity observed on plain radiograph is due to an unusually high aortic arch *(solid arrows)* that buckled in its descending portion so as to produce a prominent notch on its posterior and left lateral aspects.

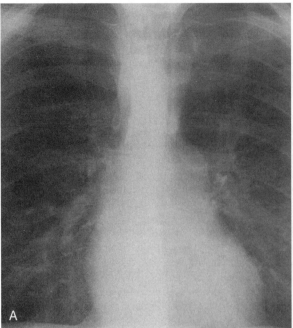

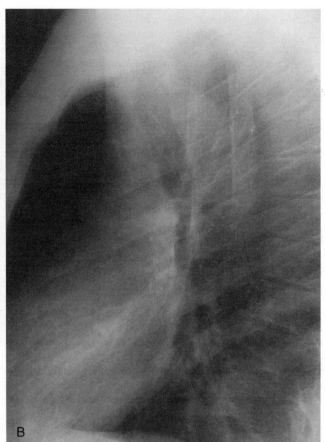

Figure 22–59. Right Aortic Arch. Close-up views from posteroanterior *(A)* and lateral *(B)* chest radiographs from a 33-year-old man show a right aortic arch causing smooth deviation of the trachea anteriorly and to the left. The patient was asymptomatic.

grees as indeterminate, and an arc greater than 90 degrees as highly suggestive of invasion;[425] however, use of these criteria is associated with many indeterminate cases.[421] As a result, other investigators have considered arcs less than 90 degrees as excluding invasion and arcs greater than 90 degrees as suggestive of it.[426, 428] Although several workers

have shown CT to have a high degree of accuracy in the assessment of aortic invasion,[425, 429, 499] others have found it to be considerably less accurate;[430, 431] the reported sensitivity of CT in the detection of aortic invasion ranged from 6% to 100%, the specificity from 52% to 96%, and the accuracy from 55% to 96%.[421]

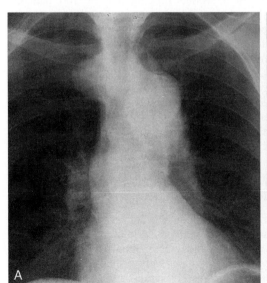

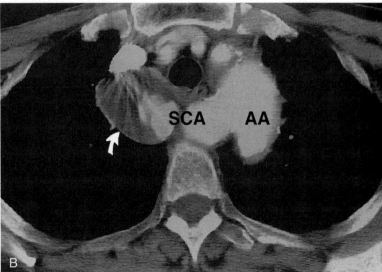

Figure 22–60. Diverticulum of Kommerell. Close-up view from posteroanterior chest radiograph *(A)* from a 74-year-old woman shows a soft tissue opacity in the superior mediastinum. Contrast-enhanced CT scan *(B)* shows the upper aspect of the aortic arch (AA) and the aberrant right subclavian artery (SCA). The proximal portion of the latter is ectatic (diverticulum of Kommerell) and contains thrombus *(curved arrow)*.

Findings suggestive of tracheobronchial invasion include posterior indentation of the airway and focal thickening of the airway wall. The reported sensitivity of CT in the detection of tracheobronchial involvement in various studies ranged from 31% to 100%, the specificity from 86% to 98%, and the accuracy from 74% to 97%.[421] Similarly, there has been considerable variation in the reported efficacy of CT in the detection of metastases to regional lymph nodes, its sensitivity ranging from 34% to 61%, specificity from 88% to 97%, and accuracy from 51% to 70%.[421]

The results of these studies indicate that CT is helpful in identifying advanced local disease and the presence of metastases to the lungs, liver, and intra-abdominal lymph nodes.[421, 430] CT has limited value in the detection of early periesophageal tumor extension or involvement of mediastinal lymph nodes, however.[430] Several investigators have shown that endoscopic ultrasound examination is superior in the detection of local tumor spread.[426, 428, 432] It also has been shown that the combination of CT and endoscopic ultrasound examination provides greater diagnostic accuracy than either modality alone.[426, 432] MR imaging has not been found to have any significant advantages over CT and plays a limited role in assessment.[433, 434] Preliminary results suggest that positron emission tomography (PET) using 2-(^{18}F)-fluoro-2-deoxy-d-glucose (FDG) has a greater than 90% sensitivity in the detection of primary esophageal cancers.[503] However, because of its low intrinsic spatial resolution (approximately 5 mm), FDG PET is not helpful in the assessment of local invasion. FDG PET, like CT, also has a low sensitivity in the detection of local nodal metastases.[503] PET is superior to CT in the detection of metastases to the lungs, liver, and skeleton and in the diagnosis of tumor recurrence.[503, 435]

Mesenchymal Neoplasms. Leiomyosarcomas constitute fewer than 1% of malignant esophageal tumors.[436, 437] Benign neoplasms of the esophagus consist mostly of leiomyomas, fibromas, and lipomas. The appearance of leiomyomas and fibromas is that of a nonspecific intramural soft tissue mass. Lipomas have a characteristic appearance on CT scans consisting of homogeneous fat attenuation.[284]

Diverticula

Diverticula occur in the pharyngeal region (Zenker's diverticulum), in the midthoracic region as a result of cicatricial contraction from healed infected lymph nodes (traction diverticula), and in the lower esophagus as a result of outpouching of the mucosa through defects in the muscular wall at the point of entry of blood vessels (pulsion diverticula). In contrast to the other two varieties, traction diverticula are seldom, if ever, visible on plain radiographs.

Zenker's diverticulum may become large enough to be identified in the superior mediastinum on plain radiographs, in which case it frequently contains an air-fluid level. Barium studies not only outline the sac, but also reveal the degree of anterior displacement of the proximal esophagus. The diagnosis can be made using CT. Symptoms include dysphagia, chronic cough owing to aspiration, and recurrent pneumonia.

Diverticula arising from the lower third of the esophagus almost always are congenital in origin and present as round, cystlike structures to the right of the midline just above the diaphragm. An air-fluid level is usually present. Barium studies are diagnostic.[438]

Megaesophagus

Esophageal dilation has many causes, including stenosis secondary to reflux esophagitis or fibrosing mediastinitis, progressive systemic sclerosis, carcinoma, and achalasia. Among these, achalasia causes the most severe generalized dilation. Symptoms of the latter abnormality include dysphagia, pain on swallowing, and chronic cough; recurrent pneumonia may result from aspiration.

The dilated esophagus usually is apparent radiographically as a shadow projecting entirely to the right side of the mediastinum. Because it is behind the heart, it does not cause a silhouette sign with that structure. The trachea may be displaced anteriorly (Fig. 22–61). Depending on the underlying cause, an air-fluid level may be observed in the dilated esophagus, most frequently in achalasia and seldom in progressive systemic sclerosis. Although a barium study is the diagnostic procedure of choice, CT also enables diagnosis, even in patients in whom the condition is not suspected.[439, 440] On conventional chest radiographs, an air-containing esophagus may be identified in some patients who have progressive systemic sclerosis and, in the appropriate clinical context, is suggestive of the diagnosis. Air in the esophagus can be seen postoperatively[441] and in patients who employ esophageal speech after laryngectomy.[442]

Esophageal Varices

Paraesophageal varices occasionally result in abnormalities on chest radiograph (Fig. 22–62).[443, 444] In one review of 352 patients who had portal hypertension, varices were evident in 17 (5%);[444] they included middle-posterior mediastinal or paravertebral opacities, a soft tissue opacity adjacent to the descending thoracic aorta, and obscuration of the aorta.[444] In a second investigation of 100 patients, abnormalities consistent with esophageal varices were seen on chest radiographs in 20 and on CT in 38;[445] most of the varices detected on radiographs were greater than 2.5 cm in diameter. Rarely, blood flows from the abdomen through the diaphragm into the thorax and drains into the pericardiophrenic vein;[446, 447] such a portosystemic shunt can result in an abnormal soft tissue shadow at the level of the left cardiophrenic angle.[447] The diagnosis of esophageal varices and transdiaphragmatic portosystemic shunt can be made by CT.[447, 448]

MASSES SITUATED PREDOMINANTLY IN THE PARAVERTEBRAL REGION

The paravertebral region is bounded in the front by the anterior surface of the vertebral column and in the back by the chest wall. It is in a sense almost a potential space because it normally contains only a small amount of connective tissue, blood vessels, sympathetic nerve chains, and peripheral nerves. Neoplasms that originate in the last two structures as well as abnormalities related to the spinal canal can expand to present as masses in this region (Table

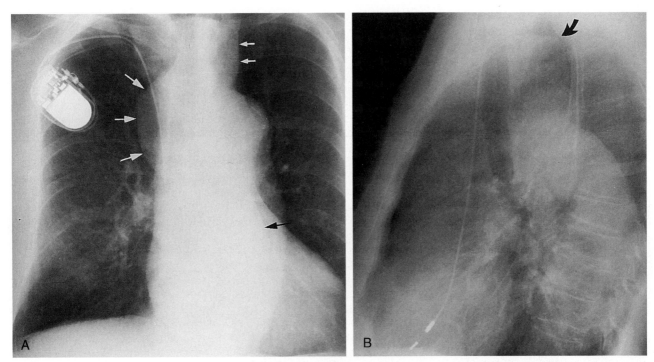

Figure 22–61. Achalasia. Posteroanterior *(A)* and lateral *(B)* chest radiographs from a 74-year-old man show marked dilation of the esophagus *(straight arrows),* which contains an air-fluid level *(curved arrow)* and displaces the trachea anteriorly. The patient had long-standing achalasia.

22–3). Although herniation of abdominal contents through a posterior diaphragmatic defect and infectious, traumatic, or neoplastic diseases of the thoracic spine can be manifested by a paravertebral mass, for convenience these are discussed in Chapter 23.

Tumors and Tumor-Like Conditions of Neural Tissue

Neoplasms of neural tissue account for about 20% of all primary mediastinal neoplasms in adults[452, 453] and 35%

in children;[453] they are the most common type in the paravertebral compartment.[454] From a histogenetic point of view, there are two basic types: tumors arising from the peripheral nerves and tumors originating from sympathetic ganglia.

Tumors Arising from Peripheral Nerves

Most neural tumors that arise in the thorax originate in an intercostal nerve in the paravertebral region. Several

Table 22–3. PARAVERTEBRAL MASSES

Etiology	Radiographic Manifestations	CT Findings
Developmental		
Meningocele and meningomyelocele	Sharply circumscribed. Frequently spine and rib deformities	Communication with subarachnoid space; homogeneous water density
Infectious		
Suppurative or tuberculous spondylitis	Smooth, fusiform mass. Erosion or destruction of vertebrae at level of paravertebral mass	Inhomogeneous paravertebral soft tissue; erosion or destruction of adjacent vertebrae
Neoplastic		
Neurogenic tumors; neurofibroma and neurilemoma most common	Round or oval, well-defined margins	Can have homogeneous soft tissue attenuation or contain cystic areas; often show inhomogeneous contrast enhancement
Bone and cartilage neoplasms	Round mass. Destruction of affected bone, often associated with soft tissue mass protruding into and compressing lung	CT and MR imaging used to assess tumor characteristics and extension into adjacent structures
Traumatic		
Fracture of vertebra with hematoma	Smooth paravertebral swelling, usually bilateral	CT diagnostic
Miscellaneous causes		
Bochdalek's hernia. Focal defects in diaphragm leading to Bochdalek's hernia in the adult increase in frequency with age	Round or oval retrocardiac or paravertebral	CT diagnostic; shows discontinuity of diaphragm and herniation of omental fat and, less commonly in the adult, abdominal viscera
Extramedullary hematopoiesis	Smooth or lobulated, usually bilateral. Spleen may be enlarged	Homogeneous soft tissue attenuation; fatty replacement can occur after resolution of the causative hemolytic disorder

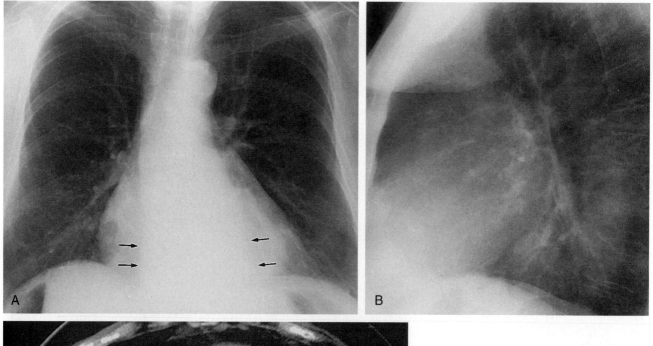

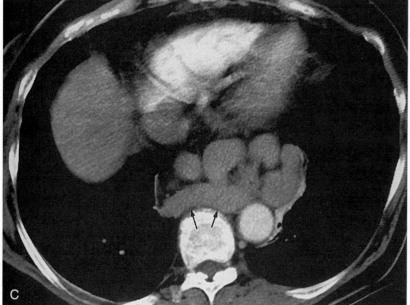

Figure 22–62. Paraesophageal Varices. Postero-anterior chest radiograph *(A)* from a 66-year-old woman who had long-standing cirrhosis of the liver shows increased opacity in the lower paraspinal region *(arrows)*. Lateral view *(B)* shows increased opacity in the retrocardiac region. Contrast-enhanced CT scan *(C)* shows the characteristic serpiginous appearance of esophageal varices *(arrows)*.

histologic forms can be seen, including neurilemoma (schwannoma), neurofibroma (plexiform and nonplexiform types), and neurogenic sarcoma (malignant schwannoma); neurilemoma is the most common. Most tumors are discovered in young adults. Many do not cause symptoms and are discovered on screening chest radiograph; in one series of 49 patients, 32 (65%) were asymptomatic.[192]

In most cases, neurilemomas and neurofibromas are manifested radiographically as sharply defined round, smooth, or lobulated paraspinal masses.[87, 455] They typically span only one or two posterior rib interspaces but can become quite large.[87, 455] In approximately 50% of cases, they are associated with bone abnormalities, such as expansion of the neural foramina, erosion of the vertebral bodies, and erosion or deformity of the ribs.[87] On CT scans, both

forms of tumor can have homogeneous or heterogeneous attenuation; in most cases, attenuation is slightly lower than that of chest wall muscle (Fig. 22–63).[456, 457] Tumors usually show heterogeneous enhancement after intravenous administration of contrast medium (Fig. 22-64),[456–458] a feature related to the presence of lipid within myelin and to areas of hypocellularity, cystic degeneration, or hemorrhage.[456, 457] Punctate foci of calcification are seen in 10% of cases.[465] Plexiform neurofibroma may be manifested on CT as a mass that has poorly defined margins and diffusely infiltrates the mediastinum along the distribution of the sympathetic chains and various large nerves (including the phrenic, recurrent laryngeal, and vagus nerves).[459]

On MR imaging, schwannomas and neurofibromas have low to intermediate signal intensity on T1-weighted images

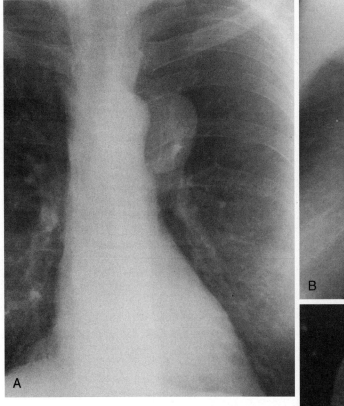

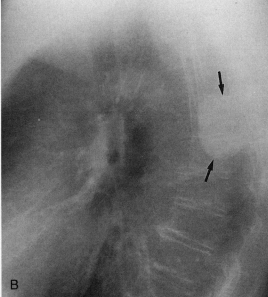

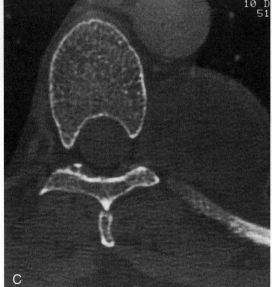

Figure 22–63. Neurilemoma. Close-up views from posteroanterior *(A)* and lateral *(B)* chest radiographs show a left paraspinal mass *(arrows)*. On thin-section CT scan *(C)*, the mass has lower attenuation than the paraspinal muscles. The patient was a 58-year-old asymptomatic man.

and focal areas with intermediate to high signal intensity on T2-weighted images (Fig. 22–65).[460] The procedure is particularly helpful in determining the nerve of origin for tumors in the thoracic inlet.[461]

Neurogenic sarcomas usually present radiographically as round masses greater than 5 cm in diameter.[87, 462] CT typically shows areas of low attenuation related to hemorrhage and necrosis.[87, 463] The tumors may have well-defined smooth margins[87, 463] or poorly defined margins because of infiltration of the chest wall or adjacent mediastinal structures.[456, 457] Calcification is evident in some cases.[87]

Tumors Arising from Sympathetic Ganglia

Ganglioneuroma, ganglioneuroblastoma, and neuroblastoma are tumors that arise from the sympathetic ganglia and represent a continuum whose histologic appearance varies from mature, fully differentiated tissue in the first-named to immature tissue in the last-named. Neuroblastomas and ganglioneuroblastomas occur most commonly in infants and children, whereas ganglioneuromas tend to occur in adolescents and young adults.[464] Many patients are asymptomatic; some have chest wall pain.

Radiographic appearance consists of sharply defined oblong masses located along the anterolateral surface of the thoracic spine (Fig. 22–66).[455, 465] These tumors usually can be distinguished from neurogenic tumors by their vertical orientation and elongated, tapering appearance. Calcification occurs in approximately 25%.[466] The ribs or vertebrae are eroded in some cases, just as often by benign as by malignant forms; such erosion can be striking in neuroblastoma but tends to be more subtle in ganglioneuroma.[465] The tumors can exhibit homogeneous or heterogeneous attenuation on CT.[87] MR imaging usually shows homoge-

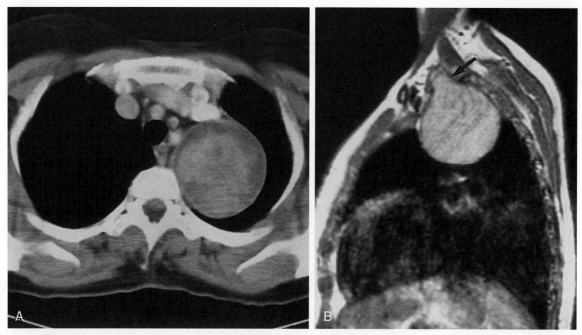

Figure 22–64. Neurilemoma. Contrast-enhanced CT scan *(A)* from a 39-year-old woman who presented with left arm pain shows a sharply marginated mass in the left upper chest. The mass has inhomogeneous attenuation, a finding commonly seen in neurogenic tumors. Sagittal MR image (TR/TE, 1,700/30) *(B)* shows that the mass has a pedicle *(arrow)* extending to the brachial plexus. At surgery, a neurilemoma was found to arise from the left T1 nerve root.

neous, intermediate signal intensity on T1-weighted and T2-weighted images.[87, 467] Occasionally, curvilinear bands of low signal intensity are seen on T1-weighted and T2-weighted images, causing a whorled appearance.[460] As discussed previously *(see* page 714), intrathoracic paragangliomas usually occur in the middle mediastinum in relation to the aortopulmonary paraganglia or in the paravertebral region in relation to the aorticosympathetic paraganglia.

Meningocele and Meningomyelocele

Meningocele and meningomyelocele are rare anomalies that consist of herniation of the leptomeninges through an intervertebral foramen; a meningocele contains cerebrospinal fluid only, whereas a meningomyelocele also contains neural tissue. The abnormalities occur slightly more often on the right side than on the left and can be situated anywhere between the thoracic inlet and the diaphragm. Approximately 75% of patients present between the ages of 30 and 60 years;[468] many have neurofibromatosis.[469]

On conventional radiographs, the lesions show no specific features that distinguish them from neurogenic neoplasms. The diagnosis usually can be made on CT or MR imaging, both of which show continuity between the cerebrospinal fluid in the thecal sac and the meningocele (Fig. 22–67).[87, 469] Kyphoscoliosis is frequent, being ob-

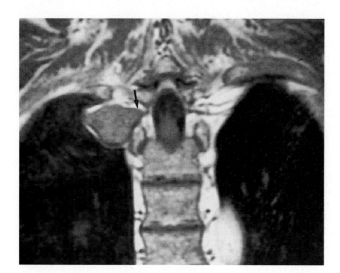

Figure 22–65. Neurofibroma. Coronal MR image obtained using T1-weighted spin-echo technique (TR/TE, 800/15) shows a paraspinal tumor. The mass has heterogeneous signal intensity and can be seen to originate from a nerve root *(arrow).*

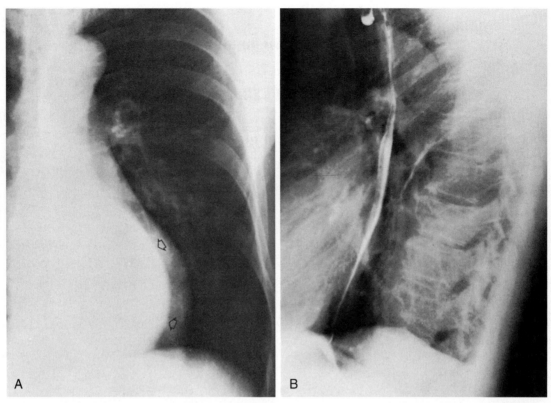

Figure 22–66. Ganglioneuroma. Close-up views of the left hemithorax from posteroanterior *(A)* and lateral *(B)* radiographs from a 42-year-old asymptomatic man show a smooth, well-defined, homogeneous mass in the paravertebral region *(arrows).* It contains no visible calcium. The thoracic spine showed no abnormality.

served in 47 of 70 patients in one series;[468] the meningocele usually was situated at the apex of the curvature on its convex side. Enlargement of the intervertebral foramen is present in most patients.[468] An association with vertebral and rib anomalies is fairly frequent and should suggest the diagnosis.[470, 471]

Gastroenteric (Neurenteric) Cyst

Gastroenteric cysts are lined in whole or in part by gastric or small intestinal epithelium; when such a cyst is associated with anomalies of the spinal column (e.g., spina bifida and hemivertebrae), the designation *neurenteric* usually is applied. The latter typically produce symptoms and manifest themselves early in life;[475] most are diagnosed in the first year of life.[87, 476]

The radiographic appearance is that of a sharply defined, round or lobulated opacity of homogeneous density.[87, 472] Because of their fluid content, the cysts tend to mold themselves to surrounding structures. They often are connected by a stalk to the meninges and commonly to a portion of the gastrointestinal tract.[288, 473] If attachment is to the esophagus, communication is rare; however, if it is to the gastrointestinal tract, there is usually communication, permitting gas to enter the cyst. The cyst may opacify with barium during examination of the upper gastrointestinal tract. Approximately 50% of cases are associated with incomplete closure of the neural tube (spinal dysraphism) or with butterfly vertebrae or hemi-

vertebrae.[87, 474] MR imaging is required to exclude intraspinal extension.[87]

Extramedullary Hematopoiesis

Extramedullary hematopoiesis occurs as a compensatory phenomenon in various diseases in which there is inadequate production or excessive destruction of blood cells. Most cases are associated with congenital hemolytic anemia (usually hereditary spherocytosis) or thalassemia (most often thalassemia major or intermedia).[477, 489] The most common sites of extramedullary hematopoiesis are the liver and spleen; however, foci can occur in many other organs and tissues, including the paravertebral areas of the thorax.[477]

The characteristic radiographic finding is one or several smooth but often lobulated masses situated in the lower chest (Fig. 22–68).[478–480] Less commonly, masses occur at multiple levels or involve the entire paravertebral region.[478, 479] On CT scans, the masses usually have homogeneous soft tissue density;[480–482] occasionally, there is a large fatty component.[483, 484] In some tumors, fatty replacement appears to be the result of adipocytic metaplasia after resolution of the underlying hemolytic disorder.[485] Other features include widening of the ribs as a result of expansion of the medullary cavity, a lacy appearance of the vertebrae, and absence of bone erosion.[480] Radionuclide bone marrow scans may[480, 486, 487] or may not[488] show uptake within the mass.

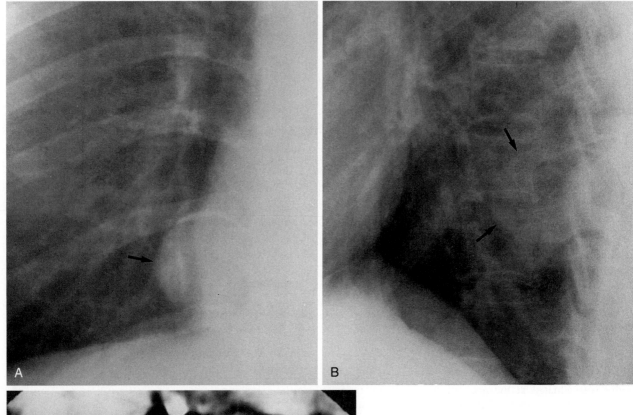

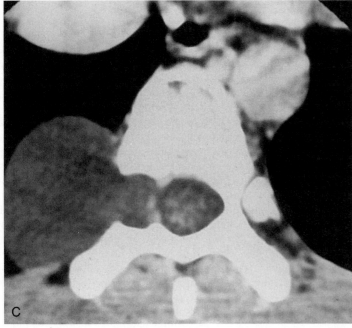

Figure 22–67. Meningocele. Close-up views from postero-anterior *(A)* and lateral *(B)* chest radiographs show a para-spinal opacity *(arrows)* at the level of T10. CT scan *(C)* shows characteristic fluid attenuation of the meningocele, which communicates with the thecal sac. The patient was a 29-year-old man.

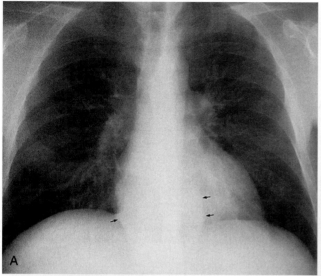

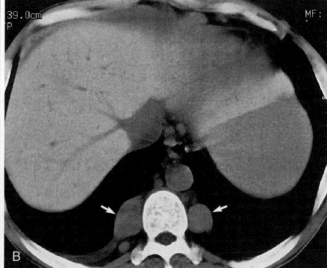

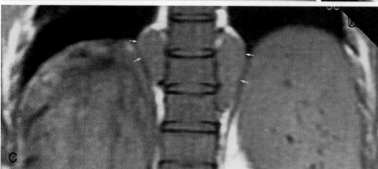

Figure 22–68. Extramedullary Hematopoiesis. Posteroanterior chest radiograph *(A)* from a 39-year-old man shows displacement of the paraspinal interfaces *(arrows).* CT scan obtained without intravenous contrast material *(B)* shows paraspinal soft tissue masses *(arrows).* The increased attenuation of the liver is a result of hemosiderosis. Coronal T1-weighted MR image *(C)* better shows the extent of the extramedullary hematopoiesis *(arrows).* The patient had thalassemia intermedia.

References

1. Goldstein LA, Thompson WR: Esophageal perforation: A 15 year experience. Am J Surg 143:495, 1982.
2. Burnett CM, Rosemurgy AS, Pfeiffer EA: Life-threatening acute posterior mediastinitis due to esophageal perforation. Ann Thorac Surg 49:979, 1990.
3. Carrol CL, Jeffrey B Jr, Federle MP, et al: CT evaluation of mediastinal infections. J Comput Assist Tomogr 11:449, 1987.
4. El Oakley RM, Wright JE: Postoperative mediastinitis: Classification and management. Ann Thorac Surg 61:1030, 1996.
5. Watanabe M, Ohshika Y, Aoki T, et al: Empyema and mediastinitis complicating retropharyngeal abscess. Thorax 49:1179, 1994.
6. Pollack MS: Staphylococcal mediastinitis due to sternoclavicular pyarthrosis: CT appearance. J Comput Assist Tomogr 14:924, 1990.
7. Breatnach E, Nath PH, Delany DJ: The role of computed tomography in acute and subacute mediastinitis. Clin Radiol 37:139, 1986.
8. Kushihashi T, Munechika H, Motoya H: CT and MR findings in tuberculous mediastinitis. J Comput Assist Tomogr 19:379, 1995.
9. Swensen SJ, Aughenbaugh GL, Brown LR: Chest case of the day. Am J Roentgenol 160:1318, 1993.
10. Tocino IM, Miller MH: Mediastinal trauma and other acute mediastinal conditions. J Thorac Imaging 2:79, 1987.
11. LaBerge JM, Kerlan RK Jr, Pogany AC, et al: Esophageal rupture: Complication of balloon dilatation. Radiology 157:56, 1985.
12. Rogers LF, Puig AW, Dooley BN, et al: Diagnostic considerations in mediastinal emphysema: A pathophysiologic-roentgenologic approach to Boerhaave's syndrome and spontaneous pneumomediastinum. Am J Roentgenol 115:495, 1972.
13. Gray JM, Hanson GC: Mediastinal emphysema: Aetiology, diagnosis, and treatment. Thorax 21:325, 1966.
14. Christoforidis A, Nelson SW: Spontaneous rupture of the esophagus with emphasis on the roentgenologic diagnosis. Am J Roentgenol 78:574, 1957.
15. Appleton DS, Sandrasagra FA, Flower CDR: Perforated oesophagus: Review of twenty-eight consecutive cases. Clin Radiol 30:493, 1979.
16. Han SY, McElvein RB, Aldrete JS, et al: Perforation of the esophagus: Correlation of site and cause with plain film findings. Am J Roentgenol 145:537, 1985.
17. Gollub MJ, Bains MS: Barium sulfate: A new (old) contrast agent for diagnosis of postoperative esophageal leaks. Radiology 202:360, 1997.
18. Dodds WJ, Stewart ET, Vlymen WJ: Appropriate contrast media for evaluation of esophageal disruption. Radiology 144:439, 1982.
19. Reich SB: Production of pulmonary edema by aspiration of water-soluble nonabsorbable contrast media. Radiology 92:367, 1969.
20. Gobien RP, Stanley JH, Gobien BS, et al: Percutaneous catheter aspiration and draining of suspected mediastinal abscesses. Radiology 151:69, 1984.
21. Backer CL, LoCicero JD, Hartz RS, et al: Computed tomography in patients with esophageal perforation. Chest 98:1078, 1990.
22. White CS, Templeton PA, Attar S: Esophageal perforation: CT findings. Am J Roentgenol 160:767, 1993.
23. Lee S, Mergo PJ, Ros PR: The leaking esophagus: CT patterns of esophageal rupture, perforation, and fistulization. Crit Rev Diagn Imaging 37:461, 1996.
24. Craddock DR, Logan A, Mayell M: Traumatic rupture of the oesophagus and stomach. Thorax 23:657, 1968.
25. Sherrick AD, Brown LR, Harms GF, et al: The radiographic findings of fibrosing mediastinitis. Chest 106:484, 1994.
26. Schowengerdt CG, Suyemoto R, Main FB: Granulomatous and fibrous mediastinitis—a review and analysis of 180 cases. J Thorac Cardiovasc Surg 57:365, 1969.
27. Mole TM, Glober J, Sheppard MN: Sclerosing mediastinitis: A report on 18 cases. Thorax 50:280, 1995.
28. Dozois RR, Bernatz PE, Woolner LB, et al: Sclerosing mediastinitis involving major bronchi. Mayo Clin Proc 43:557, 1968.
29. Katzenstein ALA, Mazur MT: Pulmonary infarct: An unusual manifestation of fibrosing mediastinitis. Chest 77:521, 1980.
30. Feigin DS, Eggleston JC, Siegelman SS: The multiple roentgen manifestations of sclerosing mediastinitis. Johns Hopkins Med J 144:1, 1979.

31. Weinstein JB, Aronberg DJ, Sagel SS: CT of fibrosing mediastinitis: Findings and their utility. Am J Roentgenol 141:247, 1983.

32. Kountz PD, Molina PL, Sagel S: Fibrosing mediastinitis in the posterior thorax. Am J Roentgenol 153:489, 1989.

33. Dunn EJ, Ulicny KS Jr, Wright CB, et al: Surgical implication of sclerosing mediastinitis: A report of six cases and review of the literature. Chest 97:338, 1990.

34. Wieder S, White TJ III, Salazar J, et al: Pulmonary artery occlusion due to histoplasmosis. Am J Roentgenol 138:243, 1982.

35. Mendelson EB, Mintzer RA, Hidvegi DF: Veno-occlusive pulmonary infarct: An unusual complication of fibrosing mediastinitis. Am J Roentgenol 141:175, 1983.

36. Mallin WH, Silberstein EB, Shipley RT, et al: Fibrosing mediastinitis causing nonvisualization of one lung on pulmonary scintigraphy. Clin Nucl Med 18:594, 1993.

37. Farmer DW, Moore E, Amparo E, et al: Calcific fibrosing mediastinitis: Demonstration of pulmonary vascular obstruction by magnetic resonance imaging. Am J Roentgenol 143:1189, 1984.

38. Rholl KS, Levitt RG, Glazer HS: Magnetic resonance imaging of fibrosing mediastinitis. Am J Roentgenol 145:255, 1985.

39. Williams SM, Jones ET: General case of the day. Radiographics 17:1324, 1997.

40. Mathisen DJ, Grillo HC: Clinical manifestation of mediastinal fibrosis and histoplasmosis. Ann Thorac Surg 54:1053, 1992.

41. Lillard RL, Allen RP: The extrapleural air sign in pneumomediastinum. Radiology 85:1093, 1965.

42. Cyrlak D, Milne EN, Imray TJ: Pneumomediastinum: A diagnostic problem. Crit Rev Diagn Imaging 23:75, 1984.

43. Rouby JJ, Lherm T, deLassale EM, et al: Histologic aspects of pulmonary barotrauma in critically ill patients with acute respiratory failure. Intensive Care Med 19:383, 1993.

44. Jamadar DA, Kazerooni EA, Hirschl RB: Pneumomediastinum: Elucidation of the anatomic pathway by liquid ventilation. J Comput Assist Tomogr 20:309, 1996.

45. Campbell RE, Boggs TR Jr, Kirkpatrick JA: Early neonatal pneumoperitoneum from progressive massive tension pneumomediastinum. Radiology 114:121, 1975.

46. Kakitsubata Y, Inatsu H, Kakitsubata S, et al: CT manifestations of intraspinal air associated with pneumomediastinum. Acta Radiol 35:305, 1994.

47. Drevelengas A, Kalaitzoglou I, Petridis A: Pneumorrhachis associated with spontaneous pneumomediastinum. Eur J Radiol 18:122, 1994.

48. Fultz PJ, Melville D, Ekanej A, et al: Nontraumatic rupture of the thoracic aorta: Chest radiographic features of an often unrecognized condition. Am J Roentgenol 171:351, 1998.

49. Munsell WP: Pneumomediastinum: A report of 28 cases and review of the literature. JAMA 202:689, 1967.

50. Morgan EJ, Henderson DA: Pneumomediastinum as a complication of athletic competition. Thorax 36:155, 1981.

51. Varkey B, Kory RC: Mediastinal and subcutaneous emphysema following pulmonary function tests. Am Rev Respir Dis 108:1393, 1973.

52. Karson EM, Saltzman D, Davis MR: Pneumomediastinum in pregnancy: Two case reports and a review of the literature, pathophysiology, and management. Obstet Gynecol 64(3 Suppl):395, 1984.

53. Bejvan SM, Godwin JD: Pneumomediastinum: Old signs and new signs. Am J Roentgenol 166:1041, 1996.

54. Miller WE, Spiekerman RE, Hepper NG: Pneumomediastinum resulting from performing Valsalva maneuvers during marihuana smoking. Chest 62:233, 1972.

55. Eurman DW, Potash HI, Eyler WR, et al: Chest pain and dyspnea related to "crack" cocaine smoking: Value of chest radiography. Radiology 172:459, 1989.

56. Dattwyler RJ, Goldman MA, Bloch KJ: Pneumomediastinum as a complication of asthma in teenage and young adult patients. J Allergy Clin Immunol 63:412, 1979.

57. Ruttley M, Mills RA: Subcutaneous emphysema and pneumomediastinum in diabetic ketoacidosis. Br J Radiol 44:672, 1971.

58. Rohlfing BM, Webb WR, Schlobohm RM: Ventilator-related extraalveolar air in adults. Radiology 121:25, 1976.

59. Altman AR, Johnson TH: Pneumoperitoneum and pneumoretroperitoneum: Consequences of positive end-expiratory pressure therapy. Arch Surg 114:208, 1979.

60. Marcy TW: Barotrauma: Detection, recognition, and management. Chest 104:578, 1993.

61. Thorsøe H: Mediastinal emphysema due to perforation of the intestinal tract. Nord Med 59:286, 1958.

62. Landay MJ, Cohen DJ, Deaton CW Jr: Another look at the "ring-around-the-artery" in pneumomediastinum. J Can Assoc Radiol 36:343, 1985.

63. Friedman AC, Lautin EM, Rothenberg L: Mach bands and pneumomediastinum. J Can Assoc Radiol 32:232, 1981.

64. Naclerio E: The "V" sign in the diagnosis of spontaneous rupture of the esophagus (an early roentgen clue). Am J Surg 93:291, 1957.

65. Levin B: The continuous diaphragm sign: A newly recognized sign of pneumomediastinum. Clin Radiol 24:337, 1973.

66. Felson B: The mediastinum. Semin Roentgenol 4:40, 1969.

67. Tsuji H, Takazakura E, Terade Y, et al: CT demonstration of spinal epidural emphysema complicating bronchial asthma and violent coughing. J Comput Assist Tomogr 13:38, 1989.

68. Yoshimura T, Takeo G, Souda M, et al: Case report: CT demonstration of spinal epidural emphysema after strenuous exercise. J Comput Assist Tomogr 14:303, 1990.

69. Unger JM, England DM, Bogust GA: Interstitial emphysema in adults: Recognition and prognostic implications. J Thorac Imaging 4:86, 1989.

70. Satoh K, Kobayashi T, Kawase Y, et al: CT appearance of interstitial pulmonary emphysema. J Thorac Imaging 11:153, 1996.

71. Mirvis SE, Bidwell JK, Buddemeyer EU, et al: Value of chest radiography in excluding traumatic aortic rupture. Radiology 163:487, 1987.

72. Creasy JD, Chiles C, Routh WD, et al: Overview of traumatic injury of the thoracic aorta. Radiographics 17:27, 1997.

73. Gavant ML, Menke PG, Fabian T, et al: Blunt traumatic aortic rupture: Detection with helical CT of the chest. Radiology 197:125, 1995.

74. Mirvis SE, Shanmuganathan K, Miller BH, et al: Traumatic aortic injury: Diagnosis with contrast-enhanced thoracic CT-five-year experience at a major trauma center. Radiology 200:413, 1996.

75. Gomelsky A, Barry MJ, Wagner RB: Spontaneous mediastinal hemorrhage: A case report with a review of the literature. Md Med J 46:83, 1997.

76. Bethancourt B, Pond GD, Jones SE, et al: Mediastinal hematoma simulating recurrent Hodgkin disease during systemic chemotherapy. Am J Roentgenol 142:1119, 1984.

77. Ellison R, Carrao W, Fox M, et al: Spontaneous mediastinal hemorrhage in patients on chronic hemodialysis. Ann Intern Med 95:704, 1981.

78. MacDonald R, Kelly J: Cervico-mediastinal hematoma following sneezing. Anesthesia 30:50, 1975.

79. Stilwell M, Weisbrod G, Ilves R: Spontaneous mediastinal hematoma. J Assoc Can Radiol 32:60, 1981.

80. Singh S, Ptacin MJ, Bamrah VS: Spontaneous mediastinal hemorrhage: A complication of intracoronary streptokinase infusion for coronary thrombosis. Arch Intern Med 143:562, 1983.

81. Woodring JH, Loh FK, Kryscio RJ: Mediastinal hemorrhage: An evaluation of radiographic manifestations. Radiology 151:15, 1984.

82. Panicek DM, Ewing DK, Markarian B, et al: Interstitial pulmonary hemorrhage from mediastinal hematoma secondary to aortic rupture. Radiology 162(1 Pt 1):165, 1987.

83. Kucich VA, Vogelzang RL, Hartz RS, et al: Ruptured thoracic aneurysm: Unusual manifestation and early diagnosis using CT. Radiology 160:87, 1986.

84. Swensen SJ, McLeod RA, Stephens DH: CT of extracranial hemorrhage and hematomas. Am J Roentgenol 143:907, 1984.

85. Glazer HS, Molina PL, Siegel MJ, et al: High-attenuation mediastinal masses on unenhanced CT. Am J Roentgenol 156:45, 1991.

86. Strollo DC, Rosado-de-Christenson ML, Jett JR: Primary mediastinal tumors: Part 1. Tumors of the anterior mediastinum. Chest 112:511, 1997.

87. Strollo DC, Rosado-de-Christenson ML, Jett JR: Primary mediastinal tumors: Part II. Tumors of the middle and posterior mediastinum. Chest 112:1344, 1997.

88. Landay MJ: Anterior clear space: How clear? How often? How come? Radiology 192:165, 1994.

89. Felson B: Chest Roentgenology. Philadelphia, WB Saunders, 1973.

90. Marchevsky A: The mediastinum. Pathology 3:339, 1996.

91. Wychulis AR, Payne WS, Clagett OT, et al: Surgical treatment of mediastinal tumors: A 40-year experience. J Thorac Cardiovasc Surg 62:379, 1971.

92. Linegar AG, Odell JA, Fennell WM, et al: Massive thymic hyperplasia. Ann Thorac Surg 55:1197, 1993.

93. Langer CJ, Keller SM, Erner SM: Thymic hyperplasia with hemorrhage simulating recurrent Hodgkin disease after chemotherapy-induced complete remission. Cancer 70:2082, 1992.

94. Düe W, Dieckmann K-P, Stein H: Thymic hyperplasia following chemotherapy of a testicular germ cell tumor: Immunohistological evidence for a simple rebound phenomenon. Cancer 63:446, 1989.

95. Kissin CM, Husband JE, Nicholas D, et al: Benign thymic enlargement in adults after chemotherapy: CT demonstration. Radiology 163:67, 1987.

96. Simmonds P, Silberstein M, McKendrick J: Thymic hyperplasia in adults following chemotherapy for malignancy. Aust N Z J Med 23:264, 1993.

97. Tabarin A, Catargi B, Chanson P, et al: Pseudo-tumors of the thymus after correction of hypercortisolism in patients with ectopic ACTH syndrome: A report of five cases. Clin Endocrinol 42:207, 1995.

98. Mizuno T, Hashimoto T, Masaoka A, et al: Thymic follicular hyperplasia manifested as an anterior mediastinal mass. Surg Today 27:275, 1997.

99. Doppman JL, Oldfield EH, Chrousos GP, et al: Rebound thymic hyperplasia after treatment of Cushing's syndrome. Am J Roentgenol 147:1145, 1986.

100. Sidhu US, Malhotra V, Chhina GS: Roentgenogram of the month: An unusual case of pseudocardiomegaly. Chest 113:1711, 1998.

101. Choyke PL, Zeman RK, Gootenberg JE, et al: Thymic atrophy and regrowth in response to chemotherapy: CT evaluation. Am J Roentgenol 149:269, 1987.

102. Moul JW, Fernandez EB, Bryan MG, et al: Thymic hyperplasia in newly diagnosed testicular germ cell tumors. J Urol 152:1480, 1994.

103. Levine GD, Rosai J: Thymic hyperplasia and neoplasia: A review of current concepts. Hum Pathol 9:495, 1978.

104. Fyfe B, Dominguez F, Poppiti RJ: Thymic hyperplasia: A clue to the diagnosis of hyperthyroidism. Am J Forensic Med Pathol 11:257, 1990.

105. Bergman TA, Mariash CN, Oppenheimer JH: Anterior mediastinal mass in a patient with Graves' disease. J Clin Endocrinol Metab 55:587, 1982.

106. Pendlebury SC, Boyages S, Koutts J, et al: Thymic hyperplasia associated with Hodgkin disease and thyrotoxicosis. Cancer 70:1985, 1992.

107. Freundlich IM, McGavran MH: Abnormalities of the thymus. J Thorac Imaging 11:58, 1996.

108. Baron RL, Lee JKT, Sagel SS, et al: Computed tomography of the normal thymus. Radiology 142:121, 1982.

109. Nicolaou S, Müller NL, Li DKB, et al: Thymus in myasthenia gravis: Comparison of CT and pathologic findings and clinical outcome after thymectomy. Radiology 201:471, 1996.

110. Front D, Ben-Haim S, Israel O, et al: Lymphoma: Predictive value of Ga-67 scintigraphy after treatment. Radiology 182:359, 1992.

111. Israel O: Benign mediastinal and parahilar uptake of gallium-67 in treated lymphoma: Do we have all the answers? J Nucl Med 34:1330, 1993.

112. Small EJ, Venook AP, Damon LE: Gallium-avid thymic hyperplasia in an adult after chemotherapy for Hodgkin disease. Cancer 72:905, 1993.

113. Rosai J, Levine GD: Atlas of Tumor Pathology: Tumors of the Thymus. Second Series, Fascicle 13. Washington, DC, Armed Forces Institute of Pathology, 1976.

114. Wong KF, Chau KF, Chan JK, et al: Pure red cell aplasia associated with thymic lymphoid hyperplasia and secondary erythropoietin resistance. Am J Clin Pathol 103:346, 1995.

115. Batra P, Herrmann C Jr, Mulder D: Mediastinal imaging in myasthenia gravis: Correlation of chest radiography, CT, MR and surgical findings. Am J Roentgenol 148:515, 1987.

116. Chen J, Weisbrod GL, Herman SJ: Computed tomography and pathologic correlations of thymic lesions. J Thorac Imaging 3:61, 1988.

117. Teplick JG, Nedwich A, Haskin ME: Roentgenographic features of thymolipoma. Am J Roentgenol 117:873, 1973.

118. Nishimura O, Naito Y, Noguchi Y, et al: Thymolipoma: A report of three cases. Jpn J Surg 20:234, 1990.

119. Moran CA, Rosado-de-Christenson M, Suster S: Thymolipoma: Clinicopathologic review of 33 cases. Mod Pathol 8:741, 1995.

120. Rosado-de-Christenson M, Pugatch RD, Moran CA, et al: Thymolipoma: Analysis of 27 cases. Radiology 193:121, 1994.

121. Yeh H-C, Gordon A, Kirschner PA, et al: Computed tomography and sonography of thymolipoma. Am J Roentgenol 140:1131, 1983.

122. Faerber EN, Balsara RK, Schidlow DV, et al: Thymolipoma: Computed tomographic appearances. Pediatr Radiol 20:196, 1990.

123. Shirkhoda A, Chasen MH, Eftekhari F, et al: MR imaging of mediastinal thymolipoma. J Comput Assist Tomogr 11:364, 1987.

124. Molina PL, Siegel MJ, Glazer HS: Thymic masses on MR imaging. Am J Roentgenol 155:495, 1990.

125. Ahn JM, Lee KS, Goo JM, et al: Predicting the histology of anterior mediastinal masses: Comparison of chest radiography and CT. J Thorac Imaging 11:265, 1996.

126. McCafferty MH, Bahnson HT: Thymic cyst extending into the pericardium: A case report and review of thymic cysts. Ann Thorac Surg 33:503, 1982.

127. Indeglia RA, Shea MA, Grage TB: Congenital cysts of the thymus gland. Arch Surg 94:149, 1967.

128. Bieger RC, McAdams AJ: Thymic cysts. Arch Pathol 82:535, 1966.

129. Jaramillo D, Perez-Atayde A, Griscom NT: Apparent association between thymic cysts and prior thoracotomy. Radiology 172:207, 1989.

130. Borgna-Pignatti C, Andreis IB, Rugolotto S, et al: Thymic cyst appearing after treatment of mediastinal non-Hodgkin lymphoma. Med Pediatr Oncol 22:70, 1994.

131. Mishalani SH, Lones MA, Said JW: Multilocular thymic cyst: A novel thymic lesion associated with human immunodeficiency virus infection. Arch Pathol Lab Med 119:467, 1995.

132. Avila NA, Mueller BU, Carrasquillo JA, et al: Multilocular thymic cysts: Imaging features in children with human immunodeficiency virus infection. Radiology 201:130, 1996.

133. Brown LR, Aughenbaugh GL: Masses of the anterior mediastinum: CT and MR imaging. Am J Roentgenol 157:1171, 1991.

134. Hoffman OA, Gillespie DJ, Aughenbaugh GL, et al: Primary mediastinal neoplasms (other than thymoma). Mayo Clin Proc 68:880, 1993.

135. Verley JM, Hollmann KH: Thymoma: A comparative study of clinical stages, histologic features, and survival in 200 cases. Cancer 55:1074, 1985.

136. Lewis JE, Wick MR, Scheithauer BW, et al: Thymoma: A clinicopathologic review. Cancer 60:2727, 1987.

137. Pan C-C, Wu H-P, Yang C-F, et al: The clinicopathological correlation of epithelial subtyping in thymoma: A study of 112 consecutive cases. Hum Pathol 25:893, 1994.

138. Quintanilla-Martinez L, Wilkins EW Jr, Choi N, et al: Histologic subclassification is an independent prognostic factor. Cancer 74:606, 1994.

139. Rosado-de-Christenson ML, Galobardes J, Moran CA: Thymoma: Radiologic-pathologic correlation. Radiographics 12:151, 1992.

140. Tan A, Holdener GP, Hecht A, et al: Malignant thymoma in an ectopic thymus: CT appearance. J Comput Assist Tomogr 15:842, 1991.

141. Hofmann W, Möller P, Manke HG, et al: Thymoma: A clinicopathologic study of 98 cases with special reference to three unusual cases. Pathol Res Pract 179:337, 1985.

142. Morgenthaler TI, Brown LR, Colby TV, et al: Thymoma. Mayo Clin Proc 68:1110, 1993.

143. Brown LR, Muhm JR, Gray JE: Radiographic detection of thymoma. Am J Roentgenol 134:1181, 1980.

144. Dixon AK, Hilton CJ, Williams GT: Computed tomography and histological correlation of the thymic remnant. Clin Radiol 32:255, 1981.

145. Baron RL, Lee JKT, Sagel SS, et al: Computed tomography of the abnormal thymus. Radiology 142:127, 1982.

146. Keen SJ, Libshitz HI: Thymic lesions: Experience with computed tomography in 24 patients. Cancer 59:1520, 1987.

147. Zerhouni EA, Scott WW Jr, Baker RR, et al: Invasive thymomas: Diagnosis and evaluation by computed tomography. J Comput Assist Tomogr 6:92, 1982.

148. Do YS, Im J-G, Lee BH, et al: CT findings in malignant tumors of thymic epithelium. J Comput Assist Tomogr 19:192, 1995.

149. Verstandig AG, Epstein DM, Miller WT, et al: Thymoma: Report of 71 cases and a review. Crit Rev Diagn Imaging 33:201, 1992.

150. Scatarige JC, Fishman EK, Zerhouni EA, et al: Transdiaphragmatic extension of invasive thymoma. Am J Roentgenol 144:31, 1985.

151. Sakai F, Sone S, Kiyono K, et al: MR imaging of thymoma: Radiologic-pathologic correlation. Am J Roentgenol 158:751, 1992.

152. Hale DA, Cohen AJ, Schaefer P, et al: Computerized tomography in the evaluation of myasthenia gravis. South Med J 83:414, 1990.
153. Fon GT, Bein ME, Mancuso AA, et al: Computed tomography of the anterior mediastinum in myasthenia gravis: A radiologic-pathologic correlative study. Radiology 142:135, 1982.
154. Brown LR, Muhm JR, Sheedy PF II, et al: The value of computed tomography in myasthenia gravis. Am J Roentgenol 140:31, 1983.
155. Ellis K, Austin JHM, Ill AJ: Radiologic detection of thymoma in patients with myasthenia gravis. Am J Roentgenol 151:873, 1988.
156. Venegas RJ, Sun NCJ: Cardiac tamponade as a presentation of malignant thymoma. Acta Cytol 32:257, 1988.
157. Shishido M, Yano K, Ichiki H, et al: Pericarditis as the initial manifestation of malignant thymoma: Disappearance of pericardial effusion with corticosteroid therapy. Chest 106:313, 1994.
158. Dib HR, Friedman B, Khouli HI, et al: Malignant thymoma: A complicated triad of SVC syndrome, cardiac tamponade, and DIC. Chest 105:941, 1994.
159. Futami S, Yamasaki T, Minami R, et al: Intracaval and intracardiac extension of malignant thymoma. Intern Med 32:257, 1993.
160. Rosenthal T, Hertz M, Samra Y, et al: Thymoma: Clinical and additional radiologic signs. Chest 65:428, 1974.
161. Masaoka A, Hashimoto T, Shibata K, et al: Thymomas associated with pure red cell aplasia: Histologic and follow-up studies. Cancer 64:1872, 1989.
162. Bailey RO, Dunn HG, Rubin AM, et al: Myasthenia gravis with thymoma and pure red blood cell aplasia. Am J Clin Pathol 89:687, 1988.
163. De Giacomo T, Rendina EA, Venuta F, et al: Pancytopenia associated with thymoma resolving after thymectomy and immunosuppressive therapy: Case report. Scand J Thorac Cardiovasc Surg 29:149, 1995.
164. Postiglione K, Ferris R, Jaffe JP, et al: Immune mediated agranulocytosis and anemia associated with thymoma. Am J Hematol 49:336, 1995.
165. Athanassiou P, Ioakimidis D, Weston J, et al: Type 1 cryoglobulinaemia associated with a thymic tumour: Successful treatment with plasma exchange. Br J Rheumatol 34:285, 1995.
166. Honda T, Hayasaka M, Hachiya T, et al: Invasive thymoma with hypogammaglobulinemia spreading within the bronchial lumen. Respiration 62:294, 1995.
167. Lishner M, Ravid M, Shapira J, et al: Delta-T-lymphocytosis in a patient with thymoma. Cancer 74:2924, 1994.
168. Friedman HD, Inman DA, Hutchison RE, et al: Concurrent invasive thymoma and T-cell lymphoblastic leukemia and lymphoma: A case report with necropsy findings and literature review of thymoma and associated hematologic neoplasm. Am J Clin Pathol 101:432, 1994.
169. Nickels J, Franssila K: Thymoma metastasizing to extrathoracic sites. Acta Pathol Microbiol Scand Sect A 84:331, 1976.
170. Suster S, Moran CA: Thymic carcinoma: Spectrum of differentiation and histologic types. Pathology 30:111, 1998.
171. Kirchner T, Schalke B, Buchwald J, et al: Well-differentiated thymic carcinoma: An organotypical low-grade carcinoma with relationship to cortical thymoma. Am J Surg Pathol 16:1153, 1992.
172. Suster S, Rosai J: Thymic carcinoma: A clinicopathologic study of 60 cases. Cancer 67:1025, 1991.
173. Lee JD, Choe KO, Kim SJ, et al: CT findings in primary thymic carcinoma. J Comput Assist Tomogr 15:429, 1991.
174. Wick MR, Weiland LH, Scheithauer BW, et al: Primary thymic carcinomas. Am J Surg Pathol 6:613, 1982.
175. Hsu CP, Chen CY, Chen CL, et al: Thymic carcinoma: Ten years' experience in twenty patients. J Thorac Cardiovasc Surg 107:615, 1994.
176. Chang HK, Wang CH, Liaw CC, et al: Prognosis of thymic carcinoma: Analysis of 16 cases. J Formos Med Assoc 91:764, 1992.
177. Sungur A, Ruacan S, Gungen Y, et al: Myasthenia gravis and primary squamous cell carcinoma of the thymus. Arch Pathol Lab Med 117:937, 1993.
178. Negron-Soto JM, Cascade PN: Squamous cell carcinoma of the thymus with paraneoplastic hypercalcemia. Clin Imaging 19:122, 1995.
179. Ilhan I, Kutluk T, Gogus S, et al: Hypertrophic pulmonary osteoarthropathy in a child with thymic carcinoma: An unusual presentation in childhood. Med Pediatr Oncol 23:140, 1994.
180. Wick MR, Rosai J: Neuroendocrine neoplasms of the mediastinum. Semin Diagn Pathol 8:35, 1991.

181. Rosai J, Levine G, Weber WR, et al: Carcinoid tumors and oat cell carcinomas of the thymus. Pathol Ann 11:201, 1976.
182. Viebahn R, Hiddemann W, Klinke F, et al: Thymus carcinoid. Pathol Res Pract 180:445, 1985.
183. Gartner LA, Voorhess ML: Adrenocorticotropic hormone-producing thymic carcinoid in a teenager. Cancer 71:106, 1993.
184. Brown LR, Aughenbaugh GL, Wick MR, et al: Roentgenologic diagnosis of primary corticotropin-producing carcinoid tumors of the mediastinum. Radiology 142:143, 1982.
185. Felson B, Castleman B, Levinsohn EM, et al: Cushing syndrome associated with mediastinal mass. Am J Roentgenol 138:815, 1982.
186. Wang DY, Chang DB, Kuo SH, et al: Carcinoid tumours of the thymus. Thorax 49:357, 1994.
187. Economopoulos GC, Lewis JW Jr, Lee MW, et al: Carcinoid tumors of the thymus. Ann Thorac Surg 50:58, 1990.
188. Hughes JP, Ancalmo N, Leonard GL, et al: Carcinoid tumour of the thymus gland: Report of a case. Thorax 30:470, 1975.
189. Lowenthal RM, Gumpel JM, Kreel L, et al: Carcinoid tumour of the thymus with systemic manifestations: A radiological and pathological study. Thorax 29:553, 1974.
190. Kimura N, Ishikawa T, Sasaki Y, et al: Expression of prohormone convertase, PC2, in adrenocorticotropin-producing thymic carcinoid with elevated plasma corticotropin-releasing hormone. J Clin Endocrinol Metab 81:390, 1996.
191. Moran CA, Suster S: Primary germ cell tumors of the mediastinum: I. Analysis of 322 cases with special emphasis on teratomatous lesions and a proposal for histopathologic classification and clinical staging. Cancer 80:681, 1997.
192. Benjamin SP, McCormack LJ, Effler DB, et al: Critical review—"Primary tumours of the mediastinum." Chest 62:297, 1972.
193. Nichols CR: Mediastinal germ cell tumors. Semin Thorac Cardiovasc Surg 4:45, 1992.
194. Knapp RH, Hurt RD, Payne WS, et al: Malignant germ cell tumors of the mediastinum. J Thorac Cardiovasc Surg 89:82, 1985.
195. Dulmet EM, Macchiarini P, Suc B, et al: Germ cell tumors of the mediastinum: A 30-year experience. Cancer 72:1894, 1993.
196. Albuquerque KV, Mistry RC, Deshpande RK, et al: Primary germ cell tumours of the mediastinum. Indian J Cancer 31:250, 1994.
197. Rosado-de-Christenson ML, Templeton PA, Moran CA: Mediastinal germ cell tumors: Radiologic and pathologic correlation. Radiographics 12:1013, 1992.
198. Lee KS, Im J-G, Han CH, et al: Malignant primary germ cell tumors of the mediastinum: CT features. Am J Roentgenol 153:947, 1989.
199. Templeton AW: Malignant mediastinal teratoma with bone metastases: A case report. Radiology 76:245, 1961.
200. Schlumberger HG: Teratoma of the anterior mediastinum in the group of military age. Arch Pathol 41:398, 1946.
201. Le Roux BT: Mediastinal teratomata. Thorax 15:333, 1960.
202. Moeller KH, Rosado-de-Christenson ML, Templeton PA: Mediastinal mature teratoma: Imaging features. Am J Roentgenol 169:985, 1997.
203. Fulcher AS, Proto AV, Jolles H: Cystic teratoma of the mediastinum: Demonstration of fat/fluid level. Am J Roentgenol 154:259, 1990.
204. Sasaka K, Kurihara Y, Nakajima Y, et al: Spontaneous rupture: A complication of benign mature teratomas of the mediastinum. Am J Roentgenol 170:323, 1998.
205. Yeoman LJ, Dalton HR, Adam EJ: Fat-fluid level in pleural effusion as a complication of a mediastinal dermoid: CT characteristics. J Comput Assist Tomogr 14:305, 1990.
206. Moran CA, Suster S, Przygodzki RM, et al: Primary germ cell tumors of the mediastinum: II. Mediastinal seminomas—a clinicopathologic and immunohistochemical study of 120 cases. Cancer 80:691, 1997.
207. Choi S-J, Lee JS, Song KS, et al: Mediastinal teratoma: CT differentiation of ruptured and unruptured tumors. Am J Roentgenol 171:591, 1998.
208. Aygun C, Slawson RG, Bajaj K, et al: Primary mediastinal seminoma. Urology 23:109, 1984.
209. Shin MS, Ho KJ: Computed tomography of primary mediastinal seminomas. J Comput Assist Tomogr 7:990, 1983.
210. Truong LD, Harris L, Mattioli C, et al: Endodermal sinus tumor of the mediastinum: A report of seven cases and review of the literature. Cancer 58:730, 1986.
211. Sandhaus L, Strom RL, Mukai K: Primary embryonal-choriocarci-

noma of the mediastinum in a woman: A case report with immuno-histochemical study. Am J Clin Pathol 75:573, 1981.

212. Knapp RH, Fritz SR, Reiman HM: Primary embryonal carcinoma and choriocarcinoma of the mediastinum. Arch Pathol Lab Med 106:507, 1982.

213. Moran CA, Suster S: Primary mediastinal choriocarcinomas: A clinicopathologic and immunohistochemical study of eight cases. Am J Surg Pathol 21:1007, 1997.

214. Waldron JA Jr, Dohring EJ, Farber LR: Primary large cell lymphomas of the mediastinum: An analysis of 20 cases. Semin Diagn Pathol 2:281, 1985.

215. Levitt LJ, Aisenberg AC, Harris NL, et al: Primary non-Hodgkin's lymphoma of the mediastinum. Cancer 50:2486, 1982.

216. Yokose T, Kodama T, Matsuno Y, et al: Low-grade B cell lymphoma of mucosa-associated lymphoid tissue in the thymus of a patient with rheumatoid arthritis. Pathol Int 48:74, 1998.

217. Suematsu N, Watanabe S, Shimosato Y: A case of large "thymic granuloma": Neoplasm of T-zone histiocyte. Cancer 54:2480, 1984.

218. Szporn AH, Dikman S, Jagirdar J: True histiocytic lymphoma of the thymus: Report of a case and a study of the distribution of histiocytic cells in the fetal and adult thymus. Am J Clin Pathol 82:734, 1984.

219. Martin JJ: The Nisbet Symposium: Hodgkin's disease: Radiological aspects of the disease. Australas Radiol 11:206, 1967.

220. Fisher AMH, Kendall B, Van Leuven BD: Hodgkin's disease: A radiological survey. Clin Radiol 13:115, 1962.

221. Keller AR, Castleman B: Hodgkin's disease of the thymus gland. Cancer 33:1615, 1974.

222. Wernecke K, Vassallo P, Rutsch F, et al: Thymic involvement in Hodgkin's disease: CT and sonographic findings. Radiology 181:375, 1991.

223. Lahey FH: Intrathoracic goiters. Surg Clin North Am 25:609, 1945.

224. Nielsen VM, Lvgreen NA, Elbrnd O: Intrathoracic goitre: Surgical treatment in an ENT department. J Laryngol Otol 97:1039, 1983.

225. Katlic MR, Wang C, Grillo HC: Substernal goiter. Ann Thorac Surg 39:391, 1985.

226. Karadeniz A, Hacihanefioglu U: Abscess formation in an intrathoracic goitre. Thorax 37:556, 1982.

227. Irwin RS, Pratter MR, Hamolsky MW: Chronic persistent cough: An uncommon presenting complaint of thyroiditis. Chest 81:386, 1982.

228. Ward MJ, Davies D: Riedel's thyroiditis with invasion of the lungs. Thorax 36:956, 1981.

229. Rietz K-A, Werner B: Intrathoracic goiter. Acta Chir Scand 119:379, 1960.

230. Fragomeni LS, Ceratti de Zambuja P: Intrathoracic goitre in the posterior mediastinum. Thorax 35:638, 1980.

231. Spinner RJ, Moore KL, Gottfried MR, et al: Thoracic intrathymic thyroid. Ann Surg 220:91, 1994.

232. Bashist B, Ellis K, Gold RP: Computed tomography of intrathoracic goiters. Am J Roentgenol 140:455, 1983.

233. Glazer GM, Axel L, Moss AA: CT diagnosis of mediastinal thyroid. Am J Roentgenol 138:495, 1982.

234. Tecce PM, Fishman EK, Kuhlman JE: CT evaluation of the anterior mediastinum: Spectrum of disease. Radiographics 14:973, 1994.

235. Mori K, Eguchi K, Moriyama H, et al: Computed tomography of anterior mediastinal tumors. Acta Radiol 28:395, 1987.

236. Takashima S, Morimoto S, Ikezoe J, et al: CT evaluation of anaplastic thyroid carcinoma. Am J Roentgenol 154:1079, 1990.

237. Gefter WB, Spritzer CE, Eisenberg B, et al: Thyroid imaging with high-field-strength surface-coil MR. Radiology 164:483, 1987.

238. Noma S, Nishimura K, Togashi K, et al: Thyroid gland: MR imaging. Radiology 164:495, 1987.

239. Park H-M, Tarver RD, Siddiqui AR, et al: Efficacy of thyroid scintigraphy in the diagnosis of intrathoracic goiter. Am J Roentgenol 148:527, 1987.

240. Irwin RS, Braman SS, Arvanitidis AN, et al: ^{131}I thyroid scanning in preoperative diagnosis of mediastinal goiter. Ann Intern Med 89:73, 1978.

241. Irwin RS: Two asymptomatic patients with mediastinal disease. Chest 112:1677, 1997.

242. Schneider JA, Divgi CR, Scott AM, et al: Hiatal hernia on whole-body radioiodine survey mimicking metastatic thyroid cancer. Clin Nucl Med 18:751, 1993.

243. Willis LL, Cowan RJ: Mediastinal uptake of I-131 in a hiatal hernia mimicking recurrence of papillary thyroid carcinoma. Clin Nucl Med 18:961, 1993.

244. Vermiglio F, Baudin E, Travagli JP, et al: Iodine concentration by the thymus in thyroid carcinoma. J Nucl Med 37:1830, 1996.

245. Murphy MN, Glennon PG, Diocee MS, et al: Nonsecretory parathyroid carcinoma of the mediastinum: Light microscopic, immunocytochemical, and ultrastructural features of a case, and review of the literature. Cancer 58:2468, 1986.

246. Leigh TF, Weens HS: Roentgen aspects of mediastinal lesions. Semin Roentgenol 4:59, 1969.

247. Lee YT, Hutcheson JK: Mediastinal parathyroid carcinoma detected on routine chest film. Chest 65:354, 1974.

248. Braxel C, Haemers S, van der Straeten M: Mediastinal parathyroid adenoma detected on a routine chest X-ray. Scand J Respir Dis 60:367, 1979.

249. Hanson DJ Jr: Unusual radiographic manifestations of parathyroid adenoma: Report of a case. N Engl J Med 267:1080, 1962.

250. Stark DD, Gooding GAW, Moss AA, et al: Parathyroid imaging: Comparison of high-resolution CT and high-resolution sonography. Am J Roentgenol 141:633, 1983.

251. Yousem DM, Scheff AM: Thyroid and parathyroid gland pathology. Otolaryngol Clin North Am 28:621, 1995.

252. Kang YS, Rosen K, Clark OH, et al: Localization of abnormal parathyroid glands of the mediastinum with MR imaging. Radiology 189:137, 1993.

253. Doppman JL, Skarulis MC, Chen CC, et al: Parathyroid adenomas in the aortopulmonary window. Radiology 201:456, 1996.

254. Hauet EJ, Paul MA, Salu MK: Compression of the trachea by a mediastinal parathyroid cyst. Ann Thorac Surg 64:851, 1997.

255. Auffermann W, Gooding GA, Okerlung MD, et al: Diagnosis of recurrent hyperparathyroidism: Comparison of MR imaging and other imaging techniques. Am J Roentgenol 150:1027, 1988.

256. Lee VS, Spritzer CE: MR imaging of abnormal parathyroid glands. Am J Roentgenol 170:1097, 1998.

257. Seelos KC, DeMarco R, Clark OH, et al: Persistent and recurrent hyperparathyroidism: Assessment with gadopentetate dimeglumine-enhanced MR imaging. Radiology 177:373, 1990.

258. Wei J, Burke GJ, Mansberger AR: Preoperative imaging of abnormal parathyroid glands in patients with hyperparathyroid disease using combination Tc-99m-pertechnetate and Tc-99m-sestamibi radionuclide scans. Ann Surg 219:568, 1994.

259. Gordon BM, Gordon L, Hoang K, et al: Parathyroid imaging with 99mTc-sestamibi. Am J Roentgenol 167:1563, 1996.

260. Udelsman R: Parathyroid imaging: The myth and the reality. Radiology 201:317, 1996.

261. Lee VS, Spritzer CE, Coleman RE, et al: The complementary roles of fast spin-echo MR imaging and double-phase 99mTc-sestamibi scintigraphy for localization of hyperfunctioning parathyroid glands. Am J Roentgenol 167:1555, 1996.

262. Krudy AG, Doppman JL, Brennan MF, et al: The detection of mediastinal parathyroid glands by computed tomography, selective arteriography and venous sampling: An analysis of 17 cases. Radiology 140:739, 1981.

263. Krudy AG, Doppman JL, Miller DL, et al: Detection of mediastinal parathyroid glands by nonselective digital arteriography. Am J Roentgenol 142:693, 1984.

264. Doppman JL, Skarulis MC, Chang R, et al: Hypocalcemic stimulation and nonselective venous sampling for localizing parathyroid adenomas: Work in progress. Radiology 208:145, 1998.

265. Gibbs AR, Johnson NF, Giddings JC, et al: Primary angiosarcoma of the mediastinum: Light and electron microscopic demonstration of factor VIII-related antigen in neoplastic cells. Hum Pathol 15:687, 1984.

266. Swanson PE: Soft tissue neoplasms of the mediastinum. Semin Diagn Pathol 8:14, 1991.

267. Pachter MR, Lattes R: Mesenchymal tumors of the mediastinum: I. Tumors of fibrous tissue, adipose tissue, smooth muscle, and striated muscle. Cancer 16:74, 1963.

268. Wilson ES: Radiolucent mediastinal lipoma. Radiology 118:44, 1976.

269. Mendez G Jr, Isikoff MB, Isikoff SK, et al: Fatty tumors of the thorax demonstrated by CT. Am J Roentgenol 133:207, 1979.

270. Santini LC, Williams JL: Mediastinal widening (presumably lipomatosis) in Cushing's syndrome. N Engl J Med 284:1357, 1971.

271. Koerner HJ, Sun DI-C: Mediastinal lipomatosis secondary to steroid therapy. Am J Roentgenol 98:461, 1966.

272. Teates CD: Steroid-induced mediastinal lipomatosis. Radiology 96:501, 1970.

273. van de Putte LBA, Wagenaar JPM, San KH: Paracardiac lipomatosis in exogenous Cushing's syndrome. Thorax 28:653, 1973.

274. Lee WJ, Fattal G: Mediastinal lipomatosis in simple obesity. Chest 70:308, 1976.

275. Streiter ML, Schneider HJ, Proto AV: Steroid-induced thoracic lipomatosis: Paraspinal involvement. Am J Roentgenol 139:679, 1982.

276. Chalaoui J, Sylvestre J, Dussault RG, et al: Thoracic fatty lesions: Some usual and unusual appearances. J Can Assoc Radiol 32:197, 1981.

277. Summer TE, Volberg FM, Kiser PE, et al: Mediastinal cystic hygroma in children. Pediatr Radiol 11:160, 1981.

278. Topcu S, Soysal O, Balkan E, et al: Mediastinal cystic lymphangioma: Report of two cases. Thorac Cardiovasc Surg 45:209, 1997.

279. Pannell TL, Jolles H: Adult cystic mediastinal lymphangioma simulating a thymic cyst. J Thorac Imaging 7:86, 1991.

280. Pilla TJ, Wolverson MK, Sundaram M, et al: CT evaluation of cystic lymphangiomas of the mediastinum. Radiology 144:841, 1982.

281. Shaffer K, Rosado-de-Christenson ML, Patz EF Jr, et al: Thoracic lymphangioma in adults: CT and MR imaging features. Am J Roentgenol 162:283, 1994.

282. Miyake H, Shiga M, Takaki H, et al: Mediastinal lymphangiomas in adults: CT findings. J Thorac Imaging 11:83, 1996.

283. Khoury GH, Demong CV: Mediastinal cystic hygroma in childhood. J Pediatr 62:432, 1963.

284. Glazer HS, Wick MR, Anderson DJ, et al: CT of fatty thoracic masses. Am J Roentgenol 159:1181, 1992.

285. Rodríguez E, Soler R, Gayol A, et al: Massive mediastinal and cardiac fatty infiltration in a young patient. J Thorac Imaging 10:225, 1995.

286. Peterson DT, Katz LM, Popp RL: Pericardial cyst 10 years after acute pericarditis. Chest 67:719, 1975.

287. Stoller JK, Shaw C, Matthay RA: Enlarging, atypically located pericardial cyst: Recent experience and literature review. Chest 89:402, 1986.

288. Ochsner JL, Ochsner SF: Congenital cysts of the mediastinum: 20-year experience with 42 cases. Ann Surg 163:909, 1966.

289. Pader E, Kirschner PA: Pericardial diverticulum. Dis Chest 55:344, 1969.

290. Snyder SN: Massive pericardial coelomic cyst: Diagnostic features and unusual presentation. Chest 71:100, 1977.

291. Pugatch RD, Braver JH, Robbins AH, et al: CT diagnosis of pericardial cysts. Am J Roentgenol 131:515, 1978.

292. Ikezoe J, Sone S, Morimoto S, et al: Computed tomography reveals atypical localization of benign mediastinal tumors. Acta Radiol 30:175, 1989.

293. Vinee P, Stover B, Sigmund G, et al: MR imaging of the pericardial cyst. J Magn Reson Imaging 2:593, 1992.

294. Padder FA, Conrad AR, Manzar KJ, et al: Echocardiographic diagnosis of pericardial cyst. Am J Med Sci 313:191, 1997.

295. Rogers CI, Seymour EQ, Brock JG: Atypical pericardial cyst location: The value of computed tomography: Case report. J Comput Assist Tomogr 4:683, 1980.

296. Brunner DR, Whitley NO: A pericardial cyst with high CT numbers. Am J Roentgenol 142:279, 1984.

297. Aronberg DJ, Peterson RP, Glazer HS, et al: Superior diaphragmatic lymph nodes: CT assessment. J Comput Assist Tomogr 10:937, 1986.

298. Schwartz EE, Wechsler RJ: Diaphragmatic and paradiaphragmatic tumors and pseudotumors. J Thorac Imaging 4:19, 1989.

299. Vock P, Hodler J: Cardiophrenic angle adenopathy: Update of causes and significance. Radiology 159:395, 1986.

300. Cho CS, Blank N, Castellino RA: CT evaluation of cardiophrenic angle lymph nodes in patients with malignant lymphoma. Am J Roentgenol 143:719, 1984.

301. Castellino RA, Blank N: Adenopathy of the cardiophrenic angle (diaphragmatic) lymph nodes. Am J Roentgenol 114:509, 1972.

302. Fayos JV, Lampe I: Cardiac apical mass in Hodgkin's disease. Radiology 99:15, 1971.

303. Strollo DC, Rosado-de-Christenson ML, Jett JR: Primary mediastinal tumors: Part II. Tumors of the middle and posterior mediastinum. Chest 112:1344, 1997.

304. Azizkhan RG, Dudgeon DL, Buck JR, et al: Life-threatening airway obstruction as a complication to the management of mediastinal masses in children. J Pediatr Surg 20:816, 1985.

305. Castleman B (ed): Case records of the Massachusetts General Hospital, case 40011. N Engl J Med 250:26, 1954.

306. Keller AR, Hochholzer L, Castleman B: Hyaline-vascular and plasma-cell types of giant lymph node hyperplasia of the mediastinum and other locations. Cancer 29:670, 1972.

307. Frizzera G: Castleman's disease: More questions than answers. Hum Pathol 16:202, 1985.

308. Kirsch CFE, Webb EM, Webb WR: Multicentric Castleman's disease and POEMS syndrome: CT findings. J Thorac Imaging 12:75, 1997.

309. Johkoh T, Müller NL, Ichikado K, et al: Intrathoracic multicentric Castleman's disease: CT findings in 12 patients. Radiology 209:477, 1998.

310. Kim JH, Jun TG, Sung SW, et al: Giant lymph node hyperplasia (Castleman's disease) in the chest. Ann Thorac Surg 59:1162, 1995.

311. Moon WK, Im J-G, Kim JS, et al: Mediastinal Castleman disease: CT findings. J Comput Assist Tomogr 18:43, 1994.

312. McAdams HP, Rosado-de-Christenson M, Fishback NF, et al: Castleman disease of the thorax: Radiologic features with clinical and histopathologic correlation. Radiology 209:221, 1998.

313. Moon WK, Im J-G, Han MC: Castleman's disease of the mediastinum: MR imaging features. Clin Radiol 49:466, 1994.

314. Khan J, von Sinner W, Akhtar M, et al: Castleman's disease of the chest: Magnetic resonance imaging features. Chest 105:1608, 1994.

315. Glenner GG, Grimley PM: Atlas of Tumor Pathology: Second Series, Fascicle 9. Tumors of the Extra-Adrenal Paraganglion System (Including Chemoreceptors). Washington, DC, Armed Forces Institute of Pathology, 1974.

316. Lack EE, Stillinger RA, Colvin DB, et al: Aorticopulmonary paraganglioma: Report of a case with ultrastructural study and review of the literature. Cancer 43:269, 1979.

317. Ros PR, Rosado-de-Christenson ML, Buetow PC, et al: The Radiological Society of North America 83rd Scientific Assembly and Annual Meeting: Image interpretation session: 1997. Radiographics 18:195, 1998.

318. Hamilton BH, Francis IR, Gross BH, et al: Intrapericardial paragangliomas (pheochromocytomas): Imaging features. Am J Roentgenol 168:109, 1997.

319. Ogawa J, Inoue H, Koide S, et al: Functioning paraganglioma in the posterior mediastinum. Ann Thorac Surg 33:507, 1982.

320. Drucker EA, McLoud TC, Dedrick CG, et al: Mediastinal paraganglioma: Radiologic evaluation of an unusual vascular tumor. Am J Roentgenol 148:521, 1987.

321. Bomanji J, Conry BG, Britton KE, et al: Imaging neural crest tumors with ^{123}I-meta-iodobenzylguanidine and x-ray computed tomography: A comparative study. Clin Radiol 39:502, 1988.

322. van Gils AP, Falke TA, van Erkel AR, et al: MR imaging and MIBG scintigraphy of pheochromocytomas and extra-adrenal functioning paragangliomas. Radiographics 11:37, 1991.

323. Kwekkeboom DJ, van Urk H, Pauw BK, et al: Octreotide scintigraphy for the detection of paragangliomas. J Nucl Med 34:873, 1993.

324. van Gelder T, Verhoeven GT, de Jong P, et al: Dopamine-producing paraganglioma not visualized by iodine-123-MIBG scintigraphy. J Nucl Med 36:620, 1995.

325. Rappaport DC, Herman SJ, Weisbrod GL: Congenital bronchopulmonary diseases in adults: CT findings. Am J Roentgenol 162:1295, 1994.

326. Kawashima A, Fishman EK, Kuhlman JE, et al: CT of posterior mediastinal masses. Radiographics 11:1045, 1991.

327. Murayama S, Murakami J, Watanabe H, et al: Signal intensity characteristics of mediastinal cystic masses on T1-weighted MRI. J Comput Assist Tomogr 19:188, 1995.

328. Endo S, Sohara Y, Yamaguchi T, et al: The effectiveness of transesophageal ultrasonography in preoperatively diagnosing an esophageal cyst in a 75-year-old woman: Report of a case. Surg Today 24:356, 1994.

329. Zeilender S, Turner MA, Glauser FL: Mediastinal pseudocyst associated with chronic pleural effusion. Chest 97:1014, 1990.

330. Sambrook Gowar FJ: Mediastinal thoracic duct cyst. Thorax 33:800, 1978.

331. Tsuchiya R, Sugiura Y, Ogata T, et al: Thoracic duct cyst of the mediastinum. J Thorac Cardiovasc Surg 79:856, 1980.

332. Hori S, Harada K, Morimoto S, et al: Lymphangiographic demonstration of thoracic duct cyst. Chest 78:652, 1980.

333. Morettin LB, Allen TE: Thoracic duct cyst: Diagnosis with needle aspiration. Radiology 161:437, 1986.

334. Buckingham WB, Sutton GC, Meszaros WT: Abnormalities of the pulmonary artery resembling intrathoracic neoplasms. Dis Chest 40:698, 1961.

335. Hom M, Jolles H: Traumatic mediastinal lymphocele mimicking other thoracic injuries: Case report. J Thorac Imaging 7:78, 1992.

336. Fleming JS, Gibson RV: Absent right superior vena cava as an isolated anomaly. Br J Radiol 37:696, 1964.

337. White CS, Baffa JM, Haney PJ, et al: MR imaging of congenital anomalies of the thoracic veins. Radiographics 17:595, 1997.

338. Webb WR, Gamsu G, Speckman JM, et al: Computed tomographic demonstration of mediastinal venous anomalies. Am J Roentgenol 139:157, 1982.

339. Kellman GM, Alpern MB, Sandler MA, et al: Computed tomography of vena caval anomalies with embryologic correlation. Radiographics 8:533, 1988.

340. Cormier MG, Yedlicka JW, Gray RJ, et al: Congenital anomalies of the superior vena cava: A CT study. Semin Roentgenol 24:77, 1989.

341. Voci P, Luzi G, Agati L: Diagnosis of persistent left superior vena cava by multiplane transesophageal echocardiography. Cardiologia 40:273, 1995.

342. Dillon EH, Camputaro C: Partial anomalous pulmonary venous drainage of the left upper lobe vs duplication of the superior vena cava: Distinction based on CT findings. Am J Roentgenol 160:375, 1993.

343. Escalante CP: Causes and management of superior vena cava syndrome. Oncology 7:61, 1993.

344. Lochridge SK, Knibbe WP, Doty DB: Obstruction of the superior vena cava. Surgery 85:14, 1979.

345. Schraufnagel DE, Hill R, Leech JA, et al: Superior vena caval obstruction: Is it a medical emergency? Am J Med 70:1169, 1981.

346. Davies PF, Shevland JE: Superior vena caval obstruction: An analysis of seventy-six cases, with comments on the safety of venography. Angiology 36:354, 1985.

347. Kastner RJ, Fisher WG, Blacky AR, et al: Pacemaker-induced superior vena cava syndrome with successful treatment by balloon venoplasty. Am J Cardiol 77:789, 1996.

348. Dhondt E, Hutse W, Vanmeerhaeghe X, et al: Superior vena cava syndrome after implantation of a transvenous cardioverter defibrillator. Eur Heart J 16:716, 1995.

349. Richmond G, Handwerger S, Schoenfeld N, et al: Superior vena cava syndrome: A complication of Hickman catheter insertion in patients with the acquired immunodeficiency syndrome. N Y State J Med 92:65, 1992.

350. Doty DB: Bypass of superior vena cava: 6 years' experience with spiral vein graft for obstruction of superior vena cava due to benign and malignant disease. J Thorac Cardiovasc Surg 83:326, 1982.

351. Brown G, Husband JE: Mediastinal widening: A valuable radiographic sign of superior vena cava thrombosis. Clin Radiol 47:415, 1993.

352. Engel IA, Auh YH, Rubenstein WA, et al: CT diagnosis of mediastinal and thoracic inlet venous obstruction. Am J Roentgenol 141:521, 1983.

353. Kim H-J, Kim HS, Chung SH: CT diagnosis of superior vena cava syndrome: Importance of collateral vessels. Am J Roentgenol 161:539, 1993.

354. Gosselin MV, Rubin GD: Altered intravascular contrast material flow dynamics: Clues for refining thoracic CT diagnosis. Am J Roentgenol 169:1597, 1997.

355. Weinreb JC, Mootz A, Cohen JM: MRI evaluation of mediastinal and thoracic inlet venous obstruction. Am J Roentgenol 146:679, 1986.

356. Preger L, Hooper TI, Steinbach HL, et al: Width of azygos vein related to central venous pressures. Radiology 93:521, 1969.

357. Doyle FH, Read AE, Evans KT: The mediastinum in portal hypertension. Clin Radiol 12:114, 1961.

358. Steinberg I: Dilatation of the hemiazygos veins in superior vena caval occlusion simulating mediastinal tumor. Am J Roentgenol 87:248, 1962.

359. Floyd GD, Nelson WP: Developmental interruption of the inferior vena cava with azygos and hemiazygos substitution: Unusual radiographic features. Radiology 119:55, 1976.

360. Rockoff SD, Druy EM: Tortuous azygos arch simulating a pulmonary lesion. Am J Roentgenol 138:577, 1982.

361. Allen HA, Haney PJ: Left-sided inferior vena cava with hemiazygos continuation: Case report. J Comput Assist Tomogr 5:917, 1981.

362. Breckenridge JW, Kinlaw WB: Azygos continuation of inferior vena cava: CT appearance. J Comput Assist Tomogr 4:392, 1980.

363. Ball JB Jr, Proto AV: The variable appearance of the left superior intercostal vein. Radiology 144:445, 1982.

364. Friedman AC, Chambers E, Sprayregen S: The normal and abnormal left superior intercostal vein. Am J Roentgenol 131:599, 1978.

365. Hatfield MK, Vyborny CJ, MacMahon H, et al: Congenital absence of the azygos vein: A cause for "aortic nipple" enlargement. Am J Roentgenol 149:273, 1987.

366. Guthaner DF, Wexler L, Harell G: CT demonstration of cardiac structures. Am J Roentgenol 133:75, 1979.

367. Hirose Y, Hamade S, Takamiya M, et al: Aortic aneurysms: Growth rates measured with CT. Radiology 185:249, 1992.

368. Godwin JD: Conventional CT of the aorta. J Thorac Imaging 5:18, 1990.

369. Chen JTT: Plain radiographic evaluation of the aorta. J Thorac Imaging 5:1, 1990.

370. Posniak HV, Olson MC, Demos TC, et al: CT of thoracic aortic aneurysms. Radiographics 10:839, 1990.

371. Pressler V, McNamara JJ: Thoracic aortic aneurysm: Natural history and treatment. J Thorac Cardiovasc Surg 79:489, 1980.

372. Moreno-Cabral CE, Miller DC, Mitchell RS, et al: Degenerative and atherosclerotic aneurysms of the thoracic aorta: Determinants of early and late surgical outcome. J Thorac Cardiovasc Surg 88:1020, 1984.

373. Johansen K, Devin J: Mycotic aortic aneurysms: A reappraisal. Arch Surg 118:583, 1983.

374. Felson B, Akers PV, Hall GS, et al: Mycotic tuberculous aneurysm of the thoracic aorta. JAMA 237:1104, 1977.

375. Adachi H, Ino T, Mizuhara A, et al: Assessment of aortic disease using three-dimensional CT angiography. J Card Surg 9:673, 1994.

376. Chung JW, Park JH, Im J-G, et al: Spiral CT angiography of the thoracic aorta. Radiographics 16:811, 1996.

377. Alley MT, Shifrin RY, Pelc NJ, et al: Ultrafast contrast-enhanced three-dimensional MR angiography: State-of-the-art. Radiographics 18:273, 1998.

378. Ho VB, Prince MR: Thoracic MR aortography: Imaging techniques and strategies. Radiographics 18:287, 1998.

379. Kamp O, van Rossum AC, Torenbeek R: Transesophageal echocardiography and magnetic resonance imaging for the assessment of saccular aneurysm of the transverse thoracic aorta. Int J Cardiol 33:330, 1991.

380. Cramer M, Foley WD, Palmer TE, et al: Compression of the right pulmonary artery by aortic aneurysms: CT demonstration. J Comput Assist Tomogr 9:310, 1985.

381. Duke RA, Barrett MR, Payne SD, et al: Compression of left main bronchus and left pulmonary artery by thoracic aortic aneurysm. Am J Roentgenol 149:261, 1987.

382. Heiberg E, Wolverson MK, Sundaram M, et al: CT characteristics of aortic atherosclerotic aneurysm versus aortic dissection. J Comput Assist Tomogr 9:78, 1985.

383. Wilson SK, Hutchins GM: Aortic dissecting aneurysms: Causative factors in 204 subjects. Arch Pathol Lab Med 106:175, 1982.

384. Fisher ER, Stern EJ, Godwin JD: Acute aortic dissection: Typical and atypical imaging features. Radiographics 14:1263, 1994.

385. Roberts WC: Aortic dissection: Anatomy, consequences, and causes. Am Heart J 101:195, 1981.

386. Yamada T, Tada S, Harada J: Aortic dissection without intimal rupture: Diagnosis with MR imaging and CT. Radiology 168:347, 1988.

387. Hirst AE Jr, Johns VJ Jr, Kime SW Jr: Dissecting aneurysm of the aorta: A review of 505 cases. Medicine 37:217, 1958.

388. Wolff KA, Herold CJ, Tempany CM, et al: Aortic dissection: Atypical patterns seen at MR imaging. Radiology 181:489, 1991.

389. Nienaber CA, von Kodolitsch Y, Nicolas V, et al: The diagnosis of thoracic aortic dissection by noninvasive imaging procedures. N Engl J Med 328:1, 1993.

390. DeBakey ME, McCollum H, Crawford ES, et al: Dissection and dissecting aneurysms of the aorta: Twenty-year follow-up of five hundred twenty-seven patients treated surgically. Surgery 92:1118, 1982.

391. Petasnick JP: Radiologic evaluation of aortic dissection. Radiology 180:297, 1991.

392. Sakamoto I, Hayashi K, Matsunaga N, et al: Aortic dissection caused by angiographic procedures. Radiology 191:467, 1994.

393. Beachley MC, Ranniger K, Roth FJ: Roentgenographic evaluation of dissecting aneurysms of the aorta. Am J Roentgenol 121:617, 1974.

394. Demos TC, Posniak HV, Marsan RE: CT of aortic dissection. Semin Roentgenol 24:22, 1989.

395. Luker GD, Glazer HS, Eagar G, et al: Aortic dissection: Effect of prospective chest radiographic diagnosis on delay to definitive diagnosis. Radiology 193:813, 1994.

396. Vasile N, Mathieu D, Keita K, et al: Computed tomography of thoracic aortic dissection: Accuracy and pitfalls. J Comput Assist Tomogr 10:211, 1986.

397. Sommer T, Fehske W, Holzknecht N, et al: Aortic dissection: A comparative study of diagnosis with spiral CT, multiplanar transesophageal echocardiography, and MR imaging. Radiology 199:347, 1996.

398. Torres WE, Maurer DE, Steinberg HV, et al: CT of aortic aneurysms: The distinction between mural and thrombus calcification. Am J Roentgenol 150:1317, 1988.

399. DeSanctis RW, Doroghazi RM, Austen WG, et al: Aortic dissection. N Engl J Med 317:1060, 1987.

400. Cigarroa JE, Isselbacher EM, DeSanctis RW, et al: Medical progress: Diagnostic imaging in the evaluation of suspected aortic dissection: Old standards and new directions. Am J Roentgenol 161:485, 1993.

401. Shuford WH, Sybers RG, Weens HS: Problems in the aortographic diagnosis of dissecting aneurysm of the aorta. N Engl J Med 280:225, 1969.

402. Wilbers CRH, Carrol CL, Hnilica MA: Optimal diagnostic imaging of aortic dissection. Tex Heart Inst J 17:271, 1990.

403. Eagle KA, DeSanctis RW: Aortic dissection. Curr Prob Cardiol 14:225, 1989.

404. Green RA: Enlargement of the innominate and subclavian arteries simulating mediastinal neoplasm. Am Rev Tuberc 79:790, 1959.

405. Hallman GL, Cooley DA: Congenital aortic vascular ring: Surgical considerations. Arch Surg 88:666, 1964.

406. Lam CR, Kabbani S, Arciniegas E: Symptomatic anomalies of the aortic arch. Surg Gynecol Obstet 147:673, 1978.

407. Idbeis B, Levinsky L, Srinivasan V, et al: Vascular rings: Management and a proposed nomenclature. Ann Thorac Surg 31:255, 1981.

408. Engelman RM, Madayag M: Aberrant right subclavian artery aneurysm: A rare cause of a superior mediastinal tumor. Chest 62:45, 1972.

409. VanDyke CW, White RD: Congenital abnormalities of the thoracic aorta presenting in the adult. J Thorac Imaging 9:230, 1994.

410. Gaupp RJ, Fagan CJ, Davis M, et al: Pseudocoarctation of the aorta: Case report. J Comput Assist Tomogr 5:571, 1981.

411. Kennard DR, Spigos DG, Tan WS: Cervical aortic arch: CT correlation with conventional radiologic studies. Am J Roentgenol 141:295, 1983.

412. Salomonowitz E, Edwards JE, Hunter DW, et al: The three types of aortic diverticula. Am J Roentgenol 142:673, 1984.

413. Shuford WH, Sybers RG, Edwards FK: The three types of right aortic arch. Am J Roentgenol 109:67, 1970.

414. Raymond GS, Miller RM, Müller NL, et al: Congenital thoracic lesions that mimic neoplastic disease on chest radiographs of adults. Am J Roentgenol 168:763, 1997.

415. Bevelaqua F, Schicchi JS, Haas F, et al: Aortic arch anomaly presenting as exercise-induced asthma. Am Rev Respir Dis 140:805, 1989.

416. Branscom JJ, Austin JHM: Aberrant right subclavian artery: Findings seen on plain chest roentgenograms. Am J Roentgenol 119:539, 1973.

417. Kommerell B: Verlagerung des Oesophagus durch eine abnorm verlaufende Arteria subclavia dextra (Arteria lusoria). Fortschr Geb Rontgenstr Nuklearmed 54:590, 1936.

418. Lindell MM Jr, Hill CA, Libshitz HI: Esophageal cancer: Radiographic chest findings and their prognostic significance. Am J Roentgenol 133:461, 1979.

419. Daffner RH, Postlethwait RW, Putman CE: Retrotracheal abnormalities in esophageal carcinoma: Prognostic implications. Am J Roentgenol 130:719, 1978.

420. Yrjana J: The posterior tracheal band and recurrent esophageal carcinoma. Radiology 146:433, 1983.

421. Wolfman NT, Scharling ES, Chen MYM: Esophageal squamous carcinoma. Radiol Clin North Am 32:1183, 1994.

422. Levine MS: Esophageal cancer: Radiologic diagnosis. Radiol Clin North Am 35:265, 1997.

423. Reinig JW, Stanley JH, Schabel SI: CT evaluation of thickened esophageal walls. Am J Roentgenol 140:931, 1983.

424. Rankin S, Mason R: Staging of oesophageal carcinoma. Clin Radiol 46:373, 1992.

425. Picus D, Balfe DM, Koehler RE, et al: Computed tomography in the staging of esophageal carcinoma. Radiology 146:433, 1983.

426. Botet JF, Lightdale CJ, Zauber AG, et al: Preoperative staging of esophageal cancer: Comparison of endoscopic US and dynamic CT. Radiology 181:419, 1991.

427. Noh HM, Fishman EK, Forastiere AA, et al: CT of the esophagus: Spectrum of disease with emphasis on esophageal carcinoma. Radiographics 15:1113, 1995.

428. Vilgrain V, Mompoint D, Palazzo L, et al: Staging of esophageal carcinoma: Comparison of results with endoscopic sonography and CT. Am J Roentgenol 155:277, 1990.

429. Sharma OP, Chandermohan M, Mashankar AS, et al: Role of computed tomography in preoperative evaluation of esophageal carcinoma. Indian J Cancer 31:12, 1994.

430. Maerz LL, Deveney CW, Lopez RR, et al: Role of computed tomographic scans in the staging of esophageal and proximal gastric malignancies. Am J Surg 165:558, 1993.

431. Crawford ES, Svensson LG, Coselli JS, et al: Aortic dissection and dissecting aortic aneurysms. Ann Surg 208:254, 1988.

432. Armengol Miro JR, Benjamin S, Binmoeller K, et al: Clinical applications of endoscopic ultrasonography in gastroenterology: State of the art 1993. Results of a Consensus Conference, Orlando, Florida, 19 January 1993. Endoscopy 25:358, 1993.

433. Takashima S, Takeuchi N, Shiozaki H, et al: Carcinoma of the esophagus: CT vs MR imaging in determining resectability. Am J Roentgenol 156:297, 1991.

434. Thompson WM, Halvorsen RA Jr: Staging esophageal carcinoma: II. CT and MRI. Semin Oncol 21:447, 1994.

435. Rankin SC, Taylor H, Cook GJR, et al: Computed tomography and positron emission tomography in the pre-operative staging of oesophageal carcinoma. Clin Radiol 53:659, 1998.

436. Rainer WG, Brus R: Leiomyosarcoma of the esophagus. Surgery 58:343, 1965.

437. Choh JH, Khazei AH, Ihm HJ: Leiomyosarcoma of the esophagus: Report of a case and review of the literature. J Surg Oncol 32:223, 1986.

438. Jalundhwala JM, Shah RC: Epiphrenic esophageal diverticulum. Chest 57:97, 1970.

439. Tishler JM, Shin MS, Stanley RJ, et al: CT of the thorax in patients with achalasia. Dig Dis Sci 28:692, 1983.

440. Rabushka LS, Fishman EK, Kuhlman JE: CT evaluation of achalasia. J Comput Assist Tomogr 15:434, 1991.

441. Blomquist G, Mahoney PS: Noncollapsing air-filled esophagus in diseased and postoperative chests. Acta Radiol 55:32, 1961.

442. Schabel SI, Stanley JH: Air esophagram after laryngectomy. Am J Roentgenol 136:19, 1981.

443. Moult PJA, Waite DW, Dick W: Posterior mediastinal venous masses in patients with portal hypertension. Gut 16:57, 1975.

444. Ishikawa T, Saeki M, Tsukune Y, et al: Detection of paraesophageal varices by plain films. Am J Roentgenol 144:701, 1985.

445. Lee SJ, Lee KS, Kim SA, et al: Computed radiography of the chest in patients with paraesophageal varices: Diagnostic accuracy and characteristic findings. Am J Roentgenol 170:1527, 1998.

446. Arakawa A, Nagata Y, Miyagi S, et al: Case report: Interruption of inferior vena cava with anomalous continuations. J Comput Assist Tomogr 11:341, 1987.

447. Minami M, Kawauchi N, Itai Y, et al: Transdiaphragmatic portosystemic shunt to the pericardiacophrenic vein. Am J Roentgenol 161:569, 1993.

448. Wachsberg RH, Yaghmai V, Javors BR, et al: Cardiophrenic varices in portal hypertension: Evaluation with CT. Radiology 195:553, 1995.

449. Blendis LM, Laws JW, Williams R, et al: Calcified collateral veins and gross dilatation of the azygos vein in cirrhosis. Br J Radiol 41:909, 1968.

450. Milner LB, Marchan R: Complete absence of the inferior vena cava presenting as a paraspinous mass. Thorax 35:798, 1980.

451. Schneeweiss A, Bleiden LC, Deutsch V, et al: Uninterrupted inferior vena cava with azygos continuation. Chest 80:114, 1981.

452. Ingels GW, Campbell DC, Giampetro AM, et al: Malignant schwannomas of the mediastinum. Cancer 27:1190, 1971.

453. Azarow KS, Pearl RH, Zurcher R, et al: Primary mediastinal masses: A comparison of adult and pediatric populations. J Thorac Cardiovasc Surg 106:67, 1993.

454. Saenz NC, Schnitzer JJ, Eraklis AE, et al: Posterior mediastinal masses. J Pediatr Surg 28:172, 1993.

455. Reed JC, Kagan-Hallett K, Feigin DS: Neural tumors of the thorax: Subject review from the AFIP. Radiology 126:9, 1978.

456. Kumar AJ, Kuhajda FP, Martinez CR, et al: Computed tomography of the extracranial nerve sheath tumors with pathological correlation. J Comput Assist Tomogr 7:857, 1983.

457. Ko S-F, Lee T-Y, Lin J-W, et al: Thoracic neurilemomas: An analysis of computed tomography findings in 36 patients. J Thorac Imaging 13:21, 1998.

458. Cohen LM, Schwartz AM, Rockoff SD: Benign schwannomas: Pathologic basis for CT inhomogeneities. Am J Roentgenol 147:141, 1986.

459. Bourgouin PM, Shepard JO, Moore EH, et al: Plexiform neurofibromatosis of the mediastinum: CT appearance. Am J Roentgenol 151:461, 1988.

460. Sakai F, Sone S, Kiyono K, et al: Intrathoracic neurogenic tumors: MR-pathologic correlation. Am J Roentgenol 159:279, 1992.

461. Sakai F, Sone S, Kiyono K, et al: Magnetic resonance imaging of neurogenic tumors of the thoracic inlet: Determination of the parent nerve. J Thorac Imaging 11:272, 1996.

462. Ducatman BS, Scheithauer BW, Piepgras DG, et al: Malignant peripheral nerve sheath tumors: A clinicopathologic study of 120 cases. Cancer 57:2006, 1986.

463. Coleman BG, Arger PH, Dalinka MK, et al: CT of sarcomatous degeneration in neurofibromatosis. Am J Roentgenol 140:383, 1983.

464. Adam A, Hochholzer L: Ganglioneuroblastoma of the posterior mediastinum: A clinicopathologic review of 80 cases. Cancer 47:373, 1981.

465. Bar-Ziv J, Nogrady MB: Mediastinal neuroblastoma and ganglioneuroma: The differentiation between primary and secondary involvement on the chest roentgenogram. Am J Roentgenol 125:380, 1975.

466. Schweisguth O, Mathey J, Renault P, et al: Intrathoracic neurogenic tumors in infants and children: A study of forty cases. Ann Surg 150:29, 1959.

467. Wang YM, Li YW, Sheih CP, et al: Magnetic resonance imaging of neuroblastoma, ganglioneuroblastoma and ganglioneuroma. Acta Paediatr Sin 36:420, 1995.

468. Miles J, Pennybacker J, Sheldon P: Intrathoracic meningocele: Its development and association with neurofibromatosis. J Neurol Neurosurg Psychiatry 32:99, 1969.

469. Glazer HS, Siegel MJ, Sagel SS: Low-attenuation mediastinal masses on CT. Am J Roentgenol 152:1173, 1989.

470. Wychulis AR, Payne WS, Clagett OT, et al: Surgical treatment of mediastinal tumors: A 40-year experience. J Thorac Cardiovasc Surg 62:379, 1971.

471. Cabooter M, Bogaerts Y, Javaheri S, et al: Intrathoracic meningocele. Eur J Respir Dis 63:347, 1982.

472. Ochsner JL, Ochsner SF: Congenital cysts of the mediastinum: 20-year experience with 42 cases. Ann Surg 163:909, 1966.

473. Leigh TF: Mass lesions of the mediastinum. Radiol Clin North Am 1:377, 1963.

474. Kirwan WO, Walbaum PR, McCormack RJM: Cystic intrathoracic derivatives of the foregut and their complications. Thorax 28:424, 1973.

475. Benton C, Silverman FN: Some mediastinal lesions in children. Semin Roentgenol 4:91, 1969.

476. Snyder ME, Luck SR, Hernandez R, et al: Diagnostic dilemmas of mediastinal cysts. J Pediatr Surg 20:810, 1985.

477. Verani R, Olson J, Moake JL: Intrathoracic extramedullary hematopoiesis: Report of a case in a patient with sickle cell disease-β-thalassemia. Am J Clin Pathol 73:133, 1980.

478. Gumbs R, Ford EAH, Tea JS, et al: Intrathoracic extramedullary hematopoiesis in sickle cell disease. Am J Roentgenol 149:889, 1987.

479. Papavasiliou C, Gouliamos A, Andreou J: The marrow heterotopia in thalassemia. Eur J Radiol 6:92, 1986.

480. Alam R, Padmanabhan K, Rao H: Paravertebral mass in a patient with thalassemia intermedia. Chest 112:265, 1997.

481. Long JA Jr, Doppman JL, Nienhuis AW: Computed tomographic studies of thoracic extramedullary hematopoiesis. J Comput Assist Tomogr 4:67, 1980.

482. Fielding JR, Owens M, Naimark A: Intrathoracic extramedullary hematopoiesis secondary to B_{12} and folate deficiency: CT appearance. J Comput Assist Tomogr 15:308, 1991.

483. Yamato M, Fuhrman CR: Computed tomography of fatty replacement in extramedullary hematopoiesis. J Comput Assist Tomogr 11:541, 1987.

484. Joy G, Logan PM: Intrathoracic extramedullary hematopoiesis secondary to idiopathic myelofibrosis. Can Assoc Radiol J 49:200, 1998.

485. Martin J, Palacio A, Petit J, et al: Fatty transformation of thoracic extramedullary hematopoiesis following splenectomy: CT features. J Comput Assist Tomogr 14:477, 1990.

486. Stebner FC, Bishop CR: Bone marrow scan and radioiron uptake of an intrathoracic mass. Clin Nucl Med 7:86, 1982.

487. Coates GG, Eisenberg B, Dail DH: Tc-99m sulfur colloid demonstration of diffuse pulmonary interstitial extramedullary hematopoiesis in a patient with myelofibrosis: A case report and review of the literature. Clin Nucl Med 19:1079, 1994.

488. Harnsberger HR, Datz FL, Knockel JQ, et al: Failure to detect extramedullary hematopoiesis during bone marrow imaging with indium-111 to technetium-99m sulphur colloid. J Nucl Med 23:589, 1982.

489. Papavasiliou CG: Tumor simulating intrathoracic extramedullary hemopoiesis: Clinical and roentgenologic considerations. Am J Roentgenol 93:695, 1965.

490. Cartier Y, Nogueira HA, Müller NL: Fibrosing mediastinitis associated with Riedel's thyroiditis: Computed tomographic findings. Can Assoc Radiol J 49:408, 1998.

491. Grewal RG, Prager K, Austin JHM, et al: Long term survival in non-encapsulated primary liposarcoma of the mediastinum. Thorax 48:1276, 1993.

492. Eisenstat R, Bruce D, Williams LE, et al: Primary liposarcoma of the mediastinum with coexistent mediastinal lipomatosis. Am J Roentgenol 174:572, 2000.

493. Finn JP, Zisk JHS, Edelman RR, et al: Central venous occlusion: MR angiography. Radiology 187:245, 1993.

494. Arpasi PJ, Bis KG, Shetty AN, et al: MR angiography of the thoracic aorta with an electrocardiographically triggered breath-hold contrast-enhanced sequence. Radiographics 20:107, 2000.

495. Ramakantan R, Shah P: Dysphagia due to mediastinal fibrosis in advanced pulmonary tuberculosis. Am J Roentgenol 154:61, 1990.

496. Sandler CM, Libshitz HI, Marks G: Pneumoperitoneum, pneumomediastinum and pneumopericardium following dental extraction. Radiology 115:539, 1975.

497. Dontas NS: Intrathoracic goitre. Br J Tuberc 52:154, 1958.

498. Drasin GF, Lynch T, Temes GP: Ectopic ACTH production and mediastinal lipomatosis. Radiology 127:610, 1978.

499. Thompson WM, Halvorsen RA, Foster WL Jr, et al: Computed tomography for staging esophageal and gastroesophageal cancer: Reevaluation. Am J Roentgenol 141:951, 1983.

500. Jung K-J, Lee KS, Han J, et al: Malignant thymic epithelioid tumors CT-pathologic correlation. Am J Roentgenol 176:433, 2001.

501. Lemay K, Gray R, Numerow L: Mediastinal pancreatic pseudocyst. Can Assoc Radiol J 51:358, 2000.

502. Hartnell GG; Imaging of aortic aneurysms and dissection: CT and MRI. J Thorac Imaging 16:35, 2001.

503. Skelan SJ, Brown AL, Thompson M, et al: Imaging features of primary and recurrent esophageal cancer at FDG PET. Radiographics 20:713, 2000.

CHAPTER 23

Disease of the Diaphragm and Chest Wall

THE DIAPHRAGM

Abnormalities of Diaphragmatic Position or Motion

Unilateral Diaphragmatic Paralysis

Paralysis of a hemidiaphragm usually results from interruption of transmission of the nerve impulses through the phrenic nerve and is associated with many causes. The most common is invasion of the nerve by a neoplasm, usually of pulmonary origin. The second most frequent category is paralysis of unknown etiology; in these idiopathic cases, the paralysis is almost invariably right-sided and usually occurs in males.

Unilateral diaphragmatic paralysis can occur as a complication of radical neck[9] or thoracic[10] surgery, especially coronary artery bypass surgery.[11, 12] The mechanism by which the hemidiaphragm is paralyzed has not been definitely determined in the latter circumstance; however, there is evidence that it may be the result of cold topical cardioplegia. During cardiopulmonary bypass and aortocoronary bypass grafting, ice slush cooled to subfreezing temperatures by the addition of salt is sometimes packed into the pericardial cavity around the heart. The left phrenic nerve runs within the posterior pericardium on the left side; thus, temporary cold-induced injury can theoretically occur.[13, 14]

Patients who have a paralyzed hemidiaphragm usually do not have symptoms; however, some complain of dyspnea on effort or (rarely) orthopnea.[8] The severity of either symptom relates to the rapidity of development of the paralysis and to the presence or absence of underlying pulmonary disease.

Radiologically, an elevated, paralyzed hemidiaphragm presents an accentuated dome configuration in both posteroanterior and lateral projections. The peripheral points of attachment of the diaphragm are fixed; thus, costophrenic and costovertebral sulci tend to be deepened, narrowed, and sharpened (Fig. 23–1). If the paralysis is left-sided, the stomach and splenic flexure of the colon relate to the inferior surface of the elevated hemidiaphragm and usually contain more gas than normal. Invasion or compression of the phrenic nerve by abnormalities such as pulmonary carcinoma or calcified lymph nodes can be clarified by computed tomography (CT) should the nature of the abnormalities be unclear from conventional radiographic studies.[15]

In a review of the radiographic manifestations of unilateral diaphragmatic paralysis, four cardinal signs were described:[1] (1) elevation of a hemidiaphragm above the normal range; (2) diminished, absent, or paradoxical motion during respiration; (3) paradoxical motion under conditions of augmented load, such as sniffing; and (4) mediastinal swing during respiration. There are several potential pitfalls in the assessment of these signs:[16] (1) the judgment that there is an abnormal elevation may be erroneous because of the considerable variation in the normal height of the

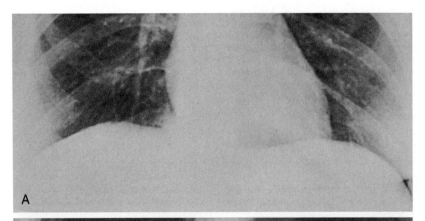

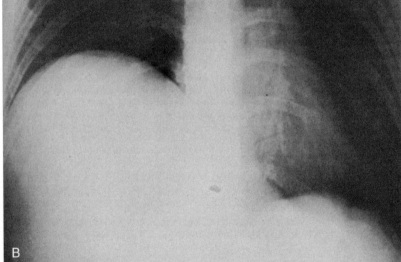

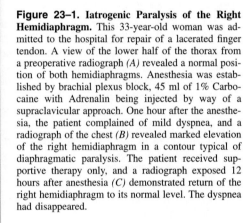

Figure 23–1. Iatrogenic Paralysis of the Right Hemidiaphragm. This 33-year-old woman was admitted to the hospital for repair of a lacerated finger tendon. A view of the lower half of the thorax from a preoperative radiograph *(A)* revealed a normal position of both hemidiaphragms. Anesthesia was established by brachial plexus block, 45 ml of 1% Carbocaine with Adrenalin being injected by way of a supraclavicular approach. One hour after the anesthesia, the patient complained of mild dyspnea, and a radiograph of the chest *(B)* revealed marked elevation of the right hemidiaphragm in a contour typical of diaphragmatic paralysis. The patient received supportive therapy only, and a radiograph exposed 12 hours after anesthesia *(C)* demonstrated return of the right hemidiaphragm to its normal level. The dyspnea had disappeared.

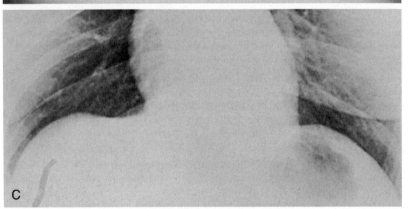

Table 23–1. UNILATERAL DIAPHRAGMATIC PARALYSIS

Most common cause: invasion of phrenic nerve by pulmonary carcinoma
Radiologic manifestations:
Elevation of hemidiaphragm
Diminished, absent, or paradoxical motion during respiration
Paradoxical motion with increased load; e.g., sniffing
Reversed excursion of 2 cm or more required for diagnosis
Motion best assessed by fluoroscopy or ultrasound

hemidiaphragms; (2) mediastinal swing during respiration is a totally unreliable sign in the presence of bronchial obstruction or atelectasis; (3) motion may be absent or paradoxical during respiration in various pulmonary, pleural, and subphrenic diseases, which makes this sign unreliable unless such diseases can be excluded; and (4) sniffing can cause paradoxical motion of one hemidiaphragm in some normal individuals, and in order for it to be considered pathologic it should consist of a reverse excursion of at least 2 cm. Despite these observations, with reasonable care, the diagnosis of unilateral diaphragmatic paralysis can be made radiologically in most cases (Table 23–1).

The most reliable radiologic maneuver for detecting hemidiaphragmatic paralysis is the sniff test. Normally, both hemidiaphragms descend sharply during a sniff; with unilateral diaphragmatic paralysis, there is paradoxical upward motion of the affected side. Although significant paradoxical motion provides strong evidence of diaphragmatic paralysis or eventration, the incidence of false-positive results is about 5%; in addition, false-negative results can be recorded if the patient uses the abdominal musculature to elevate the diaphragm during the expiratory phase of breathing.[1]

Preliminary results suggest that ultrasound is superior to fluoroscopy in the demonstration of abnormalities of hemidiaphragmatic motion.[4] One investigation of the diaphragm in 30 individuals included 5 who had bilateral diaphragmatic paralysis, 7 who had unilateral paralysis, 3 who had inspiratory weakness but normally functioning diaphragm, and 5 who were healthy.[6] In this study, the thickness of the diaphragm at functional residual capacity (FRC) was significantly less in patients who had bilateral diaphragmatic paralysis (1.8 ± 0.2 mm) than in normal subjects (2.8 ± 0.4 mm; $P < 0.001$); paralyzed diaphragms showed no change in thickness during inspiration compared to a change in thickness (delta thickness from FRC to total lung capacity [TLC]) of $37\% \pm 9\%$ in the normal subjects. In patients who had unilateral paralysis, the thickness of the paralyzed hemidiaphragm at FRC (1.7 ± 0.2 mm) was significantly less than that of the normally functioning hemidiaphragm (2.7 ± 0.5 mm; $P < 0.01$), and the change in thickness with inspiration was significantly lower ($-8.5\% \pm 13\%$ compared to $65\% \pm 26\%$).

Bilateral Diaphragmatic Paralysis

Patients who have bilateral paralysis have profound respiratory symptoms and functional derangement.[17] Most eventually develop ventilatory failure and hypercapnia; some present with evidence of cor pulmonale and right ventricular failure. Dyspnea that occurs when the patient exerts himself and when he assumes the supine position is characteristic. The most common cause of bilateral diaphragmatic paralysis is spinal cord injury.

The radiographic appearance of bilateral diaphragmatic paralysis consists of elevated hemidiaphragms in both posteroanterior and lateral projections.[1] Linear atelectasis may be present at the lung bases. Paradoxical upward motion of both hemidiaphragms during an inspiratory effort or sniff is usually observed on fluoroscopic examination, although recruitment of abdominal expiratory muscles can cause a false-negative test.[17, 18] Some patients actively expire to a lung volume below true FRC and then use the elastic recoil forces of the abdominothoracic structures to assist the next inspiration passively; the sudden downward motion of the diaphragm coincident with abdominal muscle relaxation may be misinterpreted as diaphragmatic contraction when one views it fluoroscopically. Despite these potential pitfalls, fluoroscopy can be effectively used to evaluate the condition.[19] The characteristic findings consist of cephalad movement of the paralyzed diaphragm during inspiration, accompanied by outward chest wall and inward abdominal wall motion, a phenomenon known as "thoracoabdominal paradox."[19]

Diaphragmatic motion can also be monitored by ultrasonography.[20, 21] The fact that ultrasound also permits assessment of diaphragmatic thickness and changing thickness with respiration[5, 6] makes it possibly superior to fluoroscopy.

Eventration

Eventration is a congenital anomaly consisting of failure of muscular development of part or all of one or both hemidiaphragms.[22] In some cases, it is difficult or impossible to distinguish it from diaphragmatic paralysis (Table 23–2).[23, 24] When marked diaphragmatic elevation can be attributed to a specific cause (e.g., interruption of the phrenic nerve by invasive neoplasm or surgical section), it is clearly possible to employ specific terminology in describing the situation. Sometimes, however, there is no way of knowing whether elevation is caused by congenital absence of muscle or by phrenic nerve paralysis (Fig. 23–2). In an extensive radiographic survey of individuals older than nursery school age, a group of Japanese investigators showed that the incidence of partial eventration of the right hemidiaphragm increased with age, particularly among women older than the age of 60 years.[25]

Pathologically, a totally eventrated hemidiaphragm consists of a thin membranous sheet attached peripherally to normal muscle at points of origin from the rib cage. It occurs almost exclusively on the left side, a point that may be of value in its differentiation from diaphragmatic

Table 23–2. DIAPHRAGMATIC EVENTRATION

Failure of muscular development of hemidiaphragm
Most commonly partial: typically anteromedial right hemidiaphragm
Occasionally may be complete: usually left hemidiaphragm
Radiologic manifestations:
Complete failure of muscular development: signs similar to paralysis
Partial failure of muscular development:
Smaller than normal inspiratory excursion
May have inspiratory lag but shows downward motion

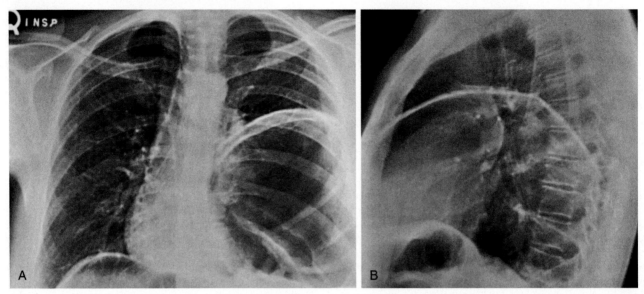

Figure 23–2. Paralysis or Eventration of the Left Hemidiaphragm Associated with Severe Colonic Dilation Secondary to Sigmoid Volvulus. Posteroanterior *(A)* and lateral *(B)* radiographs reveal a remarkable degree of elevation of the left hemidiaphragm. Severely dilated loops of colon are situated beneath this hemidiaphragm and to a lesser extent beneath the right one. The mediastinum is displaced considerably into the right hemithorax.

paralysis. The latter has an approximately equal incidence on the two sides, except in idiopathic cases in which it occurs almost invariably on the right side.[7] Partial eventration is more common than the total form and is usually present in the anteromedial portion of the right hemidiaphragm; it occurs with equal frequency in men and women,[27] rarely on the left, and occasionally in the central portion of either cupola.[27]

Characteristically, eventration is unassociated with symptoms and is discovered on a screening chest radiograph. However, symptoms may be present in obese patients as the result of raised intra-abdominal pressure. Although these symptoms are usually related to the gastrointestinal tract, respiratory embarrassment and, rarely, cardiac distress have been attributed to the anomaly.[31]

A confident diagnosis of partial eventration can be established by CT[2, 29] or ultrasonography.[2, 30] The main value of these procedures is in distinguishing partial eventration from a focal bulge on the diaphragmatic contour due to a tumor or a diaphragmatic hernia. In eventration, the diaphragm, although thin, can be seen as a continuous layer above the elevated abdominal viscera and retroperitoneal or omental fat. On fluoroscopy and real-time ultrasound, the focal area of eventration can be seen to move downward with the normal portions of the hemidiaphragm, although it may have a slight lag in its inspiratory excusion.[2]

The radiologic signs of complete eventration are identical to those described for diaphragmatic paralysis. In patients in whom there is only partial failure of muscular development of one hemidiaphragm, the affected hemidiaphragm shows a smaller than normal inspiratory excursion. On fluoroscopy or real-time ultrasound, it may have an initial inspiratory lag or small paradoxical motion; however, later in inspiration it has downward motion.[2]

Restriction of Diaphragmatic Motion

A great variety of diseases of the lungs, pleura, intra-abdominal organs, and of the diaphragm itself, may lead to restriction of diaphragmatic motion. In some, the limitation of motion is imposed by the character of the disease itself—for example, the severe pulmonary overinflation and air trapping that categorize diffuse emphysema or asthma prevent normal ascent of the diaphragm during expiration. In other diseases, local irritation causes "splinting" of a hemidiaphragm that is manifested not only by reduced excursion but also by elevation; such splinting can be caused by acute lower lobe pneumonia or infarction, acute pleuritis, rib fractures, and acute intra-abdominal processes, such as subphrenic abscess, cholecystitis, and peritonitis.

Although other skeletal muscle groups react to irritation or injury by spasm, the diaphragm appears to react by relaxation; this is the only way of explaining the elevation that characteristically accompanies local inflammation. The mechanism by which the diaphragm is splinted in the postoperative period is thought to be neural inhibition of diaphragmatic activation,[32, 33] possibly caused by stimulation of diaphragmatic or splanchnic afferents. Diaphragmatic dysfunction is maximal in patients 8 hours after upper abdominal surgery, with function improving over the subsequent 2 to 7 days.[32]

Diaphragmatic Hernias

Herniation of abdominal or retroperitoneal organs or tissues into the thorax may occur through congenital or acquired weak areas in the diaphragm or through rents resulting from trauma (the latter are discussed in Chapter 18). The most common diaphragmatic hernia occurs through the esophageal hiatus; less common forms include those through the pleuroperitoneal hiatus (Bochdalek's hernias) and through the parasternal hiatus (Morgagni's hernias).

Hernia Through the Esophageal Hiatus

Although a congenital weakness of the esophageal hiatus may be partly responsible for the development of hiatus hernia, there is little doubt that acquired factors play a significant role, the most important being obesity and pregnancy. The prevalence increases with age; in one investigation of 120 patients, the hernias were seen in 2 of 40 (5%) patients younger than the age of 40 years, 12 of 40 (30%) between the ages of 40 and 59 years, and 26 of 40 (65%) between the ages of 60 and 79 years.[35] Most patients do not have symptoms, and the abnormality is discovered on a screening chest radiograph or examination of the upper gastrointestinal tract for unrelated complaints.

Plain radiographs of the chest often show a retrocardiac mass, usually containing air or an air-fluid level (Fig. 23–3). Definitive diagnosis, however, sometimes requires barium study of the esophagogastric junction or the use of CT.[35, 36] Occasionally, large hernias are located predominantly on one side of the hemithorax and mimic a lung abscess on the radiograph (Fig. 23–4). In cases in which most of the stomach has herniated through the hiatus, the stomach may undergo volvulus within the mediastinum and present as a large mass, sometimes containing a double air-fluid level; incarceration of such hernial contents is common, and strangulation may occur.[37] There have also been reports of a number of cases of strangulation of contents that have herniated through the diaphragmatic incision made for repair of hiatus hernia.[38] The development of acute upper gastrointestinal tract symptoms in a patient who has a herniated stomach should immediately raise the suspicion of strangulation;[39] the complication is life-threatening and necessitates immediate surgical intervention.

Although the stomach is the most common hernial content, other structures are seen occasionally, including a portion of the transverse colon, a pancreatic pseudocyst,[40] omentum, or liver.[41] In addition, ascitic fluid can extend from the peritoneal cavity into the posterior mediastinum through the esophageal hiatus, an occurrence that can be demonstrated to excellent advantage with CT.[42]

Hernia Through the Foramen of Bochdalek

In infants, herniation through a persistent embryonic pleuroperitoneal hiatus is not only the most common form

Table 23–3. BOCHDALEK'S HERNIAS

Congenital
    Herniation through persistent pleuroperitoneal hiatus
    Incidence 1:2,200 live births
    75%–90% left-sided
    Associated with severe respiratory distress
Acquired
    Herniation through small acquired diaphragmatic defects
    Seen in 5%–10% of adults
    Incidence increases with age
        Not seen before 40 years of age
        Incidence increases to 35% in patients older than 70 years of age
    Herniation usually limited to omental fat
    Patients usually asymptomatic

of diaphragmatic hernia but also, by far, the most serious. Its incidence is 1 in 2,200 live births.[2, 44] A total of 75% to 90% occur on the left side.[45] When large, the hernias are associated with high mortality unless surgically corrected. Even with surgery, the mortality is about 30% as the result of hypoplasia of the underlying lung and pulmonary arterial hypertension.[45]

The size of the defect ranges widely. When large, as with complete or almost complete absence of a hemidiaphragm, almost the entire abdominal contents, including the stomach, may be in the left hemithorax, thereby interfering with normal lung development and resulting in hypoplasia.[46, 47] In most large hernias, there is no peritoneal sac, and communication between the pleural and the peritoneal cavities is wide open. When the defect is small, a sac lined by pleura and containing retroperitoneal fat, a portion of the spleen or kidney,[49] or omentum may be the only discernible abnormality.[50]

In adults, small Bochdalek's hernias are much more common than in infants and are almost always unassociated with symptoms (Table 23–3). Their incidence increases with age, suggesting that they are acquired. In one review of CT scans of the chest and abdomen performed in 940 adult patients, 60 Bochdalek's hernias were found in 52, a prevalence of 6%.[51] Thirty-nine (65%) were left-sided, and

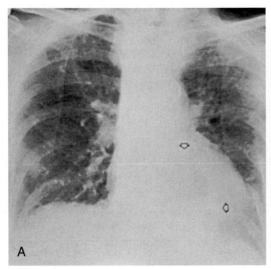
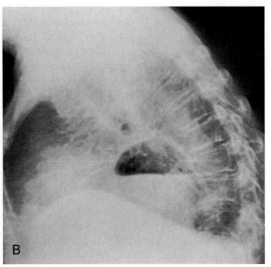

Figure 23–3. Large Hiatus Hernia. Posteroanterior *(A)* and lateral *(B)* radiographs of the chest of an 87-year-old woman reveal a large soft-tissue mass containing a prominent air-fluid level occupying the posteroinferior portion of the mediastinum *(arrows in A)*. The patient had no symptoms referable to this hernia.

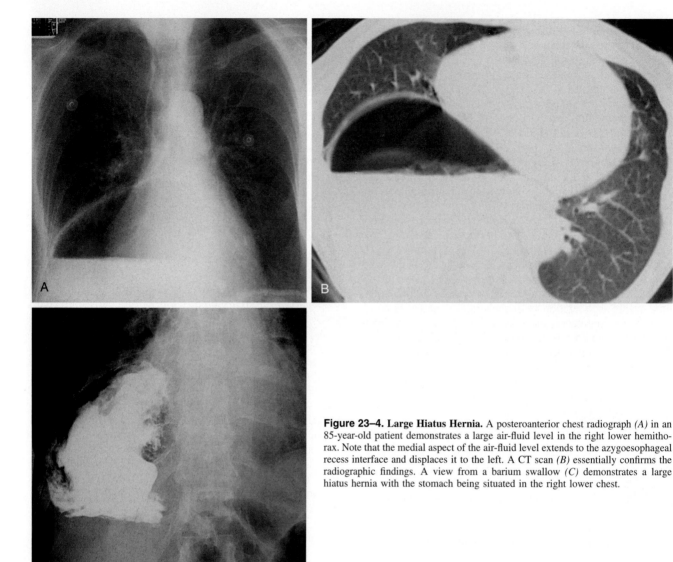

Figure 23–4. Large Hiatus Hernia. A posteroanterior chest radiograph *(A)* in an 85-year-old patient demonstrates a large air-fluid level in the right lower hemithorax. Note that the medial aspect of the air-fluid level extends to the azygoesophageal recess interface and displaces it to the left. A CT scan *(B)* essentially confirms the radiographic findings. A view from a barium swallow *(C)* demonstrates a large hiatus hernia with the stomach being situated in the right lower chest.

21 (35%) right-sided. In all cases, the hernias contained only fat and were unassociated with symptoms. Another group of investigators correlated the frequency of diaphragmatic defects seen on CT with age in 120 patients ranging from 20 to 79 years of age.[35] Bochdalek's hernias were seen in 14 patients (12%). They were present in 1 of 20 (5%) patients between 40 and 49 years of age, 3 of 20 (15%) between 50 and 59 years, 3 of 20 (15%) between 60 and 69 years of age, and 7 of 20 (35%) between 70 and 79 years old; none were present in patients younger than 40 years of age.

A total of 65% of the defects involved the left hemidiaphragm; 60% involved the posterior diaphragm; 27% were at the junction of the lateral arm of the crus and the posterior diaphragm; and 13% were located in the crus or laterally near the costal region of the diaphragm. The frequency of diaphragmatic defects did not correlate with the amount of skeletal muscle or with obesity, but was greater in patients who had emphysema.

On the chest radiograph, Bochdalek's hernias can present as a focal bulge in the hemidiaphragm or as a mass adjacent to the posteromedial aspect of either hemidiaphragm (Fig. 23–5). Although the diagnosis can often be suspected on the radiograph by the typical location and by the lower-than-soft-tissue density of the mass due to its fat content, the appearance can mimic that of pulmonary, mediastinal, or paravertebral masses.[52] The diagnosis is readily made on CT.[52] Occasionally, spiral CT, coronal or sagittal re-formations, may be required to demonstrate small diaphragmatic defects.[53, 54]

Hernia Through the Foramen of Morgagni

Morgagni's (retrosternal or parasternal) hernia is uncommon. The left foramen relates to the heart; thus, most herniations occur on the right; in one series of 50 cases, 4 were bilateral and only 1 was solely left-sided.[55] Although the defects are developmental in origin, hernias are more commonly seen in adults than in children and are often associated with obesity, severe effort, or other causes of increased intra-abdominal pressure or trauma;[2, 56] in fact, affected patients are usually overweight, middle-aged

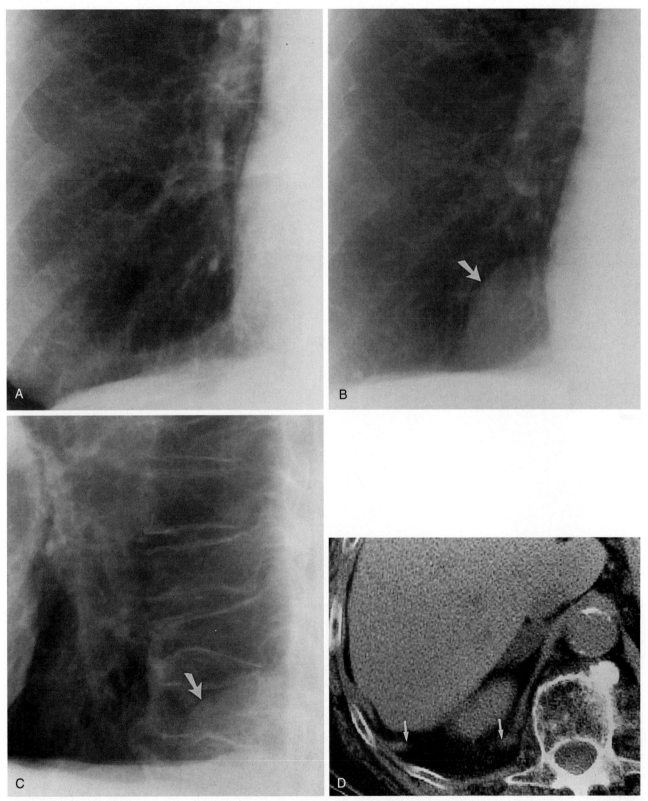

Figure 23–5. Development of a Bochdalek Hernia in an Elderly Patient. A view of the right lower chest from a posteroanterior radiograph *(A)* in a 78-year-old woman is unremarkable. Views from posteroanterior *(B)* and lateral *(C)* radiographs performed 5 years later demonstrate a large mass adjacent to the posteromedial aspect of the right hemidiaphragm *(arrows)*. The mass has lower opacity than the heart and soft tissues of the abdomen, consistent with fat. A view of the right hemidiaphragm from a CT scan *(D)* demonstrates focal defect *(arrows)* in the posterior aspect of the right hemidiaphragm with herniation of omental fat. The patient had no symptoms related to the hernia.

women. In contrast with Bochdalek's hernias, a peritoneal sac is present in most cases. The content of the hernial sac is usually omentum, and sometimes liver or bowel; rarely, other structures, such as a stone-filled gallbladder,[57] stomach,[58] or a congenital hepatic cyst,[59] have been identified. Cases have been reported in which the defect has extended into the pericardial sac, allowing displacement of abdominal contents into this site.[60]

Most hernias through the foramen of Morgagni do not give rise to symptoms. The minority of adults who have symptoms complain of epigastric or lower sternal pressure and discomfort and, sometimes, cardiorespiratory and gastrointestinal symptoms.[63]

Radiologically, the typical appearance is that of a smooth, well-defined opacity in the right cardiophrenic angle (Fig. 23–6). In most patients, the shadow is of homogeneous density. Occasionally, it is inhomogeneous as the result of either an air-containing loop of bowel or the predominantly fatty nature of the hernial contents. In the latter situation, the hernia is likely to contain omentum, and CT or barium enema reveals the transverse colon to be situated high in the abdomen with a peak situated anteriorly and superiorly, a finding that is virtually diagnostic. Bilateral anteromedial defects in the diaphragm produce a characteristic radiographic pattern when abdominal organs herniate through a single midline opening.[61] In the rare case in which the hernia penetrates into the pericardial sac, loops of air-containing bowel may be identified anterior to the cardiac shadow.[60] The diagnosis of Morgagni's hernia can be readily made on CT,[3, 52] or magnetic resonance imaging (MRI).[2]

Neoplasms of the Diaphragm

Primary Neoplasms

Primary neoplasms of the diaphragm are rare.[64, 65] In a review of the literature from 1868 to 1968, one group of investigators identified only 84 cases.[65] Most develop from

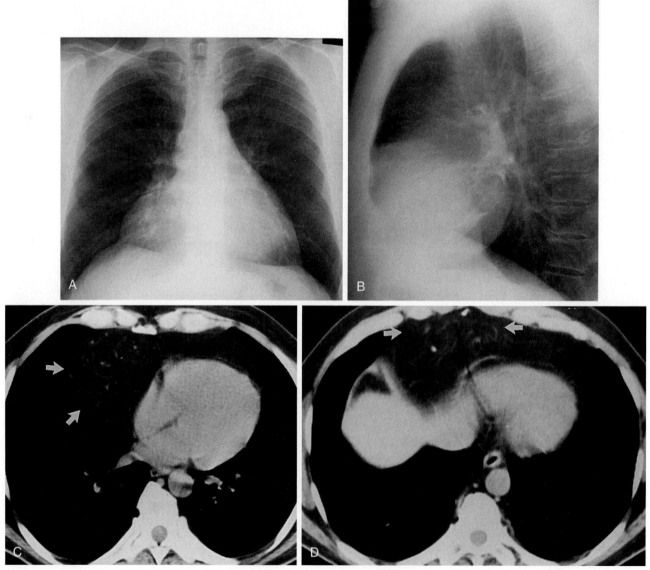

Figure 23–6. Morgagni's Hernia. Posteroanterior *(A)* and lateral *(B)* chest radiographs demonstrate a mass in the right costophrenic sulcus. The mass has a lower-than-soft-tissue density consistent with fat. Computed tomography scans *(C* and *D)* demonstrate herniation of omental fat *(arrows)* through the right lower parasternal region *(arrows)* diagnostic of Morgagni's hernia. The patient was a 49-year-old man.

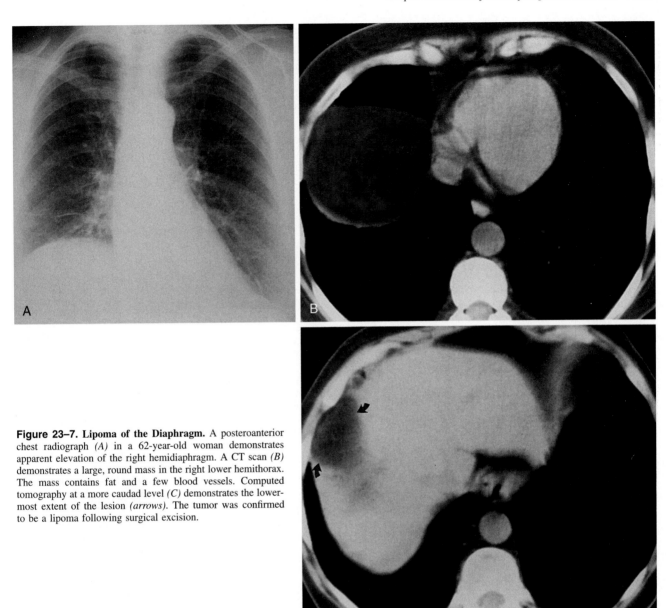

Figure 23–7. Lipoma of the Diaphragm. A posteroanterior chest radiograph *(A)* in a 62-year-old woman demonstrates apparent elevation of the right hemidiaphragm. A CT scan *(B)* demonstrates a large, round mass in the right lower hemithorax. The mass contains fat and a few blood vessels. Computed tomography at a more caudad level *(C)* demonstrates the lowermost extent of the lesion *(arrows)*. The tumor was confirmed to be a lipoma following surgical excision.

the tendinous or anterior muscular portion. Benign and malignant forms occur with relatively equal frequency. The former include lipoma, the most common;[67, 163] angiofibroma; neurofibroma; neurilemoma;[69] leiomyoma; teratoma;[70] and desmoid tumor, fibromatosis.[71] Fat pads and herniations of omental fat are common in the region of the diaphragm; thus, a diagnosis of lipoma requires demonstration of a true capsule.[68] Malignant neoplasms include fibrosarcoma, the most common;[68, 72] malignant fibrous histiocytoma;[73] hemangiopericytoma;[74] germ cell tumors;[75] pheochromocytoma;[76] epithelioid hemangioendothelioma;[77] leiomyosarcoma;[66, 78] and chondrosarcoma.[79, 80] Various non-neoplastic abnormalities that form localized tumors, such as lymphangioma and endometrioma,[64] are also occasionally found.

Characteristically, benign neoplasms occasion no symptoms; by contrast, the majority of patients who have primary malignant neoplasms complain of epigastric or lower chest pain, cough, dyspnea, and gastrointestinal discomfort.[64, 65]

Radiologically, most diaphragmatic tumors present as smooth or lobulated soft-tissue masses protruding into the inferior portion of the lung (Fig. 23–7). Benign neoplasms may calcify. In many cases, malignant tumors involve much of one hemidiaphragm and thus simulate diaphragmatic elevation; associated pleural effusion is common. The presence of an intradiaphragmatic mass can be established most easily by CT.[2, 68, 70] When the tumor is large, it may not be possible to determine whether it arose from the diaphragm, pleura, lungs, or liver.[68] Variations in diaphragmatic thickness on CT occasionally mimic an intradiaphragmatic mass or a tumor in an adjacent organ.[81] The distinction can be readily made by careful analysis of sequential images. Rarely, muscular hypertrophy of a diaphragmatic crus may simulate a paraspinal mass on the radiograph.[82]

Secondary Neoplasms

Secondary neoplastic involvement of the diaphragm occurs most frequently by direct extension of neoplasm from the basal pleura in cases of pulmonary carcinoma or mesothelioma; however, any neoplasm that metastasizes to the pleura or that involves the basal lung, liver, or subphrenic peritoneum can spread into the diaphragm. Ovarian carcinoma is particularly likely to be the cause when the initial site of involvement is the peritoneum.[83] Discrete diaphragmatic metastases, derived from either lymphatic or hematogenous spread, are rare. Radiographic features and clinical manifestations are usually related to the presence of neoplasm in contiguous structures or elsewhere, rather than in the diaphragm itself.

Miscellaneous Abnormalities of the Diaphragm

An accessory diaphragm is a rare anomaly in which the right hemithorax is partitioned into two compartments by a musculotendinous membrane resembling a diaphragm.[84] About 30 cases had been reported by 1995.[85] The accessory leaf is usually situated within the oblique fissure, separating the lower lobe from the remainder of the right lung. Radiologically, it may be mistaken for a somewhat thickened major fissure.

Diaphragmatic defects too small to allow passage of a hernial sac may explain the pleural effusions that develop in patients who have conditions such as Meigs' syndrome or cirrhosis and ascites.[86, 87] Such defects may be congenital or acquired and can be demonstrated either directly at autopsy or surgery, or indirectly by the development of pneumothorax following intraperitoneal administration of gas.[87] Similar small defects have been postulated as the entry sites for tissue or air in some cases of pleural endometriosis and catamenial pneumothorax.[88, 89]

Intradiaphragmatic cysts are rare and usually represent extralobar sequestration. The abnormality is presumably caused by entrapment of the accessory lung bud within the diaphragm during its development. In most cases, the cyst receives its blood supply from the abdominal aorta or one of its branches and characteristically drains by way of the systemic veins.[90] The anomaly relates to the left hemidiaphragm in 90% of cases and is usually associated with diaphragmatic eventration.[91] Occasionally, intradiaphragmatic cysts are the result of degenerated traumatic hematomas.[2]

THE CHEST WALL

Abnormalities of the Pectoral Girdle and Adjacent Structures

The most common congenital anomaly of the clavicle is cleidocranial dysostosis, a syndrome characterized by incomplete ossification associated with defective development of the pubic bones, vertebral column, and long bones.

Sprengel's deformity is characterized by a failure of the scapula to descend normally so that its superior angle lies on a plane higher than the neck of the first rib. It is frequently associated with fusion of two or more cervical vertebrae, resulting in a short, wide neck with considerably limited movement (the Klippel-Feil deformity).[92]

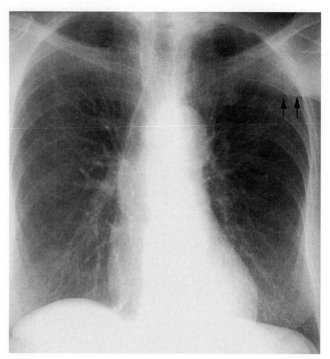

Figure 23–8. Congenital Absence of the Pectoralis Muscle. A posteroanterior chest radiograph demonstrates increased radiolucency of the left hemithorax. The course of the left anterior axillary fold *(arrows)* is horizontal, as the result of absence of the left pectoralis muscle. Note that the breast shadows are symmetric. The patient was a 67-year-old woman.

Poland's syndrome is a congenital anomaly consisting of hypoplasia or aplasia of the pectoralis major muscle and ipsilateral syndactyly;[93] rarely, the hypoplasia-aplasia is bilateral.[94] Unilateral absence of the pectoralis muscles results in unilateral hyperlucency on the chest radiograph, not to be confused with the Swyer-James syndrome (Fig. 23–8).

A pulmonary hernia occurs when there is a protrusion of the lung beyond the confines of the thoracic cage. It is an uncommon abnormality, only approximately 300 cases having been reported by 1996.[95] Approximately 20% are congenital and 80% are acquired.[95] The hernias can be classified as cervical (approximately one-third), intercostal (two-thirds), or diaphragmatic (about 1%).[95, 96] The majority of acquired hernias develop following penetrating injury, blunt trauma associated with multiple rib fractures, thoracotomy, or insertion of multiple chest tubes.[95, 96] Most patients are asymptomatic. Occasionally, a painless, local bulge can be palpated during cough. The radiographic manifestations include a well-circumscribed lucency extending beyond the rib cage or an air collection in the tissues overlying the chest wall.[95, 96] Unless the hernia is tangential to the x-ray beam, it may not be apparent on the radiograph. The diagnosis can be readily made on CT (Fig. 23–9).[96, 97]

Abnormalities of the Ribs

Cervical Rib

An anomalous accessory rib in the cervical region is a relatively common finding, being seen in about 0.5% of

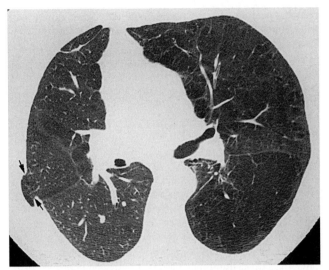

Figure 23–9. Lung Hernia. An HRCT scan demonstrates focal defect in right chest wall *(arrows)* with associated lung hernia. The patient was a 64-year-old woman who had undergone right lung transplantation for emphysema.

Table 23–4. CAUSES OF INFERIOR RIB NOTCHING

ARTERIAL
   Aortic obstruction
      Coarctation of the aortic arch
      Thrombosis of the abdominal aorta
   Subclavian artery obstruction
      Blalock-Taussig operation
      Takayasu's arteritis
   Widened arterial pulse pressure
   Decreased pulmonary blood flow
      Tetralogy of Fallot
      Pulmonary atresia (pseudotruncus)
      Ebstein's malformation
      Pulmonary valve stenosis
      Unilateral absence of the pulmonary artery
      Pulmonary emphysema
VENOUS
   Superior vena cava obstruction
ARTERIOVENOUS
   Pulmonary arteriovenous fistula
   Intercostal arteriovenous fistula
NEUROGENIC
   Intercostal neurogenic tumor
OSSEOUS
   Hyperparathyroidism
IDIOPATHIC

the general population.[98] It usually arises from the seventh cervical vertebra. Both the anomaly and the symptoms that derive therefrom are said to be more common in women in a ratio of approximately 2.5 to 1.[98] In about 90% of cases, the ribs do not cause symptoms; however, when they compress the cervical spinal cord,[99] the subclavian vessels, or the brachial plexus (thoracic outlet syndrome), symptoms can be present and are sometimes disabling.[100, 101]

Rib Notching and Erosion

Notching of ribs is most frequent on the inferior aspect and has many causes (Table 23–4).[102] By far the most common—coarctation of the aorta—typically produces notching several centimeters lateral to the costovertebral junction on ribs 3 to 9 (Fig. 23–10). The notches result

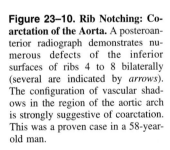

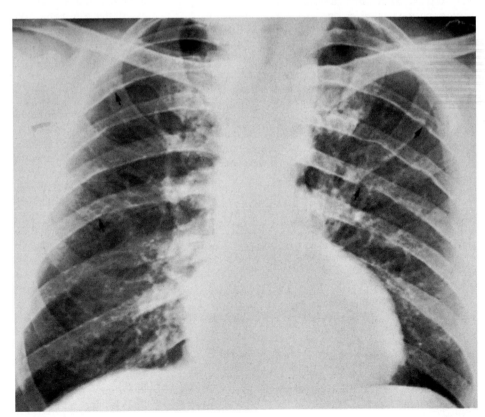

Figure 23–10. Rib Notching: Coarctation of the Aorta. A posteroanterior radiograph demonstrates numerous defects of the inferior surfaces of ribs 4 to 8 bilaterally (several are indicated by *arrows*). The configuration of vascular shadows in the region of the aortic arch is strongly suggestive of coarctation. This was a proven case in a 58-year-old man.

from erosion by dilated intercostal arteries taking part in collateral arterial flow. These arteries may become extremely tortuous and may even extend to and erode the superior aspects of contiguous ribs. Rib notching secondary to coarctation of the aorta seldom is seen in patients before the age of 6 or 7 years and usually is not well developed until the early teens.[103]

Notching or erosion of the superior aspects of the ribs is considerably less common than that of the inferior aspect; however, we suspect that it may be present more often than is generally recognized because its more subtle radiographic appearance may hinder its appreciation. The causes of superior marginal rib defects can be classified into three groups:[104] (1) those associated with a disturbance of osteoblastic activity (decreased or deficient bone formation); (2) those associated with a disturbance of osteoclastic activity (increased bone resorption); and (3) idiopathic (Table 23–5). The radiographic appearance typically consists of shallow indentations ranging from 1 to 4 cm in length on ribs 3 to 9 posterolaterally.

Osteomyelitis

Primary infection of the ribs is rare and may be difficult to appreciate radiologically until bone destruction is advanced. More commonly, osteomyelitis is secondary to infectious processes in the lung (usually the result of *Mycobacterium tuberculosis*, *Actinomyces israelii*, or *Nocardia asteroides*) or to empyema (empyema necessitatis).

Costochondral Osteochondritis

Costochondral osteochondritis (Tietze's syndrome) is characterized by painful, nonsuppurative swelling of one or more costochondral or sternochondral joints.[105]

Although the majority of affected patients undoubtedly manifest no radiologic changes, hypertrophy and excess calcification of the costal cartilages can be identified in some.[106] The second ribs are the most commonly involved. The affected ribs may show evidence of periosteal reaction and increased size and density anteriorly. When subperiosteal new bone formation develops, it tends to occur along the superior aspects of the affected ribs. Enlargement and alteration of the trabecular pattern of the anterior portion of the first ribs can also occur and may lead to an extremely

Table 23–5. CAUSES OF SUPERIOR RIB NOTCHING

DISTURBANCE OF OSTEOBLASTIC ACTIVITY (DECREASED OR DEFICIENT BONE FORMATION)
    Connective tissue diseases (rheumatoid arthritis, progressive systemic sclerosis, lupus erythematosus, Sjögren's syndrome)
    Localized pressure (rib retractors, chest tubes, multiple hereditary exostoses, neurofibromatosis, thoracic neuroblastoma, coarctation of the aorta)
    Osteogenesis imperfecta
    Marfan's syndrome
    Radiation damage
DISTURBANCE OF OSTEOCLASTIC ACTIVITY (INCREASED BONE RESORPTION)
    Hyperparathyroidism
    Hypervitaminosis D
IDIOPATHIC

dense appearance of the bone. Computed tomography can sometimes help to distinguish the swelling of Tietze's syndrome from more serious disease:[107, 108] for example, in six patients who had Tietze's syndrome in one series, CT showed no abnormality in two, ventral angulation of the involved costal cartilage in two, and enlargement of the costal cartilage at the site of the complaint in two.[108]

Abnormalities of the Sternum

Pectus Excavatum

Pectus excavatum ("funnel chest") is a common deformity that consists of depression of the sternum so that the ribs on each side protrude anteriorly more than the sternum itself. It is generally believed to result from a genetically determined abnormality of the sternum and related portions of the diaphragm; the condition can occur either sporadically or with a dominant pattern of inheritance.[109, 110] The prevalence in the general population has been estimated to range from 0.13% to 0.4%.[109] The vast majority of patients are free from symptoms.

The radiographic manifestations are easily recognized (Fig. 23–11). In posteroanterior projection, the heart is displaced to the left and rotated. The parasternal soft tissues of the anterior chest wall, which are seen in profile rather than straight on, are apparent as increased density over the inferomedial portion of the right hemithorax and should not be mistaken for disease of the right middle lobe, even though the right heart border is obscured (see Fig. 23–11). The degree of sternal depression is easily seen on a lateral radiograph. Possibly as the result of upward compression deformity of the heart and great vessels, the abnormality is occasionally associated with an unusual mediastinal configuration that can simulate a mediastinal mass;[111] in such cases, the true nature of the configuration can usually be readily clarified by CT.

Infection of the Sternum and Its Articulations

Inflammatory diseases affecting the sternum and sternal articulations are uncommon and occur most frequently as a complication of median sternotomy for heart surgery. Local infection occurs in 0.5% to 5% of patients undergoing sternotomy.[113, 114] Occasionally, evidence of sternal osteomyelitis or a retrosternal abscess is apparent on the lateral radiograph;[115, 116] however, CT is the imaging method of choice in the assessment of patients suspected of having poststernotomy complications.[114, 116] Findings include irregularity of the bony sternotomy margins, periosteal new bone formation, bony sclerosis, and peristernal soft-tissue masses that may contain areas of low attenuation due to abscess formation.[114, 116, 117] Early sternal osteomyelitis is difficult to distinguish from the normal sternal irregularities following the surgical procedure.[114] Bone scintigraphy or the sequential use of bone scintigraphy and gallium-67 scintigraphy can also be helpful in evaluating these patients.[114, 116]

Abnormalities of the Thoracic Spine

Kyphoscoliosis

Abnormalities of curvature of the thoracic spine may be predominantly lateral (scoliosis) or predominantly posterior

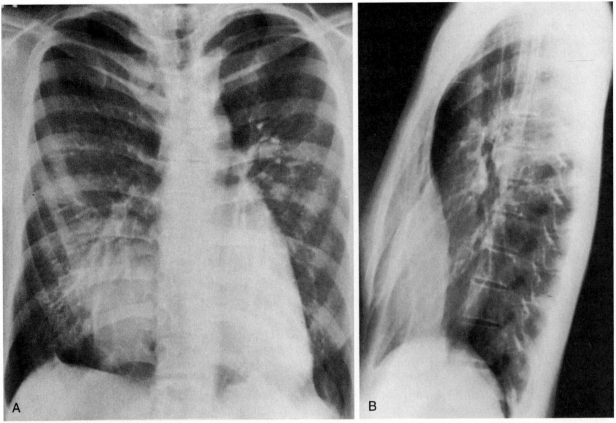

Figure 23–11. Severe Pectus Excavatum. Posteroanterior *(A)* and lateral *(B)* radiographs of the chest reveal a fairly large opacity projected over the lower portion of the right hemithorax contiguous with the shadow of the thoracic spine. The pulmonary arteries to the right lower lobe are displaced laterally and the heart is displaced to the left. The severe deformity of the sternum can be readily identified in lateral projection and is of sufficient degree to displace the heart posteriorly so that the contour of the left ventricle is projected over the thoracic vertebral bodies. The patient was a young woman who had no symptoms.

(kyphosis), or a combination of the two (kyphoscoliosis). Although such abnormalities are common, particularly scoliosis, deformity of a degree sufficient to cause symptoms and signs of cardiac or pulmonary disease is rare.

The causes of the abnormal curvature can be considered in three groups: (1) congenital, including anomalies of the thoracic spine such as hemivertebrae, and various hereditary disorders in which spinal deformity constitutes only a part of the clinical picture (e.g., neurofibromatosis, Friedreich's ataxia, muscular dystrophy, Ehlers-Danlos syndrome, and Marfan's syndrome);[112, 118, 119] (2) paralytic, including poliomyelitis, muscular dystrophy, or cerebral palsy; and (3) idiopathic. Patients in the last group constitute approximately 80% of those who have severe kyphoscoliosis; this variety shows a female sex predominance of 4 to 1.

Ankylosing Spondylitis

Ankylosing spondylitis is an immunologic disorder that develops in approximately 1 in 2,000 persons in the general population. It is strongly associated with the histocompatibility antigen HLA-B27;[120, 121] 20% of HLA-B27–positive individuals will develop the disease,[122] and approximately 90% of patients who have ankylosing spondylitis have the antigen.[121] Although the disease has been reported to occur four to eight times more frequently in males than in females, the distribution of HLA-B27–positive individuals is

equal in the two sexes.[123] The discrepancy in sex incidence is related to the fact that the disease in women tends to be milder and therefore is diagnosed less often.[123] In any event, the typical patient is a man who has a history of onset of symptoms early in the third decade of life.

In addition to the characteristic changes in the thoracic skeleton, approximately 1% to 2% of patients develop pleuropulmonary manifestations,[124, 125] most commonly in the form of upper lobe fibrobullous disease.[126–128] The bullae can be secondarily infected and associated with significant hemoptysis;[129] usually, this is related to the formation of a fungus ball and, occasionally, to nontuberculous mycobacterial infection. Computed tomography, particularly high-resolution computed tomography (HRCT), is useful in characterizing the extent and nature of the upper lobe changes as well as detecting or excluding an intracavitary fungus ball.[130, 131] In one review of 26 patients who had ankylosing spondylitis, 19 (70%) showed an abnormality on HRCT compared with only 4 (15%) on chest radiography.[132] The most frequently detected abnormalities were bronchial wall thickening and bronchiectasis, paraseptal emphysema, apical fibrosis, and interstitial lung disease. In another series of 2,080 patients, an unexpected number manifested evidence of pleuritis with effusion.[124]

The clinical picture is characterized by intermittent or continuous low back pain, sometimes associated with constitutional symptoms such as fatigue, weight loss, anorexia, and low-grade fever. The back pain can be distinguished from that of a mechanical or nonspecific type by its insidious onset, its duration (usually more than 3 months before the patient seeks medical help), its association with morning stiffness, and its improvement with exercise.[122]

Infectious Spondylitis

Pyogenic or tuberculous spondylitis can result in destruction of the vertebral body and intervertebral disc and the development of a paraspinal mass evident on the chest radiograph. The mass is often fusiform and has its maximal diameter at the point of major bone destruction (Fig. 23–12). Tuberculous spondylitis shows a predilection for the lower thoracic and upper lumbar spine.[134, 135] Computed tomography demonstrates bony destruction and associated soft-tissue masses which usually contain areas of low attenuation and show rim enhancement following intravenous

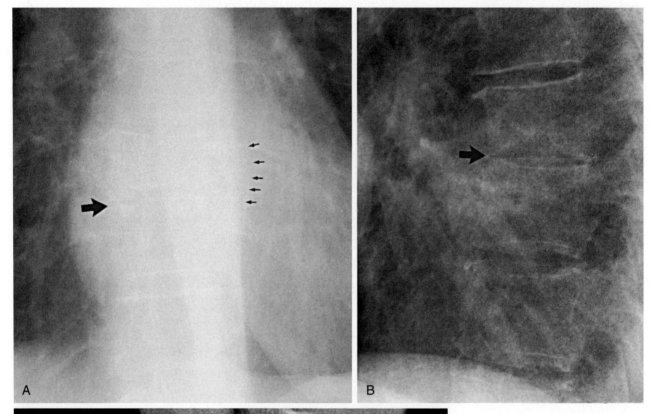

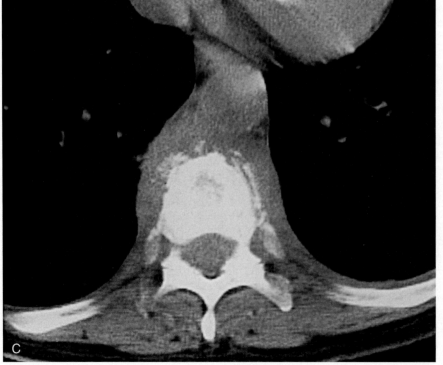

Figure 23–12. Staphylococcal Diskitis and Osteomyelitis. Views from posteroanterior *(A)* and lateral *(B)* chest radiographs in a 54-year-old intravenous drug abuser show narrowing of the T9-10 intervertebral disc space *(large arrows),* mild anterior wedging of the T9 vertebral body, and focal displacement of the left paraspinal interface *(small arrows).* Computed tomography *(C)* demonstrates bony erosion of the T9 vertebral body, paravertebral inflammatory tissue, and small left pleural effusion. Biopsy and blood cultures grew *Staphylococcus aureus.*

administration of contrast medium.[135] Foci of calcification are frequently present within the soft-tissue masses.[135]

The extent of bony destruction and paraspinal abscess formation are particularly well seen on MRI.[136] Early vertebral osteomyelitis and disc space infection are more readily apparent on MRI than on the plain radiograph or CT.[136–138] The MR findings consist of decreased signal intensity in the disc space and adjacent vertebra on T1-weighted images and increased signal intensity on T2-weighted images.[136–138] With disease progression, there is gradual loss in disc space and increasing bone destruction. Gadolinium enhancement is helpful in assessing extraosseous extension of the inflammatory process, including extension into the epidural space.[139, 140]

Neoplasms and Non-Neoplastic Tumors of the Chest Wall

Neoplasms of Soft Tissue

Primary neoplasms of the soft tissues of the chest wall are rare. In adults, the most common benign lesion is lipoma; other benign tumors include neurogenic neoplasms of the intercostal nerves (neurofibroma and schwannoma), fibromas and angiofibromas of the intercostal muscles, and desmoid tumors (fibromatosis).[142] The most common primary malignant neoplasms are fibrosarcoma, malignant fibrohistiocytoma, and peripheral neuroectodermal tumor; however, virtually any form of mesenchymal tumor can be seen.[144] Lymphoma and plasmacytomas are almost always secondary to adjacent skeletal or pleural disease; however, chest wall involvement is rarely the presenting manifestation of Hodgkin's disease, in which it probably represents direct spread from internal mammary lymph nodes.[145]

Lipoma

The point of origin of a lipoma in the chest wall establishes its mode of presentation: when it originates adjacent to the parietal pleura, it causes a soft-tissue mass that indents the lung and possesses a contour characteristic of its extrapulmonary origin; when it arises outside the rib cage, it presents as a palpable soft-tissue mass that may be visualized radiographically if viewed in profile or, if of sufficient size, even en face. Most lipomas that arise between the ribs have a dumbbell or hourglass configuration, part projecting inside and part outside the thoracic cage (Fig. 23–13).

As a result of the specificity of CT in identifying fat-containing structures, this technique is especially valuable in the diagnosis of these tumors.[146, 147] The characteristic appearance consists of a well-defined mass that has homogeneous fat attenuation. The presence of soft-tissue strands should suggest the possibility of liposarcoma (Fig. 23–14).[147] Foci of calcification may be present in areas of fat necrosis.[147, 148] The diagnosis can also be made on MRI, which shows signal intensities characteristic of fat on all pulse sequences (high-signal intensity on T1-weighted images, lower-signal intensity on T2-weighted images, and low-signal intensity on fat-saturation images).[148, 149]

Neurogenic Tumors

Neurogenic tumors may involve the thoracic spine roots, the paraspinal ganglions of the sympathetic chain, the intercostal nerves along the thoracic cage, or the peripheral nerves on the chest wall. Plexiform neurofibromas, seen in patients who have neurofibromatosis, can involve the chest wall extensively.[147] Tumors arising from the intercostal

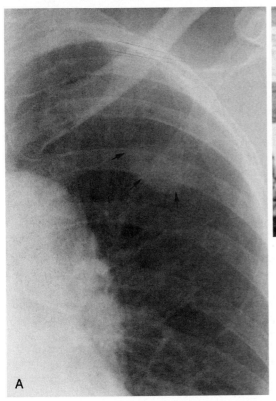

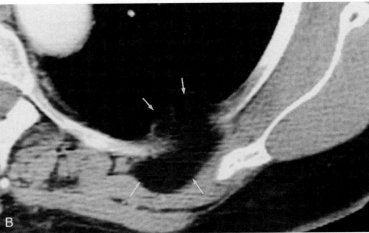

Figure 23–13. Lipoma. A view of the left upper chest from a posteroanterior chest radiograph *(A)* shows soft-tissue opacity *(arrows)* projecting over the left posterior fifth rib. The opacity has well-defined lower margins and poorly defined upper margins, suggesting that it abuts the lung and the chest wall. A CT scan *(B)* demonstrates that the mass *(arrows)* has homogeneous fat attenuation and an hourglass configuration. The findings are diagnostic of a lipoma, presumably originating from the extrapleural fat. The patient was a 22-year-old woman who presented with focal chest wall pain. The patient's symptoms necessitated the resection of the tumor, which was confirmed to be a lipoma.

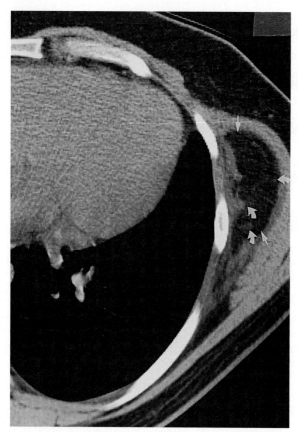

Figure 23–14. Liposarcoma. A CT scan demonstrates a left chest wall tumor displacing the adjacent muscles. The tumor contains large areas of fat attenuation *(straight arrows)* and focal areas of soft-tissue attenuation *(curved arrows)*. The appearance is characteristic of low-grade liposarcoma. The patient was a 32-year-old man.

nerves can result in rib erosion, notching, and sclerosis (Fig. 23–15).[147] On CT, neurogenic tumors usually present as well-circumscribed cylindrical masses. They may have homogeneous or heterogeneous attenuation that may be lower than or equal to that of chest wall muscle.[150, 151] They usually show inhomogeneous enhancement following intravenous administration of contrast medium and often contain single or multiple areas that have low attenuation.[147]

On MRI, neurogenic tumors usually have low to intermediate signal intensity on T1-weighted images and inhomogeneously high signal intensity on T2-weighted images.[147, 152] Neurilemomas often have peripheral high-signal intensity on T2-weighted images and contain central areas with low signal intensity. Ganglioneuromas typically have a whorled appearance on both T1- and T2-weighted images caused by the presence of curvilinear or nodular bands of low-signal intensity.[152]

Neoplasms and Non-Neoplastic Tumors of Bone

Neoplasms of the thoracic skeleton are uncommon, accounting for only 5% of all neoplasms of bones and joints in one large series.[154] Of the 134 cases of thoracic bone tumors in this series, 84 (63%) were primary (48 benign and 36 malignant), and the remainder metastatic.[154] The majority of the latter were from primaries in the lung and

breast. The average age of the patients who had malignant neoplasms was 48 years, and that of patients with benign neoplasms 26 years. The most common primary malignant chest wall tumor is chondrosarcoma.[153]

Most neoplasms occur in the ribs. For example, in one series of 100 patients, tumor was localized to the ribs in 78 and to the sternum in 22;[155] in the review of 134 patients cited previously, 72 involved the ribs, 26 the scapulae, 15 the thoracic vertebrae, 14 the clavicles, and 7 the sternum.[154] In the latter study, the following characteristics were noted: (1) rib lesions were most commonly metastatic; (2) the majority of lesions arising in the sternum were malignant, most often chondrosarcoma; (3) involvement of the clavicles was most often by metastases, with benign neoplasms the next most common; (4) primary neoplasms in the scapulae were more numerous than metastatic ones, with the majority benign; and (5) involvement of the thoracic vertebrae was almost invariably metastatic in nature.

The clinical manifestations of these neoplasms are varied. A pathologic fracture occasionally causes a patient to seek medical advice. Malignant neoplasms may cause pain and, if extensive, respiratory insufficiency. Tumors of the vertebrae may compress the cord and result in neurologic signs and symptoms.[141] Radiologic assessment may be useful in suggesting the diagnosis; however, definitive diagnosis requires correlation between the histologic and the radiologic appearances of the neoplasm. Computed tomography and MRI are helpful in characterizing the tumor and in assessing its extent. Computed tomography is superior to MRI in the demonstration of the foci of calcification seen in chondrosarcomas and osteosarcomas.[116, 147, 149] However, because of its greater ability to distinguish tumor from normal soft tissue, MRI is the modality of choice in the assessment of the extent of chest wall tumors and their relationship to adjacent structures.[116, 147, 149]

Benign Tumors and Tumor-Like Lesions

Osteochondroma is the most common benign neoplasm of the thoracic skeleton. Approximately 0.5% to 2% undergo malignant transformation.[157] The most common non-neoplastic tumor of the thoracic skeleton is fibrous dysplasia (Fig. 23–16). The lesion is usually monostotic and asymptomatic; rarely, multiple lesions are sufficient to result in progressive restrictive lung disease, pulmonary hypertension, and cor pulmonale.[143] Involvement of the rib cage by Paget's disease represents a typical radiographic appearance similar to that in any other bone.

Malignant Neoplasms

Sternal metastases most frequently originate in the breast, thyroid, or lung and may be associated with pathologic fractures.[158] Hodgkin's disease can also involve the sternum and parasternal chest wall as the result of contiguous spread from retrosternal lymph nodes.[159] A wide variety of primary neoplasms can involve the thoracic spine; however, metastatic carcinoma is much more common.

The most common primary malignant mesenchymal neoplasm is chondrosarcoma.[156] Radiographically, the tumor usually appears as a mass on the lateral chest wall;

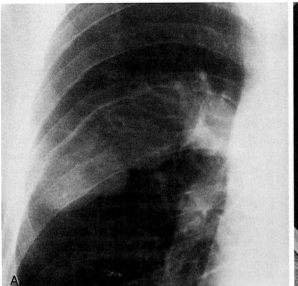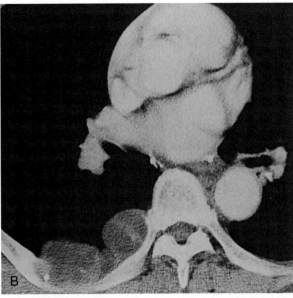

Figure 23–15. Intercostal Neurilemoma. A close-up view of the right chest from an anteroposterior chest radiograph *(A)* in a 69-year-old man demonstrates soft-tissue tumor adjacent to and parallel to the right seventh rib. Also note notching and sclerosis of the undersurface of the rib and widening of the interspace between the seventh and the eighth ribs. A contrast-enhanced CT scan *(B)* shows the tumor to have nonhomogeneous attenuation and to contain cystic areas. Note erosion of the posterior seventh rib. Proven intercostal neurilemoma. (Case courtesy of Dr. Eun-Young Kang, Department of Radiology, Korea University Guro Hospital, Seoul, South Korea.)

sometimes, it arises in the posterior aspect of a rib, in which case it may appear as a paravertebral mass.[160] Chondrosarcomas are usually large masses with indistinct margins and soft-tissue involvement.[153] Foci of calcification may be seen within the cartilaginous matrix. The latter as well as soft-tissue extension are better seen on CT. The

MRI signal characteristics are nonspecific, with intermediate signal intensity on T1-weighted images and inhomogeneous areas of high signal intensity on T2-weighted images.[153]

Multiple myeloma and, occasionally, solitary plasmacytoma are the most frequent malignant lymphoid neoplasms,

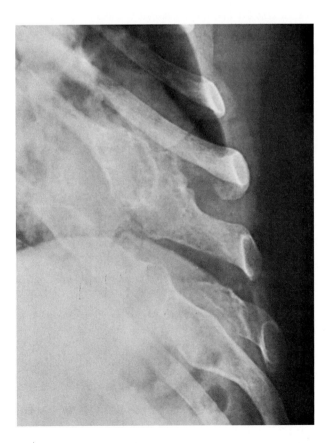

Figure 23–16. Polyostotic Fibrous Dysplasia of the Left Rib Cage. Oblique view of the left rib cage reveals considerable expansion and distortion of ribs along the lower axillary lung zone. The left innominate bone and left tibia were affected in a similar manner. Bone involvement is thus unilateral, representing the osseous manifestation of Albright's syndrome.

followed by Hodgkin's and non-Hodgkin's lymphoma.[154, 162] In older patients, particularly men, the association of a destructive lesion of one or more ribs with a soft-tissue mass that protrudes into the thorax and indents the lung is highly suggestive of myeloma. However, a similar appearance can be seen in association with a primary pulmonary carcinoma that invades the chest wall and with other primary or metastatic chest wall neoplasms. Advanced myelomatosis of the rib cage may be associated with expansion of bone. Pathologic fractures, particularly of the sternum, may result in severe deformity of the chest wall.

References

1. Alexander C: Diaphragm movements and the diagnosis of diaphragmatic paralysis. Clin Radiol 17:79, 1966.
2. Tarver RD, Conces DJ Jr, Cory DA, et al: Imaging the diaphragm and its disorders. J Thorac Imaging 4:1, 1989.
3. Graham NJ, Müller NL: The diaphragm. Can Assoc Radiol J 43:250, 1992.
4. Houston JG, Fleet M, Cowan MD, et al: Comparison of ultrasound with fluoroscopy in the assessment of suspected hemidiaphragmatic movement abnormality. Clin Radiol 50:95, 1995.
5. Ueki J, De Bruin PF, Pride NB: In vivo assessment of diaphragm contraction by ultrasound in normal subjects. Thorax 50:1157, 1995.
6. Gottesman E, McCool FD: Ultrasound evaluation of the paralyzed diaphragm. Am J Respir Crit Care Med 155:1570, 1997.
7. Riley EA: Idiopathic diaphragmatic paralysis: A report of eight cases. Am J Med 32:404, 1962.
8. Ridyard JB, Stewart RM: Regional lung function in unilateral diaphragmatic paralysis. Thorax 31:438, 1976.
9. Moorthy SS, Gibbs PS, Losasso AM, et al: Transient paralysis of the diaphragm following radical neck surgery. Laryngoscope 93:642, 1983.
10. Heine MF, Asher EF, Roy TM, et al: Phrenic nerve injury following scalenectomy in a patient with thoracic outlet obstruction. J Clin Anesth 7:75, 1995.
11. Markand ON, Moorthy S, Mahomed Y, et al: Postoperative phrenic nerve palsy in patients with open heart surgery. Ann Thorac Surg 39:68, 1985.
12. Wilcox P, Baile EM, Hards J, et al: Phrenic nerve function and its relationship to atelectasis after coronary artery bypass surgery. Chest 93:693, 1988.
13. Benjamin JJ, Cascade PN, Reubenfire N, et al: Left lower atelectasis and consolidation following cardiac surgery: The effect of topical cooling on the phrenic nerve. Radiology 142:11, 1982.
14. Rousou JA, Parker T, Angelman RM, et al: Phrenic nerve paresis associated with the use of iced slush and the cooling jacket for topical hypothermia. J Thorac Cardiovasc Surg 89:921, 1985.
15. Shin MS, Ho K-J: Computed tomographic evaluation of the pathologic lesion for the idiopathic diaphragmatic paralysis. J Comput Tomogr 6:257, 1982.
16. Arborelius M, Lilja B, Senyk J: Regional and total lung function studies in patients with hemidiaphragmatic paralysis. Respiration 32:253, 1975.
17. Newsom Davis J, Goldman M, Loh L, et al: Diaphragm function and alveolar hypoventilation. QJM 45:87, 1976.
18. Loh L, Goldman M, Newsom Davis J: The assessment of diaphragm function. Medicine 56:165, 1977.
19. Ch'en IY, Armstrong JD II: Value of fluoroscopy in patients with suspected bilateral hemidiaphragmatic paralysis. Am J Roentgenol 160:29, 1993.
20. Ambler R, Gruenewald SJ: Ultrasound monitoring of diaphragm activity in bilateral diaphragmatic paralysis. Arch Dis Child 60:170, 1985.
21. Diament MJ, Boechat MI, Kangarloo H: Real-time sector ultrasound in the evaluation of suspected abnormalities of diaphragmatic motion. J Clin Ultrasound 13:539, 1985.
22. Prasad R, Nath J, Mukerji PK: Eventration of diaphragm. J Indian Med 84:187, 1986.
23. Tamas A, Dunbar JS: Eventration of the diaphragm. J Can Assoc Radiol 8:1, 1957.
24. Paris F, Blasco E, Canto A, et al: Diaphragmatic eventration in infants. Thorax 28:66, 1973.
25. Okuda K, Nomura F, Kawai M, et al: Age-related gross changes of the liver and right diaphragm, with special reference to partial eventration. Br J Radiol 52:870, 1979.
26. Avnet NL: Roentgenologic features of congenital bilateral anterior diaphragmatic eventration. Am J Roentgenol 88:743, 1962.
27. Tarver RD, Godwin JD, Putman CE: The diaphragm. Radiol Clin North Am 22:615, 1984.
28. Rubinstein ZJ, Solomon A: CT findings in partial eventration of the right diaphragm. J Comput Assist Tomogr 5:719, 1981.
29. Brink JA, Heiken JP, Semenkovich J, et al: Abnormalities of the diaphragm and adjacent structures: Findings on multiplanar spiral CT scans. Am J Roentgenol 163:307, 1994.
30. Yeh H-C, Halton KP, Gray CE: Anatomic variations and abnormalities in the diaphragm seen with US. RadioGraphics 10:1019, 1990.
31. Symbas PN, Hatcher CR, Waldon W: Diaphragmatic eventration in infancy and childhood. Ann Thorac Surg 4:113, 1977.
32. Ford GT, Whitelaw WA, Rosenal TW, et al: Diaphragm function after upper abdominal surgery in humans. Am Rev Respir Dis 127:431, 1983.
33. Road JD, Burgess KR, Whitelaw WA, et al: Diaphragm function and respiratory response after upper abdominal surgery in dogs. J Appl Physiol 57:576, 1984.
34. Simonneau G, Vivien A, Sartene R, et al: Diaphragm dysfunction induced by upper abdominal surgery: Role of postoperative pain. Am Rev Respir Dis 128:899, 1983.
35. Caskey CI, Zerhouni EA, Fishman EK, et al: Aging of the diaphragm: A CT study. Radiology 171:385, 1989.
36. Bogaert JA, Weemaes K, Verschakelen JA, et al: Spiral CT findings in a postoperative intrathoracic gastric herniation: A case report. Eur Radiol 5:192, 1995.
37. Pearson S: Strangulated diaphragmatic hernia: Report of four cases. Arch Surg 66:155, 1953.
38. Hoffman E: Strangulated diaphragmatic hernia. Thorax 23:541, 1968.
39. Menuck L: Plain film findings of gastric volvulus herniating into the chest. Am J Roentgenol 126:1169, 1976.
40. Johnston RH Jr, Owensby LC, Vargas GM, et al: Pancreatic pseudocyst of the mediastinum. Ann Thorac Surg 41:210, 1986.
41. Poe RG, Schowengerdt CG: Two cases of atraumatic herniation of the liver. Am Rev Respir Dis 105:959, 1972.
42. Godwin JD, MacGregor JM: Extension of ascites into the chest with hiatal hernia: Visualization on CT. Am J Roentgenol 148:31, 1987.
43. Graham JC Jr, Blanchard IT, Scatliff JH: Calcified gastric leiomyoma presenting as a mediastinal mass. Am J Roentgenol 1114:529, 1972.
44. Naeye RL, Shochat SJ, Whitman V, et al: Unsuspected pulmonary abnormalities associated with diaphragmatic hernia. Pediatrics 58:902, 1976.
45. Mallik K, Rodgers BM, McGahren ED: Congenital diaphragmatic hernia: Experience in a single institution from 1978 through 1994. Ann Thorac Surg 60:1331, 1995.
46. Vanamo K: A 45-year perspective of congenital diaphragmatic hernia. Br J Surg 83:1758, 1996.
47. Muraskas JK, Husain A, Myers TF, et al: An association of pulmonary hypoplasia with unilateral agenesis of the diaphragm. J Pediatr Surg 28:999, 1993.
48. Jasnosz KM, Hermansen MC, Snider C, et al: Congenital complete absence (bilateral agenesis) of the diaphragm: A rare variant of congenital diaphragmatic hernia. Am J Perinatol 11:340, 1994.
49. Lundius B: Intrathoracic kidney. Am J Roentgenol 125:678, 1975.
50. Le Roux BT: Supraphrenic herniation of perinephric fat. Thorax 20:376, 1965.
51. Gale ME: Bochdalek hernia: Prevalence and CT characteristics. Radiology 156:449, 1985.
52. Raymond GS, Miller RM, Müller NL, Logan PM: Congenital thoracic lesions that mimic neoplastic disease on chest radiographs of adults. Am J Roentgenol 168:763, 1997.
53. Yamana D, Ohba S: Three-dimensional image of Bochdalek diaphragmatic hernia: A case report. Radiat Med 12:39, 1994.
54. Van Hise ML, Primack SL, Israel RS, Müller NL: CT in blunt chest trauma: Indications and limitations. RadioGraphics 18:1071, 1998.
55. Cormer TP, Clagett OT: Surgical treatment of hernia of the foramen of Morgagni. J Thorac Cardiovasc Surg 52:461, 1966.

56. Paris F, Tarazona V, Casillas M, et al: Hernia of Morgagni. Thorax 28:631, 1973.
57. Fischel RE, Joel EM: Herniation of a stone-filled gallbladder through the diaphragm. Acta Radiol (Diagn) 2:172, 1964.
58. Vaughan BF: Diaphragmatic hernia as a finding in the chest radiograph. Proc Coll Radiol Aust 3:42, 1959.
59. Chu DY, Olson AL, Mishaalany HG: Congenital liver cyst presenting as congenital diaphragmatic hernia. J Pediatr Surg 21:897, 1986.
60. Wallace DB: Intrapericardial diaphragmatic hernia. Radiology 122:596, 1977.
61. Robinson AE, Gooneratne NS, Blackburn WR, et al: Bilateral anteromedial defect of the diaphragm in children. Am J Roentgenol 135:301, 1980.
62. Panicek DM, Benson CB, Gottlieb RH, et al: The diaphragm: Anatomic, pathologic, and radiologic considerations. RadioGraphics 8:385, 1988.
63. Boyd DP, Wooldridge BF: Diaphragmatic hernia through the foramen of Morgagni. Surg Gynecol Obstet 104:727, 1957.
64. Anderson LS, Forrest JV: Tumors of the diaphragm. Am J Roentgenol 119:259, 1973.
65. Olafsson G, Rausing A, Holen O: Primary tumors of the diaphragm. Chest 59:568, 1971.
66. Blondeel PN, Christiaens MR, Thomas J, et al: Primary leiomyosarcoma of the diaphragm. Eur J Surg 21:429, 1995.
67. Ferguson DD, Westcott JL: Lipoma of the diaphragm: Report of a case. Radiology 118:527, 1976.
68. Schwartz EE, Wechsler RJ: Diaphragmatic and paradiaphragmatic tumors and pseudotumors. J Thorac Imaging 4:19, 1989.
69. McHenry CR, Pickleman J, Winters G, et al: Diaphragmatic neurilemoma. J Surg Oncol 37:198, 1988.
70. Müller NL: CT features of cystic teratoma of the diaphragm. J Comput Assist Tomogr 10:325, 1986.
71. Soysal O, Libshitz HI: Diaphragmatic desmoid tumor. Am J Roentgenol 166:1496, 1996.
72. Sbokos CG, Salama FD, Powell V, et al: Primary fibrosarcoma of the diaphragm. Br J Dis Chest 71:49, 1977.
73. Yamamoto H, Watanabe K, Takayama W, et al: Primary malignant fibrous histiocytoma of the diaphragm: Report of a case. Surg Today 24:744, 1994.
74. Seaton D: Primary diaphragmatic haemangiopericytoma. Thorax 29:595, 1974.
75. Kekomaki M, Ekfors TO, Nikkanen V, et al: Intrapleural endodermal sinus tumor arising from the diaphragm. J Pediatr Surg 19:312, 1984.
76. Buckley KM, Whitman GJ, Chew FS: Radiologic-pathologic conferences of the Massachusetts General Hospital: Diaphragmatic pheochromocytoma. Am J Roentgenol 165:260, 1995.
77. Bevelaqua FA, Valensi Q, Hulnick D: Epithelioid hemangioendothelioma: A rare tumor with variable prognosis presenting as a pleural effusion. Chest 93:665, 1988.
78. Parker MC: Leiomyosarcoma of the diaphragm: A case report. Eur J Surg Oncol 11:171, 1985.
79. Ujiki GT, Method HL, Putong PB, et al: Primary chondrosarcoma of the diaphragm. Am J Surg 122:132, 1971.
80. Gordon LF, Ramchandani P, Goldenberg NC, et al: Thoraco-abdominal mass: Roentgenologic CPC. Invest Radiol 16:451, 1981.
81. Federle MP, Mark AS, Guillaumin ES: CT of subpulmonic pleural effusions and atelectasis: Criteria for differentiation from subphrenic fluid. Am J Roentgenol 146:685, 1986.
82. Woodring JH, Bognar B: Muscular hypertrophy of the left diaphragmatic crus: An unusual cause of a paraspinal "mass." J Thorac Imaging 13:144, 1998.
83. Kapnick SJ, Griffiths CT, Finkler NJ: Occult pleural involvement in stage III ovarian carcinoma: Role of diaphragm resection. Gynecol Oncol 39:135, 1990.
84. Nigogosyan G, Ozarda A: Accessory diaphragm: A case report. Am J Roentgenol 85:309, 1961.
85. Becmeur F, Horta P, Donato L, et al: Accessory diaphragm: Review of 31 cases in the literature. Eur J Pediatr Surg 5:43, 1995.
86. Lieberman FL, Hidemura R, Peters RL, et al: Pathogenesis and treatment of hydrothorax complicating cirrhosis with ascites. Ann Intern Med 64:341, 1966.
87. Lieberman FL, Peters RL: Cirrhotic hydrothorax: Further evidence that an acquired diaphragmatic defect is at fault. Arch Intern Med 125:114, 1970.
88. Müller NL, Nelems B: Postcoital catamenial pneumothorax: Report of a case not associated with endometriosis and successfully treated with tubal ligation. Am Rev Respir Dis 134:803, 1986.
89. Shiraishi T: Catamenial pneumothorax: Report of a case and review of the Japanese and non-Japanese literature. Thorac Cardiovasc Surg 39:304, 1991.
90. Ranniger K, Valvassori GE: Angiographic diagnosis of intralobar pulmonary sequestration. Am J Roentgenol 92:540, 1964.
91. Wier JA: Congenital anomalies of the lung. Ann Intern Med 52:330, 1960.
92. Greenspan A, Cohen J, Szabo RM: Klippel-Feil syndrome: An unusual association with Sprengel deformity, omovertebral bone, and other skeletal, hematologic, and respiratory disorders: A case report. Bull Hosp Joint Dis Orthop Inst 51:54, 1991.
93. Pearl M, Chow TF, Friedman E: Poland's syndrome. Radiology 101:619, 1976.
94. Karnak I, Tanyel C, Tuncbilek E, et al: Bilateral Poland anomaly. Am J Med Genet 75:505, 1998.
95. Moncada R, Vade A, Gimenez C, et al: Congenital and acquired lung hernias. J Thorac Imaging 11:75, 1996.
96. Bhalla M, Leitman BS, Forcade C, et al: Lung hernia: Radiographic features. Am J Roentgenol 154:51, 1990.
97. Tamburro F, Grassi R, Romano S, et al: Acquired spontaneous intercostal hernia of the lung diagnosed on helical CT. Am J Roentgenol 174:876, 2000.
98. Fisher MS: Eve's rib (letters to the editor). Radiology 140:841, 1981.
99. Rock JP, Spickler EM: Anomalous rib presenting as cervical myelopathy: A previously unreported variant of Klippel-Feil syndrome: Case Report. J Neurosurg 75:465, 1991.
100. Novak CB, Mackinnon SE: Thoracic outlet syndrome. Orthop Clin North Am 27:747, 1996.
101. Mackinnon SE, Patterson GA, Novak CB: Thoracic outlet syndrome: A current overview. Semin Thorac Cardiovasc Surg 8:176, 1996.
102. Boone ML, Swenson BE, Felson B: Rib notching: Its many causes. Am J Roentgenol 91:1075, 1964.
103. Ferris RA, LoPresti JM: Rib notching due to coarctation of the aorta: Report of a case initially observed at less than one year of age. Br J Radiol 47:357, 1974.
104. Sargent EN, Turner AF, Jacobson G: Superior marginal rib defects: An etiologic classification. Am J Roentgenol 106:491, 1969.
105. Aeschlimann A, Kahn MF: Tietze's syndrome: A critical review. Clin Exp Rheumatol 8:407, 1990.
106. Skorneck AB: Roentgen aspects of Tietze's syndrome: Painful hypertrophy of costal cartilage and bone—osteochondritis? Am J Roentgenol 83:748, 1960.
107. Edelstein G, Levitt RG, Slaker DP, et al: CT observation of rib abnormalities: Spectrum of findings. J Comput Assist Tomogr 9:65, 1985.
108. Edelstein G, Levitt RG, Slaker DP, et al: Computed tomography of Tietze syndrome. J Comput Assist Tomogr 8:20, 1984.
109. Guller B, Hable K: Cardiac findings in pectus excavatum in children: Review and differential diagnosis. Chest 66:165, 1974.
110. Leung AKC, Hoo JJ: Familial congenital funnel chest. Am J Med Genet 26:887, 1987.
111. Soteropoulos GC, Cigtay OS, Schellinger D: Pectus excavatum deformities simulating mediastinal masses. J Comput Assist Tomogr 3:596, 1979.
112. Zorab PA: Chest deformities. BMJ 1:1155, 1966.
113. Goodman LR, Kay HR, Teplick SK, et al: Complications of median sternotomy: Computer tomographic evaluation. Am J Roentgenol 141:225, 1983.
114. Templeton PA, Fishman EK: CT evaluation of poststernotomy complications. Am J Roentgenol 159:45, 1992.
115. Biesecker GL, Aaron BL, Mullen JT: Primary sternal osteomyelitis. Chest 63:236, 1973.
116. Franquet T, Giménez A, Alegret X, et al: Imaging findings of sternal abnormalities. Eur Radiol 7:492, 1997.
117. Kay HR, Goodman LR, Teplick SK, et al: Use of computed tomography to assess mediastinal complications after median sternotomy. Ann Thorac Surg 36:706, 1983.
118. Joseph KN, Bowen JR, MacEwen GD: Unusual orthopedic manifestations of neurofibromatosis. Clin Orthop 278:17, 1992.
119. Pope FM, Nicholls AC, Palan A, et al: Clinical features of an affected father and daughter with Ehlers-Danlos syndrome type VIIB. Br J Dermatol 126:77, 1992.

120. Brewerton DA, Caffrey M, Hart FD, et al: Ankylosing spondylitis and HLA 27. Lancet 1:904, 1973.

121. Schlosstein L, Terasaki PI, Bluestone R, et al: High association of an HLA antigen, W27, with ankylosing spondylitis. N Engl J Med 288:704, 1973.

122. Calin A, Porta J, Fried JF, et al: Clinical history as a screening test for ankylosing spondylitis. JAMA 237:2613, 1977.

123. Calin A, Fries JF: Striking prevalence of ankylosing spondylitis in "healthy" W27 positive males and females: A controlled study. N Engl J Med 293:835, 1975.

124. Rosenow EC III, Strimlan CV, Muhm JR, et al: Pleuropulmonary manifestations of ankylosing spondylitis. Mayo Clin Proc 52:641, 1977.

125. Luthra HS: Extra-articular manifestations of ankylosing spondylitis. Mayo Clin Proc 52:655, 1977.

126. Jessamine AG: Upper lobe fibrosis in ankylosing spondylitis. Can Med Assoc J 98:25, 1968.

127. Campbell AH, MacDonald CB: Upper lobe fibrosis associated with ankylosing spondylitis. Br J Dis Chest 59:90, 1965.

128. Ferdoutsis M, Bouros D, Meletis G, et al: Diffuse interstitial lung disease as an early manifestation of ankylosing spondylitis. Respiration 62:286, 1995.

129. Strobel ES, Fritschka E: Case report and review of the literature: Fatal pulmonary complication in ankylosing spondylitis. Clin Rheumatol 16:617, 1997.

130. Rumancik WM, Firooznia H, Davis MS, et al: Fibrobullous disease of the upper lobes: An extraskeletal manifestation of ankylosing spondylitis. J Comput Tomogr 8:225, 1984.

131. Fenlon HM, Casserly I, Sant SM, et al: Plain radiographic and thoracic high-resolution CT in patients with ankylosing spondylitis. Am J Roentgenol 168:1067, 1997.

132. Casserly IP, Fenlon HM, Breatnach E, et al: Lung findings on high-resolution computed tomography in idiopathic ankylosing spondylitis—correlation with clinical findings, pulmonary function testing and plain radiography. Br J Rheumatol 36:677, 1997.

133. Kinnear WJ, Shneerson JM: Acute pleural effusions in inactive ankylosing spondylitis. Thorax 40:150, 1985.

134. Weaver P, Lifeso RM: The radiological diagnosis of tuberculosis of the adult spine. Skeletal Radiol 12:178, 1984.

135. Coppola J, Müller NL, Connell DG: Computed tomography of musculoskeletal tuberculosis. J Can Assoc Radiol 38:199, 1987.

136. de Roos A, van Persijn van Meerten EL, Bloem JL, et al: MRI of tuberculous spondylitis. Am J Roentgenol 146:9, 1986.

137. Modic MT, Feiglin DH, Paraino DW, et al: Vertebral osteomyelitis: Assessment using MR. Radiology 157:157, 1985.

138. Smith AS, Weinstein MA, Mizushima A, et al: MR imaging characteristics of tuberculous osteomyelitis vs vertebral osteomyelitis. AJNR Am J Neuroradiol 153:399, 1989.

139. Post MJD, Sze G, Quencer RM, et al: Gadolinium-enhanced MR in spinal infection. J Comput Assist Tomogr 14:721, 1990.

140. Hlavin ML, Kaminski HY, Ross JS, et al: Spinal epidural abscess: A ten-year perspective. Neurosurgery 27:177, 1990.

141. Morisaki Y, Takagi K, Ishii Y, et al: Periosteal chondroma developing in a rib at the side of a chest wall wound from a previous thoracotomy: Report of a case. Surg Today 26:57, 1996.

142. Rami-Porta R, Bravo-Bravo JL, Aroca-Gonzalez MJ, et al: Tumours and pseudotumours of the chest wall. Scand J Thorac Cardiovasc Surg 19:97, 1985.

143. King RM, Payne WS, Olafsson S, et al: Surgical palliation of respiratory insufficiency secondary to massive exuberant polyostotic fibrous dysplasia of the ribs. Ann Thorac Surg 39:185, 1985.

144. Jain SK, Afzal M, Mathew M, et al: Malignant mesenchymoma of the chest wall in an adult. Thorax 48:407, 1993.

145. Meis JM, Butler JJ, Osborne BM: Hodgkin's disease involving the breast and chest wall. Cancer 57:1859, 1986.

146. Castillo M, Shirkhoda A: Computed tomography of diaphragmatic lipoma. J Comput Assist Tomogr 9:167, 1985.

147. Kuhlman JE, Bouchardy L, Fishman EK, et al: CT and MR imaging evaluation of chest wall disorders. RadioGraphics 14:571, 1994.

148. Sulzer MA, Goei R, Bollen EC, et al: Lipoma of the external thoracic wall. Eur Respir J 7:207, 1994.

149. Fortier M, Mayo JR, Swensen SJ, et al: MR imaging of chest wall lesions. RadioGraphics 14:597, 1994.

150. Cohen LM, Schwartz AM, Rockoff SD: Benign schwannomas: Pathologic basis for CT inhomogeneities. Am J Roentgenol 147:141, 1986.

151. Ko S-F, Lee T-Y, Lin J-W, et al: Thoracic neurilemomas: An analysis of computed tomography findings in 36 patients. J Thorac Imaging 13:21, 1998.

152. Sakai F, Sone S, Kiyono K, et al: Intrathoracic neurogenic tumors: MR-pathologic correlation. Am J Roentgenol 159:279, 1992.

153. Meyer CA, White CS: Cartilaginous disorders of the chest. RadioGraphics 18:1109, 1998.

154. Ochsner A Jr, Lucas GL, McFarland GB Jr: Tumors of the thoracic skeleton: Review of 134 cases. J Thorac Cardiovasc Surg 52:311, 1966.

155. Pairolero PC, Arnold PG: Chest wall tumors: Experience with 100 consecutive patients. J Thorac Cardiovasc Surg 90:367, 1985.

156. Marcove RC, Huvos AG: Cartilaginous tumors of the ribs. Cancer 27:794, 1971.

157. Meyer CA, White CS: Cartilaginous disorders of the chest. RadioGraphics 18:1109, 1998.

158. Urovitz EPM, Fornasier VL, Czitrom AA: Sternal metastases and associated pathological fractures. Thorax 32:444, 1977.

159. Goldman JM: Parasternal chest wall involvement in Hodgkin's disease. Chest 59:133, 1971.

160. Ishida T, Kuwada Y, Motoi N, et al: Dedifferentiated chondrosarcoma of the rib with a malignant mesenchymomatous component: An autopsy case report. Pathol Int 47:397, 1997.

161. Ogose A, Motoyama T, Hotta T, et al: Clear cell chondrosarcomas arising from rare sites. Pathol Int 45:684, 1995.

162. Eygelaar A, Homan Van Der Heide JN: Diagnosis and treatment of primary malignant costal and sternal tumors. Dis Chest 52:683, 1967.

163. Tihansky DP, Lopez G: Bilateral lipomas of the diaphragm. NY State J Med 88:151, 1988.

Index